European Handbook of Neurological Management
Volume 1

EDITED BY

Nils Erik Gilhus MD PhD

Professor, Department of Clinical Medicine, University of Bergen and Department of Neurology,
Haukeland University Hospital, Bergen, Norway

Michael P. Barnes MD, FRCP

Professor of Neurological Rehabilitation, University of Newcastle, Medical Director,
Hunters Moor Neurorehabilitation Ltd, Newcastle upon Tyne, UK

Michael Brainin MD

Professor, Department of Clinical Medicine and Prevention, and Center for Clinical Neurosciences
Donau-Universität Krems and Head, Department of Neurology, Landesklinikum Donauregion Tulln
Tulln, Austria

SECOND EDITION

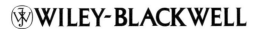

WILEY-BLACKWELL

A John Wiley & Sons, Ltd., Publication

This edition first published 2011, © 2006, 2011 by Blackwell Publishing Ltd

Blackwell Publishing was acquired by John Wiley & Sons in February 2007. Blackwell's publishing program has been merged with Wiley's global Scientific, Technical and Medical business to form Wiley-Blackwell.

Registered office: John Wiley & Sons Ltd, The Atrium, Southern Gate, Chichester, West Sussex PO19 8SQ, UK

Editorial offices: 9600 Garsington Road, Oxford OX4 2DQ, UK
111 River Street, Hoboken, NJ 07030-5774, USA
The Atrium, Southern Gate, Chichester, West Sussex, PO19 8SQ, UK

For details of our global editorial offices, for customer services and for information about how to apply for permission to reuse the copyright material in this book please see our website at www.wiley.com/wiley-blackwell

Library of Congress Cataloging-in-Publication Data

European handbook of neurological management / edited by Nils Erik Gilhus, Michael P. Barnes, Michael Brainin. – 2nd ed.
p. ; cm.
Includes bibliographical references and index.
ISBN 978-1-4051-8533-2
1. Nervous system–Diseases–Treatment–Europe–Handbooks, manuals, etc. I. Gilhus, Nils Erik. II. Barnes, Michael P. III. Brainin, M. (Michael), 1952–
[DNLM: 1. Nervous System Diseases–therapy–Practice Guideline.   WL 140 E885 2010]
RC346.E97 2010
616.8–dc22

2010023982

A catalogue record for this book is available from the British Library.

Set in 9/12 pt Minion by Toppan Best-set Premedia Limited
Printed in Singapore by Markono Print Media Pte Ltd

1   2011

Contents

Section 6 Sleep Disorders

Section 7 Rehabilitation

Introduction

N. E. Gilhus,[1] *M. P. Barnes,*[2] *M. Brainin*[3]

[1]University of Bergen and Department of Neurology, Haukeland University Hospital, Bergen, Norway; [2]Professor of Neurological Rehabilitation Hunters Moor Neurorehabilitation Ltd; [3]Center of Clinical Neurosciences, Donau-Universität Krems, and Landesklinikum Tulln, Austria

This second edition of the *European Handbook of Neurological Management* includes peer-reviewed guidelines on topics highly relevant for all areas of neurological practice. The first edition of this Handbook was published in 2006. Since then there has been an ongoing development in all fields of neurology, making a revision necessary. All authors have revised and updated their chapters, and the newly submitted guidelines have gone through an extensive peer review. All guideline chapters had previously also been published in the *European Journal of Neurology*. Of the revised documents, only 15 will be published in the journal, having been selected mainly due to the anticipated interest of the topic and the extent of revision due to new developments in their field. The remaining revisions are published in this Handbook only. Thus, the revised Handbook is the new and complete compendium for all EFNS guidelines.

The guidelines in this *European Handbook of Neurological Management* are produced according to the rules given by EFNS and the EFNS Scientific Committee. All 24 EFNS Scientist Panels (www.efns.org/Scientist-Panels.15.0.html) are continuously encouraged to establish such task forces with the aim of producing guidelines relevant in their field.

The search for and evaluation of scientific evidence is for all guidelines undertaken according to the EFNS guidance paper [1]. The classification of evidence is explained in the enclosed tables for therapeutic intervention and for diagnostic measures, respectively (tables 1 and 2). As for the recommendations, these are graded from A to C. The scheme for this grading is explained in tables 3 and 4, for therapeutic and diagnostic measures. For several important neurological questions, no high-class scientific evidence is available. The recommendation of 'Good Practice Point' can be given when only Class IV evidence has been published.

The aim of developing, publishing, and disseminating European guidelines is to improve neurological practice. The preliminary work and extensive drafting of recommendations, based on evaluation of clinical trials and meta-analyses by a group of leading experts is not visible in the end product. It is therefore justified to note that the process of establishing high-quality guidelines is based on the right mix of experts, usually from a wider selection of European countries. This is what the Scientific Committee of the EFNS does. It reviews task forces from these panels to develop such guidelines and reviews their performance as well as their final recommendations. Invariably, external reviewers are also involved. Attention is given to conflict of interest declarations by all members of the guideline group. The product is what the current President of the EFNS, Richard Hughes, once called the 'first peer-reviewed book in the world'. We cannot think of a better characterization.

This Handbook is primarily written for European neurologists, but should be helpful also for other groups of health professionals treating patients with disorders of the brain, spine, nerve, and muscle. Clinical experience and present practice do not always give good guidance for best treatment. The guideline chapters in this Handbook are among the most frequently cited articles that have been published in *European Journal of Neurology*.

A challenge for quality control in neurology, as well as in medicine in general, is how to promote the implementation of guidelines in the daily, patient-related work. A first prerequisite is the awareness of their existence, and then their availability. This second edition of the

European Handbook of Neurological Management: Volume 1, 2nd edition. Edited by N. E. Gilhus, M. P. Barnes and M. Brainin.
© 2011 Blackwell Publishing Ltd.

Table 1 Evidence classification scheme for a therapeutic intervention.

Class I An adequately powered prospective, randomized, controlled clinical trial with masked outcome assessment in a representative population *or* an adequately powered systematic review of prospective randomized controlled clinical trials with masked outcome assessment in representative populations. The following are required:
(a) randomization concealment;
(b) primary outcome(s) is/are clearly defined;
(c) exclusion/inclusion criteria are clearly defined;
(d) adequate accounting for dropouts and crossovers with numbers sufficiently low to have minimal potential for bias;
(e) relevant baseline characteristics are presented and substantially equivalent among treatment groups or there is appropriate statistical adjustment for differences.
Class II Prospective matched group cohort study in a representative population with masked outcome assessment that meets a–e above *or* a randomized, controlled trial in a representative population that lacks one criteria a–e.
Class III All other controlled trials (including well-defined natural history controls or patients serving as own controls) in a representative population, where outcome assessment is independent of patient treatment.
Class IV Evidence from uncontrolled studies, case series, case reports, or expert opinion.

Table 2 Evidence classification scheme for a diagnostic measure.

Class I A prospective study in a broad spectrum of persons with the suspected condition, using a 'gold standard' for case definition, where the test is applied in a blinded evaluation, and enabling the assessment of appropriate tests of diagnostic accuracy.
Class II A prospective study of a narrow spectrum of persons with the suspected condition, or a well-designed retrospective study of a broad spectrum of persons with an established condition (by 'gold standard') compared to a broad spectrum of controls, where the test is applied in a blinded evaluation, and enabling the assessment of appropriate tests of diagnostic accuracy.
Class III Evidence provided by a retrospective study where either persons with the established condition or controls are of a narrow spectrum, and where the test is applied in a blinded evaluation.
Class IV Any design where the test is not applied in blinded evaluation or evidence is provided by expert opinion alone or in descriptive case series (without controls).

Table 3 Evidence classification scheme for the rating of recommendations for a therapeutic intervention.

Level A (established as effective, ineffective, or harmful) requires at least one convincing Class I study or at least two consistent, convincing Class II studies.
Level B (probably effective, ineffective, or harmful) requires at least one convincing Class II study or overwhelming Class III evidence.
Level C (possibly effective, ineffective, or harmful) requires at least two convincing Class III studies.

Table 4 Evidence classification scheme for the rating of recommendations for a diagnostic measure.

Level A (established as useful/predictive or not useful/predictive) requires at least one convincing Class I study or at least two consistent, convincing Class II studies.
Level B (established as probably useful/predictive or not useful/predictive) requires at least one convincing Class II study or overwhelming Class III evidence.
Level C (established as possibly useful/predictive or not useful/predictive) requires at least two convincing Class III studies.

Handbook should help with this aspect. We recommend that the guidelines are used widely, and also for retrospective and prospective quality control studies, to check if actual therapeutic and diagnostic procedures are undertaken in accordance with best clinical practice. Too little attention is often given to the effective dissemination, adoption, and implementation strategies for clinical guidelines.

Several of the guidelines in this Handbook represent joint projects between EFNS and more disease-specific European neurological societies. Such co-operation between general neurological societies and disease-specific organizations is an aim for EFNS both regarding guideline production and in general. The European Stroke Organisation has produced the guideline on stroke in this Handbook. The Movement Disorder Society – European Section and the International Peripheral Nerve Society have contributed to the guideline production. In the future, we hope for more co-operation with European and international societies regarding all aspects of the guideline production, from defining the topic and membership to approval of the final guideline.

Better treatment and more exact diagnosis is needed in European neurology. There is often a gap between best practice and what is actually carried out for the individual patient. Guidelines represent an important tool to minimize this gap. Suboptimal treatment may sometimes be due to lack or resources, especially in poor countries. In arguing for sufficient resources, requirements as listed in the guidelines of this European Handbook may be helpful. Diseases of the brain and nervous system represent one-third of the total burden of disease in Europe, and they incur huge costs on the society. The direct costs of treatment and diagnosis represent only a small part of the total cost, so that real improvements for patients' function and ability will usually be highly cost-effective.

These guidelines clearly demonstrate the need for more research. Even for several established treatments and diagnostic procedures there frequently is only weak scientific evidence. There is no doubt that practice is going on in all European departments that would not have been continued if properly controlled studies had been undertaken. Research is needed to select the best treatment and diagnostic options. Although the big breakthroughs usually come from basic research, there is room for much improvement by optimizing what is already available to most neurologists. EFNS intends to support multinational European initiatives to help in this process.

Guidelines represent recommendations. They should not have legally binding implications. In disputed cases, actual practice will be compared with approved guidelines. For the individual patient, there may, however, be reasons to deviate from guideline recommendations. Still, there is a clear and wanted development towards a stronger quality control of neurological practice, including the systematic use of international guidelines.

The editors thank all the authors who have contributed to this second edition of the *European Handbook of Neurological Management*. Their work to evaluate and update all new scientific and controlled information in their field as a joint effort within the task force is highly appreciated. Lisa Müller, executive director of the EFNS, has done a formidable job in following up the task forces. We will especially thank Professor Richard Hughes, President of EFNS, who was the leading editor of the first edition of this Handbook and a key person in initiating and organizing the guideline work within EFNS.

Reference

1. Brainin M, Barnes M, Baron JC, et al. Guidance for the preparation of neurological management guidelines by EFNS scientific task forces – revised recommendations 2004. *Eur J Neurol* 2004;**11**:577–81.

CHAPTER 1

Routine cerebrospinal fluid (CSF) analysis

*F. Deisenhammer,[1] A. Bartos,[2] R. Egg,[1] N. E. Gilhus,[3] G. Giovannoni,[4] S. Rauer,[5]
F. Sellebjerg,[6] H. Tumani[7]*

[1]Innsbruck Medical University, Austria; [2]Charles University, Prague, Czech Republic; [3]University of Bergen, and Haukeland University Hospital, Bergen, Norway; [4]University College London, Queen Square, London, UK; [5]Albert-Ludwigs University, Freiburg, Germany; [6]Copenhagen University Hospital, Denmark; [7]University of Ulm, Germany

Introduction

The cerebrospinal fluid (CSF) is a dynamic, metabolically active substance that has many important functions. It is invaluable as a diagnostic aid in the evaluation of inflammatory conditions, infectious or non-infectious, involving the brain, spinal cord, and meninges, as well as in CT-negative subarachnoidal haemorrhage and in leptomeningeal metastases. CSF is obtained with relative ease by lumbar puncture (LP). Alterations in CSF constituents may be similar in different pathologic processes and cause difficulties in interpretation. Combining a set of CSF variables referred to as routine parameters (i.e. determination of protein, albumin, immunoglobulin, glucose, lactate, and cellular changes, as well as specific antigen and antibody testing for infectious agents) will increase the diagnostic sensitivity and specificity.

The aim of this guideline paper was to produce recommendations on how to use this set of CSF parameters in different clinical settings and to show how different constellations of these variables correlate with diseases of the nervous system (table 1.1) [1].

Search strategy

A MEDLINE search using the search terms cerebrospinal fluid (CSF), immunoglobulin G (IgG) immunoglobulin M (IgM), immunoglobulin A (IgA), and albumin was conducted. Also, the key words 'cerebrospinal fluid' or 'CSF' were cross-referenced with 'glucose', 'lactate', 'cytology', 'cell* in title' excluding 'child*'. Furthermore, a search for 'cerebrospinal fluid' and 'immunoglobulin' and 'diagnosis' and 'electrophoresis' or 'isoelectric focusing' was performed limited to the time between 1 January 1980 and 1 January 2005, and returned only items with abstracts, and English language (274 references). A search for 'cerebrospinal fluid' AND 'infectious' limited for time (1 January 1980 until now) returned 560 abstracts. Abstracts that primarily did not deal with diagnostic issues and infectious CSF (e.g. non-infectious inflammatory diseases, vaccination, general CSF parameters, pathophysiology, cytokines and therapy) were excluded, resulting in 60 abstracts. Searching the items 'cerebrospinal fluid' AND 'serology' limited for time (1 January 1980 until now) and excluding abstracts not directly related to the topic returned 35 abstracts and a search for 'cerebrospinal fluid' AND 'bacterial culture' limited for time (1 January 1980 until now) resulted in 28 abstracts.

For the current update (deadline October 2009) all the above search terms and selection criteria were applied for the time between 2005 and now.

Because this was not included in the first edition an additional MEDLINE search for the items 'cerebrospinal fluid analysis' AND 'quality assurance' from 1981 until now returned 87 references. Only 15 of these references dealt primarily with quality assurance aspects of cerebrospinal fluid analysis.

The abstracts were selected by the author in charge of the respective topic.

In addition, textbooks and articles identified in reference lists of individual papers were selected if considered appropriate.

European Handbook of Neurological Management: Volume 1, 2nd edition. Edited by N. E. Gilhus, M. P. Barnes and M. Brainin.
© 2011 Blackwell Publishing Ltd.

Table 1.1 Typical constellation of CSF parameters in some neurological diseases.

	Total protein (g/l)	Glucose ratio	Lactate (mmol/l)	Cell count (per 3.2 μl)	Typical cytology
Normal values[a]	<0.45	>0.4–0.5	<1.0–2.9	<15	MNC
Disease					
Acute bacterial meningitis	↑	↓	↑	>1000	PNC
Viral neuro-infections (meningo/ encephalitis)	=/↑	=/↓	=	10–1000	PNC/MNC
Autoimmune polyneuropathy	↑	=	=	=	
Infectious polyneuropathy	↑	=	=	↑	MNC
Subarachnoidal haemorrhage	↑	=	=	↑	erythrocytes, macrophages, siderophages MNC
Multiple sclerosis	=	=	=	=/↑	MNC
Leptomeningeal metastases	↑	=/↓	NA	=/↑	malignant cells, mononuclears

CSF, cerebrospinal fluid; MNC, mononuclear cells; PNC, polymorphonuclear cells. ↑/↓, increased/decreased; =, within normal limits; NA, evidence not available.
[a]Normal values are given for lumbar CSF in adults.

There are no guidelines for CSF analysis published by the American Academy of Neurology (AAN). Individual task force members prepared draft statements for various parts of the manuscript. Evidence was classified as Class I–IV and recommendations as Level A–C according to the scheme agreed for EFNS guidelines [1]. When only Class IV evidence was available but consensus could be reached, the task force has offered advice as Good Practice Points (GPP) [1]. The statements were revised and adapted into a single document that was then revised until consensus was reached.

Quantitative analysis of total protein and albumin

The blood–CSF barrier is a physical barrier, consisting of different anatomical structures, for the diffusion and filtration of macromolecules from blood to CSF. The integrity of these barriers and CSF bulk flow determine the protein content of the CSF [2, 3]. In newborns, CSF protein concentrations are high, but decrease gradually during the first year of life, and are maintained at low levels in childhood. In adults, CSF protein concentrations increase with age [4, 5] (Class I). The CSF to serum albumin concentration quotient (Q_{alb}) can also be used to evaluate blood–CSF barrier integrity [6]. The Q_{alb} is not influenced by intrathecal protein synthesis, is corrected for the plasma concentration of albumin, and is an integral part of intrathecal immunoglobulin synthesis formulae. The Q_{alb} is a method-independent measure, allowing the use of the same reference values in different laboratories [7, 8]. However, there are no conclusive data on how the Q_{alb} performs compared to total protein as a measure of blood–CSF barrier function in large cohorts of unselected patients.

There is a concentration gradient for total protein and the Q_{alb} along the neuraxis, with the lowest concentrations in the ventricular fluid and the highest concentrations in the lumbar sac [2, 9]. A significant decrease of the Q_{alb} was observed from the first 0–4 ml of CSF to the last 21–24 ml of CSF obtained by LP [7] (Class I). The Q_{alb} is also influenced by body weight, sex, degenerative lower back disease, hypothyroidism, alcohol consumption (Class II), and smoking (Class III) [10–13]. Posture and physical activity may influence the CSF protein concentration, resulting in higher CSF protein concentrations in inactive, bed-ridden patients [13] (Class III). Elevated CSF protein concentrations can be found in the majority of patients with bacterial (0.4–4.4 g/l), cryptococcal (0.3–3.1 g/l), tuberculous (0.2–1.5 g/l) meningitis and neuroborreliosis [14–17] (Class II). A concentration of >1.5 g/l is specific (99%), but insensitive (55%) for bacterial meningitis as compared to a variety of other inflammatory diseases [18] (Class I).

In viral neuroinfections, CSF protein concentrations are raised to a lesser degree (usually <0.95 g/l) [16] (Class II). The concentration in herpes simplex virus encephalitis is normal in half of the patients during the first week of illness [19] (Class IV).

Non-infectious causes for an increased CSF protein and sometimes with an increased cell count include subarachnoidal haemorrhage, central nervous system (CNS) vasculitis, and CNS neoplasm [20] (Class IV). Elevated total protein concentration with normal CSF cell count (albuminocytologic dissociation) is a hallmark in acute and chronic inflammatory demyelinating polyneuropathies but protein levels may be normal during the first week [21, 22] (Class IV). Total CSF protein is elevated in 80% of patients with leptomeningeal metastases with a range of a median concentrations between 1 and 2.4 g/l and even wider individual ranges [23, 24] (Class III). In addition, normal pressure, hydrocephalus, spinal stenosis, polyneuropathy, and high body weight and body mass index have been associated with increased CSF-serum albumin quotients [25] (Class III).

In conclusion, there is Class I evidence that increased Q_{alb} and total CSF protein concentrations are mainly supportive of bacterial, cryptococcal, and tuberculous meningitis as well as leptomingeal metastases. As Q_{alb} or protein is usually not the only CSF investigation, the combination with other CSF variables will increase the diagnostic specificity, like albuminocytologic dissociation in Gullain–Barré syndrome.

Quantitative intrathecal immunoglobulin synthesis

Intrathecal Ig synthesis is found in various, mainly inflammatory CNS diseases (table 1.2). There is a close correlation between the Q_{alb} and the CSF-serum IgG concentration quotient (Q_{IgG}), which led to the development of the IgG index (Q_{IgG}/Q_{alb}) [26–28]. Reiber's hyperbolic formula and Öhman's extended immunoglobulin indices are based on the demonstration of non-linear relationships between the Q_{alb} and CSF-serum concentration quotients for IgG, IgA, and IgM [3, 29, 30]. For the detection of intrathecal IgG synthesis, the detection of IgG oligoclonal bands is superior to the IgG index and the non-linear formulae both in terms of diagnostic sensitivity and specificity. However, the detection of IgG oligoclonal bands is technically more demanding than the quantitative measures, and it has been suggested that in the setting of suspected multiple sclerosis (MS), oligoclonal bands analysis may be omitted in patients with an IgG-index value above 1.1, as almost 100% of such patients turn out to have intrathecally synthesized IgG oligoclonal bands (F. Deisenhammer, unpublished data).

In studies comparing CSF findings in patients with MS and other neurological diseases, non-linear formulae were superior [33, 34]. Intrathecal IgA, IgG, and IgM synthesis formulae may be helpful in discriminating between different infectious diseases of the nervous system [36, 37] (Class III). However, one study suggested that increased values of the Reiber formula do not always reflect intrathecal IgM synthesis as increased values were observed in several patients with non-inflammatory diseases without IgM oligoclonal bands in CSF [38] (Class II). In conclusion, there is no evidence to support the routine use of quantitative assessment of intrathecal immunoglobulin synthesis in the diagnosis of neurological diseases, but in the setting of suspected MS, the IgG index may be used as a screening procedure to determine intrathecal IgG synthesis.

Qualitative (oligoclonal) intrathecal IgG synthesis

The detection of intrathecal oligoclonal IgG in the CSF is useful diagnostically, particularly as it is one of the laboratory criteria supporting the clinical diagnosis of MS [39]. In addition, it can be used to assist in the diagnosis of other putative autoimmune disorders of the CNS, such as paraneoplastic disorders and CNS infections [40–42].

Using electrophoresis techniques it is possible to classify the humoral responses according to the number of antibody clones produced (i.e. monoclonal, oligoclonal,

Table 1.2 Percentage of patients in different categories of disease with elevated IgA-index, IgG-index, IgM-index, or non-linear intrathecal synthesis formula values (data from [31–35]). Unexpected increases are more common with the IgA index, IgG index, and IgM index than with corresponding non-linear formulae.

	IgG (%)	IgA (%)	IgM (%)
No inflammatory and no CNS disease	<5	<5	<5
Non-inflammatory CNS disease (including degenerative and vascular diseases)	<25[a]	<5	<5
Infections of the nervous system	25–50	25	25
Bacterial infections	25–50	25–50	<25
Viral infections	25–50	<25	<25
Lyme neuroborreliosis	25–50	<25	75
Multiple sclerosis	70–80	<25	<25
Clinically isolated syndromes	40–60	<10	<25
Inflammatory neuropathies	25–50[a]	25–50[a]	25–50[a]
Neoplastic disorders (in general)	<25[a]	ND	ND
Paraneoplastic syndromes	<25	ND	ND
Meningeal carcinomatosis	25–50	ND	ND
Other neuroinflammatory diseases	25–50[b]	ND[c]	ND

CNS, central nervous system; ND, not determined in larger studies using non-linear immunoglobulin formulae.
[a]Usually not associated with oligoclonal bands (artefact in presence of barrier impairment);
[b]rare in biopsy-proven neurosarcoidosis;
[c]prominent IgA synthesis in adrenoleukodystrophy.

and polyclonal responses; figure 1.1). Earlier methods have now been superseded by the development of the more sensitive technique of isoelectric focusing (IEF) and immunofixation [6].

Isoelectric focusing uses a pH gradient to separate IgG populations on the basis of charge, which are then transferred onto a nitro-cellulose or other membrane before immunostaining using an anti-human immunoglobulin [43]. Some laboratories continue to use silver staining to detect oligoclonal bands (OCBs) with good results [44].

As CSF is an ultrafiltrate of plasma, it contains immunoglobulins that are passively transferred from the plasma, as well as immunoglobulins synthesized locally. Any systemic pattern of immunoglobulin production seen in plasma or serum will therefore be mirrored in the CSF. It is imperative that any CSF analysis for oligoclonal bands is accompanied by a paired blood analysis.

An oligoclonal intrathecal IgG antibody response is not specific. Table 1.3 provides a list with the proportion of cases with oligoclonal bands (for a more detailed list please see [32]). Local synthesis of oligoclonal bands is therefore not diagnostic and has to be interpreted in the clinical context. A recently published recommendation regarding detection of oligoclonal bands concluded as follows [45]:

The single most informative analysis is a qualitative assessment of CSF for IgG, best performed using IEF together with some form of immunodetection (blotting or fixation). This qualitative analysis should be performed using unconcentrated CSF and must be compared directly with serum run simultaneously in the same assay in an adjacent track. Optimal runs utilize similar amounts of IgG from paired serum and CSF. Recognised positive and negative controls should be run with each set of samples.

In putative non-infectious inflammatory disorders of the CNS there is Class I evidence to support the use of

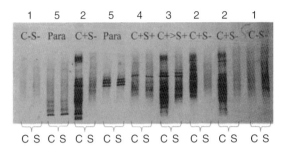

Figure 1.1. IEF immunoblots of the five consensus patterns of various CSF and serum isoelectric focusing patterns for local/systemic synthesis. The pattern number is given above the paired samples.

Type 1 (C–S–): No bands in CSF and serum. Normal.

Type 2 (C+S–): Oligoclonal IgG is present in the CSF with no apparent corresponding abnormality in serum, indicating local intrathecal synthesis of IgG. Typical example: MS.

Type 3 (C+>S+): There are IgG bands in both the CSF and serum, with additional bands present in the CSF. The oligoclonal bands that are common to both CSF and serum imply a systemic inflammatory response, whereas the bands that are restricted to the CNS suggest that there is an additional CNS-only response. Typical examples: MS, systemic lupus erythematosus (SLE), sarcoid, etc.

Type 4 (C+S+): There are oligoclonal bands present in the CSF, which are identical to those in serum. This is not indicative of local synthesis, but rather, the pattern is consistent with passive transfer of oligoclonal IgG from a systemic inflammatory response. Typical examples: Guillain–Barré syndrome, acute disseminated encephalomyelitis (ADEM), and systemic infections.

Type 5 (Para): There is a monoclonal IgG pattern in both CSF and serum, the source of which lies outside the CNS. Typical examples: Myeloma, monoclonal gammopathy of undetermined significance (MGUS).

CSF IEF for both predictive and diagnostic testing in the diagnosis of MS. In other non-infectious inflammatory disorders of the CNS, Class II and III evidence exists to support the use of CSF IEF to supplement other diagnostic tests (table 1.3).

CSF glucose concentration, CSF/serum glucose ratio and lactate

As glucose is actively transported across the blood–brain barrier the CSF glucose levels are directly proportional to the plasma levels and therefore simultaneous measurement in CSF and blood is required. Normal CSF glucose concentration is 50–60% of serum values [20] (Class IV).

A CSF/serum glucose ratio less than 0.4–0.5 is considered to be pathological [48] (Class IV). CSF glucose takes several hours to equilibrate with plasma glucose; therefore, in unusual circumstances, levels of CSF glucose can actually be higher than plasma levels for several hours. During CSF storage glucose is degraded. Therefore, glucose determination must be performed immediately after CSF collection.

A high CSF glucose concentration has no specific diagnostic importance and is related to an elevated blood glucose concentration, for example in diabetics.

The behaviour of the CSF/serum glucose ratio in different neurological diseases is shown in table 1.1.

The relevance of CSF lactate is similar to that of the CSF/serum glucose ratio. CSF lactate is independent of blood concentration [49] (Class IV). The normal value is considered to be <2.8–3.5 mmol/l [50] (Class II). Except for mitochondrial disease, CSF lactate correlates inversely with CSF/serum glucose ratio. An increased level can be detected earlier than the reduced glucose concentration.

Decreased CSF/serum glucose ratio or increased CSF lactate indicates bacterial and fungal infections or leptomeningeal metastases.

Cytological examination

Cytological evaluation should be performed within 2 h after puncture, preferably within 30 min because of a lysis of both red blood cells and white blood cells [51] (Class IV).

Cerebrospinal fluid leukocytes are usually counted in a Fuchs-Rosenthal chamber (volume 3.2 μl) and therefore counts are reported as '/3' cells to correct for a standard volume of 1 μl. A cytocentrifuge (cytospin), the Sayk sedimentation chamber, or membrane filtration can be used to obtain a sufficient number of cells for cytology [52]. For cellular differentiation May–Gruenwald–Giemsa staining is widely used but specific methods may be performed, especially for the detection of malignant cells [53, 54] (Class II).

Lymphocytes and monocytes at the resting phase and occasionally ependymal cells are found in normal CSF.

An increased number of neutrophilic granulocytes can be found in bacterial and acute viral CNS infections [54, 55] (Class II). In the postacute phase a mononuclear transformation occurs.

Table 1.3 Inflammatory diseases of the CNS associated with CSF oligoclonal IgG bands [32].

Disorder	Incidence of oligoclonal bands (%)	Evidence
Multiple sclerosis	95	Class I[a]
Auto-immune		
Neuro-SLE	50	Class III
Neuro-Behçet's	20	Class II
Neuro-sarcoid	40	Class III
Harada's meningitis-uveitis	60	Class III
Infectious		
Acute viral encephalitis (<7 days)	<5	Class II
Acute bacterial meningitis (<7 days)	<5	Class II
Subacute sclerosing panencephalitis (SSPE)	100	Class I
Progressive rubella panencephalitis	100	Class I
Neurosyphilis	95	Class I
Neuro-AIDS	80	Class II
Neuro-borrelliosis	80	Class I
Tumour	<5	Class III
Hereditary		
Ataxia-telangiectasia	60	Class III
Adrenoleukodystrophy (encephalitic)	100	Class II

CNS, central nervous system; CSF, cerebrospinal fluid; IgG, immunoglobulin G; SLE, systemic lupus erythematosus.
[a]This is based on studies using the Poser diagnostic criteria [46] that were validated against the original Schumacher criteria [47]. None of these criteria has been validated using population-based studies. Therefore, it could be argued that the diagnostic 'gold standard' is a flawed standard.

Upon activation, lymphocytes can enlarge or become plasma cells indicating an unspecific inflammatory reaction [54, 56] (Class IV). Resting monocytes enlarge and display vacuoles when activated. Macrophages are the most activated monocytes. These cell forms can occur in a great variety of diseases.

Erythrophages occur 12–18h after haemorrhage. Siderophages containing haemosiderin are seen as early as 1–2 days after haemorrhage and may persist for weeks. Macrophages containing haematoidin (crystallized bilirubin) degraded from haemoglobin may appear about 2 weeks after bleeding and are a sign of a previous subarachnoid bleeding [54] (Class IV). However, spectrophotometry of CSF involving bilirubin quantitation has been recommended as the method of choice to prove CT-negative subarachnoid bleeding up to 2 weeks after onset [57].

Lipophages indicate CNS tissue destruction. The presence of macrophages without detectable intracellular material is a non-specific finding, occurring in disc herniation, malignant meningeal infiltration, spinal tumours, head trauma, stroke, MS, vasculitis, infections, and subarachnoid haemorrhage [54] (Class IV).

Eosinophils are normally not present in CSF. The presence of 10 or more eosinophils/μl in CSF or eosinophilia of at least 10% of the total CSF leukocyte count is associated with a limited number of diseases, including parasitic infections and coccidioiodomycosis. It can occur in malignancies and react to medication and ventriculoperitoneal shunts [58].

Malignant CSF cells indicate leptomeningeal metastases. False-positive results often occur when inflammatory cells are mistaken for tumour cells or due to contamination with peripheral blood [59]. False-negative detection of malignant cells on cytologic examination of CSF is common. Factors increasing the detection rate of malignant cells include a volume of at least 10.5 ml and repeating this procedure once if the cytology is negative. The detection rate of 50–70% after the first investigation can be increased to 85–92% after a second puncture [60] (Class III). Further LPs will only slightly increase the diagnostic sensitivity [61, 62] (Class III).

In conclusion, cell count is generally useful because most of the indications for CSF analysis include diseases that are associated with elevated numbers of various cells. Cytological staining can be helpful in distinguishing CNS diseases when the cell count is increased.

Investigation of infectious CSF

There are many small to medium-sized studies investigating the diagnostic sensitivity and specificity of tests for various infectious agents but no controlled study evaluating a work-up of infectious CSF in general. Therefore, there are no valid data on the indication, sensitivity, and specificity of microbiological procedures in general (i.e. how to proceed with CSF in obvious CNS infections). Existing proposals for the general work-up of infectious CSF are based on clinical practice and theoretically plausible procedures [63–65].

There are a great number of methods for antigen or specific antibody detection and their use depends mainly on the type of antigen (table 1.4).

Table 1.4 List of infectious agents responsible for the vast majority of infectious CNS diseases.

Pathogen	Symptoms, Comments	Recommended diagnostic method*
Bacteria		
Should be considered in first line		
Neisseria meningitides	–	Microscopy, culture**
Streptococcus pneumoniae	–	Microscopy, culture**
Haemophilus influenzae	Rare due to vaccination	Microscopy, culture**
Staphylococcus aureus	Neurosurgical intervention, trauma	Microscopy, culture**
Escherichia coli	Newborns	Microscopy, culture**
Borrelia burgdorferi sensu lato	–	Serology
Treponema pallidum	Syphilis in the past	Serology
Mycobacterium tuberculosis	–	PCR[a], culture**, microscopy, positive tuberculin test
Mycobacteria other than tuberculosis (MOTT, 'atypical Mykobacteria')	–	PCR[a], culture**, microscopy, positive tuberculin test
Should be considered especially in immunosuppressed patients		
Actinobacter species	–	Culture**
Bacteroides fragilis	–	Culture***
Listeria monocytogenes	–	Microscopy, culture
Nocardia asteroides	–	Microscopy (modified Ziehl-Neelsen stain and culture from brain biopsy)
Pasteurella multocida	–	Culture
Streptococcus mitis	–	Culture
Should be considered in special situations		
Brucella spp.	Ingestion of raw milk (products) from cows, sheep, or goats	Culture
Campylobacter fetus		Microscopy, culture
Coxiella burnetti (Q-fever)	Contact with infected parturient animals (sheep, goat, cattle) or inhalation of dust contaminated by the excrement of infected animals or ticks	Serology
Leptospira interrogans	Exposure to contaminated water or rodent urine	Culture, serology
Mycoplasma pneumoniae	Children and young adults	Serology
Rickettsia	Tick exposure, exanthema	Serology
Coagulase-negative staphylococci	Patients with ventricular shunts or drainages	Culture
Group B streptococci	(preterm) newborns	Microscopy, culture
Tropheryma whipplei	(M. Whipple) Patients with gastrointestinal symptoms (malabsorption)	PCR

Table 1.4 continued

Pathogen	Symptoms, Comments	Recommended diagnostic method*
Viruses		
Should be considered in first line		
Herpes simplex virus (HSV) type 1 and 2	–	PCR, serology
Varicella–Zoster virus (VZV)	–	PCR, serology
Enteroviruses (Echovirus, Coxsackievirus A, B)	Usually mild symptoms, favourable prognosis	PCR, serology
Human immunodeficiency virus (HIV) type 1 and 2	–	PCR, serology
Tick-borne encephalitis virus (TBE)	In endemic regions only	Serology
Cytomegalovirus (CMV)	Very rare in immunocompetent patients	PCR
Should be considered in special situations		
Adenovirus	Children and young adults	PCR, culture, antigen detection
Epstein–Barr virus (EBV)	Lymphadenitis, splenomegaly, causes very rare CNS-infections	PCR
Human T-cell leukaemia virus type I (HTLV-I)	Spastic paraparesis	Serology
Influenza and Parainfluenza virus	–	Serology
JC virus	Progressive multifocal leukoencephalopathy, associated with immunosuppression and/ or immunomodulatory therapy (e.g. natalizumab, rituximab)	PCR, brain biopsy
Lymphocytic chorio-meningitis (LCM)	–	Serology
Measles virus	–	Serology
Mumps virus	–	Serology
Poliovirus	Flaccid paresis	PCR
Rabies virus	Contact with rabies-infected animals	PCR from CSF, root of hair, cornea
Rotavirus	Diarrhoea, febrile convulsions in children	Antigen detection in stool specimens
Rubella virus	–	Serology
Sandfly fever	Endemic region: Italy	Serology
Fungi		
Aspergillus fumigatus	–	Where required, culture from brain biopsy
Cryptococcus neoformans	–	Antigen detection in CSF, india ink stain, less sensitive than antigen detection, culture
Candida spp.	–	Antigen detection
Parasites		
Echinococcus granulosus, Echinococcus multilocularis	–	Serology
Toxoplasma gondii	–	CSF: PCR, serology; brain biopsy: PCR
Strongyloides stercoralis	–	Pathogen detection in stool

The following pathogens should be considered in acute myelitis [Recommendation Level B]: HSV type 1 and 2 (PCR), VZV (PCR), enteroviruses (PCR), *Borrelia burgdorferi sensu latu* (serology, AI), HIV (serology), tick-borne encephalitis virus (only in endemic areas) (serology, AI).
[a]Nested PCR technique has been shown to be substantially more sensitive and specific than conventional single step PCR techniques [66].
**Culture from CSF and blood;
***aerobic and anaerobic culture from abscess aspirate, CSF, and blood.

In neuroinfections specific antigen or antibody detection should be performed depending on the clinical presentation and the results of basic CSF analysis. The formula for the estimation of the relative intrathecal synthesis of specific antibodies in the CSF (Antibody Index [AI] is as follows:

Estimation of intrathecal synthesis of specific antibodies in the CSF (Antibody Index [AI])

$$\text{Antibody ratio} = \frac{\text{Antibody-concentration}_{CSF}}{\text{Antibody-concentration}_{serum}}$$

$$\text{IgG ratio} = \frac{\text{IgG-concentration}_{CSF}}{\text{IgG-concentration}_{serum}}$$

$$\text{AI} = \text{Antibody ratio}/\text{IgG ratio}(\text{postive} > 1, 5)$$

Cerebrospinal fluid polymerase chain reaction can be performed rapidly and inexpensively and has become an integral component of diagnostic medical practice. A patient with a positive PCR result is 88 times more likely to have a definite diagnosis of viral infection of the CNS as compared to a patient with a negative PCR result. A negative PCR result can be used with moderate confidence to rule out a diagnosis of viral infection of the CNS (the probability of a definite viral CNS infection was 0.1 in case of a negative PCR result compared to a positive PCR result) [67]. It should be considered that false-negative results are most likely if the CSF sample is taken within the first 3 days after the illness or 10 days and more after the onset of the disease [68, 69].

In general, PCR is indicated in the following situations:

• when microscopy, culture or serology is insensitive or inappropriate;
• when culture does not yield a result despite clinical suspicion of infectious meningitis/meningoencephalitis; and
• in immunodeficient patients.

Quality assurance in CSF diagnostics

Some CSF quality assurance programmes have been published showing that to ensure optimal performance and results, standardized protocols should be in place for the spinal tap and sample processing [8] (Class 1). Furthermore it is important to analyse the CSF in a specialized laboratory which is routinely evaluated for its performance and uses standardized analytical techniques and interpretation of the laboratory findings in the clinical context [8] (Class 1); [70] (Class 4). If proteins are measured that potentially originate from blood or brain compartments, CSF and serum samples should be run in parallel in the same assay to minimize variability [8] (Class I, Level A).

A cytology training programme resulted in an increase of the number of correctly identified CSF cells from as low as 11% to 93% [71]. In a recent study investigating inter-laboratory variation of neurofilament light chain detection, it turned out that the lack of preparation of accurate and consistent protein standards was the main reason for a very poor inter-laboratory accordance [72] (Class I).

Recommendations

CSF should be analysed immediately (i.e. <1 h) after collection. If storage is required for later investigation this can be done at 4–8°C (short term) or at −20°C (long term). Only protein components and RNA (after appropriate preparation) can be analysed from stored CSF (GPP).

The Level B recommendation regarding CSF partitioning and storage states that 12 ml of CSF should be partitioned into three to four sterile tubes. It is important that the CSF is not allowed to sediment before partitioning. Store 3–4 ml at 4°C for general investigations, cultivation and microscopic investigation of bacteria and fungi, antibody testing, polymerase chain reaction (PCR), and antigen detection. Larger volumes (10–15 ml) are necessary for certain pathogens like *Mycobacterium tuberculosis*, fungi, or parasites.

Normal CSF protein concentration should be related to the patient's age (higher in the neonate period and after age of 60 years) and the site of LP (Level B). Exact upper normal limits of protein concentration differ according to the technique and the examining laboratory.

The Q_{alb} should be preferred to total protein concentrations, partly because reference levels are more clearly defined and partly because it is not confounded by changes in other CSF proteins (Level B).

The glucose concentration in CSF should be related to the blood concentration. Therefore CSF glucose/serum ratio is preferable. Pathological changes in this ratio or in lactate concentration are supportive for bacterial or fungal meningitis or leptomeningeal metastases (Level B).

Intrathecal IgG synthesis can be measured by various quantitative methods, but at least for the diagnosis of MS, the detection of oligoclonal bands by appropriate methods is superior to any existing formula (Level A). Patients with other diseases associated with intrathecal inflammation, for example patients with CNS infections, may also have intrathecal IgA and IgM synthesis as assessed by non-linear formulae (Reiber hyperbolic formulae or extended indices), which should be preferred to the linear IgA and IgM indices (Level B).

Cellular morphology (cytological staining) should be evaluated whenever pleocytosis is found or leptomeningeal metastases or pathological bleeding is suspected (Level B). If cytology is inconclusive in case of query CSF bleeding, measurement of bilirubin is recommended up to 2 weeks after the clinical event.

For standard microbiological examination sedimentation at 3000×g for 10 min is recommended (Level B). Microscopy should be performed using Gram or methylene blue, Auramin O or Ziehl-Nielsen (*M. tuberculosis*), or Indian ink stain (*Cryptococcus*). Depending on the clinical presentation,

incubation with bacterial and fungal culture media can be useful. Anaerobic culture media are recommended only if there is suspicion of brain abscess. A viral culture is generally not recommended. A list of infectious agents and their association with different diseases as well as the recommended method of detection is provided in table 1.4. The results of bacterial antigen detection have to be interpreted with respect to the microscopical CSF investigation and culture results. It is not routinely recommended in cases of negative microscopy. A diagnosis of bacterial nervous system infection based on antigen detection alone is not recommended (risk of contamination).

CSF laboratories need to participate in regular internal and external quality assessment (Level A). In addition, to avoid possible erroneous differential diagnostic interpretations due to inadequate CSF findings, clinicians should make sure that the co-operating laboratory adheres to the essential quality standards (proof of education and training, certification of the CSF laboratory, continuous participation in internal and external controls) [70] (GPP).

Conflicts of interest

The authors have reported no conflicts of interest.

Acknowledgement

We are grateful to Professor Christian Bogdan (Director of the Department for Microbiology and Hygiene, Albert Ludwigs-Universität Freiburg, Germany) and to Professor Rüdiger Dörries (Head of the Department of Virology, Institute of Medical Microbiology und Hygiene Ruprecht-Karls-Universität Heidelberg, Germany) for critical review of the microbiological part of the manuscript (infectious CSF).

References

1. Brainin M, Barnes M, Baron JC, *et al*. Guidance for the preparation of neurological management guidelines by EFNS scientific task forces – revised recommendations 2004. *Eur J Neurol* 2004;**11**:577–81.

2. Thompson EJ. *The CSF Proteins: A Biochemical Approach*. Amsterdam, Netherlands: Elsevier, 1988.

3. Reiber H. Flow rate of cerebrospinal fluid (CSF) – a concept common to normal blood–CSF barrier function and to dysfunction in neurological diseases. *J Neurol Sci* 1994;**122**: 189–203.

4. Eeg-Olofson O, Link H, Wigertz A. Concentrations of CSF proteins as a measure of blood brain barrier function and synthesis of IgG within the CNS in 'normal' subjects from the age of 6 months to 30 years. *Acta Paediatr Scand* 1981;**70**:167–70.

5. Statz A, Felgenhauer K. Development of the blood–CSF barrier. *Develop Med Child Neurol* 1983;**25**:152–61.

6. Andersson M, Alvarez-Cermeño J, Bernadi G, *et al*. Cerebrospinal fluid in the diagnosis of multiple sclerosis: a consensus report. *J Neurol Neurosurg Psychiatry* 1994;**57**:897–902.

7. Blennow K, Fredman P, Wallin A, Gottfries C-G, Långström G, Svennerholm L. Protein analyses in cerebrospinal fluid. I. Influence of concentration gradients for proteins on cerebrospinal fluid/serum albumin ratio. *Eur Neurol* 1993; **33**:126–8.

8. Reiber H. External quality assessment in clinical neurochemistry: survey of analysis for cerebrospinal fluid (CSF) proteins based on CSF/serum quotients. *Clin Chem* 1995; **41**:256–63.

9. Kornhuber J, Kaiserauer CH, Kornhuber AW, Kornhuber ME. Alcohol consumption and blood–cerebrospinal fluid barrier dysfunction in man. *Neurosci Lett* 1987;**79**:218–22.

10. Skouen JS, Larsen JL, Vollset SE. Cerebrospinal fluid protein concentrations related to clinical findings in patients with sciatica caused by disk herniation. *J Spinal Disord* 1994;**7**: 12–8.

11. Nyström E, Hamberger A, Lindstedt G, Lundquist C, Wikkelsö C. Cerebrospinal fluid proteins in subclinical and overt hypothyroidism. *Acta Neurol Scand* 1997;**95**:311–4.

12. Seyfert S, Kunzmann V, Schwertfeger N, Koch HC, Faulstich A. Determinants of lumbar CSF protein concentration. *J Neurol* 2002;**249**:1021–6.

13. Stockstill MT, Kauffman CA. Comparison of cryptococcal and tuberculous meningitis. *Arch Neurol* 1983;**40**:81–5.

14. Kaiser R. Neuroborreliosis. *J Neurol* 1998;**245**:247–55.

15. Negrini B, Kelleher KJ, Wald ER. Cerebrospinal fluid findings in aseptic versus bacterial meningitis. *Pediatrics* 2000;**105**:316–9.

16. Lindquist L, Linne T, Hansson LO, Kalin M, Axelsson G. Value of cerebrospinal fluid analysis in the differential diagnosis of meningitis: a study in 710 patients with suspected central nervous system infection. *Eur J Clin Microbiol Infect Dis* 1988;**7**:374–80.

17. Koskiniemi M, Vaheri A, Taskinen E. Cerebrospinal fluid alterations in herpes simplex virus encephalitis. *Rev Infect Dis* 1984;**6**:608–18.

18. Jerrard DA, Hanna JR, Schindelheim GL. Cerebrospinal fluid. *J Emerg Med* 2001;**21**:171–8.

19. Segurado OG, Kruger H, Mertens HG. Clinical significance of serum and CSF findings in the Guillain-Barre syndrome and related disorders. *J Neurol* 1986;**233**:202–8.

20. Twijnstra A, Ongerboer de Visser BW, van Zanten AP, Hart AA, Nooyen WJ. Serial lumbar and ventricular cerebrospinal fluid biochemical marker measurements in patients with leptomeningeal metastases from solid and hematological tumors. *J Neurooncol* 1989;**7**:57–63.

21. Bruna J, González L, Miró J, Velasco R, Gil M, Tortosa A. Neuro-Oncology Unit of the Institute of Biomedical Investigation of Bellvitge. Leptomeningeal carcinomatosis: prognostic implications of clinical and cerebrospinal fluid features. *Cancer* 2009;**115**:381–9.

22. Brettschneider J, Claus A, Kassubek J, Tumani H. Isolated blood–cerebrospinal fluid barrier dysfunction: prevalence and associated diseases. *J Neurol* 2005;**252**:1067–73.

23. Delpech B, Lichtblau E. Étude quantitative des immuno-globulines G et de l'albumine du liquide cephalo rachidien. *Clin Chim Acta* 1972;**37**:15–23.

24. Ganrot K, Laurell C-B. Measurement of IgG and albumin content of cerebrospinal fluid, and its interpretation. *Clin Chem* 1974;**20**:571–3.

25. Link H, Tibbling G. Principles of albumin and IgG analyses in neurological disorders. III. Evaluation of IgG synthesis within the central nervous system in multiple sclerosis. *Scand J Clin Lab Invest* 1977;**37**:397–401.

26. Schipper HI, Bardosi A, Jacobi C, Felgenhauer K. Meningeal carcinomatosis: origin of local IgG production in the CSF. *Neurology* 1988;**38**:413–6.

27. McLean BN, Luxton RW, Thompson EJ. A study of immunoglobulin G in the cerebrospinal fluid of 1007 patients with suspected neurological disease using isoelectric focusing and the Log IgG-Index. A comparison and diagnostic applications. *Brain* 1990;**113**:1269–89.

28. Öhman S, Ernerudh J, Forsberg P, Henriksson A, von Schenck H, Vrethem M. Comparison of seven formulae and isoelectrofocusing for determination of intrathecally produced IgG in neurological diseases. *Ann Clin Biochem* 1992;**29**:405–10.

29. Sellebjerg F, Christiansen M, Rasmussen LS, Jaliachvili I, Nielsen PM, Frederiksen JL. The cerebrospinal fluid in multiple sclerosis. Quantitative assessment of intrathecal immunoglobulin synthesis by empirical formulae. *Eur J Neurol* 1996;**3**:548–59.

30. Korenke GC, Reiber H, Hunneman DH, Hanefeld F. Intrathecal IgA synthesis in X-linked cerebral adrenoleukocystrophy. *J Child Neurol* 1997;**12**:314–20.

31. Felgenhauer K. Differentiation of the humoral immune response in inflammatory diseases of the central nervous system. *J Neurol* 1982;**228**:223–37.

32. Felgenhauer K, Schädlich H-J. The compartmental IgM and IgA response within the central nervous system. *J Neurol Sci* 1987;**77**:125–35.

33. Sharief MK, Keir G, Thompson EJ. Intrathecal synthesis of IgM in neurological diseases: a comparison between detection of oligoclonal bands and quantitative estimation. *J Neurol Sci* 1990;**96**:131–43.

34. McDonald WI, Compston A, Edan G, *et al.* Recommended diagnostic criteria for multiple sclerosis: guidelines from the international panel on the diagnosis of multiple sclerosis. *Ann Neurol* 2001;**50**:121–7.

35. Rauer S, Kaiser R. Demonstration of anti-HuD specific oligoclonal bands in the cerebrospinal fluid from patients with paraneoplastic neurological syndromes. Qualitative evidence of anti-HuD specific IgG-synthesis in the central nervous system. *J Neuroimmunol* 2000;**111**:241–4.

36. Stich O, Graus F, Rasiah C, Rauer S. Qualitative evidence of anti-Yo-specific intrathecal antibody synthesis in patients with paraneoplastic cerebellar degeneration. *J Neuroimmunol* 2003;**141**:165–9.

37. Storstein A, Monstad SE, Honnorat J, Vedeler CA. Paraneoplastic antibodies detected by isoelectric focusing of cerebrospinal fluid and serum. *J Neuroimmunol* 2004; **155**:150–4.

38. Keir G, Luxton RW, Thompson EJ. Isoelectric focusing of cerebrospinal fluid immunoglobulin G: an annotated update. *Ann Clin Biochem* 1990;**27**:436–43.

39. Blennow K, Fredman P. Detection of cerebrospinal fluid leakage by isoelectric focusing on polyacrylamide gels with silver staining using the PhastSystem. *Acta Neurochir* 1995;**136**:135–9.

40. Freedman MS, Thompson EJ, Deisenhammer F, *et al.* Recommended standard of cerebrospinal fluid analysis in the diagnosis of multiple sclerosis. *Arch Neurol* 2005;**62**: 865–70.

41. Poser CM, Paty W, Scheinberg LC, *et al.* New diagnostic criteria for multiple sclerosis: guidelines for research protocols. *Ann Neurol* 1983;**13**:227–31.

42. Schumacher FA, Beebe GW, Kibler RF, *et al.* Problems of experimental trials of therapy in multiple sclerosis. *Ann N Y Acad Sci* 1965;**122**:552–68.

43. Feigin RD, McCracken GH Jr, Klein JO. Diagnosis and management of meningitis. *Pediatr Infect Dis J* 1992;**11**: 785–814.

44. Watson MA, Scott MG. Clinical utility of biochemical analysis of cerebrospinal fluid. *Clin Chem* 1995;**41**:343–60.

45. Steele RW, Marmer DJ, O'Brien MD, Tyson ST, Steele CR. Leukocyte survival in cerebrospinal fluid. *J Clin Microbiol* 1986;**23**:965–6.

46. Lamers KJB, Wevers RA. Cerebrospinal fluid diagnostics: biochemical and clinical aspects. *Klin Biochem Metab* 1995;**3**:63–75.

47. Roma AA, Garcia A, Avagnina A, Rescia C, Elsner B. Lymphoid and myeloid neoplasms involving cerebrospinal fluid: comparison of morphologic examination and immunophenotyping by flow cytometry. *Diagn Cytopathol* 2002;**27**:271–5.

48. Adam P, Taborsky L, Sobek O, *et al.* Cerebrospinal fluid. *Adv Clin Chem* 2001;**36**:1–62.

49. Spanos A, Harrell FE Jr, Durack DT. Differential diagnosis of acute meningitis. An analysis of the predictive value of initial observations. *JAMA* 1989;**262**:2700–7.

50. Zeman D, Adam P, Kalistova H, Sobek O, Andel J, Andel M. Cerebrospinal fluid cytologic findings in multiple sclerosis. A comparison between patient subgroups. *Acta Cytol* 2001;**45**:51–9.

51. UK National External Quality Assessment Scheme for Immunochemistry Working Group. National guidelines for analysis of cerebrospinal fluid for bilirubin in suspected subarachnoid haemorrhage. *Ann Clin Biochem* 2003;**40**: 481–8.

52. Twijnstra A, Ongerboer de Visser BW, van Zanten AP. Diagnosis of leptomeningeal metastasis. *Clin Neurol Neurosurg* 1987;**89**:79–85.

53. Glantz MJ, Cole BF, Glantz LK, et al. Cerebrospinal fluid cytology in patients with cancer: minimizing false-negative results. *Cancer* 1998;**82**:733–9.

54. Wasserstrom WR, Glass JP, Posner JB. Diagnosis and treatment of leptomeningeal metastases from solid tumors: experience with 90 patients. *Cancer* 1982;**49**:759–72.

55. Kaplan JG, DeSouza TG, Farkash A, et al. Leptomeningeal metastases: comparison of clinical features and laboratory data of solid tumors, lymphomas and leukemias. *J Neurooncol* 1990;**9**:225–9.

56. Schlossberg D. *Infections of the Nervous System.* Berlin: Springer-Verlag, 1990.

57. Kaiser R. Entzündliche und infektiöse Erkrankungen. In: Hufschmidt A, Lücking CH (eds) *Neurologie Compact, Leitlinie Für Klinik Und Praxis.* Stuttgart: Georg Thieme Verlag, 2002; pp. 121–172.

58. Takahashi T, Nakayama T, Tamura M, et al. Nested polymerase chain reaction for assessing the clinical course of tuberculous meningitis. *Neurology* 2005;**64**:1789–93.

59. Jeffery KJ, Read SJ, Peto TE, Mayon-White RT, Bangham CR. Diagnosis of viral infections of the central nervous system: clinical interpretation of PCR results. *Lancet* 1997; **349**:313–7.

60. Davies NW, Brown LJ, Gonde J, *et al.* Factors influencing PCR detection of viruses in cerebrospinal fluid of patients with suspected CNS infections. *J Neurol Neurosurg Psychiatry* 2005;**76**:82–7.

61. Kennedy PG. Viral encephalitis. *J Neurol* 2005;**252**:268–72.

62. Reiber H, Thompson EJ, Grimsley G, *et al.* Quality assurance for cerebrospinal fluid protein analysis: international consensus by an internet-based group discussion. *Clin Chem Lab Med* 2003;**41**:331–7. Available at: www.teamspace.net/CSF.

63. Linke E, Wieczorek V, Zimmermann K. Qualitätskontrolle in der Liquorzytodiagnostik. In: Zettl UK, Lehmitz R, Mix E (eds) *Klinische Liquordiagnostik*, 2nd edn. Berlin/New York: Walter de Gruyter, 2005; pp. 380–91.

64. Petzold A, Altintas A, Andreonie L, *et al.* Neurofilament ELISA validation. *J Immunol Methods* 2009; Oct 24. **352**: 23–31; [Epub ahead of print] doi:10.1016/j.jim.2009.09.014.

65. Fishman RA. *Cerebrospinal Fluid in Diseases of the Nervous System.* Philadelphia, PA: W.B. Saunders, 1992.

66. Jordan GW, Statland B, Halsted C. CSF lactate in diseases of the CNS. *Arch Intern Med* 1983;**143**:85–7.

67. Kniehl ER, Dörries HK, Geiss B, *et al.* In: Mauch H, Lütticken R (eds) *MiQ 17: Qualitätsstandards in Der Mikrobiologisch-Infektiologischen Diagnostik.* München, Jena: Urban & Fischer, 2001; pp. 1–77.

68. Lo Re V 3rd, Gluckman SJ. Eosinophilic meningitis. *Am J Med* 2003;**114**:217–23.

69. Öhman S, Forsberg P, Nelson N, Vrethem M. An improved formula for the judgement of intrathecally produced IgG in

the presence of blood brain barrier damage. *Clin Chim Acta* 1989;**181**:265–72.

70. Öhman S, Ernerudh J, Forsberg P, von Schenck H, Vrethem M. Improved formulae for the judgement of intrathecally produced IgA and IgM in the presence of blood CSF barrier damage. *Ann Clin Biochem* 1993;**30**:454–62.

71. Sabetta JR, Andriole VT. Cryptococcal infection of the central nervous system. *Med Clin North Am* 1985;**69**:333–44.

72. Seneviratne U. Guillain-Barré syndrome. *Postgrad Med J* 2000;**76**:774–82.

CHAPTER 2

Use of imaging in cerebrovascular disease

P. Irimia,[1] S. Asenbaum,[2] M. Brainin,[3] H. Chabriat,[4] E. Martínez-Vila,[1] K. Niederkorn,[5] P. D. Schellinger,[6] R. J. Seitz,[7] J. C. Masdeu[1]

[1]University of Navarra, Pamplona, Spain; [2]Medical University of Vienna, Austria; [3]Donauklinikum and Donau-Universität, Maria Gugging, Austria; [4]Lariboisiere Hospital, University of Paris, France; [5]Karl Franzens University, Graz, Austria; [6]University Clinic at Erlangen, Germany; [7]University Hospital Düsseldorf, Germany

Objectives

The objective of the task force is to actualize the EFNS Guideline on the use of neuroimaging for the management of acute stroke published in 2006. The Guideline is based on published scientific evidence as well as the consensus of experts. The resulting report is intended to provide updated and evidence-based recommendations regarding the use of diagnostic neuroimaging techniques, including cerebrovascular ultrasonography (US), in patients with stroke and thus guide neurologists, other healthcare professionals, and healthcare providers in clinical decision making and in the elaboration of clinical protocols. It is not intended to have legally binding implications in individual situations.

Background

Stroke is the second most common cause of death worldwide, and one of the major determining factors of hospital admission and permanent disability in the developed countries [1]. The proportion of the population over the age of 65 years is growing and this trend is likely to increase stroke incidence in the next decades [2]. Major advances in the understanding of the mechanisms of stroke and its management have been made thanks to the substantial progress in neuroimaging techniques. However, the multiplicity and continuous advances of neuroimaging techniques available for the evaluation of stroke patients has increased the complexity of decision making for physicians. Neurologists, who have been educated to manage acute stroke patients, should be trained in the use of neuroimaging, which allows for the development of a pathophysiologically oriented treatment.

Successful care of acute stroke patients requires a rapid and accurate diagnosis because the time window for treatment is narrow. In the case of intravenous thrombolysis for ischaemic stroke, the treatment is safer and more effective the earlier it is given [3]. Current recommendations call for a 4.5-h time limit for intravenous thrombolysis [4] that can be extended to 6 h for intra-arterial thrombolysis [5]. Thus, the neuroimaging protocol designed to determine the cause of stroke should delay treatment as little as possible. Neuroimaging can provide information about the presence of ischaemic but still viable and thus salvageable tissue (penumbra tissue) and vessel occlusion in the hyperacute phase of ischemic stroke. This information is critical for an improved selection of patients who could be treated with intravenous thrombolysis up to the 4.5-h limit and beyond [5]. Thus, neuroimaging criteria have been used for patient selection and outcome in different trials, using thrombolysis beyond 3 h after stroke onset [6, 7]. Determining stroke type using neuroimaging goes well beyond separating ischaemic from haemorrhagic stroke. For instance, the depiction of multiple cortical infarcts may lead to a fuller work-up for cardiogenic emboli [8, 9]. In arterial dissection, the characteristic semilunar high-intensity signal in the vessel wall on high-resolution T1-weighted magnetic resonance imaging (MRI) alerts to the presence of this cause of stroke [10].

European Handbook of Neurological Management: Volume 1, 2nd edition. Edited by N. E. Gilhus, M. P. Barnes and M. Brainin.

Search strategy

The Cochrane Library was consulted and no studies were found regarding the use of neuroimaging techniques in stroke. A comprehensive literature review using the MEDLINE database has been conducted by searching for the period 1965–2009. Relevant literature in English, including existing guidelines, meta-analyses, systematic reviews, randomized controlled trials, and observational studies have been critically assessed. Selected articles have been rated based on the quality of study design, and clinical practice recommendations have been developed and stratified to reflect the quality and the content of the evidence according to EFNS criteria [11].

Method for reaching consensus

The author panel critically assessed the topic through analysis of the medical literature. A draft guideline with specific recommendations was circulated to all panel members. Each panellist studied and commented in writing on this draft, which was revised to progressively accommodate the panel consensus. After the approval of the panellists, two independent experts gave their opinion on the final version.

Results

Imaging of the brain

The primary objectives of brain imaging in acute stroke are to exclude a non-vascular lesion as the cause of the symptoms and to determine whether the stroke is caused by an ischaemic infarction or a haemorrhage. It is not possible to exclude stroke mimics, such as a neoplasm, and distinguish between ischaemic and haemorrhagic stroke based exclusively on the history and physical examination [12]. Determining the nature of the lesion by brain imaging is necessary before starting any treatment, particularly thrombolysis and antithrombotic drugs (Class I, Level A).

Secondary objectives of brain imaging are to facilitate the identification of stroke mechanisms, to detect salvageable tissue, and to improve the selection of patients who could be candidates for reperfusion therapies.

Computed tomography (CT)

Conventional CT of the head is the examination most frequently used for the emergent evaluation of patients with acute stroke because of its wide availability and usefulness (Class II, Level B). It has been utilized as a screening tool in most of the major therapeutic trials conducted to date [3]. It is useful to distinguish between ischaemic stroke and intracerebral or subarachnoid haemorrhage (SAH), and can also rule out other conditions that could mimic stroke, such as brain tumours. Signs of early ischemia may be identified as early as 2 hrs from stroke onset, although they may appear much later [13]. Early infarct signs include the hyperdense middle cerebral artery (MCA) sign [14, 15] (indicative of a thrombus or embolus in the M1 segment of the vessel), the MCA dot sign [16, 17] (indicating thrombosis of M2 or M3 MCA branches), the loss of grey-white differentiation in the cortical ribbon [18] or the lentiform nucleus [19], and sulcal effacement [20]. The presence of some of these signs has been associated with poor outcome [20–22]. In the European Cooperative Acute Stroke Study (ECASS) I trial those patients with signs of early infarction involving more than one-third of the territory of the MCA had an increased risk of haemorrhagic transformation following treatment with thrombolysis [23]. A secondary analysis of other thrombolytic trials with a 6-h time window (ECASS II and Multicentre Acute Stroke Trial – Europe (MAST-E)) demonstrated that the presence of early CT changes was a risk factor for intracerebral haemorrhage (ICH) [24, 25], and similar results have been observed in larger series of patients [26]. However, in the National Institute of Neurological Disease and Stroke (NINDS) trial and the Australian Streptokinase Trial there was no relation between intracranial haemorrhage and early CT changes [27, 28], and it has been argued that the poorer outcome in patients with CT changes may have more to do with delayed treatment than with the changes themselves, with additional damage of the potentially salvageable tissue in the larger, CT-visible infarcts [29]. Because ischaemic changes are difficult to detect for clinicians without an adequate training in reading CT [30, 31], scoring systems have been developed to quantify early CT changes, such as the Alberta Stroke Programme Early CT Score (ASPECTS). More extensive early changes using ASPECTS correlate with high rates of intracranial haemorrhage and poor outcome at long term. Therefore, its use could improve the identification of ischaemic stroke patients who would particularly benefit from thrombolysis and those at risk of symptomatic haemorrhage [32, 33]. However, given the conflicting evidence, the presence of decreased attenuation on early CT, even affecting more than one-third of the MCA territory, cannot be construed as an absolute contraindication for the use of thrombolytic therapy in the first 3 h after stroke (Class IV, Good Clinical Practice Point (GCPP)).

Conventional CT contrast enhancement is not indicated for the acute diagnosis of stroke, and seldom may be helpful to show the infarcted area in the subacute stage (2–3 weeks after stroke onset) when there may be obscuration of the infarction by the 'fogging effect' [34, 35] (Class IV, Level C).

Computed tomography shows acute ICHs larger than 5 mm in diameter as areas of increased attenuation. Not depicted by CT are petechial haemorrhages and bleedings in patients with very low haemoglobin levels [36], because the high density of blood on CT is a function of haemoglobin concentration. CT demonstrates the size and topography of the haemorrhage and gives information about the presence of mass effect, hydrocephalus, and intraventricular extension of the bleeding. In addition, it may identify (although not as well as MRI) possible structural abnormalities (aneurysms, arteriovenous malformations, or tumours) that caused the haemorrhage. The characteristic hyperdensity of ICH on CT disappears with time, becoming hypodense after approximately 8–10 days [37, 38]. For this reason, CT is not a useful technique to distinguish between old haemorrhage and infarction. With newer CT helical units, SAH can be detected in 98–100% of patients in the first 12 h from the onset of symptoms [39, 40] and in 93% of patients studied within the first 24 h [41, 42].

CT is the imaging procedure of choice to diagnose SAH (Class I, Level A). Some experts recommend performing the study with thin cuts (3 mm in thickness) through the base of the brain, because small collections of blood may be missed with thicker cuts [39, 43] (Class IV, GCPP). CT cannot identify SAH in patients with low haemoglobin levels, because blood may appear isodense, and in those scanned after 3 weeks of the bleeding, when blood has usually been metabolized [44]. Lumbar puncture with CSF analysis should be performed when CT scan is negative or doubtful [45].

Cerebral venous thrombosis (CVT) is an uncommon cause of stroke [46, 47]. CT can show direct signs of venous thrombosis and other indirect non-specific signs, but in about one-third of cases CT is normal [48, 49]. Direct signs on unenhanced CT are the cord sign, corresponding to thrombosed cortical veins, and the dense triangle sign, corresponding to a thrombus in the superior sagittal sinus, and, on enhanced CT of the sagittal sinus, the delta sign [50]. Indirect signs such as local hypodensities caused by oedema or infarction, hyperdensities secondary to haemorrhagic infarction, or brain swelling and small ventricles suggest the diagnosis of CVT. CT venography has emerged as a good procedure to detect CVT [51–53] (Class III, Level C).

Perfusion-CT (PCT) techniques, despite being less sensitive than diffusion-weighted (DWI) MRI can show the area of ischaemia [54, 55]. Also, may it help distinguish between reversible (ischaemic penumbra) and irreversible (infarction) areas of ischaemia with standardized methodology [56–58]. Different preliminary studies comparing PCT with MRI have shown comparable results to depict penumbra tissue [59–62]. There is only one study to date (in which the primary end point was negative) demonstrating that perfusion CT may be used for the selection of candidates to thrombolytic therapy beyond the 3-h window [63]. Pregnancy, diabetes, renal failure, and allergy to contrast material are relative contraindications to performing a perfusion brain CT. Perfusion CT may be useful to characterize the presence of marginally perfused tissue (Class II, Level B).

Magnetic resonance imaging (MRI)

Magnetic resonance imaging has a higher sensitivity than conventional CT and results in lower inter-rater variability in the diagnosis of ischaemic stroke within the first hours of stroke onset [64–69] (Class I, Level A). MRI is particularly useful to show lesions in the brain stem or cerebellum, identify lacunar infarcts, and document vessel occlusion and brain oedema [65, 66, 68] (Class I, Level A).

In addition, MRI techniques can provide information about tissue viability. DWI and perfusion (PI) MRI studies may inform about the presence of reversibly and irreversibly damaged ischaemic tissues in the hyperacute phase of stroke [70–78] (Class II, Level B). DWI may demonstrate deeply ischaemic or infarcted brain tissue within minutes of symptom onset [77]. However, areas of abnormal DWI signal are not always infarcted and the finding may disappear spontaneously or after thrombolysis [79–81]. PI requires the intravenous administration of gadolinium and provides information about brain tissue perfusion at a given time. Different perfusion parameters give different perfusion lesion volumes in the same patient [82, 83]. The absolute volume difference or ratio of the PI area and the DWI area (diffusion–perfusion mismatch) is a useful method to estimate the presence of ischaemic penumbra tissue [84]. Not only the volume of abnormally perfused tissue but also the degree of perfusion drop predict the extent of ischaemic brain damage [85]. PI/DWI mismatch has been evaluated in several studies as a selection tool for thrombolytic therapy beyond 3 h [86–89] and in a phase II trial it was used as a selection tool and surrogate parameter for thrombolysis within 3–9 h [63]. A proposal for the standardization of perfusion and penumbral imaging techniques has been published [56]

Some neuroimaging findings on MRI, such as the presence of leukoaraiosis [90] and large DWI lesions [91], are associated with an increased risk for symptomatic intracerebral haemorrhage associated with thrombolytic treatment.

MRI may be useful to predict which patients will develop massive swelling with an MCA infarct. The measurement of infarct volume on DWI allows the prediction of malignant infarction [92, 93], and may be helpful for early management of these patients [94, 95].

MRI can help identify occluded intracranial arteries by the loss of the normal intravascular flow voids [65]. Some sequences, such as T2*-weighted MRI or fluid-attenuated inversion recovery (FLAIR; hyperintense artery sign), may demonstrate acute MCA thromboembolism with a higher sensitivity than CT, but the type of arterial change on MRI does not predict recanalization, clinical outcome, or ICH after intravenous thrombolysis [96, 97].

Intracranial haemorrhage is easily detectable on MRI using T2*-weighted images [98–100]. MRI can identify intraparenchymal haemorrhage within the first 6 h after symptom onset as accurately as CT [100, 101] (Class I, Level A). Susceptibility-weighted T2* sequences (gradient echo) can also detect clinically silent parenchymal microbleeds, not visible on CT, which may leave enough local haemosiderin to remain detectable for months or years after the bleeding. Microbleeds are associated with a history of ICH and prospectively have been shown to pose a 3% risk of ICH [102]. Although some retrospec-

tive studies reported an increased risk of symptomatic haemorrhage after thrombolysis [103, 104], this risk was not found in more recent studies [82, 105, 106]. The risk of bleeding after thrombolysis in patients with microbleeds is small [106] and their presence is not a contraindication to the use of thrombolytic therapy in the first 3 h after stroke (Class III, Level C).

MRI is also useful to date the haemorrhagic event accurately and to detect lesions (as tumours, vascular malformations, or aneurysms) that may underlie the ICH [107]. To detect these lesions, repeated studies may be needed after some of the swelling and vasospasm have subsided.

Subarachnoid haemorrhage (SAH) can be detected using T2* [108] and FLAIR [109, 110] MR sequences, but at present CT remains the imaging method of choice for this diagnosis (Class I, Level A).

Arterial dissection is a leading cause of stroke in young persons [47]. MRI is the initial procedure of choice [66, 68, 111, 112], replacing conventional angiography as the gold standard (Class II, Level B), because MRI can show the mural haematoma of the dissected vessel on the axial images [112] (high signal in the wall). Visualization of these changes in the vertebral artery is more difficult than for the larger carotid artery, making diagnosis of vertebral dissection less reliable. The study can be completed with magnetic resonance angiography (MRA) to visualize occlusion of the artery, pseudoaneurysms, or a long stenotic segment with tapered ends [113, 114]. Other techniques, including US [115–117] or CT angiography [113, 114, 118, 119], may be useful for the non-invasive diagnosis of arterial dissection.

MRI combined with MRA is the method of choice for the diagnosis and follow-up of CVT [49, 120–123]. MRI is more sensitive than CT to show parenchymal abnormalities and the presence of thrombosed veins.

In summary, MRI is very helpful in the clinical setting for the management of acute stroke and to guide decisions regarding thrombolysis (Class I, Level A). It is particularly helpful for the study of stroke patients for whom perfusion CT may be dangerous, such as those with renal failure or diabetes. However, MRI in the acute phase of stroke is not widely available at European hospitals [124]. Other limitations and contraindications for the use of MRI are: claustrophobia, agitation, morbid obesity, the presence of intracranial ferromagnetic elements, an aneurysm recently clipped or coiled, otic or cochlear implants, some old prosthetic heart valves, pacemakers, and some, not all, neurostimulators.

SPECT and PET

Single photon emission computed tomography (SPECT) and positron emission tomography (PET) are functional neuroimaging techniques based on the principles of tracer technology using radiolabelled substances as systemically administered tracers. In the setting of stroke, SPECT has been used for the evaluation of cerebral perfusion. Earlier perfusion SPECT studies failed to show any advantage of SPECT over the structured clinical evaluation (NIH, Canadian, Scandinavian stroke scales) in the prediction of the evolution of acute stroke [125]. However, using ethyl cysteinate dimer (ECD) SPECT in the first 6 h after stroke, Barthel et al. [126] were able to determine which patients would develop massive MCA-territory necrosis, with hemispheric herniation. These patients have a high risk of haemorrhage following thrombolysis and could potentially be helped by early decompressive hemicraniectomy [127]. Complete MCA infarctions were predicted with significantly higher accuracy with early SPECT compared with early CT and clinical parameters. The predictive value increased when the findings on CT, clinical examination, and SPECT were considered [126]. Other studies have found SPECT to add predictive value to the clinical score on admission [128–130]. Those studies suggest that a patient with a normal SPECT study performed within 3 h of stroke onset will most likely recover spontaneously and therefore may not benefit from thrombolysis. A patient with a dense deficit in the entire MCA distribution has a high risk of haemorrhage with thrombolysis, and, depending on age and other factors, should be considered for decompressive hemicraniectomy. The patients most likely to benefit from thrombolysis are the ones with less massive lesions [126, 128]. Thus, SPECT is helpful in the evaluation of acute stroke (Class III, Level C). Unfortunately, the need to perform either CT or MRI in acute stroke renders the performance of SPECT difficult within the time frame allotted for the evaluation of these patients. SPECT is also helpful in the evaluation of cerebral perfusion in non-acute cerebrovascular disease, for instance in the days after a SAH [131] (Class III, Level C).

PET can be used to evaluate a large variety of physiological variables including cerebral blood flow, cerebral blood volume, and cerebral glucose metabolism, as well as the density of neurotransmitters and neuroreceptors, such as benzodiazepine receptors with flumazenil, an accurate marker of neuronal loss [132]. As PET has been considered the gold standard for these kinds of measurements in humans, it is also extremely well suited to help identify the degree of ischaemic damage in the brain. Heiss et al. compared ^{15}O-water PET and MRI in patients with acute ischaemic stroke. They observed that DW/PW–MRI mismatch overestimates the penumbra defined by PET [133]. Although PET is the reference method for quantitative perfusion imaging, it does not allow for the reliable identification of lesions in the vessels or non-vascular lesions giving rise to the stroke syndrome. This, coupled with the cost and current lack of availability of this technique, renders it less useful than MRI and CT for most practising neurologists.

Imaging of the extracranial vessels

Imaging of the extracranial and intracranial vessels will help identify the underlying mechanism of the stroke (atherothrombotic, embolic, dissection, or other). Non-invasive imaging methods are increasingly accepted as replacements of digital substraction angiography (DSA) in the evaluation of carotid stenosis prior to endarterectomy [134] (Class IV, GCPP). US, comprising Doppler sonography and colour-coded duplex sonography, is probably the most common non-invasive imaging examination performed to aid in the diagnosis of carotid disease. The peak systolic velocity and the presence of plaque on greyscale and/or colour Doppler/Duplex US images are the main parameters that should be used when diagnosing and grading internal carotid artery (ICA) stenosis [135]. The examination may be limited by the presence of extensive plaque calcifications, vessel tortuosity and in patients with tandem lesions. In addition, Doppler US is both technician- and equipment-dependent and all sonographers should be able to demonstrate that they have validated their testing procedures. Meta-analyses of published criteria for US have demonstrated sensitivities of 98% and specificities of 88% for detecting > 50% ICA stenosis; and 94% and 90% respectively for detecting > 70% ICA stenosis [136].

Magnetic resonance angiography using time-of-flight angiography (TOF) and contrast-enhanced MRA (CEMRA) are powerful means to assess vascular pathology. Either technique provides specific information:

while TOF visualizes changes of flow in the arteries or veins depending on imaging parameters, CEMRA visualizes the vascular lumen. MRA and US have yielded comparable findings. Two meta-analyses [137, 138] and several reviews [139, 140] have compared the diagnostic value of Doppler US, MRA, and conventional DSA for the diagnosis of carotid artery stenosis. The meta-analysis published by Blakeley et al. [137] in 1995 concluded that Doppler US and MRA had similar diagnostic performance in predicting carotid artery occlusion and >70% stenosis. In the systematic review performed by Nederkoorn et al. [139] for the diagnosis of 70–99% stenosis, MRA had a pooled sensitivity of 95% and a pooled specificity of 90%, and US 86% and 87% respectively. For recognising occlusion, MRA had a sensitivity of 98% and a specificity of 100%, and DUS had a sensitivity of 96% and a specificity of 100%. A meta-analysis comparing the accuracy of TOF or CEMRA for the detection of ICA disease against intra-arterial angiography showed that CEMRA is slightly more precise than TOF for the detection of ICA high-grade (≥70 to 99%) stenosis and occlusion, and appears to achieve a higher sensitivity for the detection of moderate (50–69%) stenosis [141]. Computed tomography angiography, a contrast-dependent technique, has been compared with DSA for the detection and quantification of carotid stenosis and occlusions [142–147]. A systematic review concludes that this technique has demonstrated a good sensitivity and specificity for occlusion (97%), but the pooled sensitivity and specificity for detection of a 70–99% stenosis by CTA were 85% and 93% respectively [146] (Class II, Level B). In a systematic review, CEMRA is more accurate than CTA to adequately evaluate 70–99% carotid stenosis [148], especially when there is an excess of calcium in the plaque [149]. The difference among these modalities is small, and other factors, such as availability and quality of US performance, may render one procedure more useful than the other (Class II, Level B).

Similarly to carotid stenosis, CEMRA and CTA may be more sensitive in diagnosing vertebral artery stenosis than DUS [150].

Digital substraction angiography is the reference method to determine the degree of carotid and vertebral artery stenosis. Endarterectomy trials for symptomatic [151–153] and asymptomatic [154] patients were performed using this method. However, angiography carries the risk of stroke and death [134, 155], and many centres are not using DSA prior to carotid endarterectomy [135, 156–159], particularly when non-invasive methods are concordant (Class IV, GCPP). When non-invasive methods are inconclusive or there is a discrepancy between them, DSA is necessary.

Imaging of the intracranial vessels

Transcranial Doppler (TCD) and transcranial colour-coded duplex (TCCD) are non-invasive ultrasonographic procedures that measure local blood flow velocity and direction but also permit visualization of blood vessels (TCCD) in the proximal portions of large intracranial arteries [160, 161]. These methods are useful for the screening of intracranial stenosis [162–164] and occlusion [165, 166] in patients with cerebrovascular disease (Class II, Level B). In children with sickle cell disease, detection of asymptomatic intracerebral stenoses using TCD allows selection of a group at high risk of future stroke, who benefit from exchange transfusion [167] (Class II, Level B). It is also useful for the detection and monitoring of intracranial artery vasospasm after SAH, particularly in the MCA [168] (Class I, Level A). TCD can be used to monitor recanalization during thrombolysis in acute MCA occlusions [169] (Class II, Level B). There is increasing interest in its therapeutic use. In vitro studies demonstrate it has an additive effect on clot lysis when used with recombinant tissue plasminogen activator (rtPA), and clinical studies have suggested that continuous TCD monitoring in patients with acute MCA occlusion treated with intravenous thrombolysis may improve both early recanalization and clinical outcome [170]. TCD allows for the documentation of a right-to-left shunt in patients with ischaemic stroke (Class II, Level A). TCD discloses a shower of air bubbles in the MCA after the intravenous injection of saline mixed with air bubbles [171–173].

TCD is the only imaging technique that allows detection of circulating emboli, even in asymptomatic patients (Class II, Level A). Emboli cause short-duration, high-intensity signals, because they reflect and backscatter more ultrasound than the surrounding red blood cells. Studies have shown that asymptomatic embolization is common in acute stroke, particularly in patients with carotid artery disease [174, 175]. In this group the presence of embolic signals has been shown to predict the risk of stroke and transient ischaemic attack (TIA) [176–178] (Class II, Level A). Embolic signals have also been used as surrogate markers to evaluate antiplatelet agents in both single-centre studies [179] and in the multicentre international Clopidogrel and Aspirin for Reduction of Emboli in Symptomatic Carotid Stenosis trial [180]. Embolic signal monitoring is used to monitor embolization following carotid endarterectomy; the presence of frequent embolic signals in this setting predicts early postoperative stroke [181] and can be reduced by more aggressive antiplatelet treatment, including dextran [182] and clopidogrel [183]. TCD can also be used to evaluate cerebrovascular reserve by determining the extent to which MCA flow velocity can increase in response to the vasodilator carbon dioxide or acetazolamide. Reserve is reduced in a proportion of patients with carotid occlusion and tight stenosis, and impaired reserve predicts recurrent TIA and stroke risk, particularly in the group with carotid occlusion [184, 185] (Class III, Level B).

Transcranial Doppler examination cannot be performed in about 10–15% of patients, particularly older women, because they lack a transtemporal window due to the thickness of the skull [186]. The use of intravenous echo contrast agents may improve detection of flow velocities in patients with limited transtemporal window [187]. TCD velocities may be altered in patients with cardiac pump failure (low velocities) or anaemia (increased velocities).

Magnetic resonance angiography (MRA) can identify intracranial steno-occlusive lesions mainly in the proximal segments. Both TCD ultrasound and MRA non-invasively identify 50–99% of intracranial large vessel stenoses with substantial negative predictive value (86% and 91% respectively) [188]. Compared with DSA, MRA has a higher sensitivity and specificity (superior to 80%)

for the identification of proximal intracranial arterial stenosis [189, 190] (Class II, Level B).

CT angiography is another useful technique with high sensitivity and specificity (superior to 90%) for the diagnosis of occlusion and intracranial stenosis [191, 192], with the exception of stenosis in the cavernous portion of the internal carotid or in arteries with circumferential wall calcification [189, 193] (Class II, Level B).

Magnetic resonance and CT angiography can be used to show large aneurysms (Class II, Level B), but these techniques fail to identify aneurysm of less than 5 mm in diameter, those located in the intracranial carotid artery, and cannot clearly establish the critical relationship of the neck of the aneurysm(s) with arterial branches [194–197]. Therefore non–invasive techniques have not replaced DSA for aneurysm identification and localization. The sensitivity of 3-dimensional time-of-flight MRA for cerebral aneurysms ≥5 mm after SAH is between 85% and 100% [198–200], with lower percentages for aneurysms <5 mm [45, 198, 200]. CT angiography has a sensitivity for aneurysms ≥5 mm between 95% and 100% and a specificity between 79% and 100% [45, 201–203]. Some authors suggest that CT angiography can be used as a reliable alternative to DSA after SAH, particularly in cases in which the risk of delaying surgery does not justify the performance of a catheter study [45, 204] (Class II, Level B).

MR and CT angiography have been used for screening individuals with a history of intracranial aneurysm or SAH in first-degree relatives [205, 206] (Class II, Level B). Overall reported sensitivity for both techniques was 76–98% and specificity was 85–100% [207].

DSA is needed to demonstrate small aneurysms and before surgery or endovascular treatment (Class I, Level A).

Recommendations

Imaging of the brain

- Either non-contrast computed tomography (CT) or magnetic resonance imaging (MRI) should be used for the definition of stroke type and treatment of stroke (Class I, Level A).

- The presence of early CT infarct signs cannot be construed as an absolute contraindication to thrombolysis in the first 3 h after stroke (Class IV, GCPP).

- MRI has a higher sensitivity than conventional CT for the documentation of infarction within the first hours of stroke onset, lesions in the posterior fossa, identification of small

lesions, and documentation of vessel occlusion and brain oedema (Class I, Level A).

- In conjunction with MRI and magnetic resonance angiography (MRA), perfusion and diffusion MR are very helpful for the evaluation of patients with acute ischaemic stroke (Class I, Level A).

- Single photon emission computed tomography (SPECT) is helpful to predict the malignant course of brain swelling with large hemispheric infarctions (Class III, Level C). SPECT is also helpful in the evaluation of cerebral perfusion in non-acute cerebrovascular disease, for instance in the days after a subarachnoid haemorrhage (SAH) (Class III, Level C).

Detection of haemorrhagic stroke

- MRI can detect acute and chronic intracerebral haemorrhage (Class I, Level A).
- Although the detection of SAH is possible with MRI, currently CT scan is the diagnostic procedure of choice (Class I, Level A). In case of doubt or negative CT scan, lumbar puncture and cerebrospinal fluid (CSF) analysis is recommended (Class I, Level B)

Imaging of extracranial vessels

- Although MRA has slightly higher sensitivity and specificity than ultrasonography (US) to determine carotid stenosis and occlusion, the usefulness of either procedure may be determined by other factors, such as availability (Class II, Level B).
- Computed tomography angiography (CTA) has a sensitivity and specificity similar to MR for carotid occlusion and similar to US for the detection of severe stenosis (Class II, Level B).
- Digital substraction angiography (DSA) is generally recommended for grading carotid stenosis prior to endarterectomy (Class I, Level A), but when there is concordance of non-invasive methods cerebral arteriography may not be necessary (Class IV, GCPP).

Imaging of intracraneal vessels

- Transcranial Doppler (TCD) is very useful for assessing stroke risk of children aged 2–16 years with sickle cell disease (Class II, Level B), detection and monitoring of vasospasm after SAH (Class I, Level A), diagnosis of intracranial steno-occlusive disease (Class II, Level B), diagnosis of right-to-left shunts (Class II, Level A), and for monitoring arterial recanalization after thrombolysis of acute middle cerebral artery (MCA) occlusions (Class II, Level B).
- TCD can detect cerebral emboli and impaired cerebral haemodynamics. The presence of embolic signals with carotid stenosis predicts early recurrent stroke risk (Class II, Level A). The detection of impaired cerebral haemodynamics in carotid occlusion may identify a group at high risk of recurrent stroke (Class III, Level B).
- MRA and CTA are very useful for the diagnosis of intracranial stenosis and cerebral aneurysms >5 mm (Class II, Level B). MRA and CTA are the recommended techniques for screening cerebral aneurysms in individuals with a history of aneurysms or SAH in a first-degree relative (Class II, Level B).
- DSA is the recommended technique for the diagnosis of cerebral aneurysm as the cause of SAH (Class I, Level A). CTA can be used as a reliable alternative to DSA in patients with SAH, particularly in cases in which the risk of delaying surgery for a catheter study is not justified (Class II, Level B).
- MRI with MRA is recommended for the diagnosis and follow-up of cerebral venous thrombosis (Class II, Level B). Alternatively, CT venography is accurate and can be used for the same purpose (Class III, Level C).

Conflicts of interest

J. Masdeu received an honorarium as Editor-in-Chief of the *Journal of Neuroimaging*. With regard to this manuscript there is no conflict of interest.

P. D. Schellinger has received travel stipends, advisory board and speakers honoraria from Boehringer Ingelheim, the manufacturers of Alteplase.

The rest of authors have reported no conflicts of interest relevant to this manuscript.

References

1. World Health Organization. *The Global Burden of Disease: 2004 Update*. Geneva, Switzerland: World Health Organization, 2008.

2. Truelsen T, Piechowski-Jozwiak B, Bonita R, Mathers C, Bogousslavsky J, Boysen G. Stroke incidence and prevalence in Europe: a review of available data. *Eur J Neurol* 2006;**13**(6):581–98.

3. Hacke W, Donnan G, Fieschi C, *et al*. Association of outcome with early stroke treatment: pooled analysis of ATLANTIS, ECASS, and NINDS rt-PA stroke trials. *Lancet* 2004;**363**(9411):768–74.

4. Hacke W, Kaste M, Bluhmki E, *et al*. Thrombolysis with alteplase 3 to 4.5 hours after acute ischemic stroke. *N Engl J Med* 2008;**359**(13):1317–29.

5. Furlan A, Higashida R, Wechsler L, *et al*. Intra-arterial prourokinase for acute ischemic stroke: the PROACT II Study: a randomized controlled trial. *JAMA* 1999;**282**(21): 2003–11.

6. Schellinger PD, Fiebach JB, Hacke W. Imaging-based decision making in thrombolytic therapy for ischemic stroke: present status. *Stroke* 2003;**34**(2):575–83.

7. Donnan GA, Baron JC, Ma H, Davis SM. Penumbral selection of patients for trials of acute stroke therapy. *Lancet Neurol* 2009;**8**(3):261–9.

8. Wessels T, Wessels C, Ellsiepen A, *et al.* Contribution of diffusion-weighted imaging in determination of stroke etiology. *AJNR Am J Neuroradiol* 2006;**27**(1):35–9.

9. Caso V, Budak K, Georgiadis D, Schuknecht B, Baumgartner RW. Clinical significance of detection of multiple acute brain infarcts on diffusion weighted magnetic resonance imaging. *J Neurol Neurosurg Psychiatry* 2005;**76**(4): 514–8.

10. Lanczik O, Szabo K, Hennerici M, Gass A. Multiparametric MRI and ultrasound findings in patients with internal carotid artery dissection. *Neurology* 2005;**65**(3):469–71.

11. Brainin M, Barnes M, Baron JC, *et al.* Guidance for the preparation of neurological management guidelines by EFNS scientific task forces – revised recommendations 2004. *Eur J Neurol* 2004;**11**(9):577–81.

12. Britton M, Hindmarsh T, Murray V, Tyden SA. Diagnostic errors discovered by CT in patients with suspected stroke. *Neurology* 1984;**34**(11):1504.

13. von Kummer R, Nolte PN, Schnittger H, Thron A, Ringelstein EB. Detectability of cerebral hemisphere ischaemic infarcts by CT within 6 h of stroke. *Neuroradiology* 1995;**38**(1):31–3.

14. Gacs G, Fox AJ, Barnett HJ, Vinuela F. CT visualization of intracranial arterial thromboembolism. *Stroke* 1983;**14**(5): 756–62.

15. Bastianello S, Pierallini A, Colonnese C, *et al.* Hyperdense middle cerebral artery CT sign. *Neuroradiology* 1991;**33**(3): 207–11.

16. Barber PA, Demchuk AM, Hudon ME, Pexman JH, Hill MD, Buchan AM. Hyperdense sylvian fissure MCA "Dot" sign: a CT marker of acute ischemia. *Stroke* 2001;**32**(1): 84–8.

17. Leary MC, Kidwell CS, Villablanca JP, *et al.* Validation of computed tomographic middle cerebral artery "dot"sign: an angiographic correlation study. *Stroke* 2003;**34**(11): 2636–40.

18. Truwit CL, Barkovich AJ, Gean-Marton A, Hibri N, Norman D. Loss of the insular ribbon: another early CT sign of acute middle cerebral artery infarction. *Radiology* 1990;**176**(3):801–6.

19. Tomura N, Uemura K, Inugami A, Fujita H, Higano S, Shishido F. Early CT finding in cerebral infarction: obscuration of the lentiform nucleus. *Radiology* 1988;**168**(2): 463–7.

20. Moulin T, Cattin F, Crepin-Leblond T, *et al.* Early CT signs in acute middle cerebral artery infarction: predictive value for subsequent infarct locations and outcome. *Neurology* 1996;**47**(2):366–75.

21. Kharitonova T, Ahmed N, Thoren M, *et al.* Hyperdense middle cerebral artery sign on admission CT scan – prognostic significance for ischaemic stroke patients treated with intravenous thrombolysis in the safe implementation of thrombolysis in Stroke International Stroke Thrombolysis Register. *Cerebrovasc Dis* 2009;**27**(1):51–9.

22. von Kummer R, Allen KL, Holle R, *et al.* Acute stroke: usefulness of early CT findings before thrombolytic therapy. *Radiology* 1997;**205**(2):327–33.

23. Hacke W, Kaste M, Fieschi C, *et al.* Intravenous thrombolysis with recombinant tissue plasminogen activator for acute hemispheric stroke. The European Cooperative Acute Stroke Study (ECASS). *JAMA* 1995;**274**(13):1017–25.

24. Larrue V, von Kummer RR, Muller A, Bluhmki E. Risk factors for severe hemorrhagic transformation in ischemic stroke patients treated with recombinant tissue plasminogen activator: a secondary analysis of the European-Australasian Acute Stroke Study (ECASS II). *Stroke* 2001;**32**(2):438–41.

25. Jaillard A, Cornu C, Durieux A, *et al.* Hemorrhagic transformation in acute ischemic stroke: the MAST-E study. *Stroke* 1999;**30**(7):1326–32.

26. Tanne D, Kasner SE, Demchuk AM, *et al.* Markers of increased risk of intracerebral hemorrhage after intravenous recombinant tissue plasminogen activator therapy for acute ischemic stroke in clinical practice: the multicenter rt-PA acute stroke survey. *Circulation* 2002;**105**(14): 1679–85.

27. Patel SC, Levine SR, Tilley BC, *et al.* Lack of clinical significance of early ischemic changes on computed tomography in acute stroke. *JAMA* 2001;**286**(22):2830–8.

28. Gilligan AK, Markus R, Read S, *et al.* Baseline blood pressure but not early computed tomography changes predicts major hemorrhage after streptokinase in acute ischemic stroke. *Stroke* 2002;**33**(9):2236–42.

29. Grotta J. NIHSS/EIC mismatch explains the >1/3 MCA conundrum. *Stroke* 2003;**34**:e148–9.

30. von Kummer R, Holle R, Gizyska U, *et al.* Interobserver agreement in assessing early CT signs of middle cerebral artery infarction. *AJNR Am J Neuroradiol* 1996;**17**(9): 1743–8.

31. von Kummer R. Effect of training in reading CT scans on patient selection for ECASS II. *Neurology* 1998;**51**(3 Suppl 3):S50–2.

32. Hill MD, Rowley HA, Adler F, *et al.* Selection of acute ischemic stroke patients for intra-arterial thrombolysis with pro-urokinase by using ASPECTS. *Stroke* 2003;**34**(8): 1925–31.

33. Barber PA, Demchuk AM, Zhang J, Buchan AM. Validity and reliability of a quantitative computed tomography

score in predicting outcome of hyperacute stroke before thrombolytic therapy. *Lancet* 2000;**355**(9216):1670–4.

34. Wing SD, Norman D, Pollock JA, Newton TH. Contrast enhancement of cerebral infarcts in computed tomography. *Radiology* 1976;**121**(1):89–92.

35. Becker H, Desch H, Hacker H, Pencz A. CT fogging effect with ischemic cerebral infarcts. *Neuroradiology* 1979;**18**(4):185–92.

36. New PF, Aronow S. Attenuation measurements of whole blood and blood fractions in computed tomography. *Radiology* 1976;**121**(3):635–40.

37. Dennis M, Bamford JM, Molyneux AJ, Warlow CP. Rapid resolution of signs of primary intracerebral haemorrhage in computed tomograms of the brain. *Br Med J (Clin Res Ed)* 1987;**295**:379–81.

38. Wardlaw J, Keir SL, Seymour J, *et al.* What is the best imaging strategy for acute stroke? *Health Technol Assess* 2004;**8**(iii, ix–iii):1–180.

39. Sidman R, Connolly E, Lemke T. Subarachnoid hemorrhage diagnosis: lumbar puncture is still needed when the computed tomography scan is normal. *Acad Emerg Med* 1996;**3**(9):827–31.

40. van der Wee N, Rinkel GJ, Hasan D, van Gijn J. Detection of subarachnoid haemorrhage on early CT: is lumbar puncture still needed after a negative scan? *J Neurol Neurosurg Psychiatry* 1995;**58**(3):357–9.

41. Sames T, Storrow AB, Finkelstein JA, Magoon MR. Sensitivity of new-generation computed tomography in subarachnoid hemorrhage. *Acad Emerg Med* 1996;**3**(1):16–20.

42. Morgenstern L, Luna-Gonzales H, Huber JC Jr, *et al.* Worst headache and subarachnoid hemorrhage: prospective, modern computed tomography and spinal fluid analysis. *Ann Emerg Med* 1998;**32**(3Pt 1):297–304.

43. Edlow JA, Caplan LR. Avoiding pitfalls in the diagnosis of subarachnoid hemorrhage. *N Engl J Med* 2000;**342**(1):29–36.

44. van Gijn J, van Dongen KJ. The time course of aneurysmal haemorrhage on computed tomograms. *Neuroradiology* 1982;**23**(3):153–6.

45. Bederson JB, Connolly ES Jr, Batjer HH, *et al.* Guidelines for the management of aneurysmal subarachnoid hemorrhage: a statement for healthcare professionals from a special writing group of the Stroke Council, American Heart Association. *Stroke* 2009;**40**(3):994–1025.

46. Arboix A, Bechich S, Oliveres M, García-Eroles L, Massons J, Targa C. Ischemic stroke of unusual cause: clinical features, etiology and outcome. *Eur J Neurol* 2001;**8**(2):133–9.

47. Bogousslavsky J, Pierre P. Ischemic stroke in patients under age 45. *Neurol Clin* 1992;**10**(1):113–24.

48. Bousser MG, Chiras J, Bories J, Castaigne P. Cerebral venous thrombosis – a review of 38 cases. *Stroke* 1985;**16**(2):199–213.

49. Renowden S. Cerebral venous sinus thrombosis. *Eur Radiol* 2004;**14**(2):215–26.

50. Virapongse C, Cazenave C, Quisling R, Sarwar M, Hunter S. The empty delta sign: frequency and significance in 76 cases of dural sinus thrombosis. *Radiology* 1987;**162**(3):779–85.

51. Casey SO, Alberico RA, Patel M, *et al.* Cerebral CT venography. *Radiology* 1996;**198**(1):163–70.

52. Gaikwad AB, Mudalgi BA, Patankar KB, Patil JK, Ghongade DV. Diagnostic role of 64-slice multidetector row CT scan and CT venogram in cases of cerebral venous thrombosis. *Emerg Radiol* 2008;**15**(5):325–33.

53. Linn J, Ertl-Wagner B, Seelos KC, *et al.* Diagnostic value of multidetector-row CT angiography in the evaluation of thrombosis of the cerebral venous sinuses. *AJNR Am J Neuroradiol* 2007;**28**(5):946–52.

54. Kohrmann M, Schellinger PD. Acute stroke triage to intravenous thrombolysis and other therapies with advanced CT or MR imaging: pro MR imaging. *Radiology* 2009;**251**(3):627–33.

55. Wintermark M, Rowley HA, Lev MH. Acute stroke triage to intravenous thrombolysis and other therapies with advanced CT or MR imaging: pro CT. *Radiology* 2009;**251**(3):619–26.

56. Wintermark M, Albers GW, Alexandrov AV, *et al.* Acute stroke imaging research roadmap. *AJNR Am J Neuroradiol* 2008;**29**(5):e23–30.

57. Schaefer PW, Roccatagliata L, Ledezma C, *et al.* First-pass quantitative CT perfusion identifies thresholds for salvageable penumbra in acute stroke patients treated with intra-arterial therapy. *AJNR Am J Neuroradiol* 2006;**27**(1):20–5.

58. Wintermark M, Flanders AE, Velthuis B, *et al.* Perfusion-CT assessment of infarct core and penumbra: receiver operating characteristic curve analysis in 130 patients suspected of acute hemispheric stroke. *Stroke* 2006;**37**(4):979–85.

59. Wintermark M, Reichhart M, Cuisenaire O, *et al.* Comparison of admission perfusion computed tomography and qualitative diffusion- and perfusion-weighted magnetic resonance imaging in acute stroke patients. *Stroke* 2002;**33**(8):2025–31.

60. Eastwood JD, Lev MH, Wintermark M, *et al.* Correlation of early dynamic CT perfusion imaging with whole-brain MR diffusion and perfusion imaging in acute hemispheric stroke. *AJNR Am J Neuroradiol* 2003;**24**(9):1869–75.

61. Schramm P, Schellinger PD, Klotz E, *et al.* Comparison of perfusion computed tomography and computed tomography angiography source images with perfusion-

weighted imaging and diffusion-weighted imaging in patients with acute stroke of less than 6 hours' duration. *Stroke* 2004;**35**(7):1652–8.

62. Schaefer PW, Barak ER, Kamalian S, *et al.* Quantitative assessment of core/penumbra mismatch in acute stroke: CT and MR perfusion imaging are strongly correlated when sufficient brain volume is imaged. *Stroke* 2008; **39**(11):2986–92.

63. Hacke W, Furlan AJ, Al-Rawi Y, *et al.* Intravenous desmoteplase in patients with acute ischaemic stroke selected by MRI perfusion-diffusion weighted imaging or perfusion CT (DIAS-2): a prospective, randomised, double-blind, placebo-controlled study. *Lancet Neurol* 2009;**8**(2):141–50.

64. Fiebach JB, Schellinger PD, Jansen O, *et al.* CT and diffusion-weighted MR imaging in randomized order: diffusion-weighted imaging results in higher accuracy and lower interrater variability in the diagnosis of hyperacute ischemic stroke. *Stroke* 2002;**33**(9):2206–10.

65. Bryan RN, Levy LM, Whitlow WD, Killian JM, Preziosi TJ, Rosario JA. Diagnosis of acute cerebral infarction: comparison of CT and MR imaging. *AJNR Am J Neuroradiol* 1991;**12**(4):611–20.

66. Culebras A, Kase CS, Masdeu JC, *et al.* Practice guidelines for the use of imaging in transient ischemic attacks and acute stroke: a report of the stroke council, American Heart Association. *Stroke* 1997;**28**(7):1480–97.

67. Shuaib A, Lee D, Pelz D, Fox A, Hachinski VC. The impact of magnetic resonance imaging on the management of acute ischemic stroke. *Neurology* 1992;**42**(4):816.

68. European Stroke Organization (ESO) Executive Committee. Guidelines for management of ischaemic stroke and transient ischaemic attack 2008. *Cerebrovasc Dis* 2008;**25**(5): 457–507.

69. Chalela JA, Kidwell CS, Nentwich LM, *et al.* Magnetic resonance imaging and computed tomography in emergency assessment of patients with suspected acute stroke: a prospective comparison. *Lancet* 2007;**369**(9558):293–8.

70. Rohl L, Ostergaard L, Simonsen CZ, *et al.* Viability thresholds of ischemic penumbra of hyperacute stroke defined by perfusion-weighted MRI and apparent diffusion coefficient. *Stroke* 2001;**32**(5):1140–6.

71. Warach S, Mosley M, Sorensen AG, Koroshetz W. Time course of diffusion imaging abnormalities in human stroke. *Stroke* 1996;**27**:1254–6.

72. Sorensen AG, Buonanno FS, Gonzalez RG, *et al.* Hyperacute stroke: evaluation with combined multisection diffusion-weighted and hemodynamically weighted echo-planar MR imaging. *Radiology* 1996;**199**(2): 391–401.

73. Barber PA, Darby DG, Desmond PM, *et al.* Prediction of stroke outcome with echoplanar perfusion-

and diffusion-weighted MRI. *Neurology* 1998;**51**(2): 418–26.

74. Warach S, Dashe JF, Edelman RR. Clinical outcome in ischemic stroke predicted by early diffusion-weighted and perfusion magnetic resonance imaging: a preliminary analysis. *J Cereb Blood Flow Metab* 1996;**16**(1): 53–9.

75. Beaulieu C, de Crespigny A, Tong DC, Moseley ME, Albers GW, Marks MP. Longitudinal magnetic resonance imaging study of perfusion and diffusion in stroke: evolution of lesion volume and correlation with clinical outcome. *Ann Neurol* 1999;**46**(4):568–78.

76. Schlaug G, Benfield A, Baird AE, *et al.* The ischemic penumbra: operationally defined by diffusion and perfusion MRI. *Neurology* 1999;**53**(7):1528.

77. Warach S, Chien D, LiW, Ronthal M, Edelman RR. Fast magnetic resonance diffusion-weighted imaging of acute human stroke. *Neurology* 1992;**42**(9):1717.

78. Wittsack H-J, Ritzl A, Fink GR, *et al.* MR imaging in acute stroke: diffusion-weighted and perfusion imaging parameters for predicting infarct size. *Radiology* 2002;**222**(2): 397–403.

79. Fiehler J, Foth M, Kucinski T, *et al.* Severe ADC decreases do not predict irreversible tissue damage in humans. *Stroke* 2002;**33**(1):79–86.

80. Fiehler J, Knudsen K, Kucinski T, *et al.* Predictors of apparent diffusion coefficient normalization in stroke patients. *Stroke* 2004;**35**(2):514–9.

81. Oppenheim C, Lamy C, Touze E, *et al.* Do transient ischemic attacks with diffusion-weighted imaging abnormalities correspond to brain infarctions? *AJNR Am J Neuroradiol* 2006;**27**(8):1782–7.

82. Kane I, Carpenter T, Chappell F, *et al.* Comparison of 10 different magnetic resonance perfusion imaging processing methods in acute ischemic stroke: effect on lesion size, proportion of patients with diffusion/perfusion mismatch, clinical scores, and radiologic outcomes. *Stroke* 2007;**38**(12):3158–64.

83. Kane I, Sandercock P, Wardlaw J. Magnetic resonance perfusion diffusion mismatch and thrombolysis in acute ischaemic stroke: a systematic review of the evidence to date. *J Neurol Neurosurg Psychiatry* 2007;**78**(5):485–91.

84. Latchaw RE, Yonas H, Hunter GJ, *et al.* Guidelines and recommendations for perfusion imaging in cerebral ischemia: a scientific statement for healthcare professionals by the writing group on perfusion imaging, from the council on cardiovascular radiology of the American Heart Association. *Stroke* 2003;**34**(4):1084–104.

85. Seitz RJ, Meisel S, Weller P, Junghans U, Wittsack HJ, Siebler M. Initial ischemic event: perfusion-weighted MR imaging and apparent diffusion coefficient for stroke evolution. *Radiology* 2005;**237**(3):1020–8.

86. Rother J, Schellinger PD, Gass A, *et al.* Effect of intravenous thrombolysis on MRI parameters and functional outcome in acute stroke <6 hours. *Stroke* 2002;**33**(10): 2438–45.

87. Davis SM, Donnan GA, Parsons MW, *et al.* Effects of alteplase beyond 3 h after stroke in the Echoplanar Imaging Thrombolytic Evaluation Trial (EPITHET): a placebo-controlled randomised trial. *Lancet Neurol* 2008;**7**(4): 299–309.

88. Albers GW, Thijs VN, Wechsler L, *et al.* Magnetic resonance imaging profiles predict clinical response to early reperfusion: the diffusion and perfusion imaging evaluation for understanding stroke evolution (DEFUSE) study. *Ann Neurol* 2006;**60**(5):508–17.

89. Schellinger PD, Thomalla G, Fiehler J, *et al.* MRI-based and CT-based thrombolytic therapy in acute stroke within and beyond established time windows: an analysis of 1210 patients. *Stroke* 2007;**38**(10):2640–5.

90. Neumann-Haefelin T, Hoelig S, Berkefeld J, *et al.* Leuko-araiosis is a risk factor for symptomatic intracerebral hemorrhage after thrombolysis for acute stroke. *Stroke* 2006;**37**(10):2463–6.

91. Singer OC, Humpich MC, Fiehler J, *et al.* Risk for symptomatic intracerebral hemorrhage after thrombolysis assessed by diffusion-weighted magnetic resonance imaging. *Ann Neurol* 2008;**63**(1):52–60.

92. Oppenheim C, Samson Y, Manai R, *et al.* Prediction of malignant middle cerebral artery infarction by diffusion-weighted imaging. *Stroke* 2000;**31**(9):2175–81.

93. Thomalla GJ, Kucinski T, Schoder V, *et al.* Prediction of malignant middle cerebral artery infarction by early perfusion- and diffusion-weighted magnetic resonance imaging. *Stroke* 2003;**34**(8):1892–9.

94. Vahedi K, Vicaut E, Mateo J, *et al.* Sequential-design, multicenter, randomized, controlled trial of early decompressive craniectomy in malignant middle cerebral artery infarction (DECIMAL Trial). *Stroke* 2007;**38**(9):2506–17.

95. Juttler E, Schwab S, Schmiedek P, *et al.* Decompressive Surgery for the Treatment of Malignant Infarction of the Middle Cerebral Artery (DESTINY): a randomized, controlled trial. *Stroke* 2007;**38**(9):2518–25.

96. Schellinger PD, Chalela JA, KangDW, Latour LL, Warach S. Diagnostic and prognostic value of early mr imaging vessel signs in hyperacute stroke patients imaged <3 hours and treated with recombinant tissue plasminogen activator. *AJNR Am J Neuroradiol* 2005;**26**(3):618–24.

97. Flacke S, Urbach H, Keller E, *et al.* Middle Cerebral Artery (MCA) susceptibility sign at susceptibility-based perfusion MR imaging: clinical importance and comparison with hyperdense MCA sign at CT. *Radiology* 2000;**215**(2): 476–82.

98. Linfante I, Llinas RH, Caplan LR, Warach S. MRI features of intracerebral hemorrhage within 2 hours from symptom onset. *Stroke* 1999;**30**(11):2263–7.

99. Schellinger PD, Jansen O, Fiebach JB, Hacke W, Sartor K. A standardized MRI stroke protocol: comparison with CT in hyperacute intracerebral hemorrhage. *Stroke* 1999;**30**(4):765–8.

100. Fiebach JB, Schellinger PD, Gass A, *et al.* Stroke magnetic resonance imaging is accurate in hyperacute intracerebral hemorrhage: a multicenter study on the validity of stroke imaging. *Stroke* 2004;**35**(2):502–6.

101. Kidwell CS, Chalela JA, Saver JL, *et al.* Comparison of MRI and CT for detection of acute intracerebral hemorrhage. *JAMA* 2004;**292**(15):1823–30.

102. Tsushima Y, Aoki J, Endo K. Brain microhemorrhages detected on T2*-weighted gradient-echo MR images. *AJNR Am J Neuroradiol* 2003;**24**(1):88–96.

103. Kidwell CS, Saver JL, Villablanca JP, *et al.* Magnetic resonance imaging detection of microbleeds before thrombolysis: an emerging application. *Stroke* 2002;**33**(1):95–8.

104. Nighoghossian N, Hermier M, Adeleine P, *et al.* Old microbleeds are a potential risk factor for cerebral bleeding after ischemic stroke: a gradient-echo T2*-weighted brain MRI study. *Stroke* 2002;**33**(3):735–42.

105. Derex L, Nighoghossian N, Hermier M, *et al.* Thrombolysis for ischemic stroke in patients with old microbleeds on pretreatment MRI. *Cerebrovasc Dis* 2004;**17**(2–3):238–41.

106. Fiehler J, Albers GW, Boulanger JM, *et al.* Bleeding risk analysis in stroke imaging before thromboLysis (BRASIL): pooled analysis of T2*-weighted magnetic resonance imaging data from 570 patients. *Stroke* 2007;**38**(10): 2738–44.

107. Dul K, Drayer B. CT and MRI imaging of intracerebral hemorrhage. In: Kase CS, Caplan LR (eds) *Intracerebral Hemorrhage*. Boston, MA: Butterworth-Heinemann, 1994; pp. 73–93.

108. Fiebach JB, Schellinger PD, Geletneky K, *et al.* MRI in acute subarachnoid haemorrhage; findings with a standardised stroke protocol. *Neuroradiology* 2004;**46**(1): 44–8.

109. Noguchi K, Ogawa T, Inugami A, *et al.* Acute subarachnoid hemorrhage: MR imaging with fluid-attenuated inversion recovery pulse sequences. *Radiology* 1995;**196**(3): 773–7.

110. Noguchi K, Ogawa T, Seto H, *et al.* Subacute and chronic subarachnoid hemorrhage: diagnosis with fluid-attenuated inversion-recovery MR imaging. *Radiology* 1997;**203**(1):257–62.

111. Oelerich M, Stogbauer F, Kurlemann G, Schul C, Schuierer G. Craniocervical artery dissection: MR imaging and MR angiographic findings. *Eur Radiol* 1999;**9**(7):1385–91.

112. Kirsch E, Kaim A, Engelter S, *et al.* MR angiography in internal carotid artery dissection: improvement of diagnosis by selective demonstration of the intramural haematoma. *Neuroradiology* 1998;**40**(11):704–9.

113. Bousson V, Levy C, Brunereau L, Djouhri H, Tubiana JM. Dissections of the internal carotid artery: three-dimensional time-of-flight MR angiography and MR imaging features. *AJR Am J Roentgenol* 1999;**173**(1):139–43.

114. Levy C, Laissy JP, Raveau V, *et al.* Carotid and vertebral artery dissections: three-dimensional time-of- flight MR angiography and MR imaging versus conventional angiography. *Radiology* 1994;**190**(1):97–103.

115. de Bray JM, Lhoste P, Dubas F, Emile J, Saumet JL. Ultrasonic features of extracranial carotid dissections: 47 cases studied by angiography. *J Ultrasound Med* 1994;**13**(9):659–64.

116. Bartels E, Flugel KA. Evaluation of extracranial vertebral artery dissection with duplex color-flow imaging. *Stroke* 1996;**27**(2):290–5.

117. Benninger DH, Georgiadis D, Gandjour J, Baumgartner RW. Accuracy of color duplex ultrasound diagnosis of spontaneous carotid dissection causing ischemia. *Stroke* 2006;**37**(2):377–81.

118. Vertinsky AT, Schwartz NE, Fischbein NJ, Rosenberg J, Albers GW, Zaharchuk G. Comparison of multidetector CT angiography and MR imaging of cervical artery dissection. *AJNR Am J Neuroradiol* 2008;**29**(9):1753–60.

119. Chen CJ, Tseng YC, Lee TH, Hsu HL, See LC. Multisection CT angiography compared with catheter angiography in diagnosing vertebral artery dissection. *AJNR Am J Neuroradiol* 2004;**25**(5):769–74.

120. Mattle HP, Wentz KU, Edelman RR, *et al.* Cerebral venography with MR. *Radiology* 1991;**178**(2):453–8.

121. Ameri A, Bousser M. Cerebral venous thrombosis. *Neurol Clin* 1992;**10**(1):87–111.

122. Bousser MG, Ferro JM. Cerebral venous thrombosis: an update. *Lancet Neurol* 2007;**6**(2):162–70.

123. Idbaih A, Boukobza M, Crassard I, Porcher R, Bousser MG, Chabriat H. MRI of clot in cerebral venous thrombosis: high diagnostic value of susceptibility-weighted images. *Stroke* 2006;**37**(4):991–5.

124. Thomassen L, Brainin M, Demarin V, Grond M, Toni D, Venables GS. Acute stroke treatment in Europe: a questionnaire-based survey on behalf of the EFNS Task Force on acute neurological stroke care. *Eur J Neurol* 2003;**10**(3):199–204.

125. Bowler JV, Wade JP, Jones BE, Nijran K, Steiner TJ. Single-photon emission computed tomography using hexamethylpropyleneamine oxime in the prognosis of acute cerebral infarction. *Stroke* 1996;**27**(1):82–6.

126. Barthel H, Hesse S, Dannenberg C, *et al.* Prospective value of perfusion and X-Ray attenuation imaging with single-photon emission and transmission computed tomography in acute cerebral ischemia. *Stroke* 2001;**32**(7):1588–97.

127. Berrouschot J, Barthel H, von Kummer R, Knapp WH, Hesse S, Schneider D. 99mTechnetium-ethyl-cysteinate-dimer single-photon emission CT can predict fatal ischemic brain edema. *Stroke* 1998;**29**(12):2556–62.

128. Alexandrov AV, Masdeu JC, Devous M, Sr., Black SE, Grotta JC. Brain single-photon emission CT with HMPAO and safety of thrombolytic therapy in acute ischemic stroke: proceedings of the meeting of the SPECT safe thrombolysis study collaborators and the members of the brain imaging council of the society of nuclear medicine. *Stroke* 1997;**28**(9):1830–4.

129. Mahagne M, David O, Darcourt J, *et al.* Voxel-based mapping of cortical ischemic damage using Tc 99 m L,L-ethyl cysteinate dimer SPECT in acute stroke. *J Neuroimaging* 2004;**14**(1):23–32.

130. Hirano T, Read SJ, Abbott DF, *et al.* Prediction of the final infarct volume within 6 h of stroke using single photon emission computed tomography with technetium-99m hexamethylpropylene amine oxime. *Cerebrovasc Dis* 2001;**11**(2):119–27.

131. Sviri GE, Lewis DH, Correa R, Britz GW, Douville CM, Newell DW. Basilar artery vasospasm and delayed posterior circulation ischemia after aneurysmal subarachnoid hemorrhage. *Stroke* 2004;**35**(8):1867–72.

132. Heiss W-D, Sobesky J, Smekal V, *et al.* Probability of cortical infarction predicted by flumazenil binding and diffusion-weighted imaging signal intensity: a comparative positron emission tomography/magnetic resonance imaging study in early ischemic stroke. *Stroke* 2004;**35**(8):1892–8.

133. Sobesky J, Zaro Weber O, Lehnhardt FG, *et al.* Does the mismatch match the penumbra? Magnetic resonance imaging and positron emission tomography in early ischemic stroke. *Stroke* 2005;**36**(5):980–5.

134. Hankey GJ, Warlow CP, Sellar RJ. Cerebral angiographic risk in mild cerebrovascular disease. *Stroke* 1990;**21**(2):209–22.

135. Grant EG, Benson CB, Moneta GL, *et al.* Carotid artery stenosis: gray-scale and doppler us diagnosis – society of radiologists in ultrasound consensus conference. *Radiology* 2003;**229**(2):340–6.

136. Jahromi AS, Cina CS, Liu Y, Clase CM. Sensitivity and specificity of color duplex ultrasound measurement in the estimation of internal carotid artery stenosis: a systematic review and meta-analysis. *J Vasc Surg* 2005;**41**(6):962–72.

137. Blakeley DD, Oddone EZ, Hasselblad V, Simel DL, Matchar DB. Noninvasive carotid artery testing: a meta-analytic review. *Ann Intern Med* 1995;**122**(5):360–7.

138. Kallmes DF, Omary RA, Dix JE, Evans AJ, Hillman BJ. Specificity of MR angiography as a confirmatory test of carotid artery stenosis. *AJNR Am J Neuroradiol* 1996;**17**(8):1501–6.

139. Nederkoorn PJ, van der Graaf Y, Hunink MGM. Duplex ultrasound and magnetic resonance. Angiography compared with digital subtraction angiography in carotid artery stenosis: a systematic review. *Stroke* 2003;**34**(5):1324–31.

140. Westwood ME, Kelly S, Berry E, *et al.* Use of magnetic resonance angiography to select candidates with recently symptomatic carotid stenosis for surgery: systematic review. *BMJ* 2002;**324**(7331):198.

141. Debrey SM, Yu H, Lynch JK, *et al.* Diagnostic accuracy of magnetic resonance angiography for internal carotid artery disease: a systematic review and meta-analysis. *Stroke* 2008;**39**(8):2237–48.

142. Marianne C, Christopher TL, Hanh P, Andrew L, Samuel Eric W, Ian G. Helical CT angiography in the preoperative evaluation of carotid artery stenosis. *J Vasc Surg* 1998;**28**(2):290–300.

143. Schwartz RB, Jones KM, Chernoff DM, *et al.* Common carotid artery bifurcation: evaluation with spiral CT. Work in progress. *Radiology* 1992;**185**(2):513–9.

144. Leclerc X, Godefroy O, Pruvo JP, Leys D. Computed tomographic angiography for the evaluation of carotid artery stenosis. *Stroke* 1995;**26**(9):1577–81.

145. Cumming MJ, Morrow IM. Carotid artery stenosis: a prospective comparison of CT angiography and conventional angiography. *Am J Roentgenol* 1994;**163**(3):517–23.

146. Koelemay MJW, Nederkoorn PJ, Reitsma JB, Majoie CB. Systematic review of computed tomographic angiography for assessment of carotid artery disease. *Stroke* 2004;**35**(10):2306–12.

147. Sameshima T, Futami S, Morita Y, *et al.* Clinical usefulness of and problems with three-dimensional CT angiography for the evaluation of arteriosclerotic stenosis of the carotid artery: comparison with conventional angiography, MRA, and ultrasound sonography. *Surg Neurol* 1999;**51**(3):301–8.

148. Wardlaw JM, Chappell FM, Best JJ, Wartolowska K, Berry E. Non-invasive imaging compared with intra-arterial angiography in the diagnosis of symptomatic carotid stenosis: a meta-analysis. *Lancet* 2006;**367**(9521):1503–12.

149. Alvarez-Linera J, Benito-Leon J, Escribano J, Campollo J, Gesto R. Prospective evaluation of carotid artery stenosis: elliptic centric contrast-enhanced MR angiography and spiral CT angiography compared with digital subtraction angiography. *AJNR Am J Neuroradiol* 2003;**24**(5):1012–9.

150. Khan S, Cloud GC, Kerry S, Markus HS. Imaging of vertebral artery stenosis: a systematic review. *J Neurol Neurosurg Psychiatry* 2007;**78**(11):1218–25.

151. North American Symptomatic Carotid Endarterectomy Trial Collaborators. Beneficial effect of carotid endarterectomy in symptomatic patients with high-grade carotid stenosis. *N Engl J Med* 1991;**325**(7):445–53.

152. ECST Collaborators. Randomised trial of endarterectomy for recently symptomatic carotid stenosis: final results of the MRC European Carotid Surgery Trial (ECST). *Lancet* 1998;**351**(9113):1379–87.

153. Barnett HJM, Taylor DW, Eliasziw M, *et al.* Benefit of carotid endarterectomy in patients with symptomatic moderate or severe stenosis. *N Engl J Med* 1998;**339**(20):1415–25.

154. Executive Committee for the Asymptomatic Carotid Atherosclerosis Study. Endarterectomy for asymptomatic carotid artery stenosis. Executive Committee for the Asymptomatic Carotid Atherosclerosis Study. *JAMA* 1995;**273**(18):1421–8.

155. Willinsky RA, Taylor SM, TerBrugge K, Farb RI, Tomlinson G, Montanera W. Neurologic complications of cerebral angiography: prospective analysis of 2,899 procedures and review of the literature. *Radiology* 2003;**227**(2):522–8.

156. Long A, Lepoutre A, Corbillon E, Branchereau A, Kretz JG. Modalities of preoperative imaging of the internal carotid artery used in France. *Ann Vasc Surg* 2002;**16**(3):261–5.

157. David LD, Christopher AR, Roy MF. Preoperative testing before carotid endarterectomy: a survey of vascular surgeons' attitudes. *Ann Vasc Surg* 1997;**11**(3):264–72.

158. Barth A, Arnold M, Mattle HP, Schroth G, Remonda L. Contrast-enhanced 3-D MRA in decision making for carotid endarterectomy: a 6-year experience. *Cerebrovasc Dis* 2006;**21**(5-6):393–400.

159. Osarumwense D, Pararajasingam R, Wilson P, Abraham J, Walker SR. Carotid artery imaging in the United Kingdom: a postal questionnaire of current practice. *Vascular* 2005;**13**(3):173–7.

160. Babikian V, Feldmann E, Wechsler LR, *et al.* Transcranial Doppler ultrasonography: year 2000 update. *J Neuroimaging* 2000;**10**:101–15.

161. Sloan MA, Alexandrov AV, Tegeler CH, *et al.* Assessment: transcranial doppler ultrasonography: report of the therapeutics and technology assessment subcommittee of the American Academy of Neurology. *Neurology* 2004;**62**(9):1468–81.

162. Rorick MB, Nichols FT, Adams RJ. Transcranial Doppler correlation with angiography in detection of intracranial stenosis. *Stroke* 1994;**25**(10):1931–4.

163. Demchuk A, Christou I, Wein TH, *et al.* Accuracy and criteria for localizing arterial occlusion with transcranial Doppler. *J Neuroimaging* 2000;**10**(1):1–12.

164. Baumgartner RW, Mattle HP, Schroth G. Assessment of >/=50% and <50% intracranial stenoses by transcranial color-coded duplex sonography. *Stroke* 1999;**30**(1):87–92.

165. Zanette EM, Fieschi C, Bozzao L, *et al.* Comparison of cerebral angiography and transcranial Doppler sonography in acute stroke. *Stroke* 1989;**20**(7):899–903.

166. Gerriets T, Goertler M, Stolz E, *et al.* Feasibility and validity of transcranial duplex sonography in patients with acute stroke. *J Neurol Neurosurg Psychiatry* 2002;**73**(1):17–20.

167. Adams RJ, McKie VC, Hsu L, *et al.* Prevention of a first stroke by transfusions in children with sickle cell anemia and abnormal results on transcranial doppler ultrasonography. *N Engl J Med* 1998;**339**(1):5–11.

168. Lysakowski C, Walder B, Costanza MC, Tramer MR. Transcranial Doppler versus angiography in patients with vasospasm due to a ruptured cerebral aneurysm: a systematic review. *Stroke* 2001;**32**(10):2292–8.

169. Burgin WS, Malkoff M, Felberg RA, *et al.* Transcranial Doppler ultrasound criteria for recanalization after thrombolysis for middle cerebral artery stroke. *Stroke* 2000;**31**(5):1128–32.

170. Alexandrov AV, Molina CA, Grotta JC, *et al.* Ultrasound-enhanced systemic thrombolysis for acute ischemic stroke. *N Engl J Med* 2004;**351**(21):2170–8.

171. Job F, Ringelstein EB, Grafen Y, *et al.* Comparison of transcranial contrast Doppler sonography and transesophageal contrast echocardiography for the detection of patent foramen ovale in young stroke patients. *Am J Cardiol* 1994;**74**(4):381–4.

172. Klotzsch C, Janssen G, Berlit P. Transesophageal echocardiography and contrast-TCD in the detection of a patent foramen ovale: experiences with 111 patients. *Neurology* 1994;**44**(9):1603.

173. Serena J, Segura T, Perez-Ayuso MJ, Bassaganyas J, Molins A, Davalos A. The need to quantify right-to-left shunt in acute ischemic stroke: a case-control study. *Stroke* 1998;**29**(7):1322–8.

174. Markus HS, Thomson ND, Brown MM. Asymptomatic cerebral embolic signals in symptomatic and asymptomatic carotid artery disease. *Brain* 1995;**118**(4):1005–11.

175. Siebler M, Sitzer M, Rose G, Bendfeldt D, Steinmetz H. Silent cerebral embolism caused by neurologically symptomatic high-grade carotid stenosis: event rates before and after carotid endarterectomy. *Brain* 1993;**116**(5):1005–15.

176. Molloy J, Markus HS. Asymptomatic embolization predicts stroke and TIA risk in patients with carotid artery stenosis. *Stroke* 1999;**30**(7):1440–3.

177. Siebler M, Nachtmann A, Sitzer M, *et al.* Cerebral microembolism and the risk of ischemia in asymptomatic high-grade internal carotid artery stenosis. *Stroke* 1995;**26**(11):2184–6.

178. Markus HS, MacKinnon A. Asymptomatic embolization detected by doppler ultrasound predicts stroke risk in symptomatic carotid artery stenosis. *Stroke* 2005;**36**(5):971–5.

179. Kaposzta Z, Martin JF, Markus HS. Switching off embolization from symptomatic carotid plaque using S-nitrosoglutathione. *Circulation* 2002;**105**(12):1480–4.

180. Markus HS, Droste DW, Kaps M, *et al.* Dual antiplatelet therapy with clopidogrel and aspirin in symptomatic carotid stenosis evaluated using Doppler embolic signal detection: the Clopidogrel and Aspirin for Reduction of Emboli in Symptomatic Carotid Stenosis (CARESS) trial. *Circulation* 2005;**111**(17):2233–40.

181. Levi CR, O'Malley HM, Fell G, *et al.* Transcranial Doppler detected cerebral microembolism following carotid endarterectomy. High microembolic signal loads predict postoperative cerebral ischaemia. *Brain* 1997;**120**(4):621–9.

182. Levi CR, Stork JL, Chambers BR, *et al.* Dextran reduces embolic signals after carotid endarterectomy. *Ann Neurol* 2001;**50**(4):544–7.

183. Payne DA, Jones CI, Hayes PD, *et al.* Beneficial effects of clopidogrel combined with aspirin in reducing cerebral emboli in patients undergoing carotid endarterectomy. *Circulation* 2004;**109**(12):1476–81.

184. Markus H, Cullinane M. Severely impaired cerebrovascular reactivity predicts stroke and TIA risk in patients with carotid artery stenosis and occlusion. *Brain* 2001;**124**(3):457–67.

185. Silvestrini M, Vernieri F, Pasqualetti P, *et al.* Impaired cerebral vasoreactivity and risk of stroke in patients with asymptomatic carotid artery stenosis. *JAMA* 2000;**283**(16):2122–7.

186. Jarquin-Valdivia A, McCartney J, Palestrant D, *et al.* The thickness of the temporal squama and its implication for transcranial sonography. *J Neuroimaging* 2004;**14**(2):139–42.

187. Hansberg T, Wong KS, Droste DW, Ringelstein EB, Kay R. Effects of the ultrasound contrast-enhancing agent Levovist on the detection of intracranial arteries and stenoses in Chinese by transcranial Doppler ultrasound. *Cerebrovasc Dis* 2002;**14**(2):105–8.

188. Feldmann E, Wilterdink JL, Kosinski A, *et al.* The stroke outcomes and neuroimaging of intracranial atherosclerosis (SONIA) trial. *Neurology* 2007;**68**(24):2099–106.

189. Hirai T, Korogi Y, Ono K, *et al.* Prospective evaluation of suspected stenoocclusive disease of the intracranial artery: combined MR angiography and CT angiography

compared with digital subtraction angiography. *AJNR Am J Neuroradiol* 2002;**23**(1):93–101.

190. Korogi Y, Terae S, Katoh C, *et al.* Intracranial vascular stenosis and occlusion: MR angiographic findings. *AJNR Am J Neuroradiol* 1997;**18**(1):135–43.

191. Bash S, Villablanca JP, Jahan R, *et al.* Intracranial vascular stenosis and occlusive disease: evaluation with CT angiography, MR angiography, and digital subtraction angiography. *AJNR Am J Neuroradiol* 2005;**26**(5):1012–21.

192. Nguyen-Huynh MN, Wintermark M, English J, *et al.* How accurate is CT angiography in evaluating intracranial atherosclerotic disease? *Stroke* 2008;**39**(4):1184–8.

193. Skutta B, Furst G, Eilers J, Ferbert A, Kuhn FP. Intracranial stenoocclusive disease: double-detector helical CT angiography versus digital subtraction angiography. *AJNR Am J Neuroradiol* 1999;**20**(5):791–9.

194. Chung T-S, Joo JY, Lee SK, Chien D, Laub G. Evaluation of cerebral aneurysms with high-resolution MR angiography using a section-interpolation technique: correlation with digital subtraction angiography. *AJNR Am J Neuroradiol* 1999;**20**(2):229–35.

195. White PM, Teasdale EM, Wardlaw JM, Easton V. Intracranial aneurysms: CT angiography and MR angiography for detection—prospective blinded comparison in a large patient cohort. *Radiology* 2001;**219**(3):739–49.

196. Villablanca JP, Jahan R, Hooshi P, Detection and characterization of very small cerebral aneurysms by using 2D and 3D helical CT angiography. *AJNR Am J Neuroradiol* 2002;**23**(7):1187–98.

197. Kouskouras C, Charitanti A, Giavroglou C, *et al.* Intracranial aneurysms: evaluation using CTA and MRA. Correlation with DSA and intraoperative findings. *Neuroradiology* 2004;**46**(10):842–50.

198. Huston J 3rd, Nichols DA, Luetmer PH, *et al.* Blinded prospective evaluation of sensitivity of MR angiography to known intracranial aneurysms: importance of aneurysm size. *AJNR Am J Neuroradiol* 1994;**15**(9):1607–14.

199. Schuierer G, Huk WJ, Laub G. Magnetic resonance angiography of intracranial aneurysms: comparison with intra-arterial digital subtraction angiography. *Neuroradiology* 1992;**35**(1):50–4.

200. Anzalone N, Triulzi F, Scotti G. Acute subarachnoid haemorrhage: 3D time-of-flight MR angiography versus intra-arterial digital angiography. *Neuroradiology* 1995;**37**(4): 257–61.

201. Korogi Y, Takahashi M, Katada K, *et al.* Intracranial aneurysms: detection with three-dimensional CT angiography with volume rendering – comparison with conventional angiographic and surgical findings. *Radiology* 1999;**211**(2): 497–506.

202. Alberico RA, Patel M, Casey S, Jacobs B, Maguire W, Decker R. Evaluation of the circle of Willis with three-dimensional CT angiography in patients with suspected intracranial aneurysms. *AJNR Am J Neuroradiol* 1995;**16**(8):1571–8.

203. Velthuis BK, Rinkel GJ, Ramos LM, *et al.* Subarachnoid hemorrhage: aneurysm detection and preoperative evaluation with CT angiography. *Radiology* 1998;**208**(2): 423–30.

204. Hoh BL, Cheung AC, Rabinov JD, Pryor JC, Carter BS, Ogilvy CS. Results of a prospective protocol of computed tomographic angiography in place of catheter angiography as the only diagnostic and pretreatment planning study for cerebral aneurysms by a combined neurovascular team. *Neurosurgery* 2004;**54**(6):1329–40.

205. Masaryk T, Drayer BP, Anderson RE, *et al.* Cerebrovascular disease. American College of Radiology. ACR Appropriateness Criteria. *Radiology* 2000;**215**(Suppl): 415–35.

206. The Magnetic Resonance Angiography in Relatives of Patients with Subarachnoid Hemorrhage Study Group. Risks and benefits of screening for intracranial aneurysms in first-degree relatives of patients with sporadic subarachnoid hemorrhage. *N Engl J Med* 1999;**341**(18):1344–50.

207. Wardlaw JM, White PM. The detection and management of unruptured intracranial aneurysms. *Brain* 2000;**123**(Pt 2): 205–21.

CHAPTER 3

Use of imaging in multiple sclerosis

M. Filippi,[1] M. A. Rocca,[1] D. L. Arnold,[2] R. Bakshi,[3] F. Barkhof,[4] N. De Stefano,[5] F. Fazekas,[6] E. Frohman,[7] D. H. Miller,[8] J. S. Wolinsky[9]

[1]Institute of Experimental Neurology, Scientific Institute and University Ospedale San Raffaele, Milan, Italy; [2]Montreal Neurological Institute, Canada; [3]Partners MS Center, Brigham and Women's Hospital, Harvard Medical School, Boston, MA, USA; [4]VU Medical Centre, Amsterdam, The Netherlands; [5]Institute of Neurological Sciences, University of Siena, Italy; [6]Medical University, Graz, Austria; [7]University of Texas Southwestern Medical Center at Dallas, USA; [8]Institute of Neurology, Queen Square, London, UK; [9]University of Texas Health Science Center, Houston, USA

Introduction

Conventional magnetic resonance imaging (cMRI) has proven to be sensitive for detecting multiple sclerosis (MS) lesions and their changes over time [1]. This exquisite sensitivity has made cMRI the most important paraclinical tool in supporting a diagnosis of MS and establishing a prognosis at the clinical onset of the disease. These are the main reasons why cMRI findings have a major role in the International Panel (IP) diagnostic criteria for MS proposed during the past few years [2, 3]. Many research groups have subsequently taken steps to validate and refine these recommendations. However, for clinicians, it still remains unclear how and when cMRI should be used, not only at the onset of the disease, but also during the subsequent disease phases. In addition, despite the sensitivity of cMRI for detecting MS lesions, the correlation between cMRI metrics (i.e. hyperintense lesions on T2- and post-contrast T1-weighted images, hypointense lesions on T1-weighted images and atrophy measurements) and clinical findings of MS is still limited [1]. Among the likely reasons for this clinical/MRI discrepancy, a major one is the low pathological specificity of the abnormalities seen on cMRI scans and the inability of cMRI metrics to detect and quantify the extent of damage in normal-appearing brain tissues (NABT). These inherent limitations of cMRI have prompted the development and application of quantitative MR 'non-conventional' techniques (MR spectroscopy [^{1}H-MRS], magnetization transfer [MT] MRI, diffusion weighted [DW] MRI and functional MRI [fMRI]) to the study of MS. Although these techniques have provided important insight into the pathobiology of MS, their practical value in the assessment of MS patients in clinical practice has yet to be realized.

Aim of the European Federation of Neurological Society (EFNS) task force

The aim of the 'EFNS Expert Panel of Neuroimaging of MS' is to define guidelines for the application of conventional and non-conventional MR techniques for the diagnosis and monitoring of patients with MS in clinical practice. In addition, they review the current status and clinical role of non-conventional MR techniques. The present guidelines are an update and a revision of the previous ones, which were published in 2006 [4].

Search strategy: data for this review were identified by searches of MEDLINE and references from relevant articles from 1965 to August 2009. The search terms 'multiple sclerosis', 'magnetic resonance imaging', 'diagnosis', 'prognosis', 'atrophy', 'magnetization transfer MRI', 'diffusion weighted MRI', 'diffusion tensor MRI', 'proton magnetic resonance spectroscopy', 'disability' and 'treatment' were used. Only papers published in English were reviewed.

European Handbook of Neurological Management: Volume 1, 2nd edition. Edited by N. E. Gilhus, M. P. Barnes and M. Brainin.

MRI assessment of patients at presentation with clinically isolated syndromes suggestive of MS

In about 85% of patients with MS, the clinical onset of the disease is a clinically isolated syndrome (CIS) involving the optic nerve, brainstem, or spinal cord [5]. Approximately 50–80% of these patients already have lesions on cMRI, consistent with prior disease activity [6–8]. As several randomised controlled trials [9–12] have shown a treatment effect in patients with a CIS and MRI abnormalities suggestive of MS, it has become critical to expedite the identification of those patients with a high risk for developing a multiphasic inflammatory demyelinating disorder consistent with MS. Equally compelling has been the desire to characterize those factors that have the ability to prospectively predict which patients will be at highest risk for rapid and substantial disability accrual.

Conventional MRI

Diagnosis

All of the diagnostic criteria proposed for MS [2, 3, 13, 14] require the demonstration of disease dissemination in space (DIS) and time (DIT). The central principle advanced in each of these diagnostic schemes requires the confirmation of two or more clinical attacks, separated in time, which involve at least two distinct areas of the central nervous system (CNS). Another key requirement in each of the diagnostic criteria is the exclusion of alternative diagnostic considerations that can mimic MS by appropriate tests [15]. The Poser criteria, published in 1983, were the first set of criteria that integrated findings from paraclinical and laboratory tests (including cerebrospinal fluid [CSF] analysis, evoked potentials [EP] and MRI) to demonstrate spatial dissemination of the disease and to increase diagnostic confidence.

A critical feature in the diagnostic evaluation of patients suspected of having MS is the characterization of lesions profiles that are suggestive of the disease. Brain MS lesions are frequently located in the periventricular and juxtacortical white matter (WM) regions, the corpus callosum, and infratentorial areas (with the pons and cerebellum more frequently affected than the medulla and midbrain), and are sometimes characterized by oval or elliptical shapes [16]. Consensus has also been reached on criteria useful to identify T2-hyperintense [17] and T1-enhancing lesions [18]. Considering the frequent involvement of the spinal cord by MS, MRI features of MS cord lesions have also been identified [19]. Cord MS lesions are more frequently observed within the cervical than in other regions, are usually peripheral, limited to two vertebral segments in length or less, occupy less than half the cross-sectional area of the cord, and are not seen as T1-hypointensities. Acute plaques can produce swelling of the cord and enhancement after gadolinium (Gd) administration.

Recently, the application of a double-inversion recovery (DIR) sequence [20] has contributed to imaging lesions of the grey matter (GM). These lesions have been detected in the major disease clinical phenotypes, including those with CIS [21]. The sensitivity and utility of GM lesions detection in the context of MS diagnosis requires further investigation.

The optic nerve is also frequently involved in the course of MS. When an attack of optic neuritis (ON) is suspected to be the onset manifestation of MS, the principal role of MRI is to assess the brain for asymptomatic lesions [22–24], whereas optic nerve MRI can be useful in ruling out alternative diagnoses. The sensitivity of MRI for detecting optic nerve lesions in patients with ON is high: a seminal study using a short-tau inversion recovery (STIR) sequence showed lesions in 84% of symptomatic nerves and 20% of asymptomatic nerves [25]. The use of fat-saturated fast spin echo [26] and selective partial inversion recovery pre pulse (SPIR)-FLAIR [27] sequences has led to increases in sensitivity for detecting lesions in patients with an ON. In MS patients, increased T2 signal can be seen for a long time after an episode of ON, despite improvements in vision and visual EP, and even in the absence of acute attacks of ON [28]. T1-hypointense lesions are not usually seen in the optic nerve, whereas Gd enhancement is a consistent feature of acute ON [29].

A number of MRI criteria have been proposed [7, 30, 31] to increase the confidence in rendering a diagnosis of MS:

• Criteria of Paty et al. [31]: presence of at least four T2-hyperintense lesions, or three T2 lesions, of which one is periventricular. These criteria are characterized by high sensitivity but relatively low specificity [32] (Class I evidence).

• Criteria of Fazekas et al. [30]: presence of at least three T2-hyperintense lesions with two of the following characteristics: an infratentorial lesion, a periventricular lesion, and a lesion larger than 6 mm. These criteria showed both high sensitivity and high specificity when evaluated retrospectively in definite MS [33], but have limited predictive value when applied prospectively in patients with CIS [34] (Class II evidence).

• Criteria of Barkhof *et al.* [7]: presence of at least three of the four following features: at least one Gd enhancing lesion, at least one juxtacortical lesion, at least one infratentorial lesion, and three or more periventricular lesions (Class I evidence). In 2000, Tintorè *et al.* [35] slightly modified these criteria by allowing for nine T2 lesions to be an alternative for the presence of an enhancing lesion and reported a high specificity of these criteria to predict conversion from CIS to clinically definite (CD) MS (class I evidence).

In 2001, an IP of MS specialists [2] proposed the use of MRI to generate objective evidence of lesion DIS and DIT. For the demonstration of DIS, the IP decided to apply the modified Barkhof-Tintoré criteria [7, 35]. When these imaging criteria were not fulfilled, the IP considered the presence of at least two T2 lesions plus the presence of oligoclonal bands in the CSF as equivalent. However, this alternative combination of criteria may result in a decreased diagnostic accuracy [36] (Class III evidence).

In the 2001 IP criteria [2], DIT can be demonstrated either by the presence of at least one enhancing lesion on an MRI scan performed 3 months or more after the onset of the clinical event or by the presence of one new T2 lesion which develops with reference to a prior scan obtained at least 3 months after the onset of the clinical event. The major advantage of the McDonald criteria is that they facilitate the early diagnosis of MS in patients with a clinically isolated attack before a second clinical relapse has occurred. Several studies have evaluated the ability of the IP criteria to predict conversion to CDMS and found a sensitivity ranging from 74 to 83% and a specificity of 83 to 85% [36, 37] (Class III evidence). Several studies have also assessed whether accurate pieces of information on DIS and DIT could be obtained with spinal cord MRI and serial T2-weighted images alone, respectively. The presence of asymptomatic cord lesions was found to contribute to the demonstration of DIS in recently diagnosed MS patients [38] (Class IV evidence), but the substitution of a brain lesion with a cord lesion did not impact significantly on the subsequent diagnosis

in patients presenting with ON [39] (Class III evidence). When a new T2-lesion was allowed as evidence for DIT, one study showed that 82% of CIS patients who fulfilled the IP MRI criteria for MS after 3 months had developed CDMS within 3 years [39] (Class III evidence), and another found that 80% of those CIS who fulfilled the same criteria after 1 year developed CDMS within 3 years [36] (Class III evidence).

The IP criteria have been challenged by a consensus report of the Therapeutics and Technology Assessment Subcommittee of the AAN [40] that performed a systematic analysis of studies on the use of MRI in the diagnosis of MS and concluded that the presence of three WM lesions in CIS patients represents a more sensitive predictor of the subsequent development of CDMS than the IP criteria. The specificity of the IP criteria and of that proposed by the Subcommittee of the AAN [40] have been assessed in patients suspected of having MS, but who ultimately had another diagnosis [41]. Whereas the IP criteria for DIS had a good specificity (89%), those proposed by the Subcommittee of the AAN had a much lower specificity (29%), indicating an increased risk of a false-positive diagnosis (Class III evidence).

To simplify and make an even earlier diagnosis, while maintaining adequate sensitivity and specificity, the IP criteria have been revised recently [3] (table 3.1). The main changes derived from this revision pertain to: (a) the demonstration of DIT, which can be obtained by the detection of a new T2 lesion, if it appears at any time compared with a reference scan done at least 30 days after the onset of the first clinical event; (b) the use of spinal cord MRI to demonstrate DIS. In this context, a cord lesion can be considered equivalent to a brain infratentorial lesion, an enhancing cord lesion is equivalent to an enhancing brain lesion, and individual cord lesions can contribute together with individual brain lesions to reach the required number of T2 lesions; (c) the diagnosis of primary progressive (PP) MS, which can be made in the presence of typical clinical evolution when accompanied by suggestive MRI changes in both brain and spinal cord, even in the absence of positive CSF findings.

Meanwhile several proposals have been made to simplify the revised McDonald criteria. According to the Swanton criteria [42], at least one subclinical T2 lesion in at least two of four locations defined as characteristic for MS in the McDonald criteria (i.e. juxtacortical, periventricular, infratentorial, and spinal-cord) is required

Table 3.1 Diagnostic criteria for multiple sclerosis: 2005 revisions to the 'McDonald Criteria' [3].

Dissemination in space	Three of the following: • at least 1 Gd-enhancing lesion or 9 T2 lesions • at least 3 periventricular lesions • at least 1 juxtacortical lesion • at least 1 infratentorial lesion A spinal cord lesion equivalent to a brain infratentorial lesion; can contribute along with individual brain lesions to reach required lesion number
Dissemination in time	**(a)** Detection of Gd enhancement at least 3 months after onset of initial clinical event (if not at site of event) **(b)** Detection of a new T2 lesion if it appears at any time compared to a reference scan done at least 30 days after onset of initial clinical event
Diagnosis of MS in disease with progression from onset	**(a)** One year of disease progression (retrospectively or prospectively determined). **(b)** *Plus* two of the following • Positive brain MRI (nine T2 lesions or four or more T2 lesions with positive VEP) • Positive spinal cord MRI (two focal T2 lesions) • Positive CSF (isoelectric focusing evidence of oligoclonal IgG bands or increased IgG index, or both)

Gd = gadolinium, MS = multiple sclerosis, MRI = magnetic resonance imaging, VEP = visual evoked potentials, CSF = cerebrospinal fluid.

for DIS, while DIT requires a new T2 lesion on a follow-up scan irrespective of the timing of a baseline scan. Such interpretation can be done on T2-weighted images alone and does not require Gd enhancement. These criteria have been found to be slightly more sensitive (72%) than the original and revised McDonald criteria, while maintaining high specificity (87%) [42, 43] (Class II evidence). These criteria may lose differential diagnostic information, due to the absence of Gd administration. Recently, Rovira *et al.* [44] suggested that a single brain MRI study performed early (i.e. <3 months) after the onset of CIS is highly specific for predicting the development of CDMS in the presence of both Gd-enhancing and non-enhancing lesions, which, when present, suggest DIT (Class II evidence).

Individuals without overt clinical symptoms but with MRI features highly suggestive of MS (i.e. subclinical demyelinating lesions) have been recently defined 'radiologically isolated syndromes' (RIS). Although routinely encountered in clinical practice, only limited data exist on the natural history or evolution of such individuals. Okuda *et al.* acquired MRI data from 41 RIS subjects [45]. While radiologic progression was identified in 59% of the cases, only 10 patients converted to either CIS or CDMS [45]. The presence of Gd-enhancing lesions on the initial MRI was predictive of DIT on repeat imaging of the brain [45]. During a mean follow-up of 5.2 years,

the rate of clinical conversions of 70 RIS patients who had DIS on MRI was 33% [46] (Class II evidence). Examination of pejorative markers for clinical conversion showed that sex, number of T2 lesions, presence of oligoclonal bands, and IgG index were not statistically different in patients with MS determined by MRI compared with CDMS [46]. Visual evoked potential abnormalities, young age, and Gd enhancement on follow-up MRI scans more frequent in CDMS than in MS determined by MRI [46].

Prognosis

Several authors have investigated the prognostic role of MR-derived metrics in patients presenting with CIS. The MRI findings that showed the strongest predictive value for the subsequent development of CDMS on short- to medium-term follow-up were the number and extent of T2-visible brain lesions at disease onset [6, 8, 22, 47] (Class II evidence), the presence of infratentorial lesions [47] (Class III evidence) and the presence of Gd-enhancing lesions [7] (Class I evidence),[9] (Class IV evidence)]. For patients with CIS and brain MRI lesions, the chance of developing CDMS was > 80% over the next 14–20 years, in the longest follow-up study to date [8, 22]. Several studies also showed the baseline MRI pattern is a strong predictor of disability accumulation over time in these patients [8, 48] (Class IV evidence).

During the past decades, several quantitative MR techniques have been developed for the assessment of brain damage in patients with MS. Even if the application of these techniques in everyday clinical practice is, at the moment, still premature, as these techniques often require dedicated personnel and specific software for the analysis, it is likely that with augmented availability their use in clinical practice will increase.

The progressive development of brain and spinal cord atrophy is a well-known neuroimaging feature of MS [49]. Objective quantification of CNS atrophy has been recognized as a potentially useful marker of the destructive and irreversible components of MS-related tissue damage. Recent MRI studies have confirmed that irreversible tissue loss/damage occurs early in the course of the disease and it is likely that the extent of such irreversible tissue damage conveys important prognostic information. In CIS patients who evolved to MS, the development of regional or global brain atrophy over a period of up to 3 years [50–52], as well as progressive brain GM atrophy, was observed [50]. In CIS patients, a low dose of interferon (IFN) beta-1a given subcutaneously once a week has been shown to reduce the rate of brain atrophy by about 30% over 2 years [51]. Conversely, compared to normal controls, cord area was found to be only slightly reduced in patients presenting with CIS and an abnormal MRI scan, and cord area remained stable over 1 year after disease onset [53].

Non-conventional MRI

(1) MT-MRI. Reduced MT ratio (MTR) values have been detected in the normal-appearing WM (NAWM) and GM from patients at presentation with CIS [54–56].

While a seminal study suggested that the extent of these abnormalities might be an independent predictor of subsequent disease evolution [56], subsequent studies did not confirm this observation [44, 55]. No MT MRI abnormalities have been detected in the cervical cord of CIS patients [57].

(2) DT MRI. DT MRI has disclosed subtle abnormalities in the NAWM of CIS patients [58], which were not predictive of DIT (as defined by McDonald criteria) at 3 and 12 months [58]. Recently, a significant increase of GM diffusivity has been described in these patients, which was unrelated to clinical activity [59].

(3) ¹H-MRS. Metabolic abnormalities, consisting of a reduction of the concentration of N-acetylasparate (NAA) of the whole brain [60] and in an increase of myo-inositol (mI) and creatine (Cr) in NAWM [61] have been shown in CIS patients, suggesting that widespread axonal pathology, glial injury, and an increase in cell turnover or metabolism are rather early phenomena in the course of the disease. Metabolic abnormalities in CIS patients have been found to be more pronounced in those patients with evolution to CDMS over a relatively short period of time [62].

(4) Functional MRI. Using fMRI, an abnormal pattern of movement-associated cortical activation has also been described in CIS patients within 3 months of disease onset [63, 64]. In a 1-year follow-up study of CIS patients [65], those who developed CDMS had a different motor fMRI response at first presentation when compared with those who did not, suggesting that, in CIS patients, the extent of early cortical reorganization following tissue injury might be a factor associated to a different disease evolution.

Recommendations

In patients at presentation with CIS suggestive of MS (i.e. neurological findings typically seen in the setting of MS), after appropriate exclusion of alternative diagnostic considerations that can mimic MS, the following recommendations should be considered.

(1) cMRI of the brain (dual-echo, FLAIR, and post-contrast T1-weighted scans) should be obtained as soon as possible in all patients presenting with an isolated demyelinating syndrome involving the CNS, not only to collect additional evidence for DIS, but also to exclude other possible neurological conditions. As suggested by the guidelines from the AAN [40], the finding in these

patients of three or more T2-hyperintense lesions with the imaging characteristics underlined by the IP guidelines [2, 3] (Level A recommendation) and the presence of two or more Gd-enhancing lesions at baseline are sensitive predictors of the subsequent development of CDMS within the next 7–10 years (Level B recommendation).

(2) The presence of three or more WM lesions on brain T2-weighted MRI in patients suspected of having MS is not diagnostic, especially when their location and appearance is non-characteristic for demyelination. In this context, the IP criteria [2, 3] should be applied. Incidental WM lesions are not an infrequent observation even in

the young normal population. Note that with ageing (at least > 50 years) incidental WM lesions may also show progression [66] (Good Clinical Practice Point, GCPP).

(3) In the case of corticosteroid treatment, which is known to dramatically suppress Gd enhancement, one of the possible markers of inflammation, cMRI should be performed before treatment or, at least, 1 month after treatment termination (GCPP).

(4) cMRI of the spinal cord is useful in those circumstances when brain MRI is normal or equivocal, and in patients with non-specific brain T2-abnormalities (especially when older than 50 years), because, contrary to what happens for the brain, cord lesions rarely develop with ageing per se [67]. In patients presenting with a spinal cord syndrome, spinal cord MRI is highly recommended to rule out other conditions that may mimic MS, such as compressive lesions (GCPP).

(5) In patients with acute ON, although it will not always be required, MRI of the optic nerve can be useful in ruling out alternative diagnosis. In this case, STIR sequences should be used (GCPP).

(6) Follow-up MRIs are required to demonstrate DIT. In this perspective, the appearance of Gd-enhancing lesions 3 months after the clinical episode or new T2 or Gd-enhancing lesions 30 days after the clinical episode (and after a baseline MRI assessment) is highly recommended. Follow-up scans should be performed with the same machinery and scanning parameters, and identical slice positions are required for exact comparison (Level B recommendation). A scanner with at least 1.0 Tesla should be used to optimize image quality and tissue contrast.

(7) Repeat scanning beyond the two initial studies needs to be considered by the neurologist individually according to the clinical circumstances that are appropriate for each patient [is not routinely recommended as the disease becomes more likely to manifest clinically in the longer term [68]] (GCPP).

(8) Nephrogenic systemic fibrosis (NSF) is a medical condition that has come to be associated with exposure to the Gd [69, 70]. Normal renal function has to be confirmed prior to Gd administration (GCPP).

(9) Although non-conventional MRI techniques may provide essential and critical information about patients with CIS, and their application for monitoring treatment might provide a more accurate assessment of efficacy on inflammation, axonal protection, and demyelination/remyelination, their use in clinical practice is currently not recommended. All these techniques are yet to be adequately compared to cMRI for sensitivity and specificity in detecting tissue damage in MS and for predicting the development of MS and disability. At present, these quantitative techniques show differences at a group level, but do not allow inferences at an individual level (GCPP).

(10) In patients with insidious neurological progression over at least one year, PPMS [71] can be diagnosed reliably in the absence of positive CSF findings (when typical brain and spinal cord MRI changes are present). Even if in these patients a positive CSF finding increases the level of confidence for a diagnosis of MS, such a finding is not specific and may be commonly detected in patients with progressive myelopathies of other causes (GCPP).

MRI in patients with CDMS

In patients with relapsing-remitting (RR) and secondary progressive (SP) MS, disease activity is detected five to 10 times more frequently on cMRI scans than with clinical assessment of relapses. This, coupled with the fact that cMRI provides objective and sensitive measures of disease activity, led to the use of cMRI as an established tool for assessing the natural history of MS progression and for monitoring response to treatment. In a clinical trial context, cMRI is used as a primary outcome measure in phase II studies, where serial scans (usually monthly) are acquired to detect disease activity (new or enlarged T2-lesion counts, total enhancing and new enhancing lesion counts, and enhancing lesion volume) [72]. In phase III trials, given the uncertainty of cMRI in predicting clinical benefit, surrogate imaging methods are used as secondary outcome measures to detect disease pro-

gression, usually on yearly scans, specifically in terms of increase in total T2-hyperintense lesion load [73].

Conventional MRI

The cMRI sequences typically used for studying MS patients are dual-echo and post-contrast T1-weighted scans. Lesion burden on T2 MRI increases by about 5–10% per year. Several cross-sectional studies evaluated differences in T2-lesion load among different MS phenotypes. T2-lesion load is higher in SPMS in comparison to benign, RRMS, and PPMS [74]. However, the magnitude of the correlation between T2-lesion measures and disability within various disease phenotypes in cross-sectional studies has been rather disappointing [75]. This poor relationship is likely related to the many limitations of the clinical scales used to measure impairment and disability in MS and to the inability of cMRI to characterize and quantify the extent and severity of MS pathology beyond T2-visible lesions [1]. Furthermore, albeit not confirmed by a subsequent study [76], a plateauing relationship between dual-echo lesion load and disability has been shown, indicating that for Expanded Disability Status Scale (EDSS) higher than 4.5, metrics different from T2-lesion loads should be taken into account [77]. Serial MRI studies have shown that enhancement occurs in almost all new lesions in patients with RRMS or SPMS and can be sometimes detected even before the onset of clinical symptoms [78]. The burden of MRI activity can be stratified on the basis of clinical phenotype, being higher in RRMS [79] and SPMS [80] in comparison with PPMS [80] and benign MS [79]. Severely disabled SPMS patients exhibit a substantially lower incidence of enhancing lesions when compared to those with mildly disabled RRMS [81]. Several studies have investigated the prognostic role of enhancing MRI on corresponding clinical parameters. The number of enhancing lesions increases shortly before and during clinical relapses and predicts subsequent MRI activity [82–84]. A moderate correlation has been demonstrated between the degree of clinical disability and the mean frequency of enhancing lesions in patients with RRMS [85] and SPMS [86].

A rigorous and valid strategy for the MR-based longitudinal monitoring of MS (either natural or modified by treatment) must involve the use of standardized imaging protocols (including consistency in slice thickness and imaging planes, field strength, and patient repositioning). Several guidelines have emphasized the importance of accurate patient positioning inside the magnet to define landmarks for achieving effective co-registration on serial scans. Such procedures facilitate the accurate interpretation of follow-up studies [73, 87]. Several reviews provide detailed analysis of the advantages and disadvantages of the application of different pulse sequences for characterizing the disease burden in MS [73]. In addition, considering the importance of active lesion detection for assessing disease activity, several strategies have been suggested to increase enhancing lesion detection, including increased post-injection delay, increased Gd dose, and the application of MT saturation pulses to reduce background signal and increase lesion identification [88]. However, despite the increased sensitivity of these strategies, the application of higher doses of Gd and MT pulsing in the routine assessment of MS patients is still not advisable due to an unfavourable cost-benefit ratio. On the contrary, there is general agreement that an interval of

5–7 min between the injection of contrast material and the acquisition of post-contrast sequences should be maintained routinely to optimize the sensitivity and create standardization within and between centres [89].

Over the past decade, a large number of parallel group, placebo-controlled, and baseline-versus-treatment trials have clearly shown the ability of several immunomodulating and immunosuppressive treatments to reduce both MRI-measured inflammation and the consequent increase of accumulated lesion burden in patients with CIS [9–12] (Class I evidence), RRMS [90–119] (Class I evidence) and SPMS [106, 120–125] (Class I evidence). The long-term effects of some of these treatments on MRI-accumulated disease burden have also been documented ([126–128] (Class I evidence). A few studies in patients treated with IFN-beta, have explored whether MRI disease activity measured with Gd or new T2 lesions at the beginning of the treatment identifies better subsequent therapeutic response than clinical activity [129–132] (Class I evidence). Patients with rapidly evolving severe RRMS, defined by two or more disabling relapses in one year, and with one or more Gd-enhancing lesions on brain MRI or a significant increase in T2 lesion load as compared to a previous recent MRI, have been shown to have a greater treatment effect in the natalizumab trial [102]. Following the European Medicines Agency (EME) guidelines, natalizumab is indicated as single disease modifying therapy in highly active RRMS for the following patient groups: (a) patients with high disease activity (including at least one Gd-enhancing lesion) despite treatment with a IFN-beta, or (b) patients with rapidly evolving severe RRMS (including new T2 lesions or at least one new Gd-enhancing lesion compared with a recent MRI). Even if these data suggest that MRI classification may facilitate rational therapeutic decisions, they need to be replicated before being applied in clinical practice.

Persistently hypointense lesions on enhanced T1-weighted images (known as 'black holes') correspond to areas where chronic severe tissue disruption has occurred. At present, there is a general tendency to consider the assessment of the extent of chronic black holes as a surrogate marker to monitor MS evolution. T1-hypointense lesion load is higher and increases more rapidly over time in SPMS and PPMS than in RRMS [133]. In addition, T1-hypointense lesion load correlates better with clinical disability than T2-lesion load, particularly in SPMS patients. A few trials have investigated the effect of treatment in preventing the accumulation of T1 black holes [134–137] in RRMS and SPMS and have consistently shown that the effect, if any, of all the tested treatments in reducing the rate of accumulation of black holes is moderate at best. A greater effect has been shown in patients treated with natalizumab: median T1-hypointense lesion volume decreased by 1.5% in the placebo group and by 23.5% in the natalizumab group [102]. Several studies have also evaluated the effects of available treatments [138–140] on the probability of newly formed MS lesions to evolve into chronically T1-hypointense lesions. Although this approach is highly time-consuming, it is promising for assessing in a relatively short time the ability of a given treatment to favourably alter the mechanisms leading to irreversible tissue loss.

Measurement of brain and cord atrophy has also been applied to assess the extent of tissue loss in MS [49, 141]. In MS patients with different disease phenotypes, on average, brain volume decreases by about 1% yearly [49], despite evidence of highly variable disease activity. Although it appears to be more pathologically specific than T2-lesion load, brain atrophy is at best only moderately correlated with disability in RRMS and SPMS [49, 142]. The strength of the correlation increases when neuropsychological impairment is considered [143] and with a longitudinal study design [144, 145]. Also, in patients with MS, particularly in those with the progressive phenotypes of the disease, changes at a given time point and over time of cord cross-sectional area correlate better with clinical disability than changes in cord T2-visible lesions [19].

Good correlations have been found between regional brain atrophy and disability in MS patients. GM atrophy has been demonstrated by cross-sectional and longitudinal studies [146, 147] from the early stages of the disease. Such a GM atrophy tends to worsen over time [148], and is correlated with worsening of disability progression [149]. In addition, brain atrophy appears to evolve by involving different structures in different phases of the disease, with ventricular enlargement predominant in RRMS and cortical atrophy more important in the progressive forms of the disease [150, 151].

As shown for T1-hypointense lesions, the effect of treatment in preventing the development of brain atrophy in patients with RRMS and SPMS was at best

moderate and not seen at all in some studies [84, 102, 121, 152–156]. Overall, treatment effects on T1-hypointense lesions are more impressive than those seen on brain atrophy and are more in line with treatment effects observed on T2 lesions. The T1 lesion putatively investigates axonal loss only in a subgroup of visible WM lesions; whereas whole brain atrophy will be sensitive to neuroaxonal loss wherever it occurs in brain GM or WM. To refine the reproducibility of brain atrophy measurements, several recommendations have been provided [49, 142], including: (1) the acquisition of 3D T1-weighted sequences; (2) the use of automated segmentation algorithms for images segmentation; (3) the development of a quality assurance programme to confirm the stability of the measurement system over time.

Non-conventional MRI

MT-MRI, DT-MRI, and ¹H-MRS provide quantitative and continuous measures that can assess global (whole brain) as well as specific CNS structures, including the optic nerve and spinal cord, and various compartments (i.e. macroscopic lesions, NABT, NAWM, and GM) [157–159]. Using these techniques, microscopic abnormalities beyond the resolution of cMRI have been detected in patients with different MS phenotypes and have been shown to correlate better with the degree of disability and cognitive impairment than cMRI measures [157–159]. Longitudinal studies have shown significant worsening of non-conventional MRI metrics over time in MS patients. These techniques provide useful prognostic information for the medium-term clinical disease evolution [160–162].

Although the optimization and standardization across multiple sites and over time of MT sequences might be challenging, and long-term longitudinal studies using MT MRI are lacking, MT MRI holds substantial promise to provide good surrogate measures for MS evolution. This is witnessed by the fact that several MS trials have already incorporated MT MRI quantities as additional outcome measures, with a view to assessing the impact of treatment on demyelination and axonal loss. MT MRI has been used in phase II and phase III trials for RRMS (injectable and oral IFN beta-1a, IFN beta-1b, and oral glatiramer acetate [GA]) and SPMS (IFN beta-1b and immunoglobulins). In these phase III trials, MT MRI acquisition has been limited to highly specialized MR centres and only subgroups of patients (about 50–100 per trial) have been studied using this technique. Two phase II studies have shown that treatment with IFN beta-1b [163] or IFN beta-1a [164] favourably modifies the recovery of MT ratio values which follows the cessation of Gd enhancement in newly formed lesions from RRMS patients (Class II evidence). On the contrary, Richert et al. [163] did not find any significant difference in the MTR values of NAWM regions of interest before and during IFN beta-1b therapy, as well as in the parameters derived from whole-brain MTR histograms [165] in RRMS patients (Class II evidence). In patients with SPMS, a lack of effect of IFN beta-1b [166] on MT-MRI-derived quantities of the whole-brain tissue and NAWM was reported and the findings with intravenous immunoglobulins were equivocal [167] (Class II evidence).

An international consensus conference of the White Matter Study Group of the International Society for MR in Medicine has provided several guidelines for using MT-MRI for monitoring treatment in MS [168]. Among the suggestions provided in these guidelines, are the recommended use of scanners with field strength of 1.5 T, gradient-echo sequences, and the standardization of magnetization saturation among centres. Corrections for scanner properties like variations in the B_1 field may also serve to reduce the variability of MT measurements between sites [169]. Quality assurance procedures and centralized analysis of the data represent additional important requirements.

^{1}H-MRS is relatively time-consuming and requires experienced personnel, which limits its use in the context of multicentre studies. Nevertheless, a few studies have been conducted to evaluate the effect of disease-modifying treatments on ^{1}H-MRS-derived parameters.

Using monthly ^{1}H-MRS scans, Sarchielli et al. [170] found that treatment with IFN beta-1a has an impact on Cho peaks in spectra of lesions from RRMS patients, suggesting an increase in lesion membrane turnover during the first period of treatment. Narayanan et al. [171] found an increase of NAA/Cr in a small group of RRMS patients after 1 year of treatment with IFN beta-1b, suggesting a potential effect of treatment in preventing chronic, sublethal axonal injury. Schubert et al. [172] showed a stability of metabolite concentration over time in patients with RRMS treated with IFN beta-1b. Khan and co-workers [173] showed that patients receiving GA therapy for 4 years had an increase in NAA in the NAWM. One study used multicentre ^{1}H-MRS data to assess PPMS patients [174]. This study reported comparable cross-sectional ^{1}H-MRS values in healthy controls from different centres, indicating that ^{1}H-MRS data can be highly reproducible across sites, when factors such as data acquisition, position and size of the volume of interest, postprocessing, and quantification procedures are standardized. A 3-year follow-up [175] showed no significant difference in metabolite ratios between patients treated with GA and those of the placebo group in lesions, NAWM and GM. However, there were also no detectable temporal changes in metabolite ratios in the two groups of patients relative to baseline values during the study period. As a consequence, ^{1}H-MRS sensitivity to MS-related changes in clinical trials remains to be established. A panel of MS experts has recently reviewed the current clinical applications of ^{1}H-MRS in MS, discussed the potential and limitations of the technique, and suggested recommendations for the application of ^{1}H-MRS to clinical trials [176].

Recommendations

In patients with established MS, the following recommendations should be considered:

(1) cMRI scans (dual-echo and post-contrast T1-weighted images) should be obtained using standardized protocols and accurate procedures for patients' repositioning to facilitate the interpretation of follow-up studies. Post-contrast T1-weighted scans should be acquired after an interval of 5–7 min from the injection of contrast material. Considering the weak correlation with clinical finding and the low predictive value of cMRI metrics for the subsequent worsening of clinical disability, the use of surveillance MRI for the purpose of making treatment

decisions cannot be generally recommended. Serial MRI scans should be considered when diagnostic issues arise (GCPP).

(2) Repetition of MRI of the spinal cord is advisable only if suspicion arises concerning the evolution of an alternate process (e.g. mechanical compression) or atypical symptoms develop (GCPP).

(3) Although preliminary work based on clinical trial data has suggested that the presence and amount of MRI-detected disease activity may identify IFN response status in terms of relapse rate and accumulated disability in MS patients at a group level, there are no validated methods for monitoring disease-modifying therapy in individual patients (Class I evidence).

(4) Metrics derived from cMRI are not enough to provide a complete picture of the MS pathological process. Although cMRI has undoubtedly improved our ability to assess the efficacy of experimental MS therapies and, at least partially, our understanding of MS evolution, it provides only limited information on MS pathology in terms of accuracy and specificity and it has limited correlations with clinical metrics. This implies that the ability of a given treatment to modify metrics derived from cMRI does not mean that the treatment will necessarily be able to prevent the progressive accumulation of clinical disability, especially at an individual patient level.

(5) Measurements of T1-hypointense lesions loads and brain and cord atrophy in clinical practice continue to be considered at a preliminary stage of development, as they need to be standardized in terms of acquisition and post-processing. Conversely, these metrics should be included as an end-point in disease-modifying agents trials, to further elucidate the mechanisms responsible for disability (GCPP).

(6) The application of non-conventional MRI techniques in monitoring patients with established MS in clinical practice is, at the moment, not advisable. All these techniques still need to be evaluated for sensitivity and specificity in detecting tissue damage in MS and its changes over time (GCPP).

(7) MT-MRI should be incorporated into new clinical trials to gain additional insights into disease pathophysiology and into the value of this technique in the assessment of MS (Class II evidence). The performance and contribution of DT MRI and ^{1}H-MRS in multicentre trials still have to be evaluated.

Conflicts of interest

D. L. Arnold has served on advisory boards for Genentech and Biogen Idec, and received speaker honoraria from Genentech, MS Forum, Biogen Idec, Serono Symposia, Teva & Sanofi Aventis, Teva Neuroscience, Bayer HealthCare Pharmaceuticals, and EMD Serono. He has received consultant's fees from Biogen Idec, Teva Neuroscience, MS Forum, Genentech, Bayer HealthCare Pharmaceuticals, Novartis, and Eisai Medical Research, and grants from Multiple Sclerosis Society of Canada and Canadian Institutes of Health Research.

R. Bakshi has received speaker honoraria and grants from Biogen Idec, Teva Neuroscience, and EMD Serono.

F. Barkhof has received consultancy fees from Bayer-Schering Pharma, Sanofi-Aventis, Biogen-Idec, UCB, Merck-Serono, Novartis, and Roche.

N. De Stefano has served on advisory boards for Merck-Serono and received speaker honoraria from Merck-Serono, Teva, Biogen, and Bayer. He has received a consultant's fee from Merck-Serono and travel grants from Merck-Serono and Biogen.

F. Fazekas has served on advisory boards and received speaker honoraria from Biogen Idec, Teva Sanofi Aventis, Merck-Serono, and Bayer Schering. He has received grants from Bayer Schering, Biogen Idec, Teva Sanofi Aventis, Baxter, and Merck-Serono.

M. Filippi has received speaker honoraria and grants from Teva, Merck-Serono, Bayer Schering, Biogen-Dompè, and Genmab. He has received a consultant's fee from Pepgen and travel grants from Teva, Merck-Serono, Bayer Schering, and Biogen-Dompè.

M. A. Rocca has received speaker honoraria and travel grants from Biogen-Dompè.

The other authors have reported no conflicts of interest.

References

1. Bakshi R, Thompson AJ, Rocca MA, *et al*. MRI in multiple sclerosis: current status and future prospects. *Lancet Neurol* 2008;**7**:615–25.
2. McDonald WI, Compston A, Edan G, *et al*. Recommended diagnostic criteria for multiple sclerosis: guidelines from the International Panel on the diagnosis of multiple sclerosis. *Ann Neurol* 2001;**50**:121–7.
3. Polman CH, Reingold SC, Edan G, *et al*. Diagnostic criteria for multiple sclerosis: 2005 revisions to the 'McDonald Criteria'. *Ann Neurol* 2005;**58**:840–6.
4. Filippi M, Rocca MA, Arnold DL, *et al*. EFNS guidelines on the use of neuroimaging in the management of multiple sclerosis. *Eur J Neurol* 2006;**13**:313–25.
5. Noseworthy JH, Lucchinetti C, Rodriguez M, Weinshenker BG. Multiple sclerosis. *N Engl J Med* 2000;**343**: 938–52.
6. Filippi M, Horsfield MA, Morrissey SP, *et al*. Quantitative brain MRI lesion load predicts the course of clinically isolated syndromes suggestive of multiple sclerosis. *Neurology* 1994;**44**:635–41.

7. Barkhof F, Filippi M, Miller DH, *et al.* Comparison of MRI criteria at first presentation to predict conversion to clinically definite multiple sclerosis. *Brain* 1997;**120**:(Pt 11): 2059–69.

8. Fisniku LK, Brex PA, Altmann DR, *et al.* Disability and T2 MRI lesions: a 20-year follow-up of patients with relapse onset of multiple sclerosis. *Brain* 2008;**131**:808–17.

9. Jacobs LD, Beck RW, Simon JH, *et al.* Intramuscular interferon beta-1a therapy initiated during a first demyelinating event in multiple sclerosis. CHAMPS Study Group. *N Engl J Med* 2000;**343**:898–904.

10. Comi G, Filippi M, Barkhof F, *et al.* Effect of early interferon treatment on conversion to definite multiple sclerosis: a randomised study. *Lancet* 2001;**357**:1576–82.

11. Achiron A, Kishner I, Sarova-Pinhas I, *et al.* Intravenous immunoglobulin treatment following the first demyelinating event suggestive of multiple sclerosis: a randomized, double-blind, placebo-controlled trial. *Arch Neurol* 2004;**61**:1515–20.

12. Kappos L, Polman CH, Freedman MS, *et al.* Treatment with interferon beta-1b delays conversion to clinically definite and McDonald MS in patients with clinically isolated syndromes. *Neurology* 2006;**67**:1242–9.

13. Schumacher GA. Problems of multiple sclerosis. *N Y State J Med* 1966;**66**:1743–52.

14. Poser CM, Paty DW, Scheinberg L, *et al.* New diagnostic criteria for multiple sclerosis: guidelines for research protocols. *Ann Neurol* 1983;**13**:227–31.

15. Miller DH, Weinshenker BG, Filippi M, *et al.* Differential diagnosis of suspected multiple sclerosis: a consensus approach. *Mult Scler* 2008;**14**:1157–74.

16. Ormerod IE, Miller DH, McDonald WI, *et al.* The role of NMR imaging in the assessment of multiple sclerosis and isolated neurological lesions. A quantitative study. *Brain* 1987;**110**:(Pt 6):1579–616.

17. Filippi M, Gawne-Cain ML, Gasperini C, *et al.* Effect of training and different measurement strategies on the reproducibility of brain MRI lesion load measurements in multiple sclerosis. *Neurology* 1998;**50**:238–44.

18. Barkhof F, Filippi M, van Waesberghe JH, *et al.* Improving interobserver variation in reporting gadolinium-enhanced MRI lesions in multiple sclerosis. *Neurology* 1997;**49**: 1682–8.

19. Bot JC, Barkhof F. Spinal-cord MRI in multiple sclerosis: conventional and nonconventional MR techniques. *Neuroimaging Clin N Am* 2009;**19**:81–99.

20. Geurts JJ, Pouwels PJ, Uitdehaag BM, Polman CH, Barkhof F, Castelijns JA. Intracortical lesions in multiple sclerosis: improved detection with 3D double inversion-recovery MR imaging. *Radiology* 2005;**236**:254–60.

21. Calabrese M, De Stefano N, Atzori M, *et al.* Detection of cortical inflammatory lesions by double inversion recovery magnetic resonance imaging in patients with multiple sclerosis. *Arch Neurol* 2007;**64**:1416–22.

22. Brex PA, Ciccarelli O, O'Riordan JI, Sailer M, Thompson AJ, Miller DH. A longitudinal study of abnormalities on MRI and disability from multiple sclerosis. *N Engl J Med* 2002;**346**:158–64.

23. Hickman SJ, Dalton CM, Miller DH, Plant GT. Management of acute optic neuritis. *Lancet* 2002;**360**:1953–62.

24. The Optic Neuritis Study Group. Multiple sclerosis risk after optic neuritis: final optic neuritis treatment trial follow-up. *Arch Neurol* 2008;**65**:727–32.

25. Miller DH, Newton MR, van der Poel JC, *et al.* Magnetic resonance imaging of the optic nerve in optic neuritis. *Neurology* 1988;**38**:175–9.

26. Gass A, Moseley IF, Barker GJ, *et al.* Lesion discrimination in optic neuritis using high-resolution fat-suppressed fast spin-echo MRI. *Neuroradiology* 1996;**38**:317–21.

27. Jackson A, Sheppard S, Laitt RD, Kassner A, Moriarty D. Optic neuritis: MR imaging with combined fat- and water-suppression techniques. *Radiology* 1998;**206**:57–63.

28. Davies MB, Williams R, Haq N, Pelosi L, Hawkins CP. MRI of optic nerve and postchiasmal visual pathways and visual evoked potentials in secondary progressive multiple sclerosis. *Neuroradiology* 1998;**40**:765–70.

29. Rocca MA, Hickman SJ, Bo L, *et al.* Imaging the optic nerve in multiple sclerosis. *Mult Scler* 2005;**11**:537–41.

30. Fazekas F, Offenbacher H, Fuchs S, *et al.* Criteria for an increased specificity of MRI interpretation in elderly subjects with suspected multiple sclerosis. *Neurology* 1988;**38**:1822–5.

31. Paty DW, Oger JJ, Kastrukoff LF, *et al.* MRI in the diagnosis of MS: a prospective study with comparison of clinical evaluation, evoked potentials, oligoclonal banding, and CT. *Neurology* 1988;**38**:180–5.

32. Lee KH, Hashimoto SA, Hooge JP, *et al.* Magnetic resonance imaging of the head in the diagnosis of multiple sclerosis: a prospective 2-year follow-up with comparison of clinical evaluation, evoked potentials, oligoclonal banding, and CT. *Neurology* 1991;**41**:657–60.

33. Offenbacher H, Fazekas F, Schmidt R, *et al.* Assessment of MRI criteria for a diagnosis of MS. *Neurology* 1993;**43**: 905–9.

34. Tas MW, Barkhof F, van Walderveen MA, Polman CH, Hommes OR, Valk J. The effect of gadolinium on the sensitivity and specificity of MR in the initial diagnosis of multiple sclerosis. *AJNR Am J Neuroradiol* 1995;**16**: 259–64.

35. Tintore M, Rovira A, Martinez MJ, *et al.* Isolated demyelinating syndromes: comparison of different MR imaging

criteria to predict conversion to clinically definite multiple sclerosis. *AJNR Am J Neuroradiol* 2000;**21**:702–6.

36. Tintore M, Rovira A, Rio J, *et al.* New diagnostic criteria for multiple sclerosis: application in first demyelinating episode. *Neurology* 2003;**60**:27–30.

37. Dalton CM, Brex PA, Miszkiel KA, *et al.* Application of the new McDonald criteria to patients with clinically isolated syndromes suggestive of multiple sclerosis. *Ann Neurol* 2002;**52**:47–53.

38. Bot JC, Barkhof F, Lycklama a Nijeholt G, *et al.* Differentiation of multiple sclerosis from other inflammatory disorders and cerebrovascular disease: value of spinal MR imaging. *Radiology* 2002;**223**:46–56.

39. Dalton CM, Brex PA, Miszkiel KA, *et al.* New T2 lesions enable an earlier diagnosis of multiple sclerosis in clinically isolated syndromes. *Ann Neurol* 2003;**53**:673–6.

40. Frohman EM, Goodin DS, Calabresi PA, *et al.* The utility of MRI in suspected MS: report of the Therapeutics and Technology Assessment Subcommittee of the American Academy of Neurology. *Neurology* 2003;**61**:602–11.

41. Nielsen JM, Korteweg T, Barkhof F, Uitdehaag BM, Polman CH. Overdiagnosis of multiple sclerosis and magnetic resonance imaging criteria. *Ann Neurol* 2005;**58**:781–3.

42. Swanton JK, Fernando K, Dalton CM, *et al.* Modification of MRI criteria for multiple sclerosis in patients with clinically isolated syndromes. *J Neurol Neurosurg Psychiatry* 2006;**77**:830–3.

43. Swanton JK, Rovira A, Tintore M, *et al.* MRI criteria for multiple sclerosis in patients presenting with clinically isolated syndromes: a multicentre retrospective study. *Lancet Neurol* 2007;**6**:677–86.

44. Rovira A, Swanton J, Tintore M, *et al.* A single, early magnetic resonance imaging study in the diagnosis of multiple sclerosis. *Arch Neurol* 2009;**66**:587–92.

45. Okuda DT, Mowry EM, Beheshtian A, *et al.* Incidental MRI anomalies suggestive of multiple sclerosis: the radiologically isolated syndrome. *Neurology* 2009;**72**:800–5.

46. Lebrun C, Bensa C, Debouverie M, *et al.* Association between clinical conversion to multiple sclerosis in radiologically isolated syndrome and magnetic resonance imaging, cerebrospinal fluid, and visual evoked potential: follow-up of 70 patients. *Arch Neurol* 2009;**66**:841–6.

47. Minneboo A, Barkhof F, Polman CH, Uitdehaag BM, Knol DL, Castelijns JA. Infratentorial lesions predict long-term disability in patients with initial findings suggestive of multiple sclerosis. *Arch Neurol* 2004;**61**:217–21.

48. Tintore M, Rovira A, Rio J, *et al.* Baseline MRI predicts future attacks and disability in clinically isolated syndromes. *Neurology* 2006;**67**:968–72.

49. Miller DH, Barkhof F, Frank JA, Parker GJ, Thompson AJ. Measurement of atrophy in multiple sclerosis: pathological basis, methodological aspects and clinical relevance. *Brain* 2002;**125**:1676–95.

50. Dalton CM, Chard DT, Davies GR, *et al.* Early development of multiple sclerosis is associated with progressive grey matter atrophy in patients presenting with clinically isolated syndromes. *Brain* 2004;**127**:1101–7.

51. Filippi M, Rovaris M, Inglese M, *et al.* Interferon beta-1a for brain tissue loss in patients at presentation with syndromes suggestive of multiple sclerosis: a randomised, double-blind, placebo-controlled trial. *Lancet* 2004;**364**:1489–96.

52. Dalton CM, Brex PA, Jenkins R, *et al.* Progressive ventricular enlargement in patients with clinically isolated syndromes is associated with the early development of multiple sclerosis. *J Neurol Neurosurg Psychiatry* 2002;**73**:141–7.

53. Brex PA, Leary SM, O'Riordan JI, *et al.* Measurement of spinal cord area in clinically isolated syndromes suggestive of multiple sclerosis. *J Neurol Neurosurg Psychiatry* 2001;**70**:544–7.

54. Fernando KT, Tozer DJ, Miszkiel KA, *et al.* Magnetization transfer histograms in clinically isolated syndromes suggestive of multiple sclerosis. *Brain* 2005;**128**:2911–25.

55. Rocca MA, Agosta F, Sormani MP, *et al.* A three-year, multi-parametric MRI study in patients at presentation with CIS. *J Neurol* 2008;**255**:683–91.

56. Iannucci G, Tortorella C, Rovaris M, Sormani MP, Comi G, Filippi M. Prognostic value of MR and magnetization transfer imaging findings in patients with clinically isolated syndromes suggestive of multiple sclerosis at presentation. *AJNR Am J Neuroradiol* 2000;**21**:1034–8.

57. Rovaris M, Gallo A, Riva R, *et al.* An MT MRI study of the cervical cord in clinically isolated syndromes suggestive of MS. *Neurology* 2004;**63**:584–5.

58. Gallo A, Rovaris M, Riva R, *et al.* Diffusion-tensor magnetic resonance imaging detects normal-appearing white matter damage unrelated to short-term disease activity in patients at the earliest clinical stage of multiple sclerosis. *Arch Neurol* 2005;**62**:803–8.

59. Rovaris M, Judica E, Ceccarelli A, *et al.* A 3-year diffusion tensor MRI study of grey matter damage progression during the earliest clinical stage of MS. *J Neurol* 2008;**255**:1209–14.

60. Filippi M, Bozzali M, Rovaris M, *et al.* Evidence for widespread axonal damage at the earliest clinical stage of multiple sclerosis. *Brain* 2003;**126**:433–7.

61. Fernando KT, McLean MA, Chard DT, *et al.* Elevated white matter myo-inositol in clinically isolated syndromes suggestive of multiple sclerosis. *Brain* 2004;**127**:1361–9.

62. Wattjes MP, Harzheim M, Lutterbey GG, *et al.* Prognostic value of high-field proton magnetic resonance spectroscopy in patients presenting with clinically isolated syndromes suggestive of multiple sclerosis. *Neuroradiology* 2008;**50**:123–9.

63. Rocca MA, Mezzapesa DM, Falini A, *et al.* Evidence for axonal pathology and adaptive cortical reorganization in patients at presentation with clinically isolated syndromes suggestive of multiple sclerosis. *Neuroimage* 2003;**18**: 847–55.

64. Filippi M, Rocca MA, Mezzapesa DM, *et al.* Simple and complex movement-associated functional MRI changes in patients at presentation with clinically isolated syndromes suggestive of multiple sclerosis. *Hum Brain Mapp* 2004;**21**: 108–17.

65. Rocca MA, Mezzapesa DM, Ghezzi A, *et al.* A widespread pattern of cortical activations in patients at presentation with clinically isolated symptoms is associated with evolution to definite multiple sclerosis. *AJNR Am J Neuroradiol* 2005;**26**:1136–9.

66. Longstreth WT Jr, Arnold AM, Beauchamp NJ Jr, *et al.* Incidence, manifestations, and predictors of worsening white matter on serial cranial magnetic resonance imaging in the elderly: the Cardiovascular Health Study. *Stroke* 2005;**36**:56–61.

67. Kidd D, Thorpe JW, Thompson AJ, *et al.* Spinal cord MRI using multi-array coils and fast spin echo. II. Findings in multiple sclerosis. *Neurology* 1993;**43**:2632–7.

68. Miller DH, Filippi M, Fazekas F, *et al.* Role of magnetic resonance imaging within diagnostic criteria for multiple sclerosis. *Ann Neurol* 2004;**56**:273–8.

69. Kanal E, Barkovich AJ, Bell C, *et al.* ACR guidance document for safe MR practices: 2007. *AJR Am J Roentgenol* 2007;**188**:1447–74.

70. Thomsen HS. European Society of Urogenital Radiology guidelines on contrast media application. *Curr Opin Urol* 2007;**17**:70–6.

71. Thompson AJ, Montalban X, Barkhof F, *et al.* Diagnostic criteria for primary progressive multiple sclerosis: a position paper. *Ann Neurol* 2000;**47**:831–5.

72. Barkhof F, Filippi M, Miller DH, Tofts P, Kappos L, Thompson AJ. Strategies for optimizing MRI techniques aimed at monitoring disease activity in multiple sclerosis treatment trials. *J Neurol* 1997;**244**:76–84.

73. Filippi M, Horsfield MA, Ader HJ, *et al.* Guidelines for using quantitative measures of brain magnetic resonance imaging abnormalities in monitoring the treatment of multiple sclerosis. *Ann Neurol* 1998;**43**:499–506.

74. Thompson AJ, Miller DH, MacManus DG, McDonald WI. Patterns of disease activity in multiple sclerosis. *BMJ* 1990;**301**:44–5.

75. Filippi M, Rocca MA. Conventional MRI in multiple sclerosis. *J Neuroimaging* 2007;**17**(Suppl. 1):3S–9S.

76. Sormani MP, Rovaris M, Comi G, Filippi M. A composite score to predict short-term disease activity in patients with relapsing-remitting MS. *Neurology* 2007;**69**:1230–5.

77. Li DK, Held U, Petkau J, *et al.* MRI T2 lesion burden in multiple sclerosis: a plateauing relationship with clinical disability. *Neurology* 2006;**66**:1384–9.

78. Kermode AG, Thompson AJ, Tofts P, *et al.* Breakdown of the blood-brain barrier precedes symptoms and other MRI signs of new lesions in multiple sclerosis. Pathogenetic and clinical implications. *Brain* 1990;**113**(Pt 5): 1477–89.

79. Thompson AJ, Miller D, Youl B, *et al.* Serial gadolinium-enhanced MRI in relapsing/remitting multiple sclerosis of varying disease duration. *Neurology* 1992;**42**:60–3.

80. Thompson AJ, Kermode AG, Wicks D, *et al.* Major differences in the dynamics of primary and secondary progressive multiple sclerosis. *Ann Neurol* 1991;**29**:53–62.

81. Filippi M, Rossi P, Campi A, Colombo B, Pereira C, Comi G. Serial contrast-enhanced MR in patients with multiple sclerosis and varying levels of disability. *AJNR Am J Neuroradiol* 1997;**18**:1549–56.

82. Koudriavtseva T, Thompson AJ, Fiorelli M, *et al.* Gadolinium enhanced MRI predicts clinical and MRI disease activity in relapsing-remitting multiple sclerosis. *J Neurol Neurosurg Psychiatry* 1997;**62**:285–7.

83. Molyneux PD, Filippi M, Barkhof F, *et al.* Correlations between monthly enhanced MRI lesion rate and changes in T2 lesion volume in multiple sclerosis. *Ann Neurol* 1998;**43**:332–9.

84. Simon JH. From enhancing lesions to brain atrophy in relapsing MS. *J Neuroimmunol* 1999;**98**:7–15.

85. Stone LA, Smith ME, Albert PS, *et al.* Blood-brain barrier disruption on contrast-enhanced MRI in patients with mild relapsing-remitting multiple sclerosis: relationship to course, gender, and age. *Neurology* 1995;**45**:1122–6.

86. Losseff NA, Kingsley DP, McDonald WI, Miller DH, Thompson AJ. Clinical and magnetic resonance imaging predictors of disability in primary and secondary progressive multiple sclerosis. *Mult Scler* 1996;**1**:218–22.

87. Simon JH, Li D, Traboulsee A, *et al.* Standardized MR imaging protocol for multiple sclerosis: Consortium of MS Centers consensus guidelines. *AJNR Am J Neuroradiol* 2006;**27**:455–61.

88. Filippi M, Rocca MA. MRI aspects of the 'inflammatory phase' of multiple sclerosis. *Neurol Sci* 2003;**24**(Suppl. 5):S275–8.

89. Fazekas F, Barkhof F, Filippi M, *et al.* The contribution of magnetic resonance imaging to the diagnosis of multiple sclerosis. *Neurology* 1999;**53**:448–56.

90. PRISMS (Prevention of Relapses and Disability by Interferon beta-1a Subcutaneously in Multiple Sclerosis) Study Group. Randomised double-blind placebo-controlled study of interferon beta-1a in relapsing/remitting multiple sclerosis. *Lancet* 1998;**352**:1498–504.

91. Simon JH, Jacobs LD, Campion M, *et al*. Magnetic resonance studies of intramuscular interferon beta-1a for relapsing multiple sclerosis. The Multiple Sclerosis Collaborative Research Group. *Ann Neurol* 1998;**43**:79–87.

92. Li DK, Paty DW. Magnetic resonance imaging results of the PRISMS trial: a randomized, double-blind, placebo-controlled study of interferon-beta1a in relapsing-remitting multiple sclerosis. Prevention of Relapses and Disability by Interferon-beta1a Subcutaneously in Multiple Sclerosis. *Ann Neurol* 1999;**46**:197–206.

93. Sorensen PS, Wanscher B, Jensen CV, *et al*. Intravenous immunoglobulin G reduces MRI activity in relapsing multiple sclerosis. *Neurology* 1998;**50**:1273–81.

94. O'Connor P, Comi G, Montalban X, *et al*. Oral fingolimod (FTY720) in multiple sclerosis: two-year results of a phase II extension study. *Neurology* 2009;**72**:73–9.

95. Kappos L, Antel J, Comi G, *et al*. Oral fingolimod (FTY720) for relapsing multiple sclerosis. *N Engl J Med* 2006;**355**:1124–40.

96. Mikol DD, Barkhof F, Chang P, *et al*. Comparison of subcutaneous interferon beta-1a with glatiramer acetate in patients with relapsing multiple sclerosis (the REbif vs Glatiramer Acetate in Relapsing MS Disease [REGARD] study): a multicentre, randomised, parallel, open-label trial. *Lancet Neurol* 2008;**7**:903–14.

97. Comi G, Filippi M, Wolinsky JS. European/Canadian multiticenter, double-blind, randomized, placebo-controlled study of the effects of glatiramer acetate on magnetic resonance imaging – measured disease activity and burden in patients with relapsing multiple sclerosis. European/Canadian Glatiramer Acetate Study Group. *Ann Neurol* 2001;**49**:290–7.

98. Clanet M, Radue EW, Kappos L, *et al*. A randomized, double-blind, dose-comparison study of weekly interferon beta-1a in relapsing MS. *Neurology* 2002;**59**:1507–17.

99. Comi G, Pulizzi A, Rovaris M, *et al*. Effect of laquinimod on MRI-monitored disease activity in patients with relapsing-remitting multiple sclerosis: a multicentre, randomised, double-blind, placebo-controlled phase IIb study. *Lancet* 2008;**371**:2085–92.

100. Miller DH, Khan OA, Sheremata WA, *et al*. A controlled trial of natalizumab for relapsing multiple sclerosis. *N Engl J Med* 2003;**348**:15–23.

101. Goodman AD, Rossman H, Bar-Or A, *et al*. GLANCE: results of a phase 2, randomized, double-blind, placebo-controlled study. *Neurology* 2009;**72**:806–12.

102. Miller DH, Soon D, Fernando KT, *et al*. MRI outcomes in a placebo-controlled trial of natalizumab in relapsing MS. *Neurology* 2007;**68**:1390–401.

103. Metz LM, Zhang Y, Yeung M, *et al*. Minocycline reduces gadolinium-enhancing magnetic resonance imaging lesions in multiple sclerosis. *Ann Neurol* 2004;**55**:756.

104. Rose JW, Watt HE, White AT, Carlson NG. Treatment of multiple sclerosis with an anti-interleukin-2 receptor monoclonal antibody. *Ann Neurol* 2004;**56**:864–7.

105. Vollmer T, Key L, Durkalski V, *et al*. Oral simvastatin treatment in relapsing-remitting multiple sclerosis. *Lancet* 2004;**363**:1607–8.

106. O'Connor PW, Li D, Freedman MS, *et al*. A Phase II study of the safety and efficacy of teriflunomide in multiple sclerosis with relapses. *Neurology* 2006;**66**:894–900.

107. Kappos L, Gold R, Miller DH, *et al*. Efficacy and safety of oral fumarate in patients with relapsing-remitting multiple sclerosis: a multicentre, randomised, double-blind, placebo-controlled phase IIb study. *Lancet* 2008;**372**:1463–72.

108. Paty DW, Li DK. Interferon beta-1b is effective in relapsing-remitting multiple sclerosis. II. MRI analysis results of a multicenter, randomized, double-blind, placebo-controlled trial. UBC MS/MRI Study Group and the IFNB Multiple Sclerosis Study Group. *Neurology* 1993;**43**:662–7.

109. Jacobs LD, Cookfair DL, Rudick RA, *et al*. Intramuscular interferon beta-1a for disease progression in relapsing multiple sclerosis. The Multiple Sclerosis Collaborative Research Group (MSCRG). *Ann Neurol* 1996;**39**:285–94.

110. Panitch H, Goodin DS, Francis G, *et al*. Randomized, comparative study of interferon beta-1a treatment regimens in MS: The EVIDENCE Trial. *Neurology* 2002;**59**:1496–506.

111. Rudick RA, Stuart WH, Calabresi PA, *et al*. Natalizumab plus interferon beta-1a for relapsing multiple sclerosis. *N Engl J Med* 2006;**354**:911–23.

112. Smith DR, Weinstock-Guttman B, Cohen JA, *et al*. A randomized blinded trial of combination therapy with cyclophosphamide in patients-with active multiple sclerosis on interferon beta. *Mult Scler* 2005;**11**:573–82.

113. Polman CH, O'Connor PW, Havrdova E, *et al*. A randomized, placebo-controlled trial of natalizumab for relapsing multiple sclerosis. *N Engl J Med* 2006;**354**:899–910.

114. Andersen O, Lycke J, Tollesson PO, *et al*. Linomide reduces the rate of active lesions in relapsing-remitting multiple sclerosis. *Neurology* 1996;**47**:895–900.

115. Millefiorini E, Gasperini C, Pozzilli C, *et al*. Randomized placebo-controlled trial of mitoxantrone in relapsing-remitting multiple sclerosis: 24-month clinical and MRI outcome. *J Neurol* 1997;**244**:153–9.

116. Hauser SL, Waubant E, Arnold DL, *et al*. B-cell depletion with rituximab in relapsing-remitting multiple sclerosis. *N Engl J Med* 2008;**358**:676–88.

117. Fazekas F, Lublin FD, Li D, *et al*. Intravenous immunoglobulin in relapsing-remitting multiple sclerosis: a dose-finding trial. *Neurology* 2008;**71**:265–71.

118. Segal BM, Constantinescu CS, Raychaudhuri A, Kim L, Fidelus-Gort R, Kasper LH. Repeated subcutaneous injections of IL12/23 p40 neutralising antibody, ustekinumab, in patients with relapsing-remitting multiple sclerosis: a phase II, double-blind, placebo-controlled, randomised, dose-ranging study. *Lancet Neurol* 2008;**7**:796–804.

119. Coles AJ, Compston DA, Selmaj KW, *et al*. Alemtuzumab vs. interferon beta-1a in early multiple sclerosis. *N Engl J Med* 2008;**359**:1786–801.

120. Miller DH, Molyneux PD, Barker GJ, MacManus DG, Moseley IF, Wagner K. Effect of interferon-beta1b on magnetic resonance imaging outcomes in secondary progressive multiple sclerosis: results of a European multicenter, randomized, double-blind, placebo-controlled trial. European Study Group on Interferon-beta1b in secondary progressive multiple sclerosis. *Ann Neurol* 1999;**46**:850–9.

121. Paolillo A, Coles AJ, Molyneux PD, *et al*. Quantitative MRI in patients with secondary progressive MS treated with monoclonal antibody Campath 1H. *Neurology* 1999;**53**: 751–7.

122. Rice GP, Filippi M, Comi G. Cladribine and progressive MS: clinical and MRI outcomes of a multicenter controlled trial. Cladribine MRI Study Group. *Neurology* 2000;**54**: 1145–55.

123. Rose JW, Burns JB, Bjorklund J, Klein J, Watt HE, Carlson NG. Daclizumab phase II trial in relapsing and remitting multiple sclerosis: MRI and clinical results. *Neurology* 2007;**69**:785–9.

124. Garren H, Robinson WH, Krasulova E, *et al*. Phase 2 trial of a DNA vaccine encoding myelin basic protein for multiple sclerosis. *Ann Neurol* 2008;**63**:611–20.

125. Bar-Or A, Calabresi PA, Arnold D, *et al*. Rituximab in relapsing-remitting multiple sclerosis: a 72-week, open-label, phase I trial. *Ann Neurol* 2008;**63**:395–400.

126. Panitch H, Miller A, Paty D, Weinshenker B. Interferon beta-1b in secondary progressive MS: results from a 3-year controlled study. *Neurology* 2004;**63**:1788–95.

127. Kappos L, Traboulsee A, Constantinescu C, *et al*. Long-term subcutaneous interferon beta-1a therapy in patients with relapsing-remitting MS. *Neurology* 2006;**67**:944–53.

128. Rovaris M, Comi G, Rocca MA, *et al*. Long-term follow-up of patients treated with glatiramer acetate: a multicentre, multinational extension of the European/Canadian double-blind, placebo-controlled, MRI-monitored trial. *Mult Scler* 2007;**13**:502–8.

129. Rudick RA, Lee JC, Simon J, Ransohoff RM, Fisher E. Defining interferon beta response status in multiple sclerosis patients. *Ann Neurol* 2004;**56**:548–55.

130. Rio J, Rovira A, Tintore M, *et al*. Relationship between MRI lesion activity and response to IFN-beta in relapsing-remitting multiple sclerosis patients. *Mult Scler* 2008;**14**: 479–84.

131. Prosperini L, Gallo V, Petsas N, Borriello G, Pozzilli C. One-year MRI scan predicts clinical response to interferon beta in multiple sclerosis. *Eur J Neurol* 2009;**16**:1202–9.

132. Tomassini V, Paolillo A, Russo P, *et al*. Predictors of long-term clinical response to interferon beta therapy in relapsing multiple sclerosis. *J Neurol* 2006;**253**:287–93.

133. Fazekas F, Soelberg-Sorensen P, Comi G, Filippi M. MRI to monitor treatment efficacy in multiple sclerosis. *J Neuroimaging* 2007;**17**(Suppl. 1):50S–5S.

134. Simon JH, Lull J, Jacobs LD, *et al*. A longitudinal study of T1 hypointense lesions in relapsing MS: MSCRG trial of interferon beta-1a. Multiple Sclerosis Collaborative Research Group. *Neurology* 2000;**55**:185–92.

135. Barkhof F, van Waesberghe JH, Filippi M, *et al*. T(1) hypointense lesions in secondary progressive multiple sclerosis: effect of interferon beta-1b treatment. *Brain* 2001;**124**:1396–402.

136. Filippi M, Rovaris M, Rice GP, *et al*. The effect of cladribine on T(1) 'black hole' changes in progressive MS. *J Neurol Sci* 2000;**176**:42–4.

137. Patti F, Amato MP, Filippi M, Gallo P, Trojano M, Comi GC. A double blind, placebo-controlled, phase II, add-on study of cyclophosphamide (CTX) for 24 months in patients affected by multiple sclerosis on a background therapy with interferon-beta study denomination: CYCLIN. *J Neurol Sci* 2004;**223**:69–71.

138. Filippi M, Rovaris M, Rocca MA, Sormani MP, Wolinsky JS, Comi G. Glatiramer acetate reduces the proportion of new MS lesions evolving into 'black holes'. *Neurology* 2001;**57**:731–3.

139. Dalton CM, Miszkiel KA, Barker GJ, *et al*. Effect of natalizumab on conversion of gadolinium enhancing lesions to T1 hypointense lesions in relapsing multiple sclerosis. *J Neurol* 2004;**251**:407–13.

140. Brex PA, Molyneux PD, Smiddy P, *et al*. The effect of IFNbeta-1b on the evolution of enhancing lesions in secondary progressive MS. *Neurology* 2001;**57**:2185–90.

141. Bermel RA, Bakshi R. The measurement and clinical relevance of brain atrophy in multiple sclerosis. *Lancet Neurol* 2006;**5**:158–70.

142. Giorgio A, Battaglini M, Smith SM, De Stefano N. Brain atrophy assessment in multiple sclerosis: importance and limitations. *Neuroimaging Clin N Am* 2008;**18**:675–86.

143. Lanz M, Hahn HK, Hildebrandt H. Brain atrophy and cognitive impairment in multiple sclerosis: a review. *J Neurol* 2007;**254**(Suppl. 2):II43–8.

144. Fisher E, Rudick RA, Simon JH, *et al*. Eight-year follow-up study of brain atrophy in patients with MS. *Neurology* 2002;**59**:1412–20.

145. Khaleeli Z, Ciccarelli O, Manfredonia F, *et al*. Predicting progression in primary progressive multiple sclerosis: a 10-year multicenter study. *Ann Neurol* 2008;**63**:790–3.

146. Chard DT, Griffin CM, Parker GJ, Kapoor R, Thompson AJ, Miller DH. Brain atrophy in clinically early relapsing-remitting multiple sclerosis. *Brain* 2002;**125**:327–37.

147. De Stefano N, Matthews PM, Filippi M, *et al*. Evidence of early cortical atrophy in MS: relevance to white matter changes and disability. *Neurology* 2003;**60**:1157–62.

148. Valsasina P, Benedetti B, Rovaris M, Sormani MP, Comi G, Filippi M. Evidence for progressive gray matter loss in patients with relapsing-remitting MS. *Neurology* 2005;**65**:1126–8.

149. Fisher E, Lee JC, Nakamura K, Rudick RA. Gray matter atrophy in multiple sclerosis: a longitudinal study. *Ann Neurol* 2008;**64**:255–65.

150. Pagani E, Rocca MA, Gallo A, *et al*. Regional brain atrophy evolves differently in patients with multiple sclerosis according to clinical phenotype. *AJNR Am J Neuroradiol* 2005;**26**:341–6.

151. Ceccarelli A, Rocca MA, Pagani E, *et al*. A voxel-based morphometry study of grey matter loss in MS patients with different clinical phenotypes. *Neuroimage* 2008;**42**:315–22.

152. Rudick RA, Fisher E, Lee JC, Simon J, Jacobs L. Use of the brain parenchymal fraction to measure whole brain atrophy in relapsing-remitting MS. Multiple Sclerosis Collaborative Research Group. *Neurology* 1999;**53**:1698–704.

153. Filippi M, Rovaris M, Iannucci G, Mennea S, Sormani MP, Comi G. Whole brain volume changes in patients with progressive MS treated with cladribine. *Neurology* 2000;**55**:1714–8.

154. Molyneux PD, Kappos L, Polman C, *et al*. The effect of interferon beta-1b treatment on MRI measures of cerebral atrophy in secondary progressive multiple sclerosis. European Study Group on Interferon beta-1b in secondary progressive multiple sclerosis. *Brain* 2000;**123**(Pt 11):2256–63.

155. Rovaris M, Comi G, Rocca MA, Wolinsky JS, Filippi M. Short-term brain volume change in relapsing-remitting multiple sclerosis: effect of glatiramer acetate and implications. *Brain* 2001;**124**:1803–12.

156. Sormani MP, Rovaris M, Valsasina P, Wolinsky JS, Comi G, Filippi M. Measurement error of two different tech-niques for brain atrophy assessment in multiple sclerosis. *Neurology* 2004;**62**:1432–4.

157. Ropele S, Fazekas F. Magnetization transfer MR imaging in multiple sclerosis. *Neuroimaging Clin N Am* 2009;**19**:27–36.

158. Rovaris M, Agosta F, Pagani E, Filippi M. Diffusion tensor MR imaging. *Neuroimaging Clin N Am* 2009;**19**:37–43.

159. Sajja BR, Wolinsky JS, Narayana PA. Proton magnetic resonance spectroscopy in multiple sclerosis. *Neuroimaging Clin N Am* 2009;**19**:45–58.

160. Rovaris M, Agosta F, Sormani MP, *et al*. Conventional and magnetization transfer MRI predictors of clinical multiple sclerosis evolution: a medium-term follow-up study. *Brain* 2003;**126**:2323–32.

161. Agosta F, Absinta M, Sormani MP, *et al*. In vivo assessment of cervical cord damage in MS patients: a longitudinal diffusion tensor MRI study. *Brain* 2007;**130**:2211–9.

162. Agosta F, Rovaris M, Pagani E, Sormani MP, Comi G, Filippi M. Magnetization transfer MRI metrics predict the accumulation of disability 8 years later in patients with multiple sclerosis. *Brain* 2006;**129**:2620–7.

163. Richert ND, Ostuni JL, Bash CN, Leist TP, McFarland HF, Frank JA. Interferon beta-1b and intravenous methylpred-nisolone promote lesion recovery in multiple sclerosis. *Mult Scler* 2001;**7**:49–58.

164. Kita M, Goodkin DE, Bacchetti P, Waubant E, Nelson SJ, Majumdar S. Magnetization transfer ratio in new MS lesions before and during therapy with IFNbeta-1a. *Neurology* 2000;**54**:1741–5.

165. Richert ND, Ostuni JL, Bash CN, Duyn JH, McFarland HF, Frank JA. Serial whole-brain magnetization transfer imaging in patients with relapsing-remitting multiple sclerosis at baseline and during treatment with interferon beta-1b. *AJNR Am J Neuroradiol* 1998;**19**:1705–13.

166. Inglese M, van Waesberghe JH, Rovaris M, *et al*. The effect of interferon beta-1b on quantities derived from MT MRI in secondary progressive MS. *Neurology* 2003;**60**:853–60.

167. Filippi M, Rocca MA, Pagani E, *et al*. European study on intravenous immunoglobulin in multiple sclerosis: results of magnetization transfer magnetic resonance imaging analysis. *Arch Neurol* 2004;**61**:1409–12.

168. Horsfield MA, Barker GJ, Barkhof F, Miller DH, Thompson AJ, Filippi M. Guidelines for using quantitative magnetization transfer magnetic resonance imaging for monitoring treatment of multiple sclerosis. *J Magn Reson Imaging* 2003;**17**:389–97.

169. Ropele S, Filippi M, Valsasina P, *et al*. Assessment and correction of B1-induced errors in magnetization transfer ratio measurements. *Magn Reson Med* 2005;**53**:134–40.

170. Sarchielli P, Presciutti O, Tarducci R, *et al*. 1H-MRS in patients with multiple sclerosis undergoing treatment with interferon beta-1a: results of a preliminary study. *J Neurol Neurosurg Psychiatry* 1998;**64**:204–12.

171. Narayanan S, De Stefano N, Francis GS, *et al*. Axonal metabolic recovery in multiple sclerosis patients treated with interferon beta-1b. *J Neurol* 2001;**248**:979–86.

172. Schubert F, Seifert F, Elster C, *et al*. Serial 1H-MRS in relapsing-remitting multiple sclerosis: effects of interferon-beta therapy on absolute metabolite concentrations. *MAGMA* 2002;**14**:213–22.

173. Khan O, Shen Y, Bao F, *et al*. Long-term study of brain 1H-MRS study in multiple sclerosis: effect of glatiramer acetate therapy on axonal metabolic function and feasibility of long-Term H-MRS monitoring in multiple sclerosis. *J Neuroimaging* 2008;**18**:314–9.

174. Narayana PA, Wolinsky JS, Rao SB, He R, Mehta M. Multicentre proton magnetic resonance spectroscopy imaging of primary progressive multiple sclerosis. *Mult Scler* 2004;**10**(Suppl. 1):S73–8.

175. Sajja BR, Narayana PA, Wolinsky JS, Ahn CW. Longitudinal magnetic resonance spectroscopic imaging of primary progressive multiple sclerosis patients treated with glatiramer acetate: multicenter study. *Mult Scler* 2008;**14**: 73–80.

176. De Stefano N, Filippi M, Miller D, *et al*. Guidelines for using proton MR spectroscopy in multicenter clinical MS studies. *Neurology* 2007;**69**:1942–52.

CHAPTER 4

Neurophysiological tests and neuroimaging procedures in non-acute headache

G. Sandrini,[1] L. Friberg,[2] G. Coppola,[3] W. Jänig,[4] R. Jensen,[5] M. Kruit,[6] P. Rossi,[7] D. Russell,[8] M. Sanchez del Rìo,[9] T. Sand,[10] J. Schoenen[11]

[1]IRCCS C. Mondino Foundation, Pavia, Italy; [2]Bispebjerg Hospital, Copenhagen, Denmark; [3]G.B. Bietti Eye Foundation IRCCS, Rome, Italy; [4]Physiologisches Institut, Christian-Albrechts-Universität, Kiel, Germany; [5]Glostrup Hospital, University of Copenhagen, Glostrup, Denmark; [6]Leiden University Medical Center, The Netherlands; [7]INI Grottaferrata, UCADH, Pavia-Roma, Italy; [8]Rikshospitalet, Oslo, Norway; [9]Hospital Ruber Internacional, Madrid, Spain; [10]Norwegian University of Science and Technology, Trondheim, Norway; [11]CHR Citadelle, Liege, Belgium

Introduction

The most important tools in the diagnosis and treatment of headache disorders are, without doubt, careful clinical neurological examinations and detailed reports on the patient's history and symptoms. Application of the diagnostic criteria of the International Headache Society (IHS Classification 2nd edition [1]), can lead to a probable diagnosis that allows adequate treatment. However, in many cases, particularly when the headache presents as atypical with changing clinical features or as a symptom of another primary illness, neurologists find it necessary to supplement the clinical work-up of the patient with para-clinical tests. The differential diagnosis of acute headache (e.g. primary thunderclap headache) versus symptomatic headache presents several difficulties and neuroimaging investigations are mandatory. This report is an update of the first edition of these guidelines [2] and is based on a critical review of the literature on the application of neurophysiological tests and imaging procedures in non-acute headache patients. In addition to evaluating the clinical usefulness of these tests and procedures in the diagnostic setting, we present updated guidelines for their use, as attempted previously by

various authors [3–5]. Of all the available techniques, neuroimaging, particularly magnetic resonance imaging (MRI), is still the most suitable and cost-effective para-clinical testing method used in headache patients, with the highest rate of diagnosis. Finally, we consider the potential use of these methods in headache research. An extensive review of the main references in the literature, together with an update on the most important contributions made by neurophysiological studies to our understanding of the pathogenesis of primary headache, was published in connection with the publication of the first edition of these guidelines [2, 6].

Aims and methods

The intention in compiling the information in this document was to develop guidelines to help physicians make appropriate choices regarding the use of instrumental tests in non-acute headache patients. Reviews of published clinical evidence (from 1988 to July 2009) were evaluated. Key literature references pre-dating the first edition of the IHS Classification [7] were particularly carefully examined as these studies applied different diagnostic criteria for headache.

The guidelines were prepared according to the EFNS criteria [8, 9] and the level of evidence and grade of recommendation are expressed in accordance with this reference.

Main findings for the different techniques

Electroencephalography (EEG)

The usefulness of EEG in the diagnosis of headache is debated. Early EEG studies of migraine emphasized the frequent abnormal recordings, contemporary reviewers have criticized most of them for various methodological omissions and flaws [10, 11]). The American Academy of Neurology concluded that 'EEG is not useful in the routine evaluation of patients with headache (guideline)', admitting, however, that EEG may be used in headache patients with associated symptoms suggesting a seizure disorder [12].

EEG is the best laboratory investigation to support the clinical diagnosis of epilepsy, showing good sensitivity (80–90% in serial recordings) and specificity (false-positive rates in 0.2–3.5% of healthy subjects) [13]. It also plays an important role in the evaluation of other focal and diffuse central nervous system (CNS) disorders.

Quantitative frequency analysis of EEG (QEEG), with or without topographic mapping, is a more objective method than conventional EEG interpretation, although there are a number of possible methodological pitfalls that should be avoided. The use of QEEG is generally recommended only in conjunction with visual EEG interpretation performed by a skilled observer [14].

Evoked potentials

Evoked potentials (EPs) are cortical EEG potentials temporally linked to a specific sensory input. Although all sensory stimuli contribute to the overall EEG activity, EPs cannot be identified in the normal EEG because they are not separable from ongoing EEG activity. However, when clear temporal definition of the stimulus is possible (i.e. in the case of a sudden onset), short stretches of post-stimulus EEG can be averaged. Any activity that is not time-locked to the stimulus disappears from the average, while the EEG response to the stimulus remains. In this way, the cortical response to very specific stimuli can be investigated in spatial and temporal detail. In migraine, much attention has been paid to visual stimuli, which is not surprising given the presence of visual auras and photophobia in this disorder. EPs have made it possible to document cortical excitability,

as well as habituation and gating phenomena in migraine [15].

Reflex responses

Several electrophysiological techniques have been used to explore polysynaptic reflexes in headache patients. The blink reflex (BR) and corneal reflex (CR) are reflected in the bilateral closure of the eyelids in response to a stimulus; in laboratory settings, that is usually an electrical stimulation of the supraorbital nerve. The BR consists of three components: an ipsilateral early component (R1), a bilateral late component (R2), and a bilateral ultralate component (R3). The precise nature of R1 and R2 is still debated, while R3 is considered to be a nociceptive component. The CR is composed of two late bilateral symmetrical components, probably equivalent to the R2 component.

Several BR and CR abnormalities have been described in primary headaches, but data documenting the specificity and sensitivity of these tests [16–19] are scarce. The exteroceptive suppression (ES) of masticatory muscle activity is a trigemino–trigeminal reflex consisting of biphasic (ES1 and ES2) inhibition of voluntary contraction (of variable duration) that occurs bilaterally in response to various exteroceptive stimuli. The inhibitory effect is mediated by interneurones located in the propriobulbar and pontine reticular formation, close to the trigeminal motor nucleus on each side. The literature contains conflicting data on ES abnormalities in tension-type headaches [20].

Recent evidence suggests the nociceptive blink reflex (nBR) could be a useful tool for evidencing sensitization phenomena induced by nitroglycerin [21]. Using nBR and pain-related evoked potentials (PREP) Obermann *et al.* [22] evidenced an impairment of the trigeminal nociceptive system due to demyelination and/or axonal dysfunction on the symptomatic side and locate this defect close to the root entry zone in the brainstem in trigeminal neuralgia.

Nociceptive flexion reflexes (NFRs), evoked at the biceps femoral muscle by electrical stimulation of the sural nerve, are thought to constitute a useful tool for exploring the pain control system in human beings, but only a few NFR studies have been conducted in headache patients [18]. NFRs allow the documentation sensitization phenomena and impairment of diffuse noxious inhibitory controls in migraine and chronic tension type headache [23, 24].

Autonomic tests

The autonomic nervous system (ANS) consists of three parts: the sympathetic, parasympathetic, and enteric nervous systems. Each of these is divided into subsystems according to the effector organs innervated by the terminal neurons. 'Sympathetic' and 'parasympathetic' neurons are actually defined on the basis of anatomical rather than functional criteria; thus, afferent neurones innervating visceral organs are not denoted as sympathetic or parasympathetic, but as visceral [25, 26]. When considering the role of the ANS in the different types of headache, there are three questions that should be borne in mind [27, 28]).

1 Is the ANS involved in the generation and maintenance of pain? Hypotheses regarding the mechanisms of possible sympathetic nervous system involvement in the generation and maintenance of pain have been formulated and tested in animal and human experimental models [27, 29, 30]).

2 Are functional autonomic abnormalities associated with different types of headache, the consequence of and therefore secondary to headache? This question addresses the observation that all pain is accompanied by autonomic reactions that are based on central reflex pathways in the neuraxis, and on the central integration of nociceptive with autonomic systems. In normal biological conditions, these autonomic reactions are primarily protective for the organism, but this may not necessarily continue to be the case in pathobiological conditions [27].

3 Are headache and functional autonomic abnormalities parallel events and therefore the consequence of possible central abnormalities? If they are, it could be useful to investigate these autonomic abnormalities in an attempt to elucidate the central pathophysiological changes that may underlie both headache and autonomic disturbances.

The diagnosis and management of autonomic disorders are highly dependent on the testing procedures used [31]. Neurophysiological techniques have revealed several autonomic disturbances in primary headache, in cluster headache, in trigeminal autonomic cephalgias in particular [32], but the clinical relevance of these findings is doubtful.

Clinical tests in headache

Central sensitization is thought to play an important role in the maintenance and exacerbation of the acute migraine headache attack, and in the development of the chronic form of migraine, as well as in TTH [33–36]. Clinically, central sensitization may result in allodynia of the face and scalp [33–35] during the headache attack, whereas pain sensitivity seems to be normal between attacks [34, 35]. Central sensitization is also associated with cortical plastic changes in the chronic subforms [36]. Clinical tests to demonstrate central sensitization are still unspecific and cannot yet be used to discriminate between different coexisting primary or secondary headaches. The ICHD-I and II divided TTH arbitrarily into two subgroups in order to study the pathophysiological relevance of pericranial muscles in this disorder. The subdivision was motivated by the clinical observation that many TTH patients have increased tension, tenderness, and stiffness in their neck and shoulder muscles, whereas some, a smaller group and much more difficult to treat, lack muscle tenderness. The IHS classification did not lay down specific diagnostic methods and although several studies have been carried out since then [19, 33, 37–39], it is still not clear whether different pathophysiological mechanisms subtend the headache in these two subgroups. The recording of tenderness has been a widely debated subject but methodological studies now show manual palpation to be an easy and reliable method of studying myofascial pain sensitivity in a clinical setting, providing the intensity of the applied pressure is controlled [39]. Most, but not all, systematic studies of pressure pain threshold (PPT) demonstrate that patients with chronic TTH have increased pain sensitivity due to central sensitization [19, 33, 36, 39, 40]. Nevertheless, neither PPT nor surface EMG recordings from the pericranial muscles provide additional diagnostic information in the clinical setting. Therefore, although the level of evidence is restricted, only manual palpation, preferably as pressure controlled palpation, can be recommended to divide the three subtypes of TTH (infrequent episodic, episodic, and chronic TTH) and no clinical test can yet be recommended for migraine.

Neuroimaging

Radiological examinations are often sought in patients with headache. Most headache sufferers seeking medical attention fear they may have a serious illness and often request a radiological investigation. As radiological examinations are not particularly invasive or uncomfortable, and as they detect any intracranial diseases present, the threshold for requesting them is low. However, when deciding whether or not to use radiological techniques, one should consider the likelihood of detecting underlying diseases in headache patients [41]. In the medical literature, studies that use radiological techniques in populations of headache patients can be divided into three categories. First, studies investigating the aetiology and pathophysiological mechanisms of headache; second, studies focusing on the pathological sequelae of headache; and third, studies on the role of radiological techniques in the work-up of headache patients. As one of the aims of this paper was to provide guidelines on the usefulness of radiological techniques in the evaluation of headache patients with normal neurological examinations, we reviewed a subset of the third category.

The current literature has been reviewed with a view to establishing guidelines for the future use of radiological methods in headache patients [42], and the methods were found to present certain limitations. Although there is a need for further systematic studies on this topic, some conclusions can, nevertheless, be drawn [42].

There is no role for conventional roentgen techniques (skull films) in the work-up of headache patients, as the conditions underlying headache in these subjects are generally located inside the skull and therefore not detectable using these methods. Digital subtraction angiography (DSA) is an invasive procedure associated with a significant morbidity and mortality rate. DSA still seems to be superior to other radiological techniques in detecting intracranial arteriovenous malformations (AVMs) and fistulas. However, it is relatively rare for any of these conditions to underlie the headache and, furthermore, some lesions of this kind are also visible using non-invasive techniques (computerized tomography (CT) and MRI). Therefore, it is not appropriate to use DSA in the screening of headache patients for intracranial disease.

Both CT and MRI can be performed with and without the application of intravenous contrast agents. MRI is more sensitive to the presence of intracranial disease than CT, and the sensitivity of both techniques is increased when they are used in conjunction with intravenous contrast agents.

Detection of the presence of a recent intracranial haemorrhage is straightforward on CT. However, it has been demonstrated that MRI is at least as sensitive as CT in detecting bleeding in the subarachnoid space, if adequate sequences such as fluid attended inversion recovery (FLAIR) are used [43]. Recently, functional MRI (fMRI) of the brain also allowed very interesting studies of brain time perfusion, water molecular diffusion, and cerebral cortical activation. However, these techniques and applications are still in a state of evolution. The extent to which they can be applied in the examination of headache is not yet clear, although they may prove to be helpful in differentiating between ischaemic insult and prolonged migraine aura in select patients during migraine attacks [44].

A large prospective consecutive study by AP Sempere *et al.* [45] included 1,876 patients with non-acute headache. Neuroimaging was performed with MRI or CT. Significant intracranial lesions were found in 22 patients (1.2%). The rate of significant intracranial abnormalities in patients with headache and normal neurological examination was 0.9%. However, the only clinical variable associated with a higher probability of intracranial abnormalities was neurological examination. The authors conclude that the proportion of patients with headache and intracranial lesions was relatively small, but neither neurological examination nor the features in the clinical history provide a basis on which to rule out such abnormalities.

Very recently a population-based MRI study demonstrated that migraine is associated with an increased risk of deep white matter lesions, but further investigations are need to define the long-term functional correlates [46].

The relevance of neuroimaging in trigeminal autonomic cephalalgia (TACs) has been just revised by Wilbrink *et al.* [47] and it was recommended that neuroimaging should be carefully considered in all patients with TACs(-like) syndromes.

SPECT and PET

Single-photon emission computerized tomography (SPECT) and positron emission tomography (PET) are nuclear medicine imaging methods [48], both of which require the administration of radioactive tracers to the patient. SPECT involves the sampling of emitted radiation by means of a gamma camera, with the camera heads or their collimators moving around the subject's head during data acquisition. Because SPECT cameras are versatile, less expensive, and less costly to run than PET cameras, SPECT brain scans are carried out at most large hospitals.

The most commonly performed type of brain SPECT reveals regional cerebral blood flow (rCBF) changes. Following inhalation or intravenous injection of Xe^{133}, it is possible to quantify the rCBF, although at the expense of spatial resolution [49]. Tc^{99m}-labelled rCBF tracers are the ones most frequently used because Tc^{99m} is readily available in all nuclear medical departments. SPECT rCBF investigations can provide information about acute changes in regional perfusion that often arise in relation to the neurological symptoms associated with the aura phase of migraine [6, 50]. SPECT combined with transcranial Doppler (TCD) can, in addition, provide information about changes in diameter of the larger intracranial arteries [51].

Positron emission tomography is a cumbersome and more expensive technique than SPECT. With the exception of F^{18}-labelled tracers ($t_{1/2} = 110 \, min$), most isotopes for PET decay very quickly. Therefore PET requires an in-house cyclotron and online radiochemistry production unit [52]. Positron emitting isotopes, such as C^{11}, O^{15} and F^{18}, are naturally incorporated into biologically active molecules. This has facilitated the synthesis of a large number of radioactive labelled tracers for PET, for example receptor-specific ligands and metabolism markers. However, only a fraction of these are used in clinical scans. As a result of the high cost of establishing and running a PET unit, the availability of PET scans is limited. Most countries in Europe have only a few PET centres, located in university hospitals.

Transcranial Doppler

The Doppler principle is utilized in medicine in the following way: an ultrasound signal is transmitted into the body and the changes in sound frequency that occur when it is reflected or scattered from the moving blood cells are observed. The accuracy of TCD velocity recordings is influenced by the angle of insonation, which in turn is determined by the technique adopted and the local vessel anatomy. Assuming the angle of insonation is constant, velocity (V) is dependent on volume flow (F) through the vessel and on the vessel cross-sectional area (A), according to the formula $F = V \times A$. It will, therefore, be influenced by factors that cause changes in CBF, vessel diameter, or both. Simultaneous TCD and rCBF measurements may contribute to determining vascular changes in headache patients, as each cerebral vessel supplies a defined volume of cerebral tissue [53]. TCD is mainly used to evaluate vascular reactivity in migraine [6].

Recommendations

Electroencephalogram

Routine EEG with intermittent photic stimulation and standard visual interpretation

Interictal EEG is not routinely indicated in the diagnostic evaluation of headache patients. Interictal EEG is only indicated if the clinical history suggests a possible diagnosis of epilepsy, e.g. in the case of: (a) unusually brief headache episodes; (b) unusual aura symptoms (e.g. gastric/olfactory sensations, circular visual symptoms); (c) headache associated with unusually brief auras or aura-like phenomena; (d) headache associated with severe neurological deficits; (e) other risk factors for epilepsy. Ictal EEG is indicated when headache is suspected to be a symptom of an epileptic seizure or an encephalopathy. Ictal EEG is indicated during episodes suggesting complicated aura and during auras associated with decreased consciousness or confusion.

Quantitative EEG methods (frequency analysis with or without topographic mapping)

Spectral bandpower abnormalities have recently been reported before and during headache in migraineurs [54]. The utility of advanced methods based on coherence and neural networks [55] has not yet been independently confirmed. Current QEEG methods are still not routinely indicated in the diagnostic evaluation of headache patients.

QEEG must always be recorded with EEG raw data and interpreted by a skilled physician to avoid misinterpretation of technical artifacts, normal state fluctuations and various physiological rhythms.

Analysis of photic driving

Photic driving amplitude may be increased in migraine and tension headache patient groups as compared to headache-free subjects. The specificity of the method is not yet sufficiently documented.

There is not enough evidence to suggest that the photic driving methods that are currently in use can reliably discriminate either between migraine and non-migraine primary headache patients or between primary headache patients and headache-free subjects.

Evoked potentials

The literature data, often conflicting, failed to demonstrate the usefulness of EPs as a diagnostic tool in migraine. Findings should therefore be replicated before visually evoked potentials (VEPs) can be recommended in the diagnosis of migraine (not enough data are available for other types of headache). In conclusion, we do not recommend the use of EPs in the diagnosis of headache disorders.

This is a Class II level of evidence, but the literature contains contrasting data and the clinical significance of abnormalities is poorly understood. The grade of recommendation is B.

Reflex responses

Most of the reflex response investigations have only limited usefulness in the diagnosis of headache. Further research in large populations is needed to establish which electrophysiological markers could be relevant in clinical practice.

This is a Class IV level of evidence for nociceptive flexion reflex (not blinded studies), and Class III for corneal reflex and blink reflex. The grade of recommendation is C for corneal and blink reflex. As for exteroceptive suppression of masticatory muscle activity, only a few blinded studies (Class III) fail to confirm previous investigations. The grade of recommendation is C.

Autonomic tests

Studies of autonomic functions in migraine and cluster headache were mostly focused on autonomic systems innervating specific target organs which, anatomically and functionally, are not necessarily related to the supposed autonomic origin of the pain. Autonomic parameters are confounded by effector organ response characteristics.

Therefore, there is no clear evidence justifying the recommendation of autonomic tests for the routine clinical examination of headache patients (Class IV, Level C).

Clinical tests in headache

Tenderness recorded by manual palpation is the most specific and sensitive test in patients with tension-type headache, and can therefore be recommended as a routine clinical test in contrast to EMG and pressure pain thresholds. This manual

palpation is, however, non-specific and cannot be used to discriminate between different co-existing primary or secondary headaches. In migraine, no clinical test can, yet, be recommended (Class II, Level B).

Neuroimaging

1 In adult and paediatric patients with migraine, with no recent change in pattern, no history of seizures, and no other focal neurological signs or symptoms, the routine use of neuroimaging is not warranted.

2 In patients with atypical headache patterns, a history of seizures, neurological signs or symptoms, or symptomatic illness such as tumours, acquired immunodeficiency syndrome (AIDS) and neurofibromatosis, MRI may be indicated (to be carefully evaluated in each case).

When neuroimaging is warranted, the most sensitive method should be used, and we recommend MRI and not CT in these cases.

This is a class III recommendation, as most studies are non-analytical and although there exist a few randomized clinical trials, some of them are not directly relevant to these recommendations (the grade of recommendation is B).

SPECT and PET

If attacks can be fully accounted for by the standard headache classification (IHS), a PET or SPECT scan will generally be of no further diagnostic value.

Nuclear medicine examinations of cerebral circulation and metabolism can be carried out in subgroups of headache patients for diagnosis and evaluation of complications. rCBF can be of particular value in patients in whom the standard classification (IHS) cannot be fully applied, when patients experience unusually severe attacks, or the quality or severity of attacks has changed. In such situations rCBF recordings should be carried out both during an attack (if possible several repeated scans) and interictally (at a time interval of >5 days after an attack). Quantifiable rCBF measurements are preferable to distribution images.

This is a Class IV level of evidence, that is most studies are case reports or case series. There is insufficient evidence to make specific recommendations.

Transcranial Doppler

Transcranial Doppler examination is not helpful in headache diagnosis. It is, however, a non-invasive examination with an excellent temporal resolution that is useful for studying the vascular aspects of the headache pathophysiology and the vascular effects of anti-headache medication. The information obtained using this method is easier to interpret if side-to-side comparisons are made or if it is combined with rCBF measurements (This is a class IV level of evidence and the grade of recommendation is C).

Appendix

Neurophysiological tests and genetics

Emerging evidence increasingly supports the notion that a predisposition to the common migraine phenotypes is transmitted from parent to offspring. Studies analysing the familial distribution of migraine suggest a complex mode of inheritance, probably because genetic effects (susceptibility genes) and environmental factors are interrelated.

Migraine is a recurrent disorder in which genetic influences not only determine a critical biological threshold to migraine attack, but may also disturb sensory information processing in the central nervous system (CNS) during the interictal period. The subtle subclinical signs related to disturbed CNS sensory processing may be useful biological markers for identifying persons genetically predisposed to migraine disorder.

Neurophysiological studies in patients with migraine typically disclose high-intensity dependence of auditory potentials (IDAPs) and reduced habituation to all cortical sensory evoked potentials. During the past decade researchers have therefore investigated whether these abnormalities in sensory information processing have a migraine-specific familial prevalence and, whether they can be considered as endophenotypic markers for presymptomatic migraine.

Investigating IDAP slopes and visual evoked potential (VEP) habituation in pairs of migraineur parents and their offspring, Sándor et al. [56] observed that children tended to have more abnormal auditory and VEP values than parents. In a later study, Siniatchkin et al. [57] observed that children suffering from migraine have steeper IDAP slopes than age-matched healthy subjects and also steeper slopes than adult migraineurs. The same authors [58] later observed a considerable familial component in the amplitude and habituation of early-wave contingent negative variation (iCNV) in migraine. For example, they found strong iCNV amplitude and habituation correlations between children with migraine and their parents with migraine, and between young migraineurs and their healthy parents who have a family history of migraine. The same investigators subsequently found no iCNV habituation in asymptomatic subjects with a family history of migraine, defined as 'at risk', and the iCNV amplitude correlated significantly with the number of migraine sufferers among first- and second-

degree relatives [59]. Others studying a group of healthy asymptomatic subjects having a first-degree relative affected by migraine reported a similar habituation deficit also in the nociceptive blink reflex [60].

Collectively, these findings strongly suggest a link between the underlying genetic load and the interictal abnormal sensory information processing in migraineurs. Hence, in subjects with a familial predisposition to migraine, abnormal evoked cortical potential amplitudes and habituation may be neurophysiological markers indicating presymptomatic migraine.

Implementation of the first edition of EFNS guidelines on the use of neurophysiological tests in non-acute headache patients

In a recently published paper [61], a cohort of 150 Italian headache specialists, neurologists, and general practitioners (GPs) were surveyed, with the following aims: (a) to investigate the diffusion, use, and perception of usefulness of the EFNS guidelines on the use of neurophysiological tests in non-acute headache patients [2]; (b) to survey the frequency of recommendation of the different neurophysiological tests in non-acute migraine patients by guideline-aware and unaware headache specialists, neurologists, and general practitioners; (c) to evaluate the motivation for recommending neurophysiological tests and to verify their appropriateness and concordance with EFNS guidelines; and (d) to survey the perception of usefulness of neurophysiological testing in the differential diagnosis of migraine.

The results obtained in this study are used here as the basis of an optimisation process that aims to improve the dissemination, production, and implementation of the above-mentioned guidelines.

The most important findings may be summarized as follows.

(a) At least in Italy, the level of diffusion of the EFNS guidelines and recommendations on neurophysiological tests is variable, being optimal among headache specialists and very limited among neurologists (the real target of the guidelines) and GPs. These data suggest that there is a need to improve the strategy for the diffusion of the EFNS guidelines on neurophysiological tests in headache among non-headache specialists.

(b) The great majority of guideline-aware physicians commented positively on the EFNS guidelines and said they used them in their everyday clinical practice. Specifically, they considered EFNS guidelines on neurophysiological testing to be easy to apply, useful, effective in improving the appropriateness of recommending neurophysiological tests, and without weak points. All the guideline-unaware physicians declared an interest in knowing the guidelines. This possibly reflects the good quality (clarity of the message, strong evidence-based support) and utility of the guideline document.

(c) Guideline-aware physicians (headache specialists) were found to recommend neurophysiological tests to migraine patients less frequently and more appropriately than guideline-unaware physicians. The majority of guideline-aware physicians had a correct perception (i.e. in accordance with the EFNS guidelines) of the usefulness of neurophysiological tests for diagnosing migraine. These data suggest that application of the EFNS guidelines could lead to more rational use of neurophysiological tests in the diagnostic work-up of migraine patients. Alternatively, it could be that the suggestions contained in the EFNS guidelines reflect what is already the usual practice of headache specialists. Prospective randomized controlled trials are needed before definitive conclusions can be drawn about the effectiveness of the guidelines in producing changes in physicians' behaviour.

(d) The most important deviation from EFNS guidelines observed in the guideline-conscious physicians concerned the recommendation of transcranial Doppler (TCD), which was frequent and often inappropriate (TCD was recommended for the differential diagnosis with secondary headaches or for deciding about the necessity of recommending a neuroimaging exam). EFNS guidelines should be more explicit in establishing that neurophysiological tests are not helpful in discriminating between migraine and secondary headaches, or migraine and primary headaches, are not useful to confirm the diagnosis of migraine and for orienting toward an appropriate recommendation of a neuroimaging procedure.

Conflicts of interest

The authors have no conflicts of interest to declare in connection with this work.

Acknowledgements

We wish to thank Ms Catherine Wrenn for the linguistic revision of the manuscript.

This is a Continuing Medical Education paper and can be found with corresponding questions on the internet at: http://www.blackwellpublishing.com/products/journals/ene/mcqs. Certificates for correctly answering the questions will be issued by the EFNS.

References

1. Headache Classification Committee of the International Headache Society. Classification and diagnostic criteria for headache disorders, cranial neuralgias and facial pain. *Cephalalgia* 2004;**24**(Suppl. 1):1–160.
2. Sandrini G, Friberg L, Janig W, *et al.* Neurophysiological tests and neuroimaging procedures in non-acute headache: guidelines and recommendations. *Eur J Neurol* 2004;**11**:217–24.
3. Silberstein SD. Practice parameter: evidence-based guidelines for migraine headache (an evidence-based review): report of the Quality Standards Subcommittee of the American Academy of Neurology. [Erratum appears in *Neurology* **56**(1):142]. *Neurology* 2000;**55**:754–62.
4. Lewis DW, Ashwal S, Dahl G, *et al.* Practice parameter. Evaluation of children and adolescents with recurrent headaches: report of the Quality Standards Subcommittee of the American Academy of Neurology and the Practice Committee of the Child Neurology Society. *Neurology* 2002;**59**:490–8.
5. Evans RW. Diagnostic testing for migraine and other primary headaches. *Neurol Clin* 2009;**27**(2):393–415.
6. Friberg L, Sandrini G, Jänig W, *et al.* Instrumental investigations in primary headache. An updated review and new perspectives. *Funct Neurol* 2003;**8**:27–44.
7. Headache Classification Committee of the International Headache Society. (Olesen J *et al.*).Classification and Diagnostic criteria for headache disorders, cranial neuralgias and facial pain. *Cephalalgia* 1988;**8**(Suppl. 7):1–96.
8. Hughes RAC, Barnes MP, Baron JC, Brainin M. Guidance for the preparation of neurological management guidelines by EFNS scientific task forces. *Eur J Neurol* 2001;**8**:549–50.
9. Brainin M, Barnes M, Baron J-C, *et al.* Guidance for the preparation of neurological management guidelines by EFNS scientific task forces. *Eur J Neurol* 2004;**1**:577–81.
10. Sand T. EEG in migraine: a review of the literature. *Funct Neurol* 1991;**6**:722.
11. Sand T. Electroencephalography in migraine: a review with focus on quantitative electroencephalography and the migraine vs. epilepsy relationship. *Cephalalgia* 2003;**23**(Suppl. 1):5–11.

12. Rosenberg J, Alter M, Byrne TD, *et al.* Practice parameter: the electroencephalogram in the evaluation of headache. Report of the Quality Standards Subcommittee of the American Academy of Neurology. *Neurology* 1995;**45**: 1411–3.

13. Walczak T, Jayakar P. Interictal EEG in epilepsy. In: Engel J, Pedley T (eds) *A Comprehensive Textbook.* Philadelphia, New York: Lippincott Raven, 1998; pp. 831–48.

14. Nuwer M. Assessment of digital EEG, quantitative EEG and EEG brain mapping. Report of the American Academy of Neurology and the American Clinical Neurophysiology Society. *Neurology* 1997;**49**:277–92.

15. Ambrosini A, Maertens de Noordhout A, Sandor P, Schoenen J. Electrophysiological studies in migraine: a comprehensive review of their interest and limitations. *Cephalalgia* 2003;**23**(Suppl. 1):13–31.

16. Sandrini G, Friberg L, Schoenen J, Nappi G. Exploring pathophysiology of headache. *Cephalalgia* 2003;**23**(Suppl. 1):152.

17. Sandrini G, Alfonsi E, Ruiz L, *et al.* Impairment of corneal pain perception in cluster headache. *Pain* 1991;**3**:299–304.

18. Sandrini G, Arrigo A, Bono G, Nappi G. The nociceptive flexion reflex as a tool for exploring pain control systems in headache and other pain syndromes. *Cephalalgia* 1993;**13**: 21–7.

19. Sandrini G, Proietti Cecchini A, Milanov I, Tassorelli C, Buzzi MG, Nappi G. Electrophysiological evidence for trigeminal neuron sensitization in patients with migraine. *Neurosci Lett* 2002;**317**:135–8.

20. Schoenen J, Bendtsen L. Neurophysiology of tension-type headache. In: Olesen J, Tfelt-Hansen P, Welch KMA (eds) *The Headaches*, 2nd edn. Philadelphia, PA: Lippincott Williams & Wilkins, 2000; pp. 463–70.

21. Di Clemente L, Coppola G, Magis D, et al. Nitroglycerin sensitises in healthy subjects CNS structures involved in migraine pathophysiology: evidence from a study of nociceptive blink reflexes and visual evoked potentials. *Pain* 2009;**144**(1–2):156–61.

22. Obermann M, Yoon MS, Ese D, *et al.* Impaired trigeminal nociceptive processing in patients with trigeminal neuralgia. *Neurology* 2007;**28**(69)(9):835–41.

23. Sandrini G, Rossi P, Milanov I, Serrao M, Cecchini AP, Nappi G. Abnormal modulatory influence of diffuse noxious inhibitory controls in migraine and chronic tension-type headache patients. *Cephalalgia* 2006;**26**(7):782–9.

24. Perrotta A, Serrao M, Sandrini G, et al. Sensitisation of spinal cord pain processing in medication overuse headache involves supraspinal pain control. *Cephalalgia* 2009;**30**(2): 272–284.

25. Jänig W, McLachlan EM. Neurobiology of the autonomic nervous system. In: Bannister R, Mathias CJ (eds) *Auto-* *nomic Failure*, 4th edn. Oxford: Oxford University Press, 2002; pp. 3–15.

26. Jänig W. *The Integrative Action of the Autonomic Nervous System. Neurobiology of Homeostasis.* Cambridge New York: Cambridge University Press, 2006.

27. Jänig W. Autonomic nervous system and pain. In: Bushnell MC, Basbaum AI (eds) *The Senses: A Comprehensive Reference* (ed. by Basbaum AI, Kaneko A, Shepherd GM, Westheimer G). Vol. **5**, San Diego: Pain. Academic Press, 2008; pp. 193–226.

28. Jänig W. Relationship between pain and autonomic phenomena in headache and other pain syndromes. *Cephalalgia* 2003;**23**(Suppl. 1):43–8.

29. Jänig W, Baron R. Complex regional pain syndrome: mystery explained? *Lancet Neurol* 2003;**2**:687–97.

30. Jänig W, Baron R. Complex regional pain syndrome is a disease of the central nervous system. *Clin Auton Res* 2002;**12**:150–64.

31. Mathias CJ, Bannister R. Investigation of autonomic disorders. In: Bannister R, Mathias CJ (eds) *Autonomic Failure*, 4th edn. Oxford: Oxford University Press, 1999; pp. 232–44.

32. Goadsby PJ. Primary neurovascular headache. In: McMahon SB, Koltzenburg M (eds) *Wall and Melzack's Textbook of Pain*, 5th edn. Edinburgh: Elsevier Churchill Livingstone, 2006; pp. 851–74.

33. Bendtsen L. Sensitization: its role in primary headache. *Curr Opin Investig Drugs* 2002;**3**:449–53.

34. Burstein R, Cutrer MF, Yarnitsky D. The development of cutaneous allodynia during a migraine attack clinical evidence for the sequential recruitment of spinal and supraspinal nociceptive neurons in migraine. *Brain* 2000;**123**: 1703–9.

35. Burstein R, Yarnitsky D, Goor-Aryeh I, Ransil BJ, Bajwa ZH. An association between migraine and cutaneous allodynia. *Ann Neurol* 2000;**47**:614–24.

36. Buchgreitz L, Egsgaard LL, Jensen R, Arendt-Nielsen L, Bendtsen L. Abnormal pain processing in chronic tension-type headache: a high-density EEG brain mapping study. *Brain* 2008;**131**:3232–8.

37. Schoenen J, Gerard P, de Pasqua V, Sianard-Gainko J. Multiple clinical and paraclinical analyses of chronic tension-type headache associated or unassociated with disorder of pericranial muscles. *Cephalalgia* 1991;**11**:135–9.

38. Jensen R, Rasmussen BK. Muscular disorders in tension-type headache. *Cephalalgia* 1996;**16**:97–103.

39. Bendtsen L, Jensen R, Jensen NK, Olesen J. Pressure-controlled palpation: a new technique which increases the reliability of manual palpation. *Cephalalgia* 1995;**15**:205–10.

40. Lindelof K, Ellrich J, Jensen R, Bendtsen L. Central pain processing in chronic tension-type headache. Clinical Neurophysiology. *Clin Neurophysiol* 2009;**120**(7):1364–70.

41. Mitchell CS, Osborn RE, Grosskreutz SR. Computed tomography in the headache patient: is routine evaluation really necessary? *Headache* 1993;**33**:82–6.

42. Frishberg BM. The utility of neuroimaging in the evaluation of headache in patients with normal neurological examinations. *Neurology* 1994;**44**:1191–7.

43. Noguchi K, Ogawa T, Seto H, *et al.* Subacute and chronic subarachnoid hemorrhage: diagnosis with fluid-attenuated inversion-recovery MR imaging. *Radiology* 1997;**203**:257–62.

44. Ay H, Buonanno FS, Rordorf G, *et al.* Normal diffusion-weighted MRI during stroke-like deficits. *Neurology* 1999;**52**:1784–92.

45. Sempere Ap, Porta-Etessam J, Medrano V, et al. Neuroimaging in the evaluation of patients with non-acute headache. *Cephalalgia* 2004;**25**:30–5.

46. Kruit M, van Buchem M, Launer L, Terwindt G, Ferrari M. Migraine is associated with an increased risk of deep white matter lesions, subclinical posterior circulation infarcts and brain iron accumulation: the population-based MRI CAMERA study. *Cephalalgia* 2009;**30**(2):129–36.

47. Wilbrink LA, Ferrari MD, Kruit MC, Haan J. Neuroimaging in trigeminal autonomic cephalgias: when, how, and of what? *Curr Opin Neuro* 2009;**22**(3):247–53.

48. De Deyn PP, Nagels G, Pickut BA, *et al.* SPECT in neurology and psychiatry. In: De Deyn PP, Dierckx RA, Alavi A, Pickut BA (eds) *SPECT in Headache with Special Reference to Migraine*, 1st edn. Vol. **54**, London: John Libbey & Co., 1997; pp. 455–66.

49. Croft BY. Instrumentation and computers for brain single photon emission computed tomography. *J Nucl Med* 1990;**20**:281–9.

50. Friberg L. Migraine pathophysiology and its relation to cerebral hemodynamic changes. In: Edvinsson L (ed.) *Migraine and Headache Pathophysiology*. London: Martin Dunitz, 1999; pp. 133–40.

51. Friberg L, Olesen J, Iversen HK, Sperling B. Migraine pain associated with middle cerebral artery dilatation: reversal by sumatripan. *Lancet* 1991;**338**:13–7.

52. Saha GB, MacIntyre WJ, Go RT. Cyclotrons and positron emission tomography radiopharmaceuticals for clinical imaging. *Semin Nucl Med* 1992;**22**:150–61.

53. Dahl A, Russell D, Nyberg-Hansen R, Rootwelt K. Cluster headache: transcranial Doppler ultrasound and rCBF studies. *Cephalalgia* 1990;**10**:87–94.

54. Bjørk M, Sand T. Quantitative EEG power and asymmetry increase 36 h before a migraine attack. *Cephalalgia* 2008; **28**(9):960–8.

55. Bellotti R, De Carlo F, de Tommaso M, Lucente M. Migraine detection through spontaneous EEG analysis. *Conf Proc IEEE Eng Med Biol Soc* 2007;**29**:1834–7.

56. Sándor PS, Afra J, Proietti-Cecchini A, Albert A, Schoenen J. Familial influences on cortical evoked potentials in migraine. *Neuroreport* 1999;**10**:1235–8.

57. Siniatchkin M, Kropp P, Neumann M, Gerber WD, Stephani U. Intensity dependence of auditory evoked cortical potentials in migraine families. *Pain* 2000;**85**:247–54.

58. Siniatchkin M, Kirsch E, Kropp P, Stephani U, Gerber WD. Slow cortical potentials in migraine families. *Cephalalgia* 2000;**20**:881–92.

59. Siniatchkin M, Kropp P, Gerber WD. Contingent negative variation in subjects at risk for migraine without aura. *Pain* 2001;**94**(2):159–67.

60. Di Clemente L, Coppola G, Magis D, *et al.* Interictal habituation deficit of the nociceptive blink reflex: an endophenotypic marker for presymptomatic migraine? *Brain* 2007;**130**: 765–70.

61. Rossi P, Schoenen J, Bolla M, Tassorelli C, Sandrini G, Nappi G. Implementation and evaluation of existing guidelines on the use of neurophysiological tests in non-acute migraine patients: a questionnaire survey of neurologists and primary care physicians. *Eur J Neurol* 2009;**16**: 937–42.

CHAPTER 5

Use of anti-interferon beta antibody measurements in multiple sclerosis

P. Soelberg Sørensen,[1] F. Deisenhammer,[2] P. Duda,[3] R. Hohlfeld,[4] K.-M. Myhr,[5] J. Palace,[6] C. Polman,[7] C. Pozzilli,[8] C. Ross[9]

[1]Copenhagen Danish Multiple Sclerosis Research Center, Copenhagen University Hospital, Rigshospitalet, Denmark; [2]University of Innsbruck, Austria; [3]University Hospitals, Basel, Switzerland; [4]Institute for Clinical Neuroimmunology, University of Munich, Klinikum Grosshadern, Germany; [5]Haukeland University Hospital, Bergen, Norway; [6]Multiple Sclerosis Group, Radcliffe Infirmary, Oxford, UK; [7]VU University Medical Center, Amsterdam, The Netherlands; [8]II Faculty of Medicine, University 'La Sapienza', Rome, Italy; [9]Institute for Inflammation Research, Copenhagen University Hospital, Rigshospitalet, Denmark

Background and objectives

Interferon (IFN)β is a first-line therapy for relapsing–remitting multiple sclerosis (MS). In recent years, several publications have concordantly reported that binding antibodies (BABs) and neutralizing antibodies (NABs) occur during treatment with recombinant IFNβ products. The frequencies and titres of anti-IFNβ antibodies vary considerably depending on the IFNβ preparation, the frequency and route of administration, and the type of assay being used. There is no generally accepted standardized assay for measuring BABs and NABs. Clinical studies in patients with MS have demonstrated that when NABs to IFNβ develop, the therapeutic benefits of IFNβ are reduced or abolished.

The objectives of our task force were to: (i) evaluate differences in immunogenicity of IFNβ products; (ii) evaluate the reliability and give recommendations on BABs and NABs assays; (iii) evaluate the impact of NABs on clinical efficacy and give recommendations on the clinical use of measurement of IFNβ antibodies; and (iv) review the evidence on prevention of NAB development and the management of patients with NABs.

European Handbook of Neurological Management: Volume 1, 2nd edition. Edited by N. E. Gilhus, M. P. Barnes and M. Brainin.
© 2011 Blackwell Publishing Ltd.

Search strategy and consensus

The task force systematically searched the MEDLINE database for available information published in English up to September 2004. Key words included: interferon beta, multiple sclerosis, immunogenicity, antibodies, binding antibody assays, and NAB assays. Articles related to this topic from the authors' personal literature databases were also included. For each specific issue at least one member of the task force assessed all published papers and omitted those that did not fulfil given criteria, and read and rated the remaining articles according to the guidance for preparation of neurological management guidelines by EFNS scientific task force's revised recommendations 2004 [1]. Each paragraph of the guidelines was drafted by one member of the task force and circulated to the other members. After appropriate revision the guidelines were finalized and consensus was reached among all task force members at a meeting.

Immunogenicity

It is entirely predictable that patients treated with long-term recombinant IFNβ produce antibodies against the product. This observation follows in the wake of other biological products troubled by the production of antibodies, including IFN-α, erythropoietin, factor VIII, and human insulin. Understandably, the closer a product is to the species' natural antigen the less likely it is to provoke antibodies.

Immunogenicity of IFNβ products

The three commercially available IFNβ products vary substantially in their immunogenicity. The first licensed product, FNβ-1b, is produced from *Escherichia. coli* and it differs from the natural human product by methionine-1 deletion, cysteine-17 to serine mutation, and lack of glycosylation. There is about a tenfold increase in the weight of protein present in a single IFNβ-1b dose compared to the IFNβ-1a versions to reach a suitable specific activity level. This is likely to lead to increased aggregation [2], which may enhance its antigenicity. IFNβ-1a in contrast is identical in primary and secondary structure to the native form and is produced in mammalian cells – a system associated with fewer host cell contaminants. The proportion of patients reported to have neutralizing antibodies range from 2% to greater than 40% and table 5.1 summarizes the data from the initial pivotal relapsing–remitting and secondary progressive placebo controlled trials. The immunogenicity of Avonex after the initial studies was profoundly reduced for reasons that either are not clear or confidential, but it is possible that the tendency for aggregation was reduced.

Dynamics of NABs

The majority of patients destined to become NAB-positive do so within 6–18 months of treatment. Patients on IFNβ-1b tend to become positive earlier than those on IFNβ-1a. However, the percentage becoming positive on IFNβ-1a (Rebif) has been reported to catch up in frequency [10, 11]. It is likely that tolerance may occur over the long term during continued IFNβ therapy [12, 13]. For NAB-positive patients, the probability of reverting to NAB-negative status was significantly higher in patients treated with IFNβ-1b than in patients treated with IFNβ-1a (Rebif) when followed over 36–48 months [13, 14]. Thus it seems that tolerance is an earlier feature with the IFNβ-1b formulation than with the IFNβ-1a formulation. Antibody titre appears to be predictive, with lower NAB titres more likely to revert to a NAB-negative state [12, 14].

Influence of dosage and route of administration

It is difficult to separate the relative influence of: (i) dosage frequency; (ii) total weekly dosage; and (iii) method of administration from the present available evidence.

Intramuscular administration (im) of IFNβ-1b once weekly at 250 μg delayed the appearance and reduced the levels of BABs detected by ELISA when compared to the standard regime [15]. However, NABs were present in 41% of patients treated with repeated im IFNβ-1b and 38% of those treated by the subcutaneous route [3, 16]. IFNβ-1a (Rebif) 22 μg administered subcutaneously (sc) once weekly was significantly less immunogenic than three times weekly [10]. However, IFNβ-1a (Rebif) 22 μg im once or twice weekly was not obviously different to

Table 5.1 Frequency of NAB-positive patients in initial pivotal placebo-controlled trials

Study	IFN-β product and dosage	Frequency of NAB-positive patients (%)
The IFNB Multiple Sclerosis Study Group (1993)	IFN-β-1b (Betaferon) 250 μg b.i.d.	42
European Study Group on interferon beta-1b in secondary progressive MS (1998)	IFN-β-1b (Betaferon) 250 μg b.i.d.	28
Jacobs *et al.* (1996)	IFN-β-1a (Avonex) 30 μg weekly	22
PRISMS Study Group (1998)	IFN-β-1a (Rebif) 22 μg thrice weekly	24
PRISMS Study Group (1998)	IFN-β-1a (Rebif) 44 μg thrice weekly	13
SPECTRIMS Study Group (2001)	IFN-β-1a (Rebif) 22 μg thrice weekly	21
SPECTRIMS Study Group (2001)	IFN-β-1a (Rebif) 44 μg thrice weekly	15
Clanet *et al.* (2002)	IFN-beta 1a (Avonex) 60 μg weekly	3.3
The North Amercian Study Group on Interferon beta-1b in Secondary Progressive MS (2004)	IFN-beta 1b 250 μg b.i.d.	23
The North American Study Group on Interferon beta-1b in Secondary Progressive MS (2004)	IFN-beta 1b 160 μg/m² b.i.d.	33

conventional treatment [15, 17]. No effect on antibody frequency was seen with two different doses of IFNβ-1b (1.6 and 8 MIU). An increase in NAB frequency was seen with an increased dose of Avonex [8]. However, the higher dose of IFNβ-1a (Rebif 44 μg) was associated with a lower proportion of patients developing NABs than the lower dose (22 μg) in the pivotal relapsing–remitting and secondary progressive studies (see table 5.1). The presence of a drug in the serum tested could reduce the sensitivity of the assay leading to an apparent but false reduction in antibody positive rates [10, 18]. Oddly, this Rebif dose effect was not noted in those 2-year placebo patients who were subsequently randomized to either IFNβ-1a (Rebif) 22 or 44 μg, or in the EVIDENCE study where IFNβ-1a (Rebif) 44 μg three times weekly was associated with a high rate of NAB-positive patients (>20%) [19]. Thus doubt exists as to whether Rebif 44 μg really does stimulate less antibody production than 22 μg three times weekly.

Evidence regarding immmunogenicity

Overall, the immunogenicity of the recombinant IFNβ appears to be most influenced by the formulation itself, although increasing the frequency of injections also appears to be important. The influence of the intramuscular versus the subcutaneous route appears minimal. The effect of different doses is less clear. There is general agreement that the IFNβ-1a (Avonex) is the least immunogenic. There is Class I evidence that the majority of patients with two consecutive NAB-positive tests remain NAB-positive for more than 2 years, although a substantial number of patients who become NAB-positive may revert to NAB-negative status during continuous IFNβ-1b therapy.

Measurements of binding and neutralizing antibodies

Binding antibodies

A Pub-Med search using 'binding antibodies assay interferon beta' found that 21 of the 55 articles were relevant for detection of BABs with IFNβ treatment.

Although BABs against IFNβ are induced in a majority of such treated patients, only a subset develop NABs causing loss of bioactivity. As the method of NAB detection is cumbersome, many laboratories use a simpler

binding assay for screening purposes and only BAB-positive samples are further analysed by the NAB assay. The different assays can be divided into three basic methods: ELISA, Western Blotting (WB), and radio-immunoprecipitation (RIPA) or affinity chromatography (ACA) assays (table 5.2).

ELISA methods

The ELISA methods most commonly used are direct binding (i.e. direct coating of test wells with IFNβ) assays or capture (i.e. coating of test wells with a capture anti-IFNβ antibody) assays. ELISA titres generally correlated only weakly with NAB titres, but BAB-negative samples measured by ELISA reliably predict NAB-negativity. Only one study compared different BAB assays and demonstrated that cELISA is superior to dELISA with respect to specificity for NABs and the correlation between the BAB and NAB titre.

Western blot

This method gave similar results to the ELISA and had a low false-negative rate when screening for NAB positivity. BAB titres cannot be calculated using WB.

Affinity chromatography and radio-immunoprecipitation assay

The advantage of affinity chromatography assay (ACA) and radio-immunoprecipitation assay (RIPA) is that the antigen is in solution and, therefore, no epitopes are obscured by binding to a solid phase. Radioactive isotopes usage limits the use of these assays. Affinity chromatography was very sensitive, with up to 97% of treated patients being BAB-positive depending on the IFNβ preparation and time on treatment. In the RIPA, no NAB-positive sample was negative and there was a moderate correlation with the NAB titre. RIPA state correlated better with MRI lesion burden change than NAB titres (table 5.2).

Conclusion and recommendations

There are no existing recommendations on BAB assays. There is Class 1 evidence that IFNβ BAB assays have a very high sensitivity and specificity, and can be used reliably for IFNβ antibody screening before performing a NAB assay (Level A recommendation). Different BAB assays should be evaluated and compared using a large number of serum samples to identify the method with

Table 5.2 Methods used for BAB detection: the ELISA method, the Western Blot (WB) method, and the radio-immunoprecipitation (RIPA) or affinity chromatography (ACA) assays.

Method	Type* and concentration of IFN	Validation/cut-off	Reference
dELISA	IFNβ-1a or 1b/0.2 μg	Mean + 3x SD of normal	[20]
ELISA	IFNβ-1b/concentration not given	NAB (MxA induction)	[21]
dELISA, cELISA	IFNβ-1a and 1b/1.5 μg/ml	NAB assay	[22]
dELISA	IFNβ-1a/1b/human IFNβ	Mean + 3x SD of normal	[23]
dELISA	IFNβ-1b/1000 IU per ml	NAB assay	[24]
dELISA	IFNβ/1 μg/ml	2x background of uncoated wells	[25]
dELISA	IFNβ-1a/1 μg/ml	Mean + 3x SD of baseline sera	[26]
	IFNβ/1.2 μg/ml		
dELISA	IFNβ-1a/1 μg/ml	3x OD of background	[27]
dELISA	IFNβ-1a and 1b/1 μg/ml	Arbitrary (OD > 0.5)	[28]
Affinity chromatography	Radio-labelled IFNβ-1a/3000 cpm	Mean + 3x SD of controls	[10]
cELISA	IFNβ-1a and 1b/10₄U/ml	Standard curve†	[29]
dELISA	IFNβ-1a and 1b/1–312ng per well	Mean + 2x SD of controls	[30]
WB, dELISA	IFNβ-1b/5000 IU/well (ELISA)	NAB assay/detection limit of WB	[31]
	IFNβ-1b/2.5 μg per gel		
dELISA	IFNβ-1b/2 μg/ml	Control placebo samples/39 binding units	[32]
dELISA	IFNβ-1a and 1b/1000 IU per ml	Mean of control + 2x SD	[33]
dELISA	IFNβ-1b/1 μg/ml	Mean of control + 3x SD	[34]
RIPA	Radio-labelled IFNβ-1a and 1b/10 μg	NAB assay/mean of control + 3x SD	[35]
			[36]

dELISA: direct enzyme-linked immunosorbent assay; cELISA: capture ELISA; WB: western blot; RIPA: radio-immunoprecipitation assay. *This column refers to the antigen used in the assay. IFNβ-1a is a recombinant human glycosylated IFNβ preparation whereas IFNβ-1b is not glycosylated. †For the standard curve an internal positive control was used which in turn was compared to a WHO reference antibody (G038-501-572).

the best sensitivity and specificity for NAB detection (Level B recommendation).

Neutralizing antibodies

PubMed was searched using the terms 'neutralizing antibodies interferon beta assay'. Thirty-four of 54 articles covered methods of NAB detection and were included. About 50% of patients who develop BABs also develop NABs. There is no standardized assay for NAB detection and, although the principle of NAB measurement is more or less unique, the materials used vary immensely between different laboratories.

Test systems

Almost all reported NAB assays used cultured cell lines responsive to IFNβ. Test samples are incubated with IFNβ prior to addition of the cells. If the test samples

contain NABs, receptor activation is blocked and antiviral proteins will not be induced.

In most cases, one of two different methods are used: either to measure the antiviral effect of IFNβ by challenging the cells with viruses, i.e. the CPE, or to measure IFNβ-induced gene products, namely the MxA protein (a specific marker of Class 1 IFNs), i.e. the MxA induction assay. The assays vary with respect to several variables including the cell line, the virus, the IFNβ preparations and dosage, the incubation times, and the methods of MxA detection (table 5.3).

A few alternative methods have been reported. Measurement of IFNβ bioactivity showed that NAB-positive patients had significantly lower levels of in vivo IFNβ-inducible genes at the mRNA and protein level. Although the different markers were not compared to each other directly, MxA mRNA appears to be the most sensitive

Table 5.3 Overview of assays for NAB detection showing cell lines, viruses, IFNβ preparations and doses, incubation times, and methods of MxA detection.

Type of assay (read-out)	Cells/Virus	IFNβ type/ concentration	Titre calculation/Cut-off for NAB positivity	Validation/QC	Reference
MxA protein	Human whole blood	Betaferon/1000IU/ml	MxA increase < 22.5 ng/ml	NAB assay [32] Standard curve with rMxA	[37]
MxA RNA	Human PBMC	Avonex, Betaferon, Rebif, therapeutic dose	MxA RNA < 132 fg/ pgGAPDH	CPE assay [39]	[38]
MxA protein (Meditest)	Human lung carcinoma cells (A549)	Betaferon 10IU	>20 neutralizing units	CPE assay [32]	[40]
CPE	A549/EMCV	rIFNβ1a and 1b/10LU	Kawade titre > 80	Internal positive and negative controls	[26]
CPE/MxA protein by FACS	WISH/VSV PBMC	IFNβ-1a/10 experimental units	Titre > 20 for bioassay MxA protein < 2 × mean of baseline	Not stated	[27]
CPE	A549/EMCV	IFN type?/3,10,100LU	% reduction of IFN activity		[10]
CPE	A549/EMCV	Avonex, Betaferon, Rebif/10IU/ml	Kawade titre > 20	Internal positive and negative controls	[39]
CPE	A549/EMCV	IFNβ-1a	Kawade/50% CPE		[41]
CPE	WISH/VSV	IFNβ-1b/100IU/ml	Kawade titre > 20	Reference ab G038-501-572	[29]
CPE	Sindbis virus	IFNβ-1a and 1b/20U/ml	Kawade/10LU	Not stated	[30]
CPE	FL-cells/Sindbis virus	IFNβ?/10U/ml	6 × serum dilution of EC50	Not stated	[42]
MxA protein	A549	IFNβ-1b (Betaser) 10LU	Kawade > 20	CPE assay using EMCV	[32]
CPE	Human fibroblasts/VSV	IFNβ1-a and 1-b/100U/ml	50% of CPE	Not stated	[33]
CPE	A549/EMCV	IFNβ-1a/10IU	Kawade, different cut-off values compared to neopterin as bioactivity marker	Internal positive and negative controls	[43]
CPE	WISH/VSV	IFNβ-1a/10EU/ml	Kawade/titre > 4	Controlled for cell survival	[44]
CPE	FS-4 fibroblasts/EMCV	Fiblaferon (natural IFNβ) and IFNβ-1a	NU as difference between original and remaining IFNβ activity	Not stated	[45]
Cell proliferation	Melanoma cells		Relative reduction of proliferation		
Cell proliferation	Daudi cells	IFNβ 10IU	50% inhibition of proliferation	CPE	[46]
CPE	FS-4 fibroblasts/EMCV	Fiblaferon (natural IFNβ)/100U/ml	Neutralizing unit = one unit of neutralized IFNβ	Not stated	[47]
CPE	A549/EMCV	Betaser	Kawade		[48]
CPE	Human fibroblasts	Betaser	Serum dilution that reduces activity of 3 to 1LU/ml/ Once > 100NU/ml or 3 consecutive times > 20NU	Reference antibody no G023-902-527	

CPE: cytopathic effect; FACS: fluorescence activated cell sorter; LU: laboratory unit; NU: neutralizing unit; PBMC: peripheral blood mononuclear cells; EMCV: encephalomyocarditis virus; VSV: vesicular stomatitis virus.

and specific marker of NABs. Low MxA levels indicated the presence of NABs.

Validation

The MxA induction assay is one of the most thoroughly validated NAB assays and has been used by several authors. It was validated using a CPE assay as gold-standard and two different IFNβ preparations for cell stimulation were compared. Most laboratories use internal standards for quality controls. One of these standards is the reference IFNβ antibody (NIH code GO38-501 572), which has a defined neutralizing titre of 1:1700 against ten Laboratory Units (LU) of human IFNβ. In CPE assays cell viability and viral CPE controls are widely used.

Existing recommendations

The WHO expert committee on biological standardization published informal recommendations on measurement of antibodies to interferon in the technical report series No. 725 in 1985. The reference assay in this international study group used A549 cells and the encephalo-myocarditis (EMC) virus but recommended development of simpler assays. For NAB assays the expert committee recommended that the following details should be reported: (1) final concentration of interferon and serum in the reaction mixture; (2) final volume in the reaction mixture; (3) the lowest final dilution of serum tested. For the calculation of the neutralizing titre the Kawade method was recommended. This method calculates the serum dilution that reduces the IFN potency from 10 LU/ml to 1 LU/ml [52].

Conclusion and recommendations

Measurements of binding and neutralizing antibodies against IFNβ should be performed in specialized laboratories (Level A recommendation). Measurement of NABs with a validated CPE assay is still the gold standard. It is recommended that A549 cells are used with a fixed amount of IFNβ (the preparation used by the patient) for stimulation and serial dilution of the test sera. The stimulated cells can either be challenged with EMC viruses or MxA production determined. Standard curves should be obtained using increasing amounts of IFNβ until saturation is reached. The NAB titre should be calculated using the Kawade formula (Level A recommendation).

Titres above 20–60 (depending on the IFNβ prepara-

tion used in the assay) are associated with a loss of IFNβ bioactivity (Class I evidence). As the EMEA currently validates a NAB assay based on the MxA production of A549 cells (MxA induction assay), it is recommended to use the EMEA protocol. (This recommendation is based on Class IV evidence only, but consensus was reached to offer this advice as good practice.) Validation of simpler NAB assay methods is strongly recommended, such as the vivo biological response to IFNβ administration (Level A recommendation).

Clinical use of measurements of antibodies against IFNβ

PubMed was searched for 'IFNβ antibodies and multiple sclerosis'. Of the 236 articles searched, 103 were original articles or review articles on antibodies against IFNβ or controlled clinical trials of IFNβ in which measurements of antibodies were performed. For assessment of the impact of NABs we selected controlled randomized trials of IFNβ in MS with blindly analysed NABs and controlled non-randomized studies with blind evaluation of NABs of at least 3 years' duration (table 5.4). NABs usually appear as low affinity antibodies in small concentrations and later as higher affinity antibodies in larger concentrations. Therefore, whereas the effect on antibodies on the biologic response to IFNβ may be apparent after 9–12 months, the clinical consequences of neutralizing antibodies are usually not seen until 12–18 moths after start of IFNβ therapy. Hence, only trials of sufficient duration (≥3 years) and blind evaluation of NAB status were graded as Class I evidence for effects of NABs. Trials of less sufficient duration (2–3 years) and blind evaluation of NAB status were graded as Class II evidence, and trials of inappropriate duration (<2 years) and/or no blind evaluation of NAB status were classified as Class III evidence regarding clinical effects of NABs.

It has been common to classify patients as NAB-positive after two consecutive serum samples containing NABs in a titre of 20 or more ('once positive, always positive') [3, 16]. The use of this approach will invariably result in an underestimation of the clinical consequences of NABs in studies of 2 years or shorter. Therefore, methods that account for switches between NAB-positive and NAB-negative periods ('interval positive') theoretically provide a more accurate assessment of the clinical impact of NABs on relapse rate and MRI activity [51].

Table 5.4 Effect of NABs to IFNβ on clinical and MRI outcomes in MS therapeutic trials[†].

Study	IFNβ product	No. of patients	Duration	Relapse rate[‡]	MRI Activity[‡]	Disease progression[‡]	MRI Severity[‡]	Class (primary end-point)	Class (NAB evaluation)[§]
IFNB MS Study Group [16]	Betaferon		3 years	+([)	+(ns)	+(ns)	+(ns)	I	I
Rudick et al. [43]	Avonex		2 years	−(ns)	+(ns)	+(ns)	ND	I	II
PRISMS-4 [49]	Rebif		4 years	+([)	+([[[)			I	I
SPECTRIMS [7]	Rebif		3 years	+(ns)	ND	−(ns)	ND	I	I
Durelli et al. [50]	Betaferon/ Avonex		2 years	+(ns)	ND	ND	ND	III	II
Panitch et al. [19]	Rebif/Avonex		48 weeks	+(ns)	+([[[)	ND	ND	I	III
Polman et al. [40]	Betaferon		3 years	+([)	ND	+(ns)	+([)	I	I
Sorensen et al. [51]	Betaferon/ Avonex/ Rebif		5 years	+([)	ND	+(ns)	+(ns)	III	I

†See text for selection of trials and for definition of the different clinical and MRI outcomes.
‡+ = outcome worse in the NAB-positive group than in the NAB-negative group.
− = outcome better in the NAB-positive group than in the NAB-negative group.
ND = not done.
Statistical significance is given in parentheses (ns = not significant; [= $p < 0.05$; [[= $p < 0.01$; [[[= $p < 0.001$).
§I = trials of sufficient duration (>3 years) and blind evaluation of NAB status.
II = trials of less sufficient duration (2–3 years) and blind evaluation of NAB status.
III = trials of inappropriate duration (<2 years) and/or no blind evaluation of NAB status.

Effect of NABs on relapses

In the pivotal phase III trial of IFNβ-1b, NAB-positive patients had significantly higher annual relapse rates during years 2 and 3 (1.08) than NAB-negative patients (0.56) ($p < 0.01$) and equivalent to patients given placebo (1.06) [3]. In the pivotal phase III IFNβ-1a (Rebif) trial, no significant difference in relapse rate was seen over the study duration of 2 years between NAB-positive and NAB-negative patients [6]. But in the 2-year extension phase, NABs caused a clear reduction in efficacy on relapses [49].

There was no correlation observed between NAB status and relapse rate in patients treated for 2 years in the pivotal phase III trial of IFNβ-1a (Avonex) [43].

In the secondary progressive Betaferon study [40] the 'once positive, always positive' method showed that NAB-positive patients had a 45% increase in relapse rates ($p = 0.009$) when they switched to being NAB-positive compared to their prior NAB-negative state. However,

relapse rates in NAB-positive patients showed only a trend ($p = 0.07$) to increase when the 'all switches considered' method was applied. Higher titres seemed to reduce the treatment effect more. In the secondary progressive IFNβ-1a (Rebif) study the relapse effect was reduced in NAB-positive patients (44 μg) such that the difference between NAB-positive and placebo patients was no longer statistically significant [7]. The INCOMIN-study (an open randomized study comparing IFNβ-1b (Betaferon) with IFNβ-1a (Avonex) reported that the frequency of NABs in patients with relapses was a little higher than in patients without relapses [50]. The EVIDENCE study (open randomized comparison of IFNβ-1a (Rebif) with IFNβ-1a (Avonex)) continued for 48 weeks only making this study inadequate for assessing the clinical impact of NABs [19].

In a Danish nationwide prospective study, NABs were measured blinded for up to 60 months in 541 randomly selected patients [51]. The presence of NABs had a significant effect on relapse rates. In NAB-positive periods the annual relapse rate increased more than 50% compared with NAB-negative periods. Comparing NAB-positive to NAB-negative patients the median time to first relapse was significantly reduced by 244 days ($p = 0.009$), and the proportion of relapse-free patients was significantly lower ($p = 0.0064$).

Effect on MRI outcomes

The pivotal study of IFNβ-1b (Betaferon) showed significantly more enlarging lesions in NAB-positive patients compared with NAB-negative patients during years 2 ($p = 0.03$) and 3 ($p = 0.01$) [3, 16]. In the PRISMS study there was a trend over the first 2 years towards more MRI activity in NAB-positive patients [6]. Over 4 years [49], compared with NAB-negative patients, NAB-positive patients had a nearly fivefold increase in the median number of T2 active lesions ($p < 0.001$), and a 17.6% increase compared to an 8.5% decrease in MRI burden of disease ($p < 0.001$). In the pivotal study of IFNβ-1a (Avonex) a trend was seen towards more gadolinium-enhanced lesions in NAB-positive patients ($p = 0.062$) [43]. Secondary progressive patients on IFNβ-1b (Betaferon) showed a higher percentage increase from baseline in T2 lesion volume in NAB-positive patients compared with NAB-negative patients ($p = 0.004$) [40]. Despite the short duration of the EVIDENCE study it was apparent that NAB-positive patients had more T2 active lesions than NAB-negative patients ($p = 0.0004$) [19].

Effect of NABs on disease progression

None of the randomized studies was powered to detect a NAB effect on disease progression. In the pivotal IFNβ-1b study (Betaferon), however, a strong trend was seen towards an effect of NABs on the mean change in EDSS from baseline in the third year *($p = 0.083$) [3, 16]. NAB-positive patients on high dose Rebif showed a near significant *($p = 0.051$) increase in the mean number of EDSS progressions compared with NAB-negative patients in the 4-year PRISMS trial (Rice GPA, personal communication, poster presentation ECTRIMS 2000). The Danish study also showed a strong trend towards a higher mean EDSS in NAB-positive patients compared with NAB-negative patients at month 42 and 48, and towards shorter time to disease progression in NAB-positive patients ($p = 0.10$) [51]. Neither the SPECTRIMS study (IFNβ-1a (Rebif) [53], nor the study of IFNβ-1b

(Betaferon) in secondary progressive patients found a significant difference between NAB-positive and NAB-negative patients [54].

Safety issues

The presence of NABs has not been reported to be associated with adverse events or toxicity.

Conclusions and recommendations regarding the clinical use of NAB measurements

It is recommended that patients treated with IFNβ are tested for the presence of NABs during the first 24 months of therapy (Level A recommendation). Measurement of NABs can be discontinued in those patients remaining NAB-negative during this period but should be resumed if disease activity increases (Level B recommendation). There is Class I evidence that the presence of NABs significantly hampers the effect of IFNβ on the relapse rate and on both active lesions and burden of disease seen on MRI. In patients with NABs, NAB measurements should be repeated at intervals of 3–6 months and therapeutic options should be re-evaluated (Level A recommendation). Therapy with IFNβ should be discontinued in patients with high titres of NABs (e.g. titres >100 in patients using IFNβ-1b) and sustained at repeated measurements with 3–6 months intervals (Level A recommendation).

Prevention and treatment of NABs

Steroids

Short pulses of steroids have been demonstrated to be safe, well tolerated and clinically effective for patients with MS. A clinical trial randomly assigned 161 patients to receive IFNβ-1b, either alone or in combination with 1 g of methylprednisolone (MP) administered monthly intravenously (i.v.) [55]. Using an MxA assay it was found that there was a significant reduction in NAB development in patients treated with MP, when defined as titres ≥1:20 on one occasion but not when defined as twice consecutively positive. There was no difference in the frequency of patients that developed NABs at high titres (>1:100). The development of NAB-positivity was significantly delayed in the MP group (Kaplan Meyer analysis, log-Rank test; $p < 0.05$ by month 6 of therapy). These results suggest that the chronic administration of steroids prevents or delays the formation of NABs, but does not reduce the titre in NAB-positive patients.

Other immunosuppressive agents

A number of clinical trials have been performed with either RR-MS or SP-MS patients to evaluate the use of IFNβ in association with an immunosuppressive agent [56–58]. However, the NAB data originating from these small studies are inconsistent and do not allow any definitive conclusion as to whether additional immunosuppression reduces NAB formation.

Switching IFNβ preparations or increasing the dose of IFNβ

One of the possible strategies to overcome the formation of NABs in MS could be the switching from one preparation of IFNβ to another, but unfortunately many studies have shown that NABs are cross-reactive between IFNβ-1a and IFNβ-1b [29, 33, 39]. Thus, switching to an alternative IFNβ preparation is not of clinical benefit for a NAB-positive MS patient.

It is well known that the amount of antigen to which an individual is exposed influences the magnitude of the immune response and that very large doses or repeated administrations of small amounts of antigen are often inhibitory in the production of antibodies [59]. However, at present, there is no evidence that increasing the dosage of IFNβ is of benefit to NAB-positive patients.

Other strategies

Plasmapheresis and immunoglobulins (IgG) might be considered as possible procedures to diminish NAB generation. At present, the effects of the IgG on blocking antibody production are widely accepted in patients with autoimmune diseases. However, IgG and plasmapheresis do not affect memory plasma cells [60]. Therefore, the concomitant administration of IgG or plasmapheresis may be useful in eliminating circulating NABs, but it would not be expected to impede the production of NABs once it has been triggered.

Conclusions and future considerations on prevention of NABs formation

Limited evidence is available on managements that reduce NAB formation to IFNβ in MS. One gram i.v. MP administration every month has been revealed to be safe and able to minimize the formation of NABs over time (Level C recommendation). However, no effect has been observed in reducing the amplitude of NABs titres once NABs have been formed. Further studies are warranted to strengthen these results and to expand our knowledge in such an intriguing matter.

Principal recommendations regarding measurements of antibodies against IFNβ and the clinical use of NAB measurements

• BAB assays can be reliably used for IFNβ antibody screening before performing a NAB assay (Level A recommendation).

• Measurements of binding and neutralizing antibodies against IFNβ should be performed in specialized laboratories (Level A recommendation).

• Measurement of NABs should be performed with a validated CPE assay or an MxA production assay using serial dilution of the test sera. The NAB titre should be calculated using the Kawade formula (Level A recommendation).

• Tests for the presence of NABs should be performed during the first 24 months of therapy (Level A recommendation).

• Measurements of NABs can be discontinued in those patients remaining NAB-negative during this period but should be resumed if disease activity increases (Level B recommendation).

• In patient with NABs, measurements should be repeated after 3–6 months (Level A recommendation).

• Therapy with IFNβ should be discontinued in patients with high titres of NABs and sustained at repeated measurements with 3- to 6-month intervals (Level A recommendation).

Conflicts of interest

The following authors have reported conflicts of interest as follows.

Per Soelberg Sorensen has received honoraria for lecturing and advisory councils, trial steering committees or travel expenses for attending meetings from Biogen Idec, Bayer Schering, Merck Serono, TEVA, Sanofi-aventis, Novartis, and Genmab..

F. Deisenhammer has received personal compensation and research support from Biogen Idec, Schering, Serono, Aventis, and Medacorp.

P. Duda has nothing to declare.

R. Hohlfeld has received grant support and consutancy fees from Serono, Biogen Idec, Schering, and TEVA.

K.-M. Myhr has received honoraria for lecturing and travel expenses for attending meetings, and research support from Biogen Idec, Bayer, Merck Serono and Sanofi-aventis.

J. Palace has received honoraria for lecturing and advisory councils, travel expenses for attending meetings, and financial support for her department from Biogen Idec, Schering, Serono, and TEVA.

C. Polman has received honoraria for consutancy, and for delivering lectures at scientific meetings from Biogen Idec, Schering, and Serono.

C. Pozzilli has nothing to declare.

C. Ross has nothing to declare.

References

1. Brainin M, Barnes M, Baron JC, et al. Guidance for the preparation of neurological management guidelines by EFNS scientific task forces–revised recommendations 2004. Eur J Neurol 2004;**11**:577–81.

2. Runkel L, Meier W, Pepinsky RB, et al. Structural and functional differences between glycosylated and non-glycosylated forms of human interferon-beta (IFN-beta). Pharm Res 1998;**15**:641–9.

3. The IFNB Multiple Sclerosis Study Group. Interferon beta-1b is effective in relapsing-remittingmultiple sclerosis. I. Clinical results of a multicenter, randomized, double-blind, placebo-controlled trial. Neurology 1993;**43**:655–61.

4. European Study Group on interferon beta-1b in secondary progressive MS. Placebo-controlled multicentre randomised trial of interferon beta-1b in treatment of secondary progressive multiple sclerosis. Lancet 1998;**352**:1491–7.

5. Jacobs LD, Cookfair DL, Rudick RA, et al. Intramuscular interferon beta-1a for disease progression in relapsing multiple sclerosis. The Multiple Sclerosis Collaborative Research Group (MSCRG). Ann Neurol 1996;**39**:285–94.

6. PRISMS (Prevention of Relapses and Disability by Interferon beta-1a Subcutaneously in Multiple Sclerosis) Study Group. Randomised double-blind placebo-controlled study of interferon beta-1a in relapsing/remitting multiple sclerosis. Lancet 1998;**352**:1498–504.

7. Secondary Progressive Efficacy Clinical Trial of Recombinant Interferon-beta-1a in MS (SPECTRIMS) Study Group. Randomized controlled trial of interferon- beta-1a in secondary progressive MS: Clinical results. Neurology 2001;**56**:1496–504.

8. Clanet M, Radue EW, Kappos L, et al. A randomized, double-blind, dose-comparison study of weekly interferon beta-1a in relapsing MS. Neurology 2002;**59**:1507–17.

9. The North American Study Group on interferon beta-1b in Secondary Progressive MS. Interferon beta-1b in secondary progressive MS: Results from a 3-year controlled study. Neurology 2004;**63**:1788–95.

10. Ross C, Clemmesen KM, Svenson M, et al. Immunogenicity of interferon-beta in multiple sclerosis patients: influence of preparation, dosage, dose frequency, and route of administration. Danish Multiple Sclerosis Study Group. Ann Neurol 2000;**48**:706–12.

11. Dubois BD, Keenan E, Porter BE, et al. Interferon beta in multiple sclerosis: experience in a British specialist multiple sclerosis centre. J Neurol Neurosurg Psychiatry 2003;**74**: 946–9.

12. Rice GP, Paszner B, Oger J, Lesaux J, Paty D, Ebers G. The evolution of neutralizing antibodies in multiple sclerosis patients treated with interferon beta-1b. Neurology 1999;**52**: 1277–9.

13. Sorensen PS, Koch-Henriksen N, Ross C, Clemmesen KM, Bendtzen K. Appearance and disappearance of neutralizing antibodies during interferon-beta therapy. Neurology 2005; **65**:33–99.

14. Gneiss C, Reindl M, Lutterotti A, et al. Interferon-beta: the neutralizing antibody (NAb) titre predicts reversion to NAb negativity. Mult Scler 2004;**10**:507–10.

15. Perini P, Facchinetti A, Bulian P, et al. Interferon-beta (INF-beta) antibodies in interferon-beta1a- and interferon-beta1b-treated multiple sclerosis patients. Prevalence, kinetics, cross-reactivity, and factors enhancing interferon-beta immunogenicity in vivo. Eur Cytokine Netw 2001;**12**: 56–61.

16. The IFNB Multiple Sclerosis Study Group and The University of British Columbia MS/MRI Analysis Group. Neutralizing antibodies during treatment of multiple sclerosis with interferon beta-1b: experience during the first three years. Neurology 1996;**47**:889–94.

17. Bertolotto A, Malucchi S, Sala A, et al. Differential effects of three interferon betas on neutralising antibodies in patients with multiple sclerosis: a follow up study in an independent laboratory. J Neurol Neurosurg Psychiatry 2002;**73**:148–53.

18. von Wussow P, Jakschies D, Freund M, Deicher H. Humoral response to recombinant interferon-alpha 2b in patients receiving recombinant interferon-alpha 2b therapy. J Interferon Res 1989;**9**(Suppl. 1):S25–31.

19. Panitch H, Goodin DS, Francis G, et al. Randomized, comparative study of interferon beta-1a treatment regimens in MS: The EVIDENCE Trial. Neurology 2002;**59**:1496–506.

20. Perini P, Calabrese M, Biasi G, Gallo P. The clinical impact of interferon beta antibodies in relapsing-remitting MS. *J Neurol* 2004;**251**:305–9.

21. Kremenchutzky M. Long-term evolution of anti-INFbeta antibodies in IFNbeta-treated MS patients: the London, Canada, MS Clinic experience. *Neurology* 2003;**61**:S29–30.

22. Pachner AR, Narayan K, Price N, Hurd M, Dail D. MxA gene expression analysis as an interferon-beta bioactivity measurement in patients with multiple sclerosis and the identification of antibody-mediated decreased bioactivity. *Mol Diag* 2004;**7**:17–25.

23. Bellomi F, Scagnolari C, Tomassini V, *et al*. Fate of neutralizing and binding antibodies to IFN beta in MS patients treated with IFN beta for 6 years. *J Neurol Sci* 2003;**215**:3–8.

24. Mayr M, Berek K, Deisenhammer F. Evolution of interferon-beta binding antibodies in MS patients may predict development of neutralizing antibodies. *Eur J Neurol* 2003;**10**:462–4.

25. Slavikova M, Schmeisser H, Kontsekova E, Mateicka F, Borecky L, Kontsek P. Incidence of autoantibodies against type I and type II interferons in a cohort of systemic lupus erythematosus patients in Slovakia. *J Interferon Cytokine Res* 2003;**23**:143–7.

26. Monzani F, Meucci G, Caraccio N, *et al*. Discordant effect of IFN-beta1a therapy on anti-IFN antibodies and thyroid disease development in patients with multiple sclerosis. *J Interferon Cytokine Res* 2002;**22**:773–81.

27. Vallittu AM, Halminen M, Peltoniemi J, *et al*. Neutralizing antibodies reduce MxA protein induction in interferon-beta-1a-treated MS patients. *Neurology* 2002;**58**:1786–90.

28. Fernandez O, Mayorga C, Luque G, *et al*. Study of binding and neutralising antibodies to interferon-beta in two groups of relapsing-remitting multiple sclerosis patients. *J Neurol* 2001;**248**:383–8.

29. Kivisakk P, Alm GV, Fredrikson S, Link H. Neutralizing and binding anti-interferon-beta (IFN-beta) antibodies. A comparison between IFN-beta-1a and IFN-beta-1b treatment in multiple sclerosis. *Eur J Neurol* 2000;**7**:27–34.

30. Antonelli G, Simeoni E, Bagnato F, *et al*. Further study on the specificity and incidence of neutralizing antibodies to interferon (IFN) in relapsing remitting multiple sclerosis patients treated with IFN beta-1a or IFN beta-1b. *J Neurol Sci* 1999;**168**:131–6.

31. Deisenhammer F, Reindl M, Harvey J, Gasse T, Dilitz E, Berger T. Bioavailability of interferon beta 1b in MS patients with and without neutralizing antibodies. *Neurology* 1999;**52**:1239–43.

32. Pungor E, Files JG, Gabe JD, *et al*. A novel bioassay for the determination of neutralizing antibodies to IFN-ß1b. *J Interferon Cytokine Res* 1998;**18**:1025–30.

33. Khan OA, Dhib-Jalbut SS. Neutralizing antibodies to interferon beta-1a and interferon beta-1b in MS patients are cross-reactive. *Neurology* 1998;**51**:1698–702.

34. Ferrarini AM, Sivieri S, Buttarello M, Facchinetti A, Perini P, Gallo P. Time-course analysis of CD25 and HLA-DR expression on lymphocytes in interferon-beta 1b-treated multiple sclerosis patients. *Mult Scler* 1998;**4**:174–7.

35. Lawrence N, Oger J, Aziz T, Palace J, Vincent A. A sensitive radioimmunoprecipitation assay for assessing the clinical relevance of antibodies to IFN beta. *J Neurol Neurosurg Psychiatry* 2003;**74**:1236–9.

36. Lampasona V, Rio J, Franciotta D, et al. Serial immunoprecipitation assays for interferon–(IFN)-beta antibodies in multiple sclerosis patients. *Eur Cytokine Netw* 2003;**14**:154–7.

37. Kob M, Harvey J, Schautzer F, *et al*. A novel and rapid assay for the detection of neutralizing antibodies against interferon-beta. *Mult Scler* 2003;**9**:32–5.

38. Bertolotto A, Gilli F, Sala A, *et al*. Persistent neutralizing antibodies abolish the interferon beta bioavailability in MS patients. *Neurology* 2003;**60**:634–9.

39. Bertolotto A, Malucchi S, Milano E, Castello A, Capobianco M, Mutani R. Interferon beta neutralizing antibodies in multiple sclerosis: neutralizing activity and cross-reactivity with three different preparations. *Immunopharmacology* 2000;**48**:95–100.

40. Polman C, Kappos L, White R, *et al*. Neutralizing antibodies during treatment of secondary progressive MS with interferon beta-1b. *Neurology* 2003;**60**:37–43.

41. Zang YC, Yang D, Hong J, Tejada-Simon MV, Rivera VM, Zhang JZ. Immunoregulation and blocking antibodies induced by interferon beta treatment in MS. *Neurology* 2000;**55**:397–404.

42. Kageshita T, Yamamoto A, Yamazaki N, Ishihara K, Ono T. Low frequency of neutralizing antibodies against natural interferon-beta during adjuvant therapy for Japanese patients with melanoma. *J Dermatol Sci* 1999;**19**:208–12.

43. Rudick RA, Simonian NA, Alam JA, *et al*. Incidence and significance of neutralizing antibodies to interferon beta-1a in multiple sclerosis. Multiple Sclerosis Collaborative Research Group (MSCRG). *Neurology* 1998;**50**:1266–72.

44. Abdul-Ahad AK, Galazka AR, Revel M, Biffoni M, Borden EC. Incidence of antibodies to interferon-beta in patients treated with recombinant human interferon-beta 1a from mammalian cells. *Cytokines Cell Mol Ther* 1997;**3**:27–32.

45. Fierlbeck G, Schreiner T, Schaber B, Walser A, Rassner G. Neutralizing interferon beta antibodies in melanoma patients treated with recombinant and natural interferon beta. *Cancer Immunol Immunother* 1994;**39**:263–8.

46. Prummer O, Bunjes D, Wiesneth M, *et al*. Antibodies to interferon-alpha: a novel type of autoantibody occurring

after allogeneic bone marrow transplantation. *Bone Marrow Transplant* 1996;**17**:617–23.

47. Dummer R, Muller W, Nestle F, *et al.* Formation of neutralizing antibodies against natural interferon-beta, but not against recombinant interferon-gamma during adjuvant therapy for high-risk malignant melanoma patients. *Cancer* 1991;**67**:2300–4.

48. Redlich PN, Grossberg SE. Analysis of antigenic domains on natural and recombinant human IFN-ß by the inhibition of biologic activities with monoclonal antibodies. *J Immunol* 1989;**143**:1887–93.

49. PRISMS Study Group. PRISMS-4: Long-term efficacy of interferon-beta-1a in relapsing MS. *Neurology* 2001;**56**: 1628–36.

50. Durelli L, Verdun E, Barbero P, *et al.* Every-other-day interferon beta-1b versus once-weekly interferon beta-1a for multiple sclerosis: results of a 2-year prospective randomised multicentre study (INCOMIN). *Lancet* 2002;**359**: 1453–60.

51. Sorensen PS, Ross C, Clemmesen KM, *et al.* Clinical importance of neutralising antibodies against interferon beta in patients with relapsing-remitting multiple sclerosis. *Lancet* 2003;**362**:1184–91.

52. Grossberg SE, Kawade Y, Kohase M, Klein JP. The neutralization of interferons by antibody. II. Neutralizing antibody unitage and its relationship to bioassay sensitivity: the tenfold reduction unit. *J Interferon Cytokine Res* 2001;**21**: 743–55.

53. Li DK, Zhao GJ, Paty DW. Randomized controlled trial of interferon-beta-1a in secondary progressive MS: MRI results. *Neurology* 2001;**56**:1505–13.

54. Polman CH, Kappos L, Petkau J, Thompson A. Neutralising antibodies to interferon beta during the treatment of multiple sclerosis. *J Neurol Neurosurg Psychiatry* 2003;**74**: 1162–3.

55. Pozzilli C, Antonini G, Bagnato F, *et al.* Monthly corticosteroids decrease neutralizing antibodies to IFNbeta1 b: a randomized trial in multiple sclerosis. *J Neurol* 2002;**249**: 50–6.

56. Patti F, Cataldi ML, Nicoletti F, *et al.* Combination of cyclophosphamide and interferon-beta halts progression in patients with rapidly transitional multiple sclerosis. *J Neurol Neurosurg Psychiatry* 2001;**71**:404–7.

57. Calabresi PA, Wilterdink JL, Rogg JM, Mills P, Webb A, Whartenby KA. An open-label trial of combination therapy with interferon beta-1a and oral methotrexate in MS. *Neurology* 2002;**58**:314–7.

58. Fernandez O, Guerrero M, Mayorga C, *et al.* Combination therapy with interferon beta-1b and azathioprine in secondary progressive multiple sclerosis. A two-year pilot study. *J Neurol* 2002;**249**:1058–62.

59. Dresser DW, Mitchison NA. The mechanism of immunological paralysis. *Adv Immunol* 1968;**8**:129–81.

60. Rudick RA, Goodkin DE (ed.) *Multiple Sclerosis Therapeutics.* London: Martin Dunitz, 1999; pp. 309–33.

CHAPTER 6

Use of antibody testing in nervous system disorders

H. J. Willison,[1] N. E. Gilhus,[2] F. Graus,[3] B. C. Jacobs,[4] R. Liblau,[5] C. Vedeler,[2] A. Vincent[6]

[1]Institute of Neurological Sciences, Southern General Hospital, Glasgow, UK; [2]Haukeland University Hospital and University of Bergen, Bergen, Norway; [3]Hospital Clinic de Barcelona, Spain; [4]Erasmus MC, Rotterdam, The Netherlands; [5]Hopital de la Salpetriere, Paris, France; [6]Institute of Molecular Medicine, John Radcliffe Hospital, Oxford, UK

Objective

To evaluate service provision and quality assurance schemes for clinically useful autoantibody tests in neurology.

Background

Over the past 20 years there has been a steady increase in the use of anti-nerve antibody assays to aid diagnosis or research into neurological diseases thought to have an antibody-associated or antibody-mediated autoimmune basis [1–9]. The range of antigens tested and their associated diseases includes nerve and neuromuscular junction disorders, and paraneoplastic disorders affecting the central nervous system, as listed and referenced in table 6.1. With respect to the use of the anti-acetylcholine receptor (anti-AChR) antibody assay to aid in the diagnosis in myasthenia gravis, the radioimmunoassay in standard use [29] has been thoroughly validated for many years. Both non-commercial and commercial quality assurance schemes for laboratories to participate in are available. However, the procedures in place for quality assurance in the identification of antibodies that mark paraneoplastic syndromes and for anti-ganglioside antibodies are less well developed. Efforts have been

made to produce standard protocols, exchange samples, and run workshops in both these latter areas, as manifested by the INCAT (Immune Neuropathy Cause and Treatment) group [39] and the Paraneoplastic Neurological Syndrome Euronetwork [5]. Such studies have principally involved researchers and laboratories with a specialized interest in these fields rather than clinical laboratories performing routine screening.

The anti-neuronal antibodies associated with paraneoplastic syndromes, anti-Hu anti-Yo, and anti-Ri (ANNA-1, PCA-1, ANNA-2 respectively), were initially demonstrated by immunohistochemistry of brain sections and more recently by blotting of recombinant proteins, as listed in table 6.1. The clinical utility of these investigations is considerable, and the importance of accurate identification paramount to clinical decision making. In addition, this spectrum of autoantibodies is the subject of important research developments. This has been recently discussed in a detailed workshop report [40].

The determination of anti-ganglioside and glycolipid antibodies has increasingly entered clinical practice over recent years [8]. Anti-glycolipid antibodies are associated with acute and chronic peripheral neuropathies and may be useful in diagnosis of clinical subtypes of neuropathy. They are widely measured by enzyme-linked immunosorbent assay (ELISA), dot blot, and thin layer chromatography overlay [39, 41, 42].

Both anti-neuronal and anti-glycolipid antibody assays are being conducted in laboratories throughout Europe. Until recently, this has been without any externally or independently monitored quality assurance, although

European Handbook of Neurological Management: Volume 1, 2nd edition. Edited by N. E. Gilhus, M. P. Barnes and M. Brainin.
© 2011 Blackwell Publishing Ltd.

Table 6.1 Antigens tested and their associated diseases

Antibody specificity	Associated neurological disorders	Detection method	References
Anti-Hu (ANNA-1)	Subacute sensory neuronopathy, limbic encephalitis, brain stem encephalitis, paraneoplastic encephalomyelitis, chronic pseudoobstruction	IMH/IMF, confirmed by WB on recombinant protein or neuronal extracts	10, 11
Anti-Yo (PCA-1)	Paraneoplastic cerebellar degeneration	IMH/IMF, confirmed by WB as above	12, 13
Anti-Ri (ANNA-2)	Myoclonus/opsoclonus	IMH/IMF, confirmed by WB as above	14
Anti-Tr	Paraneoplastic cerebellar degeneration	IMH/IMF (requires fixed tissue),	15
Anti-amphiphysin	Stiff person syndrome, encephalomyelitis, subacute sensory neuronopathy	IMH/IMF (requires fixed tissue), confirmed by WB as above	16, 17
Anti-CV2/CRMP5	Cerebellar degeneration, encephalomyelitis, limbic encephalitis	IMH/IMF (requires fixed tissue), confirmed by WB as above	18
Anti-VGKC	Acquired neuromyotonia, limbic encephalitis (usually not paraneoplastic)	RIA	19
Anti-VGCC	Lambert-Eaton myasthenic syndrome, paraneoplastic cerebellar degeneration	RIA	20, 21
Anti-Aquaporin 4	Neuromyelitis optica	IMH/IMF. IMF on unpermeabilized cells transfected with the antigen is most sensitive	22, 23
Anti-NMDAR	NMDAR-antibody encephalopathy	IMF on unpermeabilized cells transfected with the antigen is most sensitive	24
Anti-ganglionic AChR	Autonomic neuropathy	RIA	25
Anti-(TA) Ma2	Limbic encephalitis	IMH/IMF, confirmed by WB as above	26, 27
Anti-AChR, MuSK	Myasthenia gravis	RIA	28, 29
Anti-GM1, GD1b (IgM) Anti-GM2 (IgM)	Multifocal motor neuropathy, chronic motor neuropathy	ELISA, TLC	9, 30, 31
Anti-GM1a, GM1b GD1a, GalNAcGD1a, (IgG)	Acute motor axonal neuropathy	ELISA, TLC	8, 32
Anti-GQ1b, GT1a	Miller Fisher syndrome	ELISA, TLC	8, 33
Anti-GD3, GD1b	Acute ataxic neuropathies	ELISA, TLC	34
Anti-GD1b and other disialylated gangliosides (IgM)	Paraproteinemic neuropathies, CANOMAD	ELISA, TLC	35, 36
Anti-MAG/SGPG (IgM)	IgM paraproteinaemic neuropathy	WB of CNS myelin, ELISA	37
Anti-GAD	Stiff person syndrome/cerebellar ataxia	IMH/IMF (requires fixed tissue), confirmed by WB, RIA	17, 38

IMH/IMF, immunohistochemistry/immunofluorescence; WB, Western blot; RIA, radioimmunoassay; TLC, thin layer chromatography overlay; ELISA, enzyme-linked immunosorbent assay; MAG, myelin associated glycoprotein; SGPG, sulphated glucuronyl paragloboside; CANOMAD, chronic ataxic neuropathy, ophthalmoplegia, M protein, cold agglutinins, anti-disialosyl antibodies; VGCC, voltage-gated calcium channels; VGKC, voltage-gated potassium channel; Ach-R, acetylcholine receptor; MuSK, muscle specific kinase; GAD, glutamic acid decarboxylase; NMDAR, N-methyl-D-aspartate receptor.

such schemes are now becoming available. To investigate the scale of this issue and to identify the perceived needs of neuroimmunology laboratories in assay availability and quality, we conducted a questionnaire-based survey of European neuroimmunology centres and here report and discuss the findings.

Methods

Under the auspices of the EFNS Scientific Panel on Neuroimmunology, an anti-nerve antibody task force was established to conduct the review. Eighteen national representatives were invited to participate in a questionnaire-based survey. The questionnaire requested information on: (a) the availability of tests both within the individual's institution and nationally; (b) an approximation of the number of tests conducted annually; (c) the methodology used; (d) the availability of quality assurance schemes; (e) the availability of positive and negative control sera; (f) the interest in setting up and participating in a pan-European quality assurance scheme.

Results

The questionnaire was distributed in 1999 to 18 national members of the EFNS Scientific Panel on Neuroimmunology, of which 12 responded. The range of assays being conducted is summarized in table 6.1, as are the associated neurological disorders and key references. In addition, novel assays routinely available in 2010, e.g. anti-aquaporin 4 antibody screening to aid in the diagnosis of neuromyelitis optica [22, 23] and NMDAR antibodies for the diagnosis of a newly described encephalopathy [24] are also included in the updated table.

Antibody assays for anti-AChR antibodies are widely available, being conducted in at least one centre in most of the countries that responded (10 out of 12). Quality assurance schemes were used either nationally or internationally and the exclusive method used was the standard radioimmunoassay, using iodinated bungarotoxin bound to acetylcholine receptors extracted either from muscle or from muscle-like cell lines. Commercial kits are available for AChR and MuSK antibodies from RSR Ltd, Cardiff, UK. A recent unpublished survey of centres in Europe conducted by Euromyasthenia indicated that

most groups used these tests and all groups had concordant results.

Antibodies to glutamic acid decarboxylase (GAD), found in autoimmune stiff person syndrome [17], were conducted in five of 12 neuroimmunology laboratories in responding countries and estimated using a variety of methods including immunohistology, ELISA, radioimmunoassay, and Western blot. At present it is difficult to compare values between different laboratories despite the use of international units in some cases. Because these assays are designed principally for use in investigation of diabetes, and because titres are much higher in stiff person syndrome and some cases of cerebellar ataxia than in diabetes, it will be important to ensure that laboratories performing this test for neurological disorders use techniques designed to measure high titres.

Antibody assays to voltage-gated calcium channels (VGCC) and potassium channels (VGKC) were rarely conducted, being available in three and one surveyed centres respectively. A commercial kit for the VGCC test is now available (RSR Ltd, Cardiff, UK) and results from different laboratories should be comparable.

Antibody assays for Hu (ANNA-1) and Yo (APCA-1) were widely available and frequently conducted in many centres in most countries (nine of 12), using a combination of immunhistochemistry and Western blot analysis. Anti-Ri (ANNA-2), -Tr, and -amphiphysin antibodies were sought less frequently. The less frequent paraneoplastic antibodies, anti-Ma2/anti-Ta, anti-CV2/CRMP5, can also be detected by immunohistochemistry, but in many cases fixed rather than fresh frozen tissue is required, and not all laboratories do this routinely. There is a need to distribute positive sera to help in the recognition of these antibodies. There is increasing use of comprehensive commercial immunoblots such as those marketed by Ravo-Diagnostika (Freiburg, Germany) and Euroimmun (Lubeck, Germany) that detect antibodies to a broad panel of recombinant antigens including Hu, Yo, Ri, Ma1, Ma2/Ta, CV2/CRMP5, and amphiphysin.

Anti-myelin-associated glycoprotein (MAG) antibodies were determined in laboratories in at least one centre in seven of 12 countries, using a commercial kit that has good standardization (Buhlmann Laboratories, Basel, Switzerland), or using Western blot of myelin [43]. Measurement of anti-ganglioside antibodies was also widely available in many centres and included a wide range of gangliosides and glycolipids (e.g. GM1, GM2, GA1,

GD1a, GD1b, GQ1b, and sulphatides), but the details of the ELISAs used differ considerably between laboratories [39, 41, 42, 44, 45].

In response to questions on quality assurance, most centres reported that they conducted in-house quality assurance, although information on their precise nature was not sought. However, the only assay in which national or international quality assurance was widely used was the anti-AChR antibody assay. With respect to quality assurance schemes for other antigens, all laboratories indicated that they would join a quality assurance scheme for at least some, if not all, the investigations they were conducting.

Among the newer antibodies, AQP4 antibody testing is now conducted in several centres in Europe, but a formal survey has not been conducted. NMDAR antibodies are performed in at least two centres. Both these antibody tests have recently been established by Euroimmun (Lubeck, Germany) and there is also an ELISA for AQP4 antibodies (RSR Ltd, UK).

Discussion and Good Practice Points

It is evident from this survey that a wide variety of antibody assays used in the diagnosis of neuroimmunological diseases are being conducted in many centres throughout Europe. This survey was restricted to major antigens and their respective antibodies, but did not consider the very wide array of emerging tests that have yet to be fully validated for clinical utility. This represents a healthy perception of the value of such investigations among clinical neurologists, but also highlights the need for a high degree of inter-laboratory uniformity and standards of practice.

A number of co-operative inter-laboratory studies have previously been conducted through distribution of coded positive and negative samples to participating laboratories. These have demonstrated marked variations in the ability to detect accurately positive or negative samples for both anti-ganglioside antibodies and antibodies marking paraneoplastic syndromes, particularly for borderline samples. This particular issue was not addressed in this survey. However, information was sought on methodology and in this context it is evident that methodologies being used vary quite widely among different laboratories.

Since the survey was originally conducted there has been steady progress in understanding the nature and role of antibodies to nervous system components in neurological diseases. The clinical utility of testing remains to be determined.

The most striking finding of this survey was the lack of any organized quality assurance schemes for the great majority of these autoantibodies, the exception being for anti-AChR antibodies, and more recently some anti-neuronal and anti-glycolipid antibodies. The survey indicated a very strong demand for such quality assurance schemes to be instituted. The mechanism by which such schemes should be organized is a matter for debate. Our Good Practice Points are thus summarized as follows.

1 The determination of anti-neuronal antibodies should be conducted using protocols agreed during the course of multi-centre comparative studies, such as the INCAT study for anti-glycolipid antibodies.

2 Laboratories conducting immunassays for anti-AChR antibodies should join existing quality assurance schemes.

3 Where no official scheme is available (i.e. for the majority of assays covered in this survey) laboratories should develop arrangements for exchanging coded positive and negative samples at least biannually, to ensure sensitivity and specificity are being maintained.

4 A quality assurance scheme for the most commonly measured anti-glycolipid antibodies (GM1 and GQ1b) and paraneoplastic antibodies (Hu and Yo) should be established as a matter of priority (this has now been done).

5 The EFNS should consider how open-access quality control schemes in Europe are best established, both for laboratory and other measures, and should actively promote such schemes.

Conflicts of interest
A. Vincent and Clinical Neurology, Oxford, receive royalties and payments for antibody tests.

The other authors have reported no conflicts of interest.

References

1. Giometto B, Taraloto B, Graus F. Autoimmunity in paraneoplastic neurological syndromes. *Brain Pathol* 1999;**9**: 261–73.

2. Honnorat J, Cartalat-Carel S. Advances in paraneoplastic neurological syndromes. *Curr Opin Oncol* 2004;**16**:614–20.

3. Lang B, Vincent A. Autoantibodies to ion channels at the neuromuscular junction. *Autoimmun Rev* 2003;**2**:94–100.

4. Quarles RH, Ilyas AA, Willison HJ. Antibodies to gangliosides and myelin proteins in Guillain-Barre syndrome. *Ann Neurol* 1990;**27**(Suppl):S48–S52.

5. Vincent A, Honnorat J, Antoine JC, Giometto B, Dalmau J, Lang B. Autoimmunity in paraneoplastic neurological disorders. *J Neuroimmunol* 1998;**84**:105–9.

6. Vincent A, Lily O, Palace J. Pathogenic autoantibodies to neuronal proteins in neurological disorders. *J Neuroimmunol* 1999;**100**:169–80.

7. Vincent A. Antibodies to ion channels in paraneoplastic disorders. *Brain Pathol* 1999;**9**:285–91.

8. Willison HJ, Yuki N. Peripheral neuropathies and anti-glycolipid antibodies. *Brain* 2002;**125**:2591–625.

9. Pestronk A. Multifocal motor neuropathy: diagnosis and treatment. *Neurology* 1998;**51**(Suppl 5):S22–S24.

10. Dalmau J, Graus F, Rosenblum MK, Posner JB. Anti-Hu–associated paraneoplastic encephalomyelitis/sensory neuronopathy. A clinical study of 71 patients. *Medicine (Baltimore)* 1992;**71**:59–72.

11. Lucchinetti CF, Kimmel DW, Lennon VA. Paraneoplastic and oncologic profiles of patients seropositive for type 1 antineuronal nuclear autoantibodies. *Neurology* 1998;**50**:652–7.

12. Furneaux HM, Rosenblum MK, Dalmau J, *et al*. Selective expression of Purkinje-cell antigens in tumor tissue from patients with paraneoplastic cerebellar degeneration. *N Engl J Med* 1990;**322**:1844–51.

13. Peterson K, Rosenblum MK, Kotanides H, Posner JB. Paraneoplastic cerebellar degeneration. I. A clinical analysis of 55 anti-Yo antibody-positive patients. *Neurology* 1992;**42**:1931–7.

14. Luque FA, Furneaux HM, Ferziger R, *et al*. Anti-Ri: an antibody associated with paraneoplastic opsoclonus and breast cancer. *Ann Neurol* 1991;**29**:241–51.

15. Graus F, Dalmau J, Valldeoriola F, *et al*. Immunological characterization of a neuronal antibody (anti-Tr) associated with paraneoplastic cerebellar degeneration and Hodgkin's disease. *J Neuroimmunol* 1997;**74**:55–61.

16. Folli F, Solimena M, Cofiell R, *et al*. Autoantibodies to a 128-kd synaptic protein in three women with the stiff-man syndrome and breast cancer. *N Engl J Med* 1993;**328**:546–51.

17. Saiz A, Arpa J, Sagasta A, *et al*. Autoantibodies to glutamic acid decarboxylase in three patients with cerebellar ataxia, late-onset insulin-dependent diabetes mellitus, and polyendocrine autoimmunity. *Neurology* 1997;**49**:1026–30.

18. Honnorat J, Antoine JC, Derrington E, Aguera M, Belin MF. Antibodies to a subpopulation of glial cells and a 66 kDa developmental protein in patients with paraneoplastic neurological syndromes. *J Neurol Neurosurg Psychiatry* 1996;**61**:270–8.

19. Hart IK, Waters C, Vincent A, *et al*. Autoantibodies detected to expressed K+ channels are implicated in neuromyotonia. *Ann Neurol* 1997;**41**:238–46.

20. Mason WP, Graus F, Lang B, *et al*. Small-cell lung cancer, paraneoplastic cerebellar degeneration and the Lambert-Eaton myasthenic syndrome. *Brain* 1997;**120**:1279–300.

21. Motomura M, Johnston I, Lang B, Vincent A, Newsom-Davis J. An improved diagnostic assay for Lambert-Eaton myasthenic syndrome. *J Neurol Neurosurg Psychiatry* 1995;**58**:85–7.

22. Hinson SR, McKeon A, Lennon VA. Neurological autoimmunity targeting aquaporin-4. *Neuroscience* 2009 (in press).

23. Lennon VA, Kryzer TJ, Pittock SJ, Verkman AS, Hinson SR. IgG marker of optic-spinal multiple sclerosis binds to the aquaporin-4 water channel. *J Exp Med* 2005;**202**:473–7.

24. Dalmau J, Rosenfeld MR. Paraneoplastic syndromes of the CNS. *Lancet Neurol* 2008;**7**:327–40.

25. Vernino S, Low PA, Fealey RD, Stewart JD, Farrugia G, Lennon VA. Autoantibodies to ganglionic acetylcholine receptors in autoimmune autonomic neuropathies. *N Engl J Med* 2000;**343**:847–55.

26. Dalmau J, Graus F, Villarejo A, *et al*. Clinical analysis of anti-Ma2-associated encephalitis. *Brain* 2004;**127**:1831–44.

27. Voltz R, Gultekin SH, Rosenfeld MR, *et al*. A serologic marker of paraneoplastic limbic and brain-stem encephalitis in patients with testicular cancer. *N Engl J Med* 1999;**340**:1788–95.

28. Hoch W, McConville J, Helms S, Newsom-Davis J, Melms A, Vincent A. Auto-antibodies to the receptor tyrosine kinase MuSK in patients with myasthenia gravis without acetylcholine receptor antibodies. *Nat Med* 2001;**7**:365–8.

29. Vincent A, Newsom-Davis J. Acetylcholine receptor antibody as a diagnostic test for myasthenia gravis: results in 153 validated cases and 2967 diagnostic assays. *J Neurol Neurosurg Psychiatry* 1985;**48**:1246–52.

30. O'Hanlon GM, Veitch J, Gallardo E, Illa I, Chancellor AM, Willison HJ. Peripheral neuropathy associated with anti-GM2 ganglioside antibodies: clinical and immunopathological studies. *Autoimmunity* 2000;**32**:133–44.

31. Yuki N, Yoshino H, Sato S, Miyatake T. Acute axonal polyneuropathy associated with anti-GM1 antibodies following Campylobacter enteritis. *Neurology* 1990;**40**:1900–2.

32. Ho TW, Willison HJ, Nachamkin I, *et al*. Anti-GD1a antibody is associated with axonal but not demyelinating forms of Guillain-Barre syndrome. *Ann Neurol* 1999;**45**:168–73.

33. Chiba A, Kusunoki S, Shimizu T, Kanazawa I. Serum IgG antibody to ganglioside GQ1b is a possible marker of Miller Fisher syndrome. *Ann Neurol* 1992;**31**:677–9.

34. Kaida K, Kamakura K, Ogawa G, *et al.* GD1b-specific antibody induces ataxia in Guillain-Barre syndrome. *Neurology* 2008;**71**:196–201.

35. Willison HJ, O'Leary CP, Veitch J, *et al.* The clinical and laboratory features of chronic sensory ataxic neuropathy with anti-disialosyl IgM antibodies. *Brain* 2001;**124**:1968–77.

36. Serrano-Munuera C, Rojas-Garcia R, Gallardo E, *et al.* Antidisialosyl antibodies in chronic idiopathic ataxic neuropathy. *J Neurol* 2002;**249**:1525–8.

37. Weiss MD, Dalakas MC, Lauter CJ, Willison HJ, Quarles RH. Variability in the binding of anti-MAG and anti-SGPG antibodies to target antigens in demyelinating neuropathy and IgM paraproteinemia. *J Neuroimmunol* 1999;**95**:174–84.

38. Solimena M, Folli F, Aparisi R, Pozza G, De Camilli P. Autoantibodies to GABA-ergic neurons and pancreatic beta cells in stiff-man syndrome. *N Engl J Med* 1990;**322**:1555–60.

39. Willison HJ, Veitch J, Swan AV, *et al.* Inter-laboratory validation of an ELISA for the determination of serum anti-ganglioside antibodies. *Eur J Neurol* 1999;**6**:71–7.

40. Graus F, Delattre JY, Antoine JC, *et al.* Recommended diagnostic criteria for paraneoplastic neurological syndromes. *J Neurol Neurosurg Psychiatry* 2004;**75**:1135–40.

41. Alaedini A, Briani C, Wirguin I, Siciliano G, D'Avino C, Latov N. Detection of anti-ganglioside antibodies in Guillain-Barre syndrome and its variants by the agglutination assay. *J Neurol Sci* 2002;**196**:41–4.

42. Zielasek J, Ritter G, Magi S, Hartung HP, Toyka KV. A comparative trial of anti-glycoconjugate antibody assays: IgM antibodies to GM1. *J Neurol* 1994;**241**:475–80.

43. Kuijf ML, Eurelings M, Tio-Gillen AP, *et al.* Detection of anti-MAG antibodies in polyneuropathy associated with IgM monoclonal gammopathy. *Neurology* 2009;**73**:688–95.

44. Hirakawa M, Morita D, Tsuji S, Kusunoki S. Effects of phospholipids on antiganglioside antibody reactivity in GBS. *J Neuroimmunol* 2005;**159**:129–32.

45. Kaida K, Morita D, Kanzaki M, *et al.* Ganglioside complexes as new target antigens in Guillain-Barre syndrome. *Ann Neurol* 2004;**56**:567–71.

CHAPTER 7

Use of skin biopsy in the diagnosis of small fibre neuropathy

G. Lauria,[1] S. T. Hsieh,[2] O. Johansson,[3] W. R. Kennedy,[4] J. M. Leger,[5] S. I. Mellgren,[6] M. Nolano,[7] I. S. J. Merkies,[8] M. Polydefkis,[9] A. G. Smith,[10] C. Sommer,[11] J. Valls-Solé[12]

[1]IRCCS Foundation, 'Carlo Besta' Neurological Institute, Milan, Italy; [2]National Taiwan University College of Medicine and National Taiwan University Hospital, Taipei, Taiwan; [3]Karolinska Institute, Stockholm, Sweden; [4]University of Minnesota, Minneapolis, USA; [5]Hôpital de la Salpêtrière, Paris, France; [6]University of Tromsø, Norway; [7]Salvatore Maugeri Foundation, IRCCS, Center of Telese Terme, Italy; [8]Spaarne Hospital Hoofddorp, Spaarnepoort 1, The Netherlands; [9]The Johns Hopkins University School of Medicine, Baltimore, MD, USA; [10]University of Utah, Salt Lake City, UT, USA; [11]University of Würzburg, Germany; [12]Hospital Clinic Barcelona, Spain

Objectives

This document is written under the auspices of the European Federation of the Neurological Societies (EFNS; *www.efns.org*) and the Peripheral Nerve Society (PNS; *www.pnsociety.com*). The purpose is to revise the guidelines on the use of skin biopsy in the diagnosis of peripheral neuropathy [1]. In the past 4 years, a considerable number of new papers have been published. These are mainly focused on small fibre neuropathy (SFN). The role of skin biopsy as a diagnostic tool was analysed in the evidence-based review of the American Academy of Neurology, American Association of Neuromuscular and Electrodiagnostic Medicine, and American Academy of Physical Medicine and Rehabilitation [2]. Since skin biopsy retains a particular interest in clinical practice for the diagnosis of SFN, we focused the present guidelines on this specific subtype of neuropathy.

The revision includes recommendations on: (i) methods; (ii) safety; (iii) normative reference values; (iv) diagnostic yield; (v) correlation with other measures of neuropathy; (vi) use as outcome measure; (vii) EFNS/PNS standards; (viii) new studies to address unresolved issues.

Search strategy

The task force systematically searched the MEDLINE database from 2005, the year when the first ENFS guidelines were published [1], to 30 June 2009. For each specific issue, we stored all the articles published in English sorted by the MEDLINE search using the following keywords: skin biopsy, punch biopsy, small fibre neuropathy, painful neuropathy, normative values, intraepidermal nerve fibres, cutaneous innervation, skin nerves. We omitted those articles that were not pertinent, then read and rated the remaining articles according to the guidance for EFNS guidelines [3] and objectives of the current paper. In some cases, investigators were asked for original data and methodological details.

Method for reaching consensus

Data extraction was carried out and compared among each member of the task force. A first draft of the manuscript was prepared and diffused among the members of the task force. After revision, a second draft was prepared. Discrepancies on each topic were further discussed and settled during a consensus meeting held in Wurzburg on 7 July 2009. The third draft of the manuscript prepared after the consensus meeting was revised by an expert member of the task force (W. R. Kennedy) and two experts in the field of peripheral neuropathy (J.M. Leger) and clinical neurophysiology (J. Valls-Solé) not directly involved in the use of skin biopsy. The final version of the guidelines is presented here.

Definition of small fibre neuropathy

Definitions of SFN have been proposed and used by various authors [4–17], but conclusive diagnostic criteria are not yet available. However, the most recent papers focusing on the clinical applications of skin biopsy in SFN used similar inclusion criteria for patients, based on normal sural nerve conduction studies (NCS), clinical symptoms and signs considered suggestive, and/or altered QST findings. The authors provided data on sensitivity and sensibility, from which we derived our level of recommendations.

Methological issues

How to perform skin biopsy and choice of biopsy location

Skin biopsy is most commonly performed using a 3-mm disposable punch under sterile technique, after topical anaesthesia with lidocaine. No suture is required. A shallow biopsy (3–4 mm) is adequate to study epidermal nerve fibres, whereas a deeper biopsy (6–8 mm) is required to include sweat glands, hair follicles, and arterovenous anastomosis. To optimize the sampling of such structures and of myelinated fibres in hairy skin, particular attention should be paid to including a hair in the specimen [18].

Earlier studies were performed in healthy subjects [19] and in patients with leprosy and diabetic neuropathy [20, 21]. The current technique was developed at the Karolinska Institute [22], and later standardized at the University of Minnesota [23] and at the Johns Hopkins University [24].

A less invasive sampling method is the removal of the epidermis alone by applying a suction capsule to the skin. With this method there is no bleeding and local anaesthesia is not needed. However, the method does not provide information on dermal and sweat gland nerve fibres. Moreover, thus far it has not been systematically used to investigate patients with SFN. This technique was developed at the University of Minnesota [25].

In most studies, hairy skin biopsies were obtained from the distal part of the leg (10 cm above the lateral malleolus), in some from the calf and the paraspinal region, and in many of them also from the upper lateral aspect of the thigh (20 cm below the anterior iliac spine) or other proximal locations where normal values are available. These locations were chosen to detect the length dependent loss of nerve fibres, which is typical of axonal polyneuropathy. These sites may also be sampled in the case of a non-length-dependent ganglionopathy. More details are provided on the EFNS website.

Recommendations

For diagnostic purposes in length-dependent SFN, we recommend that a 3-mm punch skin biopsy be performed at the distal leg (10 cm above the lateral malleolus) for quantification of IENF density (Level A recommendation). An additional biopsy from the proximal thigh may provide information about both length-dependent and non-length-dependent processes (Level C recommendation). When a biopsy is taken from other body sites for evaluation of a uni-lateral process, a control biopsy from a similar non-affected region should be taken (GPP).

Tissue preparation

After skin biopsy is performed, the specimen is immediately fixed in cold fixative for approximately 24 h at 4°C, then kept in a cryoprotective solution for one night, and serially cut with a freezing microtome or a cryostat. Each biopsy yields about 50 vertical 50-μm sections. The first and last few sections should not be used for nerve examination because of possible artefacts. Most studies for bright-field microscopy used 2% paraformaldehyde-lysine periodate (2% PLP), whereas most studies for indirect immunofluorescence with or without confocal microscopy used Zamboni's (2% paraformaldehyde, picric acid) fixative.

Either bright-field immunohistochemistry or immunofluorescence with or without confocal microscopy have been used, but the technique does not affect the reliability of skin biopsy in assessing IENF loss in SFN [1]. However, no study has been designed yet to compare the two techniques. More details are provided on the EFNS website.

IENF morphometry and measurement reliability

Quantification of IENF density using bright-field immunohistochemistry was mostly based on the assessment of the number of fibres per linear measurement. Significant correlation with a stereologic technique [26] supported the reliability of linear IENF density [27]. IENF are counted either under the light microscope at high magnification (i.e. 40x objective) or using software for image analysis. The length of the epidermal surface is measured using software for biological measures (a freely available software is available at http://rsb.info.nih.gov/nih-image/index.html). The density is calculated in at least three sections as the number of IENF per length of the section (IENF/mm). Other studies reported the IENF density per skin surface area [28, 29].

Quantification of IENF density using confocal immunofluorescence technique is usually performed on images based on the stack of consecutive 2 μm optical sections (usually 16 sections) for a standard linear length of epidermis. The thickness of skin sections varies from 32 to 60 μm. Four epidermal areas are selected for confocal image acquisition, two images on each of two different sections excluding areas containing hair follicles and sweat ducts. For quantitative analysis, IENF are counted at high magnification, (i.e. 40x objective) for light microscope or (20x) for epifluorescence microscope or using a software for image analysis (e.g. Neurolucida, Microbrightfield) on digitised confocal images. Other semiquantitative methods of IENF density estimation have been previously suggested [1].

In both bright-field and immunofluorescence methods, single IENF crossing the dermal–epidermal junction are counted, whereas secondary branching is excluded from quantification. No study provided information on the rules for counting IENF fragments, which have been comprehensively reviewed by Kennedy and colleagues [30]. Intra- and inter-observer variability, and interlaboratory agreement on IENF counts has been assessed [16].

The 'skin blister' is an alternative technique to assess the epidermal innervation density. IENF density in blister roofs from foot and calf correlated with IENF density in skin biopsies from adjacent areas in 25 healthy subjects ($r = 0.64$ and $r = 0.57$ respectively) showing no systematic differences between skin blisters and biopsies ($p = 0.29$) or between pairs of blisters from the same location

($p = 0.15$)[29]. More details are provided on the EFNS website.

Recommendations

For diagnostic purposes, we recommend bright-field immunohistochemistry or immunofluorescence with rabbit polyclonal anti-PGP 9.5 antibodies in 2% PLP or Zamboni's fixed sections of 50-μm thickness. For methodological issues on bright-field immunohistochemistry we refer to McCarthy et al. [24], on immunofluorescence to Wang et al. [22], and on confocal microscopy to Kennedy and Weldelschafer-Crabb [23]. IENF should be counted at high magnification in at least three sections per biopsy. We emphasize that only single IENF crossing the dermal–epidermal junction should be counted, excluding secondary branching and fragments from quantification. The length of the section should be measured in order to calculate the exact linear epidermal innervation density (IENF/mm) (Level A recommendation). An adequate training in a well-established skin biopsy laboratory is needed. Further studies are warranted to establish the reliability of the 'blister technique' (Level C recommendation) for quantification of IENF density in SFN.

Quantification of sweat gland innervation

The quantification of sudomotor nerve fibres is technically challenging because of the complex three-dimensional structure of the sweat glands. Different methods have been proposed but none has been standardized [1]. Novel methods using an unbiased stereologic technique and automated technique for quantification of sudomotor nerve fibres have been recently proposed [31, 32]. More details are provided on the EFNS website.

Recommendations

Morphometric data on sweat gland innervation density in healthy subjects and in patients with SFN are limited and further studies are warranted. The descriptive semiquantitative approach should not be used to quantify sweat gland innervation (Level B recommendation). The unbiased stereologic technique recently proposed could be a helpful tool (Level B recommendation).

Safety

No side effects have been reported in published studies but no study focused on safety was performed. The approximate number of biopsies performed with 3-mm disposable punch and side effects recorded (in brackets)

in healthy subjects and patients with neuropathy of different aetiology in the 10 laboratories participating in this guideline are: Milan 1600 (2); Telese Terme 2000 (2); Taiwan 1700 (1); Maastricht 300 (0); Utah 2000 (3); Stockholm 1000 (0); Minneapolis 10 000 (3); Würzburg 800 (10); Tromsø 600 (1); Johns Hopkins University 15 000 (44). The most common side effect was a mild infection due to improper wound management, recovering with topical antibiotic therapy. The only other complication reported was excessive bleeding which did not need suture. The estimated frequency of side effects is 1.9 : 1000. However, this figure may be underestimated because patients with a milder infection could be treated by their general practitioner or treat themselves without reporting to the centre. Healing occurs within 7–10 days.

Recommendations

Skin biopsy performed with 3-mm disposable punch is a safe and minimally invasive procedure based on the experience of the 10 established laboratories reported here. It requires training and is safe as long as sterile procedures and haemostasis are correctly performed (GPP).

Normative reference values

Bright-field immunohistochemistry

After the publication of the first guidelines on skin biopsy, three further large studies [7, 16, 33] estimated the density of IENF at the distal leg (10 cm above the lateral malleolus) in healthy subjects. Overall, including all previously cited papers [1], value ranges from 13.8 ± 6.7/mm (mean $\pm$ SD) to 9.8 ± 3.6/mm (mean $\pm$ SD).

The largest normative study [16] included 188 healthy subjects from three different laboratories (Maastricht, Ferrara, Milan) and stratified the study population per age and gender, providing normative values per decade. The authors reported that IENF density at the distal leg is lower in males than females, that weight and height do not have any significant impact, and that values decline with age (table 7.1), thus confirming previous observations [34–36].

Immunofluorescence technique

No study specifically assessed the normative range of IENF density at the distal leg using indirect immunofluorescence with or without confocal microscopy. Overall, values obtained with confocal microscopy were higher than those found using light microscopy technique. Normal values were reviewed by Kennedy and co-authors [30]. Data from 267 healthy subjects included in 17 studies performed with and without confocal microscopy [29, 37–52] ranged between 7.6 ± 3.1 and 33 ± 7.9/mm (mean $\pm$ SD) in subjects with age 20–59 years. Density of 20.1 ± 5/mm (mean $\pm$ SD) was found in subjects over 60 years (lower 5th percentile = 11.8).

Blister technique

Panoutsopoulou and colleagues [29] reported the normative values of IENF density (expressed by number of IENF per epidermal surface area) using both blister technique and punch biopsy with confocal immunofluorescence microscopy at foot and calf in 25 healthy subjects

---

Table 7.1 Intraepidermal nerve fibre (IENF) density at the ankle: normative values for clinical use (reproduced from Bakkers et al. [16], with permission).

Age (years)	Females (n = 97)		Males (n = 91)	
	0.05 Quantile values per age span	Median values per age span	0.05 Quantile values per age span	Median values per age span
20–29	6.7	11.2	5.4	9.0
30–39	6.1	10.7	4.7	8.4
40–49	5.2	9.9	4.0	7.8
50–59	4.1	8.7	3.2	7.1
60–69	3.3	7.9	2.4	6.3
≥70	2.7	7.2	2.0	5.9

(age 35–62 years). Mean IENF density on the foot was 174 IENF/mm^2 for the punch biopsy and 162 IENF/mm^2 for the blister method. Mean IENF density on the calf was 158 IENF/mm^2 for the punch biopsy and 143 IENF/mm^2 for the blister method. Intra- and inter-blister variability was less than intra-biopsy variability. The authors found a significant correlation between the two techniques.

Recommendations

Normative reference values must consider that IENF density at the distal leg (10 cm above the lateral malleolus) declines with age (Level A recommendation) and may be lower in males than in females. However, it is not influenced by weight and height. Normative reference values are available for bright-field immunohistochemistry (Level A recommendation) but not yet for confocal immunofluorescence or blister technique.

Diagnostic yield of skin biopsy

In the first guideline paper [1], we reported specificity and sensitivity of skin biopsy for the diagnosis of SFN based on an unpublished meta-analysis of 161 patients from nine studies, two of them performed with confocal microscope technique. The same year, Koskinen and colleagues [28] reported similar values for idiopathic or secondary SFN.

In the past few years, two studies [7, 51] focused on the analysis of the diagnostic yield of skin biopsy in SFN using the receiver operating characteristic (ROC) curve that graphically describes the discrimination threshold of sensitivity versus specificity or true positives versus false positives. The IENF density cut-off of 7.63/mm and ≤8.8/mm at distal leg were associated with specificity of 90% and 79.6% and sensitivity of 82.8% and 77.2% respectively. One study [17] compared three statistical methods: (1) Z-scores, calculated from multiple regression analysis, in which cut-off values were estimated for each patient and adjusted for age and gender; (2) fifth percentile, in which cut-off value was 6.7 IENF/mm; and (3) ROC analysis, in which cut-off value was 10.3 IENF/mm. Highest specificity was obtained with Z-scores (98%) and fifth percentile (95%), which had lower sensitivity (31% and 35% respectively) compared to the ROC analysis, which showed specificity of 64% and sensitivity of 78%. The authors emphasized that the diagnostic yield of skin

biopsy depends on how the reference and cut-off values have been assessed. In most studies, skin biopsy has been used to investigate patients with SFN either idiopathic or associated to different conditions, including diabetes, infectious diseases, systemic connective tissue disorders, and genetic diseases. However, no study was designed to demonstrate whether skin biopsy can be useful for identifying the aetiology of SFN. Therefore, no data on this issue are yet available. More details are provided on the EFNS website.

Assessment of morphological changes

Morphological changes of IENF and dermal nerve fibres (swellings, weaker immunoreactivity, crawler) were reported as common findings in SFN but were also present to a lesser extend in healthy individuals [53, 54]. In three other studies evaluating SFN of different aetiologies, isolated morphological abnormality with normal IENF densities were noted in 29.1%, 20%, and 25% of cases [55–57]. Similar results were reported in 62 patients with sensory neuropathy, 29% of whom had abnormal morphology but normal IENF density [58]. More details are provided on the EFNS website.

Recommendations

Skin biopsy with linear quantification of IENF density is a reliable and efficient technique to confirm the clinical diagnosis of SFN (Level A recommendation). This conclusion derives from the examination of studies involving homogeneous groups of patients with possible SFN. However, since the definition of SFN varied in the different studies, we could not provide the range of sensitivity and sensibility values.

Immunohistochemical technique does not seem to influence the diagnostic efficiency in diagnosing SFN. However, data from comparative studies using the two techniques in homogeneous groups of SFN patients are not available yet and are warranted.

For diagnostic purposes we recommend quantitative assessment of IENF density with appropriate quality controls, which include all the steps of the procedure, in particular the aspect of intra- and inter-observer ratings. The diagnosis of SFN with skin biopsy should be based on the comparison with normative reference values adjusted by age (Level A recommendation) and possibly gender (Level B recommendation). Diffuse IENF swellings, especially if large, may have a predictive value to the progression of neuropathy (Level C recommendation). Further studies to investigate the ability of skin biopsy in differentiating patients with symptoms mimicking SFN are warranted.

Correlation between IENF density and other measures of neuropathy

Correlation with clinical measures

In the past 4 years, a number of studies investigating the correlation between skin biopsy and clinical scales have been published. However, there are no definite diagnostic criteria nor validated scales for SFN. Therefore, we report here available comparative data between skin biopsy, clinical findings, and various neuropathy scales.

IENF density was closely related to, and predicted, pin sensation loss in 106 subjects with idiopathic SFN [47]. Among subjects with diabetic neuropathy, IENF density progressively declined with increased severity of clinical neuropathy, measured using the Neurological Disability Score [59–61]. Another study in diabetic subjects with normal nerve conduction studies found a negative correlation between IENF density at the lower leg and the Neuropathy Impairment Score [62].

A recent study [16] investigated three groups of patients with sarcoidosis: (1) patients without SFN symptoms ($n = 14$); (2) patients with SFN complaints and normal IENF density findings ($n = 39$); and (3) patients with SFN complaints and abnormal IENF density values ($n = 19$). The authors found that significantly more SFN-related symptoms (as reported by a SFN-related symptoms inventory questionnaire) were present in patients with abnormal IENF density, with a gradual transition between the three subgroups.

In two studies investigating patients with systemic lupus erythematosus, IENF density negatively correlated with cutaneous vasculitis and disease activity [63, 64]. Conversely, in HIV-associated neuropathy there was no correlation between distal IENF density and Total Neuropathy Score [65], although a baseline reduction in IENF density predicted the risk of developing neuropathy symptoms over a 2.9-year period, which was 14-fold higher in patients with IENF density of fewer than 10 fibres/mm [66]. Another study failed to demonstrate a relationship with the Neuropathy Symptoms Score [17].

IENF density was lower in diabetic neuropathy patients with pain compared with those without [45, 51, 59], whereas no correlation was previously found in another study [42]. In HIV-associated sensory neuropathy, IENF density inversely correlated with pain severity assessed with both VAS and the Gracely Pain Score [65]. Conversely, a previous study found a correlation only with

patient's and doctor's evaluation scores [67], and another [56] showed that assessment of IENF density could not differentiate between symptomatic or asymptomatic HIV neuropathy patients. In patients with pure SFN of mixed aetiology, IENF density was lower in those with pure spontaneous pain than those with pure evoked pain, but it did not correlate with its intensity [7].

Correlation with sensory nerve conduction studies

Concordance between sural sensory nerve action potential (SNAP) amplitude and IENF density was investigated in several studies with different results. This is likely in keeping with the different types of neuropathy examined (i.e. large or mixed fibre versus small fibre) with most studies focusing on SFN. We have previously reported [1] that concordance between sural SNAP amplitude and IENF density was found in patients with clinical impairment of large nerve fibres, whereas skin biopsy appeared more sensitive than sural sensory nerve conduction study (NCS) in diagnosing SFN. Recent studies strengthened this assumption. In 67 patients with pure SFN, sensory NCS were normal and IENF density at distal leg was reduced in 88% of cases [7]. However, a recent study [68] confirmed the previously observed linear correlation between medial plantar SNAP amplitude and IENF density in patients with SFN [14] and found a correlation with digital plantar near-nerve needle sensory NSC at the multivariate analysis. These findings suggest that most large sensory fibres can be impaired in distal segments in some patients with a clinical picture of pure SFN. Therefore, clinically pure SFN can be part of a mixed sensory neuropathy. More details are provided on the EFNS website.

Correlation with small fibre-related evoked potentials

Few studies have examined the relationship between skin biopsy and neurophysiological tests for assessing small fibre function, and most of the available data come from single case reports. More details are provided on the EFNS website.

Correlation with quantitative sensory testing (QST) and autonomic nervous system testing

Psychophysical assessment of thermal, heat-pain, and vibratory thresholds provides information on A∂ and C, and Aß fibres, respectively. However, the correlation between QST and IENF density remains controversial. More details are provided on the EFNS website.

Although IENF have somatic functions, several studies investigated their relationship with autonomic dysfunction in neuropathy of different aetiology. Clinical signs of dysautonomia and abnormal veno-arteriolar reflex and vasodilatation induced by local heating, reflecting impaired skin axonal reflexes carried by somatic C-fibres, were found in about 70% of patients with pure SFN [7]. Another study did not find any correlation between IENF density and measures of autonomic function in SFN [51].

Correlation with sural nerve biopsy

In the past 4 years, no further study investigated the correlation between skin and nerve biopsy. Therefore, we refer to the recommendations proposed in the first EFNS skin biopsy guidelines [1].

Recommendations

Decreased IENF density reliably indicates the presence of SFN (Level A recommendation). However, correlation between IENF density, validated measures of neuropathy severity, and clinical disability needs further evaluation in patients with neuropathy of specific etiologies (Level C recommendation).

The relationship between IENF density and neuropathic pain is more complex than a simple inverse correlation. Lower IENF density may be associated with the presence of neuropathic pain, especially in pure SFN (Level B recommendation), but it does not correlate with the intensity of pain.

Quantification of IENF density can better assess the diagnosis of SFN than sural NCS and sural nerve biopsy (Level A recommendation). Concordance between IENF quantification and medial plantar SNAP amplitude in patients with normal sural NCS suggests that distal sensory nerve recording might be more sensitive than sural NCS in the diagnosis of sensory neuropathy (Level C recommendation).

IENF density correlates with psychophysical examination of small fibre dysfunction using thermal and nociceptive detection thresholds (Level A recommendation), but correlation with specific sensation (e.g. cooling, warm, heat-pain) remains uncertain (Level C recommendation). Correlation with autonomic dysfunction needs more extensive validation (Level C recommendation).

Further studies are required to determine the relative diagnostic utility of non-conventional neurophysiological methods to investigate small fibre function (e.g. laser-evoked potentials [LEPs], contact heat-evoked potentials [CHEPs], and pain-related electrically evoked potential [PREPs]) and their correlation with IENF density.

Skin biopsy as a measure of outcome

Several prospective studies and case reports have investigated the relationship between skin innervation and outcome. Overall, they showed that a lower IENF density is associated with a higher risk of progression to neuropathy [59, 66] and that IENF regeneration positively correlated with decreased neuropathic pain intensity [69]. Studies measuring the rate of IENF regeneration following capsaicin chemical denervation showed that it is slower in patients with diabetes or HIV without signs or symptoms of neuropathy [70, 71]. More details are provided on the EFNS website.

Recommendations

In SFN, the reduction of IENF density over time can be used as an index of progression of neuropathy (Level A recommendation). In HIV patients without neurological symptoms, skin biopsy with quantification of the IENF densities may predict the risk of progression to symptomatic HIV neuropathy (Level B recommendation). Regeneration of IENF may be associated with recovery of neuropathic pain and sensory symptoms (Level C recommendation). Skin biopsy may be considered as an endpoint in future neuroprotective neuropathy trials (Level B recommendation).

EFNS/PNS standards

Skin biopsy with quantification of IENF density is a reliable technique to diagnose SFN. For diagnostic purposes, we endorse 3-mm punch skin biopsy at the distal leg (10 cm above the lateral malleolus) and quantification of linear IENF density in at least three 50-μm thick sections per biopsy, fixed in 2% PLP or Zamboni's solution, by immunohistochemistry using rabbit polyclonal anti-PGP 9.5 antibodies, using either bright-field microscopy or immunofluorescence with or without confocal microscopy. Appropriate normative data from healthy subjects matched for age and gender should be always used.

We strongly recommend training in an established cutaneous nerve laboratory before performing and processing skin biopsies in the diagnosis of SFN. Quality control should include all the steps of the procedure, in particular the aspect of intra- and inter-observer ratings for qualitative assessments and for quantitative analysis of epidermal densities.

Proposal for new studies

Normative reference studies reporting age- and gender-matched values of IENF density at proximal and distal sites using indirect immunofluorescence technique with and without confocal microscopy are warranted. These studies should be collaborative and designed to compare the diagnostic yield of this technique with that of brightfield microscopy in patients with SFN.

A clinimetric approach should be used to assess the correlation between skin innervation and the clinical symptoms and signs of SFN. Such studies should include patients whose clinical picture mimics that of SFN in order to definitely assess specificity and sensitivity of skin biopsy in the diagnosis of this type of neuropathy.

A consensus definition of SFN is needed to plan new studies that will determine the sensitivity and specificity of skin biopsy and other potential diagnostic strategies.

The reliability of already tested or new methods to quantify the density of nerve fibres in the sub-epidermal dermis and autonomic structures (e.g. sweat gland nerve, erector pili muscle, and vessels) should be confirmed by further studies in patients with homogeneous types of peripheral neuropathy, including SFN. Correlative studies between skin biopsy, autonomic tests, and non-conventional neurophysiologic tools are also warranted.

Lastly, further studies should focus on the ability of skin biopsy to detect early changes of nerve fibres that predict the progression of neuropathy and that assist in assessing nerve degeneration and regeneration rates over time, to confirm the potential usefulness of the technique as an outcome measure in clinical practice and research.

Conflicts of interest

None of the authors has any conflicts of interest to declare.

References

1. Lauria G, Cornblath DR, Johansson O, et al. EFNS guidelines on the use of skin biopsy in the diagnosis of peripheral neuropathy. Eur J Neurol 2005;12(10):747–58.
2. England JD, Gronseth GS, Franklin G, et al. Practice Parameter: evaluation of distal symmetric polyneuropathy: role of autonomic testing, nerve biopsy, and skin biopsy (an evidence-based review). Report of the American Academy of Neurology, American Association of Neuromuscular and Electrodiagnostic Medicine, and American Academy of Physical Medicine and Rehabilitation. Neurology 2009; 72(2):177–84.
3. Brainin M, Barnes M, Baron JC, et al. Guidance for the preparation of neurological management guidelines by EFNS scientific task forces – revised recommendations. Eur J Neurol 2004;11(9):577–81.
4. Lacomis D. Small-fiber neuropathy. Muscle Nerve 2002; 26(2):173–88.
5. Sommer C, Lauria G. Painful small-fiber neuropathies. In: Vinken PJ, Bruyn GW (eds) Handbook of Clinical Neurology, Vol. 81, 2006;pp. 621–33.
6. Lauria G. Small fiber neuropathies. Curr Opin Neurol 2005;18(5):591–7.
7. Devigili G, Tugnoli V, Penza P, Camozzi F, Lombardi R, Melli G, et al. The diagnostic criteria for small fiber neuropathy: from symptoms to neuropathology. Brain 2008;131(Pt 7):1912–25.
8. Goodman BP. Approach to the evaluation of small fiber peripheral neuropathy and disorders of orthostatic intolerance. Semin Neurol 2007;27(4):347–55.
9. Hoitsma E, Reulen JPH, de Baets M, Drent M, Spaansa F, Faber CG. Small fiber neuropathy: a common and important clinical disorder. J Neurol Sci 2004;227:119–30.
10. Said G. Small fiber involvement in peripheral neuropathies. Curr Opin Neurol 2003;16:601–2.
11. Mendell JR, Sahenk Z. Painful sensory neuropathy. N Engl J Med 2003;348:1243–55.
12. Sommer C. Painful neuropathies. Curr Opin Neurol 2003; 16:623–628.
13. Tavee J, Zhou L. Small fiber neuropathy: a burning problem. Cleve Clin J Med 2009;76(5):297–305.
14. Herrmann DN, Ferguson ML, Pannoni V, Barbano RL, Stanton M, Logigian EL. Plantar nerve AP and skin biopsy in sensory neuropathies with normal routine conduction studies. Neurology 2004;63(5):879–85.
15. Holland NR, Crawford TO, Hauer P, Cornblath DR, Griffin JW, McArthur JC. Small-fiber sensory neuropathies: clinical course and neuropathology of idiopathic cases. Ann Neurol 1998;44:47–59.
16. Bakkers M, Merkies ISJ, Lauria G, et al. Intra-epidermal nerve fiber density normative values and its application in sarcoidosis. Neurology 2009;73:1142–8.
17. Nebuchennykh M, Loseth S, Lindal S, Mellgren SI. The value of skin biopsy with recording of intraepidermal nerve fiber density and quantitative sensory testing in the assessment of small fiber involvement in patients with different causes of polyneuropathy. J Neurol 2009;256(7):1067–75.
18. Provitera V, Nolano M, Pagano A, Caporaso G, Stancanelli A, Santoro L. Myelinated nerve endings in human skin. Muscle Nerve 2007;35(6):767–75.

19. Dalsgaard CJ, Rydh M, Haegerstrand A. Cutaneous innervation in man visualized with protein gene product 9.5 (PGP9.5) antibodies. *Histochemistry* 1989;**92**:385–90.

20. Karanth SS, Springall DR, Lucas S, *et al*. Changes in nerves and neuropeptides in skin from 100 leprosy patients investigated by immunocytochemistry. *J Pathol* 1898;**157**(1): 15–26.

21. Levy DM, Karanth SS, Springall DR, Polak JM. Depletion of cutaneous nerves and neuropeptides in diabetes mellitus: an immunocytochemical study. *Diabetologia* 1989;**32**(7): 427–33.

22. Wang L, Hilliges M, Jernberg T, Wiegleb-Edstrom D, Johansson O. Protein gene product 9.5-immunoreactive nerve fibers and cells in human skin. *Cell Tissue Res* 1990;**261**(1):25–33.

23. Kennedy WR, Wendelschafer-Crabb G. The innervation of human epidermis. *J Neurol Sci* 1993;**115**(2):184–90.

24. McCarthy BG, Hsieh ST, Stocks A, *et al*. Cutaneous innervation in sensory neuropathies: evaluation by skin biopsy. *Neurology* 1995;**45**(10):1848–55.

25. Kennedy WR, Nolano M, Wendelschafer-Crabb G, Johnson TL, Tamura E. A skin blister method to study epidermal nerves in peripheral nerve disease. *Muscle Nerve* 1999;**22**: 360–71.

26. Stocks EA, McArthur JC, Griffen JW, Mouton PR. An unbiased method for estimation of total epidermal nerve fiber length. *J Neurocytol* 1996;**25**(11):637–44.

27. McArthur JC, Stocks EA, Hauer P, Cornblath DR, Griffin JW. Epidermal nerve fiber density: normative reference range and diagnostic efficiency. *Arch Neurol* 1998;**55**(12): 1513–20.

28. Koskinen M, Hietaharju A, Kylaniemi M, *et al*. A quantitative method for the assessment of intraepidermal nerve fibers in small-fiber neuropathy. *J Neurol* 2005;**252**(7):789–94.

29. Panoutsopoulou IG, Wendelschafer-Crabb G, Hodges JS, Kennedy WR. Skin blister and skin biopsy to quantify epidermal nerves: a comparative study. *Neurology* 2009;**72**(14): 1205–10.

30. Kennedy WR, McArthur JC, Polydefkis MJ, Wendelschafer G. Pathology and quantitation of cutaneous innervation. In: Thomas PJDaPK (ed.) *Peripheral Neuropathy*. Philadelphia: Elsevier Saunders, 2005; pp. 869–95.

31. Gibbons CH, Illigens BM, Wang N, Freeman R. Quantification of sweat gland innervation: a clinical-pathologic correlation. *Neurology* 2009;**72**(17):1479–86.

32. Gibbons CH, Illigens BMW, Freeman R. Quantification of sudomotor innervation: a comparison of three methods. *Muscle Nerve* 2010 Apr 16. [Epub ahead of print].

33. Umapathi T, Tan WL, Tan NC, Chan YH. Determinants of epidermal nerve fiber density in normal individuals. *Muscle Nerve* 2006;**33**(6):742–6.

34. Pan CL, Lin YH, Lin WM, Tai TY, Hsieh ST. Degeneration of nociceptive nerve terminals in human peripheral neuropathy. *Neuroreport* 2001;**12**(4):787–92.

35. Goransson LG, Mellgren SI, Lindal S, Omdal R. The effect of age and gender on epidermal nerve fiber density. *Neurology* 2004;**62**(5):774–7.

36. Chien HF, Tseng TJ, Lin WM, *et al*. Quantitative pathology of cutaneous nerve terminal degeneration in the human skin. *Acta Neuropathol* 2001;**102**(5):455–61.

37. Periquet MI, Novak V, Collins MP, *et al*. Painful sensory neuropathy: prospective evaluation using skin biopsy. *Neurology* 1999;**53**(8):1641–7.

38. Nolano M, Provitera V, Crisci C, *et al*. Small fibers involvement in Friedreich's ataxia. *Ann Neurol* 2001;**50**(1):17–25.

39. Nolano M, Provitera V, Perretti A, *et al*. Ross syndrome: a rare or a misknown disorder of thermoregulation? A skin innervation study on 12 subjects. *Brain* 2006;**129**:(Pt 8): 2119–31.

40. Nolano M, Provitera V, Estraneo A, *et al*. Sensory deficit in Parkinson's disease: evidence of a cutaneous denervation. *Brain* 2008;**13**:1903–11.

41. Hoitsma E, Marziniak M, Faber CG, *et al*. Small fiber neuropathy in sarcoidosis. *Lancet* 2002;**359**(9323):2085–6.

42. Pittenger GL, Ray M, Burcus NI, McNulty P, Basta B, Vinik AI. Intraepidermal nerve fibers are indicators of small-fiber neuropathy in both diabetic and nondiabetic patients. *Diabetes Care* 2004;**27**(8):1974–9.

43. Boucek P, Havrdova T, Voska L, *et al*. Epidermal innervation in type 1 diabetic patients: a 2.5-year prospective study after simultaneous pancreas/kidney transplantation. *Diabetes Care* 2008;**31**(8):1611–2.

44. Boucek P, Havrdova T, Voska L, *et al*. Severe depletion of intraepidermal nerve fibers in skin biopsies of pancreas transplant recipients. *Transplant Proc* 2005;**37**(8):3574–5.

45. Sorensen L, Molyneaux L, Yue DK. The relationship among pain, sensory loss, and small nerve fibers in diabetes. *Diabetes Care* 2006;**29**(4):883–7.

46. Davis MD, Weenig RH, Genebriera J, Wendelschafer-Crabb G, Kennedy WR, Sandroni P. Histopathologic findings in primary erythromelalgia are nonspecific: special studies show a decrease in small nerve fiber density. *J Am Acad Dermatol* 2006;**55**(3):519–22.

47. Walk D, Wendelschafer-Crabb G, Davey C, Kennedy WR. Concordance between epidermal nerve fiber density and sensory examination in patients with symptoms of idiopathic small fiber neuropathy. *J Neurol Sci* 2007;**255**(1–2): 23–6.

48. Scherens A, Maier C, Haussleiter IS, *et al*. Painful or painless lower limb dysesthesias are highly predictive of peripheral neuropathy: comparison of different diagnostic modalities. *Eur J Pain* 2009;**13**(7):711–8.

49. Obermann M, Katsarava Z, Esser S, *et al.* Correlation of epidermal nerve fiber density with pain-related evoked potentials in HIV neuropathy. *Pain* 2008;**138**(1):79–86.

50. Uluc K, Temucin CM, Ozdamar SE, Demirci M, Tan E. Near-nerve needle sensory and medial plantar nerve conduction studies in patients with small-fiber sensory neuropathy. *Eur J Neurol* 2008;**15**(9):928–32.

51. Vlckova-Moravcova E, Bednarik J, Dusek L, Toyka KV, Sommer C. Diagnostic validity of epidermal nerve fiber densities in painful sensory neuropathies. *Muscle Nerve* 2008;**30**(37):50–60.

52. Wopking S, Scherens A, Haussleiter IS, *et al.* Significant difference between three observers in the assessment of intraepidermal nerve fiber density in skin biopsy. *BMC Neurol* 2009;**9**:13.

53. Wendelschafer-Crabb G, Kennedy WR, Walk D. Morphological features of nerves in skin biopsies. *J Neurol Sci* 2006;**242**(1-2):15–21.

54. Ebenezer GJ, Hauer P, Gibbons C, McArthur JC, Polydefkis M. Assessment of epidermal nerve fibers: a new diagnostic and predictive tool for peripheral neuropathies. *J Neuropathol Exp Neurol* 2007;**66**(12):1059–73.

55. Chai J, Herrmann DN, Stanton M, Barbano RL, Logigian EL. Painful small-fiber neuropathy in Sjogren syndrome. *Neurology* 2005;**65**:925–7.

56. Herrmann DN, McDermott MP, Henderson D, Chen L, Akowuah K, Schifitto G. Epidermal nerve fiber density, axonal swellings and QST as predictors of HIV distal sensory neuropathy. *Muscle Nerve* 2004;**29**(3):420–7.

57. Brannagan TH 3rd, Hays AP, Chin SS, *et al.* Small-fiber neuropathy/neuronopathy associated with celiac disease: skin biopsy findings. *Arch Neurol* 2005;**62**(10):1574–8.

58. De Sousa EA, Hays AP, Chin RL, Sander HW, Brannagan TH 3rd. Characteristics of patients with sensory neuropathy diagnosed with abnormal small nerve fibers on skin biopsy. *J Neurol Neurosurg Psychiatry* 2006;**77**(8):983–5.

59. Quattrini C, Tavakoli M, Jeziorska M, *et al.* Surrogate markers of small fiber damage in human diabetic neuropathy. *Diabetes* 2007;**56**(8):2148–54.

60. Quattrini C, Jeziorska M, Boulton AJ, Malik RA. Reduced vascular endothelial growth factor expression and intra-epidermal nerve fiber loss in human diabetic neuropathy. *Diabetes Care* 2008;**31**(1):140–5.

61. Vlckova-Moravcova E, Bednarik J, Belobradkova J, Sommer C. Small-fiber involvement in diabetic patients with neuropathic foot pain. *Diabet Med* 2008;**25**(6):692–9.

62. Loseth S, Stalberg E, Jorde R, Mellgren SI. Early diabetic neuropathy: thermal thresholds and intraepidermal nerve fiber density in patients with normal nerve conduction studies. *J Neurol* 2008;**255**(8):1197–202.

63. Tseng MT, Hsieh SC, Shun CT, *et al.* Skin denervation and cutaneous vasculitis in systemic lupus erythematosus. *Brain* 2006;**129**(Pt 4):977–85.

64. Chao CC, Hsieh ST, Shun CT, Hsieh SC. Skin denervation and cutaneous vasculitis in eosinophilia-associated neuropathy. *Arch Neurol* 2007;**64**(7):959–65.

65. Zhou L, Kitch DW, Evans SR, *et al.* Correlates of epidermal nerve fiber densities in HIV-associated distal sensory polyneuropathy. *Neurology* 2007;**68**(24):2113–9.

66. Herrmann DN, McDermott MP, Sowden JE, *et al.* Is skin biopsy a predictor of transition to symptomatic HIV neuropathy? A longitudinal study. *Neurology* 2006;**66**(6):857–61.

67. Polydefkis M, Yiannoutsos CT, Cohen BA, *et al.* Reduced intraepidermal nerve fiber density in HIV-associated sensory neuropathy. *Neurology* 2002;**58**(1):115–9.

68. Uluc K, Isak B, Borucu D, *et al.* Medial plantar and dorsal sural nerve conduction studies increase the sensitivity in the detection of neuropathy in diabetic patients. *Clin Neurophysiol* 2008;**119**(4):880–5.

69. Smith AG, Russell J, Feldman EL, *et al.* Lifestyle intervention for pre-diabetic neuropathy. *Diabetes Care* 2006;**29**(6):1294–9.

70. Hahn K, Triolo A, Hauer P, McArthur JC, Polydefkis M. Impaired reinnervation in HIV infection following experimental denervation. *Neurology* 2007;**68**:1251–6.

71. Polydefkis M, Hauer P, Sheth S, Sirdofsky M, Griffin JW, McArthur JC. The time course of epidermal nerve fiber regeneration: studies in normal controls and in people with diabetes, with and without neuropathy. *Brain* 2004;**127**:(Pt 7):1606–15.

CHAPTER 8

Assessment of neuropathic pain

G. Cruccu,[1] C. Sommer,[2] P. Anand,[3] N. Attal,[4] R. Baron,[5] L. Garcia-Larrea,[6]
M. Haanpää,[7] T. S. Jensen,[8] J. Serra,[9] R.-D. Treede[10]

[1]La Sapienza University, Rome, Italy; [2]University of Würzburg, Germany; [3]Imperial College London, UK; [4]Hôpital Ambroise Paré, APHP, Boulogne-Billancourt, France; [5]Universitatsklinikum Schleswig-Holstein, Kiel, Germany; [6]Hôpital Neurologique, Lyon, France; [7]Helsinki University Hospital, Finland; [8]Aarhus University Hospital, Denmark; [9]MC Mutual, Barcelona, Spain; [10]Heidelberg University, Mannheim, Germany

Background and objectives

Neuropathic pain is a major symptom that may be intractable in common neurological disorders such as neuropathy, spinal cord injury, multiple sclerosis, and stroke. Pain is a complex sensation strongly modulated by cognitive influences, and understanding the underlying pathophysiological mechanisms in patients remains a challenge for pain specialists. The EFNS launched a task force that published guidelines for the assessment of neuropathic pain to address an unmet clinical need [1]. The aim of this new task force was to revise the previous guidelines, in accord with evidence-based studies published thereafter. We have now done so, drawing in part on similar work in this field by the neuropathic pain special interest group (NeuPSIG) of the International Association for the Study of Pain (IASP).

Search methods

Search methods adhered to those used in previous guidelines [1], and complied with EFNS recommendations [2]. Briefly, after an initial search through the central database in the Cochrane Library, MEDLINE, and other electronic databases (2004 to the present), two task force

European Handbook of Neurological Management: Volume 1, 2nd edition. Edited by N. E. Gilhus, M. P. Barnes and M. Brainin.

participants were assigned to check the sorted material per method of assessment, i.e. screening tools and questionnaires, quantitative sensory testing, microneurography, reflexes and evoked potentials, functional neuroimaging, and skin biopsy. Pertinent studies were rated for evidence level according to EFNS rules [2] whenever applicable; in some instances, such as for statements generally accepted or demonstrated by basic neuroscience, we did not give an evidence level; adequately powered systematic reviews (SR) were considered Class I.

Considerations on the methods of assessment in light of the new definition and grading system

According to a new proposal, neuropathic pain (NP) is 'Pain arising as a direct consequence of a lesion or disease affecting the somatosensory system' [3]. This proposal represents a strengthening of the old IASP definition [4] by eliminating 'dysfunction' of the nervous system as a possible cause and by requiring a specific lesion of the somatosensory system. It is clear that NP is not a single disease but represents a syndrome, i.e. a constellation of specific symptoms and signs with multiple potential underlying aetiologies. Hence an accurate neurological history and neurological examination, including sensory testing, is most important in order to reach a diagnosis and to postulate the presence of a neuropathic pain syndrome. The elucidation of underlying disease aetiology and the dissection of pain will in practice often occur simultaneously. However, for clarification, the following is a brief description of steps in assessing a neuropathic pain syndrome.

1 The history will indicate if the character and distribution of the pain is in accord with neuropathic criteria, and if a relevant lesion or disease in the nervous system is likely to be responsible for the pain.

2 The clinical examination will determine the presence of negative (loss of function) and positive (hyperalgesia and/or allodynia) sensory signs, for one or more sensory modalities affecting the somatosensory system, and their relevance to the underlying disease or lesion.

3 Further diagnostic tests can be conducted to either document the presence of a specific underlying neurological disease (e.g. imaging of the brain to document a stroke in a patient with suspected post-stroke pain) or confirm a sensory lesion within the pain distribution (e.g. skin biopsy to document presence of small fibre loss in cases with small fibre neuropathy).

Based on this stepwise assessment, it has been suggested that patients can be categorized into possible NP (fulfilling step 1 above), probable NP (fulfilling step 1 with supporting evidence for *either* lesion/disease *or* pain distribution according to step B or C), and definite NP (fulfilling step A with supporting evidence for *both* lesion/disease *and* pain distribution according to step B or C) [3].

So far there are no studies to document the effectiveness of this diagnostic grading system. Recently, simple questionnaires and/or combinations with sensory examinations have been introduced (e.g. Class I; [5]) for these to partially substitute or contribute to diagnosing NP. In a new proposal, using standardized questions and testing a few somatosensory functions, a high degree of specificity and sensitivity has been obtained for certain types of NP; the diagnostic sensitivity of the interview and sensory examination exceeded that obtained with a relevant imaging technique (Class I; [6]).

Recommendations

History and clinical examination is a requirement to confirm the presence of a neuropathic pain syndrome, and also an important step in reaching an aetiological diagnosis for NP (Good Practice Point, GPP).

Screening and assessment tools

Several tools essentially based on pain descriptors have been proposed for the purpose of distinguishing NP from non-neuropathic pain (screening tools) or characterizing multiple neuropathic phenotypes (assessment tools).

Screening tools

The development of the McGill Pain Questionnaire (MPQ) revealed that pain quality descriptors vary across different pain conditions [7]. The lack of specificity of the MPQ for NP has led to development of screening tools for the recognition of NP. Interestingly, these tools generally share similar clinical characteristics.

The Leeds Assessment of Neuropathic Symptoms and Signs (LANSS) contains five symptom items and two clinical examination items (Class I; [8]). It has also been validated as a self-report tool, the S-LANSS (Class I; [9]). Compared to clinical diagnosis, its sensitivity and specificity ranges are 82–91% and 80–94% respectively. The S-LANSS has also been used in epidemiological studies in the general population.

The Neuropathic Pain Questionnaire (NPQ) contains 12 items (of them 10 sensory and two affective) (Class I; [10]). It demonstrated 66% sensitivity and 74% specificity compared with clinical diagnosis in the validation sample, but the aetiologies of pain were not reported. The short form of the NPQ (three items) has similar discriminative properties (Class II; [11]). It has been found able to discriminate between NP and non-NP in patients referred to a specialist pain clinic.

The Douleur Neuropathique en 4 questions (DN4) contains seven items related to symptoms and three related to clinical examination (Class I; [5]). A total score ≈ 4 out of 10 suggests NP. The DN4 showed 83% sensitivity and 90% specificity when compared with clinical diagnosis in the development study. The seven sensory descriptors can be used as a self-report questionnaire with similar results. The tool was developed and validated in French and translated into 15 languages. The DN4 has been used in epidemiological studies in general population and diabetics.

PainDETECT was developed and validated in German (Class I; [12]) and is available in several other languages. It is a self-report questionnaire with nine items. It correctly classifies 83% of patients to their diagnostic group with 85% sensitivity and 80% specificity.

ID-Pain consists of five sensory descriptor items and one item relating to whether pain is located in the joints (Class II; [13]). In the validation study, 22% of the nociceptive group, 39% of the mixed group, and 58% of the neuropathic group scored more than 3 points, the recommended cut-off score; the exact sensitivity and specificity of the tool using this cut-off compared to clinical diagnosis was not reported.

The StEP (standardized evaluation of pain) was recently validated to identify NP in patients with chronic low back pain categorized into 'axial' (non neuropathic) or 'radicular' (neuropathic) low-back pain (Class I; [6]). It contains 10 physical tests and six questions, thus emphasizing clinical examination. Several symptoms (e.g. burning pain) are scored negatively, suggesting that they are less likely in NP, which is in contrast with the other screening tools. This may reflect specificities related to low-back pain or difficulties inherent to the classification of low-back pain patients [14].

Assessment questionnaires

Although the McGill Pain Questionnaire (MPQ) [7] and the short-form McGill questionnaire (SF-MPQ) [15] have not been validated for NP assessment, the SF-MPQ has been the most commonly used quality assessment tool. However, it is not more sensitive to change than unidimensional intensity scales. To overcome this limitation, the SF-MPQ 2 [16] has been recently developed as a measure of neuropathic and non-neuropathic symptoms, but it is not fully validated.

The Neuropathic Pain Scale (NPS) (Class I; [17]), the first pain quality assessment tool devoted to NP assessment, has been translated into 24 languages and used in several NP trials. However, it lacks several pain qualities commonly seen in NP and is fully validated only in multiple sclerosis. To overcome these limitations, the Pain Quality Assessment Scale (PQAS) has been derived from the NPS [18]. To date no data exist regarding its use in blinded NP trials.

The Neuropathic Pain Symptom Inventory (NPSI) was originally validated in French (Class I; [19]) and has been submitted to linguistic validation in 50 other languages. One study found that several NP dimensions of the NPSI were particularly sensitive to treatment effect. The factorial structure of the NPSI makes it suitable to capture different aspects of NP with presumably distinct mechanisms.

Recommendations

The main advantage of screening tools is to identify potential patients with NP, particularly by non-specialists (grade A). However, these tools fail to identify 10 to 20% of patients with clinician diagnosed NP, showing that they cannot replace careful clinical judgement. They have also been used in epidemiological studies, but validation studies for this purpose are necessary. More research is also needed to clarify whether they can predict response to therapy.

Pain quality assessment measures are useful to discriminate among various pain mechanisms associated with distinct dimensions of NP experience (grade B). The NPS or NPSI are recommended to evaluate treatment effects on neuropathic symptoms or their combination (grade A), but should also be used in future trials to try to predict treatment outcome and better define responder profiles. Assessment of the sensory and affective dimensions of pain can be performed with the SF-MPQ scale, but whether such assessment is more sensitive than the pain intensity measures remains to be confirmed. The SF-MPQ-2 and the PQAS have not yet been fully evaluated in NP.

Quantitative sensory testing

Quantitative sensory testing (QST) is a psychophysiological measure of perception in response to external stimuli of controlled intensity. Detection and pain thresholds are determined by applying stimuli to the skin in an ascending and descending order of magnitude. Mechanical sensitivity for tactile stimuli is measured using von Frey hairs or Semmes-Weinstein monofilaments, pinprick sensation with weighted needles, and vibration sensitivity with a tuning fork or an electronic vibrameter; thermal perception and thermal pain are measured using a probe that operates on the Peltier principle (for references see previous guidelines [1]).

The main problem with studies using QST as a diagnostic tool remains that of blinding, with only four studies (out of some 50 new studies) being prospective, in a broad spectrum of patients and controls, and having blinded examiners (Class I/II; [20–23]). The variability of methods, results and patient population (diabetic neuropathy, spinal cord injury, radiculopathy) prevents any conclusion. We must also emphasize that QST changes were also found in non-neuropathic pain states, such as rheumatoid arthritis, inflammatory arthromyalgias, and fibromyalgia (although all these studies are Class IV, e.g. [24]).

Most QST studies are still dedicated to the assessment of sensory small-fibre function only, assuming that large fibre function was probably documented by standard clinical neurophysiology. This bias precludes any analysis on the relative importance of small versus large sensory fibre function deficits in neuropathic pain syndromes. However, extensive validation data for all somatosensory submodalities have now been published by the German Research Network on Neuropathic Pain [25, 26]. QST is used for diagnosis and follow-up of small fibre neuropathy (all Class IV; e.g. [27, 28]) and its usefulness is agreed in the early diagnosis of diabetic neuropathy (SR Class I; [1]).

QST is particularly appropriate to quantify positive sensory phenomena, such as mechanical and thermal allodynia and hyperalgesia, which may help characterize painful neuropathic syndromes and predict or monitor treatment effects. In particular, pharmacological and non-pharmacological treatment trials using QST found effects on dynamic mechanical allodynia, pinprick hyperalgesia, and sensory loss, whereas treatment efficacy was predicted by thermal detection thresholds, vibration detection thresholds, heat hyperalgesia, and dynamic mechanical allodynia (Class I/II; [29–36]).

Recommendations

QST can be used in the clinic along with bedside testing to document the sensory profile. Because abnormalities have often been reported in non-neuropathic pains as well, QST cannot be considered sufficient to separate differential diagnoses (GPP). QST is helpful to quantify the effects of treatments on allodynia and hyperalgesia and may reveal a differential efficacy of treatments on different pain components (grade A). To evaluate mechanical allodynia/hyperalgesia, we recommend the use of simple tools such as a brush and at least one high-intensity weighted pinprick or von Frey filament (e.g. 128 mN). The evaluation of pain in response to thermal stimuli is best performed using the computerized thermotest, but we do not recommend the systematic measure of thermal stimuli except for pathophysiological research or treatment trials. A simple and sensitive tool to quantify pain induced by thermal stimuli in clinical practice is still lacking.

Neurophysiology

We wish to remind readers that our previous guidelines recommended the standard nerve conduction study,

although it does not provide information on small-fibre function, as a most useful tool for documenting and assessing peripheral neuropathies.

Microneurography

Microneurography is a minimally invasive technique in which single-axon recordings from peripheral nerves are made in awake subjects and provides valuable information on the physiology and pathophysiology of all nerve fibre groups. Because it can discriminate individual action potentials in single, identified peripheral fibres, microneurography is nowadays the only technique able to record and quantify positive sensory phenomena mediated by large-myelinated fibres (tactile paresthesias and dysesthesias) or small-myelinated and unmyelinated fibres (spontaneous pains). The possibility of performing intraneural microstimulation may provide a direct link between activity in peripheral nerve fibres and pain perception [37]. Because prospective studies monitoring side effects of the technique did not find overt or persistent nerve damage [38, 39], microneurography is considered a relatively safe technique if performed by experienced examiners [40].

Microneurography is time-consuming and requires both an expert investigator and a collaborative patient. Furthermore, microneurography is currently performed only in a few centres around the world. For these reasons it has only been used on very few occasions to study neuropathic pain patients. There are no published normative data for healthy subjects, and published reports are unblinded group comparisons only (Class IV).

New developments in analysis software now allow multiple simultaneous recordings of C-fibres, thus enhancing the possibility of studying ongoing abnormal activity arising from peripheral nociceptors, which is considered a possible cause for spontaneous pain in patients with peripheral neuropathies [41–44].

Pain-related reflexes

Pain-related reflexes appear to be diagnostically useful only for facial pains. Two Class I studies [45, 46] and the recent AAN-EFNS guidelines on trigeminal neuralgia management (SR Class I: [47, 48]) confirmed that the Aβ-mediated trigeminal reflexes (early R1 blink reflex and early SP1 masseter inhibitory reflex) are efficient tools to reveal symptomatic forms of trigeminal neuralgia, yielding an overall specificity of 94% and sensitivity of 87% in over 600 patients. Six other studies used blink reflexes in facial pains. Although four studies were Class IV, one Class I study in patients with ophthalmic postherpeutic neuralgia (PHN) yielded a specificity of 100% and sensitivity of 73% for the early R1 blink reflex [49] and one Class III study found that the nociceptive blink reflex (elicited by the concentric electrode) was delayed in patients with atypical odontalgia, thus supporting the view that this condition is neuropathic [50].

For the upper limb, the cutaneous silent period (CSP, an inhibitory reflex recorded from the small hand muscles after noxious stimulation of the fingers) was assessed in two studies, one in distal symmetric polyneuropathy (Class III; [51]) and the other in carpal tunnel syndrome (Class I; [52]). In neither study did CSP differentiate patients with and without pain, and this measure did not correlate with pain. This confirms the conclusions of the previous guidelines [1], that the CSP is not an adequate tool for assessing nociception. Regarding the lower limb, the nociceptive flexion reflex (RIII) is still being used in physiological and pharmacological studies of modulation of nociception, but not in patients with neuropathic pain.

Pain-related evoked potentials

According to the previous EFNS guidelines on neuropathic pain assessment (SR Class I; [1]), and the Recommendations from the International Federation of Clinical Neurophysiology (SR Class I; [53]), laser-evoked potentials (LEPs) are the easiest and most reliable of the neurophysiological methods for assessing function of nociceptive pathways.

Many new studies have investigated Aδ-mediated fibre pathways in a total of more than 300 patients with neuropathic pain: five studies used LEPs, three the contact-heat evoked potentials [54], and three evoked potentials elicited by a surface concentric electrode that provides a preferential activation of superficial terminals (i.e. small-diameter afferents) [55]. Although all techniques revealed significant sensory abnormalities when compared with controls or contralateral side, and several showed significant correlations with pain, only three studies – all using LEPs – were Class I; those using other techniques were all Class III/IV. The LEP studies investigated patients with sensory neuropathy [56], PHN [49], and carpal tunnel syndrome [52]. A cumulated analysis of these three Class I studies revealed a highly significant difference to con-

trols, with high specificity but low sensitivity (considering the responses to be certainly abnormal only when absent; sensitivity would increase considerably if the recently recommended normal limits of amplitude were used [SR Class I; [53]]).

One study only dealt with C-fibre-related LEPs (elicited from the trigeminal territory) (Class I; [49]). The recording of C-LEPs after limb stimulation is probably still technically difficult for reliable clinical applications.

Recommendations

Thus far, microneurography cannot be suggested as a routine procedure for the assessment of patients with peripheral neuropathic pain (GPP). However, we encourage new studies in selected groups of patients with neuropathic pain to understand the frequency and pathophysiological role of spontaneous ectopic activity, and the potential efficacy of drugs in reducing ectopic impulse generation in peripheral nociceptors.

The trigeminal reflexes mediated by Aδ-mediated fibres are useful in the diagnosis of trigeminal pain disorders as they are abnormal in patients with structural damage, in conditions such as trigeminal neuropathy and PHN, and normal in patients with classic trigeminal neuralgia (grade A). The cutaneous silent period is probably inadequate for neuropathic pain assessment (grade B).

Laser-evoked potentials are useful for assessing function of the Aδ-mediated fibre pathways in patients with neuropathic pain (grade A). Other evoked potential techniques that do not use laser stimulators are not supported by evidence-based studies that demonstrate their diagnostic value.

The available evidence regarding evoked potentials for assessing the C-fibre pathways (with any method of stimulation) is so far insufficient to make recommendations.

Functional neuroimaging

Positron emission tomography (PET) and functional magnetic resonance imaging (fMRI) use different methods to measure cerebral blood flow or metabolic activity in defined brain regions. Activation studies investigate local synaptic changes specifically associated with a given task or a particular stimulus by comparing statistically activated and control conditions. Functional neuroimaging has disclosed a network of brain regions jointly activated by noxious stimuli (labelled 'pain matrix'). Activation of the lateral thalamus, SI-SII, and posterior insula are thought to be related to the sensory–discriminative aspects of pain processing, while mid-anterior cingulate, posterior parietal, and prefrontal cortices participate in the affective and attentional concomitants of pain sensation [57, 58]. In unilateral spontaneous neuropathic pain, moderate but converging evidence from independent groups indicates decreased resting rCBF in contralateral thalamus, and reversal of this abnormality by analgesic procedures (but only case reports or small series with fewer than than 20 patients; [59–62]). Should this be confirmed in larger series, thalamic hypoperfusion might be used in the future as a marker of neuropathic pain, and restoration of thalamic blood flow for treatment monitoring. In patients with provoked neuropathic pain, allodynia and hyperalgesia have been associated with amplification of the thalamic, insular, SI, SII, and prefrontal-orbitofrontal responses, but not anterior-perigenual cingulate [58, 62–65]. Neuropathic allodynia has been shown to enhance insular activity ipsilateral to pain [64, 66, 67] suggesting that a shift in hemispheric balance might contribute to the allodynic experience. Again, the total number of reported patients ($n=80$) is still too small to support any diagnostic application; however, neuropathic allodynia has shown a different activation pattern than non-neuropathic allodynia (e.g. CRPS-I; [68]), which may open diagnostic perspectives. Opioid-receptor imaging has demonstrated different abnormalities in central and peripheral neuropathic pain [69–71] but the predictive value of these findings remains unknown. Assessing the effect of analgesic drugs on pain-related brain activity will provide a better understanding of pain and analgesia and hence the development of novel therapeutic strategies.

However, data in patients are still scarce and in most studies examiners were unblinded. Hence no graded recommendation could be drawn in the frame of the EFNS classification for diagnostic procedures. The comments below represent our expert opinion.

Recommendations

Studies in neuropathic pain patients have lagged far behind equivalent studies in acute pain. There is converging evidence that chronic spontaneous neuropathic pain is associated with decreased activity in the contralateral thalamus, whereas provoked neuropathic pain is associated with increased activity in the thalamic, insular, and somatosensory regions. In view of the potential relevance of these data, we encourage functional neuroimaging studies in patients with neuropathic pain.

Skin biopsy

A punch biopsy of the skin in the painful area allows immunostaining and visualisation of the intraepidermal terminals of Aä and C nerve fibres, and thus measurement of the intra-epidermal nerve fibre density (IENFD). Standardized counting rules for IENFD are required to obtain reproducible results (SR Class I; [72, 73]). In experienced centres, the sensitivity and specificity of IENFD are 88% (SR Class I; [72], Class II; [27]).

In patients with painful feet and a normal nerve conduction study, a small-fibre neuropathy can be demonstrated by IENFD (Class II/III; [27, 74–76]). Several studies have investigated the correlation between skin biopsy findings and other tests of small-fibre function. Contact heat-evoked potentials correlated significantly with IENFD (Class III; [77]). In small-fibre neuropathy, the sensitivity of IENFD may be higher that that of QST (Class II/III; [27, 75, 78]) and LEPs (Class II; [27]). Although in patients with diabetic or HIV neuropathy, IENFD was inversely correlated with pain (Class III; [75, 79]), in other conditions it was not (Class II; [27]).

Old and recent studies in PHN patients showed that IENFD in the area of pain is lower than in contralateral mirror-image skin (Class II; [80, 81]), and that the relative sparing of cutaneous innervation was associated with allodynia, thus suggesting that allodynia was related to the surviving 'irritable' nociceptors (Class II; [81, 82]).

Quantitative and qualitative changes in skin innervation have been reported in CRPS (Class III/IV; [83, 84]).

Recommendations

Skin biopsy should be performed in patients with painful/burning feet of unknown origin and clinical impression of small-fibre dysfunction (grade B). In PHN, skin innervation is reduced (grade B), and higher numbers of preserved fibres are associated with allodynia (grade B). IENFD shows only a weak negative correlation with the severity of pain, and cannot be used to measure pain in individual patients (grade C).

Conclusions

The majority of previous recommendations were reinforced by recent studies. The new definition of neuropathic pain and the diagnostic grading system will

Table 8.1 Summary of choice methods of assessing nerve function per sensation.

Fibres	Sensation	Clinical testing	QST[1]	Laboratory
Aβ	Touch	Piece of cotton wool	von Frey filaments	Nerve conduction studies,
	Vibration	Tuning fork (128 Hz)	[2]Vibrameter	[3]SEPs
Aδ	Pinprick	Cocktail stick	weighted needles	[4]LEPs
	Cold	Thermoroller	[5]Thermotest	–
C	Warmth	Thermoroller	[5]Thermotest	Skin biopsy
	Burning	–	[5]Thermotest	

[1]Quantitative Sensory Testing;
[2]or other device providing graded vibratory stimuli;
[3]somatosensory evoked potentials;
[4]laser evoked potentials;
[5]or other device providing graded thermal stimuli. Note the lack of suitable methods of assessing burning in a clinical setting and cold with a laboratory tool.

probably lead to more accurate diagnosis in clinical practice and research studies. History and bedside examination are still fundamental to a correct diagnosis. The previous lack of questionnaires and screening tools explicitly dedicated to neuropathic pain has been resolved by a number of new validated tools. Laboratory techniques methods that were restricted to research, such as QST, LEPs, and IEFND, are being used more widely in clinical practice and trials. Among these methods of assessment, QST is the best for provoked pains and the response to treatment, LEPs are the best for Aä pathways, and IEFND for C-fibre loss in distal axonal neuropathies (table 8.1).

Conflicts of interest

The authors did not receive specific funding to write this article, or any financial support from sources with a commercial interest in this subject. The authors also declare that they have no competing interests.

References

1. Cruccu G, Anand P, Attal N, *et al*. EFNS guidelines on neuropathic pain assessment. *Eur J Neurol* 2004;**11**: 153–62.

2. Brainin M, Barnes M, Baron JC, *et al*. Guideline Standards Subcommittee of the EFNS Scientific Committee. Guidance for the preparation of neurological management guidelines by EFNS scientific task forces – revised recommendations. *Eur J Neurol* 2004;**11**:577–81.

3. Treede RD, Jensen TS, Campbell JN, *et al*. Neuropathic pain: redefinition and a grading system for clinical and research purposes. *Neurology* 2008;**70**:1630–5.

4. Merskey H, Bogduk N. *Classification of Chronic Pain: Descriptions of Chronic Pain Syndromes and Definitions of Pain Terms*. Seattle: IASP Press, 1994.

5. Bouhassira D, Attal N, Alchaar H, *et al*. Comparison of pain syndromes associated with nervous or somatic lesions and development of a new neuropathic pain diagnostic questionnaire (DN4). *Pain* 2005;**114**:29–36.

6. Scholz J, Mannion RJ, Hord DE, *et al*. A novel tool for the assessment of pain: validation in low back pain. *Plos Med* 2009;e1000047.

7. Melzack R. The MacGill Pain Questionnaire: major properties and scoring methods. *Pain* 1975;**1**:275–99.

8. Bennett MI, Smith BH, Torrance N, Potter J. The S-LANSS score for identifying pain of predominantly neuropathic origin: validation for use in clinical and postal research. *J Pain* 2005;**6**:149–58.

9. Bennett MI. The LANSS Pain Scale: the Leeds assessment of neuropathic symptoms and signs. *Pain* 2001;**92**:147–57.

10. Krause SJ, Backonja M. Development of a neuropathic pain questionnaire. *Clin J Pain* 2003;**19**:306–14.

11. Backonja MM, Krause SJ. Neuropathic Pain Questionnaire – short form. *Clin J Pain* 2003;**19**:315–6.

12. Freynhagen R, Baron R, Gockel U, Tolle T. PainDetect: a new screeing questionnaire to detect neuropathic components in patients with back pain. *Curr Med Res Opin* 2006;**22**:1911–20.

13. Portenoy R for the ID Pain Steering Committee. Development and testing of a neuropathic pain screening questionnaire: ID Pain. *Curr Med Res Opin* 2006;**22**:1555–65.

14. Cruccu G, Truini A. Tools for assessing neuropathic pain. *Plos Med* 2009;(6):e1000045.

15. Melzack R. The short-form McGill Pain Questionnaire. *Pain* 1987;**30**:191–7.

16. Dworkin RH, Turk DC, Revicki DA, *et al*. Development and initial validation of an expanded and revised version of the Short-form McGill Pain Questionnaire (SF-MPQ-2). *Pain* 2009;**144**:35–42.

17. Galer BS, Jensen MP. Development and preliminary validation of a pain measure specific to neuropathic pain: the Neuropathic Pain Scale. *Neurology* 1997;**48**:332–8.

18. Jensen MP, Friedman M, Bonzo D, Richards P. The validity of the neuropathic pain scale for assessing diabetic neuropathic pain in a clinical trial. *Clin J Pain* 2006;**22**:97–103.

19. Bouhassira D, Attal N, Fermanian J, *et al*. Development and validation of the neuropathic pain symptom inventory. *Pain* 2004;**108**:248–57.

20. Chien A, Eliav E, Sterling M. Whiplash (grade II) and cervical radiculopathy share a similar sensory presentation: an investigation using quantitative sensory testing. *Clin J Pain* 2008;**24**:595–603.

21. Finnerup NB, Sørensen L, Biering-Sørensen F, Johannesen IL, Jensen TS. Segmental hypersensitivity and spinothalamic function in spinal cord injury pain. *Exp Neurol* 2007;**207**:139–49.

22. Freynhagen R, Rolke R, Baron R, *et al*. Pseudoradicular and radicular low-back pain – a disease continuum rather than different entities? Answers from quantitative sensory testing. *Pain* 2008;**135**:65–74.

23. Rader AJ. Surgical decompression in lower-extremity diabetic peripheral neuropathy. *J Am Podiatr Med Assoc* 2005;**95**:446–50.

24. Geber C, Magerl W, Fondel R, *et al*. Numbness in clinical and experimental pain – a cross-sectional study exploring the mechanisms of reduced tactile function. *Pain* 2008;**139**:73–81.

25. Rolke R, Baron R, Maier C, *et al*. Quantitative sensory testing in the German Research Network on Neuropathic Pain (DFNS): standardized protocol and reference values. *Pain* 2006;**123**:231–43.

26. Rolke R, Magerl W, Campbell KA, *et al*. Quantitative sensory testing: a comprehensive protocol for clinical trials. *Eur J Pain* 2006;**10**:77–88.

27. Devigili G, Tugnoli V, Penza P, *et al*. The diagnostic criteria for small fibre neuropathy: from symptoms to neuropathology. *Brain* 2008;**131**:1912–25.

28. Laaksonen SM, Röyttä M, Jääskeläinen SK, Kantola I, Penttinen M, Falck B. Neuropathic symptoms and findings in women with Fabry disease. *Clin Neurophysiol* 2008;**119**:1365–72.

29. Attal N, Rouaud J, Brasseur L, Chauvin M, Bouhassira D. Systemic lidocaine in pain due to peripheral nerve injury and predictors of response. *Neurology* 2004;**62**:218–25.

30. Edwards RR, Haythornthwaite JA, Tella P, Max MB, Raja S. Basal heat pain thresholds predict opioid analgesia in patients with postherpetic neuralgia. *Anesthesiology* 2006;**104**:1243–8.

31. Finnerup NB, Biering-Sorensen F, Johannesen IL, *et al*. Intravenous lidocaine relieves spinal cord injury pain:a randomized controlled trial. *Anesthesiology* 2005;**102**:1023–30.

32. Herrmann DN, McDermott MP, Sowden JE, *et al*. Is skin biopsy a predictor of transition to symptomatic HIV neuropathy? A longitudinal study. *Neurology* 2006;**66**:857–61.

33. Krämer HH, Rolke R, Bickel A, Birklein F. Thermal thresholds predict painfulness of diabetic neuropathies. *Diabetes Care* 2004;**27**:2386–91.

34. Stiasny-Kolster K, Magerl W, Oertel WH, Möller JC, Treede RD. Static mechanical hyperalgesia without dynamic tactile allodynia in patients with restless legs syndrome. *Brain* 2004;**127**:773–82.

35. Wasner G, Kleinert A, Binder A, Schattschneider J, Baron R. Postherpetic neuralgia: topical lidocaine is effective in nociceptor-deprived skin. *J Neurol* 2005;**252**:677–86.

36. Yucel A, Ozyalcin S, Koknel Talu G, *et al*. The effect of venlafaxine on ongoing and experimentally induced pain in neuropathic pain patients: a double blind, placebo controlled study. *Eur J Pain* 2005;**9**:407–16.

37. Ochoa J, Torebjörk E. Sensations evoked by intraneural microstimulation of C nociceptor fibres in human skin nerves. *J Physiol* 1989;**415**:583–99.

38. Eckberg DL, Wallin BK, Fagius J, Lundberg L, Torebjörk HE. Prospective study of symptoms after human microneurography. *Acta Physiol Scand* 1989;**137**:567–9.

39. Littell H. After-effect of microneurography in humans. Part IV. *Phys Ther* 1981;**61**:1585–6.

40. Jørum E, Schmelz M. Chapter 29 Microneurography in the assessment of neuropathic pain. *Handb Clin Neurol* 2006;**81**:427–38.

41. Bostock H, Campero M, Serra J, Ochoa JL. Temperature-dependent double spikes in C-nociceptors of neuropathic pain patients. *Brain* 2005;**128**:2154–63.

42. Ochoa J, Campero M, Serra J, Bostock H. Hyperexcitable polymodal and insensitive nociceptors in painful human neuropathy. *Muscle Nerve* 2005;**32**:459–72.

43. Orstavik K, Jørum E. Microneurographic findings of relevance to pain in patients with erythromelalgia and patients with diabetic neuropathy. *Neurosci Lett* 2010;**470**:180–84.

44. Serra J, Campero M, Bostock H, Ochoa J. Two types of C nociceptors in human skin and their behavior in areas of

capsaicin-induced secondary hyperalgesia. *J Neurophysiol* 2004;**91**:2770–81.

45. Cruccu G, Biasiotta A, Di Rezze S, *et al*. Trigeminal neuralgia and pain related to multiple sclerosis. *Pain* 2009;**143**:186–91.

46. Cruccu G, Biasiotta A, Galeotti F, Iannetti GD, Truini A, Gronseth G. Diagnostic accuracy of trigeminal reflex testing in trigeminal neuralgia. *Neurology* 2006;**66**:139–41.

47. Cruccu G, Gronseth G, Alksne J, *et al*. AAN-EFNS guidelines on trigeminal neuralgia management. *Eur J Neurol* 2008;**15**:1013–28.

48. Gronseth G, Cruccu G, Alksne J, *et al*. Practice parameter: the diagnostic evaluation and treatment of trigeminal neuralgia (an evidence-based review): report of the Quality Standards Subcommittee of the American Academy of Neurology and the European Federation of Neurological Societies. *Neurology* 2008;**71**:1183–90.

49. Truini A, Galeotti F, Haanpaa M, *et al*. Pathophysiology of pain in postherpetic neuralgia: a clinical and neurophysiological study. *Pain* 2008;**140**:405–10.

50. Baad-Hansen L, List T, Kaube H, Jensen TS, Svensson P. Blink reflexes in patients with atypical odontalgia and matched healthy controls. *Exp Brain Res* 2006;**172**:498–506.

51. Truini A, Galeotti F, Biasiotta A, *et al*. Dissociation between cutaneous silent period and laser evoked potentials in assessing neuropathic pain. *Muscle Nerve* 2009;**39**:369–73.

52. Truini A, Padua L, Biasiotta A, *et al*. Differential involvement of A-delta and A-beta fibres in neuropathic pain related to carpal tunnel syndrome. *Pain* 2009;**145**:105–9.

53. Cruccu G, Aminoff MJ, Curio G, *et al*. Recommendations for the clinical use of somatosensory-evoked potentials. *Clin Neurophysiol* 2008;**119**:1705–19.

54. Granovsky Y, Matre D, Sokolik A, Lorenz J, Casey KL. Thermoreceptive innervation of human glabrous and hairy skin: a contact heat evoked potential analysis. *Pain* 2005;**115**:238–47.

55. Katsarava Z, Ayzenberg I, Sack F, Limmroth V, Diener HC, Kaube H. A novel method of eliciting pain-related potentials by transcutaneous electrical stimulation. *Headache* 2006;**46**:1511–7.

56. Lefaucheur JP, Créange A. Neurophysiological testing correlates with clinical examination according to fibre type involvement and severity in sensory neuropathy. *J Neurol Neurosurg Psychiatry* 2004;**75**:417–22.

57. Apkarian AV, Bushnell MC, Treede RD, Zubieta JK. Human brain mechanisms of pain perception and regulation in health and disease. *Eur J Pain* 2005;**9**:463–84.

58. Peyron R, Laurent B, Garcia-Larrea L. Functional imaging of pain. A review and meta-analysis. *Neurophysiol Clin* 2000;**30**:263–88.

59. Garcia-Larrea L, Maarrawi J, Peyron R, *et al*. On the relation between sensory deafferentation, pain and thalamic activity in Wallenberg's syndrome: a PET-scan study before and after motor cortex stimulation. *Eur J Pain* 2006;**10**:677–88.

60. Garcia-Larrea L, Peyron R, Mertens P, *et al*. Electrical stimulation of motor cortex for pain control: a combined PET-scan and electrophysiological study. *Pain* 1999;**83**:259–73.

61. Hsieh JC, Belfrage M, Stone-Elander S, Hansson P, Ingvar M. Central representation of chronic ongoing neuropathic pain studied by positron emission tomography. *Pain* 1995;**63**:225–36.

62. Iadarola MJ, Max MB, Berman KF, *et al*. Unilateral decrease in thalamic activity observed with positron emission tomography in patients with chronic neuropathic pain. *Pain* 1995;**63**:55–64.

63. Baron R, Baron Y, Disbrow E, Roberts TP. Brain processing of capsaicin-induced secondary hyperalgesia: a functional MRI study. *Neurology* 1999;**11**:548–57.

64. Peyron R, Schneider F, Faillenot I, *et al*. An fMRI study of cortical representation of mechanical allodynia in patients with neuropathic pain. *Neurology* 2004;**63**:1838–46.

65. Schweinhardt P, Glynn C, Brooks J, *et al*. An fMRI study of cerebral processing of brushevoked allodynia in neuropathic pain patients. *Neuroimage* 2006;**32**:256–65.

66. Ducreux D, Attal N, Parker F, Bouhassira D. Mechanisms of central neuropathic pain: a combined psychophysical and fMRI study in syringomyelia. *Brain* 2006;**129**:963–76.

67. Witting N, Kupers RC, Svensson P, Jensen TS. A PET activation study of brush-evoked allodynia in patients with nerve injury pain. *Pain* 2006;**120**:145–54.

68. Maihöfner C, Handwerker HO, Birklein F. Functional imaging of allodynia in complex regional pain syndrome. *Neurology* 2006;**66**:711–7.

69. Jones AK, Watabe H, Cunningham VJ, Jones T. Cerebral decreases in opioid receptor binding in patients with central neuropathic pain measured by [11 C] diprenorphine binding and PET. *Eur J Pain* 2004;**8**:479–85.

70. Maarrawi J, Peyron R, Mertens P, *et al*. Differential brain opioid receptor availability in central and peripheral neuropathic pain. *Pain* 2007;**127**:183–94.

71. Willoch F, Schindler F, Wester HJ, *et al*. Central poststroke pain and reduced opioid receptor binding within pain processing circuitries: a [11C]diprenorphine PET study. *Pain* 2004;**108**:213–20.

72. Lauria G, Cornblath DR, Johansson O, *et al*. EFNS guidelines on the use of skin biopsy in the diagnosis of peripheral neuropathy. *Eur J Neurol* 2005;**12**:747–58.

73. Sommer C, Lauria G. Skin biopsy in the management of peripheral neuropathy. *Lancet Neurol* 2007;**6**:632–42.

74. Gorson KC, Herrmann DN, Thiagarajan R, *et al*. Non-length dependent small fibre neuropathy/ganglionopathy. *J Neurol Neurosurg Psychiatry* 2008;**79**:163–9.

75. Scherens A, Maier C, Haussleiter IS, *et al*. Psychophysical and neuropathological findings in patients with dysaesthesias at the lower limb. *Eur J Pain* 2009;**13**:711–8.

76. Vlckova-Moravcova E, Bednarik J, Dusek L, *et al*. Diagnostic validity of epidermal nerve fiber densities in painful sensory neuropathies. *Muscle Nerve* 2008;**37**:50–60.

77. Atherton DD, Facer P, Roberts KM, *et al*. Use of the novel contact heat evoked potential stimulator (CHEPS) for the assessment of small fibre neuropathy: correlations with skin flare responses and intra-epidermal nerve fibre counts. *BMC Neurol* 2007;**7**:21.

78. Loseth S, Stalberg E, Jorde R, Mellgren SI. Early diabetic neuropathy: thermal thresholds and intraepidermal nerve fibre density in patients with normal nerve conduction studies. *J Neurol* 2008;**255**:1197–202.

79. Sorensen L, Molyneaux L, Yue DK. The relationship among pain, sensory loss, and small nerve fibers in diabetes. *Diabetes Care* 2006;**29**:883–7.

80. Oaklander AL. The density of remaining nerve endings in human skin with and without postherpetic neuralgia after shingles. *Pain* 2001;**92**:139–45.

81. Petersen KL, Fields HL, Brennum J, *et al*. Capsaicin evoked pain and allodynia in post-herpetic neuralgia. *Pain* 2000;**88**:125–33.

82. Rowbotham MC, Yosipovitch G, Connolly MK, *et al*. Cutaneous innervation density in the allodynic form of postherpetic neuralgia. *Neurobiol Dis* 1996;**3**:205–14.

83. Albrecht PJ, Hines S, Eisenberg E, *et al*. Pathologic alterations of cutaneous innervation and vasculature in affected limbs from patients with complex regional pain syndrome. *Pain* 2006;**120**:244–66.

84. Oaklander AL, Rissmiller JG, Gelman LB, *et al*. Evidence of focal small-fiber axonal degeneration in complex regional pain syndrome-I (reflex sympathetic dystrophy). *Pain* 2006;**120**:235–43.

CHAPTER 9

Ischaemic stroke and transient ischaemic attack*

P. A. Ringleb,[1] M.-G. Bousser,[2] G. Ford,[3] P. Bath,[4] M. Brainin,[5] V. Caso,[6] Á. Cervera,[7] A.l Chamorro,[7] Charlotte Cordonnier,[8] L. Csiba,[9] A. Davalos,[7] H.-C. Diener,[10] J. Ferro,[11] W. Hacke,[1] M. Hennerici,[12] M. Kaste,[13] P. Langhorne,[14] K. Lees,[14] D. Leys,[8] J. Lodder,[15] H. S. Markus,[16] J.-L. Mas,[2] H. P. Mattle,[17] K. Muir,[14] B. Norrving,[18] V. Obach,[7] S. Paolucci,[19] E. B. Ringelstein,[20] P. D. Schellinger,[21] J. Sivenius,[22] V. Skvortsova,[23] K. Stibrant Sunnerhagen,[24] L. Thomassen,[25] D. Toni,[19] R.r von Kummer,[26] N. Gunnar Wahlgren,[27] M. F. Walker,[28] J. Wardlaw[29]

[1]Heidelberg, Germany; [2]Paris, France; [3]Newcastle, UK; [4]Nottingham, UK; [5]Krems, Austria; [6]Perugia, Italy; [7]Barcelona, Spain; [8]Lille, France; [9]Debrecen, Hungary; [10]Essen, Germany; [11]Lisbon, Portugal; [12]Mannheim, Germany; [13]Helsinki, Finland; [14]Glasgow, UK; [15]Maastricht, The Netherlands; [16]London, UK; [17]Bern, Switzerland; [18]Lund, Sweden; [19]Rome, Italy; [20]Münster, Germany; [21]Erlangen, Germany; [22]Kuopio, Finland; [23]Moscow, Russia; [24]Göteborg, Sweden; [25]Bergen, Norway; [26]Dresden, Germany; [27]Stockholm, Sweden; [28]Nottingham, UK; [29]Edinburgh, UK

Preface

This article represents the update of the European Stroke Initiative (EUSI) Recommendations for Stroke Management, which were first published in 2000 [1, 2] and subsequently translated into a number of languages, including Spanish, Portuguese, Italian, German, Greek, Turkish, Lithuanian, Polish, Russian, and Mandarin Chinese. The first update of the recommendations was published in 2003 [2]. In 2006, the EUSI decided that a larger group of authors should prepare the next update. In the meantime, a new European Stroke Society, the European Stroke Organisation (ESO), was established and took over the task of updating the guidelines. Accordingly, the new recommendations have been prepared by members of both the former EUSI Recommendations Writing Committee and the ESO (see Appendix). The members of the Writing Group met in Heidelberg, Germany, for 3 days in December 2007 to finalize the new recommendations. The members of the Writing Committee were assigned to six groups covering different topics. Each group was co-chaired by two colleagues, and included up to five further experts. To avoid bias or conflict of interest none of the chairs had major involvement in clinical trials or studies discussed in their respective group. In addition, a detailed conflict of interest disclosure form is on file with the editor of the *European Journal of Neurology* and attached to the electronic version of this article. However, due to the large number of authors, the detailed disclosures are not listed in the printed article.

These guidelines cover both ischaemic stroke and transient ischaemic attacks (TIAs), which are now considered to be a single entity. If recommendations differ for the two conditions, this will be explicitly mentioned; otherwise the recommendations are valid for both conditions. Separate guidelines exist or are being prepared for intracerebral haemorrhage [3] and subarachnoid haemorrhage. The classes of evidence and levels of recommendations used in these guidelines are defined according to the criteria of the European Federation of Neurological Societies (EFNS) (table 9.1, table 9.2). The article

---

*The authors have prepared this guideline on behalf of the European Stroke Organisation (ESO) Executive Committee and the ESO Writing Committee

---

European Handbook of Neurological Management: Volume 1, 2nd edition. Edited by N. E. Gilhus, M. P. Barnes and M. Brainin.
© 2011 Blackwell Publishing Ltd.

Table 9.1 Classification of evidence for diagnostic and for therapeutic measures (from [583]).

	Evidence classification scheme for a diagnostic measure	Evidence classification scheme for a therapeutic intervention
Class I	A prospective study in a broad spectrum of persons with the suspected condition, using a 'gold standard' for case definition, where the test is applied in a blinded evaluation, and enabling the assessment of appropriate tests of diagnostic accuracy	An adequately powered, prospective, randomized, controlled clinical trial with masked outcome assessment in a representative population or an adequately powered systematic review of prospective randomized controlled clinical trials with masked outcome assessment in representative populations. The following are required: a. randomization concealment b. primary outcome(s) is/are clearly defined c. exclusion/inclusion criteria are clearly defined d. adequate accounting for dropouts and crossovers with numbers sufficiently low to have a minimal potential for bias; and e. relevant baseline characteristics are presented and substantially equivalent among treatment groups or there is appropriate statistical adjustment for differences
Class II	A prospective study of a narrow spectrum of persons with the suspected condition, or a well-designed retrospective study of a broad spectrum of persons with an established condition (by 'gold standard') compared to a broad spectrum of controls, where test is applied in a blinded evaluation, and enabling the assessment of appropriate tests of diagnostic accuracy	Prospective matched-group cohort study in a representative population with masked outcome assessment that meets a–e above or a randomized, controlled trial in a representative population that lacks one criterion a–e
Class III	Evidence provided by a retrospective study where either persons with the established condition or controls are of a narrow spectrum, and where test is applied in a blinded evaluation	All other controlled trials (including well-defined natural history controls or patients serving as own controls) in a representative population, where outcome assessment is independent of patient treatment
Class IV	Evidence from uncontrolled studies, case series, case reports, or expert opinion	Evidence from uncontrolled studies, case series, case reports, or expert opinion

Table 9.2 Definitions for levels of recommendation (from [583]).

Level A	Established as useful/predictive or not useful/predictive for a diagnostic measure or established as effective, ineffective or harmful for a therapeutic intervention; requires at least one convincing Class I study or at least two consistent, convincing Class II studies
Level B	Established as useful/predictive or not useful/predictive for a diagnostic measure or established as effective, ineffective, or harmful for a therapeutic intervention; requires at least one convincing Class II study or overwhelming Class III evidence
Level C	Established as useful/predictive or not useful/predictive for a diagnostic measure or established as effective, ineffective or harmful for a therapeutic intervention; requires at least two Class III studies
Good Clinical Practice (GCP) points	Recommended best practice based on the experience of the guideline development group. Usually based on Class IV evidence indicating large clinical uncertainty, such GCP points can be useful for health workers

covers referral and emergency management, Stroke Unit service, diagnostics, primary and secondary prevention, general stroke treatment, specific treatment including acute management, management of complications, and rehabilitation.

Changes in the guidelines necessitated by new evidence will be continuously incorporated in the online version that can be found on the ESO website (eso-stroke.org). The reader is advised to check the online version when making important treatment decisions.

Introduction

Stroke is one of the leading causes of morbidity and mortality worldwide [4]. Large differences in incidence, prevalence, and mortality have been noted between Eastern and Western Europe. This has been attributed to differences in risk factors, with higher levels of hypertension and other risk factors resulting in more severe stroke in Eastern Europe [5]. Notable regional variations have also been found within Western Europe. Stroke is the most important cause of morbidity and long-term disability in Europe, and demographic changes will result in an increase in both incidence and prevalence. It is also the second most common cause of dementia, the most frequent cause of epilepsy in the elderly, and a frequent cause of depression [6, 7].

Many guidelines and recommendations for stroke management or specific aspects of stroke care have been published during the past decade [2, 8–18]. Most recently, the updated Helsingborg Declaration focused on standards of stroke care and research needs in Europe [19]. In the future, the global harmonization of stroke guidelines will be the focus of the World Stroke Organisation, supported by the ESO and other national and regional stroke societies.

Public awareness and education

Recommendations

- Educational programmes to increase awareness of stroke at the population level are recommended (Class II, Level B).
- Educational programmes to increase stroke awareness among professionals (paramedics/emergency physicians) are recommended (Class II, Level B).

The 'time is brain' concept means that treatment of stroke should be considered as an emergency. Thus, avoiding delay should be the major aim in the pre-hospital phase of acute stroke care. This has far-reaching implications in terms of recognition of signs and symptoms of stroke by the patient or by relatives or bystanders, the nature of first medical contact, and the means of transportation to hospital.

Delays during acute stroke management have been identified at different levels [20]:
- at the population level, due to failure to recognize the symptoms of stroke and contact emergency services
- at the level of the emergency services and emergency physicians, due to a failure to prioritize transport of stroke patients
- at the hospital level, due to delays in neuroimaging and inefficient in-hospital care.

A large amount of time is lost outside the hospital [21]: for stroke patients at a Portuguese university hospital this accounted for 82% of the delay in treatment [22]. Studies that identify demographic, social, cultural, behavioural, and clinical factors associated with longer pre-hospital time may provide targets for educational campaigns [23, 24].

The interval from symptom onset to first call for medical help is the predominant part of pre-hospital delay [25–28]. Major reasons for delayed contact include lack of awareness of stroke symptoms and recognition of their severity, but also denial of the disease and the hope that symptoms would resolve. This suggests that educating the population to recognize stroke symptoms, and changing people's attitudes to acute stroke, may reduce the delay from stroke onset to emergency medical service (EMS) involvement.

Medical attention is rarely sought by the patient: in many cases contact is initially made by a family member [28–30]. Information and educational initiatives should therefore be directed both to persons at high risk of stroke and also to those around them.

Stroke awareness depends on demographic and socio-cultural factors, and on personal medical knowledge. Knowledge of stroke warning signs varies considerably, depending on the symptoms, and is dependent on the way questions are asked (e.g. open-ended or multiple-choice questions [31, 32]).

While most people agree that stroke is an emergency, and that they would seek medical help immediately, in reality only up to 50% call EMS. In many cases the first contact is with a family member or with a general practitioner; in some studies between 45% and 48% of patients were referred via a general practitioner [29, 33–36].

Most studies show that only approximately 33–50% of patients recognize their own symptoms as stroke. There are considerable discrepancies between theoretical knowledge of stroke and the reaction in case of an acute stroke. Some studies have shown that patients with better knowledge of stroke symptoms do not always arrive earlier at hospital.

The most frequently used sources of stroke information are mass media [37–39] and friends and relatives who have knowledge of stroke; only rarely is information derived from general practitioners or books [40–44]. The sources accessed vary with age: older people more often obtain information from health campaigns or their general practitioner, whereas younger people gain more information from TV [38–40].

Interventional studies have measured the effect of education on stroke knowledge. Eight non-randomized studies measured the impact of educational measures on pre-hospital time delay or thrombolysis use [45–52]. In six studies, the intervention was a combined educational programme directed at the public, paramedics, and health professionals, while in two studies education was directed only to the population. Only the TLL Temple Foundation Stroke Project included a concurrent control group [50, 51]. All studies had a pre-post design. Thrombolysis usage increased after education in the intervention group of the TLL study, but only for up to 6 months after intervention ended [51]. This suggests that public education has to be maintained to sustain stroke awareness in the population.

Education should also be directed to paramedics and emergency department (ED) staff to improve the accuracy of stroke identification and speed up transfer to the hospital [53]. Education of paramedics increases stroke knowledge, clinical skills, and communication skills, and decreases prehospital delays [54].

Educating medical students in basic stroke knowledge during their first year at medical school has been shown to be associated with a high degree of knowledge retention [55]. The value of postgraduate training is universally acknowledged, but training programmes for stroke specialists are still heterogeneous throughout Europe. To

overcome such heterogeneity and to increase the number of specialists available for stroke care, some countries (e.g. France, UK) have developed and implemented national curricula. In contrast, other countries rely on training specialization within neurology training programmes. With a view towards harmonization of training, a European Masters' Programme for Stroke Medicine (www.donau-uni.ac.at/en/studium/strokemedicine/index.php) and annual Stroke Summer Schools (www.eso-stroke.org), have been established.

Referral and patient transfer

Recommendations

- Immediate EMS contact and priority EMS dispatch are recommended (Class II, Level B).
- Priority transport with advance notification to the receiving hospital (outside and inside hospital) is recommended (Class III, Level B).
- It is recommended that suspected stroke victims should be transported without delay to the nearest medical centre with a stroke unit that can provide ultra-early treatment (Class III, Level B).
- It is recommended that dispatchers and ambulance personnel be trained to recognize stroke using simple instruments such as the Face–Arm–Speech–Test (Class IV, GCP).
- Immediate emergency room triage, clinical, laboratory and imaging evaluation, accurate diagnosis, therapeutic decision, and administration of appropriate treatments at the receiving hospital are recommended (Class III, Level B).
- It is recommended that in remote or rural areas helicopter transfer should be considered in order to improve access to treatment (Class III, Level C).
- It is recommended that in remote or rural areas telemedicine should be considered in order to improve access to treatment (Class II, Level B).
- It is recommended that patients with suspected TIA be referred without delay to a TIA clinic or to a medical centre with a stroke unit that can provide expert evaluation and immediate treatment (Class III, Level B).

Successful care of the acute stroke victim begins with the recognition by both the public and health professionals [56] that stroke is an emergency, like acute myocardial infarction or trauma. However, in practice the majority of ischaemic stroke patients do not receive recombinant tissue plasminogen activator (rtPA) because they do not reach the hospital soon enough [22, 36, 57, 58]. Emergency care of the acute stroke victim depends on a four-step chain:

- rapid recognition of, and reaction to, stroke signs and TIAs
- immediate EMS contact and priority EMS dispatch
- priority transport with notification of the receiving hospital
- immediate emergency room triage, clinical, laboratory and imaging evaluation, accurate diagnosis, and administration of appropriate treatments at the receiving hospital.

Once stroke symptoms are suspected, patients or their proxies should call EMS. The EMS system should have an electronic validated algorithm of questions to diagnose stroke during the phone interview [33, 59]. The ambulance dispatchers and paramedics should be able to diagnose stroke using simple instruments such as the Face–Arm–Speech–Test [60]. They should also be able to identify and provide appropriate help for patients who need urgent care because of early complications or comorbidities of stroke, such as impaired consciousness, seizures, vomiting, or haemodynamic instability.

Suspected stroke victims should be transported without delay to the nearest medical centre with a stroke unit that can provide ultra-early treatment. Patients with onset of stroke symptoms within 3 h should be given priority in evaluation and transportation [20]. In each community, a network of stroke units or, if stroke units are not yet available, a network of medical centres providing organized acute stroke care should be implemented and publicized to the general population, health professionals, and the emergency transport systems [61, 62].

If a doctor receives a call or consultation from a patient with suspected stroke, they should recommend or arrange transportation, preferably through the EMS system, to the nearest hospital with a stroke unit providing organized acute stroke care and ultra-early treatment. Ambulance dispatchers should inform the stroke unit and describe the patient's clinical status. Proxies who can describe symptom onset or the patient's medical history should accompany the patient.

Few intervention studies have examined the impact of decreasing the delay from symptom onset to arrival at the hospital and making ultra-early treatment accessible for a larger proportion of patients. Most such studies have used a before-and-after intervention design, were neither randomized nor masked with respect to intervention or evaluation of outcome, and lacked concurrent controls [23, 53]. The types of intervention included education and training programmes, helicopter transfer, telemedicine, and reorganization of pre-hospital and in-hospital protocols for acute stroke patients.

Direct presentation to the ED via ambulance or EMS transportation is the fastest way of referral [28, 53, 63–65]. Helicopter transport can reduce the time between referral and hospital arrival [66, 67], and also promotes access to thrombolytic therapy in remote and rural areas [68]. In mixed rural and urban areas, air and ground distances can be compared using simple rules [69]. No studies have compared air and ground transport specifically in stroke patients. In one study, predominantly in trauma patients, ground ambulances provided shorter arrival times at distances less than 10 miles ($\approx$16 km) from the hospital; even with only short delays in despatching air transport, air was faster only for distances longer than 45 miles ($\approx$72 km) [70]. One economic study showed that helicopter transfer of patients with suspected acute ischaemic stroke for potential thrombolysis is cost-effective [71].

Telemedicine using bidirectional video-conferencing equipment to provide health services or assist health care personnel at distant sites is a feasible, valid, and reliable means of facilitating thrombolysis delivery to patients in distant or rural hospitals, where timely air or ground transportation is not feasible. The quality of treatment, complication rates, and short- and long-term outcomes are similar for acute stroke patients treated with rtPA via a telemedicine consultation at local hospitals and those treated in academic centres [72–81].

Activation of the stroke code as a special infrastructure with immediate calling of a stroke neurologist at a stroke unit and priority transfer of the patients to this centre is effective in increasing the percentage of patients treated with thrombolysis, and also in shortening pre-hospital delays [82, 83].

Recent community and hospital-based studies demonstrated a high risk of stroke immediately after a TIA [6, 84]. Observational studies showed that urgent evaluation at a TIA clinic and immediate initiation of treatment reduces stroke risk after TIA [85, 86]. This underlines the need for urgent referral of TIA for expert evaluation and immediate treatment.

Emergency management

Recommendations

- Organization of pre-hospital and in-hospital pathways and systems for acute stroke patients is recommended (Class III, Level C).
- Ancillary tests, as outlined in table 9.3, are recommended (Class IV, GCP).

In-hospital delay may account for 16% of total time lost between stroke onset and computed tomography (CT) [22]. Reasons for in-hospital delays are:
- a failure to identify stroke as an emergency
- inefficient in-hospital transport
- delayed medical assessment
- delay in imaging
- uncertainty in administering thrombolysis [20, 21, 24].

Stroke care pathways may allow care to be organized more effectively, although a meta-analysis [87] did not support their routine implementation. Such pathways may reduce delays in door-to-medical department time, door-to-imaging time [88, 89], door-to-needle time [89] and, where appropriate, door-to-arteriography time.

Acute stroke care has to integrate EMS, ED staff, and stroke care specialists. Communication and collabora-

Table 9.3 Emergency diagnostic tests in acute stroke patients.

In all patients

1 Brain imaging: CT or MRI
2 ECG
3 *Laboratory tests*
    Complete blood count and platelet count, prothrombin time or INR, partial thrombin time (PTT)
    Serum electrolytes, blood glucose
    C-reactive protein (CRP) or sedimentation rate
    Hepatic and renal chemical analysis

When indicated

4 Extracranial and transcranial Duplex/Doppler ultrasound
5 MRA or CTA
6 Diffusion and perfusion MR or perfusion CT
7 Echocardiography (transthoracic and/or transoesophageal)
8 Chest X-ray
9 Pulse oximetry and arterial blood gas analysis
10 Lumbar puncture
11 EEG
12 Toxicology screen

tion between EMS, ED staff, radiologists, clinical laboratories, and neurologists are important for rapid delivery of treatment [11, 90, 91]. Integrating EMS and ED staff was found to increase the use of thrombolysis [92]. Hospitals where patients are not delivered directly to a stroke unit should implement a system allowing the ED to prenotify the acute stroke team as soon as possible. Routinely informing ED physicians or stroke physicians during transport has been shown to be associated with reduced in-hospital delay [82, 93-95], increased use of thrombolysis [92, 93], decreased length of hospital stay [95], and decreased in-hospital mortality [92].

A stroke recognition instrument with high diagnostic accuracy is necessary for rapid triage [96]; stroke mimics such as migraine and seizure might be a problem [97, 98]. Stroke recognition instruments such as Face–Arm–Speech–Test and Recognition of Stroke in the Emergency Room (ROSIER) can assist the correct recognition of stroke by ED personnel [60, 97, 99].

A neurologist or stroke physician should be involved in the acute care of stroke patients and available in the ED [98]. Comparing neurologist care to non-neurologist care, two studies in the USA found that neurologists perform more extensive and costly testing, but that their patients had lower in-hospital and 90-day mortality rates, and were less dependent on discharge [100, 101]. However, this might not be true for other contries such as the UK, where most stroke physicians are not neurologists, but are still highly skilled in management of patients with TIA and stroke.

Reorganization of stroke wards can help to avoid bottlenecks and unnecessary in-hospital transport. Brain imaging facilities should be relocated in or next to the stroke unit or the ED, and stroke patients should have priority access [90]. Neuroradiologists should be notified as early as possible [90]. In a Finnish study, in-hospital delays were decreased considerably by moving the CT scanner close to the ED and by implementing a prenotifying system [94]. Thrombolysis should be started in the CT room or in the vicinity of the scanner. Finally, an arteriography suite should be readily accessible if endovascular treatment is required.

Written care protocols for acute stroke patients should be available; centres using such protocols were found to have higher thrombolysis rates [92]. Implementing a continuous quality improvement scheme can also diminish in-hospital delays [81, 102]. Benchmarks should be defined and measured for individual institutions, and have recently been developed for regional networks and countries. As a minimum requirement, door-to-imaging and door-to-treatment times should be monitored.

While only a minority of stroke patients present in an immediately life-threatening condition, many have significant physiological abnormalities or comorbidities. Symptoms and signs that may predict later complications such as space-occupying infarction, bleeding, or recurrent stroke, and medical conditions such as hypertensive crisis, co-existing myocardial infarction, aspiration pneumonia, or cardiac and renal failure, must be recognized early. Stroke severity should be assessed by trained staff using the National Institutes of Health Stroke Scale (NIHSS) [103].

Initial examination should include:

• observation of breathing and pulmonary function
• early signs of dysphagia, preferably with a validated assessment form [104]
• evaluation of concomitant heart disease
• assessment of blood pressure (BP) and heart rate
• determination of arterial oxygen saturation using infrared pulse oximetry if available.

Simultaneously, blood samples for clinical chemistry, glucose, coagulation, and haematology studies should be drawn, and a venous line inserted. The examination should be supplemented by a medical history that includes risk factors for stroke and cardiac disease, medications, conditions that may predispose to bleeding complications, and markers for stroke mimics. A history of drug abuse, oral contraceptive use, infection, trauma, or migraine may give important clues, particularly in young patients.

Stroke services and stroke units

Recommendations

• It is recommended that all stroke patients should be treated in a stroke unit (Class I, Level A).

• It is recommended that healthcare systems ensure that acute stroke patients have access to high technology medical and surgical stroke care when required (Class III, Level B).

• The development of clinical networks, including telemedicine, is recommended to expand access to high-technology specialist stroke care (Class II, Level B).

Providing stroke services

All acute stroke patients require specialist multidisciplinary care delivered in a stroke unit, and selected patients will require additional high-technology interventions. Health services need to establish the infrastructure to deliver these interventions to all patients who require them: the only reason for excluding patients from stroke units is if their condition does not warrant active management. Recent consensus documents [11, 105] have defined the roles of primary and comprehensive stroke centres (table 9.4).

Primary stroke centres are defined as centres with the necessary staffing, infrastructure, expertise, and programmes to provide appropriate diagnosis and treatment for most stroke patients. Some patients with rare disorders, complex stroke, or multi-organ disease may need more specialized care and resources that are not available in primary stroke centres.

Comprehensive stroke centres are defined as centres that provide both appropriate diagnosis and treatment for most stroke patients, and also high-technology medical and surgical care (new diagnostic and rehabilitation methods, specialized tests, automatic monitoring of multiple physiological parameters, interventional radiology, vascular surgery, neurosurgery).

The organization of clinical networks using telemedicine is recommended to facilitate treatment options not previously available at remote hospitals. Administration of rtPA during telemedicine consultations is feasible and safe [106]. Clinical networks using telemedicine systems achieve increased use of rtPA [80, 107] and better stroke care and clinical outcomes [80].

Stroke unit care

An updated systematic review has confirmed significant reductions in death (3% absolute reduction), dependency (5% increase in independent survivors), and the need for institutional care (2% reduction) for patients treated in a stroke unit, compared with those treated in general wards. All types of patients, irrespective of gender, age, stroke subtype, and stroke severity, appear to benefit from treatment in stroke units [61, 108]. These results have been confirmed in large observational studies of routine practice [109–111]. Although stroke unit care is more costly than treatment on general neurological or medical wards, it reduces post-acute inpatient care costs [112, 113] and is cost-effective [114–117].

Table 9.4 Recommended requirements for centres managing acute stroke patients.

Primary stroke centre	Comprehensive stroke centre
Availability of 24-h CT scanning	MRI/MRA/CTA
Established stroke treatment guidelines and operational procedures, including i.v. rtPA protocols 24/7	Transoesophageal echocardiography
Close co-operation of neurologists, internists and rehabilitation experts	Cerebral angiography
Specially trained nursing personnel	Transcranial Doppler sonography
Early multidisciplinary stroke unit rehabilitation including speech therapy, occupational therapy, and physical therapy	Extracranial and intracranial colour-coded duplex sonography
Neurosonological investigations within 24 h (extracranial doppler sonography)	Specialized neuroradiological, neurosurgical and vascular surgical consultation (including telemedicine networks)
Transthoracic echocardiography	Carotid surgery
Laboratory examinations (including coagulation parameters)	Angioplasty and stenting
Monitoring of blood pressure, ECG, oxygen saturation, blood glucose, body temperature	Automated monitoring of pulse oximetry, blood pressure
Automated ECG monitoring at bedside	Established network of rehabilitation facilities to provide a continuous process of care, including collaboration with outside rehabilitation centre

A stroke unit consists of a discrete area of a hospital ward that exclusively or nearly exclusively takes care of stroke patients and is staffed by a specialist multidisciplinary team [61]. The core disciplines of the team are medicine, nursing, physiotherapy, occupational therapy, speech and language therapy, and social work [118]. The multidisciplinary team should work in a co-ordinated way through regular meetings to plan patient care. Programmes of regular staff education and training should be provided [118]. The typical components of stroke unit care in stroke unit trials [118] were:

• medical assessment and diagnosis, including imaging (CT, magnetic resonance imaging [MRI]), and early assessment of nursing and therapy needs

• early management, consisting of early mobilization, prevention of complications, and treatment of hypoxia, hyperglycaemia, pyrexia, and dehydration

• ongoing rehabilitation, involving co-ordinated multidisciplinary team care, and early assessment of needs after discharge.

Both acute and comprehensive stroke units admit patients acutely and continue treatment for several days. Rehabilitation stroke units admit patients after 1–2 weeks and continue treatment and rehabilitation for several weeks if necessary. Most of the evidence for effectiveness comes from trials of comprehensive stroke units and rehabilitation stroke units [61, 119]. Mobile stroke

teams, which offer stroke care and treatment in a number of wards, probably do not influence important outcomes and cannot be recommended [120]. Such teams have usually been established in hospitals where stroke units were not available.

The stroke unit should be of sufficient size to provide specialist multidisciplinary care for the whole duration of hospital admission. Smaller hospitals may achieve this with a single comprehensive unit, but larger hospitals may require a pathway of care incorporating separate acute and rehabilitation units.

Diagnostics

Diagnostic imaging

Recommendations

- In patients with suspected TIA or stroke, urgent cranial CT (Class I), or alternatively MRI (Class II), is recommended (Level A).

- If MRI is used, the inclusion of diffusion-weighted imaging (DWI) and T2*-weighted gradient echo sequences is recommended (Class II, Level A).

- In patients with TIA, minor stroke, or early spontaneous recovery immediate diagnostic work-up, including urgent vascular imaging (ultrasound, CT-angiography, or MR angiography) is recommended (Class I, Level A).

Imaging of the brain and supplying vessels is crucial in the assessment of patients with stroke and TIA. Brain imaging distinguishes ischaemic stroke from intracranial haemorrhage and stroke mimics, and identifies the type and often also the cause of stroke; it may also help to differentiate irreversibly damaged tissue from areas that may recover, thus guiding emergency and subsequent treatment, and may help to predict outcome. Vascular imaging may identify the site and cause of arterial obstruction, and identifies patients at high risk of stroke recurrence.

General principles

Stroke victims should have clear priority over other patients for brain imaging, because time is crucial. In patients with suspected TIA or stroke, general and neurological examination followed by diagnostic brain imaging must be performed immediately on arrival at the hospital so that treatment can be started promptly. Investigation of TIA is equally urgent, because up to 10% of these patients will suffer stroke within the next 48h. Immediate access to imaging is facilitated by pre-hospital notification and good communication with the imaging facility: stroke services should work closely with the imaging department to plan the best use of resources.

Diagnostic imaging must be sensitive and specific in detecting stroke pathology, particularly in the early phase of stroke. It should provide reliable images, and should be technically feasible in acute stroke patients. Rapid, focused neurological assessment is helpful to determine which imaging technique should be used. Imaging tests should take into account the patient's condition [121]; for example, up to 45% of patients with severe stroke may not tolerate MR examination because of their medical condition and contraindications [122–124].

Imaging in patients with acute stroke

Patients admitted within 3 h of stroke onset may be candidates for intravenous (i.v.) thrombolysis [125]; CT is usually sufficient to guide routine thrombolysis. Patients arriving later may be candidates for trials testing extended time windows for thrombolysis or other experimental reperfusion strategies.

Plain CT is widely available, reliably identifies most stroke mimics, and distinguishes acute ischaemic from haemorrhagic stroke within the first 5–7 days [126–128]. Immediate CT scanning is the most cost-effective strategy for imaging acute stroke patients [129], but is not sensitive for old haemorrhage. Overall, CT is less sensitive than MRI, but equally specific, for early ischaemic changes [130]. Two-thirds of patients with moderate to severe stroke have visible ischaemic changes within the first few hours [130–134], but no more than 50% of patients with minor stroke have a visible relevant ischaemic lesion on CT, especially within the first few hours of stroke [135]. Training in identification of early ischaemic changes on CT [134, 136, 137], and the use of scoring systems [133], improve detection of early ischaemic changes.

Early CT changes in ischaemic stroke include decreases in tissue X-ray attenuation, tissue swelling with effacement of cerebrospinal fluid spaces, and arterial hyperattenuation, which indicates the presence of intraluminal thrombus with high specificity [138]. CT is highly specific for the early identification of ischaemic brain damage [131, 139, 140]. The presence of early signs of ischaemia on CT should not exclude patients from thrombolysis within the first 3 h, though patients with a hypoattenuating ischaemic lesion which exceeds one-third of the middle cerebral artery (MCA) territory may benefit less from thrombolysis [125, 133, 134, 141, 142].

Some centres prefer to use MRI as first-line routine investigation for acute stroke. MRI with diffusion-weighted imaging (DWI) has the advantage of higher sensitivity for early ischaemic changes than CT [130]. This higher sensitivity is particularly useful in the diagnosis of posterior circulation stroke and lacunar or small cortical infarctions. MRI can also detect small and old haemorrhages for a prolonged period with T2* (gradient echo) sequences [143]. However, DWI can be negative in patients with definite stroke [144].

Restricted diffusion on DWI, measured by the apparent diffusion coefficient (ADC), is not 100% specific for ischaemic brain damage. Although abnormal tissue on DWI often proceeds to infarction it can recover, which indicates that DWI does not show only permanently damaged tissue [145, 146]. Tissue with only modestly reduced ADC values may be permanently damaged; there is as yet no reliable ADC threshold to differentiate dead from still viable tissue [147, 148]. Other MRI sequences (T2, FLAIR, T1) are less sensitive in the early detection of ischaemic brain damage.

MRI is particularly important in acute stroke patients with unusual presentations, stroke varieties, and uncommon aetiologies, or in whom a stroke mimic is suspected but not clarified on CT. If arterial dissection is suspected, MRI of the neck with fat-suppressed T1-weighted sequences is required to detect intramural haematoma.

MRI is less suited for agitated patients or for those who may vomit and aspirate. If necessary, emergency life support should be continued while the patient is being imaged, as patients (especially those with severe stroke) may become hypoxic while supine during imaging [124]. The risk of aspiration is increased in the substantial proportion of patients who are unable to protect their airway.

Perfusion imaging with CT or MRI and angiography may be used in selected patients with ischaemic stroke (e.g. unclear time window, late admission) to aid the decision on whether to use thrombolysis, although there is no clear evidence that patients with particular perfusion patterns are more or less likely to benefit from thrombolysis [149–152]. Selected patients with intracranial arterial occlusion may be candidates for intra-arterial thrombolysis, although there is only limited evidence to support this [153, 154]. Patients with combined obstructions of the internal carotid artery (ICA) and MCA have less chance of recovering with i.v. thrombolysis than patients with isolated MCA obstructions [155]. In patients with MCA trunk occlusions, the frequency of severe extracranial occlusive disease in the carotid distribution is high [156, 157].

Mismatch between the volume of brain tissue with critical hypoperfusion (which can recover after reperfusion) and the volume of infarcted tissue (which does not recover even with reperfusion) can be detected with MR diffusion/perfusion imaging with moderate reliability [158], but this is not yet a proven strategy for improving the response to thrombolysis up to 9h [159]. There is disagreement on how to best identify irreversible ischaemic brain injury and to define critically impaired blood flow [149, 152, 160]. Quantification of MR perfusion is problematic [161], and there are widely differing associations between perfusion parameters and clinical and radiological outcomes [149]. Decreases in cerebral blood flow on CT are associated with subsequent tissue damage [150, 151], but the therapeutic value of CT perfusion imaging is not yet established. Although infarct expansion may occur in a high proportion of patients with

mismatch, up to 50% of patients without mismatch may also have infarct growth and so might benefit from tissue salvage [152, 162]. The 'imaging/clinical' mismatch, i.e. the mismatch between the extent of the lesion seen on DWI or CT and the extent of the lesion as expected from the severity of the neurological deficit, has produced mixed results [163, 164]. Hence, neither perfusion imaging with CT or MRI nor the mismatch concept can be recommended for routine treatment decisions.

Microhaemorrhages are present on T2* MRI in up to 60% of patients with haemorrhagic stroke, and are associated with older age, hypertension, diabetes, leukoaraiosis, lacunar stroke, and amyloid angiopathy [165]. The incidence of symptomatic intracranial haemorrhage following thrombolysis in ischaemic stroke patients was not increased in those having cerebral microbleeds on pretreatment T2*-weighted MRI [166].

Vascular imaging should be performed rapidly to identify patients with tight symptomatic arterial stenosis who could benefit from endarterectomy or angioplasty. Non-invasive imaging with colour-coded duplex imaging of the extracranial and intracranial arteries, CT angiography (CTA), or contrast-enhanced MR angiography (CE-MRA) is widely available. These approaches are relatively risk-free, whereas intra-arterial angiography has a 1–3% risk of causing stroke in patients with symptomatic carotid lesions [167, 168]. Digital subtraction angiography (DSA) may be needed in some circumstances, for example when other tests have been inconclusive.

Carotid ultrasound, MRA, and CTA visualise carotid stenosis. Systematic reviews and individual patient data meta-analysis indicate that CE-MRA is the most sensitive and specific non-invasive imaging modality for carotid artery stenosis, closely followed by Doppler ultrasound and CTA, with non-contrast MRA being the least reliable [169, 170].

Some data suggest that vertebrobasilar TIA and minor stroke is associated with a high risk of recurrent stroke [171]. Extracranial vertebral ultrasound diagnosis is useful, but intracranial ultrasound of the vertebrobasilar system can be misleading due to low specificity. Limited data suggest that CE-MRA and CTA offer better non-invasive imaging of the intracranial vertebral and basilar arteries [172].

Unlike other imaging modalities ultrasound is fast, non-invasive, and can be administered using portable machines. It is therefore applicable to patients unable to co-operate with MRA or CTA [157]. However, Doppler studies alone often provide only limited information, are investigator-dependent and require skilled operators, although they allow repeated measurements at the bedside.

Transcranial Doppler ultrasound (TCD) is useful for the diagnosis of abnormalities in the large cerebral arteries at the base of the skull. However, between 7 and 20% of acute stroke patients, particularly elderly individuals and those from certain ethnic groups do not have an adequate acoustic window [173, 174]. This problem can be considerably reduced by using ultrasound contrast agents, which also allow perfusion studies in the acute phase [175–177] and continuous monitoring of cerebral haemodynamic responses [178]. The combination of ultrasound imaging techniques and MRA reveals excellent results equal to DSA [179]. Cerebral reactivity and cerebral autoregulation are impaired in patients with occlusive extracerebral arterial disease (particularly carotid stenosis and occlusion) and inadequate collateral supply, who are at increased risk of recurrent stroke [180, 181]. TCD is the only technique that detects circulating intracranial emboli [182], which are particularly common in patients with large artery disease. In patients with symptomatic carotid artery stenoses, they are a strong independent predictor of early recurrent stroke and TIA [183], and have been used as a surrogate marker to evaluate antiplatelet agents [184]. TCD microbubble detection can be used to identify a right-to-left shunt, which mainly results from a patent foramen ovale (PFO) [185].

Imaging in patients with TIA, minor non-disabling stroke, and stroke with spontaneous recovery

Patients presenting with TIA are at high risk of early recurrent stroke (up to 10% in the first 48 h) [186]. They therefore need urgent clinical diagnosis to treat associated general abnormalities, modify active risk factors, and identify specific treatable causes, particularly arterial stenosis and other embolic sources. Vascular imaging is a priority in those patients with TIA or minor stroke, more than in those with major stroke in whom surgery is not going to be of benefit in the short term. Immediate preventive treatment will reduce stroke, disability, and death [86, 187]. Simple clinical scoring systems can be

used to identify patients at particularly high risk [186]. Patients with minor non-disabling stroke and rapid spontaneous clinical recovery are also at high risk of recurrent stroke [58].

Patients with widely varying brain pathology may present with transient neurological deficits indistinguishable from TIA. CT reliably detects some of these pathologies (e.g. intracerebral haemorrhage, subdural haematoma, tumours) [129], but others (e.g. multiple sclerosis, encephalitis, hypoxic brain damage, etc.) are better identified on MRI, while others (e.g. acute metabolic disturbances) are not visible at all. Intracranial haemorrhage is a rare cause of TIA.

Between 20 and 50% of patients with TIAs may have acute ischaemic lesions on DWI [144, 188, 189]. These patients are at increased risk of early recurrent disabling stroke [189]. However, there is currently no evidence that DWI provides better stroke prediction than clinical risk scores [190]. The risk of recurrent disabling stroke is also increased in patients with TIA and an infarct on CT [191].

The ability of DWI to identify very small ischaemic lesions may be particularly helpful in patients presenting late or in patients with mild non-disabling stroke, in whom the diagnosis may be difficult to establish on clinical grounds [130]. T2*-MRI is the only reliable method to identify haemorrhages after the acute phase, when blood is no longer visible on CT [143].

Other diagnostic tests

Recommendations

- In patients with acute stroke and TIA, early clinical evaluation, including physiological parameters and routine blood tests, is recommended (Class I, Level A).

- For all stroke and TIA patients, a sequence of blood tests is recommended (table 9.3, table 9.5).

- It is recommended that all acute stroke and TIA patients should have a 12-lead ECG. In addition continuous ECG recording is recommended for ischaemic stroke and TIA patients (Class I, Level A).

- It is recommended that for stroke and TIA patients seen after the acute phase, 24-h Holter ECG monitoring should be performed when arrhythmias are suspected and no other causes of stroke are found (Class I, Level A).

- Echocardiography is recommended in selected patients (Class III, Level B).

Table 9.5 Subsequent laboratory tests, according to the type of stroke and suspected aetiology.

All patients	Full blood count, electrolytes, glucose, lipids, creatinine, CRP or ESR
Cerebral venous thrombosis, hypercoagulopathy	Thrombophilia screen, AT3, Factor 2, 5, mutations, factor 8, protein C, protein S, Antiphospholipid-antibodies, d-dimer, homocysteine
Bleeding disorder	INR, aPTT, fibrinogen, etc.
Vasculitis or systemic disorder	Cerebrospinal fluid, autoantibody screen, specific antibodies or PCR for HIV, syphilis, borreliosis, tuberculosis, fungi, illicit drug- screening, blood culture
Suspected genetic disorders, e. g. mitochondrial disorders (MELAS), CADASIL, sickle cell disease, Fabry disease, multiple cavernoma, etc.	Genetic testing

Cardiac evaluation

Cardiac and ECG abnormalities are common in acute stroke patients [192]. In particular, prolonged QTc, ST depression, and T wave inversion are prevalent in acute ischaemic stroke, especially if the insular cortex is involved [193, 194]. Hence, all acute stroke and TIA patients should have a 12-channel ECG.

Cardiac monitoring should be conducted routinely after an acute cerebrovascular event to screen for serious cardiac arrhythmias. It is unclear whether continuous ECG recording at the bedside is equivalent to Holter monitoring for the detection of atrial fibrillation (AF) in acute stroke patients. Holter monitoring is superior to routine ECG for the detection of AF in patients anticipated to have thromboembolic stroke with sinus rhythm [195]; however, serial 12-channel ECG might be sufficient to detect new AF in a stroke unit setting [196]. A recent systematic review found that new AF was detected by Holter ECG in 4.6% of patients with recent ischaemic stroke or TIA, irrespective of baseline ECG and clinical examination [197]. Extended duration of monitoring, prolonged event loop recording, and confining Holter monitoring to patients with non-lacunar stroke, may improve detection rates [198].

Echocardiography can detect many potential causes of stroke [199], but there is controversy about the indications for, and type of, echocardiography in stroke and TIA patients. Transoesophageal echocardiography (TOE) has been claimed to be superior to transthoracic echocardiography (TTE) for the detection of potential cardiac sources of embolism [200], independent of age [201].

Echocardiography is particularly required in patients with:

- evidence of cardiac disease on history, examination, or ECG
- suspected cardiac source of embolism (e.g. infarctions in multiple cerebral or systemic arterial territories)
- suspected aortic disease
- suspected paradoxical embolism
- no other identifiable causes of stroke.

TTE is sufficient for evaluation of mural thrombi, particularly in the apex of the left ventricle; this technique has >90% sensitivity and specificity for ventricular thrombi after myocardial infarction [202]. TOE is superior for evaluation of the aortic arch, left atrium, and atrial septum [199]. It also allows risk stratification for further thromboembolic events in patients with AF [203].

The role of cardiac CT and cardiac MRI in the detection of embolic sources in stroke patients has not been evaluated systematically.

Blood tests

Blood tests required on emergency admission are listed in table 9.3. Subsequent tests depend on the type of stroke and suspected aetiology (table 9.5).

Primary prevention

The aim of primary prevention is to reduce the risk of stroke in asymptomatic people. Relative risk (RR), absolute risk (AR), odds ratio (OR), numbers needed to treat (NNT) to avoid one major vascular event per year, and numbers needed to harm (NNH) to cause one major complication per year are provided for each intervention in tables 9.6–9.8.

Management of vascular risk factors

Recommendations

- Blood pressure should be checked regularly. It is recommended that high blood pressure should be managed with lifestyle modification and individualized pharmacological therapy (Class I, Level A) aiming at normal levels of 120/80 mmHg (Class IV, GCP). For prehypertensive (120–139/80–90 mmHg) with congestive heart failure, MI, diabetes, or chronic renal failure, antihypertensive mediation is indicated (Class 1, Level A).

- Blood glucose should be checked regularly. It is recommended that diabetes should be managed with lifestyle modification and individualized pharmacological therapy (Class IV, Level C). In diabetic patients, high blood pressure should be managed intensively (Class I, Level A) aiming for levels below 130/80 mmHg (Class IV, Level C). Where possible, treatment should include an angiotensin converting enzyme inhibitor or angiotensin receptor antagonist (Class I, Level A).

- Blood cholesterol should be checked regularly. It is recommended that high blood cholesterol (e.g. LDL> 150 mg/dl [3.9 mmol/l]) should be managed with lifestyle modification (Class IV, Level C) and a statin (Class I, Level A).

- It is recommended that cigarette smoking be discouraged (Class III, Level B).

- It is recommended that heavy use of alcohol be discouraged (Class III, Level B).

- Regular physical activity is recommended (Class III, Level B).

- A diet low in salt and saturated fat, high in fruit and vegetables and rich in fibre is recommended (Class III, Level B).

- Subjects with an elevated body mass index are recommended to take a weight-reducing diet (Class III, Level B).

- Antioxidant vitamin supplements are not recommended (Class I, Level A).

- Hormone replacement therapy is not recommended for the primary prevention of stroke (Class I, Level A).

A healthy lifestyle, consisting of abstinence from smoking, low–normal body mass index, moderate alcohol consumption, regular exercise and healthy diet, is associated with a reduction in ischaemic stroke (RR 0.29; 95% CI 0.14–0.63) [204].

Table 9.6 Number need to treat (NNT) to prevent one stroke per year in patients who undergo surgery for ICA stenosis; all percentages reflect to the NASCET method (modified from [584] and [338]).

Disease	NNT to avoid one stroke/year
Asymptomatic (60–99%)	85
Symptomatic (70–99%)	27
Symptomatic (50–69%)	75
Symptomatic (>50%) in men	45
Symptomatic (>50%) in women	180
Symptomatic (>50%) >75 years	25
Symptomatic (>50%) <65 years	90
Symptomatic (>50%) <2 weeks after the event	25
Symptomatic (>50%) >12 weeks after the event	625
Symptomatic (≤50%)	No benefit

High blood pressure

A high (>120/80 mmHg) blood pressure (BP) is strongly and directly related to vascular and overall mortality without evidence of any threshold [205]. Lowering BP substantially reduces stroke and coronary risks, depending on the magnitude of the reduction [206–208]. BP should be lowered to 140/85 mmHg or below [209]; antihypertensive treatment should be more aggressive in diabetic patients (see below) [210]. A combination of two or more antihypertensive agents is often necessary to achieve these targets.

Most studies comparing different drugs do not suggest that any class is superior [206, 207, 211]. However, the LIFE (Losartan Intervention for Endpoint reduction in hypertension) trial found that losartan was superior to atenolol in hypertensive patients with left ventricular hypertrophy (NNT to prevent stroke 270) [212, 213]. Similarly, the ALLHAT (Antihypertensive and Lipid-Lowering treatment to prevent Heart Attack) trial found that chlorthalidone was more effective than amlodipine and lisinopril [214]. Beta-blockers may still be considered an option for initial and subsequent antihypertensive treatment [209]. In elderly subjects, controlling isolated systolic hypertension (systolic blood pressure >140 mmHg and diastolic blood pressure <90 mmHg) is beneficial [207, 215].

Table 9.7 Relative risk reduction (RRR), absolute risk reduction (ARR), and number needed to treat (NNT) to avoid one major vascular event per year in patients with antithrombotic therapy (modified from [318, 321, 584]).

Disease	Treatment	RRR %	ARR % per year	NNT to avoid one event per year
Non-cardioembolic ischaemic stroke or TIA	aspirin/PCB	13	1.0	100
	aspirin + DIP/PCB	28	1.9	53
	aspirin + DIP/aspirin	18	1.0	104
	Clop/PCB	23	1.6	62
	Clop/aspirin	10	0.6	166
Atrial fibrillation (primary prevention)	warfarin/PCB	62	2.7	37
	aspirin/PCB	22	1.5	67
Atrial fibrillation (secondary prevention)	warfarin/PCB	67	8	13
	aspirin/PCB	21	2.5	40

PCB: placebo; Clop: clopidogrel; DIP: dipyridamole.

Table 9.8 Relative risk reduction (RRR), absolute risk reduction (ARR), and number needed to treat (NNT) to avoid one major vascular event per year in patients with risk factor modifications (modified from [287, 289, 293, 584]).

Clinical condition	Treatment	RRR %	ARR % per year	NNT to avoid one event per year
General population with increased blood pressure	Antihypertensive	42	0.4	250
General population with increased vascular risk	ACE inhibitor	22	0.65	154
Post-stroke/TIA with increased blood pressure	Antihypertensive	31	2.2	45
Post-stroke/TIA with normal blood pressure	ACE inhibitor ± diuretic	24	0.85	118
Post-stroke/TIA	Statins	16	0.44	230
	Smoking cessation	33	2.3	43

Diabetes mellitus

There is no evidence that improving glucose control reduces stroke [216]. In diabetic patients, blood pressure should be lowered to below 130/80 mmHg [210]. Treatment with a statin reduces the risk of major cardiovascular events, including stroke [217-219].

Hyperlipidaemia

In a review of 26 statin trials (95 000, patients), the incidence of stroke was reduced from 3.4% to 2.7% [220]. This was due mainly to a reduction in non-fatal stroke, from 2.7% to 2.1%. The review included the Heart Protection Study, which was, in part, a secondary prevention trial [221]; this trial found an excess of myopathy of one per 10 000 patients treated per annum [221]. There are no data to suggest that statins prevent stroke in patients with low-density lipoprotein (LDL) cholesterol below 150 mg/dl (3.9 mmol/l).

Cigarette smoking

Observational studies have shown cigarette smoking to be an independent risk factor for ischaemic stroke [222] in both men and women [223–227]. Spousal cigarette smoking may be associated with an increased stroke risk [228]. A meta-analysis of 22 studies indicates that smoking doubles the risk of ischaemic stroke [229]. Subjects who stop smoking reduce this risk by 50% [224]. Making workplaces smoke-free would result in considerable health and economic benefits [230].

Alcohol consumption

Heavy alcohol drinking (>60 g/day) increases the risk of ischaemic stroke (RR 1.69; 95% CI 1.34–2.15) and haemorrhagic stroke (RR 2.18; 95% CI 1.48-3.20). In contrast, light consumption (<12 g/day) is associated with a reduction in all stroke (RR 0.83; 95% CI 0.75–0.91) and ischaemic stroke (RR 0.80; 95% CI 0.67–0.96), and moderate consumption (12–24 g/day) with a reduction in ischaemic stroke (RR 0.72; 95% CI 0.57–0.91) [231]. Red wine consumption is associated with the lowest risk in comparison with other beverages [232]. Blood pressure elevation appears to be an important intermediary in the relation between alcohol consumption and stroke [233].

Physical activity

In a meta-analysis of cohort and case-control studies, physically active individuals had a lower risk of stroke or death than those with low activity (RR 0.73; 95% CI 0.67–0.79). Similarly, moderately active individuals had a lower risk of stroke, compared with those who were inactive (RR 0.80; 95% CI 0.74–0.86) [234]. This association is mediated, in part, through beneficial effects on body weight, blood pressure, serum cholesterol, and glucose tolerance. Leisure-based physical activity (2 to 5 hours per week) has been independently associated with a reduced severity of ischaemic stroke at admission and better short-term outcome [235].

Diet

Fruit, vegetable, and fish intake

In observational studies, high fruit and vegetable intake was associated with a decreased risk of stroke, compared with lower intake (RR 0.96 for each increment of two servings/day; 95% CI 0.93–1.00) [236]. The risk of ischaemic stroke was lower in people who consumed fish at least once per month (RR 0.69; 95% CI 0.48–0.99) [237]. Whole grain intake was associated with a reduction in cardiovascular disease (OR 0.79; 95% CI 0.73–0.85) but not stroke [238]. Dietary calcium intake from dairy products was associated with lower mortality from stroke in a Japanese population [239]. However, in a further study there was no interaction between the intake of total fat or cholesterol, and stroke risk in men [240].

In a randomized controlled trial in women, dietary interventions did not reduce the incidence of coronary events and stroke despite there being an 8.2% reduction of total fat intake and an increased consumption of vegetables, fruits and grains [241].

Body weight

A high body mass index (BMI ≥25) is associated with an increased risk of stroke in men [242] and women [243], mainly mediated by concomitant arterial hypertension and diabetes. Abdominal adiposity is a risk factor for stroke in men but not women [244]. Although weight loss reduces blood pressure [245], it does not lower stroke risk [246].

Vitamins

A low intake of vitamin D is associated with an increased risk of stroke [247], but supplements of calcium plus vitamin D do not reduce the risk of stroke [248]. Supplements of tocopherol and beta carotene do not reduce stroke [249]. A meta-analysis of trials with vitamin E supplementation found that it might increase mortality when used at high doses (≥400 IU/d) [250].

High homocysteine levels are associated with increased stroke risk (OR 1.19; 95% CI 1.05–1.31) [251]. Since folic acid fortification of enriched grain products was mandated by the US Food and Drug Administration there has been a reduction in stroke mortality rates, in contrast to countries without fortification [252]. A meta-analysis concluded that folic acid supplementation can reduce the risk of stroke (RR 0.82; 95% CI 0.68–1.00) [253]; the benefit was greatest in trials with long treatment durations or larger homocysteine-lowering effects, and in countries where grain was not fortified.

Postmenopausal oestrogen replacement therapy

Stroke rates rise rapidly in women after the menopause. However, in an analysis based on a 16-year follow-up of 59,337 postmenopausal women participating in the Nurses' Health Study, there was only a weak association between stroke and oestrogen replacement [254]. According to the HERS II trial, hormone replacement in healthy women is associated with an increased risk of ischaemic stroke [255]. A Cochrane systematic review [256] found hormone replacement therapy to be associated with an increased risk of stroke (RR 1.44; 95% CI 1.10–1.89). A secondary analysis of the Women's Health Initiative randomized controlled trial suggests that the risk of stroke is increased with hormone replacement therapy only in women with prolonged hormone use (> 5 years; RR 1.32; 95% CI 1.12–1.56) [257, 258].

Antithrombotic therapy

Recommendations

- Low-dose aspirin is recommended in women aged 45 years or more who are not at increased risk for intracerebral haemorrhage and who have good gastrointestinal tolerance; however, its effect is very small (Class I, Level A).

- It is recommended that low-dose aspirin may be considered in men for the primary prevention of myocardial infarction; however, it does not reduce the risk of ischaemic stroke (Class I, Level A).

- Antiplatelet agents other than aspirin are not recommended for primary stroke prevention (Class IV, GCP).

- Aspirin may be recommended for patients with non-valvular AF who are younger than 65 years and free of vascular risk factors (Class I, Level A).

- Unless contraindicated, either aspirin or an oral anticoagulant (international normalized ratio [INR] 2.0–3.0) is recommended for patients with non-valvular AF who are aged 65–75 years and free of vascular risk factors (Class I, Level A).

- Unless contraindicated, an oral anticoagulant (INR 2.0–3.0) is recommended for patients with non-valvular AF who are aged >75, or who are younger but have risk factors such as high blood pressure, left ventricular dysfunction, or diabetes mellitus (Class I, Level A).

- It is recommended that patients with AF who are unable to receive oral anticoagulants should be offered aspirin (Class I, Level A).

- It is recommended that patients with AF who have mechanical prosthetic heart valves should receive long-term anticoagulation with a target INR based on the prosthesis type, but not less than INR 2–3 (Class II, Level B).

- Low-dose aspirin is recommended for patients with asymptomatic internal carotid artery (ICA) stenosis >50% to reduce their risk of vascular events (Class II, Level B).

Low-risk subjects

Six large randomized trials have evaluated the benefits of aspirin for the primary prevention of cardiovascular (CV) events in men and women (47,293 on aspirin, 45,580 controls) with a mean age of 64.4 years [259–264]. Aspirin reduced coronary events and CV events, but not stroke, CV mortality, or all-cause mortality [265]. In women, aspirin reduced stroke (OR 0.83; 95% CI 0.70–0.97) and ischaemic stroke (OR 0.76; 95% CI 0.63–0.93) [266]. In a separate study in 39,876 healthy women aged 45 years or more, aspirin reduced stroke (RR 0.83; 95% CI 0.69–0.99) and ischaemic stroke (RR 0.76; 95% CI

0.63–0.93), and caused a non-significant increase in haemorrhagic stroke, over 10 years; it did not reduce the risk of fatal or nonfatal myocardial infarction, or cardio-vascular death [267].

No data are currently available on the use of other antiplatelet agents in primary prevention in low-risk subjects.

Subjects with vascular risk factors

A systematic review of randomized studies comparing antithrombotic agents with placebo in patients with elevated BP and no prior cardiovascular disease showed that aspirin did not reduce stroke or total cardiovascular events [266]. In the CHARISMA (Clopidogrel for High Atherothrombotic Risk and Ischemic Stabilization, Management, and Avoidance) trial, the combination of aspirin and clopidogrel was less effective than aspirin alone in the subgroup of patients with multiple vascular risk factors but no ischaemic event [268].

Large artery atheroma

Patients with atherosclerotic arterial disease have an increased risk of myocardial infarction, stroke, and cardiovascular death. Aspirin reduces MI in patients with asymptomatic carotid artery disease [269], and reduces stroke after carotid artery surgery [270].

Atrial fibrillation

AF is a strong independent risk factor for stroke. A meta-analysis of randomized trials with at least 3 months' follow-up showed that antiplatelet agents reduced stroke (RR 0.78; 95% CI 0.65–0.94) in patients with non-valvular AF [271]. Warfarin (target INR 2.0–3.0) is more effective than aspirin at reducing stroke (RR 0.36; 95% CI 0.26–0.51) [271]. As the risk of stroke in people with AF varies considerably, risk stratification should be used to determine whether patients should be given oral anticoagulation, aspirin, or nothing [14]. Oral anticoagulation is more effective in patients with AF who have one or more risk factors, such as previous systemic embolism, age over 75 years, high blood pressure, or poor left ventricular function [14]. In the meta-analysis described above, absolute increases in major extracranial haemorrhage were less than the absolute reductions in stroke [271]. The WASPO (Warfarin versus Aspirin for Stroke Prevention in Octogenarians) [272] and BAFTA (Birmingham Atrial Fibrillation Treatment of the Aged)

[273] trials showed that warfarin was safe and effective in older individuals. The ACTIVE W (Atrial fibrillation Clopidogrel Trial with Irbesartan for prevention of Vascular Events) study found that the combination of aspirin and clopidogrel was less effective than warfarin and had a similar bleeding rate [274].

Patients with a prosthetic heart valve, with or without AF, should receive long-term anticoagulation with a target INR based on the prosthesis type (bio-prosthetic valves: INR 2.0–3.0; mechanical valves: INR 3.0–4.0 [275].

Carotid surgery and angioplasty

Recommendations

- Carotid surgery is not recommended for asymptomatic individuals with significant carotid stenosis (NASCET 60–99%), except in those at high risk of stroke (Class I, Level C).
- Carotid angioplasty, with or without stenting, is not recommended for patients with asymptomatic carotid stenosis (Class IV, GCP).
- It is recommended that patients should take aspirin before and after surgery (Class I, Level A).

Trials of carotid surgery for asymptomatic carotid stenosis have concluded that although surgery reduces the incidence of ipsilateral stroke (RR 0.47–0.54) and any stroke, the absolute benefit is small (approximately 1% per annum) [276–278], whereas the perioperative stroke or death rate is 3%. Medical management is the most appropriate option for most asymptomatic subjects; only centres with a perioperative complication rate of 3% or less should contemplate surgery. Patients with a high risk of stroke (men with stenosis of more than 80% and a life expectancy of more than 5 years) may derive some benefit from surgery in appropriate centres [276, 278]. All stenosis are graded following the NASCET-method (distal stenosis)[279].

Carotid endarterectomy (CEA) is effective in younger patients, and possibly also in older individuals, but does not appear to benefit women [276]. Patients with occlusion of the internal carotid artery contralateral to the operated carotid artery do not benefit from CEA [280, 281]. The risk of ipsilateral stroke increases with the degree of stenosis [280, 282]; CEA appears to be effective irrespective of the degree of ipsilateral stenosis over the range of 60–99% [276]. CEA is not beneficial for asymp-

tomatic patients who have a life expectancy of less than 5 years. Aspirin should not be stopped in patients undergoing carotid surgery [283]. Patients should be followed up by the referring physician after surgery. There are no data from randomized trials about the benefits and risks of carotid angioplasty, compared with CEA, in asymptomatic patients [284].

Secondary prevention

Optimal management of vascular risk factors

Recommendations

- It is recommended that blood pressure be checked regularly. Blood pressure lowering is recommended after the acute phase, including in patients with normal blood pressure (Class I, Level A).
- It is recommended that blood glucose should be checked regularly. It is recommended that diabetes should be managed with lifestyle modification and individualized pharmacological therapy (Class IV, GCP).
- In patients with type 2 diabetes who do not need insulin, treatment with pioglitazone is recommended after stroke (Class III, Level B).
- Statin therapy is recommended in subjects with non-cardioembolic stroke (Class I, Level A).
- It is recommended that cigarette smoking be discouraged (Class III, Level C).
- It is recommended that heavy use of alcohol be discouraged (Class IV, GCP).
- Regular physical activity is recommended (Class IV, GCP).
- A diet low in salt and saturated fat, high in fruit and vegetables, and rich in fibre is recommended (Class IV, GCP).
- Subjects with an elevated body mass index are recommended to adopt a weight-reducing diet (Class IV, Level C).
- Antioxidant vitamin supplements are not recommended (Class I, Level A).
- Hormone replacement therapy is not recommended for the secondary prevention of stroke (Class I, Level A).
- It is recommended that sleep-disordered breathing such as obstructive sleep apnoea be treated with continuous positive airway pressure breathing (Class III, Level GCP).
- It is recommended that endovascular closure of PFO be considered in patients with cryptogenic stroke and high risk PFO (Class IV, GCP).

High blood pressure

A meta-analysis of seven randomized controlled trials showed that antihypertensive drugs reduced stroke recurrence after stroke or TIA (RR 0.76; 95% CI 0.63–0.92) [285]. This analysis included the PATS (indapamide, a diuretic), HOPE (ramipril) and PROGRESS (perindopril, with or without indapamide) studies [286–289]. The reduction in stroke occurs regardless of BP and type of stroke [289]. Hence, BP should be lowered and monitored indefinitely after stroke or TIA. The absolute target BP level and reduction are uncertain and should be individualized, but benefit has been associated with an average reduction of about 10/5 mmHg, and normal BP levels have been defined as <120/80 mmHg [290]. However, blood pressure should not be lowered intensively in patients with suspected haemodynamic stroke or in those with bilateral carotid stenosis. The angiotensin receptor antagonist eprosartan may be more effective than the calcium channel blocker nitrendipine [291].

Diabetes mellitus

The prospective, double-blind PROactive trial randomized 5238 patients with type 2 diabetes and a history of macrovascular disease to pioglitazone or placebo. In patients with previous stroke ($n = 486$ in the pioglitazone group, $n = 498$ in the placebo group), there was a trend towards benefit with pioglitazone for the combined endpoint of death and major vascular events (HR 0.78; 95% CI 0.60–1.02; $p = 0.067$). In a secondary analysis, pioglitazone reduced fatal or non-fatal stroke (HR 0.53; 95% CI 0.34–0.85; $p = 0.0085$) and cardiovascular death, non-fatal myocardial infarction, or non-fatal stroke (HR 0.72; 95% CI 0.52–1.00; $p = 0.0467$) [292].

Hyperlipidaemia

In the SPARCL (Stroke Prevention by Aggressive Reduction in Cholesterol Levels) trial, statin therapy with atorvastatin reduced stroke recurrence (HR 0.84; 95% CI 0.71–0.99) [293], while in the Heart Protection Study, simvastatin reduced vascular events in patients with prior stroke, and reduced stroke in patients with other vascular disease (RR 0.76) [221]. Neither trial assessed efficacy by stroke subtype, and SPARCL did not include patients with presumed cardioembolic stroke [221, 293]. The risk of haemorrhagic stroke was slightly increased in both trials [221, 293]. The absolute risk reduction achieved with statin therapy is low (NNT 112–143 for 1 year). Statin

withdrawal at the acute stage of stroke may be associated with an increased risk of death or dependency [294].

Cigarette smoking

There are no specific data in secondary prevention. See primary prevention.

Diet

Overweight

There are no specific data in secondary prevention. See primary prevention. Weight loss may be beneficial after stroke as it lowers blood pressure [245].

Vitamins

Beta carotene increased the risk of cardiovascular death in a meta-analysis of primary and secondary prevention trials (RR 1.10; 95% CI 1.03–1.17) [295]. Vitamin E supplementation does not prevent vascular events [296]. Fat-soluble antioxidant supplements may increase mortality [297].

Vitamins that lower homocysteine (folate, B12, B6) do not appear to reduce stroke recurrence and may increase vascular events [298–301], but further trials are ongoing [302].

Sleep-disordered breathing

Sleep-disordered breathing represents both a risk factor and a consequence of stroke and is linked with poorer long-term outcome and increased long-term stroke mortality [303]. More than 50% of stroke patients have sleep-disordered breathing, mostly in the form of obstructive sleep apnoea (OSA). This can improve spontaneously after stroke, but may need treatment. Continuous positive airway pressure is the treatment of choice for OSA. Oxygen and other forms of ventilation may be helpful in other (e.g. central) forms of SDB.

Patent foramen ovale

Case reports and case control studies indicate an association between the presence of PFO and cryptogenic stroke in both younger and older stroke patients [304, 305]. Two population-based studies pointed in the same direction but did not confirm a significant association [306, 307]. In patients with PFO alone, the overall risk of recurrence is low. However, when the PFO is combined with an atrial septal aneurysm, a Eustachian valve, a Chiari network, or in patients who have suffered more than one stroke, the risk of recurrence can be substantial [308]. Endovascular closure of PFOs with or without septal aneurysms is feasible in such patients [309] and may lower the risk of recurrent stroke compared to medical treatment [310]; however, RCTs are still lacking.

Postmenopausal oestrogen replacement therapy

Hormone replacement therapy does not protect against vascular events and may increase stroke severity [311].

Antithrombotic therapy

Recommendations

- It is recommended that patients receive antithrombotic therapy (Class I, Level A).
- It is recommended that patients not requiring anticoagulation should receive antiplatelet therapy (Class I, Level A). Where possible, combined aspirin and dipyridamole, or clopidogrel alone, should be given. Alternatively, aspirin alone or triflusal alone may be used (Class I, Level A).
- The combination of aspirin and clopidogrel is not recommended in patients with recent ischaemic stroke, except in patients with specific indications (e.g. unstable angina or non-Q-wave MI, or recent stenting); treatment should be given for up to 9 months after the event (Class I, Level A).
- It is recommended that patients who have a stroke on antiplatelet therapy should be re-evaluated for pathophysiology and risk factors (Class IV, GCP).
- Oral anticoagulation (INR 2.0–3.0) is recommended after ischaemic stroke associated with AF (Class I, Level A). Oral anticoagulation is not recommended in patients with comorbid conditions such as falls, poor compliance, uncontrolled epilepsy, or gastrointestinal bleeding (Class III, Level C). Increasing age alone is not a contraindication to oral anticoagulation (Class I, Level A).
- It is recommended that patients with cardioembolic stroke unrelated to AF should receive anticoagulants (INR 2.0–3.0) if the risk of recurrence is high (Class III, Level C).
- It is recommended that anticoagulation should not be used after non-cardioembolic ischaemic stroke, except in some specific situations, such as aortic atheromas, fusiform aneurysms of the basilar artery, cervical artery dissection, or patent foramen ovale in the presence of proven deep vein thrombosis (DVT) or atrial septal aneurysm (Class IV, GCP).
- It is recommended that combined low dose aspirin and dipyridamole should be given if oral anticoagulation is contraindicated (Class IV, GCP).

Antiplatelet therapy

Antiplatelet therapy reduces vascular events, including non-fatal myocardial infarction, nonfatal stroke and vascular death in patients with previous stroke or TIA (RR 0.78; 95% CI 0.76–0.80) [312].

Aspirin

Aspirin reduces recurrence irrespective of dose (50 to 1300 mg/d) [313–316], although high doses (>150 mg/day) increase adverse events. In patients with symptomatic intracranial atherosclerosis, aspirin is as effective as oral anticoagulation and has fewer complications [317].

Clopidogrel

Clopidogrel is slightly more effective than aspirin in preventing vascular events (RR 0.91; 95% CI 0.84–0.97) [318]. It may be more effective in high-risk patients (i.e. those with previous stroke, peripheral artery disease, symptomatic coronary disease, or diabetes) [268].

Dipyridamole

Dipyridamole reduces stroke recurrence with similar efficacy to aspirin [319].

Triflusal

Triflusal reduces stroke recurrence with similar efficacy to aspirin but with fewer adverse events [320].

Dipyridamole plus aspirin

The combination of aspirin (38–300 mg/d) and dipyridamole (200 mg extended release twice daily) reduces the risk of vascular death, stroke or MI, compared with aspirin alone (RR 0.82; 95% CI 0.74–0.91) [319, 321]. Dipyridamole may cause headache; the incidence of this may be reduced by increasing the dose gradually [322, 323].

Clopidogrel plus aspirin

Compared with clopidogrel alone, the combination of aspirin and clopidogrel did not reduce the risk of ischaemic stroke, myocardial infarction, vascular death, or re-hospitalization [324]; however, life-threatening or major bleeding were increased with the combination. Similarly, in the CHARISMA study, the combination of aspirin and clopidogrel did not reduce the risk of myocardial infarction, stroke, or death from cardiovascular causes, compared with aspirin alone [268]. In patients who have had an acute coronary event within 12 months, or coronary stenting, the combination of clopidogrel and aspirin reduces the risk of new vascular events [325].

Oral anticoagulation

Oral anticoagulation after non-cardiac ischaemic stroke is not superior to aspirin, but causes more bleeding [326–328]. Oral anticoagulation (INR 2.0–3.0) reduces the risk of recurrent stroke in patients with non-valvular AF (whether of permanent, chronic, or paroxysmal type) [329] and most other cardiac sources of emboli. Anticoagulation should be taken long term, or for at least 3 months after cardioembolic stroke due to MI [330]. There is a controversial discussion about the optimal time point to start oral anticoagulation. After TIA or minor stroke one could start immediately, but after major stroke with significant infarction on neuroimaging (e.g. above a third of the MCA territory) one should wait for some (e.g. 4) weeks. However, this decision has to be individualized.

In patients with AF and stable coronary disease, aspirin should not be added to oral anticoagulation [331]. Anticoagulation may be beneficial in patients with aortic atheroma [332], fusiform aneurysms of the basilar artery [333], or cervical dissection [334]. The ongoing ARCH trial is comparing the combination of clopidogrel plus aspirin with oral anticoagulation in secondary prevention of patients with atherosclerotic plaques in the aortic arch.

Recurrent vascular event on antiplatelet therapy

The treatment of patients who have a recurrent vascular event on antiplatelet therapy remains unclear. Alternative causes of stroke should be sought and consistent risk-factor management is mandatory especially in those patients. Alternative treatment strategies may be considered: leave unchanged, change to another antiplatelet agent, add another antiplatelet agent, or use oral anticoagulation.

Surgery and angioplasty

Recommendations

- CEA is recommended for patients with 70–99% stenosis (Class I, Level A). CEA should only be performed in centres with a perioperative complication rate (all strokes and death) of less than 6% (Class I, Level A).
- It is recommended that CEA be performed as soon as possible after the last ischaemic event, ideally within 2 weeks (Class II, Level B).
- It is recommended that CEA may be indicated for certain patients with stenosis of 50–69%; males with very recent hemispheric symptoms are most likely to benefit (Class III, Level C). CEA for stenosis of 50–69% should only be performed in centres with a perioperative complication rate (all stroke and death) of less than 3% (Class I, Level A).
- CEA is not recommended for patients with stenosis of less than 50% (Class I, Level A).
- It is recommended that patients remain on antiplatelet therapy both before and after surgery (Class I, Level A).
- Carotid percutaneous transluminal angioplasty and/or stenting (CAS) is only recommended in selected patients (Class I, Level A). It should be restricted to the following subgroups of patients with severe symptomatic carotid artery stenosis: those with contraindications to CEA, stenosis at a surgically inaccessible site, re-stenosis after earlier CEA, and post-radiation stenosis (Class IV, GCP). Patients should receive a combination of clopidogrel and aspirin immediately before and for at least 1 month after stenting (Class IV, GCP).
- It is recommended that endovascular treatment may be considered in patients with symptomatic intracranial stenosis (Class IV, GPC).

Carotid endarterectomy

The grading of stenosis should be performed according to the NASCET criteria. Although ECST (European Carotid Surgery Trialists) and NASCET use different methods of measurement, it is possible to convert the percentage stenosis derived by one method to the other [335]. CEA reduces the risk of recurrent disabling stroke or death (RR 0.52) in patients with severe (70–99%) ipsilateral internal carotid artery stenosis [279, 336, 337]. Patients with less severe ipsilateral carotid stenosis (50–69%) may also benefit [337]. Surgery is potentially harmful in patients with mild or moderate degrees of stenosis (<50%) [337].

CEA should be performed as soon as possible (ideally within 2 weeks) after the last cerebrovascular event [338].

Surgical procedure is important in preventing stroke; carotid patch angioplasty may reduce the risk of perioperative arterial occlusion and restenosis [339].

Older patients (>75 years) without organ failure or serious cardiac dysfunction benefit from CEA [338]. Women with severe (>70%) symptomatic stenosis should undergo CEA, whereas women with more moderate stenosis should be treated medically [340]. Patients with amaurosis fugax, severe stenosis, and a high-risk profile should be considered for CEA; those with amaurosis fugax and few risk factors do better with medical treatment. Patients with mild-to-moderate intracranial stenosis and severe extracranial stenosis should be considered for CEA.

The benefit from CEA is less in patients with lacunar stroke [341]. Patients with leukoaraiosis carry an increased perioperative risk [342]. Occlusion of the contralateral ICA is not a contraindication to CEA but carries a higher perioperative risk. The benefit from endarterectomy is marginal in patients with carotid near-occlusion.

Carotid angioplasty and stenting

Several trials have compared CAS and CEA in secondary stroke prevention (table 9.9) [343–346]. However, the SAPPHIRE (Stenting and Angioplasty with Protection in Patients at High Risk for Endarterectomy) trial included more than 70% asymptomatic patients, and therefore should not be used for decisions about secondary prevention [345]. In CAVATAS (Carotid and Vertebral Artery Transluminal Angioplasty Study) the majority of the patients in the endovascular group underwent angioplasty, and only 26% were treated with a stent [346]. The two most recent studies revealed different results. SPACE (Stent-protected Angioplasty versus Carotid Eendarterectomy in symptomatic patients) marginally failed to prove the non-inferiority of CAS compared to CEA; for the endpoint ipsilateral stroke or death up to day 30, the event rates after 1,200 patients were 6.8% for CAS and 6.3% for CEA-patients (absolute difference 0.5%; 95% CI −1.9% to +2.9%; $p = 0.09$) [344]. The French EVA3S (Endarterectomy versus Stenting in Patients with Symptomatic Severe Carotid Stenosis) trial was stopped prematurely after the inclusion of 527 patients because of safety concerns and lack of efficacy. The RR of any stroke or death after CAS, compared with CEA, was 2.5 (95% CI 1.2–5.1) [343]. An updated meta-analysis of these studies revealed a significantly higher risk of any stroke and death within 30 days after CAS, compared with CEA (OR 1.41; 95% CI 1.07–1.87; $p = 0.016$). However, significant heterogeneity was found in this analysis ($p = 0.035$) [347]. After the periprocedural period, few ipsilateral strokes occurred with either procedure (table 9.9).

Intracranial and vertebral artery occlusive disease

Extracranial-intracranial anastomosis
Anastomosis between the superficial temporal and middle cerebral arteries is not beneficial in preventing stroke in patients with MCA or ICA stenosis or occlusion [348].

Table 9.9 Risk of stroke or death from large-scale randomized trials comparing endovascular and surgical treatment in patients with severe carotid artery stenosis.

Outcome	Any stroke or death at 30 days		Disabling stroke or death at 30 days		Ipsilateral stroke after 30 days	
	CAS n (%)	CEA n (%)	CAS n (%)	CEA n (%)	CAS n (%)	CEA n (%)
CAVATAS [346]	25 (10.0)	25 (9.9)	16 (6.4)	15 (5.9)	6[+]	10[+]
SAPPHIRE [345]	8 (4.8)	9 (5.4)	unk	unk	unk	unk
SPACE [344, 585]	46 (7.7)	38 (6.5)	29 (4.8)	23 (3.9)	4 (0.7)*	1 (0.2)*
EVA3S [343]	25 (9.6)	10 (3.9)	9 (3.4)	4 (1.5)	2 (0.6)*	1 (0.3)*

Intention-to-treat data; unk: unknown.
[+]Follow-up duration 1.95 years in mean;
*up to 6 months.

Stenting of intracranial or vertebral artery stenoses

Patients with symptomatic intracranial stenoses of ≥50 % are at high risk of recurrent strokes, both in the anterior and posterior circulation (12% after 1 year and 15% after 2 years in the territory of the stenosed artery) [317, 349]. Severe stenoses (≥70 %) carry a higher risk than moderate stenoses (50% to <70%) [349]. After stenting, recurrent strokes are reported in about 5–7% of patients with moderate or severe stenoses after 1 year, and in around 8% after 2 years [350, 351]. However, the incidence of complications after either angioplasty or stenting may be up to 6% [352-354]. No randomized controlled trials have evaluated angioplasty, stenting, or both for intracranial stenosis. Several non-randomized trials have shown feasibility and acceptable safety of intracranial stenting, but the risk of restenosis remains high [354, 355]. Also stenting of the extracranial segments of the vertebral artery is technical feasible with a moderate periprocedural risk as demonstrated in the SSYLVIA trial for example; but especially at the origin there is a particular high rate of restenoses [355].

General stroke treatment

Recommendations

- Intermittent monitoring of neurological status, pulse, blood pressure, temperature, and oxygen saturation is recommended for 72 h in patients with significant persisting neurological deficits (Class IV, GCP).
- It is recommended that oxygen should be administered if the oxygen saturation falls below 95% (Class IV, GCP).
- Regular monitoring of fluid balance and electrolytes is recommended in patients with severe stroke or swallowing problems (Class IV, GCP).
- Normal saline (0.9%) is recommended for fluid replacement during the first 24 h after stroke (Class IV, GCP).
- Routine blood pressure lowering is not recommended following acute stroke (Class IV, GCP).
- Cautious blood pressure lowering is recommended in patients with extremely high blood pressures (>220/120 mmHg) on repeated measurements, or with severe cardiac failure, aortic dissection, or hypertensive encephalopathy (Class IV, GCP).
- It is recommended that abrupt blood pressure lowering be avoided (Class II, Level C).

- It is recommended that low blood pressure secondary to hypovolaemia or associated with neurological deterioration in acute stroke should be treated with volume expanders (Class IV, GCP).
- Monitoring serum glucose levels is recommended (Class IV, GCP).
- Treatment of serum glucose levels >180 mg/dl (>10 mmol/l) with insulin titration is recommended (Class IV, GCP).
- It is recommended that severe hypoglycaemia (<50 mg/dl [<2.8 mmol/l]) should be treated with i.v. dextrose or infusion of 10–20% glucose (Class IV, GCP points).
- It is recommended that the presence of pyrexia (temperature >37.5°C) should prompt a search for concurrent infection (Class IV, GCP).
- Treatment of pyrexia (temperature >37.5°C) with paracetamol and fanning is recommended (Class III, Level C).
- Antibiotic prophylaxis is not recommended in immunocompetent patients (Class II, Level B).

The term 'general treatment' refers to treatment strategies aimed at stabilizing the critically ill patient in order to control systemic problems that may impair stroke recovery; the management of such problems is a central part of stroke treatment [2, 105]. General treatment includes respiratory and cardiac care, fluid and metabolic management, blood pressure control, the prevention and treatment of conditions such as seizures, venous thromboembolism, dysphagia, aspiration pneumonia, other infections, or pressure ulceration, and occasionally management of elevated intracranial pressure. However, many aspects of general stroke treatment have not been adequately assessed in randomized clinical trials.

It is common practice to actively manage neurological status and vital physiological functions such as blood pressure, pulse, oxygen saturation, blood glucose, and temperature. Neurological status can be monitored using validated neurological scales such as the NIH Stroke Scale [103] or the Scandinavian Stroke Scale [356]. There is little direct evidence from randomized clinical trials to indicate how intensively monitoring should be carried out, but in stroke unit trials [118] it was common practice to have a minimum of 4-hourly observations for the first 72 h after stroke. Clinical trials using continuous telemetry [357, 358] suggest there may be some benefit from more intensive continuous monitoring in terms of improved detection of complications and reduced length of stay, but clinical outcomes are inconclusive. In practice, more intensive monitoring is often provided for subgroups of patients, such as those with reduced consciousness, progressing neurological deficits, or a history of cardiorespiratory disease. Close monitoring is also required for the first 24 h after thrombolysis. More invasive monitoring procedures, such as central venous catheters or intracranial pressure monitoring, are used only in highly selected patient groups.

Pulmonary function and airway protection

Normal respiratory function with adequate blood oxygenation is believed to be important in the acute stroke period to preserve ischaemic brain tissue. However, there is no convincing evidence that routine provision of oxygen at low flow rates to all acute stroke patients is effective [359]. Identification and treatment of hypoxia is believed to be important in individuals with extensive brainstem or hemispheric stroke, seizure activity, or complications such as pneumonia, cardiac failure, pulmonary embolism, or exacerbation of chronic obstructive pulmonary disease (COPD). Blood oxygenation is usually improved by the administration of 2–4 litres of oxygen via a nasal tube. Ventilation may be necessary in patients with severely compromised respiratory function. However, before ventilation is performed the general prognosis, coexisting medical conditions, and the presumed wishes of the patient need to be considered.

Cardiac care

Cardiac arrhythmias, particularly AF, are relatively common after stroke, and heart failure, myocardial infarction, and sudden death are also recognized complications [360, 361]. A significant minority of stroke patients show raised blood troponin levels indicative of cardiac damage [362]. Every stroke patient should have an initial ECG. Cardiac monitoring should be conducted to screen for AF. Optimizing cardiac output with maintenance of high normal blood pressure and a normal heart rate is a standard component of stroke management. The use of inotropic agents is not routine practice, but fluid replacement therapy is commonly used to correct hypovolaemia. Increases in cardiac output may increase cerebral perfusion. Restoration of normal cardiac rhythm using drugs, cardioversion, or pacemaker support may occasionally be required.

Fluid replacement therapy

Many stroke patients are dehydrated on admission to hospital, and this is associated with a poor outcome [363]. Although clinical trial evidence is limited, delivery of i.v. fluids is commonly considered part of general management of acute stroke, particularly in patients at risk of dehydration due to reduced consciousness or impaired swallowing. Experience in the management of hyperglycaemia supports the avoidance of dextrose in the early post-stroke phase [364]. More specialist fluid replacement therapy with haemodilution has not been shown to improve stroke outcomes [365].

Blood pressure management

Blood pressure monitoring and treatment is a controversial area in stroke management. Patients with the highest and lowest levels of blood pressure in the first 24 h after stroke are more likely to have early neurological decline and poorer outcomes [366]. A low or low-normal blood pressure at stroke onset is unusual [367], and may be the result of a large cerebral infarct, cardiac failure, ischaemia, hypovolaemia, or sepsis. Blood pressure can usually be raised by adequate rehydration with crystalloid (saline) solutions; patients with low cardiac output may occasionally need inotropic support. However, clinical trials of actively elevating a low blood pressure in acute stroke have yielded inconclusive results.

A systematic review covering a variety of blood pressure altering agents has not provided any convincing evidence that active management of blood pressure after acute stroke influences patient outcomes [368]. Small studies looking at surrogate markers of cerebral blood flow such as SPECT have indicated that neither perindopril nor losartan lower cerebral blood flow when given within 2–7 days of stroke onset [369]. Several ongoing trials are examining whether blood pressure should be lowered after acute stroke, and whether antihypertensive therapy should be continued or stopped in the first few days after stroke [370, 371]. In the absence of reliable evidence from clinical trials, many clinicians have developed protocols for the management of extremely high blood pressure. In some centres it is common practice to begin cautious blood pressure reduction when levels exceed 220 mmHg systolic and 120 mmHg diastolic. However, in many centres blood pressure reduction is only considered in the presence of severe cardiac insufficiency, acute renal failure, aortic arch dissection, or malignant hypertension. In patients undergoing thrombolysis it is common practice to avoid systolic blood pressures above 185 mmHg.

The use of sublingual nifedipine should be avoided because of the risk of an abrupt decrease in blood pressure [372]. Intravenous labetalol or urapadil are frequently used in North America. Sodium nitroprusside is sometimes recommended.

Blood glucose management

Hyperglycaemia occurs in up to 60% of stroke patients without known diabetes [373, 374]. Hyperglycaemia after acute stroke is associated with larger infarct volumes and cortical involvement, and with poor functional outcome [375-377]. There is limited evidence as to whether active reduction of glucose in acute ischaemic stroke improves patient outcomes. The largest randomized trial of blood glucose lowering by glucose potassium insulin infusion [364], compared with standard i.v. saline infusion, found no difference in mortality or functional outcomes in patients with mild-to-moderate blood glucose elevations (median 137 mg/dl [7.6 mmol/l]). This regime was labour-intensive and associated with episodes of hypoglycaemia. At present the routine use of insulin infusion regimes in patients with moderate hyperglycaemia cannot be recommended. However, it is common practice in stroke units to reduce blood glucose levels exceeding 180 mg/dl (10 mmol/l) [118]. The use of i.v. saline and avoidance of glucose solutions in the first 24 h after stroke is common practice, and appears to reduce blood glucose levels [364].

Hypoglycaemia (<50 mg/dl [2.8 mmol/l]) may mimic an acute ischaemic infarction, and should be treated by i.v. dextrose bolus or infusion of 10–20% glucose [378].

Body temperature management

In experimental stroke, hyperthermia is associated with increased infarct size and poor outcome [379]. Raised temperature can be centrally driven or a result of concurrent infection, and is associated with poorer clinical outcomes [380-382]. A raised body temperature should prompt a search for infection and treatment where appropriate. Studies with antipyretic medication have been inconclusive, but treatment of raised body temperature (>37.5°C) with paracetamol is common practice in stroke patients.

Specific treatment

Recommendations

- Intravenous rtPA (0.9 mg/kg body weight, maximum 90 mg), with 10% of the dose given as a bolus followed by a 60-min infusion, is recommended within 4.5 h of onset of ischaemic stroke (Class I, Level A), although treatment between 3 and 4.5 h is currently not included in the European labelling (modified January 2009).

- The use of multimodal imaging criteria may be useful for patient selection for thrombolysis but is not recommended for routine clinical practice (Class III, Level C).

- It is recommended that blood pressures of 185/110 mmHg or higher is lowered before thrombolysis (Class IV, GCP).

- It is recommended that i.v. rtPA may be used in patients with seizures at stroke onset, if the neurological deficit is related to acute cerebral ischaemia (Class IV, GCP).

- It is recommended that i.v. rtPA may also be administered in selected patients under 18 years and over 80 years of age, although this is outside the current European labelling (Class III, Level C).

- Intra-arterial treatment of acute MCA occlusion within a 6-h time window is recommended as an option (Class II, Level B).

- Intra-arterial thrombolysis is recommended for acute basilar occlusion in selected patients (Class III, Level B). Intravenous thrombolysis for basilar occlusion is an acceptable alternative even after 3 h (Class III, Level B).

- It is recommended that aspirin (160–325 mg loading dose) be given within 48 h after ischaemic stroke (Class I, Level A).

- It is recommended that if thrombolytic therapy is planned or given, aspirin or other antithrombotic therapy should not be initiated within 24 h (Class IV, GCP).

- The use of other antiplatelet agents (single or combined) is not recommended in the setting of acute ischaemic stroke.

- The administration of glycoprotein-IIb-IIIa inhibitors is not recommended (Class I, Level A).

- Early administration of unfractionated heparin, low molecular weight heparin, or heparinoids is not recommended for the treatment of patients with acute ischaemic stroke (Class I, Level A).

- Currently, there is no recommendation to treat ischaemic stroke patients with neuroprotective substances (Class I, Level A).

Thrombolytic therapy

Intravenous tissue plasminogen activator

Thrombolytic therapy with rtPA (0.9 mg/kg body weight, maximum dose 90 mg) given within 3 h after stroke onset significantly improves outcome in patients with acute ischaemic stroke [125]: the NNT to achieve a favourable clinical outcome after 3 months is 7. By contrast, the ECASS (European Cooperative Acute Stroke Study) and ECASS II studies did not show statistically significant superiority of rtPA for the primary endpoints when treatment was given within 6 h [383, 384]. Trials with rtPA, involving a total of 2,889 patients, have shown a significant reduction in the number of patients with death or dependency (OR 0.83; 95% CI 0.73–0.94) [385]. A pooled analysis of individual data of rtPA trials showed that, even within a 3-h window, earlier treatment results in a better outcome (0–90 min: OR 2.11; 95% CI 1.33 to 3.55; 90–180 min: OR 1.69; 95% CI 1.09 to 2.62) [386]. This analysis suggested a benefit up to 4.5 h.

The recently published trial European Cooperative Acute Stroke Study III (ECASS III) has shown that i.v. alteplase administered between 3 and 4.5 h (median 3 h 59 min) after the onset of symptoms significantly improves clinical outcomes in patients with acute ischemic stroke compared to placebo [387, 388]; the absolute improvement was 7.2% and the adjusted OR of favourable outcome (mRS 0–1) was 1.42, 1.02–1.98. Mortality did not differ significantly (7.7% versus 8.4%), but alteplase increased the risk of SICH (2.4% versus 0.2%). Treatment benefit is time-dependent. The number needed to treat to get one more favourable outcome drops from 2 during the first 90 min through 7 within 3 h and towards 14 between 3 and 4.5 h [387, 388].

The SITS investigators compared 664 patients with ischaemic stroke treated between 3 and 4.5 h otherwise compliant with the European summary of the product characteristics criteria with 11,865 patients treated within 3 h [389].

In the 3–4.5-h cohort, treatment was started on average 55 min later after symptom onset. There were no significant differences between the 3–4.5-h cohort and the 3-h cohort for any outcome measures, confirming that alteplase remains safe when given between 3 and 4.5 h after the onset of symptoms in ischaemic stroke patients who otherwise fulfil the European summary of product characteristics criteria [389] (modified January 2009).

The NINDS (National Institute of Neurological Disorders and Stroke) Study showed that the extent of early ischaemic changes (using the ASPECT score) had no effect on treatment response within the 3-h time window [387]. However, European regulatory agencies do not advocate rtPA treatment in patients with severe stroke (NIHSSS ≥25), extended early ischaemic changes on CT scan, or age above 80 years (unlike the US labelling). Nevertheless, observational studies suggest that rtPA given within 3 h of stroke onset is safe and effective in patients over 80 years of age [390–392], but more randomized data are pending. The effect of gender on the response to rtPA is uncertain [393].

Thrombolytic therapy appears to be safe and effective across various types of hospitals, if the diagnosis is established by a physician with stroke expertise and brain CT is assessed by an experienced physician [394-396]. Whenever possible, the risks and benefits of rtPA should be discussed with the patient and family before treatment is initiated.

Blood pressure must be below 185/110 mmHg before, and for the first 24 h after, thrombolysis. Management of high blood pressure is required [125]. Protocol violations are associated with higher mortality rates [397, 398].

Continuous transcranial ultrasound was associated with an increased rate of early recanalization after rtPA in a small randomized trial [399]; this effect may be facilitated by the administration of microbubbles [400]. However, a randomized clinical trial has recently been stopped for undisclosed reasons.

Intravenous rtPA may be of benefit also for acute ischaemic stroke beyond 3 h after onset, but is not recommended in clinical routine. The use of multimodal imaging criteria may be useful for patient selection. Several large observational studies suggest improved safety and possibly improved efficacy in patients treated with i.v. rtPA beyond 3 h based on advanced imaging findings [130, 159, 401, 402]. However, available data on mismatch, as defined by multimodal MRI or CT, are too limited to guide thrombolysis in routine practice (see also the section on imaging) [152].

Patients with seizures at stroke onset have been excluded from thrombolytic trials because of potential confusion with post-ictal Todd's phenomena. Case series have suggested that thrombolysis may be used in such patients when there is evidence for new ischaemic stroke [390].

Post hoc analyses have identified the following potential factors associated with increased risk of intracerebral bleeding complications after rtPA use [403]:
- elevated serum glucose
- history of diabetes

- baseline symptom severity
- advanced age
- increased time to treatment
- previous aspirin use
- history of congestive heart failure
- low plasminogen activator inhibitor activity
- NINDS protocol violations.

However, none of these factors reversed the overall benefit of rtPA.

Other intravenous thrombolytics

Intravenous streptokinase was associated with an unacceptable risk of haemorrhage and death [404, 405]. Intravenous desmoteplase administered 3 to 9 h after acute ischaemic stroke in patients selected on the basis of perfusion/diffusion mismatch was associated with a higher rate of reperfusion and better clinical outcome, compared with placebo, in two small randomized clinical trials (RCTs) [406, 407]. These findings were not confirmed in the phase III DIAS (Desmoteplase in Acute Ischemic Stroke)-II study, but this agent will be evaluated further.

Intra-arterial and combined (IV + IA) thrombolysis

Intra-arterial thrombolytic treatment of proximal MCA occlusion using pro-urokinase (PUK) within 6 h was significantly associated with better outcome in the PROACT II (Pro-urokinase for Acute Ischemic Stroke) trial [153]. Additional smaller RCTs with PUK (PROACT I) or urokinase (MELT) and a meta-analysis of PROACT I, PROACT II, and MELT indicate a benefit of intra-arterial thrombolytic therapy in patients with proximal MCA occlusions [408]. Pro-urokinase is not available and intra-arterial thrombolysis with tPA is not substantiated by RCTs, but observational data and non-randomised comparisons are available [154, 409].

A randomized trial comparing standard i.v. rtPA with a combined intravenous and intra-arterial approach (IMS3) has started [410].

Intra-arterial treatment of acute basilar occlusion with urokinase or rtPA has been available for more than 20 years, but has not been tested in an adequately powered RCT [411], although encouraging results have been obtained in observational studies [412, 413]. A systematic analysis found no significant differences between intravenous or intra-arterial thrombolysis for basilar occlusion [414].

Intra-arterial recanalization devices

The MERCI (Mechanical Embolus Removal in Cerebral Embolism) trial evaluated a device that removed the thrombus from an intracranial artery. Recanalization was achieved in 48% (68/141) of patients in whom the device was deployed within 8 h of the onset of stroke symptoms [415]. No RCTs with outcome data are available for any recanalization devices.

Antiplatelet therapy

The results of two large randomized, non-blinded, intervention studies indicate that aspirin is safe and effective when started within 48 h after stroke [416, 417]. In absolute terms, 13 more patients were alive and independent at the end of follow-up for every 1000 patients treated. Furthermore, treatment increased the odds of making a complete recovery from the stroke (OR 1.06; 95% CI 1.01–1.11): 10 more patients made a complete recovery for every 1000 patients treated. Antiplatelet therapy was associated with a small but definite excess of two symptomatic intracranial haemorrhages for every 1000 patients treated, but this was more than offset by a reduction of seven recurrent ischaemic strokes and about one pulmonary embolism for every 1000 patients treated.

A randomized, double-blind, placebo-controlled trial showed that aspirin (325 mg), given once daily for 5 consecutive days and starting within 48 h of stroke onset, did not significantly reduce stroke progression, compared with placebo (RR 0.95; 95% CI 0.62–1.45) in patients with incomplete paresis [418].

The use of clopidogrel, dipyridamole, or combinations of oral antiplatelet agents in acute ischaemic stroke has not been evaluated.

In a double-blind phase II, the glycoprotein-IIb-IIIa inhibitor abciximab produced a non-significant shift in favourable outcomes, as measured by modified Rankin scores (mRS) at 3 months, compared with placebo (OR 1.20; 95% CI 0.84–1.70) [419]. A phase III study evaluating the safety and efficacy of abciximab was terminated prematurely after 808 patients had been enrolled because of an increased rate of symptomatic or fatal intracranial bleeding with abciximab compared to placebo (5.5% versus 0.5%; $p = 0.002$). This trial also did not demonstrate an improvement in outcomes with abciximab [420].

Early anticoagulation

Subcutaneous unfractionated heparin (UFH) at low or moderate doses [415], nadroparin [421, 422], certoparin [423], tinzaparin [424], dalteparin [425], and i.v. danaparoid [426] have failed to show an overall benefit of anticoagulation when initiated within 24 to 48 h from stroke onset. Improvements in outcome or reductions in stroke recurrence rates were mostly counterbalanced by an increased number of haemorrhagic complications. In a meta-analysis of 22 trials, anticoagulant therapy was associated with about nine fewer recurrent ischaemic strokes per 1000 patients treated (OR 0.76; 95% CI 0.65–0.88), and with about nine more symptomatic intracranial haemorrhages per 1,000 (OR 2.52; 95% CI 1.92-3.30) [427]. However, the quality of the trials varied considerably. The anticoagulants tested were standard UFH, low molecular weight heparins, heparinoids, oral anticoagulants, and thrombin inhibitors.

Few clinical trials have assessed the risk-benefit ratio of very early administration of UFH in acute ischaemic stroke. In one study, patients with nonlacunar stroke anticoagulated within 3 h had more self-independence (38.9% versus 28.6%; $p = 0.025$), fewer deaths (16.8% versus 21.9%; $p = 0.189$), and more symptomatic brain haemorrhages (6.2% versus 1.4%; $p = 0.008$) [428]. In the RAPID (Rapid Anticoagulation Prevents Ischemic Damage) trial, patients allocated UFH had fewer early recurrent strokes and a similar incidence of serious haemorrhagic events, compared with those receiving aspirin [429]. In the UFH group, ischaemic or haemorrhagic worsening was associated with inadequate plasma levels of UFH. In view of these findings, the value of UFH administered shortly after symptom onset is still debated [430, 431].

RCTs have not identified a net benefit of heparin for any stroke subtype. A meta-analysis restricted to patients with acute cardioembolic stroke showed that anticoagulants given within 48 h of clinical onset were associated with a non-significant reduction in recurrence of ischaemic stroke, but no substantial reduction in death or disability [432]. Despite this lack of evidence, some experts recommend full-dose heparin in selected patients, such as those with cardiac sources of embolism with high risk of re-embolism, arterial dissection, or high-grade arterial stenosis prior to surgery. Contraindications for heparin treatment include large infarcts (e.g. more than 50% of MCA territory), uncontrollable arterial hypertension and advanced microvascular changes in the brain.

Neuroprotection

No neuroprotection programme has shown improved outcome on its predefined primary endpoint. Recent RCTs with the free radical trapping agent NXY-059 [433] and magnesium sulphate [434] were negative. A randomized, placebo-controlled, phase III trial of i.v. rtPA followed by antioxidant therapy with uric acid is ongoing, following a safe phase II study [435]. A meta-analysis has suggested a mild benefit with citocoline [436]; a clinical trial with this agent is in progress.

Brain oedema and elevated intracranial pressure

Recommendations

- Surgical decompressive therapy within 48 h after symptom onset is recommended in patients up to 60 years of age with evolving malignant MCA infarcts (Class I, Level A).

- It is recommended that osmotherapy can be used to treat elevated intracranial pressure prior to surgery if this is considered (Class III, Level C).

- No recommendation can be given regarding hypothermic therapy in patients with space-occupying infarctions (Class IV, GCP).

- It is recommended that ventriculostomy or surgical decompression be considered for treatment of large cerebellar infarctions that compress the brainstem (Class III, Level C).

Space-occupying brain oedema is a main cause of early deterioration and death in patients with large supratentorial infarcts. Life-threatening brain oedema usually develops between the second and fifth day after stroke onset, but up to a third of patients can have neurological deterioration within 24 h after symptom onset [437, 438].

Medical therapy

Medical therapy in patients with large space-occupying infarctions and brain oedema is based mostly on observational data. Basic management includes head positioning at an elevation of up to 30°, avoidance of noxious stimuli, pain relief, appropriate oxygenation, and normalizing body temperature. If intracranial pressure (ICP) monitoring is available, cerebral perfusion pressure should be kept above 70 mmHg [439]. Intravenous glycerol (4 × 250 ml of 10% glycerol over 30–60 minutes) or mannitol (25–50 g every 3–6 h) is first-line medical treatment if clinical or radiological signs of space-occupying oedema occur [440, 441]. Intravenous hypertonic saline solutions are probably similarly effective [442]. Hypotonic and glucose-containing solutions should be avoided as replacement fluids. Dexamethasone and corticosteroids are not useful [443]. Thiopental given as a bolus can quickly and significantly reduce ICP, and can be used to treat acute crises. Barbiturate treatment requires ICP and electroencephalography (EEG) monitoring and careful haemodynamic monitoring, as a significant blood pressure drop may occur.

Hypothermia

Mild hypothermia (i.e. brain temperature between 32 and 33°C) reduces mortality in patients with severe MCA infarcts, but may cause severe side effects, including recurrent ICP crisis during re-warming [444, 445]. In a small RCT, mild hypothermia (35°C) in addition to decompressive surgery produced a trend towards a better clinical outcome than decompressive surgery alone ($p = 0.08$) [446].

Decompressive surgery

Malignant MCA infarction

A pooled analysis of 93 patients included in the DECIMAL (decompressive craniectomy in malignant middle cerebral artery infarcts), DESTINY (decompressive surgery for the treatment of malignant infarction of the middle cerebral artery), and HAMLET (hemicraniectomy after middle cerebral artery infarction with life-threatening edema trial) trials showed that, compared with the control group, at 1 year more patients in the decompressive surgery group had a mRS ≤4 or mRS ≤3, and more survived (NNTs 2, 4 and 2 respectively) [447, 448]. There was no increase in the proportion of patients who survived surgery in a vegetative stage (mRS 5). Inclusion criteria for this combined analysis were age 18–60 years, NIHSSS >15, decrease in level of consciousness to a score of 1 or greater on item 1a of the NIHSS, infarct signs on CT of 50% or more of the MCA territory or >145 cm³ on DWI, and inclusion <45 h after onset (surgery <48 h). Follow-up of survival and functional status beyond 1 year

is currently ongoing in the DECIMAL and DESTINY studies [448].

A systematic review of 12 observational retrospective studies found age above 50 years to be a predictor of poor outcome. The timing of surgery, side of infarction, clinical signs of herniation before surgery, and involvement of other vascular territories did not significantly affect outcome [449].

Cerebellar infarction

Ventriculostomy and decompressive surgery are considered treatments of choice for space-occupying cerebellar infarctions, although RCTs are lacking. As in space-occupying supratentorial infarction, the operation should be performed before signs of herniation are present. The prognosis among survivors can be very good, even in patients who are comatose before surgery.

Prevention and management of complications

Recommendations

- It is recommended that infections after stroke should be treated with appropriate antibiotics (Class IV, GCP).
- Prophylactic administration of antibiotics is not recommended, and levofloxacin can be detrimental in acute stroke patients (Class II, Level B).
- Early rehydration and graded compression stockings are recommended to reduce the incidence of venous thromboembolism (Class IV, GCP).
- Early mobilization is recommended to prevent complications such as aspiration pneumonia, DVT, and pressure ulcers (Class IV, GCP).
- It is recommended that low-dose subcutaneous heparin or low molecular weight heparins should be considered for patients at high risk of DVT or pulmonary embolism (Class I, Level A).
- Administration of anticonvulsants is recommended to prevent recurrent post-stroke seizures (Class I, Level A). Prophylactic administration of anticonvulsants to patients with recent stroke who have not had seizures is not recommended (Class IV, GCP).
- An assessment of falls risk is recommended for every stroke patient (Class IV, GCP).
- Calcium/vitamin D supplements are recommended in stroke patients at risk of falls (Class II, Level B).
- Bisphosphonates (alendronate, etidronate, and risedronate) are recommended in women with previous fractures (Class II, Level B).

- In stroke patients with urinary incontinence, specialist assessment and management is recommended (Class III, Level C).

- Swallowing assessment is recommended but there are insufficient data to recommend a specific approach for treatment (Class III, GCP).

- Oral dietary supplements are only recommended for non-dysphagic stroke patients who are malnourished (Class II, Level B).

- Early commencement of nasogastric (NG) feeding (within 48 h) is recommended in stroke patients with impaired swallowing (Class II, Level B).

- It is recommended that percutaneous enteral gastrostomy (PEG) feeding should not be considered in stroke patients in the first 2 weeks (Class II, Level B).

Aspiration and pneumonia

Bacterial pneumonia is one of the most important complications in stroke patients [450], and is mainly caused by aspiration [451]. Aspiration is frequently found in patients with reduced consciousness and in those with swallowing disturbances. Oral feeding should be withheld until the patient has demonstrated intact swallowing with small amounts of water and intact coughing on command. Nasogastric (NG) or percutaneous enteral gastrostomy (PEG) feeding may prevent aspiration pneumonia, although reflux of liquid feed, hypostasis, diminished cough, and immobilization increase the risk. Frequent changes of the patient's position in bed and pulmonary physical therapy may prevent aspiration pneumonia. A brain-mediated immunodepressive state contributes to post-stroke infection [452, 453]. Prophylactic administration of levofloxacin (500 mg/100 ml/day for 3 days) is not better than optimal care for the prevention of infection in patients with nonseptic acute stroke and was inversely associated with outcome at day 90 (OR 0.19; 95% CI 0.04 to 0.87; $p = 0.03$) [454].

Deep vein thrombosis and pulmonary embolism

It is generally accepted that the risk of DVT and pulmonary embolism (PE) can be reduced by early hydration and early mobilization. Although graded compression stockings are effective in preventing venous thromboembolism in surgical patients, their efficacy after stroke is unproven [455]. In stroke patients low-dose LMWH reduced the incidence of both DVT (OR 0.34; 95% CI 0.19–0.59) and pulmonary embolism (OR 0.36; 95% CI 0.15–0.87), without an increased risk of intracerebral (OR 1.39; 95% CI 0.53–3.67) or extracerebral haemorrhage (OR 1.44; 95% CI 0.13–16), NNT: 7 and 38 for DVT and pulmonary embolism respectively, while low-dose UFH decreased the thrombosis risk (OR 0.17; 95% CI 0.11–0.26), but had no influence on pulmonary embolism (OR 0.83, 95% CI 0.53–1.31); the risk of ICH was not statistically significantly increased (OR 1.67; 95% CI 0.97–2.87) [456]. Nevertheless, prophylaxis with subcutaneous low-dose heparin (5000 IU twice daily) or low molecular weight heparins is indicated in patients at high risk of DVT or PE (e.g. due to immobilization, obesity, diabetes, previous stroke) [457, 458].

Pressure ulcer

In patients at high risk of developing pressure ulcers, use of support surfaces, frequent repositioning, optimizing nutritional status, and moisturizing sacral skin are appropriate preventive strategies [459]. The skin of the incontinent patient must be kept dry. For patients at particularly high risk, an air-filled or fluid-filled mattress system should be used.

Seizures

Partial or secondary generalized seizures may occur in the acute phase of ischaemic stroke. Standard anti-epileptic drugs should be used based on general principles of seizure management. There is no evidence that primary prophylactic anticonvulsive treatment is beneficial.

Agitation

Agitation and confusion may be a consequence of acute stroke, but may also be due to complications such as fever, volume depletion, or infection. Adequate treatment of the underlying cause must precede any type of sedation or antipsychotic treatment.

Falls

Falls are common (up to 25%) after stroke in the acute setting [460], during inpatient rehabilitation [461], and in the long term [462]. Likely risk factors for falls in stroke survivors [463] include cognitive impairment, depression, polypharmacy, and sensory impairment [464, 465]. A multidisciplinary prevention package that focuses on personal and environmental factors has been found to be successful in general rehabilitation settings

[466, 467]. There is a 5% incidence of serious injury [460], including hip fractures (which are four-fold more common than in age-matched controls [468]), which is associated with poor outcome [469]. Exercise [470], calcium supplements [471], and bisphosphonates [472] improve bone strength and decrease fracture rates in stroke patients. Hip protectors can reduce the incidence of fracture for high-risk groups in institutional care, but evidence is less convincing for their use in a community setting [473].

Urinary tract infections and incontinence

Intermittent catheterization has not been shown to reduce the risk of infection. Once urinary infection is diagnosed, appropriate antibiotics should be chosen; to avoid bacterial resistance developing, prophylactic antibiotics are best avoided.

Urinary incontinence is common after stroke, particularly in older, more disabled, and cognitively impaired patients [476]. Recent estimates suggest a prevalence of 40–60% in an acute stroke population, of whom 25% are still incontinent at discharge and 15% remain incontinent at one year [477]. Urinary incontinence is a strong predictor of poor functional outcome, even after correcting for age and functional status [478]. However, data from the available trials are insufficient to guide continence care of adults after stroke [475, 479]. However, there is suggestive evidence that professional input through structured assessment and management of care and specialist continence nursing may reduce urinary incontinence and related symptoms after stroke. Structured assessment and physical management have been shown to improve continence rates in both inpatients and outpatients [475, 477]. However, trials of interventions are insufficient in number and quality to make any recommendations [479].

Dysphagia and feeding

Oropharyngeal dysphagia occurs in up to 50% of patients with unilateral hemiplegic stroke [480]. The prevalence of dysphagia is highest in the acute stages of stroke, and declines to around 15% at 3 months [481]. Dysphagia is associated with a higher incidence of medical complications and increased overall mortality [480].

Withholding or limiting oral intake can worsen the catabolic state that may be associated with an acute illness

such as stroke. Estimates of the incidence of malnutrition vary from 7 to 15% at admission [482, 483] and 22 to 35% at 2 weeks [484]. Among patients requiring prolonged rehabilitation, the prevalence of malnutrition may reach 50% [485]. Malnutrition predicts a poor functional outcome [486] and increased mortality [487, 488]. However, routine supplementation for all acute stroke patients did not improve outcomes or reduce complications [489]. There are no adequately powered trials of targeting supplementation to stroke patients at high risk of malnutrition.

For patients with continuing dysphagia, options for enteral nutrition include NG or PEG feeding. A trial of early (median 48 h post-stroke) versus delayed (1 week) NG feeding found no significant benefit of early feeding, although there was a trend to fewer deaths in the early NG group [489]. In a related trial examining PEG and NG feeding within 30 days, PEG feeding was no better than NG and in fact was potentially harmful [489]. PEG feeding has also been studied in longer-term dysphagia. Two trials comparing PEG and NG feeding found a trend towards improved nutrition with PEG feeding that did not reach statistical significance [490, 491]. Studies that have addressed quality of life found it was not improved by PEG feeding [492, 493].

Rehabilitation

Even with optimal stroke unit care including thrombolysis, fewer than one-third of patients recover fully from stroke [388]. Rehabilitation aims to enable people with disabilities to reach and maintain optimal physical, intellectual, psychological, and/or social function [494]. Goals of rehabilitation can shift from initial input to minimize impairment to more complex interventions designed to encourage active participation.

Setting for rehabilitation

Recommendations

- Admission to a stroke unit is recommended for acute stroke patients to receive co-ordinated multidisciplinary rehabilitation (Class I, Level A).
- Early initiation of rehabilitation is recommended (Class III, Level C).

- It is recommended that early discharge from stroke unit care is possible in medically stable patients with mild or moderate impairment providing that rehabilitation is delivered in the community by a multidisciplinary team with stroke expertise (Class I, Level A).
- It is recommended to continue rehabilitation after discharge during the first year after stroke (Class II, Level A).
- It is recommended to increase the duration and intensity of rehabilitation (Class II, Level B).

A key characteristic of stroke units is rehabilitation delivered by a specialized multidisciplinary team [495]. The Stroke Unit Trialists' Collaboration [61] has shown improved survival and functional outcomes for patients treated in a dedicated stroke ward, and there are also long-term functional benefits of dedicated stroke unit care; follow-up at 5 and 10 years has revealed persisting efficacy compared with controls [496, 497]. The financial and social implications of prolonged hospitalization have prompted increasing interest in services to facilitate early return to the community. A multidisciplinary early supported discharge team with stroke expertise, comprising (at least) nursing, physiotherapy, and occupational therapy, can significantly reduce bed days for selected stroke patients [498] who have mild or moderate impairment at baseline [499]. However, specialist discharge services are required; mortality was substantially increased when patients were discharged early with only generic community support [500].

A meta-analysis showed that continued rehabilitation after discharge during the first year after stroke reduces the risk of deterioration in function and improves activities of daily living [501]. The interventions included occupational therapy, physiotherapy, and multidisciplinary teams, and therefore no definitive statement can be made concerning the optimal mode of service delivery.

Timing, duration and intensity of rehabilitation

The optimal timing of rehabilitation is unclear. Proponents of early therapy cite evidence from functional neuroimaging [502] and animal studies [503, 504] that define the peri-infarct period as the crucial time to begin rehabilitation. Early initiation of rehabilitation is a key component of stroke unit care [61] but there is a lack of

consensus on the definition of 'early therapy'. Trials comparing 'early' and 'late' initiation of rehabilitation have reported improved prognosis if therapy is started within 20–30 days [505, 506]. Many of the immediate complications of stroke (DVT, skin breakdown, contracture formation, constipation, and hypostatic pneumonia) are related to immobility [507], and hence mobilization is a fundamental component of early rehabilitation. The optimal timing of first mobilization is unclear, but mobilization within the first few days appears to be well tolerated [508]. Preliminary results from the ongoing AVERT study of rehabilitation within 24 h suggest that immediate physical therapy is well tolerated with no increase in adverse events [509].

There are few studies of rehabilitation beyond a year after the acute event, and data are inconclusive to make a recommendation on rehabilitation in this phase [510].

Greater intensity of rehabilitation, especially time spent working on activities of daily living (ADL), is associated with improved functional outcomes [511, 512]. A systematic review of rehabilitation therapies for improving arm function also suggests a dose–response relationship, although heterogeneity of included studies precluded a formal measure of effect size [513]. Greatest benefits were observed in studies of lower limb exercises and general ADL training.

Organisation and 'quality' of care may be more important than absolute hours of therapy [514]. In a comparison between a dedicated stroke multidisciplinary team and usual ward-based rehabilitation, the dedicated team achieved better outcomes with significantly fewer hours of therapy [515].

Elements of rehabilitation

Recommendations

- Physiotherapy is recommended, but the optimal mode of delivery is unclear (Class I, Level A).
- Occupational therapy is recommended, but the optimal mode of delivery is unclear (Class I, Level A).
- While assessment for communication deficits is recommended, there are insufficient data to recommend specific treatments (Class III, GCP).
- It is recommended that information is provided to patient and carers but evidence does not support use of a dedicated stroke liaison service for all patients (Class II, Level B).

- It is recommended that rehabilitation be considered for all stroke patients, but there is limited evidence to guide appropriate treatment for the most severely disabled (Class II, Level B).

- While assessment for cognitive deficits appears desirable, there are insufficient data to recommend specific treatments (Class I, Level A).

- It is recommended that patients be monitored for depression during hospital stay and throughout follow-up (Class IV, Level B).

- Drug therapy and non-drug interventions are recommended to improve mood (Class I, Level A).

- Drug therapy should be considered to treat post-stroke emotionalism (Class II, Level B).

- Tricyclic or anticonvulsant therapy are recommended to treat post-stroke neuropathic pain in selected patients (Class III, Level B).

- It is recommended that botulinum toxin be considered to treat post-stroke spasticity, but functional benefits are uncertain (Class III, Level B).

The results from stroke unit trials favour co-ordinated multidisciplinary teams of staff with expertise in stroke care [516]. The composition of these teams is not formally prescribed, but usually includes stroke physicians, nursing staff, physiotherapists, occupational therapists, and speech and language therapists.

Physiotherapy

There is no clearly superior model of physiotherapy for stroke rehabilitation [517, 518], but some evidence exists to support specific interventions. Several groups have shown that strength can be improved in a dose-dependent manner, without increasing spasticity [513]. Functional electrical stimulation may increase strength, but the effect on clinically relevant outcomes is uncertain [519].

A systematic review did not demonstrate efficacy of treadmill training to improve walking [520]. Electromechanical gait training in combination with physical therapy may be more effective than physiotherapy alone [521]. There are limited data to support the widespread use of orthoses and assistive devices [522].

Cardiovascular fitness can deteriorate during the recovery phase of a stroke. This physical deconditioning impairs active rehabilitation and is a risk marker for further events [523]. Meta-analysis has shown that

aerobic training can improve exercise capacity in individuals with mild to moderate motor deficit post-stroke [470].

Constraint-induced movement therapy involves intensive task-orientated exercise of the paretic limb, with restraint of the non-paretic limb. The EXCITE study reported positive results for this method 3–9 months after stroke in a group of medically stable stroke survivors, with some arm movement benefit persisting at 1 year [524].

Occupational therapy

A systematic review of nine trials comparing occupational therapy (OT)-based ADL therapy with usual care reported improved functional outcomes in the active intervention group [525]. The data do not justify conclusions on the optimal mode of OT delivery.

A meta-analysis of community-based OT trials found improved performance on ADL measures. The greatest effects were seen in older patients and with the use of targeted interventions [526]. Specific leisure-based OT therapies did not translate into improved ADL. A trial of providing OT intervention to care home residents post-stroke found less functional deterioration in the active intervention group [527]. No controlled trial data describe the effectiveness of occupational therapy beyond 1 year after stroke.

Speech and language therapy

Speech and language therapy (SLT) may optimize safe swallowing, and may assist communication. Two trials of formal SLT input for dysphagia found no significant difference to usual care [528]. A study comparing simple written instruction to graded levels of speech and language intervention for dysphagia found no difference in outcomes between the groups [529].

Aphasia and dysarthria are common symptoms after stroke, and impact on quality of life [530]. A systematic review of SLT for dysarthria in non-progressive brain damage (stroke and head injury) found no good-quality evidence for benefit [531]. Similarly, a systematic review of SLT for aphasia [532] reported insufficient good-quality evidence to recommend formal or informal interventions. The studies included in this review were community-based and had an average time to therapy of 3 months; they offer little to inform acute ward-based rehabilitation. Two related meta-analyses of studies with weaker design concluded that improvement in speech is greater if SLT is initiated early [533, 534]. Limited evidence supports the possible use of modified constraint-induced therapy for patients with aphasia [535, 536].

Stroke liaison and information provision

A recent systematic review comparing dedicated stroke liaison to usual care found no evidence of improvement in ADL, subjective health status, or carers' health [537]. On subgroup analysis, success of a stroke liaison service was predicted by younger age, less severe deficit, and an emphasis on education within the service.

Inadequate provision of information is predictive of poor quality of life in stroke patients and their families [538]. There is some evidence that combining information with educational sessions improves knowledge and is more effective than providing information alone [539]. As the patient progresses from hospital-based rehabilitation to the community, involvement of carers in rehabilitation becomes increasingly important. Formal training of caregivers in delivery of care reduces personal costs and improves quality of life [540].

Other groups

Depending on patient-specific goals, input from various other therapists may be appropriate. Such groups include dieticians, orthoptists, and social workers. Although there has been limited formal research in this area, some authors have argued that dedicated staffing creates an 'enriched environment' that encourages practice in rehabilitation activities outside periods of formal therapy [541].

Cognitive deficits

Cognitive deficits are common following stroke and impact on quality of life. At present, there is no evidence for the efficacy of specific memory rehabilitation [542]. Cognitive training for attention deficit has not resulted in meaningful clinical improvement in ADL measures [543]. Training for spatial neglect has improved impairment measures, but an effect on ADL performance has not been demonstrated [544]. A few studies have assessed rehabilitation training strategies in visual inattention and apraxia; no specific conclusions can be drawn [545].

Sexuality

Sexuality can suffer after a stroke. Underlying physical limitations and comorbid vascular disease may be com-

pounded by side effects of medications [546]. It may be desirable to discuss issues of sexuality and intimacy with patients [547]. Provision of support and information is important; many patients wrongly fear that resuming an active sex life may result in further stroke [548].

Complications affecting rehabilitation

Rehabilitation can be compromised by complications, which may be strong predictors of poor functional outcome and mortality. Common complications during inpatient rehabilitation include depression, shoulder pain, falls, urinary disturbances, and aspiration pneumonia [549]. Some of these are discussed under 'Prevention of complications'.

Post-stroke depression

Post-stroke depression is associated with poor rehabilitation results and ultimately poor outcome [550, 551]. In clinical practice, only a minority of depressed patients are diagnosed and even fewer are treated [552]. Depression has been reported in up to 33% of stroke survivors, compared with 13% of age- and sex-matched controls [553], but reliable estimates of the incidence and prevalence of depression in a stroke cohort are limited [551]. Predictors of post-stroke depression in the rehabilitation setting include increasing physical disability, cognitive impairment, and stroke severity [551]. There is no consensus on the optimal method for screening or diagnosis of post-stroke depression. Standard depression screening tools may be inappropriate for patients with aphasia or cognitive impairment [554, 555].

Antidepressant drugs such as selective serotonin reuptake inhibitors (SSRIs) and heterocyclics can improve mood after stroke [556, 557], but there is less evidence that these agents can effect full remission of a major depressive episode or prevent depression. SSRIs are better tolerated than heterocyclics [558]. There is no good evidence to recommend psychotherapy for treatment or prevention of post-stroke depression [559], although such therapy can elevate mood. There is a lack of robust evidence regarding the effect of treating post-stroke depression on rehabilitation or functional outcomes.

Emotionalism is a distressing symptom for patients and carers. SSRIs may reduce emotional outbursts but effects on quality of life are not clear [560].

Pain and spasticity

Post-stroke shoulder pain (PSSP) is common [561], especially in patients with impaired arm function and poor functional status, and is associated with poorer outcome. Passive movement of a paretic limb may be preventive [562]. Electrical stimulation is commonly used for treatment, but its efficacy is unproven [563]. A Cochrane systematic review found insufficient data to recommend the use of orthotic devices for shoulder sub-luxation, despite a trend towards efficacy for arm strap-ping of the affected limb [564].

Lamotrigine and gabapentin may be considered for neuropathic pain [565]. They appear to be well tolerated, but cognitive side effects should be considered.

Spasticity in the chronic phase may adversely affect ADL and quality of life [566]. Posture and movement therapy, relaxing therapy, splints and supports are all commonly employed, but a sound evidence base is lacking [567]. Pharmacotherapy with botulinum toxin has proven effects on muscle tone in arms and legs, but functional benefits are less well studied [568-570]. Oral agents are limited in their use because of side effects [571].

Eligibility for rehabilitation

An important predictor of rehabilitation outcome is initial stroke severity [550]. Pre-stroke disability is clearly also a strong determinant of outcome [572]. Other factors, such as sex [573], stroke aetiology [574], age [575], and topography of lesion [576], have all been studied as potential predictors of rehabilitation outcome; however, there is no evidence that these non-modifiable factors should influence decisions on rehabilitation [577]. Admission to a dedicated stroke unit improves outcomes for all strokes irrespective of age, sex, and severity [61].

Exclusion from rehabilitation on the basis of pre-stroke dependence remains a contentious issue [578, 579]. Patients with the most severe cognitive or physical impairments have been excluded from most rehabilitation trials, and therefore caution is required in extrapolating results to this group [580]. Limited data suggest that active rehabilitation allows severely disabled patients to return home [581, 582]. For those unable to participate actively, passive movements to prevent contractures or pressure sores have been recommended [2].

Appendix

ESO (EUSI) Recommendation Writing Committee
Chair: Werner Hacke, Heidelberg, Germany
Co-chairs: Marie-Germaine Bousser, Paris, France; Gary Ford, Newcastle, UK

Education, referral and emergency room
Co-chairs: Michael Brainin, Krems, Austria; José Ferro, Lisbon, Portugal
Members: Charlotte Cordonnier, Lille, France; Heinrich P. Mattle, Bern, Switzerland; Keith Muir, Glasgow, UK; Peter D. Schellinger, Erlangen, Germany
Substantial assistance received from: Isabel Henriques, Lisbon, Portugal

Stroke units
Co-chairs: Hans-Christoph Diener, Essen, Germany; Peter Langhorne, Glasgow, UK
Members: Antony Davalos, Barcelona, Spain; Gary Ford, Newcastle, UK; Veronika Skvortsova, Moscow, Russia

Imaging and diagnostics
Co-chairs: Michael Hennerici, Mannheim, Germany; Markku Kaste, Helsinki, Finland
Members: Hugh S. Markus, London, UK; E. Bernd Ringelstein, Münster, Germany; Rüdiger von Kummer, Dresden, Germany; Joanna Wardlaw, Edinburgh, UK
Substantial assistance received from: Oliver Müller, Heidelberg, Germany

Prevention
Co-chairs: Philip Bath, Nottingham, UK; Didier Leys, Lille, France
Members: Álvaro Cervera, Barcelona, Spain; László Csiba, Debrecen, Hungary; Jan Lodder, Maastricht, The Netherlands; Nils Gunnar Wahlgren, Stockholm, Sweden

General treatment
Co-chairs: Christoph Diener, Essen, Germany; Peter Langhorne, Glasgow, UK

Members: Antony Davalos, Barcelona, Spain; Gary Ford, Newcastle, UK; Veronika Skvortsova, Moscow, Russia

Acute treatment and treatment of complications

Co-chairs: Angel Chamorro, Barcelona, Spain; Bo Norrving, Lund, Sweden

Members: Valerica Caso, Perugia, Italy; Jean-Louis Mas, Paris, France; Victor Obach, Barcelona, Spain; Peter A. Ringleb, Heidelberg, Germany; Lars Thomassen, Bergen, Norway

Rehabilitation

Co-chairs: Kennedy Lees, Glasgow, UK; Danilo Toni, Rome, Italy

Members: Stefano Paolucci, Rome, Italy; Juhani Sivenius, Kuopio, Finland; Katharina Stibrant Sunnerhagen, Göteborg, Sweden; Marion F. Walker, Nottingham, UK

Substantial assistance received from: Yvonne Teuschl, Isabel Henriques, Terence Quinn

We want to thank Dr Michael Shaw for his assistance during the preparation of this manuscript.

Glossary

ADC	apparent diffusion coefficient
ADL	activities of daily living
AF	atrial fibrillation
AR	absolute risk
BP	blood pressure
CAS	carotid artery stenting
CEA	carotid endarterectomy
CE-MRA	contrast-enhanced MR angiography
CI	confidence interval
CSF	cerebral spinal fluid
CT	computed tomography
CTA	computed tomography angiography
CV	cardiovascular
DSA	digital subtraction angiograph
DVT	deep vein thrombosis
DWI	diffusion-weighted imaging
ECG	electrocardiography
ED	emergency department
EEG	electroencephalography
EFNS	European Federation of Neurological Societies
EMS	emergency medical service
ESO	European Stroke Organisation
EUSI	European Stroke Initiative
FLAIR	fluid attenuated inversion recovery
GCP	good clinical practice
HR	hazard ratio
ICA	internal carotid artery
ICP	intracranial pressure
INR	international normalized ratio
i.v.	intravenous
LDL	low density lipoprotein
MCA	middle cerebral artery
MI	myocardial infarction
MRA	magnetic resonance angiography
MRI	magnetic resonance imaging
mRS	modified Rankin score
NASCET	North American Symptomatic Carotid Endarterectomy Trial
NG	nasogastric
NIHSS	National Institutes of Health Stroke Scale
NINDS	National Institute of Neurological Disorders and Stroke
NNH	numbers needed to harm
NNT	numbers needed to treat
OSA	obstructive sleep apnoea
OR	odds ratio
OT	occupational therapy
PE	pulmonary embolism
PEG	percutaneous enteral gastrostomy
PFO	patent foramen ovale
pUK	pro-urokinase
QTc	heart rate corrected QT interval
RCT	randomized clinical trial
RR	relative risk
rtPA	recombinant tissue plasminogen activator
SLT	speech and language therapy
SSRI	selective serotonin reuptake inhibitor
TCD	transcranial Doppler
TOE	transoesophageal echocardiography
TIA	transient ischaemic attack
TTE	transthoracic echocardiography
UFH	unfractionated heparin

Conflicts of interest

P. Bath: Research support from Boehringer-Ingelheim; speakers honoraria from AZ, Boehringer-Ingelheim; consultancy/advisory board AZ, BI, Lundbeck, ReNeurone, Servier.

M. G. Bousser: Research grants and support from SANOFI Servier; research support from Novo-Nordisk, Paion; consultancy/advisory board Servier, Sanofi.

M. Brainin: Research grant from Ebewe, Novo Nordisk; research support from Boehringer-Ingelheim, Sanofi-Aventis, Solvaypharma; speakers' honoraria, Novartis, Boehringer-Ingelheim, Sanofi-Aventis, Ebewe, Solvay-pharma; consultancy/advisory board, Boehringer-Ingelheim, Ebewe.

A. Chamorro: Speaker's honoraria from BMS, Sanofi, Boehringer; consultancy/advisory board Servier, Sanofi.

L. Csiba: Research grant from UCB EGIS Zrt, Gedeon Richter, Aventis; speakers' honoraria from Boehringer-Ingelheim, PAION, Lundbeck A/S, Pfizer, EGIS Zrt, Sanofi-Aventis, Novo-Nordisk A/S, Astra-Zeneca, Johnson & Johnson, Gedeon Richter, MSD, UCB, Convex; consultancy/advisory board, Pfizer Hungary, Johnson & Johnson, Paion, Gedeon Richter, Boehringer-Ingelheim.

A. Davalos: Speakers' honoraria from Ferrer, PAION, Lundbeck, Pfizer, Astra-Zeneca, BMS, Thrombogenics, Boehringer-Ingelheim; consultancy/advisory board, Ferrer, PAION, Lundbeck, Pfizer, Astra-Zeneca, BMS, Thrombogenics, Boehringer-Ingelheim.

H. C. Diener: Research grant from AstraZeneca, GSK, Boehringer-Ingelheim, Novartis, Janssen-Cilag, Sanofi-Aventis; research support from German Research Council(DFG), German Ministry of Education and Research (BMBF), European Union, Bertelsmann Foundation, Heinz-Nixdorf Foundation; speakers' honoraria from Abbott, AstraZeneca, Bayer Vital, Boehringer-Ingelheim, D-Pharm, Fresenius, GlaxoSmithKline, Janssen Cilag, MSD, Novartis, Novo-Nordisk, Paion, Parke-Davis, Pfizer, Sanofi-Aventis, Sankyo, Servier, Solvay, Wyeth, Yamaguchi; consultancy/advisory board, Abbott, Astra-Zeneca, Bayer Vital, Boehringer-Ingelheim, D-Pharm, Fresenius, GlaxoSmithKline, Janssen Cilag, MSD, Novartis, Novo-Nordisk, Paion, Parke-Davis, Pfizer, Sanofi-Aventis, Sankyo, Servier, Solvay, Wyeth, Yamaguchi.

J. M. Ferro: Research grant from Tecnifar, Boehringer-Ingelheim; research support from Bayer, Sanofi-Aventis; speaker's honoraria from Tecnifar, Ferrer; consultancy/advisory board, Sanofi-Aventis, Uriach, Servier, Ferrer.

G. Ford: Research grant from Boehringer-Ingelheim, Servier, NTI, Lundbeck, Paion; speakers' honoraria from Boehringer-Ingelheim, AstraZeneca; consultancy/advisory board, Boehringer-Ingelheim.

W. Hacke: Research grant from DFG, BMBF; speakers' honoraria from Sanofi Aventis, Novo-Nordisk, Ferrer, Boehringer-Ingelheim; consultancy/advisory board, Sanofi Aventis, BMS, Novo-Nordisk, Boehringer-Ingelheim, Nuvelo, Novothera, Bayer, J&J, Brainsgate, Paion, Ferrer, Lilly, Centocor, ImarX.

M. G. Hennerici: Research grants from DFG, BMBF, EU specific foundations; research support from RCTs grants; speaker's honoraria, several studies from Pfizer, Boehringer, Sanofi, Bayer, Knoll, Janssen, etc; consultancy/advisory board, SPARCL, ESTAT, ECASSII, etc.

M. Kaste: Speakers' honoraria from Boehringer-Ingelheim, Sanofi-Aventis, Pfizer, Ferro; consultancy/advisory board, Bayer, BMS, Boehringer-Ingelheim, Mitsubishi, PAION, Brainsgate, Ferrer, Neurobiological Technologies, Lundbeck A/S, Orion Oy, Pfizer, Astellas, Glaxo-Wellcome, Servier, Encorium, Forest Laboratories, Concentric Medical, Sanofi-Aventis, Novo-Nordisk A/S, Astra-Zeneca, Centocor, Johnson & Johnson.

P. Langhorne: Speakers' honoraria, Previous Boehringer, Pfizer, Sanofi.

K. Lees: Research grant from MRC, Stroke Association, Lundbeck, AstraZeneca, Boehringer-Ingelheim, Servier, NTI, Brainsgate; speakers' honoraria, AstraZeneca, BMS, NTI, Sanofi, Paion, Forest, Lundbeck, Boehringer-Ingelheim, GlaxoSmithKline, Mitsubishi, Bayer, Ferrer, Novonordisk, DPharm, Brainsgate, Thrombogenics, Servier; ownership interest, NTI; consultancy/advisory board, see honoraria.

D. Leys: Research grants from BMS, Astra Zeneca, Boehringer-Ingelheim, NovoNordisk, Servier; consultancy/advisory board, Paion.

J. Lodder: Research supportand speakers' honoraria from Boehringer-Ingelheim; consultancy/advisory board, Boehringer-Ingelheim.

H. Markus: Speakers' honoraria from Sanofi; consultancy/advisory board, Sanofi, GE, Boehringer.

J. L. Mas: Research grant from Sanofi, BMS; speakers' honoraria, Sanofi, BMS, Servier, Boehringer, Johnson & Johnson; consultancy/advisory board, Sanofi, BMS, Servier.

H. Mattle: Research grant from AGA Medical, Bayer-Schering; research support from Biogen-Idec, Merck-

Serono, Sanofi-Aventis; speakers' honoraria, Servier, Pfizer, Sanofi-Aventis, Bristol Myers Squib, Boehringer-Ingelheim; ownership interest, Novartis, Roche; consultancy/advisory board, Pfizer, Merck Sharp & Dohme.

K. W. Muir. Research grants from Shire Pharmaceuticals, BMS, Sanofi; speakers' honoraria from Novo Nordisk, Sanofi; consultancy advisory board, GSK, Paion, Lilly, Novo Nordisk, ThromboGenics.

B. Norrving: Speakers' honoraria from MSD, SHIRE; consultancy/advisory board, Boehringer, Pfizer, Servier.

S. S. Paolucci: Speakers' honoraria from Boehringer-Ingelheim, Eli Lilly.

B. Ringelstein: Research grants from Novartis, NTI (Ancrod) and INC Research; speakers' honoraria, Boehringer-Ingelheim, Sanofi-Aventis, Altana, UCB, BMS; consultancy/advisory board, INC Research, Astra-Zeneca, Bayer-Schering Health Care.

P. A. Ringleb: Speakers' honoraria from Paion, Sanofi, Boehringer; consultancy/advisory board, Paion.

P. D. Schellinger: Speaker's honoraria from Boehringer-Ingelheim, Paion, Sanofi-Aventis, Ferrer, ImarX, Solvay, Altana; consultancy/advisory board, Boehringer-Ingelheim, Ferrer, ImarX.

J. Sivenius: Speakers' honoraria from Boehringer-Ingelhein, Pfizer; consultancy/advisory board, Boehringer-Ingelheim, Pfizer.

V. Skvortsova: Speakers' honoraria from Boehringer-Ingelheim, Ebewe, Sanofi Aventis; consultancy/advisory board, Boehringer-Ingelheim.

L. Thomassen: Restricted research funding from Boehringer-Ingelheim; Speakers' honoraria, Pfizer, Boehringer-Ingelheim, Sanofi, Astra Zeneca, MSD, etc.; consultancy/advisory board, Sanofi, Boehringer, Gore reduce trial.

D. Toni: Research grants from Boehringer-Ingelheim, SHIRE; speaker's honoraria from Boehringer-Ingelheim, Novo Nordisk, Sanofi-Aventis, Astra-Zeneca; consultancy/advisory board, Boehringer-Ingelheim.

R. von Kummer: Speakers' honoraria from Boehringer-Ingelheim, Bayer Schering; consultancy/advisory board, Boehringer-Ingelheim, Paion, Bayer Schering, Novo Nordisk, Nuvelo, Astellas.

N. Wahlgren: Research grant from Boehringer-Ingelheim; research support from Boehringer-Ingelheim, Bayer, AstraZeneca, Sanofi-Aventis, Novo-Nordisk, Thrombogenics, Servier; speakers' honoraria, Boehringer-Ingelheim, Bayer, Astra-Zeneca, Sanofi-Aventis, Novo-Nordisk; consultancy/advisory board, Boehringer-Ingelheim, Bayer, AstraZeneca, Sanofi-Aventis, Novo-Nordisk.

These statements were valid at the time of the publication of this guideline in the journal *Cerebrovascular Diseases* in 2008.

References

Important references for special topics are marked with asterisks.

1. European Stroke Initiative. European Stroke Initiative recommendations for stroke management. European Stroke Council, European Neurological Society and European Federation of Neurological Societies. *Cerebrovasc Dis* 2000;**10**:335–51.

2. The European Stroke Initiative Executive Committee and the EUSI Writing Committee. European stroke initiative recommendations for stroke management – update 2003. *Cerebrovasc Dis* 2003;**16**:311–37.

3. Steiner T, Kaste M, Forsting M, *et al.* Recommendations for the management of intracranial haemorrhage – part I: spontaneous intracerebral haemorrhage. The European Stroke Initiative Writing Committee and the Writing Committee for the EUSI Executive Committee. *Cerebrovasc Dis* 2006;**22**:294–316.

4. Lopez AD, Mathers CD, Ezzati M, Jamison DT, Murray CJ. Global and regional burden of disease and risk factors, 2001: systematic analysis of population health data. *Lancet* 2006;**367**:1747–57.

5. Brainin M, Bornstein N, Boysen G, Demarin V. Acute neurological stroke care in Europe: results of the European Stroke Care Inventory. *Eur J Neurol* 2000;**7**:5–10.

6. Rothwell PM, Coull AJ, Silver LE, *et al.* Population-based study of event-rate, incidence, case fatality, and mortality for all acute vascular events in all arterial territories (Oxford Vascular Study). *Lancet* 2005;**366**:1773–83.

7. O'Brien JT, Erkinjuntti T, Reisberg B, *et al.* Vascular cognitive impairment. *Lancet Neurol* 2003;**2**:89–98.

8. *Adams HP Jr, del Zoppo G, Alberts MJ, *et al.* Guidelines for the early management of adults with ischemic stroke: a guideline from the American Heart Association/American Stroke Association Stroke Council, Clinical Cardiology Council, Cardiovascular Radiology and Intervention Council, and the Atherosclerotic Peripheral Vascular Disease and Quality of Care Outcomes in Research Interdisciplinary Working Groups: the American Academy of Neurology affirms the value of this guideline as an educational tool for neurologists. *Stroke* 2007;**38**:1655–711.

9. Albers GW, Hart RG, Lutsep HL, Newell DW, Sacco RL. AHA Scientific Statement. Supplement to the guidelines for the management of transient ischemic attacks: a statement from the Ad Hoc Committee on Guidelines for the Management of Transient Ischemic Attacks, Stroke Council, American Heart Association. *Stroke* 1999;**30**:2502–11.

10. Alberts MJ, Hademenos G, Latchaw RE, *et al.* Recommendations for the establishment of primary stroke centers. Brain Attack Coalition. *JAMA* 2000;**283**:3102–9.

11. Alberts MJ, Latchaw RE, Selman WR, *et al.* Recommendations for comprehensive stroke centers: a consensus statement from the Brain Attack Coalition. *Stroke* 2005;**36**:1597–616.

12. Biller J, Feinberg WM, Castaldo JE, *et al.* Guidelines for carotid endarterectomy: a statement for healthcare professionals from a special writing group of the Stroke Council, American Heart Association. *Stroke* 1998;**29**:554–62.

13. Diener HC, Allenberg JR, Bode C, *et al.* Primär- und Sekundärprävention der zerebralen Ischämie. In: Diener HC (ed.) *Leitlinien Für Diagnostik Und Therapie in Der Neurologie.* Stuttgart, New York: Thieme, 2005.

14. Fuster V, Ryden LE, Asinger RW, *et al.* ACC/AHA/ESC guidelines for the management of patients with atrial fibrillation: Executive Summary. A report of the American College of Cardiology/American Heart Association Task Force on Practice Guidelines and the European Society of Cardiology Committee for Practice Guidelines and Policy Conferences (Committee to Develop Guidelines for the Management of Patients With Atrial Fibrillation) developed in collaboration with the North American Society of Pacing and Electrophysiology. *Circulation* 2001;**104**:2118–50.

15. Goldstein LB, Adams R, Alberts MJ, *et al.* Primary prevention of ischemic stroke: a guideline from the American Heart Association/American Stroke Association Stroke Council: cosponsored by the Atherosclerotic Peripheral Vascular Disease Interdisciplinary Working Group; Cardiovascular Nursing Council; Clinical Cardiology Council; Nutrition, Physical Activity, and Metabolism Council; and the Quality of Care and Outcomes Research Interdisciplinary Working Group: the American Academy of Neurology affirms the value of this guideline. *Stroke* 2006;**37**:1583–633.

16. Hacke W, Kaste M, Skyhoj Olsen T, Orgogozo JM, Bogousslavsky J. European Stroke Initiative (EUSI) recommendations for stroke management. The European Stroke Initiative Writing Committee. *Eur J Neurol* 2000;**7**:607–23.

17. Sacco RL, Adams R, Albers G, *et al.* Guidelines for prevention of stroke in patients with ischemic stroke or transient ischemic attack: a statement for healthcare professionals from the American Heart Association/American Stroke Association Council on Stroke: co-sponsored by the Council on Cardiovascular Radiology and Intervention: the American Academy of Neurology affirms the value of this guideline. *Stroke* 2006;**37**:577–617.

18. The National Board of Health and Welfare. Swedish National Guidelines for the Management of Stroke, Version for Health and Medical Personnel 2000. Available at: www-sosse/sosmenyehtm   2000:Article   number: 2002-2102-2001.

19. Kjellstrom T, Norrving B, Shatchkute A. Helsingborg Declaration 2006 on European stroke strategies. *Cerebrovasc Dis* 2007;**23**:231–41.

20. Kwan J, Hand P, Sandercock P. A systematic review of barriers to delivery of thrombolysis for acute stroke. *Age Ageing* 2004;**33**:116–21.

21. Evenson KR, Rosamond WD, Morris DL. Prehospital and in-hospital delays in acute stroke care. *Neuroepidemiology* 2001;**20**:65–76.

22. Ferro J, Melo T, Oliveira V, Crespo M, Canhão P, Pinto A. An analysis of the admission delay of acute stroke. *Cerebrovasc Dis* 1994;**4**:72–5.

23. Moser DK, Kimble LP, Alberts MJ, *et al.* Reducing delay in seeking treatment by patients with acute coronary syndrome and stroke: a scientific statement from the American Heart Association Council on cardiovascular nursing and stroke council. *Circulation* 2006;**114**:168–82.

24. Gil Nunez AC, Vivancos Mora J. Organization of medical care in acute stroke: importance of a good network. *Cerebrovasc Dis* 2004;**17**(Suppl. 1):113–23.

25. Keskin O, Kalemoglu M, Ulusoy RE. A clinic investigation into prehospital and emergency department delays in acute stroke care. *Med Princ Pract* 2005;**14**:408–12.

26. Chang K, Tseng M, Tan T. Prehospital delay after acute stroke in Kaohsiung, Taiwan. *Stroke* 2004;**35**:700–4.

27. Yu RF, San Jose MC, Manzanilla BM, Oris MY, Gan R. Sources and reasons for delays in the care of acute stroke patients. *J Neurol Sci* 2002;**199**:49–54.

28. Mosley I, Nicol M, Donnan G, Patrick I, Kerr F, Dewey H. The impact of ambulance practice on acute stroke care. *Stroke* 2007;**38**:2765–70.

29. Wein TH, Staub L, Felberg R, *et al.* Activation of emergency medical services for acute stroke in a nonurban population: the T.L.L. Temple Foundation Stroke Project. *Stroke* 2000;**31**:1925–8.

30. Rosamond WD, Evenson KR, Schroeder EB, Morris DL, Johnson AM, Brice JH. Calling emergency medical services for acute stroke: a study of 9-1-1 tapes. *Prehosp Emerg Care* 2005;**9**:19–23.

31. Mandelzweig L, Goldbourt U, Boyko V, Tanne D. Perceptual, social, and behavioral factors associated with delays

in seeking medical care in patients with symptoms of acute stroke. *Stroke* 2006;**37**:1248–53.

32. Montaner J, Vidal C, Molina C, Alvarez-Sabin J. Selecting the target and the message for a stroke public education campaign: a local survey conducted by neurologists. *Eur J Epidemiol* 2001;**17**:581–6.

33. Porteous GH, Corry MD, Smith WS. Emergency medical services dispatcher identification of stroke and transient ischemic attack. *Prehosp Emerg Care* 1999;**3**:211–6.

34. DeLemos CD, Atkinson RP, Croopnick SL, Wentworth DA, Akins PT. How effective are 'community' stroke screening programs at improving stroke knowledge and prevention practices? Results of a 3-month follow-up study. *Stroke* 2003;**34**:e247–9.

35. Agyeman O, Nedeltchev K, Arnold M, *et al.* Time to admission in acute ischemic stroke and transient ischemic attack. *Stroke* 2006;**37**:963–6.

36. Harraf F, Sharma AK, Brown MM, Lees KR, Vass RI, Kalra L. A multicentre observational study of presentation and early assessment of acute stroke. *BMJ* 2002;**325**:17–21.

37. Schneider AT, Pancioli AM, Khoury JC, *et al.* Trends in community knowledge of the warning signs and risk factors for stroke. *JAMA* 2003;**289**:343–6.

38. Nedeltchev K, Fischer U, Arnold M, Kappeler L, Mattle HP. Low awareness of transient ischemic attacks and risk factors of stroke in a Swiss urban community. *J Neurol* 2007;**254**:179–84.

39. Müller-Nordhorn J, Nolte C, Rossnagel K, *et al.* Knowledge about risk factors for stroke. A population-base survey with 28 090 participants. *Stroke* 2006;**37**:946–50.

40. Parahoo K, Thompson K, Cooper M, Stringer M, Ennis E, McCollam P. Stroke: awareness of the signs, symptoms and risk factors – a population-based survey. *Cerebrovasc Dis* 2003;**16**:134–40.

41. Evci ED, Memis S, Ergin F, Beser E. A population-based study on awareness of stroke in Turkey. *Eur J Neurol* 2007;**14**:517–22.

42. Sug Yoon S, Heller RF, Levi C, Wiggers J, Fitzgerald PE. Knowledge of stroke risk factors, warning symptoms, and treatment among an Australian urban population. *Stroke* 2001;**32**:1926–30.

43. Pandian JD, Jaison A, Deepak SS, *et al.* Public awareness of warning symptoms, risk factors, and treatment of stroke in northwest India. *Stroke* 2005;**36**:644–8.

44. DuBard CA, Garrett J, Gizlice Z. Effect of language on heart attack and stroke awareness among US Hispanics. *Am J Prev Med* 2006;**30**:189–96.

45. Luiz T, Moosmann A, Koch C, Behrens S, Daffertshofer M, Ellinger K. [Optimized logistics in the prehospital management of acute stroke]. *Anasthesiol Intensivmed Notfallmed Schmerzther* 2001;**36**:735–41.

46. Schmidt NK, Huwel J, Weisner B. Causes of a prolonged prehospital phase in patients admitted to a stroke unit. Can it be influenced by campaigns to educate the public? *Nervenarzt* 2005;**76**:181–5.

47. Alberts MJ, Perry A, Dawson DV, Bertels C. Effects of public and professional education on reducing the delay in presentation and referral of stroke patients. *Stroke* 1992;**23**:352–6.

48. Barsan W, Brott T, Broderick J, Haley ECJ, Levy D, Marler J. Urgent therapy for acute stroke. Effects of a stroke trial on untreated patients. *Stroke* 1994;**25**:2132–7.

49. Hodgson C, Lindsay P, Rubini F. Can mass media influence emergency department visits for stroke? *Stroke* 2007;**38**:2115–22.

50. Morgenstern L, Staub L, Chan W, *et al.* Improving delivery of acute stroke therapy: the TLL Temple Foundation Stroke Project. *Stroke* 2002;**33**:160–6.

51. Morgenstern L, Bartholomew L, Grotta J, Staub L, King M, Chan W. Sustained benefit of a community and professional intervention to increase acute stroke therapy. *Arch Intern Med* 2003;**163**:2198–202.

52. Wojner-Alexandrov AW, Alexandrov AV, Rodriguez D, Persse D, Grotta JC. Houston paramedic and emergency stroke treatment and outcomes study (HoPSTO). *Stroke* 2005;**36**:1512–8.

53. Kwan J, Hand P, Sandercock P. Improving the efficiency of delivery of thrombolysis for acute stroke: a systematic review. *QJM* 2004;**97**:273–9.

54. Behrens S, Daffertshofer M, Interthal C, Ellinger K, van Ackern K, Hennerici M. Improvement in stroke quality management by an educational programme. *Cerebrovasc Dis* 2002;**13**:262–6.

55. Billings-Gagliardi S, Fontneau NM, Wolf MK, Barrett SV, Hademenos G, Mazor KM. Educating the next generation of physicians about stroke: incorporating stroke prevention into the medical school curriculum. *Stroke* 2001;**32**:2854–9.

56. Wang MY, Lavine SD, Soukiasian H, Tabrizi R, Levy ML, Giannotta SL. Treating stroke as a medical emergency: a survey of resident physicians' attitudes toward 'brain attack' and carotid endarterectomy. *Neurosurgery* 2001;**48**:1109–15, discussion 1115-1107.

57. Derex L, Adeleine P, Nighoghossian N, Honnorat J, Trouillas P. Factors influencing early admission in a French stroke unit. *Stroke* 2002;**33**:153–9.

58. Barber PA, Zhang J, Demchuk AM, Hill MD, Buchan AM. Why are stroke patients excluded from TPA therapy? An analysis of patient eligibility. *Neurology* 2001;**56**:1015–20.

59. Camerlingo M, Casto L, Censori B, *et al.* Experience with a questionnaire administered by emergency medical

service for pre-hospital identification of patients with acute stroke. *Neurol Sci* 2001;**22**:357–61.

60. Nor AM, McAllister C, Louw SJ, *et al*. Agreement between ambulance paramedic- and physician-recorded neurological signs with Face Arm Speech Test (FAST) in acute stroke patients. *Stroke* 2004;**35**:1355–9.

61. *Stroke Unit Trialists' Collaboration. Organised inpatient (stroke unit) care for stroke. *Cochrane Database Syst Rev* 2007;(4):CD000197.

62. Stroke Unit Trialists' Collaboration. A systematic review of the randomised trials of organised impatient (stroke unit) care after stroke. *BMJ* 1997;**314**:1151–9.

63. Barsan WG, Brott TG, Broderick JP, Haley EC, Levy DE, Marler JR. Time of hospital presentation in patients with acute stroke. *Arch Intern Med* 1993;**153**:2558–61.

64. Harbison J, Massey A, Barnett L, Hodge D, Ford GA. Rapid ambulance protocol for acute stroke. *Lancet* 1999;**353**:1935.

65. Sobesky J, Frackowiak M, Zaro Weber O, *et al*. The Cologne stroke experience: safety and outcome in 450 patients treated with intravenous thrombolysis. *Cerebrovasc Dis* 2007;**24**:56–65.

66. Thomas SH, Kociszewski C, Schwamm LH, Wedel SK. The evolving role of helicopter emergency medical services in the transfer of stroke patients to specialized centers. *Prehosp Emerg Care* 2002;**6**:210–4.

67. Svenson JE, O'Connor JE, Lindsay MB. Is air transport faster? A comparison of air versus ground transport times for interfacility transfers in a regional referral system. *Air Med J* 2006;**25**:170–2.

68. Silliman SL, Quinn B, Huggett V, Merino JG. Use of a field-to-stroke center helicopter transport program to extend thrombolytic therapy to rural residents. *Stroke* 2003;**34**:729–33.

69. Diaz M, Hendey G, Winters R. How far is by air? The derivation of an air: ground coefficient. *J Emerg Med* 2003;**24**:199–202.

70. Diaz M, Hendey G, Bivins H. When is helicopter faster? A comparison of helicopter and ground ambulance transport times. *J Trauma* 2005;**58**:148–53.

71. Silbergleit R, Scott PA, Lowell MJ. Cost-effectiveness of helicopter transport of stroke patients for thrombolysis. *Acad Emerg Med* 2003;**10**:966–72.

72. Shafqat S, Kvedar JC, Guanci MM, Chang Y, Schwamm LH. Role for telemedicine in acute stroke. Feasibility and reliability of remote administration of the NIH stroke scale. *Stroke* 1999;**30**:2141–5.

73. Wiborg A, Widder B. Teleneurology to improve stroke care in rural areas: the Telemedicine in Stroke in Swabia (TESS) Project. *Stroke* 2003;**34**:2951–6.

74. Handschu R, Littmann R, Reulbach U, *et al*. Telemedicine in emergency evaluation of acute stroke: interrater agree-

ment in remote video examination with a novel multimedia system. *Stroke* 2003;**34**:2842–6.

75. Wang S, Lee SB, Pardue C, *et al*. Remote evaluation of acute ischemic stroke: reliability of National Institutes of Health Stroke Scale via telestroke. *Stroke* 2003;**34**:188–91.

76. Audebert HJ, Kukla C, Clarmann von Claranau S, *et al*. Telemedicine for safe and extended use of thrombolysis in stroke: the Telemedical Pilot Project for Integrative Stroke Care (TEMPiS) in Bavaria. *Stroke* 2005;**36**:287–91.

77. Audebert HJ, Kukla C, Vatankhah B, *et al*. Comparison of tissue plasminogen activator administration management between Telestroke Network hospitals and academic stroke centers: the Telemedical Pilot Project for Integrative Stroke Care in Bavaria/Germany. *Stroke* 2006;**37**:1822–7.

78. Hess DC, Wang S, Hamilton W, *et al*. REACH: clinical feasibility of a rural telestroke network. *Stroke* 2005;**36**: 2018–20.

79. Schwab S, Vatankhah B, Kukla C, *et al*. Long-term outcome after thrombolysis in telemedical stroke care. *Neurology* 2007;**69**:898–903.

80. Audebert HJ, Schenkel J, Heuschmann PU, Bogdahn U, Haberl RL. Effects of the implementation of a telemedical stroke network: the Telemedic Pilot Project for Integrative Stroke Care (TEMPiS) in Bavaria, Germany. *Lancet Neurol* 2006;**5**:742–8.

81. Schwamm LH, Rosenthal ES, Hirshberg A, *et al*. Virtual TeleStroke support for the emergency department evaluation of acute stroke. *Acad Emerg Med* 2004;**11**:1193–7.

82. Bélvis R, Cocho D, Martí-Fàbregas J., *et al*. Benefits of a prehospital stroke code system. Feasibility and efficacy in the first year of clinical practice in Barcelona//Spain. *Cerebrovasc Dis* 2005;**19**:96–101.

83. de la Ossa NP, Sanchez-Ojanguren J, Palomeras E, *et al*. Influence of the stroke code activation source on the outcome of acute ischemic stroke patients. *Neurology* 2008;**70**:1238–43.

84. Giles MF, Rothwell PM. Risk of stroke early after transient ischaemic attack: a systematic review and meta-analysis. *Lancet Neurol* 2007;**6**:1063–72.

85. Lavallee PC, Meseguer E, Abboud H, *et al*. A transient ischaemic attack clinic with round-the-clock access (SOS-TIA): feasibility and effects. *Lancet Neurol* 2007;**6**:953–60.

86. *Rothwell PM, Giles MF, Chandratheva A, *et al*. Effect of urgent treatment of transient ischaemic attack and minor stroke on early recurrent stroke (EXPRESS study): a prospective population-based sequential comparison. *Lancet* 2007;**370**:1432–42.

87. Kwan J, Sandercock P. In-hospital care pathways for stroke: a Cochrane systematic review. *Stroke* 2003;**34**:587–8.

88. Suzuki M, Imai A, Honda M, Kobayashi K, Ohtsuka S. Role of a critical pathway for door-to-CT-completion

interval in the management of acute ischemic stroke patients in the emergency room. *Keio J Med* 2004;**53**: 247–50.

89. Mehdiratta M, Woolfenden AR, Chapman KM, *et al*. Reduction in IV t-PA door to needle times using an Acute Stroke Triage Pathway. *Can J Neurol Sci* 2006;**33**:214–6.

90. NINDS rt-PA Stroke Study Group. A systems approach to immediate evaluation and management of hyperacute stroke. Experience at eight centers and implications for community practice and patient care. The National Institute of Neurological Disorders and Stroke (NINDS) rt-PA Stroke Study Group. *Stroke* 1997;**28**:1530–40.

91. Acker JE 3rd, Pancioli AM, Crocco TJ, *et al*. Implementation strategies for emergency medical services within stroke systems of care: a policy statement from the American Heart Association/American Stroke Association Expert Panel on Emergency Medical Services Systems and the Stroke Council. *Stroke* 2007;**38**:3097–115.

92. Douglas VC, Tong DC, Gillum LA, *et al*. Do the Brain Attack Coalition's criteria for stroke centers improve care for ischemic stroke? *Neurology* 2005;**64**:422–7.

93. Alvarez Sabín J, Molina C, Abilleira S, Montaner J, García F, Alijotas J. 'Stroke code'. Shortening the delay in reperfusion treatment of acute ischemic stroke. *Med Clin (Barc)* 1999;**113**:481–3.

94. Lindsberg PJ, Happola O, Kallela M, Valanne L, Kuisma M, Kaste M. Door to thrombolysis: ER reorganization and reduced delays to acute stroke treatment. *Neurology* 2006;**67**:334–6.

95. Hamidon BB, Dewey HM. Impact of acute stroke team emergency calls on in-hospital delays in acute stroke care. *J Clin Neurosci* 2007;**14**:831–4.

96. Goldstein LB, Simel DL. Is this patient having a stroke? *JAMA* 2005;**293**:2391–402.

97. Harbison J, Hossain O, Jenkinson D, Davis J, Louw SJ, Ford GA. Diagnostic accuracy of stroke referrals from primary care, emergency room physicians and ambulance staff using the face arm speech test. *Stroke* 2003;**34**:71–6.

98. Hand PJ, Kwan J, Lindley RI, Dennis MS, Wardlaw JM. Distinguishing between stroke and mimic at the bedside: the brain attack study. *Stroke* 2006;**37**:769–75.

99. Nor AM, Davis J, Sen B, *et al*. The Recognition of Stroke in the Emergency Room (ROSIER) scale: development and validation of a stroke recognition instrument. *Lancet Neurol* 2005;**4**:727–34.

100. Mitchell JB, Ballard DJ, Whisnant JP, Ammering CJ, Samsa GP, Matchar DB. What role do neurologists play in determining the costs and outcomes of stroke patients? *Stroke* 1996;**27**:1937–43.

101. Goldstein LB, Matchar DB, Hoff-Lindquist J, Samsa GP, Horner RD. VA Stroke Study: neurologist care is associ-

ated with increased testing but improved outcomes. *Neurology* 2003;**61**:792–6.

102. Tilley B, Lyden P, Brott T, Lu M, Levine S, Welch K. Total Quality improvement method for reduction of delays between emergency department admission and treatment of acute ischemic stroke. The National Institute of Neurological Disorders and Stroke rt-PA Stroke Study Group. *Arch Neurol* 2007;**64**:1466–74.

103. Lyden P, Brott T, Tilley B, *et al*. Improved reliability of the NIH Stroke Scale using video training. NINDS TPA Stroke Study Group. *Stroke* 1994;**25**:2220–6.

104. Trapl M, Enderle P, Nowotny M, *et al*. Dysphagia bedside screening for acute-stroke patients: the Gugging Swallowing Screen. *Stroke* 2007;**38**:2948–52.

105. Leys D, Ringelstein EB, Kaste M, Hacke W. The main components of stroke unit care: results of a European expert survey. *Cerebrovasc Dis* 2007;**23**:344–52.

106. LaMonte MP, Bahouth MN, Hu P, *et al*. Telemedicine for acute stroke: triumphs and pitfalls. *Stroke* 2003;**34**:725–8.

107. Wu O, Langhorne P. The challenge of acute-stroke management: does telemedicine offer a solution? *Int J Stroke* 2006;**1**:201–7.

108. Ronning OM, Guldvog B, Stavem K. The benefit of an acute stroke unit in patients with intracranial haemorrhage: a controlled trial. *J Neurol Neurosurg Psychiatry* 2001;**70**:631–4.

109. Seenan P, Long M, Langhorne P. Stroke units in their natural habitat: systematic review of observational studies. *Stroke* 2007;**38**:1886–92.

110. Candelise L, Gattinoni M, Bersano A, Micieli G, Sterzi R, Morabito A. Stroke-unit care for acute stroke patients: an observational follow-up study. *Lancet* 2007;**369**: 299–305.

111. Walsh T, Cotter S, Boland M, Greally T, O'Riordan R, Lyons D. Stroke unit care is superior to general rehabilitation unit care. *Ir Med J* 2006;**99**:300–2.

112. Launois R, Giroud M, Megnigbeto AC, *et al*. Estimating the cost-effectiveness of stroke units in France compared with conventional care. *Stroke* 2004;**35**:770–5.

113. Epifanov Y, Dodel R, Haacke C, *et al*. Costs of acute stroke care on regular neurological wards: a comparison with stroke unit setting. *Health Policy* 2007;**81**:339–49.

114. Patel A, Knapp M, Perez I, Evans A, Kalra L. Alternative strategies for stroke care: cost-effectiveness and cost-utility analyses from a prospective randomized controlled trial. *Stroke* 2004;**35**:196–203.

115. *Brady BK, McGahan L, Skidmore B. Systematic review of economic evidence on stroke rehabilitation services. *Int J Technol Assess Health Care* 2005;**21**:15–21.

116. Moodie M, Cadilhac D, Pearce D, *et al*. Economic evaluation of Australian stroke services: a prospective, multi-

center study comparing dedicated stroke units with other care modalities. *Stroke* 2006;**37**:2790–5.

117. Dewey HM, Sherry LJ, Collier JM. Stroke rehabilitation 2007: what should it be? *Int J Stroke* 2007;**2**:191–200.

118. Langhorne P, Pollock A. What are the components of effective stroke unit care? *Age Ageing* 2002;**31**:365–71.

119. Teasell R, Foley N, Bhogal S, Bagg S, Jutai J. Evidence-based practice and setting basic standards for stroke rehabilitation in Canada. *Top Stroke Rehabil* 2006;**13**:59–65.

120. Langhorne P, Dey P, Woodman M, *et al.* Is stroke unit care portable? A systematic review of the clinical trials. *Age Ageing* 2005;**34**:324–30.

121. Fryback D, Thornbury J. The efficacy of diagnostic imaging. *Med Decis Making* 1991;**11**:88–94.

122. Schramm P, Schellinger PD, Klotz E, *et al.* Comparison of perfusion computed tomography and computed tomography angiography source images with perfusion-weighted imaging and diffusion-weighted imaging in patients with acute stroke of less than 6 hours' duration. *Stroke* 2004;**35**:1562–8.

123. Barber PA, Hill MD, Eliasziw M, *et al.* Imaging of the brain in acute ischaemic stroke: comparison of computed tomography and magnetic resonance diffusion-weighted imaging. *J Neurol Neurosurg Psychiatry* 2005;**76**:1528–33.

124. Hand PJ, Wardlaw JM, Rowat AM, Haisma JA, Lindley RI, Dennis MS. Magnetic resonance brain imaging in patients with acute stroke: feasibility and patient related difficulties. *J Neurol Neurosurg Psychiatry* 2005;**76**:1525–7.

125. *The National Institute of Neurological Disorders and Stroke rt-PA Stroke Study Group. Tissue plasminogen activator for acute ischemic stroke. *N Engl J Med* 1995;**333**:1581–7.

126. *Wardlaw JM, Keir SL, Dennis MS. The impact of delays in computed tomography of the brain on the accuracy of diagnosis and subsequent management in patients with minor stroke. *J Neurol Neurosurg Psychiatry* 2003;**74**:77–81.

127. *Kidwell CS, Chalela JA, Saver JL, *et al.* Comparison of MRI and CT for detection of acute intracerebral hemorrhage. *JAMA* 2004;**292**:1823–30.

128. *Schellinger PD, Fiebach JB. Intracranial hemorrhage: the role of magnetic resonance imaging. *Neurocrit Care* 2004;**1**:31–45.

129. Wardlaw JM, Keir SL, Seymour J, *et al.* What is the best imaging strategy for acute stroke? *Health Technol Assess* 2004;**8**(iii, ix–x):1–180.

130. *Chalela JA, Kidwell CS, Nentwich LM, *et al.* Magnetic resonance imaging and computed tomography in emergency assessment of patients with suspected acute stroke: a prospective comparison. *Lancet* 2007;**369**:293–8.

131. von Kummer R, Bourquain H, Bastianello S, *et al.* Early prediction of irreversible brain damage after ischemic stroke at CT. *Radiology* 2001;**219**:95–100.

132. von Kummer R, Allen KL, Holle R, *et al.* Acute stroke: usefulness of early CT findings before thrombolytic therapy. *Radiology* 1997;**205**:327–33.

133. Barber PA, Demchuk AM, Zhang J, Buchan AM. Validity and reliability of a quantitative computed tomography score in predicting outcome of hyperacute stroke before thrombolytic therapy. ASPECTS Study Group. Alberta Stroke Programme Early CT Score. *Lancet* 2000;**355**:1670–4.

134. Wardlaw JM, Mielke O. Early signs of brain infarction at CT: observer reliability and outcome after thrombolytic treatment – systematic review. *Radiology* 2005;**235**:444–53.

135. Wardlaw JM, West TM, Sandercock PA, Lewis SC, Mielke O. Visible infarction on computed tomography is an independent predictor of poor functional outcome after stroke, and not of haemorrhagic transformation. *J Neurol Neurosurg Psychiatry* 2003;**74**:452–8.

136. von Kummer R. Effect of training in reading CT scans on patient selection for ECASS II. *Neurology* 1998;**51**:S50–2.

137. Wardlaw JM, Farrall AJ, Perry D, *et al.* Factors influencing the detection of early CT signs of cerebral ischemia: an internet-based, international multiobserver study. *Stroke* 2007;**38**:1250–6.

138. von Kummer R, Meyding-Lamade U, Forsting M, *et al.* Sensitivity and prognostic value of early CT in occlusion of the middle cerebral artery trunk. *AJNR Am J Neuroradiol* 1994;**15**:9–15, discussion 16-18.

139. Dzialowski I, Weber J, Doerfler A, Forsting M, von Kummer R. Brain tissue water uptake after middle cerebral artery occlusion assessed with CT. *J Neuroimaging* 2004;**14**:42–8.

140. Dzialowski I, Klotz E, Goericke S, Doerfler A, Forsting M, von Kummer R. Ischemic brain tissue water content: CT monitoring during middle cerebral artery occlusion and reperfusion in rats. *Radiology* 2007;**243**:720–6.

141. Hill MD, Rowley HA, Adler F, *et al.* Selection of acute ischemic stroke patients for intra-arterial thrombolysis with pro-urokinase by using ASPECTS. *Stroke* 2003;**34**:1925–31.

142. Patel SC, Levine SR, Tilley BC, *et al.* Lack of clinical significance of early ischemic changes on computed tomography in acute stroke. *JAMA* 2001;**286**:2830–8.

143. *Dimigen M, Keir S, Dennis M, Wardlaw J. Long-term visibility of primary intracerebral hemorrhage on magnetic resonance imaging. *J Stroke Cerebrovasc Dis* 2004;**13**:104–8.

144. Ay H, Oliveira-Filho J, Buonanno FS, *et al*. 'Footprints' of transient ischemic attacks: a diffusion-weighted MRI study. *Cerebrovasc Dis* 2002;**14**:177–86.

145. Fiehler J, Knudsen K, Kucinski T, *et al*. Predictors of apparent diffusion coefficient normalization in stroke patients. *Stroke* 2004;**35**:514–9.

146. *Oppenheim C, Lamy C, Touze E, *et al*. Do transient ischemic attacks with diffusion-weighted imaging abnormalities correspond to brain infarctions? *AJNR Am J Neuroradiol* 2006;**27**:1782–7.

147. Wardlaw JM, Keir SL, Bastin ME, Armitage PA, Rana AK. Is diffusion imaging appearance an independent predictor of outcome after ischemic stroke? *Neurology* 2002;**59**: 1381–7.

148. Hand PJ, Wardlaw JM, Rivers CS, *et al*. MR diffusion-weighted imaging and outcome prediction after ischemic stroke. *Neurology* 2006;**66**:1159–63.

149. Kane I, Carpenter T, Chappell F, *et al*. Comparison of 10 different magnetic resonance perfusion imaging processing methods in acute ischemic stroke: effect on lesion size, proportion of patients with diffusion/perfusion mismatch, clinical scores, and radiologic outcomes. *Stroke* 2007;**38**: 3158–64.

150. Wintermark M, Reichhart M, Thiran JP, *et al*. Prognostic accuracy of cerebral blood flow measurement by perfusion computed tomography, at the time of emergency room admission, in acute stroke patients. *Ann Neurol* 2002;**51**: 417–32.

151. Lev MH, Gonzalez RG, Schaefer PW, Koroshetz WJ, Dillon WP, Wintermark M. Cerebral blood flow thresholds in acute stroke triage. *Stroke* 2006;**37**:1334–9.

152. *Kane I, Sandercock P, Wardlaw J. Magnetic resonance perfusion diffusion mismatch and thrombolysis in acute ischaemic stroke: a systematic review of the evidence to date. *J Neurol Neurosurg Psychiatry* 2007;**78**:485–90.

153. *Furlan A, Higashida R, Wechsler L, *et al*. Intra-arterial prourokinase for acute ischemic stroke. The PROACT II study: a randomized controlled trial. Prolyse in Acute Cerebral Thromboembolism. *JAMA* 1999;**282**: 2003–11.

154. Mattle HP, Arnold M, Georgiadis D, *et al*. Comparison of intraarterial and intravenous thrombolysis for ischemic stroke with hyperdense middle cerebral artery sign. *Stroke* 2008;**39**:379–83.

155. Rubiera M, Ribo M, Delgado-Mederos R, *et al*. Tandem internal carotid artery/middle cerebral artery occlusion: an independent predictor of poor outcome after systemic thrombolysis. *Stroke* 2006;**37**:2301–5.

156. Fischer U, Arnold M, Nedeltchev K, *et al*. NIHSS score and arteriographic findings in acute ischemic stroke. *Stroke* 2005;**36**:2121–5.

157. Allendoerfer J, Goertler M, von Reutern G. Prognostic relevance of ultra-early doppler sonography in acute ischaemic stroke: a prospective multicentre study. *Lancet Neurol* 2005;**5**:835–40.

158. Coutts SB, Simon JE, Tomanek AI, *et al*. Reliability of assessing percentage of diffusion-perfusion mismatch. *Stroke* 2003;**34**:1681–3.

159. *Albers GW, Thijs VN, Wechsler L, *et al*. Magnetic resonance imaging profiles predict clinical response to early reperfusion: the diffusion and perfusion imaging evaluation for understanding stroke evolution (DEFUSE) study. *Ann Neurol* 2006;**60**:508–17.

160. *Bandera E, Botteri M, Minelli C, Sutton A, Abrams KR, Latronico N. Cerebral blood flow threshold of ischemic penumbra and infarct core in acute ischemic stroke: a systematic review. *Stroke* 2006;**37**:1334–9.

161. Carpenter TK, Armitage PA, Bastin ME, Wardlaw JM. DSC perfusion MRI-Quantification and reduction of systematic errors arising in areas of reduced cerebral blood flow. *Magn Reson Med* 2006;**55**:1342–9.

162. Rivers CS, Wardlaw JM, Armitage PA, *et al*. Do acute diffusion- and perfusion-weighted MRI lesions identify final infarct volume in ischaemic stroke? *Stroke* 2006;**37**: 98–104.

163. Dávalos A, Blanco M, Pedraza S, *et al*. The clinical-DWI mismatch: a new diagnostic approach to the brain tissue at risk of infarction. *Neurology* 2004;**62**:2187–92.

164. Kent DM, Hill MD, Ruthazer R, *et al*. 'Clinical-CT mismatch' and the response to systemic thrombolytic therapy in acute ischemic stroke. *Stroke* 2005;**36**:1695–9.

165. Cordonnier C, Al-Shahi Salman R, Wardlaw J. Spontaneous brain microbleeds: systematic review, subgroup analyses and standards for study design and reporting. *Brain* 2007;**130**:1988–2003.

166. Fiehler J, Albers GW, Boulanger JM, *et al*. Bleeding risk analysis in stroke imaging before thromboLysis (BRASIL): pooled analysis of T2*-weighted magnetic resonance imaging data from 570 patients. *Stroke* 2007;**38**:2738–44.

167. Forsting M, Wanke I. Funeral for a friend. *Stroke* 2003;**34**:1324–32.

168. Willinsky RA, Taylor SM, TerBrugge K, Farb RI, Tomlinson G, Montanera W. Neurologic complications of cerebral angiography: prospective analysis of 2,899 procedures and review of the literature. *Radiology* 2003;**227**:522–8.

169. *Wardlaw JM, Chappell FM, Best JJ, Wartolowska K, Berry E. Non-invasive imaging compared with intra-arterial angiography in the diagnosis of symptomatic carotid stenosis: a meta-analysis. *Lancet* 2006;**367**:1503–12.

170. Wardlaw JM, Chappell FM, Stevenson M, *et al*. Accurate, practical and cost-effective assessment of carotid stenosis in the UK. *Health Technol Assess* 2006;**10**(iii–iv, ix–x):1–182.

171. Flossmann E, Rothwell PM. Prognosis of vertebrobasilar transient ischaemic attack and minor stroke. *Brain* 2003;**126**:1940–54.

172. Khan S, Cloud GC, Kerry S, Markus HS. Imaging of vertebral artery stenosis: a systematic review. *J Neurol Neurosurg Psychiatry* 2007;**78**:1218–25.

173. Postert T, Federlein J, Przuntek H, Buttner T. Insufficient and absent acoustic temporal bone window: potential and limitations of transcranial contrast-enhanced color-coded sonography and contrast-enhanced power-based sonography. *Ultrasound Med Biol* 1997;**23**:857–62.

174. Alexandrov AV, Burgin WS, Demchuk AM, El-Mitwalli A, Grotta JC. Speed of intracranial clot lysis with intravenous tissue plasminogen activator therapy: sonographic classification and short-term improvement. *Circulation* 2001;**103**: 2897–902.

175. Droste DW, Jurgens R, Nabavi DG, Schuierer G, Weber S, Ringelstein EB. Echocontrast-enhanced ultrasound of extracranial internal carotid artery high-grade stenosis and occlusion. *Stroke* 1999;**30**:2302–6.

176. Droste DW, Jurgens R, Weber S, Tietje R, Ringelstein EB. Benefit of echocontrast-enhanced transcranial color-coded duplex ultrasound in the assessment of intracranial collateral pathways. *Stroke* 2000;**31**:920–3.

177. Droste DW, Nabavi DG, Kemeny V, et al. Echocontrast enhanced transcranial colour-coded duplex offers improved visualization of the vertebrobasilar system. *Acta Neurol Scand* 1998;**98**:193–9.

178. Ringelstein E, van Eyck S, Mertens I. Evaluation of cerebral vasomotor reactivity by various vasodilating stimuli: comparison of CO_2 to acetazolamide. *Cereb Blood Flow Metab* 1992;**12**:162–8.

179. *Nederkoorn PJ, van der Graaf Y, Hunink MG. Duplex ultrasound and magnetic resonance angiography compared with digital subtraction angiography in carotid artery stenosis: a systematic review. *Stroke* 2003;**34**:1324–32.

180. Markus H, Cullinane M. Severely impaired cerebrovascular reactivity predicts stroke and TIA risk in patients with carotid artery stenosis and occlusion. *Brain* 2001;**124**:457–67.

181. Blaser T, Hofmann K, Buerger T, Effenberger O, Wallesch CW, Goertler M. Risk of stroke, transient ischemic attack, and vessel occlusion before endarterectomy in patients with symptomatic severe carotid stenosis. *Stroke* 2002;**33**:1057–62.

182. Ringelstein EB, Droste DW, Babikian VL, et al. Consensus on microembolus detection by TCD. International Consensus Group on Microembolus Detection. *Stroke* 1998;**29**:725–9.

183. Markus HS, MacKinnon A. Asymptomatic embolization detected by Doppler ultrasound predicts stroke risk in symptomatic carotid artery stenosis. *Stroke* 2005;**36**: 971–5.

184. Markus HS, Droste DW, Kaps M, et al. Dual antiplatelet therapy with clopidogrel and aspirin in symptomatic carotid stenosis evaluated using doppler embolic signal detection: the Clopidogrel and Aspirin for Reduction of Emboli in Symptomatic Carotid Stenosis (CARESS) trial. *Circulation* 2005;**111**:2233–40.

185. Klötzsch C, Janssen G, Berlit P. Transesophageal echocardiography and contrast-TCD in the detection of a patent foramen ovale: experiences with 111 patients. *Neurology* 1994;**44**:1603–6.

186. Rothwell P, Buchan A, Johnston S. Recent advances in management of transient ischaemic attacks and minor ischaemic strokes. *Lancet Neurol* 2005;**5**:323–31.

187. Daffertshofer M, Mielke O, Pullwitt A, Felsenstein M, Hennerici M. Transient ischemic attacks are more than 'ministrokes'. *Stroke* 2004;**35**:2453–8.

188. Crisostomo RA, Garcia MM, Tong DC. Detection of diffusion-weighted MRI abnormalities in patients with transient ischemic attack: correlation with clinical characteristics. *Stroke* 2003;**34**:932–7.

189. Coutts SB, Simon JE, Eliasziw M, et al. Triaging transient ischemic attack and minor stroke patients using acute magnetic resonance imaging. *Ann Neurol* 2005;**57**:848–54.

190. Redgrave JN, Coutts SB, Schulz UG, Briley D, Rothwell PM. Systematic review of associations between the presence of acute ischemic lesions on diffusion-weighted imaging and clinical predictors of early stroke risk after transient ischemic attack. *Stroke* 2007;**38**:1482–8.

191. Douglas VC, Johnston CM, Elkins J, Sidney S, Gress DR, Johnston SC. Head computed tomography findings predict short-term stroke risk after transient ischemic attack. *Stroke* 2003;**34**:2894–8.

192. Christensen H, Fogh Christensen A, Boysen GG. Abnormalities on ECG and telemetry predict stroke outcome at 3 months. *J Neurol Sci* 2005;**234**:99–103.

193. Fure B, Bruun Wyller T, Thommessen B. Electrocardiographic and troponin T changes in acute ischaemic stroke. *J Intern Med* 2006;**259**:592–7.

194. Tatschl C, Stollberger C, Matz K, et al. Insular involvement is associated with QT prolongation: ECG abnormalities in patients with acute stroke. *Cerebrovasc Dis* 2006;**21**:47–53.

195. Gunalp M, Atalar E, Coskun F, et al. Holter monitoring for 24 hours in patients with thromboembolic stroke and sinus rhythm diagnosed in the emergency department. *Adv Ther* 2006;**23**:854–60.

196. Douen AG, Pageau N, Medic S. Serial electrocardiographic assessments significantly improve detection of atrial fibril-

lation 2.6-fold in patients with acute stroke. *Stroke* 2008;**39**:480–2.

197. Liao J, Khalid Z, Scallan C, Morillo C, O'Donnell M. Non-invasive cardiac monitoring for detecting paroxysmal atrial fibrillation or flutter after acute ischemic stroke: a systematic review. *Stroke* 2007;**38**:2935–40.

198. Jabaudon D, Sztajzel J, Sievert K, Landis T, Sztajzel R. Usefulness of ambulatory 7-day ECG monitoring for the detection of atrial fibrillation and flutter after acute stroke and transient ischemic attack. *Stroke* 2004;**35**:1647–51.

199. Lerakis S, Nicholson WJ. Part I: use of echocardiography in the evaluation of patients with suspected cardioembolic stroke. *Am J Med Sci* 2005;**329**:310–6.

200. Kapral MK, Silver FL. Preventive health care, 1999 update: 2. Echocardiography for the detection of a cardiac source of embolus in patients with stroke. Canadian Task Force on Preventive Health Care. *CMAJ* 1999;**161**:989–96.

201. de Bruijn SF, Agema WR, Lammers GJ, *et al.* Transesophageal echocardiography is superior to transthoracic echocardiography in management of patients of any age with transient ischemic attack or stroke. *Stroke* 2006;**37**: 2531–4.

202. Chiarella F, Santoro E, Domenicucci S, Maggioni A, Vecchio C. Predischarge two-dimensional echocardiographic evaluation of left ventricular thrombosis after acute myocardial infarction in the GISSI-3 study. *Am J Cardiol* 1998;**81**:822–7.

203. Zabalgoitia M, Halperin JL, Pearce LA, Blackshear JL, Asinger RW, Hart RG. Transesophageal echocardiographic correlates of clinical risk of thromboembolism in nonvalvular atrial fibrillation. Stroke Prevention in Atrial Fibrillation III Investigators. *J Am Coll Cardiol* 1998;**31**: 1622–6.

204. Kurth T, Moore S, Gaziano J, *et al.* Healthy lifestyle and the risk of stroke in women. *Arch Intern Med* 2006;**166**:1403–9.

205. Lewington S, Clarke R, Qizilbash N, Peto R, Collins R. Age-specific relevance of usual blood pressure to vascular mortality: a meta-analysis of individual data for one million adults in 61 prospective studies. *Lancet* 2002;**360**:1903–13.

206. Neal B, MacMahon S, Chapman N. Effects of ACE inhibitors, calcium antagonists, and other blood-pressure-lowering drugs: results of prospectively designed overviews of randomised trials. Blood Pressure Lowering Treatment Trialists' Collaboration. *Lancet* 2000;**356**:1955–64.

207. Staessen JA, Fagard R, Thijs L, *et al.* Randomised double-blind comparison of placebo and active treatment for older patients with isolated systolic hypertension. The Systolic Hypertension in Europe (Syst-Eur) Trial Investigators. *Lancet* 1997;**350**:757–64.

208. Gueyffier F, Bulpitt C, Boissel JP, *et al.* Antihypertensive drugs in very old people: a subgroup meta-analysis of randomised controlled trials. INDANA Group. *Lancet* 1999;**353**:793–6.

209. *Mancia G, De Backer G, Dominiczak A, *et al.* The task force for the management of arterial hypertension of the European Society of H, The task force for the management of arterial hypertension of the European Society of C: 2007 Guidelines for the management of arterial hypertension: The Task Force for the Management of Arterial Hypertension of the European Society of Hypertension (ESH) and of the European Society of Cardiology (ESC). *Eur Heart J* 2007;**28**:1462–536.

210. *Mancia G. Optimal control of blood pressure in patients with diabetes reduces the incidence of macro- and microvascular events. *J Hypertens Suppl* 2007;**25**(Suppl. 1): S7–12.

211. Black HR, Elliott WJ, Grandits G, *et al.* Principal results of the Controlled Onset Verapamil Investigation of Cardiovascular End Points (CONVINCE) trial. *JAMA* 2003;**289**: 2073–82.

212. Dahlof B, Devereux RB, Kjeldsen SE, *et al.* Cardiovascular morbidity and mortality in the Losartan Intervention For Endpoint reduction in hypertension study (LIFE): a randomised trial against atenolol. *Lancet* 2002;**359**:995–1003.

213. Kizer JR, Dahlof B, Kjeldsen SE, *et al.* Stroke reduction in hypertensive adults with cardiac hypertrophy randomized to losartan versus atenolol: the Losartan Intervention For Endpoint reduction in hypertension study. *Hypertension* 2005;**45**:46–52.

214. ALLHAT investigators. Major outcomes in moderately hypercholesterolemic, hypertensive patients randomized to pravastatin vs usual care: the Antihypertensive and Lipid-Lowering Treatment to Prevent Heart Attack Trial (ALLHAT-LLT). *JAMA* 2002;**288**:2998–3007.

215. Ekbom T, Linjer E, Hedner T, *et al.* Cardiovascular events in elderly patients with isolated systolic hypertension. A subgroup analysis of treatment strategies in STOP-Hypertension-2. *Blood Press* 2004;**13**:137–41.

216. Turner RC, Cull CA, Frighi V, Holman RR. Glycemic control with diet, sulfonylurea, metformin, or insulin in patients with type 2 diabetes mellitus: progressive requirement for multiple therapies (UKPDS 49). UK Prospective Diabetes Study (UKPDS) Group. *JAMA* 1999;**281**: 2005–12.

217. Colhoun HM, Betteridge DJ, Durrington PN, *et al.* Primary prevention of cardiovascular disease with atorvastatin in type 2 diabetes in the Collaborative Atorvastatin Diabetes Study (CARDS): multicentre randomised placebo-controlled trial. *Lancet* 2004;**364**:685–96.

218. Sever PS, Poulter NR, Dahlof B, *et al.* Reduction in cardiovascular events with atorvastatin in 2,532 patients with type 2 diabetes: Anglo-Scandinavian Cardiac Outcomes Trial – lipid-lowering arm (ASCOT-LLA). *Diabetes Care* 2005;**28**:1151–7.

219. *Kearney PM, Blackwell L, Collins R, *et al.* Efficacy of cholesterol-lowering therapy in 18,686 people with diabetes in 14 randomised trials of statins: a meta-analysis. *Lancet* 2008;**371**:117–25.

220. *Amarenco P, Labreuche J, Lavallee P, Touboul PJ. Statins in stroke prevention and carotid atherosclerosis: systematic review and up-to-date meta-analysis. *Stroke* 2004;**35**: 2902–9.

221. Heart Protection Study Collaborative Group. MRC/BHF Heart Protection Study of cholesterol lowering with simvastatin in 20,536 high-risk individuals: a randomised placebo-controlled trial. *Lancet* 2002;**360**:7–22.

222. Wolf PA, D'Agostino RB, Kannel WB, Bonita R, Belanger AJ. Cigarette smoking as a risk factor for stroke. The Framingham Study. *JAMA* 1988;**259**:1025–9.

223. Abbott RD, Yin Y, Reed DM, Yano K. Risk of stroke in male cigarette smokers. *N Engl J Med* 1986;**315**:717–20.

224. Colditz GA, Bonita R, Stampfer MJ, *et al.* Cigarette smoking and risk of stroke in middle-aged women. *N Engl J Med* 1988;**318**:937–41.

225. Kawachi I, Colditz GA, Stampfer MJ, *et al.* Smoking cessation and decreased risk of stroke in women. *JAMA* 1993;**269**:232–6.

226. Wannamethee SG, Shaper AG, Whincup PH, Walker M. Smoking cessation and the risk of stroke in middle-aged men. *JAMA* 1995;**274**:155–60.

227. Iso H, Date C, Yamamoto A, *et al.* Smoking cessation and mortality from cardiovascular disease among Japanese men and women: the JACC Study. *Am J Epidemiol* 2005;**161**:170–9.

228. Qureshi AI, Suri MF, Kirmani JF, Divani AA. Cigarette smoking among spouses: another risk factor for stroke in women. *Stroke* 2005;**36**:e74–6.

229. Shinton R, Beevers G. Meta-analysis of relation between cigarette smoking and stroke. *BMJ* 1989;**298**:789–94.

230. Ong MK, Glantz SA. Cardiovascular health and economic effects of smoke-free workplaces. *Am J Med* 2004;**117**: 32–8.

231. Reynolds K, Lewis B, Nolen JD, Kinney GL, Sathya B, He J. Alcohol consumption and risk of stroke: a meta-analysis. *JAMA* 2003;**289**:579–88.

232. Mukamal KJ, Ascherio A, Mittleman MA, *et al.* Alcohol and risk for ischemic stroke in men: the role of drinking patterns and usual beverage. *Ann Intern Med* 2005;**142**: 11–9.

233. Bazzano LA, Gu D, Reynolds K, *et al.* Alcohol consumption and risk for stroke among Chinese men. *Ann Neurol* 2007;**62**:569–78.

234. Lee C, Folsom A, Blair S. Physical activity and stroke risk: a meta-analysis. *Stroke* 2003;**34**:2475–81.

235. Deplanque D, Masse I, Lefebvre C, Libersa C, Leys D, Bordet R. Prior TIA, lipid-lowering drug use, and physical activity decrease ischemic stroke severity. *Neurology* 2006;**67**:1403–10.

236. Joshipura KJ, Ascherio A, Manson JE, *et al.* Fruit and vegetable intake in relation to risk of ischemic stroke. *JAMA* 1999;**282**:1233–9.

237. He K, Song Y, Daviglus M, *et al.* Fish consumption and incidence of stroke: a meta-analysis of cohort studies. *Stroke* 2004;**35**:1538–42.

238. Mellen PB, Walsh TF, Herrington DM. Whole grain intake and cardiovascular disease: a meta-analysis. *Nutr Metab Cardiovasc Dis* 2007;**85**:1495–502.

239. Umesawa M, Iso H, Date C, *et al.* Dietary intake of calcium in relation to mortality from cardiovascular disease: the JACC Study. *Stroke* 2006;**37**:20–6.

240. He K, Merchant A, Rimm EB, *et al.* Dietary fat intake and risk of stroke in male US healthcare professionals: 14-year prospective cohort study. *BMJ* 2003;**327**:777–82.

241. Howard BV, Van Horn L, Hsia J, *et al.* Low-fat dietary pattern and risk of cardiovascular disease: the Women's Health Initiative Randomized Controlled Dietary Modification Trial. *JAMA* 2006;**295**:655–66.

242. Kurth T, Gaziano JM, Berger K, *et al.* Body mass index and the risk of stroke in men. *Arch Intern Med* 2002;**162**: 2557–62.

243. Kurth T, Gaziano JM, Rexrode KM, *et al.* Prospective study of body mass index and risk of stroke in apparently healthy women. *Circulation* 2005;**111**:1992–8.

244. Hu G, Tuomilehto J, Silventoinen K, Sarti C, Mannisto S, Jousilahti P. Body mass index, waist circumference, and waist-hip ratio on the risk of total and type-specific stroke. *Arch Intern Med* 2007;**167**:1420–7.

245. Neter JE, Stam BE, Kok FJ, Grobbee DE, Geleijnse JM. Influence of weight reduction on blood pressure: a meta-analysis of randomized controlled trials. *Hypertension* 2003;**42**:878–84.

246. Curioni C, Andre C, Veras R. Weight reduction for primary prevention of stroke in adults with overweight or obesity. *Cochrane Database Syst Rev* 2006;(4): CD006062.

247. Marniemi J, Alanen E, Impivaara O, *et al.* Dietary and serum vitamins and minerals as predictors of myocardial infarction and stroke in elderly subjects. *Nutr Metab Cardiovasc Dis* 2005;**15**:188–97.

248. Hsia J, Heiss G, Ren H, *et al.* Calcium/vitamin D supplementation and cardiovascular events. *Circulation* 2007;**115**:846–54.

249. Tornwall ME, Virtamo J, Korhonen PA, Virtanen MJ, Albanes D, Huttunen JK. Postintervention effect of alpha tocopherol and beta carotene on different strokes: a 6-year follow-up of the Alpha Tocopherol, Beta Carotene Cancer Prevention Study. *Stroke* 2004;**35**:1908–13.

250. *Miller ER 3rd, Pastor-Barriuso R, Dalal D, Riemersma RA, Appel LJ, Guallar E. Meta-analysis: high-dosage vitamin E supplementation may increase all-cause mortality. *Ann Intern Med* 2005;**142**:37–46.

251. The Homocysteine Studies Collaboration. Homocysteine and risk of ischemic heart disease and stroke: a meta-analysis. *JAMA* 2002;**288**:2015–22.

252. Yang Q, Botto LD, Erickson JD, *et al.* Improvement in stroke mortality in Canada and the United States, 1990 to 2002. *Circulation* 2006;**113**:1335–43.

253. Wang X, Qin X, Demirtas H, *et al.* Efficacy of folic acid supplementation in stroke prevention: a meta-analysis. *Lancet* 2007;**369**:1876–82.

254. Grodstein F, Manson JE, Stampfer MJ. Postmenopausal hormone use and secondary prevention of coronary events in the nurses' health study. a prospective, observational study. *Ann Intern Med* 2001;**135**:1–8.

255. Grady D, Herrington D, Bittner V, *et al.* Cardiovascular disease outcomes during 6.8 years of hormone therapy: Heart and Estrogen/progestin Replacement Study follow-up (HERS II). *JAMA* 2002;**288**:49–57.

256. *Gabriel S, Carmona L, Roque M, Sanchez G, Bonfill X. Hormone replacement therapy for preventing cardiovascular disease in post-menopausal women. *Cochrane Database Syst Rev* 2005;(2):CD002229.

257. Brunner RL, Gass M, Aragaki A, *et al.* Effects of conjugated equine estrogen on health-related quality of life in post-menopausal women with hysterectomy: results from the Women's Health Initiative Randomized Clinical Trial. *Arch Intern Med* 2005;**165**:1976–86.

258. Rossouw JE, Prentice RL, Manson JE, *et al.* Postmenopausal hormone therapy and risk of cardiovascular disease by age and years since menopause. *JAMA* 2007;**297**:1465–77.

259. Peto R, Gray R, Collins R, *et al.* Randomised trial of prophylactic daily aspirin in British male doctors. *Br Med J (Clin Res Ed)* 1988;**296**:313–6.

260. Steering Committee of the Physicians' Health Study Research Group. Final report on the aspirin component of the ongoing Physicians' Health Study. *N Engl J Med* 1989;**321**:129–35.

261. ETDRS Investigators. Aspirin effects on mortality and morbidity in patients with diabetes mellitus. Early Treatment Diabetic Retinopathy Study report 14. *JAMA* 1992;**268**:1292–300.

262. Hansson L, Zanchetti A, Carruthers SG, *et al.* Effects of intensive blood-pressure lowering and low-dose aspirin in patients with hypertension: principal results of the Hypertension Optimal Treatment (HOT) randomised trial. HOT Study Group. *Lancet* 1998;**351**:1755–62.

263. de Gaetano G. Low-dose aspirin and vitamin E in people at cardiovascular risk: a randomised trial in general practice. Collaborative Group of the Primary Prevention Project. *Lancet* 2001;**357**:89–95.

264. Iso H, Hennekens CH, Stampfer MJ, *et al.* Prospective study of aspirin use and risk of stroke in women. *Stroke* 1999;**30**:1764–71.

265. Bartolucci AA, Howard G. Meta-analysis of data from the six primary prevention trials of cardiovascular events using aspirin. *Am J Cardiol* 2006;**98**:746–50.

266. *Berger JS, Roncaglioni MC, Avanzini F, Pangrazzi I, Tognoni G, Brown DL. Aspirin for the primary prevention of cardiovascular events in women and men: a sex-specific meta-analysis of randomized controlled trials. *JAMA* 2006;**295**:306–13.

267. Ridker PM, Cook NR, Lee IM, *et al.* A randomized trial of low-dose aspirin in the primary prevention of cardiovascular disease in women. *N Engl J Med* 2005;**352**:1293–304.

268. *Bhatt DL, Fox KA, Hacke W, *et al.* Clopidogrel and aspirin versus aspirin alone for the prevention of atherothrombotic events. *N Engl J Med* 2006;**354**:1706–17.

269. Hobson RW 2nd, Krupski WC, Weiss DG. Influence of aspirin in the management of asymptomatic carotid artery stenosis. VA Cooperative Study Group on Asymptomatic Carotid Stenosis. *J Vasc Surg* 1993;**17**:257–63, discussion 263-255.

270. Engelter S, Lyrer P. Antiplatelet therapy for preventing stroke and other vascular events after carotid endarterectomy. *Cochrane Database Syst Rev* 2003;(3):CD001458.

271. *Hart RG, Pearce LA, Aguilar MI. Meta-analysis: antithrombotic therapy to prevent stroke in patients who have nonvalvular atrial fibrillation. *Ann Intern Med* 2007;**146**:857–67.

272. *Rash A, Downes T, Portner R, Yeo WW, Morgan N, Channer KS. A randomised controlled trial of warfarin versus aspirin for stroke prevention in octogenarians with atrial fibrillation (WASPO). *Age Ageing* 2007;**36**:151–6.

273. Mant J, Hobbs FD, Fletcher K, *et al.* Warfarin versus aspirin for stroke prevention in an elderly community population with atrial fibrillation (the Birmingham Atrial Fibrillation Treatment of the Aged Study, BAFTA): a randomised controlled trial. *Lancet* 2007;**370**:493–503.

274. Connolly S, Pogue J, Hart R, *et al.* Clopidogrel plus aspirin versus oral anticoagulation for atrial fibrillation in the Atrial fibrillation Clopidogrel Trial with Irbesartan for prevention of Vascular Events (ACTIVE W): a randomised controlled trial. *Lancet* 2006;**367**:1903–12.

275. Cannegieter SC, Rosendaal FR, Wintzen AR, van der Meer FJ, Vandenbroucke JP, Briet E. Optimal oral anticoagulant therapy in patients with mechanical heart valves. *N Engl J Med* 1995;**333**:11–7.

276. *Chambers BR, Donnan GA. Carotid endarterectomy for asymptomatic carotid stenosis. *Cochrane Database Syst Rev* 2005;(4):CD001923.

277. Executive Committee for the Asymptomatic Carotid Atherosclerosis Study. Endarterectomy for asymptomatic carotid artery stenosis. *JAMA* 1995;**273**:1421–8.

278. *Halliday A, Mansfield A, Marro J, *et al.* Prevention of disabling and fatal strokes by successful carotid endarterectomy in patients without recent neurological symptoms: randomised controlled trial. *Lancet* 2004;**363**:1491–502.

279. *North American Symptomatic Carotid Endarterectomy Trial Collaborators. Beneficial effect of carotid endarterectomy in symptomatic patients with high-grade carotid stenosis. *N Engl J Med* 1991;**325**:445–53.

280. Baker WH, Howard VJ, Howard G, Toole JF. Effect of contralateral occlusion on long-term efficacy of endarterectomy in the asymptomatic carotid atherosclerosis study (ACAS). ACAS Investigators. *Stroke* 2000;**31**:2330–4.

281. Straus SE, Majumdar SR, McAlister FA. New evidence for stroke prevention: scientific review. *JAMA* 2002;**288**:1388–95.

282. The European Carotid Surgery Trialists Collaborative Group. Risk of stroke in the distribution of an asymptomatic carotid artery. *Lancet* 1995;**345**:209–12.

283. Mayo Asymptomatic Carotid Endarterectomy Study Group. Results of a randomized controlled trial of carotid endarterectomy for asymptomatic carotid stenosis. Mayo Asymptomatic Carotid Endarterectomy Study Group. *Mayo Clin Proc* 1992;**67**:513–8.

284. Derdeyn C. Carotid stenting for asymptomatic carotid stenosis: trial it. *Stroke* 2007;**38**:715–20.

285. Rashid P, Leonardi-Bee J, Bath P. Blood pressure reduction and secondary prevention of stroke and other vascular events: a systematic review. *Stroke* 2003;**34**:2741–8.

286. Group P. Post-stroke antihypertensive treatment study. A preliminary result. *Chin Med J (Engl)* 1995;**108**:710–7.

287. Yusuf S, Sleight P, Pogue J, Bosch J, Davies R, Dagenais G. Effects of an angiotensin-converting-enzyme inhibitor, ramipril, on cardiovascular events in high-risk patients. The Heart Outcomes Prevention Evaluation Study Investigators. *N Engl J Med* 2000;**342**:145–53.

288. Bosch J, Yusuf S, Pogue J, *et al.* Use of ramipril in preventing stroke: double blind randomised trial. *BMJ* 2002;**324**:699–702.

289. PROGRESS collaborative group. Randomised trial of a perindopril-based blood-pressure-lowering regimen among 6,105 individuals with previous stroke or transient ischaemic attack. *Lancet* 2001;**358**:1033–41.

290. Chobanian AV, Bakris GL, Black HR, *et al.* The Seventh Report of the Joint National Committee on Prevention, Detection, Evaluation, and Treatment of High Blood Pressure: the JNC 7 report. *JAMA* 2003;**289**:2560–72.

291. Schrader J, Luders S, Kulschewski A, *et al.* Morbidity and Mortality After Stroke, Eprosartan Compared with Nitrendipine for Secondary Prevention: principal results of a prospective randomized controlled study (MOSES). *Stroke* 2005;**36**:1218–26.

292. Wilcox R, Bousser MG, Betteridge DJ, *et al.* Effects of pioglitazone in patients with type 2 diabetes with or without previous stroke: results from PROactive (PROspective pioglitAzone Clinical Trial In macroVascular Events 04). *Stroke* 2007;**38**:865–73.

293. *Amarenco P, Bogousslavsky J, Callahan A, *et al.* High-dose atorvastatin after stroke or transient ischemic attack. *N Engl J Med* 2006;**355**:549–59.

294. *Blanco M, Nombela F, Castellanos M, *et al.* Statin treatment withdrawal in ischemic stroke: a controlled randomized study. *Neurology* 2007;**69**:904–10.

295. Vivekananthan D, Penn M, Sapp S, Hsu A, Topol E. Use of antioxidant vitamins for the prevention of cardiovascular disease: meta-analysis of randomised trials. *Lancet* 2003;**361**:2017–23.

296. Eidelman RS, Hollar D, Hebert PR, Lamas GA, Hennekens CH. Randomized trials of vitamin E in the treatment and prevention of cardiovascular disease. *Arch Intern Med* 2004;**164**:1552–6.

297. *Bjelakovic G, Nikolova D, Gluud LL, Simonetti RG, Gluud C. Mortality in randomized trials of antioxidant supplements for primary and secondary prevention: systematic review and meta-analysis. *JAMA* 2007;**297**:842–57.

298. Wald DS, Law M, Morris JK. Homocysteine and cardiovascular disease: evidence on causality from a meta-analysis. *BMJ* 2002;**325**:1202.

299. Toole JF, Malinow MR, Chambless LE, *et al.* Lowering homocysteine in patients with ischemic stroke to prevent recurrent stroke, myocardial infarction, and death: the Vitamin Intervention for Stroke Prevention (VISP) randomized controlled trial. *JAMA* 2004;**291**:565–75.

300. Bonaa KH, Njolstad I, Ueland PM, *et al.* Homocysteine lowering and cardiovascular events after acute myocardial infarction. *N Engl J Med* 2006;**354**:1578–88.

301. Bazzano LA, Reynolds K, Holder KN, He J. Effect of folic acid supplementation on risk of cardiovascular diseases: a meta-analysis of randomized controlled trials. *JAMA* 2006;**296**:2720–6.

302. VITATOPS Trial Study Group. The VITATOPS (Vitamins to Prevent Stroke) Trial: rationale and design of an international, large, simple, randomised trial of homocysteine-lowering multivitamin therapy in patients with recent transient ischaemic attack or stroke. *Cerebrovasc Dis* 2002;**13**:120–6.

303. *Bassetti CL. Sleep and stroke. *Semin Neurol* 2005;**25**: 19–32.

304. Handke M, Harloff A, Olschewski M, Hetzel A, Geibel A. Patent foramen ovale and cryptogenic stroke in older patients. *N Engl J Med* 2007;**357**:2262–8.

305. Overell JR, Bone I, Lees KR. Interatrial septal abnormalities and stroke: a meta-analysis of case-control studies. *Neurology* 2000;**55**:1172–9.

306. Di Tullio MR, Sacco RL, Sciacca RR, Jin Z, Homma S. Patent foramen ovale and the risk of ischemic stroke in a multiethnic population. *J Am Coll Cardiol* 2007;**49**: 797–802.

307. Meissner I, Khandheria BK, Heit JA, *et al.* Patent foramen ovale: innocent or guilty? Evidence from a prospective population-based study. *J Am Coll Cardiol* 2006;**47**: 440–5.

308. Mas JL, Arquizan C, Lamy C, *et al.* Recurrent cerebrovascular events associated with patent foramen ovale, atrial septal aneurysm, or both. *N Engl J Med* 2001;**345**:1740–6.

309. Wahl A, Krumsdorf U, Meier B, *et al.* Transcatheter treatment of atrial septal aneurysm associated with patent foramen ovale for prevention of recurrent paradoxical embolism in high-risk patients. *J Am Coll Cardiol* 2005;**45**: 377–80.

310. Windecker S, Wahl A, Nedeltchev K, *et al.* Comparison of medical treatment with percutaneous closure of patent foramen ovale in patients with cryptogenic stroke. *J Am Coll Cardiol* 2004;**44**:750–8.

311. *Viscoli CM, Brass LM, Kernan WN, Sarrel PM, Suissa S, Horwitz RI. A clinical trial of estrogen-replacement therapy after ischemic stroke. *N Engl J Med* 2001;**345**: 1243–9.

312. *Antithrombotic Trialists' Collaboration. Collaborative meta-analysis of randomised trials of antiplatelet therapy for prevention of death, myocardial infarction, and stroke in high risk patients. *BMJ* 2002;**324**:71–86.

313. Algra A, van Gijn J. Aspirin at any dose above 30 mg offers only modest protection after cerebral ischaemia. *J Neurol Neurosurg Psychiatry* 1996;**60**:197–9.

314. The Dutch TIA Trial Study Group. A comparison of two doses of aspirin (30 mg vs. 283 mg a day) in patients after a transient ischemic attack or minor ischemic stroke. *N Engl J Med* 1991;**325**:1261–6.

315. Farrell B, Godwin J, Richards S, Warlow C. The United Kingdom transient ischaemic attack (UK-TIA) aspirin trial: final results. *J Neurol Neurosurg Psychiatry* 1991;**54**: 1044–54.

316. Campbell CL, Smyth S, Montalescot G, Steinhubl SR. Aspirin dose for the prevention of cardiovascular disease: a systematic review. *JAMA* 2007;**297**:2018–24.

317. *Chimowitz MI, Lynn MJ, Howlett-Smith H, *et al.* Comparison of warfarin and aspirin for symptomatic intracranial arterial stenosis. *N Engl J Med* 2005;**352**:1305–16.

318. *CAPRIE Steering Committee. A randomised, blinded trial of clopidogrel versus aspirin in patients at risk of ischaemic events (CAPRIE). *Lancet* 1996;**348**:1329–39.

319. *Diener HC, Cunha L, Forbes C, Sivenius J, Smets P, Lowenthal A. European Stroke Prevention Study. 2. Dipyridamole and acetylsalicylic acid in the secondary prevention of stroke. *J Neurol Sci* 1996;**143**:1–13.

320. *Costa J, Ferro JM, Matias-Guiu J, Alvarez-Sabin J, Torres F. Triflusal for preventing serious vascular events in people at high risk. *Cochrane Database Syst Rev* 2005;(3):CD004296.

321. *Halkes PH, van Gijn J, Kappelle LJ, Koudstaal PJ, Algra A. Aspirin plus dipyridamole versus aspirin alone after cerebral ischaemia of arterial origin (ESPRIT): randomised controlled trial. *Lancet* 2006;**367**:1665–73.

322. Chang YJ, Ryu SJ, Lee TH. Dose titration to reduce dipyridamole-related headache. *Cerebrovasc Dis* 2006;**22**: 258–62.

323. Diener H, Davidai G. Dipyridamole and headache. Future. *Neurology* 2007;**2**:279–83.

324. *Diener HC, Bogousslavsky J, Brass LM, *et al.* Aspirin and clopidogrel compared with clopidogrel alone after recent ischaemic stroke or transient ischaemic attack in high-risk patients (MATCH): randomised, double-blind, placebo-controlled trial. *Lancet* 2004;**364**:331–7.

325. Yusuf S, Zhao F, Mehta S, Chrolavicius S, Tognoni G, Fox K, and the Clopidogrel in Unstable Angina to Prevent Recurrent Events Trial Investigators. Effects of clopidogrel in addition to aspirin in patients with acute coronary syndrome without ST-segment elevation. *N Engl J Med* 2001;**345**:494–502.

326. •Mohr JP, Thompson JL, Lazar RM, *et al.* A comparison of warfarin and aspirin for the prevention of recurrent ischemic stroke. *N Engl J Med* 2001;**345**:1444–51.

327. The Stroke Prevention in Reversible Ischemia Trial (SPIRIT) Study Group. A randomized trial of anticoagulants versus aspirin after cerebral ischemia of presumed arterial origin. *Ann Neurol* 1997;**42**:857–65.

328. *Algra A. Medium intensity oral anticoagulants versus aspirin after cerebral ischaemia of arterial origin (ESPRIT):

a randomised controlled trial. *Lancet Neurol* 2007;**6**: 115–24.

329. EAFT (European Atrial Fibrillation Trial) Study Group. Secondary prevention in non-rheumatic atrial fibrillation after transient ischaemic attack or minor stroke. *Lancet* 1993;**342**:1255–62.

330. Visser CA, Kan G, Meltzer RS, Lie KI, Durrer D. Long-term follow-up of left ventricular thrombus after acute myocardial infarction. A two-dimensional echocardiographic study in 96 patients. *Chest* 1984;**86**:532–6.

331. Flaker GC, Gruber M, Connolly SJ, *et al*. Risks and benefits of combining aspirin with anticoagulant therapy in patients with atrial fibrillation: an exploratory analysis of stroke prevention using an oral thrombin inhibitor in atrial fibrillation (SPORTIF) trials. *Am Heart J* 2006;**152**:967–73.

332. Dressler FA, Craig WR, Castello R, Labovitz AJ. Mobile aortic atheroma and systemic emboli: efficacy of anticoagulation and influence of plaque morphology on recurrent stroke. *J Am Coll Cardiol* 1998;**31**:134–8.

333. Echiverri HC, Rubino FA, Gupta SR, Gujrati M. Fusiform aneurysm of the vertebrobasilar arterial system. *Stroke* 1989;**20**:1741–7.

334. Engelter ST, Brandt T, Debette S, *et al*. Antiplatelets versus anticoagulation in cervical artery dissection. *Stroke* 2007;**38**:2605–11.

335. *Rothwell PM, Eliasziw M, Gutnikov SA, *et al*. Analysis of pooled data from the randomised controlled trials of endarterectomy for symptomatic carotid stenosis. *Lancet* 2003;**361**:107–16.

336. *European Carotid Surgery Trialists' Collaborative Group. Endarterectomy for moderate symptomatic carotid stenosis: interim results from the MRC European carotid surgery trial. *Lancet* 1996;**347**:1591–3.

337. *Cina C, Clase C, Haynes R. Carotid endarterectomy for symptomatic carotid stenosis. *Cochrane Database Syst Rev* 1999;(3):CD001081.

338. *Rothwell PM, Eliasziw M, Gutnikov SA, Warlow CP, Barnett HJ. Endarterectomy for symptomatic carotid stenosis in relation to clinical subgroups and timing of surgery. *Lancet* 2004;**363**:915–24.

339. Bond R, Rerkasem K, AbuRahma AF, Naylor AR, Rothwell PM. Patch angioplasty versus primary closure for carotid endarterectomy. *Cochrane Database Syst Rev* 2004;(3): CD000160.

340. Rothwell PM, Eliasziw M, Gutnikov SA, Warlow CP, Barnett HJ. Sex difference in the effect of time from symptoms to surgery on benefit from carotid endarterectomy for transient ischemic attack and nondisabling stroke. *Stroke* 2004;**35**:2855–61.

341. Inzitari D, Eliasziw M, Sharpe BL, Fox AJ, Barnett HJ. Risk factors and outcome of patients with carotid artery stenosis

presenting with lacunar stroke. North American Symptomatic Carotid Endarterectomy Trial Group. *Neurology* 2000;**54**:660–6.

342. Streifler JY, Eliasziw M, Benavente OR, *et al*. Prognostic importance of leukoaraiosis in patients with symptomatic internal carotid artery stenosis. *Stroke* 2002;**33**: 1651–5.

343. *Mas JL, Chatellier G, Beyssen B, *et al*. Ducrocq X, for the EVA-3S Investigators: endarterectomy versus stenting in patients with symptomatic severe carotid stenosis. *N Engl J Med* 2006;**355**:1660–71.

344. *Ringleb PA, Allenberg JR, Berger J, *et al*. 30-day results from the SPACE trial of stent-protected angioplasty versus carotid endarterectomy in symptomatic patients: a randomised non-inferiority trial. *Lancet* 2006;**368**:1239–47.

345. Yadav JS, Wholey MH, Kuntz RE, *et al*. Protected carotid-artery stenting versus endarterectomy in high-risk patients. *N Engl J Med* 2004;**351**:1493–501.

346. *CAVATAS Group. Endovascular versus surgical treatment in patients with carotid stenosis in the Carotid and Vertebral Artery Transluminal Angioplasty Study (CAVATAS): a randomised trial. *Lancet* 2001;**357**:1729–37.

347. Kastrup A, Groschel K. Carotid endarterectomy versus carotid stenting: an updated review of randomized trials and subgroup analyses. *Acta Chir Belg* 2007;**107**:119–28.

348. The EC/IC Bypass Study Group. Failure of extracranial-intracranial arterial bypass to reduce the risk of ischemic stroke. Results of an international randomized trial. *N Engl J Med* 1985;**313**:1191–200.

349. Kasner SE, Chimowitz MI, Lynn MJ, *et al*. Predictors of ischemic stroke in the territory of a symptomatic intracranial arterial stenosis. *Circulation* 2006;**113**:555–63.

350. Jiang WJ, Xu XT, Du B, *et al*. Long-term outcome of elective stenting for symptomatic intracranial vertebrobasilar stenosis. *Neurology* 2007;**68**:856–8.

351. Jiang WJ, Xu XT, Du B, *et al*. Comparison of elective stenting of severe vs moderate intracranial atherosclerotic stenosis. *Neurology* 2007;**68**:420–6.

352. Marks MP, Wojak JC, Al-Ali F, *et al*. Angioplasty for symptomatic intracranial stenosis: clinical outcome. *Stroke* 2006;**37**:1016–20.

353. Fiorella D, Levy EI, Turk AS, *et al*. US multicenter experience with the wingspan stent system for the treatment of intracranial atheromatous disease: periprocedural results. *Stroke* 2007;**38**:881–7.

354. *Bose A, Hartmann M, Henkes H, *et al*. A novel, self-expanding, nitinol stent in medically refractory intracranial atherosclerotic stenoses: the Wingspan study. *Stroke* 2007;**38**:1531–7.

355. *SSYLVIA Study investigators. Stenting of Symptomatic Atherosclerotic Lesions in the Vertebral or Intracranial Arteries (SSYLVIA): study results. *Stroke* 2004;**35**:1388–92.

356. Lindstrom E, Boysen G, Christiansen L, Nansen B, Nielsen P. Reliability of Scandinavian neurological stroke scale. *Cerebrosvasc Dis* 1991;**1**:103–7.

357. Sulter G, Elting JW, Langedijk M, Maurits NM, De Keyser J. Admitting acute ischemic stroke patients to a stroke care monitoring unit versus a conventional stroke unit: a randomized pilot study. *Stroke* 2003;**34**:101–4.

358. Cavallini A, Micieli G, Marcheselli S, Quaglini S. Role of monitoring in management of acute ischemic stroke patients. *Stroke* 2003;**34**:2599–603.

359. Ronning OM, Guldvog B. Should stroke victims routinely receive supplemental oxygen? A quasi-randomized controlled trial. *Stroke* 1999;**30**:2033–7.

360. Bamford J, Dennis M, Sandercock P, Burn J, Warlow C. The frequency, causes and timing of death within 30 days of a first stroke: the Oxfordshire Community Stroke Project. *J Neurol Neurosurg Psychiatry* 1990;**53**: 824–9.

361. Broderick JP, Phillips SJ, O'Fallon WM, Frye RL, Whisnant JP. Relationship of cardiac disease to stroke occurrence, recurrence, and mortality. *Stroke* 1992;**23**:1250–6.

362. Barber M, Morton JJ, Macfarlane PW, Barlow N, Roditi G, Stott DJ. Elevated troponin levels are associated with sympathoadrenal activation in acute ischaemic stroke. *Cerebrovasc Dis* 2007;**23**:260–6.

363. Bhalla A, Sankaralingam S, Dundas R, Swaminathan R, Wolfe CD, Rudd AG. Influence of raised plasma osmolality on clinical outcome after acute stroke. *Stroke* 2000;**31**: 2043–8.

364. Gray CS, Hildreth AJ, Sandercock PA, *et al.* Glucose-potassium-insulin infusions in the management of post-stroke hyperglycaemia: the UK Glucose Insulin in Stroke Trial (GIST-UK). *Lancet Neurol* 2007;**6**:397–406.

365. Asplund K, Marke LA, Terent A, Gustafsson C, Wester P. Costs and gains in stroke prevention: European perspective. *Cerebrosvasc Dis* 1993;**3**(Suppl.):34–42.

366. Castillo J, Leira R, Garcia MM, Serena J, Blanco M, Davalos A. Blood pressure decrease during the acute phase of ischemic stroke is associated with brain injury and poor stroke outcome. *Stroke* 2004;**35**:520–6.

367. Leonardi-Bee J, Bath PM, Phillips SJ, Sandercock PA. Blood pressure and clinical outcomes in the International Stroke Trial. *Stroke* 2002;**33**:1315–20.

368. Blood pressure in Acute Stroke Collaboration (BASC). Interventions for deliberately altering blood pressure in acute stroke. *Cochrane Database Syst Rev* 2001;(44): CD000039.

369. Nazir FS, Overell JR, Bolster A, Hilditch TE, Lees KR. Effect of perindopril on cerebral and renal perfusion on normotensives in mild early ischaemic stroke: a randomized controlled trial. *Cerebrovasc Dis* 2005;**19**:77–83.

370. COSSACS investigators. COSSACS (Continue or Stop post-Stroke Antihypertensives Collaborative Study): rationale and design. *J Hypertens* 2005;**23**:455–8.

371. Thomas GN, Chan P, Tomlinson B. The role of angiotensin II type 1 receptor antagonists in elderly patients with hypertension. *Drugs Aging* 2006;**23**:131–55.

372. Grossman E, Messerli FH, Grodzicki T, Kowey P. Should a moratorium be placed on sublingual nifedipine capsules given for hypertensive emergencies and pseudoemergencies? *JAMA* 1996;**276**:1328–31.

373. Kiers L, Davis SM, Larkins R, *et al.* Stroke topography and outcome in relation to hyperglycaemia and diabetes. *J Neurol Neurosurg Psychiatry* 1992;**55**:263–70.

374. van Kooten F, Hoogerbrugge N, Naarding P, Koudstaal PJ. Hyperglycemia in the acute phase of stroke is not caused by stress. *Stroke* 1993;**24**:1129–32.

375. Baird TA, Parsons MW, Phanh T, *et al.* Persistent post-stroke hyperglycemia is independently associated with infarct expansion and worse clinical outcome. *Stroke* 2003;**34**:2208–14.

376. Baird TA, Parsons MW, Barber PA, *et al.* The influence of diabetes mellitus and hyperglycaemia on stroke incidence and outcome. *J Clin Neurosci* 2002;**9**:618–26.

377. Parsons MW, Barber PA, Desmond PM, *et al.* Acute hyperglycemia adversely affects stroke outcome: a magnetic resonance imaging and spectroscopy study. *Ann Neurol* 2002;**52**:20–8.

378. Huff JS. Stroke mimics and chameleons. *Emerg Med Clin North Am* 2002;**20**:583–95.

379. Fukuda H, Kitani M, Takahashi K. Body temperature correlates with functional outcome and the lesion size of cerebral infarction. *Acta Neurol Scand* 1999;**100**: 385–90.

380. Reith J, Jorgensen HS, Pedersen PM, *et al.* Body temperature in acute stroke: relation to stroke severity, infarct size, mortality, and outcome. *Lancet* 1996;**347**:422–5.

381. Castillo J, Davalos A, Noya M. Aggravation of acute ischemic stroke by hyperthermia is related to an excitotoxic mechanism. *Cerebrovasc Dis* 1999;**9**:22–7.

382. Hajat C, Hajat S, Sharma P. Effects of poststroke pyrexia on stroke outcome: a meta-analysis of studies in patients. *Stroke* 2000;**31**:410–4.

383. Hacke W, Kaste M, Fieschi C, *et al.* Randomised double-blind placebo-controlled trial of thrombolytic therapy with intravenous alteplase in acute ischaemic stroke (ECASS II). *Lancet* 1998;**352**:1245–51.

384. Hacke W, Kaste M, Fieschi C, *et al.* Intravenous thrombolysis with recombinant tissue plasminogen activator for acute stroke. *JAMA* 1995;**274**:1017–25.

385. *Wardlaw JM, Zoppo G, Yamaguchi T, Berge E. Thrombolysis for acute ischaemic stroke. *Cochrane Database Syst Rev* 2009;(4):CD000213.

386. *Hacke W, Donnan G, Fieschi C, *et al.* Association of outcome with early stroke treatment: pooled analysis of ATLANTIS, ECASS, and NINDS rt-PA stroke trials. *Lancet* 2004;**363**:768–74.

387. Demchuk AM, Hill MD, Barber PA, Silver B, Patel SC, Levine SR. Importance of early ischemic computed tomography changes using ASPECTS in NINDS rtPA Stroke Study. *Stroke* 2005;**36**:2110–5.

388. Hacke W, Kaste M, Bluhmki E, *et al.* Thrombolysis with alteplase 3 to 4.5 hours after acute ischemic stroke. *New England Journal of Medicine* 2008;**359**:1317–29.

389. Wahlgren N, Ahmed N, Davalos A, *et al.* Thrombolysis with alteplase 3–4 center dot 5 h after acute ischaemic stroke (SITS-ISTR): an observational study. *Lancet* 2008;**372**:1303–9.

390. Sylaja PN, Cote R, Buchan AM, Hill MD. Thrombolysis in patients older than 80 years with acute ischaemic stroke: Canadian Alteplase for Stroke Effectiveness Study. *J Neurol Neurosurg Psychiatry* 2006;**77**:826–9.

391. van Oostenbrugge RJ, Hupperts RM, Lodder J. Thrombolysis for acute stroke with special emphasis on the very old: experience from a single Dutch centre. *J Neurol Neurosurg Psychiatry* 2006;**77**:375–7.

392. Ringleb PA, Schwark C, Köhrmann M, *et al.* Thrombolytic therapy for acute ischaemic stroke in octogenarians: selection by magnetic resonance imaging improves safety but does not improve outcome. *J Neurol Neurosurg Psychiatry* 2007;**78**:690–3.

393. Elkind MS, Prabhakaran S, Pittman J, Koroshetz W, Jacoby M, Johnston KC. Sex as a predictor of outcomes in patients treated with thrombolysis for acute stroke. *Neurology* 2007;**68**:842–8.

394. Hill MD, Buchan AM. Thrombolysis for acute ischemic stroke: results of the Canadian Alteplase for Stroke Effectiveness Study (CASES). *CMAJ* 2005;**172**:1307–12.

395. Bateman BT, Schumacher HC, Boden-Albala B, *et al.* Factors associated with in-hospital mortality after administration of thrombolysis in acute ischemic stroke patients: an analysis of the nationwide inpatient sample 1999 to 2002. *Stroke* 2006;**37**:440–6.

396. *Wahlgren N, Ahmed N, Davalos A, *et al.* Thrombolysis with alteplase for acute ischaemic stroke in the Safe Implementation of Thrombolysis in Stroke-Monitoring Study (SITS-MOST): an observational study. *Lancet* 2007;**369**:275–82.

397. Katzan IL, Hammer MD, Furlan AJ, Hixson ED, Nadzam DM. Quality improvement and tissue-type plasminogen activator for acute ischemic stroke: a Cleveland update. *Stroke* 2003;**34**:799–800.

398. Graham GD. Tissue plasminogen activator for acute ischemic stroke in clinical practice: a meta-analysis of safety data. *Stroke* 2003;**34**:2847–50.

399. Alexandrov AV, Molina CA, Grotta JC, *et al.* Ultrasound-enhanced systemic thrombolysis for acute ischemic stroke. *N Engl J Med* 2004;**351**:2170–8.

400. Molina CA, Ribo M, Rubiera M, *et al.* Microbubble administration accelerates clot lysis during continuous 2-MHz ultrasound monitoring in stroke patients treated with intravenous tissue plasminogen activator. *Stroke* 2006;**37**:425–9.

401. Köhrmann M, Jüttler E, Fiebach JB, *et al.* MRI versus CT-based thrombolysis treatment within and beyond the 3 h time window after stroke onset: a cohort study. *Lancet Neurol* 2006;**5**:661–7.

402. Schellinger PD, Thomalla G, Fiehler J, *et al.* MRI-based and CT-based thrombolytic therapy in acute stroke within and beyond established time windows: an analysis of 1210 patients. *Stroke* 2007;**38**:2640–5.

403. *Lansberg MG, Thijs VN, Bammer R, *et al.* Risk factors of symptomatic intracerebral hemorrhage after tPA therapy for acute stroke. *Stroke* 2007;**38**:2275–8.

404. The Multicenter Acute Stroke Trial – Europe Study Group. Thrombolytic therapy with streptokinase in acute ischemic Stroke. *N Engl J Med* 1996;**335**:145–50.

405. (MAST-I) Group. Randomised controlled trial of streptokinase, aspirin, and combination of both in treatment of acute ischaemic stroke. Multicentre Acute Stroke Trial – Italy. *Lancet* 1995;**346**:1509–14.

406. *Hacke W, Albers G, Al-Rawi Y, *et al.* The Desmoteplase in Acute Ischemic Stroke Trial (DIAS): a phase II MRI-based 9-hour window acute stroke thrombolysis trial with intravenous desmoteplase. *Stroke* 2005;**36**:66–73.

407. *Furlan AJ, Eyding D, Albers GW, *et al.* Dose Escalation of Desmoteplase for Acute Ischemic Stroke (DEDAS): evidence of safety and efficacy 3 to 9 hours after stroke onset. *Stroke* 2006;**37**:1227–31.

408. Ogawa A, Mori E, Minematsu K, *et al.* Randomized trial of intraarterial infusion of urokinase within 6 hours of middle cerebral artery stroke: the middle cerebral artery embolism local fibrinolytic intervention trial (MELT) Japan. *Stroke* 2007;**38**:2633–9.

409. Nedeltchev K, Fischer U, Arnold M, *et al.* Long-term effect of intra-arterial thrombolysis in stroke. *Stroke* 2006;**37**:3002–7.

410. IMS investigators. The Interventional Management of Stroke (IMS) II Study. *Stroke* 2007;**38**:2127–35.

411. Macleod MR, Davis SM, Mitchell PJ, *et al.* Results of a multicentre, randomised controlled trial of intra-arterial urokinase in the treatment of acute posterior

circulation ischaemic stroke. *Cerebrovasc Dis* 2005;**20**: 12–7.

412. Brandt T, von Kummer R, Muller Kuppers M, Hacke W. Thrombolytic therapy of acute basilar artery occlusion. Variables affecting recanalization and outcome. *Stroke* 1996;**27**:875–81.

413. Hacke W, Zeumer H, Ferbert A, Bruckmann H, del Zoppo GJ. Intra-arterial thrombolytic therapy improves outcome in patients with acute vertebrobasilar occlusive disease. *Stroke* 1988;**19**:1216–22.

414. *Lindsberg PJ, Mattle HP. Therapy of basilar artery occlusion: a systematic analysis comparing intra-arterial and intravenous thrombolysis. *Stroke* 2006;**37**: 922–8.

415. *Smith WS, Sung G, Starkman S, *et al.* Safety and efficacy of mechanical embolectomy in acute ischemic stroke: results of the MERCI trial. *Stroke* 2005;**36**: 1432–8.

416. *International-Stroke-Trial-Collaborative-Group. The International Stroke Trial (IST): a randomised trial if aspirin, subcutaneous heparin, both, or neither among 19,435 patients with acute ischaemic stroke. *Lancet* 1997;**349**:1569–81.

417. *CAST-Collaborative-Group. CAST: randomised placebo-controlled trial of early aspirin use in 20,000 patients with acute ischeaemic stroke. *Lancet* 1997;**349**:1641–9.

418. Rödén-Jüllig A, Britton M, Malmkvist K, Leijd B. Aspirin in the prevention of progressing stroke: a randomized controlled study. *J Intern Med* 2003;**254**:584–90.

419. *AbESST investigators. Emergency administration of abciximab for treatment of patients with acute ischemic stroke: results of a randomized phase 2 trial. *Stroke* 2005;**36**:880–90.

420. *Adams HP Jr, Effron MB, Torner J, *et al.* Emergency administration of abciximab for treatment of patients with acute ischemic stroke: results of an international phase III trial. Abciximab in Emergency Treatment of Stroke Trial (AbESTT-II). *Stroke* 2008;**39**:87–99.

421. *Kay R, Wong KS, Yu YL, *et al.* Low-molecular-weight heparin for the treatment of acute ischemic stroke. *N Engl J Med* 1995;**333**:1588–93.

422. *Wong KS, Chen C, Ng PW, *et al.* Low-molecular-weight heparin compared with aspirin for the treatment of acute ischaemic stroke in Asian patients with large artery occlusive disease: a randomised study. *Lancet Neurol* 2007;**6**:407–13.

423. *Diener HC, Ringelstein EB, von Kummer R, *et al.* Treatment of acute ischemic stroke with the low-molecular-weight heparin certoparin: results of the TOPAS trial. Therapy of Patients With Acute Stroke (TOPAS) Investigators. *Stroke* 2001;**32**:22–9.

424. *Bath PM, Lindenstrom E, Boysen G, *et al.* Tinzaparin in acute ischaemic stroke (TAIST): a randomised aspirin-controlled trial. *Lancet* 2001;**358**:702–10.

425. *Berge E, Abdelnoor M, Nakstad PH, Sandset PM. Low molecular-weight heparin versus aspirin in patients with acute ischaemic stroke and atrial fibrillation: a double-blind randomised study. HAEST Study Group. Heparin in Acute Embolic Stroke Trial. *Lancet* 2000;**355**: 1205–10.

426. *The Publications Committee for the Trial of ORG 10172 in Acute Stroke Treatment (TOAST) Investigators. Low molecular weight heparinoid, ORG 10172 (danaparoid), and outcome after acute ischemic stroke: a randomized controlled trial. *JAMA* 1998;**279**:1265–72.

427. *Gubitz G, Sandercock P, Counsell C. Anticoagulants for acute ischaemic stroke. *Cochrane Database Syst Rev* 2008;(4):CD000024.

428. Camerlingo M, Salvi P, Belloni G, Gamba T, Cesana BM, Mamoli A. Intravenous heparin started within the first 3 hours after onset of symptoms as a treatment for acute nonlacunar hemispheric cerebral infarctions. *Stroke* 2005;**36**:2415–20.

429. Chamorro A, Busse O, Obach V, *et al.* The rapid anticoagulation prevents ischemic damage study in acute stroke – final results from the writing committee. *Cerebrovasc Dis* 2005;**19**:402–4.

430. Chamorro A. Immediate anticoagulation for acute stroke in atrial fibrillation: yes. *Stroke* 2006;**37**:3052–3.

431. Sandercock P. Immediate anticoagulation for acute stroke in atrial fibrillation: no. *Stroke* 2006;**37**:3054–5.

432. *Paciaroni M, Agnelli G, Micheli S, Caso V. Efficacy and safety of anticoagulant treatment in acute cardioembolic stroke: a meta-analysis of randomized controlled trials. *Stroke* 2007;**38**:423–30.

433. *Shuaib A, Lees KR, Lyden P, *et al.* NXY-059 for the treatment of acute ischemic stroke. *N Engl J Med* 2007;**357**: 562–71.

434. *Muir KW, Lees KR, Ford I, Davis S. Magnesium for acute stroke (Intravenous Magnesium Efficacy in Stroke trial): randomised controlled trial. *Lancet* 2004;**363**:439–45.

435. Amaro S, Soy D, Obach V, Cervera A, Planas AM, Chamorro A. A pilot study of dual treatment with recombinant tissue plasminogen activator and uric acid in acute ischemic stroke. *Stroke* 2007;**38**:2173–5.

436. Davalos A, Castillo J, Alvarez-Sabin J, *et al.* Oral citicoline in acute ischemic stroke: an individual patient data pooling analysis of clinical trials. *Stroke* 2002;**33**:2850–7.

437. Hacke W, Schwab S, Horn M, Spranger M, De Georgia M, von Kummer R. 'Malignant' middle cerebral artery territory infarction: clinical course and prognostic signs. *Arch Neurol* 1996;**53**:309–15.

438. Qureshi AI, Suarez JI, Yahia AM, *et al.* Timing of neurologic deterioration in massive middle cerebral artery infarction: a multicenter review. *Crit Care Med* 2003;**31**:272–7.

439. Unterberg AW, Kiening KL, Hartl R, Bardt T, Sarrafzadeh AS, Lanksch WR. Multimodal monitoring in patients with head injury: evaluation of the effects of treatment on cerebral oxygenation. *J Trauma* 1997;**42**:S32–7.

440. Righetti E, Celani MG, Cantisani TA, Sterzi R, Boysen G, Ricci S. Glycerol for acute stroke: a Cochrane systematic review. *J Neurol* 2002;**249**:445–51.

441. Bereczki D, Liu M, do Prado GF, Fekete I. Mannitol for acute stroke. *Cochrane Database Syst Rev* 2001;(1):CD001153.

442. Schwarz S, Georgiadis D, Aschoff A, Schwab S. Effects of hypertonic (10%) saline in patients with raised intracranial pressure after stroke. *Stroke* 2002;**33**:136–40.

443. *Qizilbash N, Lewington SL, Lopez-Arrieta JM. Corticosteroids for acute ischaemic stroke. *Cochrane Database Syst Rev* 2002;(2):CD000064.

444. Schwab S, Schwarz S, Spranger M, Keller E, Bertram M, Hacke W. Moderate hypothermia in the treatment of patients with severe middle cerebral artery infarction. *Stroke* 1998;**29**:2461–6.

445. Steiner T, Ringleb P, Hacke W. Treatment options for large hemispheric stroke. *Neurology* 2001;**57**(5 Suppl. 2):S61–8.

446. Els T, Oehm E, Voigt S, Klisch J, Hetzel A, Kassubek J. Safety and therapeutical benefit of hemicraniectomy combined with mild hypothermia in comparison with hemicraniectomy alone in patients with malignant ischemic stroke. *Cerebrovasc Dis* 2006;**21**:79–85.

447. *Vahedi K, Hofmeijer J, Jüttler E, *et al.* Early decompressive surgery in malignant infarction of the middle cerebral artery: a pooled analysis of three randomised controlled trials. *Lancet Neurol* 2007;**6**:215–22.

448. Jüttler E, Schwab S, Schmiedek P, *et al.* Decompressive Surgery for the Treatment of Malignant Infarction of the Middle Cerebral Artery (DESTINY): a randomized, controlled trial. *Stroke* 2007;**38**:2518–25.

449. Gupta R, Connolly ES, Mayer S, Elkind MS. Hemicraniectomy for massive middle cerebral artery territory infarction: a systematic review. *Stroke* 2004;**35**:539–43.

450. Weimar C, Roth MP, Zillessen G, *et al.* Complications following acute ischemic stroke. *Eur Neurol* 2002;**48**:133–40.

451. Horner J, Massey EW, Riski JE, Lathrop DL, Chase KN. Aspiration following stroke: clinical correlates and outcome. *Neurology* 1988;**38**:1359–62.

452. Prass K, Meisel C, Höflich C, *et al.* Stroke-induced immunodeficiency promotes spontaneous bacterial infections and is mediated by sympathetic activation reversal by post-stroke T helper cell type 1-like immunostimulation. *J Exp Med* 2003;**198**:725–36.

453. Chamorro A, Amaro S, Vargas M, *et al.* Interleukin 10, monocytes and increased risk of early infection in ischaemic stroke. *J Neurol Neurosurg Psychiatry* 2006;**77**:1279–81.

454. Chamorro A, Horcajada JP, Obach V, *et al.* The Early Systemic Prophylaxis of Infection After Stroke study: a randomized clinical trial. *Stroke* 2005;**36**:1495–500.

455. *Mazzone C, Chiodo GF, Sandercock P, Miccio M, Salvi R. Physical methods for preventing deep vein thrombosis in stroke. *Cochrane Database Syst Rev* 2004;(4):CD001922.

456. Kamphuisen PW, Agnelli G, Sebastianelli M. Prevention of venous thromboembolism after acute ischemic stroke. *J Thromb Haemost* 2005;**3**:1187–94.

457. *Diener HC, Ringelstein EB, von Kummer R, *et al.* Prophylaxis of thrombotic and embolic events in acute ischemic stroke with the low-molecular-weight heparin certoparin: results of the PROTECT Trial. *Stroke* 2006;**37**:139–44.

458. *Sherman DG, Albers GW, Bladin C, *et al.* The efficacy and safety of enoxaparin versus unfractionated heparin for the prevention of venous thromboembolism after acute ischaemic stroke (PREVAIL Study): an open-label randomised comparison. *Lancet* 2007;**369**:1347–55.

459. Reddy M, Gill SS, Rochon PA. Preventing pressure ulcers: a systematic review. *JAMA* 2006;**296**:974–84.

460. Forster A, Young J. Incidence and consequences of falls due to stroke: a systematic inquiry. *BMJ* 1995;**311**:83–6.

461. Mackintosh SF, Goldie P, Hill K. Falls incidence and factors associated with falling in older, community-dwelling, chronic stroke survivors (>1 year after stroke) and matched controls. *Aging Clin Exp Res* 2005;**17**:74–81.

462. Mackintosh SF, Hill KD, Dodd KJ, Goldie PA, Culham EG. Balance score and a history of falls in hospital predict recurrent falls in the 6 months following stroke rehabilitation. *Arch Phys Med Rehabil* 2006;**87**:1583–9.

463. Lamb SE, Ferrucci L, Volapto S, Fried LP, Guralnik JM. Risk factors for falling in home-dwelling older women with stroke: the Women's Health and Aging Study. *Stroke* 2003;**34**:494–501.

464. Aizen E, Shugaev I, Lenger R. Risk factors and characteristics of falls during inpatient rehabilitation of elderly patients. *Arch Gerontol Geriatr* 2007;**44**:1–12.

465. Teasell R, McRae M, Foley N, Bhardwaj A. The incidence and consequences of falls in stroke patients during inpatient rehabilitation: factors associated with high risk. *Arch Phys Med Rehabil* 2002;**83**:329–33.

466. Vassallo M, Vignaraja R, Sharma JC, *et al.* The effect of changing practice on fall prevention in a rehabilitative hos-

pital: the Hospital Injury Prevention Study. *J Am Geriatr Soc* 2004;**52**:335–9.

467. Oliver D, Connelly JB, Victor CR, *et al.* Strategies to prevent falls and fractures in hospitals and care homes and effect of cognitive impairment: systematic review and meta-analyses. *BMJ* 2007;**334**:82.

468. Ramnemark A, Nyberg L, Borssen B, Olsson T, Gustafson Y. Fractures after stroke. *Osteoporos Int* 1998;**8**:92–5.

469. Ramnemark A, Nilsson M, Borssen B, Gustafson Y. Stroke, a major and increasing risk factor for femoral neck fracture. *Stroke* 2000;**31**:1572–7.

470. *Pang MY, Eng JJ, Dawson AS, Gylfadottir S. The use of aerobic exercise training in improving aerobic capacity in individuals with stroke: a meta-analysis. *Clin Rehabil* 2006;**20**:97–111.

471. Sato Y, Iwamoto J, Kanoko T, Satoh K. Low-dose vitamin D prevents muscular atrophy and reduces falls and hip fractures in women after stroke: a randomized controlled trial. *Cerebrovasc Dis* 2005;**20**:187–92.

472. Sato Y, Asoh T, Kaji M, Oizumi K. Beneficial effect of intermittent cyclical etidronate therapy in hemiplegic patients following an acute stroke. *J Bone Miner Res* 2000;**15**:2487–94.

473. Parker MJ, Gillespie LD, Gillespie WJ. Hip protectors for preventing hip fractures in the elderly. *Cochrane Database Syst Rev* 2004;(3):CD001255.

474. Gerberding JL. Hospital-onset infections: a patient safety issue. *Ann Intern Med* 2002;**137**:665–70.

475. Thomas L, Cross S, Barrett J, *et al.* Treatment of urinary incontinence after stroke in adults. *Cochrane Database Syst Rev* 2008;(1):CD004462.

476. Jorgensen L, Engstad T, Jacobsen BK. Self-reported urinary incontinence in noninstitutionalized long-term stroke survivors: a population-based study. *Arch Phys Med Rehabil* 2005;**86**:416–20.

477. Thomas LH, Barrett J, Cross S, *et al.* Prevention and treatment of urinary incontinence after stroke in adults. *Cochrane Database Syst Rev* 2005;(3):CD004462.

478. Meijer R, Ihnenfeldt DS, de Groot IJ, van Limbeek J, Vermeulen M, de Haan RJ. Prognostic factors for ambulation and activities of daily living in the subacute phase after stroke. A systematic review of the literature. *Clin Rehabil* 2003;**17**:119–29.

479. Dumoulin C, Korner-Bitensky N, Tannenbaum C. Urinary incontinence after stroke: does rehabilitation make a difference? A systematic review of the effectiveness of behavioral therapy. *Top Stroke Rehabil* 2005;**12**: 66–76.

480. Martino R, Foley N, Bhogal S, Diamant N, Speechley M, Teasell R. Dysphagia after stroke: incidence, diagnosis, and pulmonary complications. *Stroke* 2005;**36**:2756–63.

481. Mann G, Hankey GJ, Cameron D. Swallowing function after stroke: prognosis and prognostic factors at 6 months. *Stroke* 1999;**30**:744–8.

482. Dennis MS, Lewis SC, Warlow C. Routine oral nutritional supplementation for stroke patients in hospital (FOOD): a multicentre randomised controlled trial. *Lancet* 2005; **365**:755–63.

483. Axelsson K, Asplund K, Norberg A, Alafuzoff I. Nutritional status in patients with acute stroke. *Acta Med Scand* 1988;**224**:217–24.

484. Axelsson K, Asplund K, Norberg A, Eriksson S. Eating problems and nutritional status during hospital stay of patients with severe stroke. *J Am Diet Assoc* 1989;**89**: 1092–6.

485. Finestone HM, Greene-Finestone LS, Wilson ES, Teasell RW. Malnutrition in stroke patients on the rehabilitation service and at follow-up: prevalence and predictors. *Arch Phys Med Rehabil* 1995;**76**:310–6.

486. Finestone HM, Greene-Finestone LS, Wilson ES, Teasell RW. Prolonged length of stay and reduced functional improvement rate in malnourished stroke rehabilitation patients. *Arch Phys Med Rehabil* 1996;**77**:340–5.

487. Dávalos A, Ricart W, Gonzalez-Huix F, *et al.* Effect of malnutrition after acute stroke on clinical outcome. *Stroke* 1996;**27**:1028–32.

488. Food Trial Collaboration. Poor nutritional status on admission predicts poor outcomes after stroke: observational data from the FOOD trial. *Stroke* 2003;**34**:1450–6.

489. *Dennis MS, Lewis SC, Warlow C. Effect of timing and method of enteral tube feeding for dysphagic stroke patients (FOOD): a multicentre randomised controlled trial. *Lancet* 2005;**365**:764–72.

490. Norton B, Homer-Ward M, Donnelly MT, Long RG, Holmes GK. A randomised prospective comparison of percutaneous endoscopic gastrostomy and nasogastric tube feeding after acute dysphagic stroke. *BMJ* 1996;**312**: 13–6.

491. Hamidon BB, Abdullah SA, Zawawi MF, Sukumar N, Aminuddin A, Raymond AA. A prospective comparison of percutaneous endoscopic gastrostomy and nasogastric tube feeding in patients with acute dysphagic stroke. *Med J Malaysia* 2006;**61**:59–66.

492. Callahan CM, Haag KM, Weinberger M, *et al.* Outcomes of percutaneous endoscopic gastrostomy among older adults in a community setting. *J Am Geriatr Soc* 2000;**48**: 1048–54.

493. Rickman J. Percutaneous endoscopic gastrostomy: psychological effects. *Br J Nurs* 1998;**7**:723–9.

494. WHO. *International Classification of Functioning Disability and Health.* Geneva: World Health Organisation, 2001.

495. Langhorne P, Dennis MS. *Stroke Units, an Evidence Based Approach.* London: BMJ Publishing group, 1998.

496. Lincoln NB, Husbands S, Trescoli C, Drummond AE, Gladman JR, Berman P. Five-year follow up of a randomised controlled trial of a stroke rehabilitation unit. *BMJ* 2000;**320**:549.

497. Indredavik B, Slordahl SA, Bakke F, Rokseth R, Haheim LL. Stroke unit treatment. Long-term effects. *Stroke* 1997;**28**:1861–6.

498. Early Supported Discharge Trialists. Services for reducing duration of hospital care for acute stroke patients. *Cochrane Database Syst Rev* 2005;(2):CD000443.

499. Langhorne P, Taylor G, Murray G, *et al.* Early supported discharge services for stroke patients: a meta-analysis of individual patients' data. *Lancet* 2005;**365**:501–6.

500. Ronning OM, Guldvog B. Outcome of subacute stroke rehabilitation: a randomized controlled trial. *Stroke* 1998;**29**:779–84.

501. *Legg L, Langhorne P. Rehabilitation therapy services for stroke patients living at home: systematic review of randomised trials. *Lancet* 2004;**363**:352–6.

502. Baron JC, Cohen LG, Cramer SC, *et al.* Neuroimaging in stroke recovery: a position paper from the First International Workshop on Neuroimaging and Stroke Recovery. *Cerebrovasc Dis* 2004;**18**:260–7.

503. Barbay S, Plautz E, Friel KM, *et al.* Delayed rehabilitative training following a small ischaemic infarct in non-human primate primary cortex. *Soc Neurosci Abstr* 2001;**27**:931–4.

504. Biernaskie J, Chernenko G, Corbett D. Efficacy of rehabilitative experience declines with time after focal ischemic brain injury. *J Neurosci* 2004;**24**:1245–54.

505. Paolucci S, Antonucci G, Grasso MG, *et al.* Early versus delayed inpatient stroke rehabilitation: a matched comparison conducted in Italy. *Arch Phys Med Rehabil* 2000;**81**:695–700.

506. Salter K, Jutai J, Hartley M, *et al.* Impact of early vs delayed admission to rehabilitation on functional outcomes in persons with stroke. *J Rehabil Med* 2006;**38**:113–7.

507. Langhorne P, Stott DJ, Robertson L, *et al.* Medical complications after stroke: a multicenter study. *Stroke* 2000;**31**:1223–9.

508. Diserens K, Michel P, Bogousslavsky J. Early mobilisation after stroke: review of the literature. *Cerebrovasc Dis* 2006;**22**:183–90.

509. Bernhardt J, Dewey H, Thrift A, Donnan G. Inactive and alone: physical activity within the first 14 days of acute stroke unit care. *Stroke* 2004;**35**:1005–9.

510. *Aziz N, Leonardi-Bee J, Walker M, Phillips M, Gladman J, Legg L. Therapy based rehabilitation services for patients living at home more than one year after stroke – A Cochrane review. *Cochrane Database Syst Rev* 2008;(2): CD005952.

511. *Kwakkel G, van Peppen R, Wagenaar RC, *et al.* Effects of augmented exercise therapy time after stroke: a meta-analysis. *Stroke* 2004;**35**:2529–39.

512. *Langhorne P, Wagenaar R, Partridge C. Physiotherapy after stroke: more is better? *Physiother Res Int* 1996;**1**:75–88.

513. *van der Lee JH, Snels IA, Beckerman H, Lankhorst GJ, Wagenaar RC, Bouter LM. Exercise therapy for arm function in stroke patients: a systematic review of randomized controlled trials. *Clin Rehabil* 2001;**15**:20–31.

514. Evans A, Perez I, Harraf F, *et al.* Can differences in management processes explain different outcomes between stroke unit and stroke-team care? *Lancet* 2001;**358**:1586–92.

515. Kalra L, Dale P, Crome P. Improving stroke rehabilitation. A controlled study. *Stroke* 1993;**24**:1462–7.

516. *Stroke Unit Trialists' Collaboration. How do stroke units improve patient outcomes? A collaborative systematic review of the randomized trials. Stroke Unit Trialists Collaboration. *Stroke* 1997;**28**:2139–44.

517. *van Peppen RP, Kwakkel G, Wood-Dauphinee S, Hendriks HJ, Van der Wees PJ, Dekker J. The impact of physical therapy on functional outcomes after stroke: what's the evidence? *Clin Rehabil* 2004;**18**:833–62.

518. *Pollock A, Baer G, Langhorne P, Pomeroy V. Physiotherapy treatment approaches for the recovery of postural control and lower limb function following stroke: a systematic review. *Clin Rehabil* 2007;**21**:395–410.

519. *Pomeroy VM, King LM, Pollock A, Baily-Hallam A, Langhorne P. Electrostimulation for promoting recovery of movement or functional ability after stroke. Systematic review and meta-analysis. *Stroke* 2006;**37**:2441–2.

520. *Moseley AM, Stark A, Cameron ID, Pollock A. Treadmill training and body weight support for walking after stroke. *Cochrane Database Syst Rev* 2005;(4):CD002840.

521. Mehrholz J, Werner C, Kugler J, Pohl M. Electromechanical-assisted training for walking after stroke. *Cochrane Database Syst Rev* 2007;(4):CD006185.

522. de Wit DC, Buurke JH, Nijlant JM, Ijzerman MJ, Hermens HJ. The effect of an ankle-foot orthosis on walking ability in chronic stroke patients: a randomized controlled trial. *Clin Rehabil* 2004;**18**:550–7.

523. Gordon NF, Gulanick M, Costa F, *et al.* Physical activity and exercise recommendations for stroke survivors: an American Heart Association scientific statement from the Council on Clinical Cardiology, Subcommittee on Exercise, Cardiac Rehabilitation, and Prevention; the Council on Cardiovascular Nursing; the Council on Nutrition, Physical Activity, and Metabolism; and the Stroke Council. *Stroke* 2004;**35**:1230–40.

524. Wolf SL, Winstein CJ, Miller JP, *et al.* Effect of constraint-induced movement therapy on upper extremity function 3 to 9 months after stroke: the EXCITE randomized clinical trial. *JAMA* 2006;**296**:2095–104.

525. *Legg LA, Drummond AE, Langhorne P. Occupational therapy for patients with problems in activities of daily living after stroke. *Cochrane Database Syst Rev* 2006;(4): CD003585.

526. *Walker MF, Leonardi-Bee J, Bath P, *et al.* Individual patient data meta-analysis of randomized controlled trials of community occupational therapy for stroke patients. *Stroke* 2004;**35**:2226–32.

527. Sackley C, Wade DT, Mant D, *et al.* Cluster randomized pilot controlled trial of an occupational therapy intervention for residents with stroke in UK care homes. *Stroke* 2006;**37**:2336–41.

528. Bath PMW, Bath-Hextall FJ, Smithard DG. Interventions for dysphagia in acute stroke. *Cochrane Database Syst Rev* 2007;(8):19.

529. DePippo KL, Holas MA, Reding MJ, Mandel FS, Lesser ML. Dysphagia therapy following stroke: a controlled trial. *Neurology* 1994;**44**:1655–60.

530. Engelter ST, Gostynski M, Papa S, *et al.* Epidemiology of aphasia attributable to first ischemic stroke: incidence, severity, fluency, etiology, and thrombolysis. *Stroke* 2006;**37**:1379–84.

531. *Sellars C, Hughes T, Langhorne P. Speech and language therapy for dysarthria due to non-progressive brain damage. *Cochrane Database Syst Rev* 2005;(3):CD002088.

532. *Greener J, Enderby P, Whurr R. Speech and language therapy for aphasia following stroke. *Cochrane Database Syst Rev* 2000;(2):CD000425.

533. Robey RR. The efficacy of treatment for aphasic persons: a meta-analysis. *Brain Lang* 1994;**47**:582–608.

534. Robey RR. A meta-analysis of clinical outcomes in the treatment of aphasia. *J Speech Lang Hear Res* 1998;**41**: 172–87.

535. Pulvermuller F, Neininger B, Elbert T, *et al.* Constraint-induced therapy of chronic aphasia after stroke. *Stroke* 2001;**32**:1621–6.

536. Bhogal SK, Teasell R, Speechley M. Intensity of aphasia therapy, impact on recovery. *Stroke* 2003;**34**:987–93.

537. *Stroke Liaison Workers Collaboration. Meta-analysis of stroke liaison workers for patients and carers: results by intervention characteristic. *Cerebrovasc Dis* 2006;**21**:120.

538. O'Mahony PG, Rodgers H, Thomson RG, Dobson R, James OF. Satisfaction with information and advice received by stroke patients. *Clin Rehabil* 1997;**11**:68–72.

539. *Forster A, Young J, Langhorne P. Medical day hospital care for the elderly versus alternative forms of care. *Cochrane Database Syst Rev* 2008;(4):CD001730.

540. Kalra L, Evans A, Perez I, *et al.* Training carers of stroke patients: randomised controlled trial. *BMJ* 2004;**328**: 1099.

541. Johansson BB. Brain plasticity and stroke rehabilitation. The Willis lecture. *Stroke* 2000;**31**:223–30.

542. Nair RD, Lincoln NB. Cognitive rehabilitation for memory deficits following stroke. *Cochrane Database Syst Rev* 2007;(3):CD002293.

543. Lincoln NB, Majid MJ, Weyman N. Cognitive rehabilitation for attention deficits following stroke. *Cochrane Database Syst Rev* 2000;(4):CD002842.

544. Bowen A, Lincoln NB. Cognitive rehabilitation for spatial neglect following stroke. *Cochrane Database Syst Rev* 2007;(2):CD003586.

545. Cicerone KD, Dahlberg C, Malec JF, *et al.* Evidence-based cognitive rehabilitation: updated review of the literature from 1998 through 2002. *Arch Phys Med Rehabil* 2005;**86**: 1681–92.

546. Marinkovic S, Badlani G. Voiding and sexual dysfunction after cerebrovascular accidents. *J Urol* 2001;**165**:359–70.

547. Sjogren K, Fugl-Meyer AR. Adjustment to life after stroke with special reference to sexual intercourse and leisure. *J Psychosom Res* 1982;**26**:409–17.

548. Muller JE. Triggering of cardiac events by sexual activity: findings from a case-crossover analysis. *Am J Cardiol* 2000;**86**:14F–8F.

549. McLean DE. Medical complications experienced by a cohort of stroke survivors during inpatient, tertiary-level stroke rehabilitation. *Arch Phys Med Rehabil* 2004;**85**: 466–9.

550. Paolucci S, Antonucci G, Pratesi L, Traballesi M, Lubich S, Grasso MG. Functional outcome in stroke inpatient rehabilitation: predicting no, low and high response patients. *Cerebrovasc Dis* 1998;**8**:228–34.

551. Hackett ML, Anderson CS. Predictors of depression after stroke: a systematic review of observational studies. *Stroke* 2005;**36**:2296–301.

552. Paolucci S, Gandolfo C, Provinciali L, Torta R, Toso V. The Italian multicenter observational study on post-stroke depression (DESTRO). *J Neurol* 2006;**253**:556–62.

553. Linden T, Blomstrand C, Skoog I. Depressive disorders after 20 months in elderly stroke patients: a case-control study. *Stroke* 2007;**38**:1860–3.

554. Thomas SA, Lincoln NB. Factors relating to depression after stroke. *Br J Clin Psychol* 2006;**45**:49–61.

555. Kauhanen M, Korpelainen JT, Hiltunen P, *et al.* Poststroke depression correlates with cognitive impairment and neurological deficits. *Stroke* 1999;**30**:1875–80.

556. *van de Meent H, Geurts AC, Van Limbeek J. Pharmacologic treatment of poststroke depression: a systematic review of the literature. *Top Stroke Rehabil* 2003;**10**:79–92.

557. *Hackett ML, Anderson CS, House AO. Management of depression after stroke: a systematic review of pharmacological therapies. *Stroke* 2005;**36**:1098–103.

558. *Bhogal SK, Teasell R, Foley N, Speechley M. Heterocyclics and selective serotonin reuptake inhibitors in the treatment and prevention of poststroke depression. *J Am Geriatr Soc* 2005;**53**:1051–7.

559. *Anderson CS, Hackett ML, House AO. Interventions for preventing depression after stroke. *Cochrane Database Syst Rev* 2008;(3):CD003689.

560. *House AO, Hackett ML, Anderson CS, Horrocks JA. Pharmaceutical interventions for emotionalism after stroke. *Cochrane Database Syst Rev* 2010;(2):CD003690.

561. Lindgren I, Jonsson AC, Norrving B, Lindgren A. Shoulder pain after stroke: a prospective population-based study. *Stroke* 2007;**38**:343–8.

562. Vuagnat H, Chantraine A. Shoulder pain in hemiplegia revisited: contribution of functional electrical stimulation and other therapies. *J Rehabil Med* 2003;**35**:49–54.

563. *Price CI, Pandyan AD. Electrical stimulation for preventing and treating post-stroke shoulder pain: a systematic Cochrane review. *Clin Rehabil* 2001;**15**:5–19.

564. Ada L, Foongchomcheay A, Canning C. Supportive devices for preventing and treating subluxation of the shoulder after stroke. *Cochrane Database Syst Rev* 2005;(1):CD003863.

565. *Wiffen P, Collins S, McQuay H, Carroll D, Jadad A, Moore A. Anticonvulsant drugs for acute and chronic pain. *Cochrane Database Syst Rev* 2005;(2):CD001133.

566. *Satkunam LE. Rehabilitation medicine: 3. Management of adult spasticity. *CMAJ* 2003;**169**:1173–9.

567. Lannin NA, Herbert RD. Is hand splinting effective for adults following stroke? A systematic review and methodologic critique of published research. *Clin Rehabil* 2003;**17**:807–16.

568. Brashear A, Gordon MF, Elovic E, *et al.* Intramuscular injection of botulinum toxin for the treatment of wrist and finger spasticity after a stroke. *N Engl J Med* 2002;**347**: 395–400.

569. van Kuijk AA, Geurts AC, Bevaart BJ, van Limbeek J. Treatment of upper extremity spasticity in stroke patients by focal neuronal or neuromuscular blockade: a systematic review of the literature. *J Rehabil Med* 2002;**34**: 51–61.

570. Pittock SJ, Moore AP, Hardiman O, *et al.* A double-blind randomised placebo-controlled evaluation of three doses of botulinum toxin type A (Dysport) in the treatment of spastic equinovarus deformity after stroke. *Cerebrovasc Dis* 2003;**15**:289–300.

571. Meythaler JM, Guin-Renfroe S, Johnson A, Brunner RM. Prospective assessment of tizanidine for spasticity due to acquired brain injury. *Arch Phys Med Rehabil* 2001;**82**: 1155–63.

572. Shah S, Vanclay F, Cooper B. Efficiency, effectiveness, and duration of stroke rehabilitation. *Stroke* 1990;**21**:241–6.

573. Wyller TB, Sodring KM, Sveen U, Ljunggren AE, Bautz-Holter E. Are there gender differences in functional outcome after stroke? *Clin Rehabil* 1997;**11**:171–9.

574. Chae J, Zorowitz RD, Johnston MV. Functional outcome of hemorrhagic and nonhemorrhagic stroke patients after inpatient rehabilitation. *Am J Phys Med Rehabil* 1996;**75**: 177–82.

575. Falconer JA, Naughton BJ, Strasser DC, Sinacore JM. Stroke inpatient rehabilitation: a comparison across age groups. *J Am Geriatr Soc* 1994;**42**:39–44.

576. Katz N, Hartman-Maeir A, Ring H, Soroker N. Functional disability and rehabilitation outcome in right hemisphere damaged patients with and without unilateral spatial neglect. *Arch Phys Med Rehabil* 1999;**80**:379–84.

577. Ween JE, Alexander MP, D'Esposito M, Roberts M. Factors predictive of stroke outcome in a rehabilitation setting. *Neurology* 1996;**47**:388–92.

578. Gladman JR, Sackley CM. The scope for rehabilitation in severely disabled stroke patients. *Disabil Rehabil* 1998;**20**: 391–4.

579. Rodgers H. The scope for rehabilitation in severely disabled stroke patients. *Disabil Rehabil* 2000;**22**:199–200.

580. van Peppen RP, Hendriks HJ, van Meeteren NL, Helders PJ, Kwakkel G. The development of a clinical practice stroke guideline for physiotherapists in The Netherlands: a systematic review of available evidence. *Disabil Rehabil* 2007;**29**:767–83.

581. Kalra L, Eade J. Role of stroke rehabilitation units in managing severe disability after stroke. *Stroke* 1995;**26**: 2031–4.

582. Schmidt JG, Drew-Cates J, Dombovy ML. Severe disability after stroke: outcome after inpatient rehabilitation. *Neurorehab Neural Repair* 1999;**13**:199–203.

583. Brainin M, Barnes M, Baron JC, *et al.* Guidance for the preparation of neurological management guidelines by EFNS scientific task forces–revised recommendations 2004. *Eur J Neurol* 2004;**11**:577–81.

584. Hankey GJ, Warlow CP. Treatment and secondary prevention of stroke: evidence, costs, and effects on individuals and populations. *Lancet* 1999;**354**:1457–63.

585. Ringleb PA, Hacke W. [Stent and surgery for symptomatic carotid stenosis. SPACE study results]. *Nervenarzt* 2007;**78**:1130–7.

CHAPTER 10

Drug treatment of migraine

S. Evers,[1] J. Áfra,[2] A. Frese,[1,3] P. J. Goadsby,[4] M. Linde,[5] A. May,[6] P. S. Sándor[7]

[1]University of Münster, Germany; [2]National Institute of Neurosurgery, Budapest, Hungary; [3]Academy of Manual Medicine, Münster, Germany; [4]University of California, San Francisco CA, USA, and UCL, Institute of Neurology, Queen Square, London, UK; [5]Cephalea Headache Centre, Läkarhuset Södra vägen, Gothenburg, Sweden; [6]University of Hamburg, Germany; [7]University of Zurich, Switzerland

Objectives

These guidelines aim to give evidence-based recommendations for the drug treatment of migraine attacks and of migraine prophylaxis. The non-drug management (e.g. behavioural therapy) will not be included, although it is regarded as an important part of migraine treatment. Specific rare migraine syndromes will be considered as well as specific situations such as pregnancy and childhood. A brief clinical description of the headache disorders is included. The definitions follow the diagnostic criteria of the International Headache Society (IHS).

Background

The second edition of the classification of the International Headache Society (IHS) provided a new subclassification of different migraine syndromes [1]. The basic criteria for migraine attacks remained unchanged as compared to the first edition (except one semantic change). The different migraine syndromes with specific aura features, however, were classified in a new system.

The purpose of this paper is to give evidence-based treatment recommendations for migraine attacks and for migraine prophylaxis. The recommendations are based on the scientific evidence from clinical trials and on the

expert consensus by the respective task force of the EFNS. The legal aspects of drug prescription and drug availability in the different European countries will not be considered. The definitions of the recommendation levels follow the EFNS criteria [2].

Search strategy

A literature search was performed using the reference databases MEDLINE, Science Citation Index, and the Cochrane Library; the key words used were 'migraine' and 'aura' (last search in January 2009). All papers published in English, German, or French were considered when they described a controlled trial or a case series on the treatment of at least five patients. In addition, a review book [3] and the German treatment recommendations for migraine [4] were considered.

Method for reaching consensus

All authors performed an independent literature search. The first draft of the manuscript was written by the chairman of the task force. All other members of the task force read the first draft and discussed changes by email. A second draft was then written by the chairman and again discussed by email. All recommendations had to be agreed to by all members of the task force unanimously. The background of the research strategy and of reaching consensus and the definitions of the recommendation levels used in this paper have been described in the EFNS recommendations [2].

European Handbook of Neurological Management: Volume 1, 2nd edition. Edited by N. E. Gilhus, M. P. Barnes and M. Brainin.
© 2011 Blackwell Publishing Ltd.

Table 10.1 Diagnostic criteria of migraine of the IHS classification (2004).

A At least five attacks fulfilling criteria B–D
B Headache lasting 4–72 h (untreated or unsuccessfully treated)
C Headache has at least two of the following characteristics:
  1. unilateral location
  2. pulsating quality
  3. moderate or severe pain intensity
  4. aggravation by or causing avoidance of routine physical activity (e.g. walking or climbing stairs)
D During headache at least one of the following:
  1. nausea and/or vomiting
  2. photophobia and phonophobia
E Not attributed to another disorder

Table 10.2 Subclassification of migraine according to the IHS classification (2004).

1.1 Migraine without aura
1.2 Migraine with aura
  1.2.1 Typical aura with migraine headache
  1.2.2 Typical aura with non-migraine headache
  1.2.3 Typical aura without headache
  1.2.4 Familial hemiplegic migraine
  1.2.5 Sporadic hemiplegic migraine
  1.2.6 Basilar-type migraine
1.3 Childhood periodic syndromes that are commonly precursors of migraine
  1.3.1 Cyclical vomiting
  1.3.2 Abdominal migraine
  1.3.3 Benign paroxysmal vertigo of childhood
1.4 Retinal migraine
1.5 Complications of migraine
  1.5.1 Chronic migraine
  1.5.2 Status migrainosus
  1.5.3 Persistent aura without infarction
  1.5.4 Migrainous infarction
  1.5.5 Migraine-triggered seizure
1.6 Probable migraine
  1.6.1 Probable migraine without aura
  1.6.2 Probable migraine with aura
  1.6.3 Probable chronic migraine

Clinical aspects

Migraine is an idiopathic headache disorder which is characterized by usually moderate to severe, often unilateral and pulsating headache attacks aggravated by physical activity and accompanied by vegetative symptoms such as nausea, vomiting, photophobia, and phonophobia. The diagnostic criteria for migraine attacks and the migraine aura are given in table 10.1. The duration of attacks is typically 4–72 h, and at least five attacks must have occurred before the diagnosis can be established. Most of the patients suffer from migraine attacks without aura. However, there are several migraine syndromes with specific aura features and migraine syndromes with uncommon courses or complications. These syndromes have their own diagnostic criteria, the subclassification of these syndromes is given in table 10.2 [1]. The diagnostic criteria for these migraine syndromes have been published on the homepage of the IHS (www. i-h-s.org).

In children, migraine attacks can be shorter (even only 1 or 2 h) and the accompanying symptoms, such as abdominal migraine or periodic syndromes in childhood, may be predominant [5–7].

Epidemiology

Migraine is one of the most frequent headache disorders. About 6–8% of males and 12–14% of females suffer from migraine [8–11]. The lifetime prevalence of females might be even higher, up to 25% [12]. Before puberty, the prevalence of migraine is about 5%, both in boys and girls. The highest incidence of migraine attacks is in the age between 35 and 45 years, with a female preponderance of 3 to 1. The median duration of untreated migraine attacks is 18 h, the median attack frequency is one per month.

Diagnosis

The diagnosis of migraine is based on the typical history of the patient and a normal neurological examination. Apparative investigations, in particular brain imaging, is necessary if secondary headache is suspected (e.g. the headache characteristics are untypical), if the course of headache attacks changes, or if persistent neurological or psychopathological abnormalities are present [13]. In particular, magnetic resonance imaging (MRI) imaging (and not computed tomography (CT) imaging with its inferior sensitivity to detect vascular abnormalities and lesions) of the brain in migraine is recommended when:

- the neurological examination is not normal
- typical migraine attacks occur for the first time after the age of 40
- frequency or intensity of migraine attacks continuously increase
- the accompanying symptoms of migraine attacks change
- new psychiatric symptoms occur in relation to the attacks.

Drug treatment of migraine attacks

Several large randomized, placebo-controlled trials have been published to establish the best drugs for the acute management of migraine. In most of these trials, successful treatment of migraine attacks was defined by the following criteria [14]:

- pain-free after 2 h
- improvement of headache from moderate or severe to mild or none after 2 h [15]
- consistent efficacy in two out of three attacks
- no headache recurrence and no further drug intake within 24 hours after successful treatment (so-called sustained pain relief or pain free).

Analgesics

Drugs of first choice for mild or moderate migraine attacks are simple analgesics. Evidence of efficacy in migraine treatment in at least one placebo-controlled study has been obtained for acetylsalicylic acid (ASA) up to 1000 mg [16–19], for ibuprofen 200–800 mg [17, 19–21], for diclofenac 50–100 mg [22–24], for phenazon 1000 mg [25], for metamizol 1000 mg [26], for tolfenamic acid 200 mg [27], and for paracetamol 1000 mg [28]. In addition, the fixed combination of ASA, paracetamol, and caffeine is effective in acute migraine treatment and is also more effective than the single substances or combinations without caffeine [29–31]. Intravenous ASA was more effective than subcutaneous ergotamine [32]; i.v. metamizol was superior to placebo in migraine without and with aura [33]. Lysine-ASA in combination with metoclopramide had comparable efficacy as sumatriptan [18]. Effervescent ASA 1000 mg is probably as effective as ibuprofen 400 mg and as sumatriptan 50 mg [19, 34, 35].

Also, the selective COX-2 inhibitors (coxibs) have been investigated in clinical trials. Valdecoxib 20–40 mg and rofecoxib 25–50 mg, the latter one not available on the market any more, have shown efficacy in acute migraine treatment [36–39]. However, coxibs are not recommended for acute migraine treatment because of their still undetermined risk for vascular events when taken for a long period of time. Table 10.3 presents an overview of analgesics with efficacy in acute migraine treatment.

Table 10.3 Analgesics with evidence of efficacy in at least one study on the acute treatment of migraine. The level of recommendation also considers side effects and consistency of the studies.

Substance	Dose	Level of recommendation	Comment
Acetylsalicylic acid	1000 mg (oral)	A	gastrointestinal side effects,
(ASA)	1000 mg (i.v.)	A	risk of bleeding
Ibuprofen	200–800 mg	A	side effects as for ASA
Naproxen	500–1000 mg	A	side effects as for ASA
Diclofenac	50–100 mg	A	including diclofenac-K
Paracetamol	1000 mg (oral)	A	caution in liver and kidney
	1000 mg (supp.)	A	failure
ASA plus	250 mg (oral)	A	as for ASA and paracetamol plus
	200 to 250 mg		paracetamol
caffeine	50 mg		
Metamizol	1000 mg (oral)	B	risk of agranulocytosis
	1000 mg (i.v.)	B	risk of hypotension
Phenazon	1000 mg (oral)	B	see paracetamol
Tolfenamic acid	200 mg (oral)	B	side effects as for ASA

To prevent drug overuse headache, the intake of simple analgesics should be restricted to 15 days per month and the intake of combined analgesics to 10 days per month.

Antiemetics

The use of antiemetics in acute migraine attacks is recommended to treat nausea and potential emesis, and because it is assumed that these drugs improve the resorption af analgesics [40–42]. However, there are no prospective, placebo-controlled randomized trials to prove this assertion. Metoclopramide also has a genuine mild analgesic efficacy when given orally [43] and a higher efficacy when given intravenously [44]. There is no evidence that the fixed combination of an antiemetic with an analgesic or with a triptan is more effective than the analgesic or triptan alone. Metoclopramide 20 mg is recommended for adults and adolescents; in children domperidon 10 mg should be used because of the possible extrapyramidal side effects of metoclopramide. Table 10.4 presents the antiemetics recommended for the use in migraine attacks.

Ergot alkaloids

There are very few randomised, placebo-controlled trials on the efficacy of ergot alkaloids in the acute migraine treatment; although these substances have been used for a very long time, very severe events have also been reported [45]. In comparative trials, triptans showed better efficacy than ergot alkaloids [46–49]. The advantage of ergot alkaloids is a lower recurrence rate in some patients. Therefore, these substances should be restricted to patients with very long migraine attacks or with regular recurrence. The only compounds with sufficient evidence of efficacy are ergotamine tartrate and dihydroer-

gotamine 2 mg (oral and suppositories respectively). Ergot alkaloids can induce drug overuse headache very quickly and in very low doses [50]. Therefore, their use must be limited to 10 days per month. Major side effects are nausea, vomiting, paraesthesia, and ergotism. Contraindications are cardiovascular and cerebrovascular diseases, Raynaud's disease, arterial hypertension, renal failure, and pregnancy and lactation.

Triptans (5-HT$_{1B/1D}$-agonists)

The 5-HT$_{1B/1D}$ receptor agonists sumatriptan, zolmitriptan, naratriptan, rizatriptan, almotriptan, eletriptan, and frovatriptan (order in the year of marketing), so-called triptans, are specific migraine medications and should not be applied in other headache disorders except cluster headache. The different triptans for migraine therapy are presented in table 10.5. The efficacy of all triptans has been proven in large placebo-controlled trials of which meta-analyses have been published [51, 52]. For sumatriptan [18, 53] and zolmitriptan [54], comparative studies with ASA and metoclopramide exist. In these comparative studies, the triptans were not or only a little more efficacious than ASA. In about 60% of non-responders to NSAIDs, triptans are effective [55]. Sumatriptan 6 mg subcutaneously is more effective than i.v. ASA 1000 mg s.c. but has more side effects [56]. Ergotamine tartrate was less effective in comparative studies with sumatriptan [46], with eletriptan [47], and with almotriptan [48]. Dihydroergotamine imtramuscularly is comparable in efficacy to sumatriptan subcutaneously administered [57]. Triptans can be effective at any time during a migraine attack. However, there is evidence that the earlier triptans are taken the better their efficacy is [58–62], a phenomenon probably related to attack severity not timing of treatment [63]. It is still debated whether trip-

Table 10.4 Antiemetics recommended for the acute treatment of migraine attacks.

Substances	Dose	Level	Comment
Metoclopramide	10–20 mg (oral) 20 mg (suppository) 10 mg (intramuscular, intravenous, subcutaneous)	B	side effect: dyskinesia; contraindicated in childhood and in pregnancy; *also analgesic efficacy*
Domperidon	20–30 mg (oral)	B	side effects less severe than in metoclopramide; can be given to children

Table 10.5 Different triptans for the treatment of acute migraine attacks (order in the time of marketing). Not all doses or application forms are available in all European countries.

Substance	Dose	Level	Comment
Sumatriptan	25, 50, 100 mg (oral including rapid-release)	A	100 mg sumatriptan is reference to all triptans
	25 mg (suppository)	A	
	10, 20 mg (nasal spray)	A	
	6 mg (subcutaneous)	A	
Zolmitriptan	2.5, 5 mg (oral including disintegrating form)	A	
	2.5, 5 mg (nasal spray)	A	
Naratriptan	2.5 mg (oral)	A	less but longer efficacy than sumatriptan
Rizatriptan	10 mg (oral including wafer form)	A	5 mg when taking propranolol
Almotriptan	12.5 mg (oral)	A	probably fewer side effects than sumatriptan
Eletriptan	20, 40 mg (oral)	A	80 mg allowed if 40 mg not effective
Frovatriptan	2.5 mg (oral)	A	fewer but longer efficacy than sumatriptan

General side effects for all triptans: Chest symptoms, nausea, distal paraesthesia, fatigue.
General contraindications: Arterial hypertension (untreated), coronary heart disease, cerebrovascular disease, Raynaud's disease, pregnancy and lactation, age under 18 (except sumatriptan nasal spray) and age above 65, severe liver or kidney failure.

tans are less efficacious or may even fail when taken after the onset of allodynia during a migraine attack [59, 64], with randomised controlled trials not supporting a difference for allodynic patients [62, 65]. A strategy of strictly early intake can, however, lead to frequent drug treatment in certain patients. The use of triptans is restricted to maximum nine days per month by the IHS criteria; in epidemiological studies, the risk for chronification became significant at 12 days per month of triptan intake [66]. Otherwise, the induction of a drug overuse headache is possible for all triptans [50, 67, 68]. Therefore, in clinical practice, a reasonable trade-off has to be agreed on between early intake and a reasonable intake frequency.

One typical problem of attack treatment in migraine is headache recurrence. This is defined as a worsening of headache after a pain-free state or mild pain has been achieved with a drug within 24 h [69]. This problem is more obvious with triptans and NSAIDs than with ergots. About 15–40% (depending on the primary and the lasting efficacy of the drug) of the patients taking an oral triptan experience recurrence. A second dose of the triptan is effective in most cases [70]. If the first dose of a triptan is not effective, a second dose is useless. Combining an NSAID, such as naproxen with sumatriptan in the published work, reduces headache recurrence and is more efficacious than the single components [71]. This is not the case for the combination of triptans and paracetamol [72]. Interestingly, rizatriptan in combina-

tion with dexamethasone seems to be significantly more effective than rizatriptan alone, although this combination is associated with a higher rate of adverse events [73]. Alternatively, the analgesic can be given with a temporal delay; however, no placebo-controlled trials are available for this procedure. Even if a triptan is not efficacious in three consecutive attacks, another triptan can be efficacious [74, 75].

After application of sumatriptan, severe adverse events have been reported, such as myocardial infarction, cardiac arrhythmias, and stroke. The incidence of these events was about 1 in 1 000 000 [76, 77]. Reports on severe adverse events also exist for other triptans and for ergotamine tratrate. However, all of the reported patients had contraindications against triptans or the diagnosis of migraine was wrong. In population-based studies, no increased risk of vascular events could be detected for triptan users as compared to a healthy population [78, 79]. Thus, contraindications for the use of triptans are untreated arterial hypertension, coronary heart disease, Raynaud's disease, history of ischaemic stroke, pregnancy, lactation, and severe liver or renal failure.

Due to safety aspects, triptans should not be taken during the aura, although no specific severe adverse events have been reported. The best time for application is the very onset of headache. Furthermore, triptans are not efficacious when taken during the aura phase before headache has developed [80, 81].

Comparison of triptans

The triptans are a very homogenous group of acute migraine drugs with respect to efficacy, pharmacology, and safety. However, some minor differences exist which will be discussed to give guidance on which triptan to use in an individual patient. It is important to notice that a triptan can be efficacious even if another (or more than one other) triptan was not.

Subcutaneous sumatriptan has the fastest onset of efficacy of about 10 min [82]. Oral rizatriptan and eletriptan need about 30 min, oral sumatriptan, almotriptan, and zolmitriptan need about 45–60 min [51], and naratriptan and frovatriptan need up to 4 h for the onset of efficacy [83, 84]. Zolmitriptan nasal spray has a shorter duration until efficacy than oral zolmitriptan [85]. There is no evidence that different oral formulations such as rapidly disolving tablets, wafer forms, or rapid release forms [86] act earlier than others.

Pain relief after 2 h as the most important efficacy parameter is best in subcutaneous sumatripan with up to 80% responders [87]. Sumatriptan nasal spray has the same efficacy as oral sumatriptan 50 mg or 100 mg. Twenty-five milligram oral sumatriptan is less effective than the higher doses but has fewer side effects [51]. Sumatriptan suppositories are about as effective as oral sumatriptan 50 mg or 100 mg and should be given to patients with vomiting [88–90]. Naratriptan and frovatriptan (2.5 mg) are less effective than sumatriptan 50 mg or 100 mg but have fewer side effects. The duration until the onset of efficacy is longer in these two triptans as compared to all others. Rizatriptan 10 mg is a little more effective than sumatriptan 100 mg. Oral zolmitriptan 2.5 or 5 mg, almotriptan 12.5 mg and eletriptan 40 mg show a similar efficacy and similar side effects [91–93]. Eletriptan 80 mg is the most effective oral triptan but also has the most side effects [51].

Headache recurrence is a major problem in clinical practice. The recurrence rate is between 15 and 40%. The highest recurrence rate is observed after subcutaneous sumatriptan. Naratriptan and frovatriptan show the lowest recurrence rates but have poor initial response rates. Frovatriptan has been compared to sumatriptan but the recurrence data have never been made public, which at least calls the assertion that is has a lower recurrence rate into question. It might be that triptans with a longer half-life time have a lower recurrence rate [94], although if frovatriptan does not have a lower recurrence rate this argument would no longer be tenable. If migraine recurs after successful treatment with a triptan, a second dose of this triptan can be given. Another problem in clinical practice is inconsistency of efficacy. Therefore, efficacy in only two out of three attacks is regarded as good.

Other drugs

There is some evidence that the i.v. application of valproic acid in a dose of 300–800 mg is efficacious in the acute treatment of migraine attacks [95, 96], and similarly an older study for i.v. flunarizine [97]. However, these trials were small and had no power calculation. Tramadol in combination with paracetamol has also shown efficacy in acute migraine attacks [98]. However, opioids are of only minor efficacy, and no modern controlled trials are available for these substances; opioids and tranquilizers should not be used in the acute treatment of migraine. CGRP receptor antagonists are a new class of substance and have the advantage that they do not cause vasoconstriction. The first placebo-controlled clinical trials with two different substances, olcegepant [99] and telcagepant [100, 101] have been positive .

Migraine prophylaxis

Prophylactic drug treatment of migraine is possible with several drugs. Substances with good efficacy and tolerability, and evidence of efficacy, are beta-blockers, calcium channel blockers, antiepileptic drugs, NSAIDs, antidepressants, and miscellaneous drugs. The use of all these drugs, however, is based on empirical data rather than on proven pathophysiological concepts. The decision to introduce a prophylactic treatment has to be discussed carefully with the patient. The efficacy of the drugs, their potential side effects, and their interactions with other drugs have to be considered in the individual patient. There is no commonly accepted indication for starting a prophylactic treatment. In the view of the task force, prophylactic drug treatment of migraine should be considered and discussed with the patient when:

• the quality of life, business duties, or school attendance are severely impaired

• frequency of attacks per month is two or higher

• migraine attacks do not respond to acute drug treatment

• frequent, very long, or uncomfortable auras occur.

Table 10.6 Recommended substances (drugs of first choice) for the prophylactic drug treatment of migraine.

Substances	Daily dose	Level
Beta-blockers		
Metoprolol	50–200 mg	A
Propranolol	40–240 mg	A
Calcium channel blockers		
Flunarizine	5–10 mg	A
Antiepileptic drugs		
Valproic acid	500–1800 mg	A
Topiramate	25–100 mg	A

Table 10.8 Drugs of third choice for migraine prophylaxis (only probable efficacy).

Substances	Daily dose	Level
Acetylsalicylic acid	300 mg	C
Gabapentin	1200–1600 mg	C
Magnesium	24 mmol	C
Tanacetum parthenium	3 × 6.25 mg	C
Riboflavin	400 mg	C
Coenzyme Q10	300 mg	C
Candesartan	16 mg	C
Lisinopril	20 mg	C
Methysergide	4–12 mg	C

Table 10.7 Drugs of second choice for migraine prophylaxis (evidence of efficacy, but less effective or more side effects than drugs of table 10.6).

Substances	Daily dose	Level
Amitriptyline	50–150 mg	B
Venlafaxine	75–150 mg	B
Naproxen	2 × 250–500 mg	B
Petasites	2 × 75 mg	B
Bisoprolol	5–10 mg	B

A migraine prophylaxis is regarded as successful if the frequency of migraine attacks per month is decreased by at least 50% within 3 months. For therapy evaluation, a migraine diary is extremely useful. In the following paragraphs, the placebo-controlled trials in migraine prophylaxis are summarized. The recommended drugs of first choice, according to the consensus of the task force, are given in table 10.6. Tables 10.7 and 10.8 present drugs recommended as second or third choice when the drugs of table 10.6 are not effective, contraindicated, or when comorbidity of the patients suggests the respective drug of second or third choice (e.g. amitriptyline for migraine prophylaxis in depressed patients or in patients with sleep disturbances or with tension-type headache).

Beta-blockers

Beta blockers are clearly effective in migraine prophylaxis and very well studied in a lot of placebo-controlled, randomized trials. The best evidence has been obtained for the selective beta-blocker metoprolol [102–106] and for the non-selective beta-blocker propranolol [102, 103, 107–113]. Also, bisoprolol [106, 114], timolol [108, 115], and atenolol [116] might be efficacious, but evidence is less convincing compared to propranolol and metoprolol.

Calcium channel blockers

The 'non-specific' calcium channel blocker flunarizine has been shown to be effective in migraine prophylaxis in several studies [105, 113, 117–126]. The dose is 5–10 mg; female patients seem to benefit from lower doses than male patients [127]. Another 'non-specific' calcium channel blocker, cyclandelate, has also been studied but with conflicting results [122, 128–131]. Since the better-designed studies were negative, cyclandelate cannot be recommended.

Antiepileptic drugs

Valproic acid in a dose of at least 600 mg [132–135] and topiramte in a dose between 25 and 100 mg [136–139] are the two antiepileptic drugs with evidence of efficacy in more than one placebo-controlled trial. The efficacy rates are comparable to those of metoprolol, propranolol, and flunarizine. Topiramate is also efficacious in the prophylaxis of chronic migraine and may have some effect in migraine with medication overuse [140, 141]. Other antiepileptic drugs studied in migraine prophylaxis are lamotrigine and gabapentin. Lamotrigine did not reduce the frequency of migraine attacks without aura but may be efficacious in reducing the frequency of migraine with aura [142, 143]. Gabapentin showed efficacy in one placebo-controlled trial in doses between

1200 and 1600 mg using a non-intention-to-treat analysis [144]. Oxcarbazepine was without any efficacy in a very recent study [145], as was tonabersat, the GAP junction blocker with anti-convulsant properties [146].

NSAIDs

In some comparative trials, ASA was equivalent to or worse than a comparator (with known efficacy in migraine) but it has never achieved a better efficacy than placebo in direct comparison. In two large cohort trials, ASA 200–300 mg reduced the frequency of migraine attacks [147, 148]. Naproxen 1000 mg was better than placebo in three controlled trials [149–151]. Tolfenamic acid also showed efficacy in two placebo-controlled trials [152, 153]. Other NSAIDs studied were ketoprofen, mefenamic acid, indobufen, flurbiprofen, and rofecoxib [154]. However, all studies for the latter substances were small and had insufficient design.

Antidepressants

The only antidepressant with consistent efficacy in migraine prophylaxis is amitriptyline in doses between 10 and 150 mg. It has been studied in four older placebo-controlled trials, all with positive results [155–158]. Since the studies with amitriptyline were small and revealed central side effects, this drug is recommended only with Level B. For femoxetine, two small, positive placebo-controlled trials have been published [159, 160]. Fluoxetine in doses between 10 and 40 mg was effective in three [161–163] and not effective in one placebo-controlled trial [164]. Venlafaxine extended release (dose 75–150 mg) has shown efficacy in one placebo-controlled [165] and two open trials [166, 167], and can therefore be recommended as a second choice antidepressant in migraine prophylaxis.

Other antidepressants not effective in placebo-controlled trials were clomipramine and sertraline; for several further antidepressants, only open or not placebo-controlled trials are available [154].

Miscellaneous drugs

The antihypertensive drugs lisinopril [168] and candesartan [169] showed efficacy in migraine prophylaxis in one placebo-controlled trial each. However, these results have to be confirmed before the drugs can definitely be recommended. The same is true for high-dose riboflavin (400 mg) and coenzyme Q10, which have shown efficacy in one placebo-controlled trial each [170, 171]. For oral magnesium, conflicting studies (one positive, one negative) have been published [172, 173]. A herbal drug with evidence of efficacy is butterbur root extract (Petasites hybridus). This has been shown for a remedy with 75 mg (two tablets per day) in two placebo-controlled trials [174, 175]. Another herbal remedy, feverfew (Tanacetum parthenium), has been studied in several placebo-controlled trials with conflicting results. Also, the two most recent and best-designed studies showed a negative [176] and a positive [177] result; a Cochrane review resulted in a negative meta-analysis of all controlled studies on Tanacetum [178]. However, since there exist positive placebo-controlled trials, Tanacetum can be tried as a third-line drug (but only as a CO_2-extraction preparation).

In older studies, clonidine, pizotifen, and methysergide have shown efficacy in migraine prophylaxis. The more recent and better-designed studies on clonidine, however, did not confirm any efficacy (for review see [154]. Methysergide, which is clearly effective, can be recommended for short-term use only (maximum 6 months per treatment period) because of potentially severe side effects [179]; it can be re-established after a wash-out period of 4–6 weeks. Pizotifen is not generally recommended because the efficacy is not better than in the substances mentioned above and the side effects (dizziness, weight gain) are classified as very severe by the task force and limit the use too much [180]. Some experts have found it useful in childhood migraine. Ergot alkaloids have also been used in migraine prophylaxis. The evidence for dihydroergotamine is weak, since several studies reported both positive and negative results (for review see [154]). Dihydroergocryptine has also shown efficacy in one small placebo-controlled study [181].

Botulinum toxin for episodic migraine was studied in seven published placebo-controlled trials [182–188]. All these placebo-controlled trials were negative; only one study showed an efficacy for the low-dose (but not the high-dose) treatment with botulinum toxin [182]. In another study, a post hoc analysis of a subgroup of chronic migraine patients without further prophylactic treatment showed benefit from botulinum toxin A [185]. This indication is currently evaluated in a trial programme. A press release has suggested two large studies of chronic migraine were positive; these data need peer review before the treatment can be recommended.

Finally, those substances with negative, modern randomized, placebo-controlled, double-blind trials, which are not mentioned above, are listed as follows: no efficacy at all in migraine prophylaxis has been shown for homoeopathic remedies [189–191]; for the cysteinyl-leukotriene receptor antagonist montelukast [192]; for acetazolamide 500 mg per day [193]; and for the neurokinin-1 receptor antagonist lanepitant [194].

Specific situations

Emergency situation

Patients with a severe migraine attack in an emergency situation have often already tried oral medication without any success. Treatment of first choice in this situation is the i.v. application of 1000 mg ASA with or without metoclopramide [56]. Alternatively, 6 mg subcutaneous sumatriptan can be given. For the treatment of a status migrainosus, 50–100 mg prednisone or 10 mg dexamethasone is recommended by expert consensus. In placebo-controlled trials, however, no consistent efficacy of this procedure in the acute treatment of migraine attacks [195] or in the prevention of recurrence could be proven [196–199]. Also by expert consensus and supported by open-label studies, dihydroergotamine 2 mg (nasal spray or suppositories) is recommended for severe migraine attacks [38]. The i.v. application of metamizol was significantly superior to placebo but can cause severe arterial hypotension and allergic reactions [33, 200]. The i.v. application of paracetamol was not efficacious in a placebo-controlled trial in acute migraine attacks [201].

Menstrual migraine

In the recent 2nd edition of IHS diagnostic criteria, the entity of menstrual migraine is to be found in the appendix (and not the main criteria), reflecting a degree of uncertainty about the best criteria. Nevertheless, different drug regimens have been studied to treat this condition of quite some importance in clinical practice. On the one hand, acute migraine treatment with triptans has been studied, showing the same efficacy of triptans in menstrual migraine attacks as compared to non-menstrual migraine attacks. On the other hand, short-term prophylaxis of menstrual migraine has been studied.

Naproxen sodium (550 mg twice daily) has been shown to reduce pain including headache in the premenstrual syndrome [202]. Its specific effects on menstrual migraine (550 mg twice daily) have also been evaluated [203–205]. In one trial [203], patients reported fewer and less severe headaches during the week before menstruation than patients treated with placebo, but only severity was significantly reduced. In the other two placebo-controlled trials, naproxen sodium, given 1 week before and 1 week after the start of menstruation, resulted in fewer perimenstrual headaches; in one study, severity was not reduced [205], but in the other, both severity and analgesic requirements were decreased [204]. Even triptans have been used as short-term prophylaxis of menstrual migraine. For naratriptan (2 × 1 mg per day for 5 days starting 2 days prior to the expected onset of menses) and for frovatriptan (2 × 2.5 mg given for 6 days perimenstrually), superiority over placebo has been shown [206–208]; however, it can happen that the menstrual migraine attack is delayed until another time of the menstrual cycle [208].

Another prophylactic treatment regime of menstrual migraine is oestrogen replacement therapy. The best evidence, although not as effective as beta-blockers or other first-line prophylactic drugs, has been achieved for transdermal estradiol (not less than 100 μg given for 6 days perimenstrually as a gel or a patch) [209–212]. A recent study, however, did not show efficacy of hormone replacement with respect to attack frequency during the whole menstrual cycle [213].

Migraine in pregnancy

There are no specific clinical trials evaluating drug treatment of migraine during pregnancy, and most of the migraine drugs are contraindicated. Fortunately, most of the pregnant migraineurs experience fewer or even no migraine attacks. If migraine occurs during pregnancy, only paracetamol is allowed during the whole period. NSAIDs can be given in the second trimester. These recommendations are based on the advice of the regulatory authorities in most European countries. There may be differences in some respect between different countries (in particular, NDAIDs might be allowed in the first trimester).

Triptans and ergot alkaloids are contraindicated. For sumatriptan, a large pregnancy register has been established with no reports of any adverse events or complications during pregnancy that might be attributed to sumatriptan [214–218]. Similar results have been published for rizatriptan [219]. Based on the published data, administration of triptans in the first trimester of pregnancy is recommended by expert consensus if the child is more at risk from severe attacks with vomiting than from the potential impact of the triptan. For migraine prophylaxis, only magnesium and metoprolol are recommended during pregnancy (Level B recommendation) [220].

Migraine in children and adolescents

The only analgesics with evidence of efficacy for acute migraine treatment in childhood and adolescents are ibuprofen 10 mg per kg body weight and paracetamol 15 mg per kg body weight [221]. The only antiemetic licensed for the use in children up to 12 years is domperidon. Sumatriptan nasal spray 5–20 mg is the only triptan with positive placebo-controlled trials in the acute migraine treatment of children and adolescents [222–224]; the recommended dose for adolescents from the age of 12 is 10 mg. Oral triptans did not show significant efficacy in the first placebo-controlled childhood and adolescents studies [225–227]. This was in particular due to high placebo responses of about 50% in this age group. In post hoc analyses, however, 2.5–5 mg zolmitriptan was effective in adolescents from the age of 12 to 17 [228, 229]. In recent trials, oral zolmitriptan 2.5 mg [230], nasal zolmitriptan 5 mg [231], and oral rizatriptan 5–10 mg [232] have been superior to placebo in acute migraine treatment. Ergotamine should not be used in children and adolescents. Also, children and adolescents can develop drug-induced headache due to analgesic, ergotamine, or triptan overuse.

For migraine prophylaxis, flunarizine 10 mg and propranolol 40–80 mg per day showed the best evidence of efficacy in children and adolescents [6, 226]. Recently, topiramate in a dose between 15 and 200 mg also showed efficacy in children and adolescents [233, 234]. Other drugs have not been studied or did not show efficacy in appropriate studies.

Need of update

These recommendations should be updated within three years and should be complemented by recommendations for the non-drug treatment of migraine.

Conflicts of interest

The present guidelines were developed without external financial support. The authors report the following financial supports.

Stefan Evers: Salary by the University of Münster; honoraries and research grants by Addex Pharm, AGA Medical, Allergan, Almirall, AstraZeneca, Berlin Chemie, Boehringer, CoLucid, Desitin, Eisai, GlaxoSmithKline, Ipsen Pharma, Janssen Cilag, MSD, Novartis, Pfizer, Pharm Allergan, Pierre Fabre, Reckitt-Benckiser, UCB.

Judit Áfra: Salary by the Hungarian Ministry of Health.

Achim Frese: Private praxis; honorary by Berlin Chemie.

Peter J. Goadsby: Salary from University of California, San Francisco; honorarium or research grants in 2008 from Almirall, Boston Scientific, Colucid, Eli-Lilly, GSK, J&J, MAP Pharmaceuticals MSD, Medtronic, Neuralieve.

Mattias Linde: Salary by the Swedish government; honoraries by AstraZeneca, GlaxoSmithKline, MSD, Nycomed, Pfizer.

Arne May: Salary by the University Hospital of Hamburg; honoraries by Almirall, AstraZeneca, Bayer Vital, Berlin Chemie, GlaxoSmithKline, Janssen Cilag, MSD, Pfizer.

Peter S. Sándor: Salary by the University Hospital of Zurich; honoraries by AstraZeneca, GlaxoSmithKline, Janssen Cilag, Pfizer, Pharm Allergan.

References

1. Headache Classification Committee of the International Headache Society. The international classification of headache disorders, 2nd edn. *Cephalalgia* 2004;**24**(Suppl. 1):1–160.
2. Brainin M, Barnes M, Baron JC, *et al.* Guidance for the preparation of neurological management guidelines by EFNS scientific task forces – revised recommendations 2004. *Eur J Neurol* 2004;**11**:577–81.
3. Olesen J, Goadsby PJ, Ramadan NM, Tfelt-Hansen P, Welch KMA (eds) *The Headaches*, 3rd edn. Philadelphia: Lippincott, Williams & Wilkins, 2006; pp. 553–66.
4. Evers S, Kropp P, Pothmann R, Heinen F, Ebinger F. Therapie idiopathischer Kopfschmerzen im Kindes- und Jugendalter. *Nervenheilkunde* 2008;**27**:1127–37.
5. Lewis DW. Toward the definition of childhood migraine. *Curr Opin Pediatr* 2004;**16**:628–36.
6. Lewis D, Ashwal S, Hershey A, Hirtz D, Yonker M, Silberstein S, American Academy of Neurology Quality Standards Subcommittee. Practice Committee of the Child Neurology Society. Practice parameter: pharmacological treatment of migraine headache in children and adoles-

cents: report of the American Academy of Neurology Quality Standards Subcommittee and the Practice Committee of the Child Neurology Society. *Neurology* 2004;**63**: 2215–24.

7. Maytal J, Young M, Shechter A, Lipton RB. Pediatric migraine and the International Headache Society (IHS) criteria. *Neurology* 1997;**48**:602–7.

8. Rasmussen BK, Jensen R, Schroll M, Olesen J. Epidemiology of headache in a general population – a prevalence study. *J Clin Epidemiol* 1991;**44**:1147–57.

9. Rasmussen BK. Epidemiology of headache. *Cephalalgia* 2001;**21**:774–7.

10. Lipton R, Scher A, Kolodner K, Liberman J, Steiner TJ, Stewart WF. Migraine in the United States: epidemiology and patterns of health care use. *Neurology* 2002;**58**:885–94.

11. Scher A, Stewart WF, Liberman J, Lipton RB. Prevalence of frequent headache in a population sample. *Headache* 1998;**38**:497–506.

12. Stovner LJ, Hagen K, Jensen R, et al. The global burden of headache: a documentation of headache prevalence and disability worldwide. *Cephalalgia* 2007;**27**:193–210.

13. Quality Standards Subcommittee of the American Academy of Neurology. Practice parameter: the utility of neuroimaging in the evaluation of headache in patients with normal neurologic examinations. *Neurology* 1994;**44**: 1353–4.

14. Tfelt-Hansen P, Block G, Dahlöf C, *et al.* Guidelines for controlled trials of drugs in migraine: second edition. *Cephalalgia* 2000;**20**:765–86.

15. Pilgrim AJ. The methods used in clinical trials of sumatriptan in migraine. *Headache* 1993;**33**:280–93.

16. Chabriat H, Joire JE, Danchot J, Grippon P, Bousser MG. Combined oral lysine acetylsalicylate and metoclopramide in the acute treatment of migraine: a multicentre double-blind placebo-controlled study. *Cephalalgia* 1994;**14**: 297–300.

17. Nebe J, Heier M, Diener HC. Low-dose ibuprofen in self-medication of mild to moderate headache: a comparison with acetylsalicylic acid and placebo. *Cephalalgia* 1995;**15**: 531–5.

18. Tfelt-Hansen P, Henry P, Mulder LJ, Scheldewaert RG, Schoenen J, Chazot G. The effectiveness of combined oral lysine acetylsalicylate and metoclopramide compared with oral sumatriptan for migraine. *Lancet* 1995;**346**:923–6.

19. Diener HC, Bussone G, de Liano H, *et al.*, EMSASI Study Group. Placebo-controlled comparison of effervescent acetylsalicylic acid, sumatriptan and ibuprofen in the treatment of migraine attacks. *Cephalalgia* 2004;**24**:947–54.

20. Havanka-Kanniainen H. Treatment of acute migraine attack: ibuprofen and placebo compared. *Headache* 1989;**29**:507–9.

21. Kloster R, Nestvold K, Vilming ST. A double-blind study of ibuprofen versus placebo in the treatment of acute migraine attacks. *Cephalalgia* 1992;**12**:169–71.

22. Karachalios GN, Fotiadou A, Chrisikos N, Karabetsos A, Kehagioglou K. Treatment of acute migraine attack with diclofenac sodium: a double-blind study. *Headache* 1992;**32**:98–100.

23. Dahlöf C, Björkman R. Diclofenac-K (50 and 100 mg) and placebo in the acute treatment of migraine. *Cephalalgia* 1993;**13**:117–23.

24. The Diclofenac-K/Sumatriptan Migraine Study Group. Acute treatment of migraine attacks: efficacy and safety of a nonsteroidal antiinflammatory drug, diclofenac-potassium, in comparison to oral sumatriptan and placebo. *Cephalalgia* 1999;**19**:232–40.

25. Göbel H, Heinze A, Niederberger U, Witt T, Zumbroich V. Efficacy of phenazone in the treatment of acute migraine attacks: a double-blind, placebo-controlled, randomized study. *Cephalalgia* 2004;**24**:888–93.

26. Tulunay FC, Ergun H, Gulmez SE, *et al.* The efficacy and safety of dipyrone (Novalgin) tablets in the treatment of acute migraine attacks: a double-blind, cross-over, randomized, placebo-controlled, multi-center study. *Funct Neurol* 2004;**19**:197–202.

27. Myllyla VV, Havanka H, Herrala L, *et al.* Tolfenamic acid rapid release versus sumatriptan in the acute treatment of migraine: comparable effect in a double-blind, randomized, controlled, parallel-group study. *Headache* 1998;**38**: 201–7.

28. Lipton RB, Baggish JS, Stewart WF, Codispoti JR, Fu M. Efficacy and safety of acetaminophen in the treatment of migraine: results of a randomized, double-blind, placebo-controlled, population-based study. *Arch Intern Med* 2000;**160**:3486–92.

29. Lipton RB, Stewart WF, Ryan RE, Saper J, Silberstein S, Sheftell F. Efficacy and safety of acetaminophen, aspirin, and caffeine in alleviating migraine headache pain – three double-blind, randomized, placebo-controlled trials. *Arch Neurol* 1998;**55**:210–7.

30. Diener H, Pfaffenrath V, Pageler L. The fixed combination of acetylsalicylic acid, paracetamol and caffeine is more effective than single substances and dual combination for the treatment of headache: a multi-centre, randomized, double-blind, single-dose, placebo-controlled parallel group study. *Cephalalgia* 2005;**25**:776–87.

31. Goldstein J, Silberstein SD, Saper JR, Ryan RE Jr, Lipton RB. Acetaminophen, aspirin, and caffeine in combination versus ibuprofen for acute migraine: results from a multicenter, double-blind, randomized, parallel-group, single-dose, placebo-controlled study. *Headache* 2006;**46**: 444–53.

32. Limmroth V, May A, Diener HC. Lysine-acetylsalicylic acid in acute migraine attacks. *Eur Neurol* 1999;**41**:88–93.

33. Bigal ME, Bordini CA, Tepper SJ, Speciali JG. Intravenous dipyrone in the acute treatment of migraine without aura and migraine with aura: a randomized, double blind, placebo controlled study. *Headache* 2002;**42**:862–71.

34. Diener HC, Eikermann A, Gessner U, et al. Efficacy of 1,000 mg effervescent acetylsalicylic acid and sumatriptan in treating associated migraine symptoms. *Eur Neurol* 2004;**52**:50–6.

35. Lampl C, Voelker M, Diener HC. Efficacy and safety of 1,000 mg effervescent aspirin: individual patient data meta-analysis of three trials in migraine headache and migraine accompanying symptoms. *J Neurol* 2007;**254**: 705–12.

36. Kudrow D, Thomas HM, Ruoff G, et al. Valdecoxib for treatment of a single, acute, moderate to severe migraine headache. *Headache* 2005;**45**:1151–62.

37. Misra UK, Jose M, Kalita J. Rofecoxib versus ibuprofen for acute treatment of migraine: a randomised placebo controlled trial. *Postgrad Med J* 2004;**80**:720–3.

38. Saper J, Dahlöf C, So Y, Tfelt-Hansen P, et al. Rofecoxib in the acute treatment of migraine: a randomized controlled clinical trial. *Headache* 2006;**46**:264–75.

39. Silberstein S, Tepper S, Brandes J, et al. Randomised placebo-controlled trial of rofecoxib in the acute treatment of migraine. *Neurology* 2004;**62**:1552–7.

40. Ross-Lee LM, Eadie MJ, Heazlewood V, Bochner F, Tyrer JH. Aspirin pharmacokinetics in migraine. The effect of metoclopramide. *Eur J Clin Pharmacol* 1983;**24**:777–85.

41. Waelkens J. Dopamine blockade with domperidone: bridge between prophylactic and abortive treatment of migraine? A dose-finding study. *Cephalalgia* 1984;**4**:85–90.

42. Schulman E, Dermott K. Sumatriptan plus metoclopramide in triptan-nonresponsive migraineurs. *Headache* 2003;**43**:729–33.

43. Ellis GL, Delaney J, DeHart DA, Owens A. The efficacy of metoclopramide in the treatment of migraine headache. *Ann Emerg Med* 1993;**22**:191–5.

44. Friedman BW, Corbo J, Lipton RB, et al. A trial of metoclopramide vs sumatriptan for the emergency department treatment of migraines. *Neurology* 2005;**64**:463–8.

45. Tfelt-Hansen P, Saxena PR, Dahlöf C, et al. Ergotamine in the acute treatment of migraine. A review and European consensus. *Brain* 2000;**123**:9–18.

46. The Multinational Oral Sumatriptan Cafergot Comparative Study Group. A randomized, double-blind comparison of sumatriptan and Cafergot in the acute treatment of migraine. *Eur Neurol* 1991;**31**:314–22.

47. Diener HC, Reches A, Pascual J, Pascual J, Pitei D, Steiner, TJ, Eletriptan and Cafergot Comparative Study Group. Efficacy, tolerability and safety of oral eletriptan and ergotamine plus caffeine (Cafergot) in the acute treatment of migraine: a multicentre, randomised, double-blind, placebo-controlled comparison. *Europ Neurol* 2002;**47**: 99–107.

48. Lainez MJ, Galvan J, Heras J, Vila C. Crossover, double-blind clinical trial comparing almotriptan and ergotamine plus caffeine for acute migraine therapy. *Eur J Neurol* 2007;**14**:269–75.

49. Christie S, Göbel H, Mateos V, Allen C, Vrijens F, Shivaprakash M, Rizatriptan-Ergotamine/Caffeine Preference Study Group. Crossover comparison of efficacy and preference for rizatriptan 10 mg versus ergotamine/caffeine in migraine. *Eur Neurol* 2003;**49**:20–9.

50. Evers S, Gralow I, Bauer B, et al. Sumatriptan and ergotamine overuse and drug-induced headache: a clinicoepidmiologic study. *Clin Neuropharmacol* 1999;**22**:201–6.

51. Ferrari MD, Roon KI, Lipton RB, Goadsby PJ. Oral triptans (serotonin 5-HT1B/1D agonists) in acute migraine treatment: a meta-analysis of 53 trials. *Lancet* 2001;**358**: 1668–75.

52. Goadsby PB, Lipton RB, Ferrai MD. Migraine: current understanding and management. *N Engl J Med* 2002;**346**:257–70.

53. The Oral Sumatriptan and Aspirin plus Metoclopramide Comparative Study Group. A study to compare oral sumatriptan with oral aspirin plus oral metoclopramide in the acute treatment of migraine. *Eur Neurol* 1992;**32**: 177–84.

54. Geraud G, Compagnon A, Rossi A. Zolmitriptan versus a combination of acetylsalicylic acid and metoclopramide in the acute oral treatment of migraine: a double-blind, randomised, three-attack study. *Eur Neurol* 2002;**47**:88–98.

55. Diamond M, Hettiarachchi J, Hilliard B, Sands G, Nett R. Effectiveness of eletriptan in acute migraine: primary care for Excedrin nonresponders. *Headache* 2004;**44**:209–16.

56. Diener HC, for the ASASUMAMIG Study Group. Efficacy and safety of intravenous acetylsalicylic acid lysinate compared to subcutaneous sumatriptan and parenteral placebo in the acute treatment of migraine. A double-blind, double-dummy, randomized, multicenter, parallel group study. *Cephalalgia* 1999;**19**:581–8.

57. Winner P, Ricalde O, Force BL, Saper J, Margul B. A double-blind study of subcutaneous dihydroergotamine vs subcutaneous sumatriptan in the treatment of acute migraine. *Arch Neurol* 1996;**53**:180–4.

58. Pascual J, Cabarrocas X. Within-patient early versus delayed treatment of migraine attacks with almotriptan: the sooner the better. *Headache* 2002;**42**:28–31.

59. Burstein R, Collins B, Jakubowski M. Defeating migraine pain with triptans: a race against the development of cutaneous allodynia. *Ann Neurol* 2004;**55**:19–26.

60. Dowson A, Massiou H, Lainez J, Cabarrocas X. Almotriptan improves response rates when treatment is within 1 hour of migraine onset. *Headache* 2004;**44**:318–22.

61. Cady R, Martin V, Mauskop A, *et al*. Efficacy of rizatriptan 10 mg administered early in a migraine attack. *Headache* 2006;**46**:914–24.

62. Goadsby PJ, Zanchin G, Geraud G, *et al*. Early versus non-early intervention in acute migraine – 'Act when Mild – AwM'. A double-blind placebo-controlled trial of almotriptan. *Cephalalgia* 2008;**28**:383–91.

63. Diener HC, Dodick DW, Goadsby PJ, Lipton RB, Almas M, Parsons B. Identification of negative predictors of pain-free response to triptans: analysis of the eletriptan database. *Cephalalgia* 2008;**28**:35–40.

64. Linde M, Mellberg A, Dahlöf C. Subcutaneous sumatriptan provides symptomatic relief at any pain intensity or time during the migraine attack. *Cephalalgia* 2006;**26**:113–21.

65. Cady R, Martin V, Mauskop A, *et al*. Symptoms of cutaneous sensitivity pre-treatment and post-treatment: results from the rizatriptan TAME studies. *Cephalalgia* 2007;**27**:1055–60.

66. Bigal ME, Serrano D, Buse D, Scher A, Stewart WF, Lipton RB. Acute migraine medications and evolution from episodic to chronic migraine: a longitudinal population-based study. *Headache* 2008;**48**:1157–68.

67. Limmroth V, Kazarawa S, Fritsche G, Diener HC. Headache after frequent use of new serotonin agonists zolmitriptan and naratriptan. *Lancet* 1999;**353**:378.

68. Katsarava Z, Fritsche G, Muessig M, Diener HC, Limmroth V. Clinical features of withdrawal headache following overuse of triptans and other headache drugs. *Neurology* 2001;**57**:1694–8.

69. Ferrari MD. How to assess and compare drugs in the management of migraine: success rates in terms of response and recurrence. *Cephalalgia* 1999;**19**(Suppl. 23):2–8.

70. Ferrari MD, James MH, Bates D, *et al*. Oral sumatriptan: effect of a second dose, and incidence and treatment of headache recurrences. *Cephalalgia* 1994;**14**:330–8.

71. Brandes JL, Kudrow D, Stark SR, *et al*. Sumatriptan-naproxen for acute treatment of migraine: a randomized trial. *JAMA* 2007;**297**:1443–54.

72. Freitag F, Diamond M, Diamond S, Janssen I, Rodgers A, Skobieranda F. Efficacy and tolerability of coadministration of rizatriptan and acetaminophen vs rizatriptan or acetaminophen alone for acute migraine treatment. *Headache* 2008;**48**:921–30.

73. Bigal M, Sheftell F, Tepper S, Tepper D, Ho TW, Rapoport A. A randomized double-blind study comparing rizatriptan, dexamethasone, and the combination of both in the acute treatment of menstrually related migraine. *Headache* 2008;**48**:1286–93.

74. Diener HC, Gendolla A, Gebert I, Beneke M. Almotriptan in migraine patients who respond poorly to oral sumatriptan: a double-blind, randomized trial. *Headache* 2005;**45**:874–82.

75. Stark S, Spierings EL, McNeal S, Putnam GP, Bolden-Watson CP, O'Quinn S. Naratriptan efficacy in migraineurs who respond poorly to oral sumatriptan. *Headache* 2000;**40**:513–20.

76. O'Quinn S, Davis RL, Guttermann DL, *et al*. Prospective large-scale study of the tolerability of subcutaneous sumatriptan injection for the acute treatment of migraine. *Cephalalgia* 1999;**19**:223–31.

77. Welch KMA, Mathew NT, Stone P, Rosamond W, Saiers J, Gutterman D. Tolerability of sumatriptan: clinical trials and post-marketing experience. *Cephalalgia* 2000;**20**:687–95.

78. Velentgas P, Cole JA, Mo J, Sikes CR, Walker AM. Severe vascular events in migraine patients. *Headache* 2004;**44**:642–51.

79. Hall G, Brown M, Mo J, MacRae KD. Triptans in migraine: the risks of stroke, cardiovascular disease, and death in practice. *Neurology* 2004;**62**:563–8.

80. Bates D, Ashford E, Dawson R, *et al*. Subcutaneous sumatriptan during the migraine aura. *Neurology* 1994;**44**:1587–92.

81. Olesen J, Diener HC, Schoenen J, Hettiarachchi J. No effect of eletriptan administration during the aura phase of migraine. Europ. *J Neurol* 2004;**11**:671–7.

82. Tfelt-Hansen P. Sumatriptan for the treatment of migraine attacks – a review of controlled clinical trials. *Cephalalgia* 1993;**13**:238–44.

83. Goadsby PJ. Role of naratriptan in clinical practice. *Cephalalgia* 1997;**17**:472–3.

84. Markus F, Mikko K. Frovatriptan review. *Expert Opin Pharmacother* 2007;**8**:3029–33.

85. Charlesworth BR, Dowson AJ, Purdy A, Becker WJ, Boes-Hansen S, Färkkilä M. Speed of onset and efficacy of zolmitriptan nasal spray in the acute treatment of migraine: a randomised, double-blind, placebo-controlled, dose-ranging study versus zolmitriptan tablet. *CNS Drugs* 2003;**17**:653–67.

86. Dahlöf C, Cady R, Poole AC. Speed of onset and efficacy of sumatriptan fast-disintegrating/rapid release tablets: results of two replicate randomised, placebo-controlled studies. *Headache Care* 2004;**1**:277–80.

87. The Subcutaneous Sumatriptan International Study Group. Treatment of migraine attacks with sumatriptan. *N Engl J Med* 1991;**325**:316–21.

88. Ryan R, Elkind A, Baker CC, Mullican W, DeBussey S, Asgharnejad M. Sumatriptan nasal spray for the acute treatment of migraine. *Neurology* 1997;**49**:1225–30.

89. Tepper SJ, Cochran A, Hobbs S, Woessner M. Sumatriptan suppositories for the acute treatment of migraine. *Int J Clin Pract* 1998;**52**:31–5.

90. Becker WJ, on behalf of the Study Group. A placebo-controlled, dose-defining study of sumatriptan nasal spray in the acute treatment of migraine. *Cephalalgia* 1995; **15**(Suppl. 14):271–6.

91. Goldstein J, Ryan R, Jiang K, *et al.* Crossover comparison of rizatriptan 5 mg and 10 mg versus sumatriptan 25 and 50 mg in migraine. *Headache* 1998;**38**:737–47.

92. Tfelt-Hansen P, Teall J, Rodriguez F, *et al.* Oral rizatriptan versus oral sumatriptan: a direct comparative study in the acute treatment of migraine. *Headache* 1998;**38**:748–55.

93. Tfelt-Hansen P, Ryan RE. Oral therapy for migraine: comparisons between rizatriptan and sumatriptan. A review of four randomized, double-blind clinical trials. *Neurology* 2000;**55**(Suppl. 2):S19–24.

94. Geraud G, Keywood C, Senard JM. Migraine headache recurrence: relationship to clinical, pharmacological, and pharmacokinetic properties of triptans. *Headache* 2003;**43**:376–88.

95. Edwards KR, Norton J, Behnke M. Comparison of intravenous valproate versus intramuscular dihydroergotamine and metoclopramide for acute treatment of migraine headache. *Headache* 2001;**41**:976–80.

96. Leniger T, Pageler L, Stude P, Diener HC, Limmroth V. Comparison of intravenous valproate with intravenous lysine-acetylsalicylic acid in acute migraine attacks. *Headache* 2005;**45**:42–6.

97. Soyka D, Taneri Z, Oestreich W, Schmidt R. Flunarizine i.v. in the acute treatment of the migraine attack. A double-blind placebo-controlled study. *Cephalalgia* 1988;**8**(Suppl. 8):35–40.

98. Silberstein SD, Freitag FG, Rozen TD, *et al.* Tramadol/Acetaminophen for the treatment of acute migraine pain: findings of a randomized, placebo-controlled trial. *Headache* 2005;**45**:1317–27.

99. Olesen J, Diener HC, Husstedt IW, *et al.* BIBN 4096 BS Clinical Proof of Concept Study Group. Calcitonin gene-related peptide receptor antagonist BIBN 4096 BS for the acute treatment of migraine. *N Engl J Med* 2004;**350**: 1104–10.

100. Ho TW, Mannix LK, Fan X, *et al.* MK-0974 Protocol 004 study group. Randomized controlled trial of an oral CGRP receptor antagonist, MK-0974, in acute treatment of migraine. *Neurology* 2008;**70**:1304–12.

101. Ho TW, Ferrari MD, Dodick DW, *et al.* Efficacy and tolerability of MK-0974 (telcagepant), a new oral antagonist of calcitonin gene-related peptide receptor, compared with zolmitriptan for acute migraine: a randomised, placebo-controlled, parallel-treatment trial. *Lancet* 2009;**372**: 2115–23.

102. Kangasniemi P, Hedman C. Metoprolol and propranolol in the prophylactic treatment of classical and common migraine. A double-blind study. *Cephalalgia* 1984;**4**: 91–6.

103. Olsson JE, Behring HC, Forssman B, *et al.* Metoprolol and propranolol in migraine prophylaxis: a double-blind multicenter study. *Acta Neurol Scand* 1984;**70**:160–8.

104. Steiner TJ, Joseph R, Hedman C, Rose FC. Metoprolol in the prophylaxis of migraine: parallel group comparison with placebo and dose-ranging follow-up. *Headache* 1988;**28**:15–23.

105. Sorensen PS, Larsen BH, Rasmussen MJK, *et al.* Flunarizine versus metoprolol in migraine prophylaxis: a double-blind, randomized parallel group study of efficacy and tolerability. *Headache* 1991;**31**:650–7.

106. Wörz R, Reinhardt-Benmalek B, Grotemeyer KH. Bisoprolol and metoprolol in the prophylactic treatment of migraine with and without aura – a randomized double-blind cross-over multicenter study. *Cephalalgia* 1991;**11**(Suppl. 11):152–3.

107. Diamond S, Medina JL. Double blind study of propranolol for migraine prophylaxis. *Headache* 1976;**16**:24–7.

108. Tfelt-Hansen P, Standnes B, Kangasniemi P, Hakkarainen H, Olesen J. Timolol vs. propranolol vs. placebo in common migraine prophylaxis: a double-blind multicenter trial. *Acta Neurol Scand* 1984;**69**:1–8.

109. Nadelmann JW, Stevens J, Saper JR. Propranolol in the prophylaxis of migraine. *Headache* 1986;**26**:175–82.

110. Havanka-Kanniainen H, Hokkanen E, Myllylä VV. Long acting propranolol in the prophylaxis of migraine. Comparison of the daily doses of 80 mg and 160 mg. *Headache* 1988;**28**:607–11.

111. Ludin H-P. Flunarizine and propranolol in the treatment of migraine. *Headache* 1989;**29**:218–23.

112. Holroyd KA, Penzien DB, Cordingley GE. Propranolol in the management of recurrent migraine: a meta-analytic review. *Headache* 1991;**31**:333–40.

113. Gawel MJ, Kreeft J, Nelson RF, Simard D, Arnott WS. Comparison of the efficacy and safety of flunarizine to propranolol in the prophylaxis of migraine. *Can J Neurol Sci* 1992;**19**:340–5.

114. van de Ven LLM, Franke CL, Koehler PJ. Prophylactic treatment of migraine with bisoprolol: a placebo-controlled study. *Cephalalgia* 1997;**17**:596–9.

115. Stellar S, Ahrens SP, Meibohm AR, Reines SA. Migraine prevention with timolol. A double-blind crossover study. *JAMA* 1984;**252**:2576–80.

116. Johannsson V, Nilsson LR, Widelius T, *et al*. Atenolol in migraine prophylaxis a double-blind cross-over multicentre study. *Headache* 1987;**27**:372–4.

117. Louis P. A double-blind placebo-controlled prophylactic study of flunarizine in migraine. *Headache* 1981;**21**: 235–9.

118. Diamond S, Schenbaum H. Flunarizine, a calcium channel blocker, in the prophylactic treatment of migraine. *Headache* 1983;**23**:39–42.

119. Amery WK, Caers LI, Aerts TJL. Flunarizine, a calcium entry blocker in migraine prophylaxis. *Headache* 1985;**25**: 249–54.

120. Bono G, Manzoni GC, Martucci N, *et al*. Flunarizine in common migraine: Italian cooperative trial. II. Long-term follow-up. *Cephalalgia* 1985;**5**(Suppl. 2):155–8.

121. Centonze V, Tesauro P, Magrone D, *et al*. Efficacy and tolerability of flunarizine in the prophylaxis of migraine. *Cephalalgia* 1985;**5**(Suppl. 2):163–8.

122. Nappi G, Sandrini G, Savoini G, Cavallini A, de Rysky C, Micieli G. Comparative efficacy of cyclandelate versus flunarizine in the prophylactic treatment of migraine. *Drugs* 1987;**33**(Suppl. 2):103–9.

123. Freitag FG, Diamond S, Diamond M. A placebo controlled trial of flunarizine in migraine prophylaxis. *Cephalalgia* 1991;**11**(Suppl. 11):157–8.

124. Bassi P, Brunati L, Rapuzzi B, Alberti E, Mangoni A. Low dose flunarizine in the prophylaxis of migraine. *Headache* 1992;**32**:390–2.

125. Diamond S, Freitag FG. A double blind trial of flunarizine in migraine prophylaxis. *Headache Quart* 1993;**4**:169–72.

126. Balkan S, Aktekin B, Önal Z. Efficacy of flunarizine in the prophylactic treatment of migraine. *Gazi Med J* 1994;**5**: 81–4.

127. Diener H, Matias-Guiu J, Hartung E, *et al*. Efficacy and tolerability in migraine prophylaxis of flunarizine in reduced doses: a comparison with propranolol 160 mg daily. *Cephalalgia* 2002;**22**:209–21.

128. Gerber WD, Schellenberg R, Thom M, *et al*. Cyclandelate versus propranolol in the prophylaxis of migraine – a double-blind placebo-controlled study. *Funct Neurol* 1995;**10**:27–35.

129. Diener HC, Föh M, Iaccarino C, *et al*. Cyclandelate in the prophylaxis of migraine: a randomized, parallel, double-blind study in comparison with placebo and propranolol. *Cephalalgia* 1996;**16**:441–7.

130. Siniatchkin M, Gerber WD, Vein A. Clinical efficacy and central mechanisms of cyclandelate in migraine: a double-blind placebo-controlled study. *Funct Neurol* 1998;**13**: 47–56.

131. Diener H, Krupp P, Schmitt T, Steitz G, Milde K, Freytag S, on behalf of the Study Group. Cyclandelate in the prophylaxis of migraine: a placebo-controlled study. *Cephalalgia* 2001;**21**:66–70.

132. Kaniecki RG. A comparison of divalproex with propranolol and placebo for the prophylaxis of migraine without aura. *Arch Neurol* 1997;**54**:1141–5.

133. Klapper J, on behalf of the Divalproex Sodium in Migraine Prophylaxis Study Group. Divalproex sodium in migraine prophylaxis: a dose-controlled study. *Cephalalgia* 1997;**17**: 103–8.

134. Silberstein SD, Collins SD, Carlson H. Safety and efficacy of once-daily, extended-release divalproex sodium monotherapy for the prophylaxis of migraine headaches. *Cephalalgia* 2000;**20**:269.

135. Freitag F, Collins S, Carlson H, *et al*. Depakote ER Migraine Study Group. A randomized trial of divalproex sodium extended-release tablets in migraine prophylaxis. *Neurology* 2002;**58**:1652–9.

136. Brandes J, Saper J, Diamond M, *et al*., MIGR-002 Study Group. Topiramate for migraine prevention: a randomized controlled trial. *JAMA* 2004;**291**:965–73.

137. Diener H, Tfelt-Hansen P, Dahlöf C, *et al*. MIGR-003 Study Group. Topiramate in migraine prophylaxis: results from a placebo-controlled trial with propranolol as an active control. *J Neurol* 2004;**251**:943–50.

138. Mei D, Capuano A, Vollono C, *et al*. Topiramate in migraine prophylaxis: a randomised double-blind versus placebo study. *Neurol Sci* 2004;**25**:245–50.

139. Silberstein SD, Neto W, Schmitt J, Jacobs D. Topiramate in migraine prevention: results of a large controlled trial. *Arch Neurol* 2004;**61**:490–5.

140. Diener HC, Bussone G, Van Oene JC, Lahaye M, Schwalen S, Goadsby PJ. TOPMAT-MIG-201(TOP-CHROME) Study Group. Topiramate reduces headache days in chronic migraine: a randomized, double-blind, placebo-controlled study. *Cephalalgia* 2007;**27**:814–23.

141. Silberstein SD, Lipton RB, Dodick DW, *et al*. Efficacy and safety of topiramate for the treatment of chronic migraine: a randomized, double-blind, placebo-controlled trial. *Headache* 2007;**47**:170–80.

142. Steiner TJ, Findley LJ, Yuen AWC. Lamotrigine versus placebo in the prophylaxis of migraine with and without aura. *Cephalalgia* 1997;**17**:109–12.

143. Lampl C, Buzath A, Klinger D, Neumann K. Lamotrigine in the prophylactic treatment of migraine aura – a pilot study. *Cephalalgia* 1999;**19**:58–63.

144. Mathew NT, Rapoport A, Saper J, *et al*. Efficacy of gabapentin in migraine prophylaxis. *Headache* 2001;**41**:119–28.

145. Silberstein S, Saper J, Berenson F, Somogyi M, McCague K, D'Souza J. Oxcarbazepine in migraine headache: a double-blind, randomized, placebo-controlled study. *Neurology* 2008;**70**:548–55.

146. Goadsby PJ, Ferrari MD, Csanyi A, Olesen J, Mills JG. Randomized double blind, placebo-controlled proof-of-concept study of the cortical spreading depression inhibiting agent tonabersat in migraine prophylaxis. *Cephalalgia* 2009;**29**:742–50.

147. Peto R, Gray R, Collins R, Wheatly K, Hennekens C, Jamrozik K. Randomised trial of prophylactic daily aspirin in male British doctors. *BMJ* 1988;**296**:313–6.

148. Buring JE, Peto R, Hennekens CH. Low-dose aspirin for migraine prophylaxis. *JAMA* 1990;**264**:1711–3.

149. Ziegler DK, Ellis DJ. Naproxen in prophylaxis of migraine. *Arch Neurol* 1985;**42**:582–4.

150. Welch KMA, Ellis DJ, Keenan PA. Successful migraine prophylaxis with naproxen sodium. *Neurology* 1985;**35**:1304–10.

151. Bellavance AJ, Meloche JP. A comparative study of naproxen sodium, pizotyline and placebo in migraine prophylaxis. *Headache* 1990;**30**:710–5.

152. Mikkelsen BM, Falk JV. Prophylactic treatment of migraine with tolfenamic acid: a comparative double-blind crossover study between tolfenamic acid and placebo. *Acta Neurol Scand* 1982;**66**:105–11.

153. Mikkelsen B, Pedersen KK, Christiansen LV. Prophylactic treatment of migraine with tolfenamic acid, propranolol and placebo. *Acta Neurol Scand* 1986;**73**:423–7.

154. Evers S, Mylecharane E. Nonsteroidal antiinflammatory and miscellaneous drugs in migraine prophylaxis. In: Olesen J, Goadsby PJ, Ramadan N, Tfelt-Hansen P, Welch KMA (eds) *The Headaches*, 3rd edn. Philadelphia: Lippincott, 2006; pp. 553–66.

155. Gomersall JD, Stuart A. Amitriptyline in migraine prophylaxis: changes in pattern of attacks during a controlled clinical trial. *J Neurol Neurosurg Psychchiatry* 1973;**36**:684–90.

156. Couch JR, Hassanein RS. Amitriptyline in migraine prophylaxis. *Arch Neurol* 1979;**36**:695–9.

157. Ziegler DK, Hurwitz A, Hassanein RS, Kodanaz HA, Preskorn SH, Mason J. Migraine prophylaxis. A comparison of propranolol and amitriptyline. *Arch Neurol* 1987;**44**:486–9.

158. Ziegler DK, Hurwitz A, Preskorn S, Hassanein R, Seim J. Propranolol and amitriptyline in prophylaxis of migraine: pharmacokinetic and therapeutic effects. *Arch Neurol* 1993;**50**:825–30.

159. Orholm M, Honoré PF, Zeeberg I. A randomized general practice group-comparative study of femoxetine and placebo in the prophylaxis of migraine. *Acta Neurol Scand* 1986;**74**:235–9.

160. Zeeberg I, Orholm M, Nielsen JD, Honore PLF, Larsen JJV. Femoxetine in the prophylaxis of migraine – a randomised comparison with placebo. *Acta Neurol Scand* 1981;**64**:452–9.

161. Adly C, Straumanis J, Chesson A. Fluoxetine prophylaxis of migraine. *Headache* 1992;**32**:101–4.

162. Steiner TJ, Ahmed F, Findley LJ, MacGregor EA, Wilkinson M. S-fluoxetine in the prophylaxis of migraine: a phase II double-blind randomized placebo-controlled study. *Cephalalgia* 1998;**18**:283–6.

163. d'Amato CC, Pizza V, Marmolo T, Giordano E, Alfano V, Nasta A. Fluoxetine for migraine prophylaxis: a double-blind trial. *Headache* 1999;**39**:716–9.

164. Saper JR, Silberstein SD, Lake AE, Winters ME. Double-blind trial of fluoxetine: chronic daily headache and migraine. *Headache* 1994;**34**:497–502.

165. Ozyalcin SN, Talu GK, Kiziltan E, Yucel B, Ertas M, Disci R. The efficacy and safety of venlafaxine in the prophylaxis of migraine. *Headache* 2005;**45**:144–52.

166. Adelman LC, Adelman JU, von Seggern R, Mannix LK. Venlafaxine extended release (XR) for the prophylaxis of migraine and tension-type headache: a retrospective study in a clinical setting. *Headache* 2000;**40**:572–80.

167. Bulut S, Berilgen MS, Baran A, Tekatas A, Atmaca M, Mungen B. Venlafaxine versus amitriptyline in the prophylactic treatment of migraine: randomized, double-blind, crossover study. *Clin Neurol Neurosurg* 2004;**107**:44–8.

168. Schrader H, Stovner LJ, Helde G, Sand T, Bovim G. Prophylactic treatment of migraine with angiotensin converting enzyme inhibitor (lisinopril): randomised, placebo-controlled, crossover trial. *BMJ* 2001;**322**:19–22.

169. Tronvik E, Stovner LJ, Helde G, Sand T, Bovim G. Prophylactic treatment of migraine with an angiotensin II receptor blocker. A randomized controlled trial. *JAMA* 2002;**289**:65–9.

170. Schoenen J, Jacquy J, Lenaerts M. Effectiveness of high-dose riboflavin in migraine prophylaxis – a randomized controlled trial. *Neurology* 1998;**50**:466–70.

171. Sandor PS, di Clemente L, Coppola G, *et al.* Efficacy of coenzyme Q10 in migraine prophylaxis: a randomised controlled trial. *Neurology* 2005;**64**:713–5.

172. Pfaffenrath V, Wessely P, Meyer C, *et al.* Magnesium in the prophylaxis of migraine – a double-blind, placebo-controlled study. *Cephalalgia* 1996;**16**:436–40.

173. Peikert A, Wilimzig C, Köhne-Volland R. Prophylaxis of migraine with oral magnesium: results from a prospective, multi-center, placebo-controlled and double-blind randomized study. *Cephalalgia* 1996;**16**:257–63.

174. Diener HC, Rahlfs VW, Danesch U. The first placebo-controlled trial of a special butterbur root extract for the prevention of migraine: reanalysis of efficacy criteria. *Eur Neurol* 2004;**51**:89–97.

175. Lipton RB, Göbel H, Einhäupl KM, Wilks K, Mauskop A. Petasites hybridus root (butterbur) is an effective preventive treatment for migraine. *Neurology* 2004;**63**:2240–4.

176. Pfaffenrath V, Diener HC, Fischer M, Friede M, Henneicke-von Zepelin HH, Investigators. The efficacy and safety of Tanacetum parthenium (feverfew) in migraineprophylaxis – a double-blind, multicentre, randomized placebo-controlled dose-response study. *Cephalalgia* 2002;**22**:523–32.

177. Diener HC, Pfaffenrath V, Schnitker J, Friede M, Henneicke-von Zepelin HH. Efficacy and safety of 6.25 mg t.i.d. feverfew CO2-extract (MIG-99) in migraine prevention – a randomized, double-blind, multicentre, placebo-controlled study. *Cephalalgia* 2005;**25**:1031–41.

178. Pittler MH, Ernst E. Feverfew for preventing migraine. *Cochrane Database Syst Rev* 2004;(1):CD002286.

179. Silberstein SD. Methysergide. *Cephalalgia* 1998;**18**:421–35.

180. Mylecharane EJ. 5-HT2 receptor antagonists and migraine therapy. *J Neurol* 1991;**238**(Suppl. 1):S45–52.

181. Canonico PL, Scapagnini U, Genazzani E, Zanotti A. Dihydroergokryptine (DEK) in the prophylaxis of common migraine: double-blind clinical study vs placebo. *Cephalalgia* 1989;**9**(Suppl. 10):446–7.

182. Silberstein S, Mathew N, Saper J, Jenkins S. Botulinum toxin type A as a migraine preventive treatment. *Headache* 2000;**40**:445–50.

183. Brin MF, Swope DM, O'Brian C, Abbasi S, Pogoda JM. Botox for migraine: double-blind, placebo-controlled, region-specific evaluation. *Cephalalgia* 2000;**20**:421–2.

184. Evers S, Vollmer-Haase J, Schwaag S, Rahmann A, Husstedt IW, Frese A. Botulinum toxin A in the prophylactic treatment of migraine – a randomized, double-blind, placebo-controlled study. *Cephalalgia* 2004;**24**:838–43.

185. Dodick DW, Mauskop A, Elkind AH, DeGryse R, Brin MF, Silberstein SD, BOTOX CDH Study Group. Botulinum toxin type A for the prophylaxis of chronic daily headache: subgroup analysis of patients not receiving other prophylactic medications: a randomized double-blind, placebo-controlled study. *Headache* 2005;**45**:315–24.

186. Saper JR, Mathew NT, Loder EW, DeGryse R, VanDenburgh AM, BoNTA-009 Study Group. A double-blind, randomized, placebo-controlled comparison of botulinum toxin type a injection sites and doses in the prevention of episodic migraine. *Pain Med* 2007;**8**:478–85.

187. Aurora SK, Gawel M, Brandes JL, Pokta S, Vandenburgh AM, BOTOX North American Episodic Migraine Study Group. Botulinum toxin type a prophylactic treatment of episodic migraine: a randomized, double-blind, placebo-controlled exploratory study. *Headache* 2007;**47**:486–99.

188. Relja M, Poole AC, Schoenen J, Pascual J, Lei X, Thompson C, European BoNTA Headache Study Group. A multicentre, double-blind, randomized, placebo-controlled, parallel group study of multiple treatments of botulinum toxin type A (BoNTA) for the prophylaxis of episodic migraine headaches. *Cephalalgia* 2007;**27**:492–503.

189. Whitmarsh TE, Coleston-Shields DM, Steiner TJ. Double-blind randomized placebo-controlled study of homoeopathic prophylaxis of migraine. *Cephalalgia* 1997;**17**:600–4.

190. Walach H, Haeusler W, Lowes T, *et al.* Classical homeopathic treatment of chronic headaches. *Cephalalgia* 1997;**17**:119–26.

191. Straumsheim P, Borchgrevink C, Mowinckel P, Kierulf H, Hafslund O. Homeopathic treatment of migraine: a double blind, placebo controlled trial of 68 patients. *Br Homeopath J* 2000;**89**:4–7.

192. Brandes JL, Visser WH, Farmer MV, *et al.*, Protocol 125 study group. Montelukast for migraine prophylaxis: a randomized, double-blind, placebo-controlled study. *Headache* 2004;**44**:581–6.

193. Vahedi K, Taupin P, Djomby R, *et al.*, DIAMIG investigators. Efficacy and tolerability of acetazolamide in migraine prophylaxis: a randomised placebo-controlled trial. *J Neurol* 2002;**249**:206–11.

194. Goldstein DJ, Offen WW, Klein EG, *et al.* Lanepitant, an NK-1 antagonist, in migraine prevention. *Cephalalgia* 2001;**21**:102–6.

195. Friedman BW, Greenwald P, Bania TC, *et al.* Randomized trial of IV dexamethasone for acute migraine in the emergency department. *Neurology* 2007;**69**:2038–44.

196. Donaldson D, Sundermann R, Jackson R, Bastani A. Intravenous dexamethasone vs placebo as adjunctive therapy to reduce the recurrence rate of acute migraine headaches: a multicenter, double-blinded, placebo-controlled randomized clinical trial. *Am J Emerg Med* 2008;**26**:124–30.

197. Innes GD, Macphail I, Dillon EC, Metcalfe C, Gao M. Dexamethasone prevents relapse after emergency department treatment of acute migraine: a randomized clinical trial. *CJEM* 1999;**1**:26–33.

198. Rowe BH, Colman I, Edmonds ML, Blitz S, Walker A, Wiens S. Randomized controlled trial of intravenous dexamethasone to prevent relapse in acute migraine headache. *Headache* 2008;**48**:333–40.

199. Baden EY, Hunter CJ. Intravenous dexamethasone to prevent the recurrence of benign headache after discharge from the emergency department: a randomized, double-blind, placebo-controlled clinical trial. *CJEM* 2006;**8**:393–400.

200. Bigal ME, Bordini CA, Speciali JG. Intravenous metamizol (Dipyrone) in acute migraine treatment and in episodic

tension-type headache – a placebo-controlled study. *Cephalalgia* 2001;**21**:90–5.

201. Leinisch E, Evers S, Kaempfe N, *et al.* Evaluation of the efficacy of intravenous acetaminophen in the treatment of acute migraine attacks: a double-blind, placebo-controlled parallel group multicenter study. *Pain* 2005;**117**:396–400.

202. Facchinetti F, Fioroni L, Sances G, Romano G, Nappi G, Genazzani AR. Naproxen sodium in the treatment of premenstrual symptoms: a placebo-controlled study. *Gynecol Obstet Invest* 1989;**28**:205–8.

203. Sargent J, Solbach P, Damasio H, *et al.* A comparison of naproxen sodium to propranolol hydrochloride and a placebo control for the prophylaxis of migraine headache. *Headache* 1985;**25**:320–4.

204. Sances G, Martignoni E, Fioroni L, Blandini F, Facchinetti F, Nappi G. Naproxen sodium in menstrual migraine prophylaxis: a double-blind placebo controlled study. *Headache* 1990;**30**:705–9.

205. Szekely B, Merryman S, Croft H, Post G. Prophylactic effects of naproxen sodium on perimenstrual headache: a double-blind, placebo-controlled study. *Cephalalgia* 1989;**9**(Suppl. 10):452–3.

206. Newman L, Mannix LK, Landy S, *et al.* Naratriptan as short-term prophylaxis in menstrually associated migraine: a randomised, double-blind, placebo-controlled study. *Headache* 2001;**41**:248–56.

207. Silberstein SD, Elkind AH, Schreiber C, Keywood C. A randomized trial of frovatriptan for the intermittent prevention of menstrual migraine. *Neurology* 2004;**63**:261–9.

208. Mannix LK, Savani N, Landy S, *et al.* Efficacy and tolerability of naratriptan for short-term prevention of menstrually related migraine: data from two randomized, double-blind, placebo-controlled studies. *Headache* 2007;**47**:1037–49.

209. De Lignieres B, Mauvais-Javis P, Mas JML, Mas JL, Touboul PJ, Bousser MG. Prevention of menstrual migraine by percutaneous oestradiol. *BMJ* 1986;**293**:1540.

210. Dennerstein L, Morse C, Burrows G, Oats J, Brown J, Smith M. Menstrual migraine: a double blind trial of percutaneous oestradiol. *Gynecol Endocrinol* 1988;**2**:113–20.

211. Smits MG, van den Meer YG, Pfeil JPJM, Rijnierse JJMM, Vos AJM. Perimenstrual migraine: effect of Estraderm TTS and the value of contingent negative variation and exteroceptive temporalis muscle suppression test. *Headache* 1994;**34**:103–6.

212. Pradalier A, Vincent D, Beaulieu PH, Baudesson G, Launay J-M. Correlation between estradiol plasma level and therapeutic effect on menstrual migraine. *Proc 10th Migraine Trust Symp* 1994;129–32.

213. MacGregor EA, Frith A, Ellis J, Aspinall L, Hackshaw A. Prevention of menstrual attacks of migraine: a double-

blind placebo-controlled crossover study. *Neurology* 2006;**67**:2159–63.

214. O'Quinn S, Ephross SA, Williams V, Davis RL, Gutterman DL, Fox AW. Pregnancy and perinatal outcomes in migraineurs using sumatriptan: a prospective study. *Arch Gynecol Obstet* 1999;**263**:7–12.

215. Olesen C, Steffensen FH, Sorensen HT, Nielsen GL, Olsen J. Pregnancy outcome following prescription for sumatriptan. *Headache* 2000;**40**:20–4.

216. Källen B, Lygner PE. Delivery outcome in women who used drugs for migraine during pregnancy with special reference to sumatriptan. *Headache* 2001;**41**:351–6.

217. Fox AW, Chambers CD, Anderson PO, Diamond ML, Spierings EL. Evidence-based assessment of pregnancy outcome after sumatriptan exposure. *Headache* 2002;**42**:8–15.

218. Loder E. Safety of sumatriptan in pregnancy: a review of the data so far. *CNS Drugs* 2003;**17**:1–7.

219. Evans EW, Lorber KC. Use of 5-HT1 agonists in pregnancy. *Ann Pharmacother* 2008;**42**:543–9.

220. Goadsby PJ, Goldberg J, Silberstein SD. The pregnant migraineur: what can be done? *Br Med J* 2008;**336**:1502–4.

221. Evers S, May A, Fritsche G, *et al.* Akuttherapie und Prophylaxe der Migräne. Leitlinie der Deutschen Migräne- und Kopfschmerzgesellschaft und der Deutschen Gesellschaft für Neurologie. *Nervenheilkunde* 2008;**27**:933–49.

222. Überall MA, Wenzel D. Intranasal sumatriptan for the acute treatment of migraine in children. *Neurology* 1999;**52**:1507–10.

223. Winner P, Rothner AD, Saper J, *et al.* A randomized, double-blind, placebo-controlled study of sumatriptan nasal spray in the treatment of acute migraine in adolescents. *Pediatrics* 2000;**106**:989–97.

224. Ahonen K, Hämäläinen M, Rantala H, Hoppu K. Nasal sumatriptan is effective in treatment of migraine attacks in children: a randomized trial. *Neurology* 2004;**62**:883–7.

225. Hämäläinen ML, Hoppu K, Santavuori P. Sumatriptan for migraine attacks in children: a randomized placebo-controlled study. Do children with migraine attacks respond to oral sumatriptan differently from adults? *Neurology* 1997;**48**:1100–3.

226. Evers S. Drug treatment of migraine in children. A comparative review. *Paediatr Drugs* 1999;**1**:7–18.

227. Winner P, Lewis D, Visser H, Jiang K, Ahrens S, Evans JK, Rizatriptan Adolescent Study Group. Rizatriptan 5 mg for the acute treatment of migraine in adolescents: a randomized, double-blind, placebo-controlled study. *Headache* 2002;**42**:49–55.

228. Solomon GD, Cady RK, Klapper JA, Earl NL, Saper JR, Ramadan NM. Clinical efficacy and tolerability of 2.5 mg zolmitriptan for the acute treatment of migraine. *Neurology* 1997;**49**:1219–25.

229. Tepper SJ, Donnan GA, Dowson AJ, *et al.* A long-term study to maximise migraine relief with zolmitriptan. *Curr Med Res Opin* 1999;**15**:254–71.

230. Evers S, Rahmann A, Kraemer C, *et al.* Treatment of childhood migraine attacks with oral zolmitriptan and ibuprofen. *Neurology* 2006;**67**:497–9.

231. Lewis DW, Winner P, Hershey AD, Wasiewski WW, Adolescent Migraine Steering Committee. Efficacy of zolmitriptan nasal spray in adolescent migraine. *Pediatrics* 2007;**120**:390–6.

232. Ahonen K, Hämäläinen ML, Eerola M, Hoppu K. A randomized trial of rizatriptan in migraine attacks in children. *Neurology* 2006;**67**:1135–40.

233. Winner P, Pearlman EM, Linder SL, Jordan DM, Fisher AC, Hulihan J. Topiramate for migraine prevention in children: a randomized, double-blind, placebo-controlled trial. *Headache* 2005;**45**:1304–12.

234. Winner P, Gendolla A, Stayer C, *et al.* Topiramate for migraine prevention in adolescents: a pooled analysis of efficacy and safety. *Headache* 2006;**46**:1503–10.

CHAPTER 11

Cluster headache and other trigemino-autonomic cephalgias

S. Evers,[1] J. Áfra,[2] A. Frese,[1,3] P. J. Goadsby,[4] M. Linde,[5] A. May,[6] P. S. Sándor[7]

[1]University of Münster, Germany; [2]National Institute of Neurosurgery, Budapest, Hungary; [3]Academy of Manual Medicine, Münster, Germany; [4]University of California, San Francisco, CA, USA, and UCL, Institute of Neurology, Queen Square, London, UK; [5]Cephalea Headache Centre, Läkarhuset Södra vägen, Gothenburg, Sweden; [6]University of Hamburg, Germany; [7]University of Zurich, Switzerland

Objectives

These guidelines aim to give evidence-based recommendations for the treatment of cluster headache attacks, for the prophylaxis of cluster headache, for the treatment of paroxysmal hemicranias, and for the treatment of SUNCT syndrome. A brief clinical description of the headache disorders is included. The definition of the headache disorders follows the diagnostic criteria of the International Headache Society (IHS).

Background

The second edition of the classification of the IHS provided a new primary headache grouping named the trigemino-autonomic cephalgias (TAC) [1]. All these headache syndromes have two features in common: relatively short-lasting, unilateral, severe headache attacks and typical accompanying cranial autonomic symptoms (although the latter are not obligatory). These autonomic symptoms occur on the side of headache and comprise lacrimation, conjunctival injection, rhinorrhoea, miosis, and ptosis. The following syndromes belong to the TAC:
• episodic and chronic cluster headache
• episodic and chronic paroxysmal hemicrania

• SUNCT syndrome (short-lasting unilateral neuralgiform headache attacks with conjunctival injection and tearing).

These syndromes differ in duration, frequency, and rhythmicity of the attacks, and in the intensity of pain and autonomic symptoms. The pathophysiology of TAC has been in the focus of intensive research for several years [2–4].

The purpose of this paper is to give evidence-based treatment recommendations for the different TAC. The recommendations are based on the scientific evidence from clinical trials and on the expert consensus by this EFNS task force. The legal aspects of drug prescription and drug availability in the different European countries will not be considered. The definitions of the recommendation levels follow the EFNS criteria [5].

Search strategy

A literature search was performed using the reference databases MEDLINE, Science Citation Index, and the Cochrane Library; the key words used were 'cluster headache', 'paroxysmal hemicrania', 'SUNCT', 'treatment', and 'trial' (last search in March 2009). All papers published in English, German, or French were considered when they described a controlled trial or a case series on the treatment of at least five patients (or fewer in paroxysmal hemicrania or SUNCT syndrome). In addition, a review book [6] and the German treatment recommendations for cluster headache [7] were considered.

European Handbook of Neurological Management: Volume 1, 2nd edition. Edited by N. E. Gilhus, M. P. Barnes and M. Brainin.
© 2011 Blackwell Publishing Ltd.

Method for reaching consensus

All authors performed an independent literature search. The first draft of the manuscript was written by the chairman of the task force. All other members of the task force read the first draft and discussed changes by email. A second draft was then written by the chairman and was again discussed by email. All recommendations had to be agreed to by all members of the task force unanimously. The background of the research strategy and of reaching consensus and the definitions of the recommendation levels used in this paper have been described in the EFNS recommendations [5]

Table 11.1 Diagnostic criteria of cluster headache.

A At least five attacks fulfilling criteria B–D
B Severe or very severe unilateral orbital, supraorbital and/or temporal pain lasting 15–180 min if untreated
C Headache is accompanied by at least one of the following:
   1. ipsilateral conjunctival injection and/or lacrimation
   2. ipsilateral nasal congestion and/or rhinorrhoea
   3. ipsilateral eyelid oedema
   4. ipsilateral forehead and facial sweating
   5. ipsilateral miosis and/or ptosis
   6. sense of restlessness or agitation
D Attacks have a frequency from one every other day to eight per day
E Not attributed to another disorder

Clinical syndromes

The diagnosis of a headache belonging to the TAC is based on the patient's history and on a neurological examination. Electrophysiological and laboratory examinations, including examination of the cerebrospinal fluid (CSF), are not helpful. For the first diagnosis and in the case of an abnormal neurological examination, a cranial magnetic resonance imaging (MRI) or a computed tomography (CT) scan should be performed to exclude abnormalities of the brain. Particularly in older patients, mass lesions or malformations in the midline have been described to be associated with symptomatic cluster headache.

Episodic and chronic cluster headache (IHS 3.1)

The diagnostic criteria of cluster headache are presented in table 11.1. Cluster headache is defined as a paroxysmal, strongly unilateral, very severe headache, typically with a retro-orbital maximum of pain. The occurrence of cranial autonomic symptoms such as Horner's syndrome, lacrimation, and rhinorrhoea ipsilateral and simultaneous to the pain is obligatory (but can be replaced by restlessness/ agitation). The attacks occur up to eight times a day, sometimes with a nocturnal preponderance, and last between 15 and 180 min, rarely several hours. The episodic form of cluster headache occurs in 80% of patients with bouts lasting between 7 and 365 days separated by pain-free remission periods longer than one month. Sometimes, asymptomatic periods lasting even years can be observed. If the cluster attacks occur for longer than

1 year without remission periods or with remission periods lasting less than 1 month, the diagnosis is chronic cluster headache. This is the case in 15–20% of patients. The two forms do not necessarily evolve from one another. Often, the attacks start at the same time of day or night, frequently about 1–2 h after falling asleep (mostly during the first REM period in the sleep) or in the early morning. Cluster headache is regarded as a biorhythmic disorder because the attacks often occur with a strong periodicity and because the cluster bouts regularly occur during spring and autumn. Furthermore, changes of the diurnal release of hormones involved in biorhythmicity have been detected. The lifetime prevalence of cluster headache is between 0.06 [8] and 0.4% [9], with a male to female ratio between 2.5:1 and 7.1:1 [10]. In recent years, the number of female patients who report cluster headache has increased [11, 12]. It is not clear if this is a genuine change or simply increased recognition. A genetic background for cluster headache has not been described but is likely [13]. Cluster headache can be seen in children and is just as devastating in that age group. There is a familial occurrence in 2–7%. On average, the headache starts at the age of 28–30 years (but can start in every age). After 15 years, 80% of the cluster headache patients still have attacks [10].

Episodic and chronic paroxysmal hemicrania (IHS 3.2)

Paroxysmal hemicrania was first described in 1974 in its chronic form ([14]; for recent review see [15]). The paroxysmal headache attacks, the character and localization

Table 11.2 Diagnostic criteria of paroxysmal hemicrania.

A At least 20 attacks fulfilling criteria B–D

B Attacks of severe unilateral orbital, supraorbital, or temporal pain lasting 2–30 min

C Headache is accompanied by at least one of the following:
  1. ipsilateral conjunctival injection and/or lacrimation
  2. ipsilateral nasal congestion and/or rhinorrhoea
  3. ipsilateral eyelid oedema
  4. ipsilateral forehead and facial sweating
  5. ipsilateral miosis and/or ptosis

D Attacks have a frequency above five per day for more than half the time, although periods with lower frequency may occur

E Attacks are prevented completely by therapeutic doses of indomethacin

F Not attributed to another disorder

Table 11.3 Diagnostic criteria of SUNCT syndrome.

A At least five attacks fulfilling criteria B–D

B Attacks of unilateral orbital, supraorbital or temporal stabbing or pulsating pain lasting 5–240 s

C Pain is accompanied by ipsilateral conjunctival injection and lacrimation

D Attacks occur with a frequency from 3–200 per day

E Not attributed to another disorder

of pain, and the autonomic symptoms are very similar to those observed in cluster headache. In contrast to cluster headache, the attacks are shorter (2–30 min) and more frequent (more than five attacks per day). The autonomic symptoms are often less severe than in cluster headache. The diagnostic criteria of paroxysmal hemicrania are given in table 11.2. Some patients report that their attacks can be triggered by irritation of the neck, in particular in the cervical segments C2 and C3. As for cluster headache, there is an episodic and a chronic form of paroxysmal hemicrania. The criteria for this differentiation are the same as in cluster headache (see above). The most important criterion for the diagnosis of paroxysmal hemicrania is the complete response to indomethacin. Within 1 week (often within 3 days) after the initiation of indomethacin at an adequate dose the attacks disappear, and this effect is maintained long term. The prevalence is very low, exact figures are not known. It is estimated that the paroxysmal hemicranias comprise about 3–6% of all TAC. The headaches usually start between the age of 20 and 40 years, although children as young as 3 years old with clear indomethacin responses have been described [16]. In contrast to cluster headache, the male to female ratio is 1 : 3.

SUNCT syndrome (IHS 3.3)

The name of this syndrome (short-lasting unilateral neuralgiform headache attacks with conjunctival injection and tearing) describes its typical clinical features. It was first described in 1989 [17]; for review see [18]. The

diagnostic criteria are given in table 11.3. SUNCT syndrome is characterized by very short (5–240 s) attacks with neuralgiform pain quality and severe intensity. The attacks occur in a frequency of in average 60 per day (3–200 per day), are strictly unilateral (periorbital), and are often triggered by touching, speaking, or chewing. When triggerable, there is no refractory period of triggering attacks. The autonomic symptoms are mostly restricted to lacrimation and conjunctival injection. Distinct episodic and chronic forms of SUNCT syndrome are yet to be recognized in formal classifications, but both types occur. The most important differential diagnosis is classical trigeminal neuralgia. In trigeminal neuralgia, unlike in SUNCT syndrome, autonomic symptoms are not prominent and triggered attacks have a clear refractory period. SUNCT syndrome is uncommon and its true frequency is completely unclear. The male to female ratio is 1 : 4. The diagnosis of SUNCT syndrome follows the same algorithm as described for cluster headache.

Treatment of cluster headache

The treatment of cluster headache is based on empirical data rather than on a pathophysiological concept of this disorder [4, 19]. Drug treatment can be divided into acute attack abortion and prophylaxis [7, 20]. Non-drug treatment is ineffective in nearly all patients. It has, however, to be considered that drug treatment in cluster headache shows a placebo rate similar to that observed in migraine treatment [21](table 11.4).

Attack treatment

Inhalation of pure (100%) oxygen with a flow of at least 7 l/min (sometimes more than 10 l/min) is effective

Table 11.4 Treatment recommendations for cluster headache, paroxysmal hemicrania, and SUNCT syndrome. For exact doses see text. (A denotes effective, B denotes probably effective, C denotes possibly effective)

	Cluster headache	paroxysmal hemicrania	SUNCT syndrome
Attack treatment	oxygen inhalation (A) sumatriptan 6 mg s.c. (A) zolmitriptan 5 mg nasal (A) sumatriptan 20 mg nasal (A) zolmitriptan 10 mg oral (B) lidocaine nasal (B) octreotide (B)	none	none
Prophylactic treatment	verapamil (A) steroids (A) lithium (B) methysergide (B) topiramate (B) ergotamine tartrate (B) valproic acid (C) melatonin (C) baclofen (C)	indomethacin (A) verapamil (C) NSAIDs (C) topiramate (C)	lamotrigine (C)

in abortion of cluster headache attacks [22–24]. The inhalation should be for 20 min in a sitting, upright position with a face mask. There are no contraindications known for the use of oxygen. It is safe and without side effects. About 60% of all cluster headache patients respond to this treatment with a significant pain reduction within 30 min [25, 26].

In double-blind, placebo-controlled trials, the 5-HT1$_{B/D}$ agonist sumatriptan injected subcutaneously is effective in about 75% of all cluster headache patients (i.e. pain-free within 20 min) [27, 28, 29]. It is safe and without side effects in most of the patients even after frequent use [30, 31]. Contraindications are cardio- and cerebrovascular disorders and untreated arterial hypertension. The most unpleasant side effects are chest pain and distal paresthesia. In open prospective observational studies [32, 33], even 3 mg subcutaneous sumatriptan is effective in the majority of patients. Zolmitriptan 5 mg nasal spray has also been shown to be effective in two placebo-controlled trials and has recently been approved by the EMEA for the acute treatment of cluster headache [34, 35]. In single open and double-blind, placebo-controlled trials, sumatriptan nasal spray 20 mg [36, 37] and oral zolmitriptan 10 mg [38] were also effective within 30 min. In the latter

study, only patients with episodic cluster headache responded.

Oral ergotamine has been used in the treatment of cluster headache attacks for more than 50 years [39–41] and is effective when given very early in the attack. It was then recommended for the acute cluster headache attack treatment as an aerosol spray [42–45]. However, more recent trials are missing. The intranasal application of dihydroergotamine in cluster headache attacks was not superior to placebo in a single trial [46]. Very recently, the intravenous application of 1 mg dihydroergotamine over 3 days has been shown to be effective in the abortion of severe cluster attacks in an open retrospective trial [47].

For short-term prophylaxis, ergotamine has also been studied. Ergotamine suppositories need a long time until the onset of efficacy. They have been proposed in a dose of 2 mg for short-term prophylaxis, given in the evening to prevent cluster headache attacks in the night [48]. Also, regular intramuscular or subcutaneous injections of ergotamine tartrate 0.25–0.5 mg have been studied successfully in the prevention of nightly attacks [49, 50].

The nasal installation of lidocaine (1 ml with a concentration of 4–10%; the head should be reclined by 45° and rotated to the affected side by 30 to 40°) is effective in at least one-third of patients [51–55]. The use of lidocaine evolved from early observations that cocaine is effective in aborting cluster headache attacks. This has been supported in an open and not controlled trial with 10% intranasal cocaine [55].

Recently, 100 µg subcutaneous octreotide has been shown to be effective in the treatment of acute cluster headache attacks in a double-blind, placebo-controlled trial [56].

Meanwhile, also in cluster headache patients, a risk for the development of medication overuse headache has been shown, in particular if there is a comorbidity or a family history of migraine [57].

Prophylactic drug treatment

Verapamil in a daily dose of 240–960 mg has been established as drug of first choice in the prophylaxis of episodic and chronic cluster headache [7, 20], although only a few double-blind, placebo-controlled trials which are properly designed and useful for high-grade level of evidence are available. Controlled trials compared verapamil and lithium with placebo, showing an efficacy of both substances with a more rapid action of verapamil [58], or compared verapamil 360 mg with placebo showing superiority of verapamil [59]. In some cases, a daily dose of more than 720 mg can be necessary [60]. Regular ECG controls are required to control for increase in cardiac conduction time. Sometimes, echocardiography can be necessary due to the negative inotropic effects of verapamil. Side effects of verapamil are bradycardia, oedema, constipation, gastrointestinal discomfort, gingival hyperplasia, and dull headache. There is no evidence for the optimal way of dosing verapamil. An increase of 80 mg every 3 days is recommended. The full efficacy of verapamil can be expected within 2 to 3 weeks. Since verapamil is usually well tolerated, it is also drug of first choice for continuous treatment in chronic cluster headache. In the first 2 weeks of verapamil administration, corticosteroids are also administered by some clinicians. In two small open studies, nimodipine was also effective [61, 62].

There are insufficient randomized, placebo-controlled trials for the use of corticosteroids in cluster headache. Several open studies and case series have been published and reviewed by Ekbom [63]. All reported efficacy of corticosteroids given in different regimes (30 mg predni-

sone and higher; 2 × 4 mg dexamethasone per day). By expert consensus, steroids are recommended for short-term use over 2–3 weeks when rapid control of attacks is desired. However, some patients are attack-free only under steroids and rarely continuous administration of steroids is necessary. There is no evidence on which to use corticosteroids, although their high morbidity suggests caution, short courses, and avoidance in chronic cluster headache. For the beginning of corticosteroid treatment, prednisone 60–100 mg given once a day for at least 5 days is recommended, to be decreased by 10 mg every day. At high dose, about 70–80% of all cluster headache patients respond to steroids. Intravenous and oral application of steroids can successfully be combined [64]. In the experience of the task force, 500 mg methylprednisone intravenously for up to 5 days can be even more effective.

Lithium (given as lithium carbonate) has been studied in cluster headache prophylaxis in a daily dose between 600 and 1500 mg in more than 20 open trials reviewed by Ekbom [65]. An improvement in chronic cluster headache was reported to be as high as 78% (63% in episodic cluster headache). A recent placebo-controlled trial, however, did not show any efficacy of lithium in episodic cluster headache [66]. In a comparative, double-blind crossover study, lithium and verapamil showed similar efficacy with a more rapid improvement and better tolerability for verapamil [58]. Lithium should be monitored by the plasma level which should be between 0.3 and 1.2 mmol/l [67]. Regular control of liver, renal, and thyroid function and of electrolytes is required. Major side effects are hypothyroidosis, tremor, and renal dysfunction. Lithium is commonly used in cluster headache. This is, however, based on very small and open studies with the evidence being somewhat more convincing in chronic cluster headache. Therefore, lithium is recommended in particular for chronic cluster headache and only when other drugs are ineffective or contraindicated.

The antoiserotonergic drug pizotifen (3 mg per day) has been shown to be effective in cluster headache prophylaxis in a single-blind, placebo-controlled older trial [68]. However, its use is limited by side effects such as tiredness and weight gain.

Methysergide has been recommended as prophylactic drug in episodic cluster headache [7, 63]. However, no placebo-controlled, double-blind studies are available.

The efficacy rates reported in open studies were reviewed by Ekbom [63]. The number of patients with a benefit of methysergide ranged between 20 and 73%; it was more effective in episodic cluster headache. The doses applied in the open studies varied from 4 mg to 16 mg. In the experience of the task force, methysergide can be given in a daily dose of up to 12 mg (starting with 1 mg per day). Since there is small but important incidence of pulmonary and retroperitoneal fibrosis, the continuous use of methysergide is limited to a maximum of 6 months.

Valproic acid has been studied in two open trials with acceptable results [69, 70] and in one controlled study in which it did not differentiate from placebo [71]. The objective evidence, and our experience, is that valproic acid is generally ineffective in cluster headache but can be tried as drug of third choice in a daily dose between 5 and 20 mg per kg body weight.

Open studies suggest that topiramate [72–74] and gabapentin [75] are effective in the prophylaxis of cluster headache. The recommended dose is at least 100 mg per day, the starting dose should be 25 mg. Main side effects are cognitive disturbances, paraesthesias, and weight loss. It is contraindicated in nephrolithiasis.

The pre-emptive use of 5-HT$_{1B/D}$ agonists (triptans) in cluster headache remains controversial. Oral sumatriptan (100 mg) given three times a day were not effective in preventing cluster headache attacks in a placebo-controlled trial [76]. In open trials, 40 mg eletriptan per day [77] or 2.5–5 mg naratriptan per day [78] reduced the number of cluster headache attacks.

For the ipsilateral intranasal application of capsaicin, two open [79, 80] and one double-blind, placebo-controlled [81] trials have been published showing an efficacy in about two-thirds of patients after repeated application. Intranasal application of civamide showed a modest efficacy in a recent double-blind, placebo-controlled study [82]. Although such studies are claimed to be blinded, this is a major design issue given the irritating nature of the nasally applied treatment.

Oral melatonin 10 mg was effective in a single double-blind, placebo-controlled study [83]. In cluster headache refractory to other medication, however, melatonin used open-label did not produce any additional efficacy [84].

There is very weak evidence from a small open study for the efficacy of baclofen 15–30 mg [85], and insufficient evidence for the efficacy of botulinum toxin [86] or transdermal clonidine [87] in the prophylactic treatment of cluster headache. These approaches in our experience offer nothing useful to patients with cluster headache.

Hyperbaric oxygen inhalation was suggested to be effective as prophylaxis in an open trial [88]. However, a more recent placebo-controlled, double-blind trial could not confirm that hyperbaric oxygen is effective in preventing cluster headache attacks [89].

There is no evidence for a superiority of combined prophylactic drug treatment in cluster headache, although this question has not been systematically studied.

Interventional and surgical treatment

It has been observed that greater occipital nerve blockade resulted in a significant reduction of cluster headache attacks in up to two-thirds of patients [90, 91] or less [92]. This finding confirmed previous observations but needs to be replicated in controlled trials. Also, suboccipital injection of short- and long-acting steroids was shown to be effective in the prophylaxis of cluster headache in a double-blind, placebo-controlled trial [93, 94].

If all drugs are ineffective, contraindicated, or not tolerated, and a secondary cluster headache has been excluded, surgical treatment can be discussed. Surgical procedures should be approached with great caution because no reliable long-term observational data are available and because some procedures can induce trigeminal neuralgia or anaesthesia dolorosa [63]. Unlike in trigeminal neuralgia, surgical treatment of cluster headache is not a causal therapy and continuation of cluster headache after the procedure is observed regularly. Different methods have been suggested to prevent cluster headache: application of glycerrhol or local anaesthetics into the cisterna trigeminalis of the Gasserian ganglion [95]; radiofrequency rhizotomy or gamma knife treatment of the Gasserian ganglion [96] or of the trigeminal nerve [97]; microvascular decompression [98]; resection or blockade of the N. petrosus superficialis [99] or of the ganglion sphenopalatinum [100, 101]. However, there are also case reports on different surgical procedures [102–104] and one prospective study on gamma knife treatment [105, 106] showing long-term inefficacy of surgical treatment in TACs.

Given that trigeminal destructive procedures have certain morbidity and that nerve root section has a well-described morbidity, the task force sees these procedures as surplanted by neuromodulatory procedures. Deep brain stimulation of the posterior inferior hypothalamus has been shown to be effective in about half or more of patients with intractable cluster headache [107–111]. This method is only useful for prevention, not for acute attack abortion [112]. Also, electrical stimulation of the greater occipital nerve has been described as efficacious in intractable chronic cluster headache in open-label studies [113–115]. These two methods appear to be the most promising as prospective therapeutic option in patients with otherwise intractable chronic cluster headache.

Recommendations

Level A As first choice, acute attacks of cluster headache should be treated with the inhalation of 100% oxygen with at least 7 l/min over 15 min (Class II trials) or with the subcutaneous injection of 6 mg sumatriptan or the intranasal application of zolmitriptan 5 mg (Class I trials). As second choice, sumatriptan 20 mg nasal spray can be used (Class I trial with minor efficacy or more side effects).

Prophylaxis of cluster headache should be first tried with verapamil in a daily dose of at least 240 mg (maximum dose depends on efficacy or tolerability; ECG controls are obligatory with increasing doses). Although no Class I or II trials are available, steroids are clearly effective in cluster headache. Therefore, the use of at least 100 mg oral up to 500 mg i.v. per day methylprednisone (or equivalent corticosteroid) over 5 days (then tapering down) is recommended.

Level B Intranasal lidocaine (4%) can be tried in acute cluster headache attacks if Level A medication is ineffective or contraindicated. Oral zolmitriptan 10 mg is effective in some patients (Class I trial but high dose produces many side effects and limits practical use).

Methysergide and lithium are drugs of second choice if verapamil is ineffective or contraindicated. Corticosteroids can be used for short courses where bouts are short or to help establish another medicine. Topiramate is promising but only open trials exist at this point. Melatonin is useful in some patients. Except for lithium, the maximum dose depends on efficacy and tolerability. Ergotamine tartrate is recommended in short-term prophylaxis (Class III studies). In spite of positive Class II studies, pizotifen and intranasal capsaicin should not be used because of side effects.

Level C Baclofen 15–30 mg and valproic acid showed possible efficacy and can be tried as drugs of third choice. Surgical procedures are not indicated in most patients with cluster headache. Patients with intractable chronic cluster headache should be referred to centres with expertise in both destructive and neuromodulatory procedures to be offered all reasonable alternatives before a definitive procedure is conducted.

Treatment of paroxysmal hemicrania

By definition, indomethacin in a daily dose of up to 200 mg is completely effective [116–118]. For the same reason, no placebo-controlled trials exist. Indomethacin should be administered in three or more doses per day because of its short half-life time of 4 h. Many patients need a high dose of indomethacin only in the first weeks of treatment, then a lower dose can be tried. Very rarely, doses higher than 200 mg per day are required. The major contraindication is a gastrointestinal disorder. Gastrointestinal discomfort and bleedings are the major side effects. Therefore, a proton pump inhibitor should be given in addition. For diagnostic and rapid therapeutic purposes, the so-called indo-test has been suggested [119]. Intramuscular indomethacin 50 mg should result in freedom of attacks within 30 min.

There is no drug of similar efficacy to indomethacin for the treatment of paroxysmal hemicrania. However, open studies (Class IV) suggest a moderate efficacy of alternative drugs if indomethacin is not tolerated. The best evidence in these open studies has been observed for verapamil [118, 120]. Fewer positive reports have been published for acetazolamide [121], topiramate [122, 123], and the NSAIDs piroxicam [124] and acetylsalicylic acid [14, 118]. Subcutaneous sumatriptan is ineffective [125]. Anaesthetic blockades of pericranial nerves [126] are said to be ineffective, although one of us has seen excellent response to greater occipital nerve blockade.

In summary, proxysmal hemicrania is to be treated with indomethacin up to 200 mg (Level A recommendation). Alternatively, verapamil, topiramate, and different NSAIDs can be tried (Level C recommendation).

Treatment of SUNCT syndrome

There is no consistently effective treatment known for SUNCT syndrome, including high doses of indomethacin and anaesthetic blockades [127]. No controlled trials have been published, and the rareness of the syndrome makes this a difficult task. However, some case reports have been published with individual efficacy of some drugs. Because of the extreme burden caused by this disorder, all reasonable treatment options should be tried.

Among all drugs tried in SUNCT syndrome, lamotrigine was most efficacious in the published case reports (however, the majority of patients did not respond to this drug) [128–130]. Other treatment options include gabapentin [131–133], topiramate [28, 134], oxcarbazepine [135], verapamile [136], intravenous lidocaine [137], steroids [138], and intravenous phenytoin [139]. In part, these drugs were applied in combination.

Recently, also in SUNCT syndrome, stimulation of the hypothalamus has been described as efficacious in some cases [140, 141].

In summary, no recommendation can be given for the treatment of SUNCT syndrome. Treatment with lamotrigine (at least 100 mg) is considered the first-line option.

Conflicts of interest

The present guidelines were developed without external financial support. The authors report the following financial supports.

Stefan Evers: Salary by the University of Münster; honoraries and research grants by Addex Pharm, AGA Medical, Allergan, Almirall, AstraZeneca, Berlin Chemie, Boehringer, CoLucid, Desitin, Eisai, GlaxoSmithKline, Ipsen Pharma, Janssen Cilag, MSD, Novartis, Pfizer, Pharm Allergan, Pierre Fabre, Reckitt-Benckiser, UCB.

Judit Áfra: Salary by the Hungarian Ministry of Health.

Achim Frese: Private praxis; honorary by Berlin Chemie.

Peter J. Goadsby: Salary from University of California, San Francisco; honorarium or research grants in 2008 from Almirall, Boston Scientific, Colucid, Eli-Lilly, GSK, J&J, MAP Pharmaceuticals MSD, Medtronic, Neuralieve.

Mattias Linde: Salary by the Swedish government; honoraries by AstraZeneca, GlaxoSmithKline, MSD, Nycomed, Pfizer.

Arne May: Salary by the University Hospital of Hamburg; honoraries by Almirall, AstraZeneca, Bayer Vital, Berlin Chemie, GlaxoSmithKline, Janssen Cilag, MSD, Pfizer.

Peter S. Sándor: Salary by the University Hospital of Zurich; honoraries by AstraZeneca, GlaxoSmithKline, Janssen Cilag, Pfizer, Pharm Allergan.

References

1. Headache Classification Committee of the International Headache Society. The international classification of head-ache disorders, 2nd edition. *Cephalalgia* 2004;**24**(Suppl. 1): 1–160.

2. Sjaastad O. *Cluster Headache Syndrome*. London: WB Saunders, 1992.

3. Goadsby PJ. Short-lasting primary headaches: focus on trigeminal automatic cephalgias and indomethacin-sensitive headaches. *Curr Opin Neurol* 1999;**12**:273–7.

4. May A. Headaches with (ipsilateral) autonomic symptoms. *J Neurol* 2003;**250**:1273–8.

5. Brainin M, Barnes M, Baron JC, *et al.* Guidance for the preparation of neurological management guidelines by EFNS scientific task forces – revised recommendations 2004. *Eur J Neurol* 2004;**11**:577–81.

6. Olesen J, Goadsby PJ, Ramadan NM, Tfelt-Hansen P, Welch KMA (eds) *The Headaches*, 3rd edn. Philadelphia: Lippincott, Williams & Wilkins, 2006.

7. May A, Evers S, Straube A, Pfaffenrath V, Diener HC. Therapie und Prophylaxe von Clusterkopfschmerzen und anderen trigemino-autonomen Kopfschmerzen. *Nerven-heilkunde* 2004;**23**:478–90.

8. Tonon C, Guttmann S, Volpini M, Naccarato S, Cortelli P, D'Alessandro R. Prevalence and incidence of cluster headache in the Republic of San Marino. *Neurology* 2002;**58**:1407–9.

9. Sjaastad O, Bakketeig LS. Cluster headache prevalence. Vaga study of headache epidemiology. *Cephalalgia* 2003;**23**:528–33.

10. Bahra A, May A, Goadsby PJ. Cluster headache: a prospective clinical study with diagnostic implications. *Neurology* 2002;**58**:354–61.

11. Ekbom K, Svensson DA, Traff H, Waldenlind E. Age at onset and sex ratio in cluster headache: observations over three decades. *Cephalalgia* 2002;**22**:94–100.

12. Manzoni GC. Gender ratio of cluster headache over the years: a possible role of changes in lifestyle. *Cephalalgia* 1998;**18**:138–42.

13. Russell MB. Epidemiology and genetics of cluster headache. *Lancet Neurol* 2004;**3**:279–83.

14. Sjaastd O, Dale I. Evidence for a new (?) treatable headache entity. *Headache* 1974;**14**:105–8.

15. Dodick DW. Indomethacin-responsive headache syndromes. *Curr Pain Headache Rep* 2004;**8**:19–26.

16. Blankenburg M, Hechler T, Dubbel G, Wamsler C, Zernikow B. Paroxysmal hemicrania in children-symptoms, diagnostic criteria, therapy and outcome. *Cephalalgia* 2009;**29**:873–82.

17. Sjaastad O, Saunte C, Salvesen R, *et al.* Shortlasting, unilateral neuralgiform headache attacks with conjunctival injection, tearing, sweating, and rhinorrhea. *Cephalalgia* 1989;**19**:147–56.

18. Matharu MS, Cohen AS, Boes CJ, Goadsby PJ. Short-lasting unilateral neuralgiform headache with conjunctival injection and tearing syndrome: a review. *Curr Pain Headache Rep* 2003;**7**:308–18.

19. May A, Leone M. Update on cluster headache. *Curr Opin Neurol* 2003;**16**:333–40.

20. Matharu MS, Boes CJ, Goadsby PJ. Management of trigeminal autonomic cephalgias and hemicrania continua. *Drugs* 2003;**63**:1637–77.

21. Nilsson Remahl AI, Laudon Meyer E, Cordonnier C, Goadsby PJ. Placebo response in cluster headache trials: a review. *Cephalalgia* 2003;**23**:504–10.

22. Horton BT. Histaminic cephalgia: differential diagnosis and treatment. *Mayo Clin Proc* 1956;**31**:325–33.

23. Kudrow L. Response of cluster headache to oxygen inhalation. *Headache* 1981;**21**:1–4.

24. Fogan L. Treatment of cluster headache. A double-blind comparison of oxygen v air inhalation. *Arch Neurol* 1985;**42**:362–3.

25. Ekbom K. Treatment of cluster headache: clinical trials, design and results. *Cephalalgia* 1995;**15**:33–6.

26. Gallagher RM, Mueller L, Ciervo CA. Analgesic use in cluster headache. *Headache* 1996;**36**:105–7.

27. Ekbom K, Monstad I, Prusinski A, Cole JA, Pilgrim AJ, Noronha D. Subcutaneous sumatriptan in the acute treatment of cluster headache: a dose comparison study. The Sumatriptan Cluster Headache Study Group. *Acta Neurol Scand* 1993;**88**:63–9.

28. Kuhn J, Vosskaemper M, Bewermeyer H. SUNCT syndrome: a possible bilateral case responding to topiramate. *Neurology* 2005;**64**:2159.

29. The Sumatriptan Cluster Headache Study Group. Treatment of acute cluster headache with sumatriptan. *N Engl J Med* 1991;**325**:322–6.

30. Ekbom K, Krabbe A, Micieli G, *et al*. Cluster headache attacks treated for up to three months with subcutaneous sumatriptan (6 mg). Sumatriptan Cluster Headache Long-term Study Group. *Cephalalgia* 1995;**15**:230–6.

31. Göbel H, Lindner V, Heinze A, Ribbat M, Peuschl G. Acute therapy for cluster headache with sumatriptan: findings of a one-year long-term study. *Neurology* 1998;**51**:908–11.

32. Krabbe A. Early clinical experience with GR43175 in acute cluster headache attacks. *Cephalalgia* 1989;**9**(Suppl. 10): 404–5.

33. Gregor N, Schlesiger C, Akova-Oztürk E, Kraemer C, Husstedt IW, Evers S. Treatment of cluster headache attacks with less than 6 mg subcutaneous sumatriptan. *Headache* 2005;**45**:1069–72.

34. Rapoport AM, Mathew NT, Silberstein SD, *et al*. Zolmitriptan nasal spray in the acute treatment of cluster headache: a double-blind study. *Neurology* 2007;**69**:821–6.

35. Cittadini E, May A, Straube A, Evers S, Bussone G, Goadsby PJ. Effectiveness of intranasal zolmitriptan in acute cluster headache: a randomized, placebo-controlled, double-blind crossover study. *Arch Neurol* 2006;**63**:1537–42.

36. Schuh-Hofer S, Reuter U, Kinze S, Einhaupl KM, Arnold G. Treatment of acute cluster headache with 20 mg sumatriptan nasal spray – an open pilot study. *J Neurol* 2002;**249**: 94–9.

37. Van Vliet JA, Bahra A, Martin V, *et al*. Intranasal sumatriptan in cluster headache: randomized placebo-controlled double-blind study. *Neurology* 2003;**60**:630–3.

38. Bahra A, Gawel MJ, Hardebo JE, Millson D, Breen SA, Goadsby PJ. Oral zolmitriptan is effective in the acute treatment of cluster headache. *Neurology* 2000;**54**:1832–9.

39. Horton BT, Ryan R, Reynolds JL. Clinical observations of the use of E.C. 110, a new agent for the treatment of headache. *Mayo Clin Proc* 1948;**23**:104–8.

40. Kunkle EC, Pfeiffer JB, Wilhoit WM, Hamrick LW. Recurrent brief attacks in cluster pattern. *Trans Am Neurol Assoc* 1952;**77**:240–3.

41. Friedman AP, Mikropoulos HE. Cluster headaches. *Neurology* 1958;**8**:653–63.

42. Speed WG. Ergotamine tartrate inhalation: a new approach for the management of recurrent vascular headaches. *Am J Med Sci* 1960;**240**:327–31.

43. Graham JR, Malvea BP, Gramm HF. Aerosol ergotamine tartrate for migraine and Horton's syndrome. *N Engl J Med* 1960;**263**:802–4.

44. Duvoisin RC, Parker GW, Kenoyer WL. The cluster headache. *Arch Intern Med* 1961;**108**:711–6.

45. Ekbom K, Krabbe AE, Paalzow G, Paalzow L, Tfelt-Hansen P, Waldenlind E. Optimal routes of administration of ergotamine tartrate in cluster headache patients. A pharmacokinetic study. *Cephalalgia* 1983;**3**:15–20.

46. Andersson PG, Jespersen LT. Dihydroergotamine nasal spray in the treatment of attacks of cluster headache. *Cephalalgia* 1986;**6**:51–4.

47. Magnoux E, Zlotnik G. Outpatient intravenous dihydroergotamine for refractory cluster headache. *Headache* 2004;**44**:249–55.

48. Horton BT. Histaminic cephalgia. *Lancet* 1952;**ii**:92–8.

49. Schiller F. Prophylatcic and other treatment for histaminic, cluster, or limited variant migraine. *JAMA* 1960;**173**: 1907–11.

50. Symonds C. A particular variety of headache. *Brain* 1956;**79**:217–32.

51. Kittrelle JP, Grouse DS, Seybold ME. Cluster headache. Local anesthetic abortive agents. *Arch Neurol* 1985;**42**: 496–8.

52. Markley HG. Topical agents in the treatment of cluster headache. *Curr Pain Headache Rep* 2003;**7**:139–43.

53. Mills TM, Scoggin JA. Intranasal lidocaine for migraine and cluster headaches. *Ann Pharmacother* 1997;**31**:914–5.

54. Robbins L. Intranasal lidocaine for cluster headache. *Headache* 1995;**35**:83–4.

55. Costa A, Pucci E, Antonaci F, *et al.* The effect of intranasal cocaine and lidocaine on nitroglycerin-induced attacks in cluster headache. *Cephalalgia* 2000;**20**:85–91.

56. Matharu MS, Levy MJ, Meeran K, Goadsby PJ. Subcutaneous octreotide in cluster headache: randomized placebo-controlled double-blind crossover study. *Ann Neurol* 2004;**56**:488–94.

57. Paemeleire K, Bahra A, Evers S, Matharu MS, Goadsby PJ. Medication-overuse headache in patients with cluster headache. *Neurology* 2006;**67**:109–13.

58. Bussone G, Leone M, Peccarisi C, *et al.* Double blind comparison of lithium and verapamil in cluster headache prophylaxis. *Headache* 1990;**30**:411–7.

59. Leone M, D'Amico D, Frediani F, *et al.* Verapamil in the prophylaxis of episodic cluster headache: a double-blind study versus placebo. *Neurology* 2000;**54**:1382–5.

60. Gabai IJ, Spierings EL. Prophylactic treatment of cluster headache with verapamil. *Headache* 1989;**29**:167–8.

61. Meyer JS, Nance M, Walker M, Zetusky WJ, Dowell RE. Migraine and cluster headache treatment with calcium antagonists supports a vascular pathogenesis. *Headache* 1985;**25**:358–67.

62. De Carolis P, Baldrati A, Agati R, De Capoa D, D'Alessandro R, Sacquegna T. Nimodipine in episodic cluster headache: results and methodological considerations. *Headache* 1987;**27**:397–9.

63. Ekbom K, Solomon S. Management of cluster headache. In: Olesen J, Tfelt-Hansen P, Welch KMA (eds) *The Headaches.* Philadelphia: Lippincott, 2000; pp. 731–40.

64. Mir P, Alberca R, Navarro A, *et al.* Prophylactic treatment of episodic cluster headache with intravenous bolus of methylprednisolone. *Neurol Sci* 2003;**24**:318–24.

65. Ekbom K. Lithium for cluster headache: review of the literature and preliminary results of long-term treatment. *Headache* 1981;**21**:132–9.

66. Steiner TJ, Hering R, Couturier EGM, Davies PTG, Whitmarsh TE. Double-blind placebo-controlled trial of lithium in episodic cluster headache. *Cephalalgia* 1997;**17**:673–5.

67. Manzoni GC, Bono C, Lanfranchi M, Micieli G, Terzano MG, Nappi G. Lithium carbonate in cluster headache: assessment of its short- and long-term therapeutic efficacy. *Cephalalgia* 1983;**3**:109–14.

68. Ekbom K. Prophylactic treatment of cluster headache with a new serotonin antagonist, BC 105. *Acta Neurol Scand* 1969;**45**:601–10.

69. Gallagher RM, Mueller LL, Freitag FG. Divalproex sodium in the treatment of migraine and cluster headaches. *J Am Osteopath Assoc* 2002;**102**:92–4.

70. Hering R, Kuritzky A. Sodium valproate in the treatment of cluster headache: an open clinical trial. *Cephalalgia* 1989;**9**:195–8.

71. El Amrani M, Massiou H, Bousser MG. A negative trial of sodium valproate in cluster headache: methodological issues. *Cephalalgia* 2002;**22**:205–8.

72. Förderreuther S, Mayer M, Straube A. Treatment of cluster headache with topiramate: effects and side-effects in five patients. *Cephalalgia* 2002;**22**:186–9.

73. Rozen TD. Antiepileptic drugs in the management of cluster headache and trigeminal neuralgia. *Headache* 2001;**41**(Suppl. 1):25–33.

74. McGeeney BE. Topiramate in the treatment of cluster headache. *Curr Pain Headache Rep* 2003;**7**:135–8.

75. Schuh-Hofer S, Israel H, Neeb L, Reuter U, Arnold G. The use of gabapentin in chronic cluster headache patients refractory to first-line therapy. *Eur J Neurol* 2007;**14**:694–6.

76. Monstad I, Krabbe A, Micieli G, *et al.* Pre-emptive oral treatment with sumatriptan during a cluster period. *Headache* 1995;**35**:607–13.

77. Zebenholzer K, Wober C, Vigl M, Wessely P. Eletriptan for the short-term prophylaxis of cluster headache. *Headache* 2004;**44**:361–4.

78. Mulder LJ, Spierings EL. Naratriptan in the preventive treatment of cluster headache. *Cephalalgia* 2002;**22**:815–7.

79. Fusco BM, Marabini S, Maggi CA, Fiore G, Geppetti P. Preventative effect of repeated nasal applications of capsaicin in cluster headache. *Pain* 1994;**59**:321–5.

80. Sicuteri F, Fusco BM, Marabini S, *et al.* Beneficial effect of capsaicin application to the nasal mucosa in cluster headache. *Clin J Pain* 1989;**5**:49–53.

81. Marks DR, Rapoport A, Padla D, *et al.* A double-blind, placebo-controlled trial of intranasal capsaicin for cluster headache. *Cephalalgia* 1993;**13**:114–6.

82. Saper JR, Klapper J, Mathew NT, Rapoport A, Phillips SB, Bernstein JE. Intranasal civamide for the treatment of episodic cluster headaches. *Arch Neurol* 2002;**59**:990–4.

83. Leone M, D'Amico D, Moschiano F, Fraschini F, Bussone G. Melatonin versus placebo in the prophylaxis of cluster headache: a double-blind pilot study with parallel groups. *Cephalalgia* 1996;**16**:494–6.

84. Pringsheim T, Magnoux E, Dobson CF, Hamel E, Aube M. Melatonin as adjunctive therapy in the prophylaxis of cluster headache: a pilot study. *Headache* 2002;**42**:787–92.

85. Hering-Hanit R, Gadoth N. Baclofen in cluster headache. *Headache* 2000;**40**:48–51.

86. Evers S. Botulinum toxin and the management of chronic headaches. *Curr Opin Otolaryngol Nead Neck Surg* 2004;**12**:197–203.

87. Leone M, Attanasio A, Grazzi L, *et al*. Transdermal clonidine in the prophylaxis of episodic cluster headache: an open study. *Headache* 1997;**37**:559–60.

88. Di Sabato F, Fusco BM, Pelaia P, Giacovazzo M. Hyperbaric oxygen therapy in cluster headache. *Pain* 1993;**52**:243–5.

89. Nilsson Remahl AI, Ansjon R, Lind F, Waldenlind E. Hyperbaric oxygen treatment of active cluster headache: a double-blind placebo-controlled cross-over study. *Cephalalgia* 2002;**22**:730–9.

90. Anthony M. Arrest of attacks of cluster headache by local steroid injection of the occipital nerve. In: Rose C (ed.) *Migraine*. Basel: Karger, 1985; pp. 169–73.

91. Peres MF, Stiles MA, Siow HC, Rozen TD, Young WB, Silberstein SD. Greater occipital nerve blockade for cluster headache. *Cephalalgia* 2002;**22**:520–2.

92. Busch V, Jakob W, Juergens T, Schulte-Mattler W, Kaube H, May A. Occipital nerve blockade in chronic cluster headache patients and functional connectivity between trigeminal and occipital nerves. *Cephalalgia* 2007;**27**:1206–14.

93. Ambrosini A, Vandenheede M, Rossi P, *et al*. Suboccipital (GON) injection with long-acting steroids in cluster headache: a double-blind placebo-controlled study. *Cephalalgia* 2003;**23**:734.

94. Ambrosini A, Vandenheede M, Rossi P, *et al*. Suboccipital injection with a mixture of rapid- and long-acting steroids in cluster headache: a double-blind placebo-controlled study. *Pain* 2005;**118**:92–6.

95. Ekbom K, Lindgren L, Nilsson BY, Hardebo JE, Waldenlind E. Retro-Gasserian glycerol injection in the treatment of chronic cluster headache. *Cephalalgia* 1987;**7**:21–7.

96. Taha JM, Tew JM Jr. Long-term results of radiofrequency rhizotomy in the treatment of cluster headache. *Headache* 1995;**35**:193–6.

97. Ford RG, Ford KT, Swaid S, Young P, Jennelle R. Gamma knife treatment of refractory cluster headache. *Headache* 1998;**38**:3–9.

98. Lovely TJ, Kotsiakis X, Jannetta PJ. The surgical management of chronic cluster headache. *Headache* 1998;**38**:590–4.

99. Onofrio BM, Campbell JK. Surgical treatment of chronic cluster headache. *Mayo Clin Proc* 1986;**61**:537–44.

100. Sanders M, Zuurmond WW. Efficacy of sphenopalatine ganglion blockade in 66 patients suffering from cluster headache: a 12- to 70-month follow-up evaluation. *J Neurosurg* 1997;**87**:876–80.

101. Narouze S, Kapural L, Casanova J, Mekhail N. Sphenopalatine ganglion radiofrequency ablation for the management of chronic cluster headache. *Headache* 2009;**49**:571–7.

102. Matharu MS, Goadsby PJ. Persistence of attacks of cluster headache after trigeminal nerve root section. *Brain* 2002;**125**:976–84.

103. Black DF, Dodick DW. Two cases of medically and surgically intractable SUNCT: a reason for caution and an argument for a central mechanism. *Cephalalgia* 2002;**22**:201–4.

104. Jarrar RG, Black DF, Dodick DW, Davis DH. Outcome of trigeminal nerve section in the treatment of chronic cluster headache. *Neurology* 2003;**60**:1360–2.

105. Donnet A, Valade D, Regis J. Gamma knife treatment for refractory cluster headache: prospective open trial. *J Neurol Neurosurg Psychiatry* 2005;**76**:218–21.

106. McClelland S 3rd, Tendulkar RD, Barnett GH, Neyman G, Suh JH. Long-term results of radiosurgery for refractory cluster headache. *Neurosurgery* 2006;**59**:1258–62.

107. Franzini A, Ferroli P, Leone M, Broggi G. Stimulation of the posterior hypothalamus for treatment of chronic intractable cluster headaches: first reported series. *Neurosurgery* 2003;**52**:1095–101.

108. Leone M, Franzini A, Bussone G. Stereotactic stimulation of posterior hypothalamic gray matter in a patient with intractable cluster headache. *N Engl J Med* 2001;**345**:1428–9.

109. Schoenen J, Di Clemente L, Vandenheede M, *et al*. Hypothalamic stimulation in chronic cluster headache: a pilot study of efficacy and mode of action. *Brain* 2005;**128**:940–7.

110. Starr PA, Barbaro NM, Raskin NH, Ostrem JL. Chronic stimulation of the posterior hypothalamic region for cluster headache: technique and 1-year results in four patients. *J Neurosurg* 2007;**106**:999–1005.

111. Bartsch T, Pinsker MO, Rasche D, *et al*. Hypothalamic deep brain stimulation for cluster headache: experience from a new multicase series. *Cephalalgia* 2008;**28**:285–95.

112. Leone M, Franzini, A, Broggi, G, Mea, E, Cecchini, AP, Bussone, G. Acute hypothalamic stimulation and ongoing cluster headache attacks. *Neurology* 2006;**67**:1844–5.

113. Schwedt TJ, Dodick DW, Hentz J, Trentman TL, Zimmerman RS. Occipital nerve stimulation for chronic headache – long-term safety and efficacy. *Cephalalgia* 2007;**27**:153–7.

114. Magis D, Allena M, Bolla M, De Pasqua V, Remacle JM, Schoenen J. Occipital nerve stimulation for drug-resistant chronic cluster headache: a prospective pilot study. *Lancet Neurol* 2007;**6**:314–21.

115. Burns B, Watkins L, Goadsby PJ. Treatment of intractable chronic cluster headache by occipital nerve stimulation in 14 patients. *Neurology* 2009;**72**:341–5.

116. Antonaci F, Sjaastad O. Chronic paroxysmal hemicrania(CPH): a review of its clinical manifestations. *Headache* 1989;**29**:648–56.

117. Sjaastad O, Stovner LJ, Stolt Nielsen A, Antonaci F, Fredriksen TA. CPH and hemicrania continua: requirements of high indomethacin dosages – an ominous sign? *Headache* 1995;**35**:363–7.

118. Evers S, Husstedt IW. Alternatives in drug treatment of chronic paroxysmal hemicrania. *Headache* 1996;**36**: 429–32.

119. Antonaci F, Pareja JA, Caminero AB, Sjaastad O. Chronic paroxysmal hemicrania and hemicrania continua. Parenteral indomethacin: the 'indotest. *Headache* 1998;**38**:122–8.

120. Shabbir N, McAbee G. Adolescent chronic paroxysmal hemicrania responsive to verapamil monotherapy. *Headache* 1994;**34**:209–10.

121. Warner JS, Wamil AW, McLean MJ. Acetazolamide for the treatment of chronic paroxysmal hemicrania. *Headache* 1994;**34**:597–9.

122. Cohen AS, Goadsby PJ. Paroxysmal hemicrania responding to topiramate. *J Neurol Neurosurg Psychiatry* 2007;**78**: 96–7.

123. Camarda C, Camarda R, Monastero R. Chronic paroxysmal hemicrania and hemicrania continua responding to topiramate: two case reports. *Clin Neurol Neurosurg* 2008;**110**:88–91.

124. Sjaastad O, Antonaci F. A piroxciam derivative partly effective in chronic paroxysmal hemicrania and hemicrania continua. *Headache* 1995;**35**:549–50.

125. Dahlöf C. Subcutaneous sumatriptan does not abort attacks of chronic paroxysmal hemicrania (CPH). *Headache* 1993;**33**:201–2.

126. Antonaci F, Pareja JA, Caminero AB, Sjaastad O. Chronic paroxysmal hemicrania and hemicrania continua: anaesthetic blockades of pericranial nerves. *Funct Neurol* 1997;**12**:11–5.

127. Pareja JA, Kruszewski P, Sjaastad O. SUNCT syndrome: trials of drugs and anaesthetic blockades. *Headache* 1995;**35**:138–42.

128. D'Andrea G, Granella F, Ghiotto N, Nappi G. Lamotrigine in the treatment of SUNCT syndrome. *Neurology* 2001;**57**: 1723–5.

129. Malik K, Rizvi S, Vaillancourt PD. The SUNCT syndrome: successfully treated with lamotrigine. *Pain Med* 2002;**3**: 167–8.

130. Chakravarty A, Mukherjee A. SUNCT syndrome responsive to lamotrigine: documentation of the first Indian case. *Cephalalgia* 2003;**23**:474–5.

131. Hunt CH, Dodick DW, Bosch EP. SUNCT responsive to gabapentin. *Headache* 2002;**42**:525–6.

132. Etemadifar M, Maghzi AH, Ghasemi M, Chitsaz A, Kaji Esfahani M. Efficacy of gabapentin in the treatment of SUNCT syndrome. *Cephalalgia* 2008;**28**:1339–42.

133. Porta-Etessam J, Benito-Leon J, Martinez-Salio A, Berbel A. Gabapentin in the treatment of SUNCT syndrome. *Headache* 2002;**42**:523–4.

134. Rossi P, Cesarino F, Faroni J, Malpezzi MG, Sandrini G, Nappi G. SUNCT syndrome successfully treated with topiramate: case reports. *Cephalalgia* 2003;**23**:998–1000.

135. Dora B. SUNCT syndrome with dramatic response to oxcarbazepine. *Cephalalgia* 2006;**26**:1171–3.

136. Narbone MC, Gangemi S, Abbate M. A case of SUNCT syndrome responsive to verapamil. *Cephalalgia* 2005;**25**: 476–8.

137. Matharu MS, Cohen AS, Goadsby PJ. SUNCT syndrome responsive to intravenous lidocaine. *Cephalalgia* 2004;**24**: 985–92.

138. De Lourdes Figuerola M, Bruera O, Pozzo MJ, Leston J. SUNCT syndrome responding absolutely to steroids in two cases with different etiologies. *J Headache Pain* 2009;**10**:55–7.

139. Schwaag S, Frese A, Husstedt IW, Evers S. SUNCT syndrome: the first German case series. *Cephalalgia* 2003;**23**:398–400.

140. Leone M, Franzini A, D'Andrea G, Broggi, G, Casucci G, Bussone G. Deep brain stimulation to relieve drug-resistant SUNCT. *Ann Neurol* 2005;**57**:924–7.

141. Lyons MK, Dodick DW, Evidente VG. Responsiveness of short-lasting unilateral neuralgiform headache with conjunctival injection and tearing to hypothalamic deep brain stimulation. *J Neurosurg* 2009;**110**:279–81.

CHAPTER 12

Diagnosis and treatment of primary (idiopathic) dystonia

A. Albanese,[1,2] F. Asmus,[3] A. Berardelli,[4] K. Bhatia,[5] A. E. Elia,[1] B. Elibol,[6] G. Filippini,[1] T. Gasser,[2] J. K. Krauss,[7] N. Nardocci,[1] A. Newton,[8] J. Valls-Solé,[9] M. Vidailhet[10]

[1]Istituto Neurologico Carlo Besta, Milan, Italy; [2]Università Cattolica del Sacro Cuore, Milan, Italy; [3]Hertie-Institute for Clinical Brain Research, University of Tubingen, Germany; [4]Università degli Studi La Sapienza, Rome, Italy; [5]Institute of Neurology, University College London, Queen Square, London, UK; [6]Hacettepe University Hospitals, Ankara, Turkey; [7]Medical School Hannover, MHH, Germany; [8]European Dystonia Federation, Brussels, Belgium; [9]Hospital Clínic, Barcelona, Spain; [10]Pôle des Maladies du Système Nerveux, Fédération de Neurologie, Paris, France

Objectives

The objective of the task force was to provide an updated version of earlier guidelines for diagnosis and treatment of primary dystonia and dystonia-plus, and to provide evidence-based recommendations for diagnosis and treatment.

Background

Dystonia is characterized by sustained muscle contractions, frequently causing repetitive twisting movements or abnormal postures [1, 2]. Although thought to be rare, dystonia may be more common than currently evidenced due to underdiagnosis or misdiagnosis. Adult-onset primary dystonia can present mainly with tremor, which could be misdiagnosed as Parkinson's disease [3]. In those cases, results of DAT scan may help with the differential diagnosis.

Primary dystonias are diseases where dystonia is the only or the largely prevalent clinical feature. Primary dystonias encompass pure dystonia, dystonia-plus, and paroxysmal dystonias (table 12.1). Areas of specific concern include clinical diagnosis, differential diagnosis

with other movement disorders, aetiology, genetic counselling, drug treatment, surgical interventions, and rehabilitation.

Search strategy

Computerized MEDLINE and EMBASE searches (2005–July 2009) were conducted using a combination of textwords, MeSH and EMTREE terms 'dystonia', 'blepharospasm', 'torticollis', 'writer's cramp', 'Meige syndrome', 'dysphonia', and 'sensitivity and specificity' or 'diagnosis', and 'clinical trial' or 'random allocation' or 'therapeutic use' limited to human studies. The Cochrane Library and the reference lists of all known primary and review articles were searched for relevant citations. No language restrictions were applied. Studies of diagnosis, diagnostic test, and various treatments for patients suffering from dystonia were considered and rated as Level A to C according to the recommendations for EFNS scientific task forces [4]. Where only Class IV evidence was available but consensus could be achieved we have proposed Good Practice Points (GPP).

Method for reaching consensus

The results of the literature searches were circulated by email to the task force members for comments. The task force chairman prepared a first draft of the manuscript based on the results of the literature review, data

European Handbook of Neurological Management: Volume 1, 2nd edition. Edited by N. E. Gilhus, M. P. Barnes and M. Brainin.

Table 12.1 Classification of dystonia based on three axes.

By cause (aetiology)
- **Primary pure dystonia**: dystonia is the only clinical sign (apart from tremor) and there is no identifiable exogenous cause or other inherited or degenerative disease. Examples are DYT1 and DYT6 dystonias
- **Primary dystonia-plus**: dystonia is a prominent sign, but is associated with another movement disorder, for example myoclonus or parkinsonism. There is no evidence of neurodegeneration. For example, DOPA-responsive dystonia (DYT5) and myoclonus-dystonia (DYT11) belong to this category
- **Primary paroxysmal**: dystonia occurs in brief episodes with normalcy in between. These disorders are classified as idiopathic (often familial, although sporadic cases also occur) and symptomatic due to a variety of causes. Three main forms are known depending on the triggering factor. In paroxysmal kinesigenic dyskinesia (PKD; DYT9) attacks are induced by sudden movement; in paroxysmal exercise-induced dystonia (PED) by exercise such as walking or swimming; and in the non-kinesigenic form (PNKD; DYT8) by alcohol, coffee, tea, etc. A complicated familial form with PNKD and spasticity (DYT10) has also been described
- **Heredodegenerative**: dystonia is a feature, among other neurological signs, of a heredodegenerative disorder, for example Wilson's disease
- **Secondary**: dystonia is a symptom of an identified neurological condition, such as a focal brain lesion, exposure to drugs or chemicals. Examples include dystonia due to a brain tumour and off-period dystonia in Parkinson's disease

By age at onset
- **Early onset** (variably defined as ≤20–30 years): usually starts in a leg or arm and frequently progresses to involve other limbs and the trunk
- **Late onset**: usually starts in the neck (including the larynx), the cranial muscles or one arm. Tends to remain localized with restricted progression to adjacent muscles

By distribution
- **Focal**: single body region (e.g. writer's cramp, blepharospasm)
- **Segmental**: contiguous body regions (e.g. cranial and cervical, cervical and upper limb)
- **Multifocal**: non-contiguous body regions (e.g. upper and lower limb, cranial and upper limb)
- **Generalized**: both legs and at least one other body region (usually one or both arms)
- **Hemidystonia**: half of the body (usually secondary to a structural lesion in the contralateral basal ganglia)

synthesis, and comments from the task force members. The draft and the recommendations were discussed during a conference held in Florence on 12 September 2009, until consensus was reached within the task force.

Results

In addition to the previously published literature screen [5], we found 299 papers, among which 191 were primary diagnostic studies and 108 were efficacy studies.

Clinical features of dystonia

Literature search on the clinical features of dystonia identified a report of a multidisciplinary working group [6], one workshop report [7], 64 primary studies on clinically based diagnosis, and 125 primary studies on the diagnostic accuracy of different laboratory tests. The primary clinical studies encompassed four cohort studies, 15 case-control studies, 12 cross-sectional, and 33 clinical series.

The clinical features of dystonia have been summarised in the previous guidelines edition [5]. More recent reviews and new primary studies have focused on specific diagnostic features; a recent review has assembled the features of dystonia into a diagnostic flowchart [8].

Dystonia is a dynamic condition that often changes in severity depending on the posture assumed and on voluntary activity of the involved body area. The changing nature of dystonia makes the development of rating scales with acceptable clinimetric properties problematic.

Three clinical scales are available for generalised dystonia: the Fahn-Marsden rating scale [9], the Unified Dystonia Rating Scale, and the global dystonia rating scale [10]. The total scores of these three scales correlate well, they have excellent internal consistency, from good to excellent inter-rater correlation, and from fair to excellent inter-rater agreement [10]. An evidence-based review identified more than 10 rating scales for cervical dystonia [11]. However, the most frequently used ones are the Toronto Western Spasmodic Torticollis Rating Scale [12], the Tsui scale [13], and the Cervical Dystonia Severity Scale [14].

Dystonia influences various aspects of quality of life, particularly those related to physical and social functioning. Class IV studies have evaluated the predictors of quality of life in dystonia [11, 15]. Functional disability, body concept, and depression were important predictors of quality of life in dystonia.

Classification

The classification is based on three axes: (a) aetiology, (b) age at onset of symptoms, and (c) distribution of body regions affected (table 12.1). The aetiological axis defines primary (idiopathic) dystonia with no identifiable exogenous cause or evidence of neurodegeneration (i.e. no progressive loss of neural cells). In the pure form, dystonia is the only clinical sign (apart from dystonic tremor). We propose to call these forms 'primary pure dystonia' (PPD). In dystonia-plus, usually there are additional movement disorders (e.g. myoclonus or parkinsonism). In the paroxysmal form, symptoms are intermittent and provoked by identifiable triggers (e.g. kinesigenic due to sudden movement, exercise-induced or non-kinesigenic). Non-primary dystonia is due to heredodegenerative diseases or secondary (symptomatic) to known causes; these forms are characterized by the presence of additional symptoms or signs, apart from movement disorders. A number of genes and gene loci have been identified for primary as well as for other forms.

Recommendations and Good Practice Points

1 The diagnosis of dystonia is clinical, the core being abnormal postures (with or without tremor) and the recognition of specific features, e.g. *gestes antagonistes*, overflow, mirror movements [5] (GPP).

2 The classification of dystonia is important for providing appropriate management, prognostic information, genetic counselling, and treatment (GPP).

3 Because of the lack of specific diagnostic tests, expert observation is recommended. Using a structured flow chart [8] may increase diagnostic accuracy (GPP).

4 Appropriate investigations are required if the initial presentation or the course suggest heredodegenerative or secondary (symptomatic) dystonia (GPP).

5 Assessment of dystonia should be performed using a validated rating scale (GPP).

Use of genetic test in diagnosis and counselling

Two genes for primary pure dystonia (PPD) have been identified: DYT1 and DYT6 [16, 17]. Three other gene loci for autosomal-dominant PPD (DYT4, DYT7, DYT13) and two forms of recessive PPD (DYT2, DYT17) have been described, with phenotypes ranging from cranial to generalized dystonia; however, the specific gene abnormality has not yet been identified [18].

All known DYT1 mutations reside in exon 5 of the TorsinA gene, except for one in exon 3 [19]. Screening for a GAG-deletion at position 302/303 is sufficient for clinical testing (Class II) [20]. Only two PPD patients have been described with missense mutations in exon 3 (p.F205I) and exon 5 (p.R288Q), and the pathogenicity of this variant has not been proven, as no familial cosegregation has been demonstrated [19, 21].

Early-onset DYT1 dystonia typically presents in childhood and usually starts in a limb, gradually and in many patients rapidly progressing to a generalized form (Class II) [20]. Many exceptions to this typical presentation have been reported, especially in mutation carriers from DYT1 families with focal or segmental dystonia of adult onset (Class IV) [22, 23]. Family studies have assessed that the penetrance of DYT1 dystonia is around 30%.

DYT1 mutations are the most important genetic cause of early onset PPD worldwide. Phenotype-genotype correlations have been assessed in different DYT1 dystonia populations (Class II and III) [20, 24]. In Ashkenazi Jews, DYT1 testing is positive in close to 100% of patients with limb-onset dystonia before age 26 years. Recommendation 1 below is based on such evidence [20, 25]. In the Western European population, the proportion of DYT1 mutation-negative dystonia is considered higher than in North America [24]. Patients with early onset PPD not caused by the DYT1 gene tend to have later age at onset, less commonly limb onset, more frequent cervical involvement, and a slower progression than DYT1 PPD cases (Class IV) [26] In patients with generalized dystonia with cranio-cervical onset, DYT6 mutations should be considered [27]. THAP1 (thanatos associated protein) has been identified to cause autosomal-dominant DYT6, 'mixed'-type dystonia in Amish-Mennonite families with cranial or limb onset at young age (from 5 to 48 years) [17, 28]. DYT6 mutations have been described in other populations with clinical presentations from focal to generalized dystonia in a few percent of cases. In particular, early-onset generalized PPD with spasmodic dysphonia is a characteristic phenotype caused by DYT6 mutations (Class IV) [27].

Four dystonia-plus syndromes have been characterized genetically: dopa-responsive dystonia (DRD, DYT5), myoclonus-dystonia (M-D, DYT11), rapid-onset dystonia-parkinsonism (RDP, DYT12), and autosomal-recessive dystonia parkinsonism (DYT16).

The most common form is DRD linked to the GCH1 (GTPcyclohydrolase I) gene. Since this is a treatable and often misdiagnosed condition, a particular effort should be made to establish a correct diagnosis. The classical phenotype comprises onset with walking difficulties before 20 years, and progression to segmental or generalized dystonia, sometimes with additional parkinsonism and sustained response to levodopa [29, 30]. Three additional DRD categories with different courses have been recognized: (1) young-onset (<20 years) cases with episodic dystonia, toe walking or progressive scoliosis throughout life; (2) compound heterozygous GCH1 mutation carriers, who develop young-onset severe DRD with initial hypotonia similar to autosomal-recessive (AR)-DRD caused by tyrosine hydroxylase (TH) mutations; (3) adult-onset DRD patients manifesting above age 30 years with mild dystonia or resting tremor or non-tremulous parkinsonism [30, 31]. To date, numerous GCH1 mutations but no phenotype-genotype correlations to specific heterozygous GCH1 mutations have been detected (see the database cured by N. Blau, and B. Thoeny: www.biopku.org/dbsearches/BIOMDB_Start.asp).

Inclusion of screening for gene dosage alterations of GCH1 [32, 33] in addition to direct sequencing has increased the rate of detected mutations to over 80% [34, 35].

If genetic testing of GCH1 is negative, other genes of the tetrahyhdrobiopterin and dopamine synthesis pathways, such as TH and sepiapterin reductase (SPR), should be considered, especially if inheritance is recessive or atypical features like mental retardation or oculogyric crises are present (Class IV) [35, 36]. Parkin mutations are a rare differential diagnosis of DRD and the diagnosis can be made by dopamine transporter imaging (Class IV) [37]. For the TH gene, sequencing of the 3'-promoter sequence is recommended to increase mutation detection (Class IV) [38].

A therapeutic trial with levodopa has been proposed for diagnostic purposes (Class IV) [39]. Alternatively, studies on pterin and dopamine metabolites from cerebrospinal fluid (CSF) or a phenylalanine loading test have been suggested as diagnostic complements [40–42], but there is no clear evidence regarding their diagnostic accuracy and both may only be performed in specialized centres. Hence, the practical recommendation still remains that every patient with early-onset dystonia without an alternative diagnosis should have a trial with levodopa. Onset of myoclonus-dystonia (M-D) peaks in childhood; the initial symptoms usually consist of lightning jerks and dystonia mostly affecting the neck and the upper limbs, with a prevalent proximal involvement and slow progression [43]. In a subset of patients, M-D presents as a gait disorder with lower-limb onset and evolves into the typical clinical presentation until adolescence [44], [45]. Myoclonus and dystonia are strikingly alleviated by alcohol in many but not in all patients [46]. However, a response to alcohol is not specific for DYT11 (Class IV)[47–49]. In patients with the typical M-D phenotype mutations in the epsilon-sarcoglycan gene (DYT11) may be detected in more than 50%, with an age at onset generally below 20 [50–53]. As in DRD, the rate of SGCE mutation detection is increased by screening for exon or whole gene deletions (gene dosage) [49, 54–56]. Complex phenotypes with additional features may be related to chromosomal deletions and rearrangements of the 7q21 region [49, 56–58].

In DYT12, rapid-onset dystonia-parkinsonism (RDP) the mutated gene is ATP1A3. RDP is an extremely rare disease with onset in childhood or early adulthood, in which patients develop dystonia, bradykinesia, postural instability, dysarthria, and dysphagia over a period ranging from several hours to weeks with triggering factors [59]. In addition to rapid onset, features suggesting an ATP1A3 mutation are prominent bulbar symptoms and a gradient of dystonia severity with the cranial region being more severely affected than arms and legs. Tremor at onset or prominent pain could not be found in ATP1A3 mutation-positive patients [60].

PRKRA (protein-kinase RNA-dependent activator) has been identified as the DYT16 gene on chromosome 2q31.2. Mutations cause a novel form of non-degenerative, early-onset autosomal-recessive dystonia-parkinsonism [61]. The phenotypic spectrum of DYT16 has not been determined yet.

Four forms of paroxysmal dystonias have been genetically defined to date. In two, only the locus has been mapped: paroxysmal dystonic choreoathetosis with episodic ataxia and spasticity (DYT9) and paroxysmal familial kinesigenic dyskinesia (DYT10). Paroxysmal non-kinesigenic dystonia (PNKD, DYT8) is caused by mutations in the myofibrillogenesis regulator 1 (MR-1) gene in all families with a typical PNKD phenotype [62–64]. This condition is characterized by episodes of choreodystonia with onset in infancy or early childhood. Attacks typically last 10 min to 1 h and are induced by caffeine or alcohol [65].

Paroxysmal exertion-induced dyskinesia (PED) is caused by mutations in the gene for the glucose transporter 1 (SLC2A1, DYT18). In addition to PED, DYT18 patients may present with epilepsy (absence or generalized tonic-clonic seizures), migraine, cognitive deficits, haemolytic anaemia, or developmental delay. A diagnostic marker is a decreased CSF/serum glucose ratio below 0.5 (Class III) [66, 67].

Recommendations and Good Practice Points

1 Genetic testing should be performed after establishing the clinical diagnosis. Genetic testing is not sufficient to make a diagnosis of dystonia without clinical features of dystonia [25, 68, 69] (Level B). Genetic counselling is recommended.

2 DYT1 testing is recommended for patients with limb-onset, primary dystonia with onset before age 30 [69] (Level B), as well as in those with onset after age 30 if they have an affected relative with early-onset dystonia [25, 69] (Level B).

3 In dystonia families, DYT1 testing is not recommended in asymptomatic individuals (GPP).

4 DYT6 testing is recommended in early-onset dystonia or familial dystonia with cranio-cervical predominance [27, 28] or after exclusion of DYT1 (GPP).

5 A diagnostic levodopa trial is warranted in every patient with early-onset dystonia without an alternative diagnosis [39] (GPP).

6 Individuals with early-onset myoclonus affecting the arms or neck, particularly if positive for autosomal-dominant inheritance and if triggered by action, should be tested for the DYT11 gene [50] (Good Practice Point). Gene dosage is required to improve mutation detection (Level C).

7 Diagnostic testing for the PNKD gene (DYT8) is recommended in symptomatic individuals with PNKD (GPP).

8 Gene testing for mutation in GLUT1 is recommended in patients with paroxysmal exercised-induced dyskinesias, especially if involvement of GLUT1 is suggested by low CSF/serum glucose ratio, epileptic seizures, or haemolytic anaemia (GPP).

Use of neurophysiology in the diagnosis and classification of dystonia

Neurophysiological tests are helpful in the characterization of functional abnormalities in patients with dystonia. However, all neurophysiology studies are Class IV, not providing evidence-based results. The need for standardized study designs and methods to investigate the diagnostic sensitivity and specificity of neurophysiological tests in dystonia has been emphasized in a recent review [70]. A number of studies have been reviewed previously [5] and will not be dealt with here. Alterations in cerebellar functions suggest a role of the cerebellum in the pathophysiology of dystonia [71, 72]. Cortical excitability is abnormally enhanced in symptomatic and non-symptomatic DYT1 carriers, while this is not the case in DYT11 M-D syndrome [73]. The induction of plastic changes in the motor cortex by repetitive transcranial magnetic stimulation (rTMS) at theta burst frequency has been found to be excessive in patients with dystonia (either genetic or sporadic) and abnormally reduced in asymptomatic DYT1 carriers [74]. It is possible that such decreases in gene carriers with no symptoms indicates a form of protection against the propensity or susceptibility of DYT1 patients to undergo plastic changes that could eventually lead to clinical manifestations of dystonia.

Disturbed sensory processing has been for the past years recognized as one of the main pathophysiological agents of dystonia [75, 76]. Many authors have contributed recently to confirm these findings and expand the implication of altered sensory processing in disordered motor control: abnormal sensory perception has been reported with studies of mental rotation and two-point discrimination [77]. Several reports have shown abnormal enhancement of SEPs in dystonic patients [78]. Notably, however, the only study in which the assessment was done blindly showed that differences in the size of the SEPs were not significant between patients and controls or between patients before and after botulinum toxin treatment [79]. Somatosensory stimuli cause abnormally reduced inhibitory effects on the MEP to TMS, regardless of whether the stimulus is applied on homotopic or heterotopic peripheral nerves [80]. A recent study indicates that somatosensory temporal discrimination threshold abnormalities are a generalized feature of patients with primary focal dystonias and are a valid tool for screening subclinical sensory abnormalities [81]. Using the paradigm of paired associative stimulation (PAS), i.e. applying a sensory stimulus followed 15–20 ms later by a single-pulse TMS, Tamura *et al.* [78] reported a transient enhancement of cortical excitability, manifested by an increase in the P27 of the somatosensory evoked potentials tested 15 min after PAS. The same intervention was reported to cause an abnormal increase in the MEP, which is not limited to the territory depending on the nerve stimulated but includes other muscles as well [82].

In most instances, neurophysiological abnormalities are not specific but, rather, they reveal a trend towards functional defects that may or may not become clinically relevant. This is the case in non-affected relatives of patients with dystonia [77] or in non-dystonic sites of patients with focal dystonia. Changes in neuronal excitability have been found in patients with forms of dystonia akin to psychogenicity [83, 84].

Recommendations and Good Practice Points

1 Neurophysiological tests are not routinely recommended for the diagnosis or classification of dystonia; however, the observation of abnormalities typical of dystonia is an additional diagnostic tool in cases where the clinical features are considered insufficient to the diagnosis [70, 85, 86] (GPP).

Use of brain imaging in the diagnosis of dystonia

Conventional or structural magnetic resonance imaging (MRI) studies in primary dystonia are normal, and a normal MRI study is usually considered a prerequisite to state that a patient's dystonia is primary. Recent Class III [87] and Class IV [88–90] diffusion magnetic resonance studies found signal abnormalities in various brain areas (including corpus callosum, basal ganglia, pontine brainstem, and pre-frontal cortical areas) in cervical dystonia, writer's cramp, and generalized dystonia, but not in blepharospam.

Interesting prospects of understanding the pathophysiological mechanisms of primary and secondary dystonia are offered by functional MRI studies. Class IV studies conducted in series of patients with blepharospasm [91], writer's cramp [92–94], or other focal dys-

tonia of the arm [95] demonstrated that several deep structures and cortical areas may be activated in primary dystonia, depending on the different modalities of examination. A Class II study on blepharospasm and cervical dystonia demonstrated increased basal ganglia activation in a task not primarily involving the dystonic musculature [96].

Recent Class II [97] and Class IV [98–101] voxel-based morphometry studies demonstrated an increase in grey matter density or volume in various areas, including cerebellum, basal ganglia, and primary somatosensory cortex. This increase might represent plastic changes secondary to overuse, but different interpretations have been considered. Another Class IV study found that non-DYT1 adult-onset dystonia patients and asymptomatic DYT1 carriers have significantly larger basal ganglia compared with symptomatic DYT1 mutation carriers, with a significant negative correlation between severity of dystonia and basal ganglia size in DYT1 patients [102].

Positron emission tomography (PET) studies with different tracers have provided information about areas of abnormal metabolism in different types of dystonia and in different conditions (e.g. during active involuntary movement or during sleep), providing insight on the role of cerebellar and subcortical structures versus cortical areas in the pathophysiology of dystonia (all Class IV studies) [103, 104]. A significant reduction in caudate and putamen D2 receptor availability and reduced [^{11}C] raclopride binding in the ventrolateral thalamus were evident in DYT6 and DYT1 dystonia in a Class III study [105]. The changes were greater in DYT6 than DYT1 carriers without difference between manifesting and non-manifesting carriers of either genotype.

A practical approach to differentiate patients with dystonia-plus syndromes from patients with parkinsonism and secondary dystonia is to obtain a single photon emission computerized tomography (SPECT) study with ligands for dopamine transporter; this is readily available and less expensive than PET. Patients with dopa-responsive dystonia have normal studies, whereas patients with early-onset Parkinson's disease show reduction of striatal ligand uptake (Class IV) [106]. It has been suggested that patients with tremor resembling parkinsonian tremor who have normal DAT scans may be affected by dystonia [3].

Medical treatments

Botulinum toxins

Botulinum toxin treatment continues to be the first choice treatment for most types of focal dystonia. Pharmacological and neurosurgical treatments have also a role in the treatment algorithm.

It is established that botulinum neurotoxins (BoNT), in properly adjusted doses, are effective and safe treatments of cranial (excluding oromandibular) and cervical dystonia [5]. In the last years long-term studies on the efficacy and safety of BoNT/A have become available, a new formulation of BoNT/A has been marketed, and new studies on BoNT/B have been performed. Further to systematic reviews already reported in the previous guidelines version, a new evidence-based systematic review released by the American Academy of Neurology [109] recommended that BoNT injections should be offered as a treatment option for cervical dystonia (established as effective) and may be offered for blepharospasm, focal upper extremity dystonia, and adductor laryngeal dystonia (probably effective). A lower level of evidence was detected for focal lower-limb dystonia (possibly effective).

The efficacy and safety profile of BoNT treatment has been evaluated in long-term observational studies. In patients with different dystonia types followed for >12 years there was no decline of efficacy and the main side effects consisted of muscle weakness in or around the injected region [110]. Also, immunogenicity was found to be low for BoTN/A in long-term use, although might be higher for BoTN/B (Class III, [111]). Four Class I [112–115], two Class II [116, 117], two Class III [79, 118], and 29 Class IV new studies on BoNT were identified. These reports have confirmed the long-term safety of BoNT products for dystonia and other conditions. A meta-analysis performed on children with cerebral palsy found that adverse events are more frequent among children with cerebral palsy than in individuals with other conditions [119]. Occasional occurrences of botulism-like symptoms have been reported in children and in adults treated with BoNT products; therefore, the United States Food and Drug Administration has ordered the manufacturers to add a boxed warning to the prescribing information for each product about the potential for serious side effects at sites distant from injection [120]. No similar initiative has been taken by the European Medicines Agency. Furthermore, the possible occurrence of central effect following BoNT due to axonal migration and neuronal transcytosis has been recently suggested [121], but not unequivocally demonstrated.

Three recent studies compared different BoNT/A products and three compared the A and B serotypes. Two Class II trials reported that Xeomin is as effective and safe as Botox for the treatment of cervical dystonia [116] and blepharospasm [122]. A Class IV trial found that in cervical dystonia and blepharospasm, Botox is more efficacious than Dysport and has a longer duration of effect [123]. A Class IV study with longer follow-up reported that in blepharospasm the mean duration of improvement was higher for Dysport than for Botox [124]. Two Class I studies found that improvement of cervical dystonia was comparable following BoNT/A and B treatments, but dry mouth and dysphagia were more frequent with BoNT/B [113, 115]. A Class II study reported that patients treated with BoNT/B had less saliva production and more severe constipation than those treated with BoNT/A [117].

A Class IV study reported that using EMG guidance can improve outcome in patients with cervical dystonia [125]. A Class III trial evaluated that the association of ad hoc rehabilitative programme with BoNT injections in patients with cervical dystonia [118] provided more marked improvement and a longer duration effect than BoNT injections alone.

Recommendations and Good Practice Points

1 BoNT/A (or type B if there is resistance to type A) can be regarded as first-line treatment for primary cranial (excluding oromandibular) or cervical dystonia [126, 127] (Level A).

2 BoNT/A is effective for writer's cramp [114] (Level A) and is possibly effective in other types of upper-limb dystonia, but controlled dose adjustments are needed because of frequent muscle weakness (GPP).

3 BoNT/A is probably effective for adductor-type laryngeal dystonia, but there is insufficient evidence to support efficacy in abductor-type laryngeal dystonia and in muscular tension dysphonia (GPP).

4 BoNT is safe and efficacious when repeated treatments are performed over many years (GPP), but doctors and patients should be aware that excessive cumulative doses may be dangerous, particularly in children (GPP).

5 BoNT injections can be performed by direct inspection; EMG- or ultrasound-assisted targeting may improve clinical outcome (GPP).

6 BoNT should not be used in patients affected by a disorder of neuromuscular transmission or in the presence of local infection at the injection site. The recommended dosage should not be exceeded (GPP).

Other medical treatments

No new Level A or B data are available for oral medications. Therefore the previously reported recommendations and Good Practice Points are retained [5].

Neurosurgical procedures

Deep brain stimulation

Long-term electrical stimulation of the globus pallidus internus (GPi) is now established as an effective treatment for various types of dystonia [128]. The use of deep brain stimulation (DBS) for dystonia currently addresses in particular primary generalized or segmental forms, complex cervical dystonia, and tardive dystonia in patients who do not achieve sufficient relief with conservative approaches [129]. Other manifestations are still being explored, such as status dystonicus, task-specific dystonia, camptocormia, and secondary dystonias including hemidystonia, PKAN, Lesch-Nyhan, and cerebral palsy-related dystonia-choreoathetosis. DBS for dystonia is widely available in Western countries and in

Japan. After it received FDA approval in the form of a humanitarian device exemption in the United States and CE certification in Europe, it is uniformly being reimbursed by health insurance carriers.

In August 2006, the National Institute for Clinical Excellence (NICE), UK, published a guideline for treatment of tremor and dystonia with DBS [130], which was based on data from a systematic review and two primary studies. According to this evidence, GPi DBS provided marked benefit of dystonia, with improvement of dystonia motor scores ranging between 34 and 88% and disability scores between 40 and 50%. A meta-analysis using a regression analysis published in 2006 revealed that longer duration of dystonia correlated negatively with surgical outcome [131]. The German DBS Working Group recently provided recommendations on several practical issues [132].

One Class I randomized sham-controlled study with a crossover design at 3 months found that in patients with primary generalized and segmental dystonia the change from baseline in the mean dystonia motor score was significantly greater in the neurostimulation group (-15.8 ± 14.1 points) than in the sham-stimulation group (-1.4 ± 3.8 points) [133]. In addition, patients in the sham-stimulation group had a similar benefit when they switched to active treatment during the open-label phase of the study. A total of 22 adverse events occurred in 19 patients (the most frequent adverse event was dysarthria) during an overall follow-up of 6 months.

There are several studies with some form of blinded assessment, including either blinded video evaluation or double-blind assessment randomized to off or on DBS [134–137] which provide Class II–III evidence and support the efficacy and safety of DBS GPi in selected patients with primary generalized or segmental dystonia [134, 135], primary cervical dystonia [136], or tardive dystonia [137].

Numerous Class IV studies with either prospective or retrospective design have been published over the past few years. The efficacy of GPi DBS was related to disease duration in one study [138]. Quality of life was shown to improve both in patients with primary segmental and generalized dystonia [139–142]. Stimulation via contacts located directly within the posteroventral portion of the GPi provided the best overall effect [143]. While high-frequency stimulation at 130 Hz or higher has been used in most studies, stimulation <100 Hz has been shown to be a possible alternative in selected patients with dystonia [144, 145].

It is clear that improvement of dystonia after DBS frequently follows a particular pattern, with phasic, myoclonic, and tremulous elements improving earlier than tonic elements, the latter often with a delay of weeks or months [146–148]. More recently, it has also been shown that upon recurrence of dystonia after switching off DBS, phasic elements manifest again within minutes and tonic elements within hours [149]. The GPi has been used in most studies on chronic stimulation, while there is limited experience with other targets [129] such as thalamus [150], STN [151], and cortex [152].

Overall, the most beneficial results with pallidal DBS were reported in children with primary generalized dystonia. DYT1 dystonia was shown to improve in the range of 40–90% [153–155] and also adult patients with non-DYT1 primary generalized dystonia can achieve equivalent benefit [146, 147, 156]. The French Spidy Study on patients with primary generalized dystonia reported a mean motor improvement of 54%, and a mean improvement of disability of 44% at 1-year follow-up [134].

Long-term efficacy was reported to be sustained after more than 5 years of follow-up [157–160]. Bilateral pallidal stimulation did not negatively affect cognitive performance [161].

In patients with cervical dystonia, GPi DBS has been used primarily in those who were thought not to be ideal candidates for peripheral denervation, including patients with head tremor and myoclonus, or marked phasic dystonic movements [148, 162, 163]. In the past few years, however, indications have been widened. In a recent Class II trial the Toronto Western Spasmodic Torticollis Rating Scale (TWSTRS) dystonia severity score improved from a mean of 14.7 ± 4.2 before surgery to 8.4 ± 4.4 at 12 months postoperatively [136]. Disability and pain scores improved similarly.

Patients with primary craniofacial dystonia may achieve similar benefit to patients with other segmental dystonia with regard to the severity score. In a study on six patients with Meige syndrome, a mean improvement of 72% of dystonia motor scores was seen at 6 months postoperatively [164]. The impact of GPi on secondary dystonia, in general is much less pronounced. Patients with dystonia and choreoathetosis due to cerebral palsy may achieve limited benefit with motor scores improving between 10 and 40%, but nevertheless yielding acceptable

patient satisfaction in some patients [165]. Tardive dystonia, as opposed to other dystonias appears also a good indication for Gpi DBS with benefits similar to those seen in primary dystonia [137].

Safety aspects that have to be considered include surgery-related complications, stimulation-induced side effects, and hardware-related problems. Recently, it was noted that Gpi DBS in patients with segmental dystonia may induce a parkinsonian gait or bradykinesia in extremities which were not affected by dystonia at chronic stimulation with high voltage [164, 166].

Chronic stimulation in dystonia uses both higher pulse width and voltage than in Parkinson's disease (PD), which results in earlier battery depletion; replacement may be needed, sometimes every 2 years or less. Sudden battery depletion may induce acute recurrence of dystonia, sometimes resulting in a medical emergency. No study, thus far, has evaluated if rechargeable pulse generators are more useful than non-rechargeable ones for patients with dystonia.

Recommendations and Good Practice Points

1 Pallidal DBS is considered a good option, particularly for primary generalized or segmental dystonia, after medication or BoNT have failed to provide adequate improvement [133] (Level A).

2 Pallidal DBS can be considered a good option for cervical dystonia after medication or BoNT have failed to provide adequate improvement [136] (Level B).

3 Pallidal DBS, in general, is less effective in secondary dystonia with the exception of tardive dystonia [165, 167] (Level C).

4 This procedure requires a specialized expertise and a multidisciplinary team, and is not without side effects (GPP).

5 Pallidal DBS should not be used in patients with dementia or in patients with disability due to secondary fixed deformities (GPP).

Other surgical procedures

In the past five years, there have been no new studies providing Class I or II evidence for selective peripheral denervation, myectomy and myotomy, intrathecal baclofen, or radiofrequency lesioning. Therefore, the previously reported recommendations and Good Practice Points are retained [5].

Physical therapy and rehabilitation

Recently, there has been an increased number of publications showing that physical therapy and rehabilitation procedures have an important role in the care of patients with dystonia [168, 169]. A number of studies have reported motor improvement in patients with writer's cramp and other forms of focal dystonia following physical treatment, and sensory and motor retraining [170–172].

A Class II study showed that transcutaneous electrical nerve stimulation caused a significant beneficial effect in patients with writer's cramp [173]. A Class IV study of patients with primary writing tremor showed the beneficial effect of writing after training with a device that supported the hand and held the pen [174]. This evidence adds to the already reported Class III study [118] where physical therapy was combined with BoNT/A injections in patients with cervical dystonia.

Musicians with dystonia may have specific benefit from motor retraining. A Class IV study reported the long-term subjective outcome in a large series of musicians with focal dystonia after treatment with different medical and physical options: 54% of patients reported an alleviation of symptoms, 33% improved with trihexiphenidyl, 49% with BoNT, 50% with pedagogical retraining, 56% with unmonitored technical exercises, and 63% with ergonomic changes [168].

Recommendations and Good Practice Points

1 Transcutaneous electrical nerve stimulation to forearm flexor muscles administered is probably effective in patients with writer's cramp [173] (Level B).

2 We encourage the conduction of new randomized controlled studies on these potentially useful interventions, particularly for patients with upper-limb dystonia (GPP).

Conflicts of interest

F. Asmus has received speaker honoraria and grants from Allergan, Merz Pharmaceuticals, and Ipsen Pharma.

K. Bhatia has acted as advisor to and received speaker honoraria and financial support to attend meetings from GSK, Boehringer-Ingelheim, Ipsen, Merz, and Orion Pharma. He has received grants from the Dystonia Society UK and the Halley Stewart Trust.

T. Gasser has acted as consultant for Cefalon Pharma and Merck-Serono. He has received speaker honoraria from Novartis, Merck-Serono, Schwarz Pharma, Boehringer Ingelheim, and Valeant Pharma, and grants from Novartis Pharma German Research Ministry, and Helmholtz Association: Helmholtz Alliance for Health in an Ageing Society (HELMA).

J.K. Krauss is a consultant to Medtronic and has received honoraria for speaking.

The other authors have reported no conflicts of interests.

References

1. Fahn S, Marsden CD, Calne DB. Classification and investigation of dystonia. In: Marsden CD, Fahn S (eds) *Movement Disorders 2*. London: Butterworths, 1987; pp. 332–58.
2. Fahn S, Bressman S, Marsden CD. Classification of dystonia. *Adv Neurol* 1998;**78**:1–10.
3. Schneider SA, Edwards MJ, Mir P, *et al*. Patients with adult-onset dystonic tremor resembling parkinsonian tremor have scans without evidence of dopaminergic deficit (SWEDDs). *Mov Disord* 2007;**22**:2210–5.
4. Brainin M, Barnes M, Baron JC, *et al*. Guidance for the preparation of neurological management guidelines by EFNS scientific task forces – revised recommendations 2004. *Eur J Neurol* 2004;**11**:577–81.
5. Albanese A, Barnes MP, Bhatia KP, *et al*. A systematic review on the diagnosis and treatment of primary (idiopathic) dystonia and dystonia plus syndromes: report of an EFNS/MDS-ES Task Force. *Eur J Neurol* 2006;**13**: 433–44.
6. Ludlow CL, Adler CH, Berke GS, *et al*. Research priorities in spasmodic dysphonia. *Otolaryngol Head Neck Surg* 2008;**139**:495–505.
7. Hallett M, Evinger C, Jankovic J, Stacy M. Update on blepharospasm: report from the BEBRF International Workshop. *Neurology* 2008;**71**:1275–82.
8. Albanese A, Lalli S. Is this dystonia? *Mov Disord* 2009;**24**:1725–31.
9. Burke RE, Fahn S, Marsden CD, Bressman SB, Moskowitz C, Friedman J. Validity and reliability of a rating scale for the primary torsion dystonias. *Neurology* 1985;**35**:73–7.
10. Comella CL, Leurgans S, Wuu J, Stebbins GT, Chmura T. Rating scales for dystonia: a multicenter assessment. *Mov Disord* 2003;**18**:303–12.
11. Cano SJ, Hobart JC, Fitzpatrick R, Bhatia K, Thompson AJ, Warner TT. Patient-based outcomes of cervical dystonia: a review of rating scales. *Mov Disord* 2004;**19**:1054–9.

12. Consky ES, Lang AE. Clinical assessments of patients with cervical dystonia. In: Jankovic J, Hallett M (eds) *Therapy with Botulinum Toxin*. New York, NY: Marcel Dekker, 1994; pp. 211–37.

13. Tsui JK, Eisen A, Stoessl AJ, Calne S, Calne DB. Double-blind study of botulinum toxin in spasmodic torticollis. *Lancet* 1986;**2**:245–7.

14. O'Brien C, Brashear A, Cullis P, *et al*. Cervical dystonia severity scale reliability study. *Mov Disord* 2001;**16**:1086–90.

15. Lim VK. Health related quality of life in patients with dystonia and their caregivers in New Zealand and Australia. *Mov Disord* 2007;**22**:998–1003.

16. Ozelius LJ, Hewett JW, Page CE, *et al*. The early-onset torsion dystonia gene (DYT1) encodes an ATP-binding protein. *Nat Genet* 1997;**17**:40–8.

17. Fuchs T, Gavarini S, Saunders-Pullman R, *et al*. Mutations in the THAP1 gene are responsible for DYT6 primary torsion dystonia. *Nat Genet* 2009;**41**:286–8.

18. Muller U. The monogenic primary dystonias. *Brain* 2009;**132**(Pt 8):2005–25.

19. Calakos N, Patel V, Gottron M, *et al*. Functional evidence implicating a novel TOR1A mutation in idiopathic, late-onset focal dystonia. *J Med Genet* 2009 Dec 2. [Epub ahead of print].

20. Bressman SB, Raymond D, Wendt K, *et al*. Diagnostic criteria for dystonia in DYT1 families. *Neurology* 2002;**59**:1780–2.

21. Zirn B, Grundmann K, Huppke P, *et al*. Novel TOR1A mutation p.Arg288Gln in early-onset dystonia (DYT1). *J Neurol Neurosurg Psychiatry* 2008;**79**:1327–30.

22. Edwards M, Wood N, Bhatia K. Unusual phenotypes in DYT1 dystonia: a report of five cases and a review of the literature. *Mov Disord* 2003;**18**:706–11.

23. Gambarin M, Valente EM, Liberini P, *et al*. Atypical phenotypes and clinical variability in a large Italian family with DYT1-primary torsion dystonia. *Mov Disord* 2006;**21**:1782–4.

24. Valente EM, Warner TT, Jarman PR, *et al*. The role of DYT1 in primary torsion dystonia in Europe. *Brain* 1998;**121**:2335–9.

25. Bressman SB, Sabatti C, Raymond D, *et al*. The DYT1 phenotype and guidelines for diagnostic testing. *Neurology* 2000;**54**:1746–52.

26. Fasano A, Nardocci N, Elia AE, Zorzi G, Bentivoglio AR, Albanese A. Non-DYT1 early-onset primary torsion dystonia: comparison with DYT1 phenotype and review of the literature. *Mov Disord* 2006;**21**:1411–8.

27. Djarmati A, Schneider SA, Lohmann K, *et al*. Mutations in THAP1 (DYT6) and generalised dystonia with prominent spasmodic dysphonia: a genetic screening study. *Lancet Neurol* 2009;**8**:447–52.

28. Bressman SB, Raymond D, Fuchs T, Heiman GA, Ozelius LJ, Saunders-Pullman R. Mutations in THAP1 (DYT6) in early-onset dystonia: a genetic screening study. *Lancet Neurol* 2009;**8**:441–6.

29. Segawa M, Hosaka A, Miyagawa F, Nomura Y, Imai H. Hereditary progressive dystonia with marked diurnal fluctuation. *Adv Neurol* 1976;**14**:215–33.

30. Trender-Gerhard I, Sweeney MG, Schwingenschuh P, *et al*. Autosomal-dominant GTPCH1-deficient DRD: clinical characteristics and long-term outcome of 34 patients. *J Neurol Neurosurg Psychiatry* 2009;**80**:839–45.

31. Bandmann O, Wood NW. Dopa-responsive dystonia. The story so far. *Neuropediatrics* 2002;**33**:1–5.

32. Hagenah J, Saunders-Pullman R, Hedrich K, *et al*. High mutation rate in dopa-responsive dystonia: detection with comprehensive GCHI screening. *Neurology* 2005;**64**:908–11.

33. Steinberger D, Trubenbach J, Zirn B, Leube B, Wildhardt G, Muller U. Utility of MLPA in deletion analysis of GCH1 in dopa-responsive dystonia. *Neurogenetics* 2007;**8**:51–5.

34. Zirn B, Steinberger D, Troidl C, *et al*. Frequency of GCH1 deletions in Dopa-responsive dystonia. *J Neurol Neurosurg Psychiatry* 2008;**79**:183–6.

35. Clot F, Grabli D, Cazeneuve C, *et al*. Exhaustive analysis of BH4 and dopamine biosynthesis genes in patients with Dopa-responsive dystonia. *Brain* 2009;**132**:1753–63.

36. Tassin J, Durr A, Bonnet AM, *et al*. Levodopa-responsive dystonia. GTP cyclohydrolase I or parkin mutations? *Brain* 2000;**123**:1112–21.

37. Jeon BS, Jeong JM, Park SS, *et al*. Dopamine transporter density measured by [123I]beta-CIT single-photon emission computed tomography is normal in dopa-responsive dystonia. *Ann Neurol* 1998;**43**:792–800.

38. Verbeek MM, Steenbergen-Spanjers GC, Willemsen MA, *et al*. Mutations in the cyclic adenosine monophosphate response element of the tyrosine hydroxylase gene. *Ann Neurol* 2007;**62**:422–6.

39. Robinson R, McCarthy GT, Bandmann O, Dobbie M, Surtees R, Wood NW. GTP cyclohydrolase deficiency; intrafamilial variation in clinical phenotype, including levodopa responsiveness. *J Neurol Neurosurg Psychiatry* 1999;**66**:86–9.

40. Bandmann O, Goertz M, Zschocke J, *et al*. The phenylalanine loading test in the differential diagnosis of dystonia. *Neurology* 2003;**60**:700–2.

41. Hyland K, Fryburg JS, Wilson WG, *et al*. Oral phenylalanine loading in dopa-responsive dystonia: a possible diagnostic test. *Neurology* 1997;**48**:1290–7.

42. Hyland K, Nygaard TG, Trugman JM, Swoboda KJ, Arnold LA, Sparagana SP. Oral phenylalanine loading profiles in symptomatic and asymptomatic gene carriers with

dopa-responsive dystonia due to dominantly inherited GTP cyclohydrolase deficiency. *J Inherit Metab Dis* 1999;**22**:213–5.

43. Asmus F, Gasser T. Inherited myoclonus-dystonia. *Adv Neurol* 2004;**94**:113–9.

44. Foncke EM, Gerrits MC, van RF, *et al.* Distal myoclonus and late onset in a large Dutch family with myoclonus-dystonia. *Neurology* 2006;**67**:1677–80.

45. Asmus F, Langseth A, Doherty *et al.* 'Jerky' dystonia in children: spectrum of phenotypes and genetic testing. *Mov Disord* 2009;**24**:702–9.

46. Vidailhet M, Tassin J, Durif F, *et al.* A major locus for several phenotypes of myoclonus-dystonia on chromosome 7q. *Neurology* 2001;**56**:1213–6.

47. Tezenas du Montcel S, Clot F, Vidailhet M, *et al.* Epsilon sarcoglycan mutations and phenotype in French patients with myoclonic syndromes. *J Med Genet* 2006;**43**:394–400.

48. Ritz K, Gerrits MC, Foncke EM, *et al.* Myoclonus-dystonia: clinical and genetic evaluation of a large cohort. *J Neurol Neurosurg Psychiatry* 2009;**80**:653–8.

49. Grunewald A, Djarmati A, Lohmann-Hedrich K, *et al.* Myoclonus-dystonia: significance of large SGCE deletions. *Hum Mutat* 2008;**29**:331–2.

50. Valente EM, Edwards MJ, Mir P, *et al.* The epsilon-sarcoglycan gene in myoclonic syndromes. *Neurology* 2005;**64**:737–9.

51. Klein C, Schilling K, Saunders-Pullman RJ, *et al.* A major locus for myoclonus-dystonia maps to chromosome 7q in eight families. *Am J Hum Genet* 2000;**67**:1314–9.

52. Leung JC, Klein C, Friedman J, *et al.* Novel mutation in the TOR1A (DYT1) gene in atypical early onset dystonia and polymorphisms in dystonia and early onset parkinsonism. *Neurogenetics* 2001;**3**:133–43.

53. Asmus F, Zimprich A, Tezenas du MS, *et al.* Myoclonus-dystonia syndrome: epsilon-sarcoglycan mutations and phenotype. *Ann Neurol* 2002;**52**:489–92.

54. Asmus F, Salih F, Hjermind LE, *et al.* Myoclonus-dystonia due to genomic deletions in the epsilon-sarcoglycan gene. *Ann Neurol* 2005;**58**:792–7.

55. Han F, Racacho L, Yang H, *et al.* Large deletions account for an increasing number of mutations in SGCE. *Mov Disord* 2008;**23**:456–60.

56. Asmus F, Hjermind LE, Dupont E, *et al.* Genomic deletion size at the epsilon-sarcoglycan locus determines the clinical phenotype. *Brain* 2007;**130**:2736–45.

57. Bonnet C, Gregoire MJ, Vibert M, Raffo E, Leheup B, Jonveaux P. Cryptic 7q21 and 9p23 deletions in a patient with apparently balanced de novo reciprocal translocation t(7;9)(q21;p23) associated with a dystonia-plus syndrome: paternal deletion of the epsilon-sarcoglycan (SGCE) gene. *J Hum Genet* 2008;**53**:876–85.

58. Guettard E, Portnoi MF, Lohmann-Hedrich K, *et al.* Myoclonus-dystonia due to maternal uniparental disomy. *Arch Neurol* 2008;**65**:1380–5.

59. Dobyns WB, Ozelius LJ, Kramer PL, *et al.* Rapid-onset dystonia-parkinsonism. *Neurology* 1993;**43**:2596–602.

60. Brashear A, Dobyns WB, de Carvalho Aguiar P, *et al.* The phenotypic spectrum of rapid-onset dystonia-parkinsonism (RDP) and mutations in the ATP1A3 gene. *Brain* 2007;**130**:828–35.

61. Camargos S, Scholz S, Simon-Sanchez J, *et al.* DYT16, a novel young-onset dystonia-parkinsonism disorder: identification of a segregating mutation in the stress-response protein PRKRA. *Lancet Neurol* 2008;**7**:207–15.

62. Rainier S, Thomas D, Tokarz D, *et al.* Myofibrillogenesis regulator 1 gene mutations cause paroxysmal dystonic choreoathetosis. *Arch Neurol* 2004;**61**:1025–9.

63. Lee HY, Xu Y, Huang Y, *et al.* The gene for paroxysmal non-kinesigenic dyskinesia encodes an enzyme in a stress response pathway. *Hum Mol Genet* 2004;**13**:3161–70.

64. Chen DH, Matsushita M, Rainier S, *et al.* Presence of alanine-to-valine substitutions in myofibrillogenesis regulator 1 in paroxysmal nonkinesigenic dyskinesia: confirmation in 2 kindreds. *Arch Neurol* 2005;**62**:597–600.

65. Bruno MK, Lee HY, Auburger GW, *et al.* Genotype-phenotype correlation of paroxysmal nonkinesigenic dyskinesia. *Neurology* 2007;**68**:1782–9.

66. Weber YG, Storch A, Wuttke TV, *et al.* GLUT1 mutations are a cause of paroxysmal exertion-induced dyskinesias and induce hemolytic anemia by a cation leak. *J Clin Invest* 2008;**118**:2157–68.

67. Suls A, Dedeken P, Goffin K, *et al.* Paroxysmal exercise-induced dyskinesia and epilepsy is due to mutations in SLC2A1, encoding the glucose transporter GLUT1. *Brain* 2008;**131**:1831–44.

68. American Society of Human Genetics Board of Directors, American College of Medical Genetics Board of Directors. Points to consider: ethical, legal, and psychosocial implications of genetic testing in children and adolescents. *Am J Hum Genet* 1995;**57**:1233–41.

69. Klein C, Friedman J, Bressman S, *et al.* Genetic testing for early-onset torsion dystonia (DYT1): introduction of a simple screening method, experiences from testing of a large patient cohort, and ethical aspects. *Genet Test* 1999;**3**:323–8.

70. Tinazzi M, Squintani G, Berardelli A. Does neurophysiological testing provide the information we need to improve the clinical management of primary dystonia? *Clin Neurophysiol* 2009;**120**:1424–32.

71. Brighina F, Romano M, Giglia G, *et al.* Effects of cerebellar TMS on motor cortex of patients with focal dystonia: a preliminary report. *Exp Brain Res* 2009;**192**:651–6.

72. Teo JT, van De Warrenburg BP, Schneider SA, Rothwell JC, Bhatia KP. Neurophysiological evidence for cerebellar dysfunction in primary focal dystonia. *J Neurol Neurosurg Psychiatry* 2009;**80**:80–3.

73. Marelli C, Canafoglia L, Zibordi F, *et al.* A neurophysiological study of myoclonus in patients with DYT11 myoclonus-dystonia syndrome. *Mov Disord* 2008;**23**:2041–8.

74. Edwards MJ, Huang YZ, Mir P, Rothwell JC, Bhatia KP. Abnormalities in motor cortical plasticity differentiate manifesting and nonmanifesting DYT1 carriers. *Mov Disord* 2006;**21**:2181–6.

75. Murase N, Kaji R, Shimazu H, *et al.* Abnormal premovement gating of somatosensory input in writer's cramp. *Brain* 2000;**123**:1813–29.

76. Sohn YH, Hallett M. Disturbed surround inhibition in focal hand dystonia. *Ann Neurol* 2004;**56**:595–9.

77. Fiorio M, Gambarin M, Valente EM, *et al.* Defective temporal processing of sensory stimuli in DYT1 mutation carriers: a new endophenotype of dystonia? *Brain* 2007;**130**:134–42.

78. Tamura Y, Ueki Y, Lin P, *et al.* Disordered plasticity in the primary somatosensory cortex in focal hand dystonia. *Brain* 2009;**132**:749–55.

79. Contarino MF, Kruisdijk JJ, Koster L, Ongerboer de Visser BW, Speelman JD, Koelman JH. Sensory integration in writer's cramp: comparison with controls and evaluation of botulinum toxin effect. *Clin Neurophysiol* 2007;**118**:2195–206.

80. Lourenco G, Meunier S, Vidailhet M, Simonetta-Moreau M. Impaired modulation of motor cortex excitability by homonymous and heteronymous muscle afferents in focal hand dystonia. *Mov Disord* 2007;**22**:523–7.

81. Scontrini A, Conte A, Defazio G, *et al.* Somatosensory temporal discrimination in patients with primary focal dystonia. *J Neurol Neurosurg Psychiatry* 2009;**80**:1315–9.

82. Quartarone A, Morgante F, Sant'angelo A, *et al.* Abnormal plasticity of sensorimotor circuits extends beyond the affected body part in focal dystonia. *J Neurol Neurosurg Psychiatry* 2008;**79**:985–90.

83. Espay AJ, Morgante F, Purzner J, Gunraj CA, Lang AE, Chen R. Cortical and spinal abnormalities in psychogenic dystonia. *Ann Neurol* 2006;**59**:825–34.

84. Avanzino L, Martino D, van De Warrenburg BP, *et al.* Cortical excitability is abnormal in patients with the 'fixed dystonia' syndrome. *Mov Disord* 2008;**23**:646–52.

85. Deuschl G, Heinen F, Kleedorfer B, Wagner M, Lucking CH, Poewe W. Clinical and polymyographic investigation of spasmodic torticollis. *J Neurol* 1992;**239**:9–15.

86. Hughes M, McLellan DL. Increased co-activation of the upper limb muscles in writer's cramp. *J Neurol Neurosurg Psychiatry* 1985;**48**:782–7.

87. Fabbrini G, Pantano P, Totaro P, *et al.* Diffusion tensor imaging in patients with primary cervical dystonia and in patients with blepharospasm. *Eur J Neurol* 2008;**15**:185–9.

88. Carbon M, Kingsley PB, Tang C, Bressman S, Eidelberg D. Microstructural white matter changes in primary torsion dystonia. *Mov Disord* 2008;**23**:234–9.

89. Delmaire C, Vidailhet M, Wassermann D, *et al.* Diffusion abnormalities in the primary sensorimotor pathways in writer's cramp. *Arch Neurol* 2009;**66**:502–8.

90. Bonilha L, de Vries PM, Vincent DJ, *et al.* Structural white matter abnormalities in patients with idiopathic dystonia. *Mov Disord* 2007;**22**:1110–6.

91. Schmidt KE, Linden DE, Goebel R, Zanella FE, Lanfermann H, Zubcov AA. Striatal activation during blepharospasm revealed by fMRI. *Neurology* 2003;**60**:1738–43.

92. Preibisch C, Berg D, Hofmann E, Solymosi L, Naumann M. Cerebral activation patterns in patients with writer's cramp: a functional magnetic resonance imaging study. *J Neurol* 2001;**248**:10–7.

93. Oga T, Honda M, Toma K, *et al.* Abnormal cortical mechanisms of voluntary muscle relaxation in patients with writer's cramp: an fMRI study. *Brain* 2002;**125**:895–903.

94. Peller M, Zeuner KE, Munchau A, *et al.* The basal ganglia are hyperactive during the discrimination of tactile stimuli in writer's cramp. *Brain* 2006;**129**:2697–708.

95. Butterworth S, Francis S, Kelly E, McGlone F, Bowtell R, Sawle GV. Abnormal cortical sensory activation in dystonia: an fMRI study. *Mov Disord* 2003;**18**:673–82.

96. Obermann M, Yaldizli O, De GA, *et al.* Increased basal-ganglia activation performing a non-dystonia-related task in focal dystonia. *Eur J Neurol* 2008;**15**:831–8.

97. Obermann M, Yaldizli O, De GA, *et al.* Morphometric changes of sensorimotor structures in focal dystonia. *Mov Disord* 2007;**22**:1117–23.

98. Draganski B, Thun-Hohenstein C, Bogdahn U, Winkler J, May A. 'Motor circuit' gray matter changes in idiopathic cervical dystonia. *Neurology* 2003;**61**:1228–31.

99. Garraux G, Bauer A, Hanakawa T, Wu T, Kansaku K, Hallett M. Changes in brain anatomy in focal hand dystonia. *Ann Neurol* 2004;**55**:736–9.

100. Egger K, Mueller J, Schocke M, *et al.* Voxel based morphometry reveals specific gray matter changes in primary dystonia. *Mov Disord* 2007;**22**:1538–42.

101. Delmaire C, Vidailhet M, Elbaz A, *et al.* Structural abnormalities in the cerebellum and sensorimotor circuit in writer's cramp. *Neurology* 2007;**69**:376–80.

102. Draganski B, Schneider SA, Fiorio M, *et al.* Genotype-phenotype interactions in primary dystonias revealed by differential changes in brain structure. *Neuroimage* 2009;**47**:1141–7.

103. Hutchinson M, Nakamura T, Moeller JR, et al. The metabolic topography of essential blepharospasm: a focal dystonia with general implications. Neurology 2000;55: 673–7.

104. Asanuma K, Ma Y, Huang C, et al. The metabolic pathology of dopa-responsive dystonia. Ann Neurol 2005;57:596–600.

105. Carbon M, Niethammer M, Peng S, et al. Abnormal striatal and thalamic dopamine neurotransmission: Genotype-related features of dystonia. Neurology 2009;72:2097–103.

106. Marshall V, Grosset D. Role of dopamine transporter imaging in routine clinical practice. Mov Disord 2003;18: 1415–23.

107. Rutledge JN, Hilal SK, Silver AJ, Defendini R, Fahn S. Magnetic resonance imaging of dystonic states. Adv Neurol 1988;50:265–75.

108. Meunier S, Lehericy S, Garnero L, Vidailhet M. Dystonia: lessons from brain mapping. Neuroscientist 2003;9:76–81.

109. Simpson DM, Blitzer A, Brashear A, et al. Assessment: botulinum neurotoxin for the treatment of movement disorders (an evidence-based review): report of the Therapeutics and Technology Assessment Subcommittee of the American Academy of Neurology. Neurology 2008;70: 1699–706.

110. Mejia NI, Vuong KD, Jankovic J. Long-term botulinum toxin efficacy, safety, and immunogenicity. Mov Disord 2005;20:592–7.

111. Brin MF, Comella CL, Jankovic J, Lai F, Naumann M. Long-term treatment with botulinum toxin type A in cervical dystonia has low immunogenicity by mouse protection assay. Mov Disord 2008;23:1353–60.

112. Truong D, Duane DD, Jankovic J, et al. Efficacy and safety of botulinum type A toxin (Dysport) in cervical dystonia: results of the first US randomized, double-blind, placebo-controlled study. Mov Disord 2005;20:783–91.

113. Comella CL, Jankovic J, Shannon KM, et al. Comparison of botulinum toxin serotypes A and B for the treatment of cervical dystonia. Neurology 2005;65:1423–9.

114. Kruisdijk JJ, Koelman JH, Ongerboer de Visser BW, De Haan RJ, Speelman JD. Botulinum toxin for writer's cramp: a randomised, placebo-controlled trial and 1-year follow-up. J Neurol Neurosurg Psychiatry 2007;78:264–70.

115. Pappert EJ, Germanson T. Botulinum toxin type B vs. type A in toxin-naive patients with cervical dystonia: randomized, double-blind, noninferiority trial. Mov Disord 2008;23:510–7.

116. Benecke R, Jost WH, Kanovsky P, Ruzicka E, Comes G, Grafe S. A new botulinum toxin type A free of complexing proteins for treatment of cervical dystonia. Neurology 2005;64:1949–51.

117. Tintner R, Gross R, Winzer UF, Smalky KA, Jankovic J. Autonomic function after botulinum toxin type A or B: a double-blind, randomized trial. Neurology 2005;65:765–7.

118. Tassorelli C, Mancini F, Balloni L, et al. Botulinum toxin and neuromotor rehabilitation: an integrated approach to idiopathic cervical dystonia. Mov Disord 2006;21:2240–3.

119. Albavera-Hernandez C, Rodriguez JM, Idrovo AJ. Safety of botulinum toxin type A among children with spasticity secondary to cerebral palsy: a systematic review of randomized clinical trials. Clin Rehabil 2009;23:394–407.

120. Kuehn BM. FDA requires black box warnings on labeling for botulinum toxin products. JAMA 2009;301:2316.

121. Antonucci F, Rossi C, Gianfranceschi L, Rossetto O, Caleo M. Long-distance retrograde effects of botulinum neurotoxin A. J Neurosci 2008;28:3689–96.

122. Roggenkamper P, Jost WH, Bihari K, Comes G, Grafe S. Efficacy and safety of a new Botulinum Toxin Type A free of complexing proteins in the treatment of blepharospasm. J Neural Transm 2006;113:303–12.

123. Bihari K. Safety, effectiveness, and duration of effect of BOTOX after switching from Dysport for blepharospasm, cervical dystonia, and hemifacial spasm dystonia, and hemifacial spasm. Curr Med Res Opin 2005;21:433–8.

124. Bentivoglio AR, Fasano A, Ialongo T, Soleti F, Lo Fermo S, Albanese A. Fifteen-year experience in treating blepharospasm with Botox or Dysport: same toxin, two drugs. Neurotox Res 2009;15:224–31.

125. Cordivari C, Misra VP, Vincent A, Catania S, Bhatia KP, Lees AJ. Secondary nonresponsiveness to botulinum toxin A in cervical dystonia: the role of electromyogram-guided injections, botulinum toxin A antibody assay, and the extensor digitorum brevis test. Mov Disord 2006;21:1737–41.

126. Costa J, Espirito-Santo C, Borges A, et al. Botulinum toxin type A therapy for blepharospasm. Cochrane Database Syst Rev 2005;(1):CD004900.

127. American Academy of Ophthalmology. Botulinum toxin therapy of eye muscle disorders. Safety and effectiveness. Ophthalmology 1989;96(Pt 2):37–41.

128. Krauss JK, Yianni J, Loher TJ, Aziz TZ. Deep brain stimulation for dystonia. J Clin Neurophysiol 2004;21:18–30.

129. Capelle HH, Krauss JK. Neuromodulation in dystonia: current aspects of deep brain stimulation. Neuromodulation 2009;12:8–21.

130. National Institute for Health and Clinical Excellence. Deep brain stimulation for tremor and dystonia (excluding Parkinson's disease). http://www nice org uk/guidance/IPG188 2006 (accessed http://www.nice.org.uk/guidance/IPG188 (2010/06/09).).

131. Holloway KL, Baron MS, Brown R, Cifu DX, Carne W, Ramakrishnan V. Deep brain stimulation for dystonia: a meta-analysis. Neuromodulation 2006;9:253–61.

132. Schrader C, Benecke R, Deuschl G, *et al*. Tiefe Hirnstimulation bei Dystonie. Empfehlungen der Deutschen Arbeitsgemeinschaft Tiefe Hirnstimulation. *Nervenarzt* 2009;**80**:656–61.

133. Kupsch A, Benecke R, Muller J, *et al*. Pallidal deep-brain stimulation in primary generalized or segmental dystonia. *N Engl J Med* 2006;**355**:1978–90.

134. Vidailhet M, Vercueil L, Houeto JL, *et al*. Bilateral deep-brain stimulation of the globus pallidus in primary generalized dystonia. *N Engl J Med* 2005;**352**:459–67.

135. Diamond A, Shahed J, Azher S, Dat-Vuong K, Jankovic J. Globus pallidus deep brain stimulation in dystonia. *Mov Disord* 2006;**21**:692–5.

136. Kiss ZH, Doig-Beyaert K, Eliasziw M, Tsui J, Haffenden A, Suchowersky O. The Canadian multicentre study of deep brain stimulation for cervical dystonia. *Brain* 2007;**130**: 2879–86.

137. Damier P, Thobois S, Witjas T, *et al*. Bilateral deep brain stimulation of the globus pallidus to treat tardive dyskinesia. *Arch Gen Psychiatry* 2007;**64**:170–6.

138. Isaias IU, Alterman RL, Tagliati M. Outcome predictors of pallidal stimulation in patients with primary dystonia: the role of disease duration. *Brain* 2008;**131**:1895–902.

139. Pretto TE, Dalvi A, Kang UJ, Penn RD. A prospective blinded evaluation of deep brain stimulation for the treatment of secondary dystonia and primary torticollis syndromes. *J Neurosurg* 2008;**109**:405–9.

140. Blahak C, Wohrle JC, Capelle HH, *et al*. Health-related quality of life in segmental dystonia is improved by bilateral pallidal stimulation. *J Neurol* 2008;**255**:178–82.

141. Mueller J, Skogseid IM, Benecke R, *et al*. Pallidal deep brain stimulation improves quality of life in segmental and generalized dystonia: results from a prospective, randomized sham-controlled trial. *Mov Disord* 2008;**23**: 131–4.

142. Skogseid IM. Pallidal deep brain stimulation is effective, and improves quality of life in primary segmental and generalized dystonia. *Acta Neurol Scand Suppl* 2008;**188**: 51–5.

143. Tisch S, Zrinzo L, Limousin P, *et al*. Effect of electrode contact location on clinical efficacy of pallidal deep brain stimulation in primary generalised dystonia. *J Neurol Neurosurg Psychiatry* 2007;**78**:1314–9.

144. Alterman RL, Miravite J, Weisz D, Shils JL, Bressman SB, Tagliati M. Sixty Hertz pallidal deep brain stimulation for primary torsion dystonia. *Neurology* 2007;**69**:681–8.

145. Alterman RL, Shils JL, Miravite J, Tagliati M. Lower stimulation frequency can enhance tolerability and efficacy of pallidal deep brain stimulation for dystonia. *Mov Disord* 2007;**22**:366–8.

146. Coubes P, Cif L, El Fertit H, *et al*. Electrical stimulation of the globus pallidus internus in patients with primary generalized dystonia: long-term results. *J Neurosurg* 2004;**101**:189–94.

147. Krause M, Fogel W, Kloss M, Rasche D, Volkmann J, Tronnier V. Pallidal stimulation for dystonia. *Neurosurgery* 2004;**55**:1361–70.

148. Krauss JK, Pohle T, Weber S, Ozdoba C, Burgunder JM. Bilateral stimulation of globus pallidus internus for treatment of cervical dystonia. *Lancet* 1999;**354**:837–8.

149. Grips E, Blahak C, Capelle HH, *et al*. Patterns of reoccurrence of segmental dystonia after discontinuation of deep brain stimulation. *J Neurol Neurosurg Psychiatry* 2007;**78**:318–20.

150. Woehrle JC, Blahak C, Kekelia K, *et al*. Chronic deep brain stimulation for segmental dystonia. *Stereotact Funct Neurosurg* 2009;**87**:379–84.

151. Sun B, Chen S, Zhan S, Le W, Krahl SE. Subthalamic nucleus stimulation for primary dystonia and tardive dystonia. *Acta Neurochir Suppl* 2007;**97**:207–14.

152. Romito LM, Franzini A, Perani D, *et al*. Fixed dystonia unresponsive to pallidal stimulation improved by motor cortex stimulation. *Neurology* 2007;**68**:875–6.

153. Coubes P, Roubertie A, Vayssiere N, Hemm S, Echenne B. Treatment of DYT1-generalised dystonia by stimulation of the internal globus pallidus. *Lancet* 2000;**355**:2220–1.

154. Egidi M, Franzini A, Marras C, *et al*. A survey of Italian cases of dystonia treated by deep brain stimulation. *J Neurosurg Sci* 2007;**51**:153–8.

155. Borggraefe I, Mehrkens JH, Telegravciska M, Berweck S, Botzel K, Heinen F. Bilateral pallidal stimulation in children and adolescents with primary generalized dystonia – report of six patients and literature-based analysis of predictive outcomes variables. *Brain Dev* 2010 Mar; **32**(3):223–8.

156. Yianni J, Bain P, Giladi N, *et al*. Globus pallidus internus deep brain stimulation for dystonic conditions: a prospective audit. *Mov Disord* 2003;**18**:436–42.

157. Cersosimo MG, Raina GB, Piedimonte F, Antico J, Graff P, Micheli FE. Pallidal surgery for the treatment of primary generalized dystonia: long-term follow-up. *Clin Neurol Neurosurg* 2008;**110**:145–50.

158. Isaias IU, Alterman RL, Tagliati M. Deep brain stimulation for primary generalized dystonia: long-term outcomes. *Arch Neurol* 2009;**66**:465–70.

159. Loher TJ, Capelle HH, Kaelin-Lang A, *et al*. Deep brain stimulation for dystonia: outcome at long-term follow-up. *J Neurol* 2008;**255**:881–4.

160. Mehrkens JH, Botzel K, Steude U, *et al*. Long-term efficacy and safety of chronic globus pallidus internus stimulation

in different types of primary dystonia. *Stereotact Funct Neurosurg* 2009;**87**:8–17.

161. Pillon B, Ardouin C, Dujardin K, *et al.* Preservation of cognitive function in dystonia treated by pallidal stimulation. *Neurology* 2006;**66**:1556–8.

162. Krauss JK. Deep brain stimulation for cervical dystonia. *J Neurol Neurosurg Psychiatry* 2003;**74**:1598.

163. Eltahawy HA, Saint-Cyr J, Poon YY, Moro E, Lang AE, Lozano AM. Pallidal deep brain stimulation in cervical dystonia: clinical outcome in four cases. *Can J Neurol Sci* 2004;**31**:328–32.

164. Ostrem JL, Marks WJ, Jr, Volz MM, Heath SL, Starr PA. Pallidal deep brain stimulation in patients with cranial-cervical dystonia (Meige syndrome). *Mov Disord* 2007;**22**: 1885–91.

165. Vidailhet M, Yelnik J, Lagrange C, *et al.* Bilateral pallidal deep brain stimulation for the treatment of patients with dystonia-choreoathetosis cerebral palsy: a prospective pilot study. *Lancet Neurol* 2009;**8**:709–17.

166. Berman BD, Starr PA, Marks WJ, Ostrem JL. Induction of bradykinesia with pallidal deep brain stimulation in patients with cranial-cervical dystonia. *Stereotact Funct Neurosurg* 2009;**87**:37–44.

167. Gruber D, Trottenberg T, Kivi A, *et al.* Long-term effects of pallidal deep brain stimulation in tardive dystonia. *Neurology* 2009;**73**:53–8.

168. Jabusch HC, Zschucke D, Schmidt A, Schuele S, Altenmuller E. Focal dystonia in musicians: treatment strategies and long-term outcome in 144 patients. *Mov Disord* 2005;**20**:1623–6.

169. Candia V, Rosset-Llobet J, Elbert T, Pascual-Leone A. Changing the brain through therapy for musicians' hand dystonia. *Ann N Y Acad Sci* 2005;**1060**:335–42.

170. McKenzie AL, Goldman S, Barrango C, Shrime M, Wong T, Byl N. Differences in physical characteristics and response to rehabilitation for patients with hand dystonia: musicians' cramp compared to writers' cramp. *J Hand Ther* 2009;**22**:172–81.

171. Zetterberg L, Halvorsen K, Farnstrand C, Aquilonius SM, Lindmark B. Physiotherapy in cervical dystonia: six experimental single-case studies. *Physiother Theory Pract* 2008;**24**: 275–90.

172. Byl NN, Archer ES, McKenzie A. Focal hand dystonia: effectiveness of a home program of fitness and learning-based sensorimotor and memory training. *J Hand Ther* 2009;**22**(2):183–97.

173. Tinazzi M, Farina S, Bhatia K, *et al.* TENS for the treatment of writer's cramp dystonia: a randomized, placebo-controlled study. *Neurology* 2005;**64**:1946–8.

174. Espay AJ, Hung SW, Sanger TD, Moro E, Fox SH, Lang AE. A writing device improves writing in primary writing tremor. *Neurology* 2005;**64**:1648–50.

CHAPTER 13

Mild traumatic brain injury

P. E. Vos,[1] Y. Alekseenko,[2] L. Battistin,[3] E. Ehler,[4] F. Gerstenbrand,[5] D. F. Muresanu,[6] A. Potapov,[7] Ch. A. Stepan,[8] P. Traubner,[9] L. Vecsei,[10] K. von Wild[11]

[1]Radboud University Nijmegen Medical Centre, The Netherlands; [2]Vitebsk Medical University, Vitebsk, Belarus; [3]Clinica Neurologica I, Padova, Italy; [4]Neurologicka Klinika, Pradubice, Czech Republic; [5]Ludwig Boltzmann Institute for Restorative Neurology and Neuromodulation, Vienna, Austria; [6]University CFR Hospital, University of Medicine and Pharmacy 'Iuliu Hatieganu' Cluj-Napoca, Romania; [7]Institute of Neurosurgery, Russian Academy of Medical Sciences, Moscow, Russia; [8]Neurological Hospital Rosenhügel, Vienna, Austria; [9]Comenius University School of Medicine, Bratislava, Slovak Republic; [10]Szent-Györgyi University Hospital, Szeged, Hungary; [11]Medical Faculty Westphalien University Münster and International Neuroscience Institute INI, Hannover, Germany

Introduction

Traumatic brain injury (TBI) caused by sudden impact or acceleration deceleration trauma of the head is among the most frequent neurological disorders [1]. The acute phase of mild traumatic brain injury (MTBI) is characterized by a 10% risk for intracranial abnormalities like contusion, subdural or epidural hematoma, brain swelling, subarachnoid haemorrhage, or pneumocephalus; a low risk (1%) of life-threatening intracranial haematoma that needs immediate neurosurgical operation both in adults and in children; and a very low mortality of 0.1% in adults and even lower in children [2, 3]. Early management in MTBI deals with the recognition and immediate medical treatment of physiological parameters that may worsen brain pathology. Key to the acute management of mild TBI patients is the recognition of clinical signs and symptoms (risk factors) that increase the likelihood of intracranial haematoma that need neurosurgical operation. In 2002, the EFNS guideline on early management in MTBI was published. MTBI was defined as patients with head injury and a GCS 13–15 (see table 13.1 for classification). This guideline was largely based on two formal evidence-based clinical decision rules [4, 5]. In the 2002 EFNS guideline, risk factors were defined that are associated with intracranial abnormalities including life-threatening haematoma, which resulted in a set of rules for diagnostic imaging, observation, and follow-up of patients.

Since the appearance of the EFNS guideline new data have been published. Results of an independent Dutch multicentre study in 3181 patients with MTBI demonstrated that the EFNS guideline has a 100% sensitivity for the detection of intracranial abnormalities after MTBI [6]. Despite this convincing result from the patient safety perspective, it was also concluded that the specificity of the EFNS guideline is low and the number of patients needed to scan to detect abnormalities is very high.

These limitations form an important reason to update and refine the EFNS guideline; and there have also been reports that caution against the liberal use of computed tomography (CT) because of an increase in lifetime cancer mortality risks attributable to radiation from CT [7]. Second, healthcare costs form a concern in MTBI. A restrictive use of CT compared to the current guideline has been propagated. Selecting patients with MTBI for CT, i.e. ordering a CT less frequently, may be cost-effective as long as the sensitivity of such procedures for the identification of patients who require neurosurgery remains high.

In this version, based on new publications since 2001, we present updated guidelines for early management in MTBI with respect to the indication for CT and early management (admission, clinical observation and follow-up).

European Handbook of Neurological Management: Volume 1, 2nd edition. Edited by N. E. Gilhus, M. P. Barnes and M. Brainin.
© 2011 Blackwell Publishing Ltd.

Table 13.1. Classification of traumatic brain injury and indication for immediate head CT.

Classification	Characteristics	Indication for immediate head CT*
Mild	Hospital admission GCS = 13–15 Loss of consciousness if present 30 min or less	
Category		
1	GCS = 15 No risk factors or only 1 minor risk factor present (CHIP rule) Head injury, no TBI	No
2	GCS = 15 With risk factors or ≥ 1 major risk factor(s) or ≥ 2 minor risk factors (CHIP rule)	Yes
3	GCS = 13–14	Yes
Moderate	GCS = 9–12	Yes
Severe	GCS ≤ 8	Yes
Critical	GCS = 3–4, with loss of pupillary reactions and absent or decerebrate motor reactions	Yes

GCS, Glasgow Coma Scale; TBI, traumatic brain injury; CHIP, CT in Head Injury Patients. *Major and minor risk factors for indication of immediate head CT in MTBI are shown in table 13.2.

Search strategy

A systematic search of the English literature in the MEDLINE, EMBASE, Cochrane database (2001–2009) using the key words minor head injury, mild head injury, mild traumatic brain injury, traumatic brain injury, guidelines, and management. Additional articles were identified from the bibliographies of the articles retrieved, and from textbooks. Articles were included if they contained data on classification system used (i.e. admission Glasgow Coma Scale (GCS) 13–15) and outcome data (CT abnormalities, need for neurosurgical intervention, mortality) or management. Articles judged to be of historical value and existing (new) guidelines were also included and reviewed for useful data. Where appropriate, a classification of evidence level was given for interventions, diagnostic tests, and grades of recommendation for management according to the neurological management guidelines of the EFNS [8]. Where there was a lack of evidence but consensus was clear we have stated our opinion as Good Practice Points (GPP).

Clinical decision rules for CT

Adults

The 2002 version of the EFNS guideline, which weighed heavily on two prospective Class I/II studies, offered a decision rule for use of CT to demonstrate the need for neurosurgical intervention or clinically important brain injury after MTBI [4, 5, 9]. It was subsequently demonstrated that the EFNS guideline compared to other existing guidelines has a high sensitivity for the identification of patients with clinical relevant traumatic findings at CT [6, 10]. In addition, the EFNS guideline confirmed that in patients with MTBI the use of CT can be safely limited to those who have certain clinical findings. The generalizability and reliability of existing guidelines and prediction rules is in general lower than described in the original studies as was demonstrated in an independent sample of 1101 patients evaluating 11 existing guidelines [10]. For an overview of the risk factors used in existing guidelines rules and studies from which they were derived, see table 13.2. The sensitivity of the original studies forming the basis for the guidelines after external validation amounts to 85–100% for neurosurgical intervention and 85–96% for clinical important findings [10, 11].

Conclusion Various prediction rules that employ different risk factors have high sensitivity and low specificity for clinically relevant intracranial abnormalities and the need for neurosurgical operation (Evidence Level I).

Recommendation

Protocols for initial management in MTBI should include a decision scheme or prediction rule algorithm for the use of CT after MTBI (Grade A recommendation).

Table 13.2. Overview of prediction rules/guidelines for the detection of intracranial lesions and need for neurosurgical operation after MTBI in adults.

Risk factor	EFNS 2002	NOC	CCHR	CHIP	NICE	NEXUS II
	GCS = 13–15 guideline	LOC GCS = 15 $n = 909$	LOC or PTA GCS = 13–15 $n = 3121$	GCS = 13–14 GCS = 15 + risk factor $n = 3181$	GCS = 13–15 guideline	Blunt head trauma
HISTORY						
Age	+	+ (>60y)	+ (≥65y)	+ (≥60y) or minor (40–60y)	+ (>65y, if LOC)	>65
Loss of consciousness	+	Inclusion	Inclusion	Minor	–	
Headache	+	+	–	–		
Vomiting	+	+	+ (≥2)	+	+ (>1)	+
Post-traumatic seizure	+	+	Excluded	+	+	
Dizziness						
Pre-traumatic seizure	–	–	–	–	–	
Anticoagulation therapy	+	–	Excluded	+	+ if LOC	+
EXAMINATION						
GCS score < 15	+	Excluded	+ (at 2h post injury)	+	+ (2h post injury)	+
Suspicion of open or depressed skull fracture	+	+	+	+	+	+
Clinical signs of basal skull fracture	+	+	+	+	+	+
Clinical signs of skull fracture	+	+	+	+	–	
Intoxication	+	+	–	–	–	
Persistent anterograde amnesia	+	+	–	Minor	–	+
Focal neurologic deficit	+	Excluded	Excluded	Minor	+	+
Retrograde amnesia	+	–	+ (>30min)	–	+ (>30min)	
Contusion of the skull		+	–	Minor		
Signs of facial fracture	+	+	–	–	–	
Contusion of the face	–	+	–	–	–	
GCS score deterioration	+	–	+	+ (≥2 pts) or minor (1 pt)	–	
Prolonged PTA	+	–	+	+ (≥4 h) or minor (2 to <4 h)		
Multiple injuries	+	–	–	–	–	
MECHANISM						
Dangerous mechanism[a]	–	–	+	+	+ if LOC	
High-energy trauma	+	–	–	–	–	
Unclear trauma mechanism	+	–	–	–	–	

Continued post-traumatic amnesia is defined as a GCS verbal reaction of 4 and hence the GCS is by definition < 15. High-energy (vehicle) accident in EFNS defined as initial speed > 64 km/h, major auto-deformity, intrusion into passenger compartment > 30 cm, extrication time from vehicle > 20 min, falls > 6 m, roll-over, auto–pedestrian accidents, or motor cycle crash > 32 km/h or with separation of rider and bike [26, 34]. Dangerous mechanism in CHIP defined as ejected from vehicle, pedestrian or cyclist versus vehicle. Neurosurgery defined in EFNS as: death within 7 days, craniotomy, elevation of skull fracture, intracranial pressure monitoring or intubation for head injury; in NOC as craniotomy, or placing of monitoring bolt; in CCHR as death or craniotomy; in CHIP as craniotomy, elevation of depressed skull fracture, ICP monitoring. In NEXUS-II intracranial injury was defined as mass effect or sulcal effacement, signs of herniation, basal cistern compression or midline shift, substantial epidural or subdural haematomas (>1 cm in width, or causing mass effect), substantial cerebral contusion (>1 cm in diameter, or more than one site), extensive subarachnoid haemorrhage, haemorrhage in the posterior fossa, intraventricular haemorrhage, bilateral haemorrhage of any type, depressed or diastatic skull fracture, pneumocephalus, diffuse cerebral oedema, or diffuse axonal injury.

GCS, Glasgow Coma Scale; LOC, loss of consciousness; EFNS, European Federation of Neurological Societies; NOC, New Orleans Criteria; CCHR, Canadian Closed Head Injury Rule; CHIP, CT in Head Injury Patients; NICE, National Institute of Clinical Excellence.

Children

A quarter of all patients presenting to emergency departments are children. Until recently no formal prediction rule existed for the selection of children with head injury at risk for intracranial abnormalities. So it was questioned if in young patients with MTBI prediction rules originally developed for adults may apply. In a preliminary study, Haydel *et al.* determined whether a clinical decision rule developed for adults could be used in children aged 5 years and older with MTBI and a normal consciousness [12]. In 175 patients aged 5 to 17 years with minor head injury (defined as normal GCS or modified GCS in infants, plus normal brief neurologic examination) and loss of consciousness (LOC), the presence of six clinical variables: headache, vomiting, intoxication, seizure, short-term memory deficits, and physical evidence of trauma above the clavicles, was assessed. CT was obtained for all patients. Fourteen (8%) patients had intracranial injury or depressed skull fracture on CT. The presence of any of the six criteria was significantly associated with an abnormal CT scan result ($p < 0.05$) and was 100% (95% confidence interval (CI) 73–100%) sensitive for identifying patients with intracranial injury. Use of this clinical decision rule previously validated in adults could safely reduce CT use by 23% in the paediatric population older than 5 years of age with a normal consciousness at the emergency department (ED) (Evidence Level II).

In 2006 and 2009, two large studies appeared involving more than 60 000 patients that demonstrated that in children, as in adults, use of prediction rules in the selection of CT to detect life-threatening haematoma is feasible [3, 13].

The CHALICE study, a prospective multicentre diagnostic cohort study, aimed to provide a rule for selection of high-risk children with head injury for CT scanning and included all children presenting to the EDs of 10 hospitals [13]. From 40 clinical variables, defined from the literature, 14 were appointed prior to the study. Presence of one of these variables would require a CT. Of 22 772 patients with any severity of head injury that were evaluated, 96.6% had a GCS of 15 at hospital admission [13]. Clinically significant head injury was defined as death, need for neurosurgical intervention, or abnormality on a CT scan. Recursive partitioning was used to create a highly sensitive rule for the prediction of significant intracranial pathology. Of the study population 56%

were younger than 5. In 766, a CT scan was carried out, of which 281 (37.7%) showed a traumatic abnormality, 137 had a neurosurgical operation, and 15 died. The Chalice rule was 98% (95% CI 96–100%) sensitive and 87% (95% CI 86–87%) specific for the prediction of clinically significant head injury. With this rule the CT scan rate would be 14%. Although a highly sensitive clinical decision rule was derived for the identification of children who should undergo CT scanning after head injury, the rule has not been externally validated yet. A potential weakness of this study is that only patients who had a skull radiograph or CT, were admitted to hospital, or underwent neurosurgery were followed up. However, to minimize the chance of missing a poor outcome in those not followed up endpoints were verified indirectly via collection of data collected in the participating centres and two tertiary hospitals separately on every child who had a skull radiograph or CT of the brain. In addition, hospitals prospectively collected data on patients who were admitted, underwent neurosurgery, or stayed in the intensive care unit or neurorehabilitation unit from 12 centres. These data were then cross-checked with those in the study database. Finally, to verify unexpected poor outcome in patients at low risk for important injury, the Office of National Statistics provided the investigators with details of children who died, in whom head injury was any part of the cause of death.

The Chalice rule describes criteria for use of CT that may be applicable in all children 0–17 years of age, criteria yielding a high sensitivity of 97.6% (CI: 94–99.4%) in those with a GCS of 13–15 (Evidence Level I).

A second study aiming to identify children at low risk of clinically important traumatic brain injuries for whom CT might be unnecessary, enrolled 42 412 patients younger than 18 years with a GCS of 14–15 [3]. CT scans were obtained on 14 969 (35.3%), 376 (0.9%) had clinically significant head injury (death from traumatic brain injury, neurosurgery, intubation > 24 h, or hospital admission ≥ 2 nights), and 60 (0.1%) underwent neurosurgery. Prediction rules were derived and validated separately in children younger than 2 years and for children 2–18 years, for death from traumatic brain injury, neurosurgery, intubation > 24 h, or hospital admission ≥ 2 nights).

In 2216 children younger than 2 years (normal mental status, no scalp haematoma except frontal, no loss of consciousness or loss of consciousness for less than 5 s, non-severe injury mechanism, no palpable skull fracture, and acting normally according to the parents) had a negative predictive value of 100% (95% CI 99.7–100%) and sensitivity of 100% (86.3–100%). For children aged 2 years and older, in 6411 patients, a normal mental status, no loss of consciousness, no vomiting, non-severe injury mechanism, no signs of basilar skull fracture, and no severe headache, yielded a negative predictive value of 99.95% (95% CI 99.81–99.99%) and sensitivity of 96.8% (95% CI 89.0–99.6%). Both rules identified all neurosurgical operations in the validation populations.

Recommendations

- In young patients with MTBI and a normal consciousness, prediction rules originally developed for adults may apply when they are 5 years of age or older (Grade C).

- In patients under 5 years of age, prediction rules for the need of CT to detect intracranial haematoma also apply but with a different set of risk factors, such as applied in the Chalice study [13] or the North American [3] prospective cohort study (Grade A)

- In young patients under 5 years of age, CT is a gold standard for the detection of life-threatening (and other intracranial) abnormalities after MTBI (Grade B).

- In children under 2 years of age, a CT is *not* indicated if normal mental status, no scalp haematoma except frontal, no loss of consciousness or loss of consciousness for less than 5 s, non-severe injury mechanism, no palpable skull fracture, and acting normally according to the parents (Grade A).

- In children aged 2 years and older, a CT is *not* indicated if all apply: a normal mental status, no loss of consciousness, no vomiting, non-severe injury mechanism, no signs of basilar skull fracture, and no severe headache (Grade A).

Initial patient management

According to the Advanced Trauma Life Support (ATLS) and Advanced Pediatric Life Support (APLS) guidelines, any patient with trauma should be evaluated for surgical trauma (Evidence Level III) [14]. Proper triage includes assessing the airways, breathing, and circulation, and the cervical spine. A neurological examination is obligatory and should include level of consciousness, presence of anterograde or retrograde amnesia and/or disorientation, higher cognitive functions, presence of focal neurological deficit (asymmetrical motor reactions or reflexes,

unilateral paresis or cranial nerve deficit), pupillary responses, blood pressure, and pulse rate [15–17]. In addition, the presence of frontal lobe signs, cerebellar symptoms, or sensory deficits should be actively investigated. Accurate assessment of post-traumatic amnesia (PTA) is relevant to guide clinical decision making. Although, despite the importance of PTA measurement, no gold standard for PTA assessment exists, use of formal PTA method is recommended (GPP). Existing methods to assess PTA include the Galveston Orientation and Amnesia Test (GOAT) [18], the (Modified) Oxford PTA Scale (MOPTAS) [19], the Westmead PTA Scale (Westmead) [20], and the Nijmegen PTA scale.

Recommendation

Following acute TBI all patients should undergo urgent neurological examination, in addition to a surgical examination (preferably according to ATLS or APLS guidelines). Furthermore, accurate history taking (including medication), preferably with information being obtained from a witness of the accident or personnel involved in first-aid procedures outside the hospital, is important to ascertain the circumstances (mechanism of injury) under which the accident took place and to assess the duration of LOC and amnesia (GPP).

Home discharge

In MTBI, CT can also be used to decide if patients should be admitted or transferred to a neurosurgical centre or discharged home [4, 9, 11, 16, 21–23]. The majority of MTBI patients show normal CT scan findings [2, 24]. It has been shown before that in patients with a GCS = 15 and no skull fracture the absolute risk of a haematoma is 1 in 7866 in adults and 1 in 12 559 in children (Evidence Level II) [25]. It may be assumed that CT, which is much more sensitive in the detection of intracranial haematoma than the skull X-ray, is a better instrument to select patients for home discharge. Indeed, in a review involving two prospective studies and 52 studies containing over 62 000 patients investigating the safety of early CT in MTBI, only three cases were deemed to have experienced an early adverse outcome despite a normal CT, a GCS = 15, and a normal neurological examination on initial presentation. Only eight cases were identified in which the interpretation was unclear [22]. The conclusion was that the evidence available shows that a CT strategy is a safe way to triage patients for admission (Evidence Level II).

In addition, a multicentre, pragmatic, non-inferiority randomized trial involving 2602 patients aged ≥ 6 with MTBI within the past 24 h, confirmed or suspected LOC or amnesia, or both, normal results on neurological examination and a GCS of 15, and no associated injuries that required admission, demonstrated that use of CT during triage is feasible and clinical outcomes are similar to those in patients admitted for observation (Evidence Level I) [23].

Recommendation

- Patients with MTBI and a normal neurological examination (including a GCS = 15), no risk factors (in particular a normal coagulation status), and a normal CT can be safely discharged home from the ED without head injury warning instructions or considered as such if admitted for other reasons than their head injury (Grade A).

- For children under 6 years of age who are discharged home from the ED, head injury warning instructions are recommended because of the small likelihood of delayed cerebral swelling (GPP).

- Patients with a new and clinically significant traumatic lesion on CT, GCS < 15, focal neurological deficit, restlessness or agitation, intoxication with alcohol or drugs, or other extracranial injuries should be admitted to the hospital (Grade C).

- A repeat CT should be considered if the admission CT findings were abnormal or if risk factors are present (Grade C).

Clinical observation

All patients with a GCS < 15, including continued post-traumatic amnesia, abnormal neurological examination or intracerebral abnormalities, should preferably be admitted to hospital for observation (figure 13.1). Most guidelines recommend an observation period of minimally 12–24 h [16, 26–29]. The main goal of clinical observation is to detect, at an early stage, the development or worsening of extradural or subdural haematoma or diffuse cerebral oedema. A secondary goal is to determine the duration of PTA.

An extradural haematoma usually develops within 6 h, and thus the initial CT may be false-negative when per-

formed very early (within 1 h) [30–32]. Repeated neurological observation (see above) is therefore obligatory for the timely detection of clinical deterioration and other neurological deficits (such as sensory deficits, frontal lobe signs, cerebellar symptoms, etc.).

Although no studies exist as to where patients with MTBI can be best admitted and in as far qualified personnel should carry out observations, the NICE guidelines recommend that in-hospital observation of patients with a head injury should only be conducted by professionals competent in the assessment of head injury (Evidence Level III) [33].

When patients are observed in the hospital, observations should consist of general and neurological examinations, and include breathing frequency, oxygen saturation, blood pressure, pulse rate, GCS, pupil size and reaction to light, motor reactions, and temperature [33].

Recommendation

- A complete neurological examination is mandatory after admission and should include assessment of the GCS, pupillary size and reaction to light, and short-term memory. Repeat neurological examination should be carried out, its frequency being dependent on the clinical condition of the patient; if the GCS is <15 it should be every 30 min. Patients with a GCS of 15 should be examined every 30 min, for 2 h, and if no complications or deterioration occurs, every hour for 4 h, hereafter once every 2 h. The use of a neurological checklist may be helpful to document the neurological condition and its course. If deterioration occurs, possible intracranial causes should be evaluated with (repeated) CT (Grade C).

- In-hospital observation of patients with a head injury should only be conducted by professionals competent in the assessment of head injury (GPP).

Follow-up

It has been shown that regular specialized outpatient follow-up visits are effective in reducing social morbidity and the severity of symptoms after MTBI [34]. In a large randomized controlled trial, patients with a PTA shorter than 7 days who received specialist intervention had significantly less social disability and fewer post-concussion symptoms 6 months after injury than those who did not receive the service (Evidence Level II) [34].

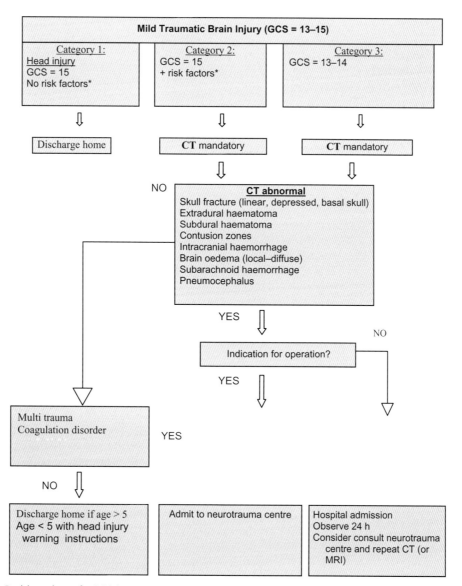

Figure 13.1. Decision scheme for initial management in Mild traumatic Brain Injury (modified from the Dutch and Scandinavian guidelines) [16, 29] GCS, Glasgow Coma Scale; LOC, loss of consciousness; PTA, post-traumatic amnesia; TBI, traumatic brain injury; CT, computed tomography; MRI, magnetic resonance imaging. *Risk factors are shown in table 13.2, no risk factor in CHIP rule includes only 1 minor risk factor.

Recommendation

It is recommended that all patients with MTBI who have been admitted to hospital should be seen at least once in the outpatient clinic in the first two weeks after discharge (Grade C) [34]. Patients who are discharged immediately should contact their general practitioners, who can decide to refer the patient to the neurologist if complaints persist (Grade C).

Conclusions

This update of the guidelines presented in this paper stress the importance of careful neurological examination, assessment of trauma history, and extensive use of CT. The use of a clinical decision rule for CT and hospital admission after MTBI is confirmed. In addition to adults, decision rules now also exist for children, including infants.

Conflicts of interest

The authors have reported no conflicts of interest relevant to this manuscript.

References

1. Hirtz D, Thurman DJ, Gwinn-Hardy K, Mohamed M, Chaudhuri AR, Zalutsky R. How common are the 'common' neurologic disorders? *Neurology* 2007;**68**:326–37.

2. af Geijerstam JL, Britton M. Mild head injury – mortality and complication rate: meta-analysis of findings in a systematic literature review. *Acta Neurochir* 2003;**145**:843–50.

3. Kuppermann N, Holmes JF, Dayan PS, *et al.* Identification of children at very low risk of clinically-important brain injuries after head trauma: a prospective cohort study. *Lancet* 2009;**374**:1160–70.

4. Stiell IG, Wells GA, Vandemheen K, *et al.* The Canadian CT Head Rule for patients with minor head injury. *Lancet* 2001;**357**:1391–6.

5. Haydel MJ, Preston CA, Mills TJ, Luber S, Blaudeau E, DeBlieux PM. Indications for computed tomography in patients with minor head injury. *New Engl J Med* 2000;**343**:100–5.

6. Smits M, Dippel DW, de Haan GG, *et al.* Minor head injury: guidelines for the use of CT. A multicenter validation study. *Radiology* 2007;**245**:831–8.

7. Brenner D, Elliston C, Hall E, Berdon W. Estimated risks of radiation-induced fatal cancer from pediatric CT. *AJR Am J Roentgenol* 2001;**176**:289–96.

8. Brainin M, Barnes M, Baron JC, *et al.* Guidance for the preparation of neurological management guidelines by EFNS scientific task forces–revised recommendations 2004. *Eur J Neurol* 2004;**11**:577–81.

9. Vos PE, Battistin L, Birbamer G, Gerstenbrand F, *et al.* EFNS guideline on mild traumatic brain injury: report of an EFNS task force. *Eur J Neurol* 2002;**9**:207–19.

10. Ibanez J, Arikan F, Pedraza S, *et al.* Reliability of clinical guidelines in the detection of patients at risk following mild head injury: results of a prospective study. *J Neurosurg* 2004;**100**:825–34.

11. Smits M, Dippel DW, de Haan GG, *et al.* External validation of the Canadian CT Head Rule and the New Orleans Criteria for CT scanning in patients with minor head injury. *JAMA* 2005;**294**:1519–25.

12. Haydel MJ, Shembekar AD. Prediction of intracranial injury in children aged five years and older with loss of conscious-

13. Dunning J, Daly JP, Lomas JP, Lecky F, Batchelor J, kway-Jones K. Derivation of the children's head injury algorithm for the prediction of important clinical events decision rule for head injury in children. *Arch Dis Child* 2006;**91**:885–91.

14. American College of Surgeons. *Advanced Trauma Life Support for Doctors*, 6th edn. Chicago, 1997.

15. Tate RL, Pfaff A, Jurjevic L. Resolution of disorientation and amnesia during post-traumatic amnesia. *J Neurol Neurosurg Psychiatry* 2000;**68**:178–85.

16. Ingebrigtsen T, Romner B, Kock-Jensen C. Scandinavian guidelines for initial management of minimal, mild, and moderate head injuries. The Scandinavian Neurotrauma Committee. *J Trauma* 2000;**48**:760–6.

17. Valadka AB, Narayan RK. Emergency room management of the head-injured patient. In: Narayan RK, Wilberger JE, Povlishock JT (eds) *Neurotrauma*. New York: McGraw-Hill, 1996; pp. 119–35.

18. Levin HS, O'Donnell VM, Grossman RG. The Galveston Orientation and Amnesia Test. A practical scale to assess cognition after head injury. *J Nerv Ment Dis* 1979;**167**:675–84.

19. Fortuny LA, Briggs M, Newcombe F, Ratcliff G, Thomas C. Measuring the duration of post traumatic amnesia. *J Neurol Neurosurg Psychiatry* 1980;**43**:377–9.

20. Shores EA, Marosszeky JE, Sandanam J, Batchelor J. Preliminary validation of a clinical scale for measuring the duration of post-traumatic amnesia. *Med J Aust* 1986;**144**:569–72.

21. The Brain Trauma Foundation. The American Association of Neurological Surgeons. The Joint Section on Neurotrauma and Critical Care. Initial management. *J Neurotrauma* 2000;**17**:463–9.

22. af Geijerstam JL, Britton M. Mild head injury: reliability of early computed tomographic findings in triage for admission. *Emerg Med J* 2005;**22**:103–7.

23. af Geijerstam JL, Oredsson S, Britton M. Medical outcome after immediate computed tomography or admission for observation in patients with mild head injury: randomised controlled trial. *BMJ* 2006;**333**:465.

24. Servadei F, Teasdale G, Merry G. Defining acute mild head injury in adults: a proposal based on prognostic factors, diagnosis, and management. *J Neurotrauma* 2001;**18**:657–64.

25. Teasdale GM, Murray G, Anderson E, *et al.* Risks of acute traumatic intracranial haematoma in children and adults: implications for managing head injuries. *BMJ* 1990;**300**:363–7.

26. Masters SJ, McClean PM, Arcarese JS, *et al.* Skull x-ray examinations after head trauma. Recommendations by a multidisciplinary panel and validation study. *N Engl J Med* 1987;**316**:84–91.

27. Bartlett J, Kett-White R, Mendelow AD, Miller JD, Pickard J, Teasdale G. Recommendations from the Society of British Neurological Surgeons. *Br J Neurosurg* 1998;**12**:349–52.

28. American Academy of Pediatrics. The management of minor closed head injury in children. Committee on Quality Improvement, American Academy of Pediatrics. Commission on Clinical Policies and Research, American Academy of Family Physicians. *Pediatrics* 1999;**104**:1407–15.

29. Twijnstra A, Brouwer OF, Keyser A, *et al. Richtlijnen voor de diagnostiek en behandeling van patienten met licht schedel-hersenletsel.* Commissie Kwaliteitsbevordering van de Nederlandse Vereniging voor Neurologie 2001;1–26.

30. Smith HK, Miller JD. The danger of an ultra-early computed tomographic scan in a patient with an evolving acute epidural hematoma. *Neurosurgery* 1991;**29**:258–60.

31. Servadei F, Vergoni G, Staffa G, *et al.* Extradural haematomas: how many deaths can be avoided? Protocol for early detection of haematoma in minor head injuries. *Acta Neurochir* 1995;**133**:50–5.

32. Frowein RA, Schiltz F, Stammler U. Early post-traumatic intracranial hematoma. *Neurosurg Rev* 1989;**12** (Suppl 1): 184–7.

33. National Institute for Clinical Excellence: *Head Injury: triage, assessment, investigation and early management of head injury in infants, children and adults.* Nice Clinical Guideline 2007;No 56 www.nice.org.uk/CG056.

34. Wade DT, King NS, Wenden FJ, Crawford S, Caldwell FE. Routine follow up after head injury: a second randomised controlled trial. *J Neurol Neurosurg Psychiatry* 1998;**65**: 177–83.

CHAPTER 14

Early (uncomplicated) Parkinson's disease

W. H. Oertel,[1] A. Berardelli,[2] B. R. Bloem,[3] U. Bonuccelli,[4] D. Burn,[5] G. Deuschl,[6] E. Dietrichs,[7] G. Fabbrini,[2] J. J. Ferreira,[8] A. Friedman,[9] P. Kanovsky,[10] V. Kostic,[11] A. Nieuwboer,[12] P. Odin,[13] W. Poewe,[14] O. Rascol,[15] C. Sampaio,[16] M. Schüpbach,[17] E. Tolosa,[18] C. Trenkwalder[19]

[1]Philipps-University of Marburg, Centre of Nervous Diseases, Germany; [2]Sapienza, Università di Roma, Italy; [3]Donders Institute for Brain, Cognition and Behavior, Radboud University Nijmegen Medical Center, The Netherlands; [4]University of Pisa, Italy; [5]Institute for Ageing and Health, Newcastle University, Newcastle upon Tyne, UK; [6]Christian-Albrechts-University Kiel, Germany; [7]Oslo University Hospital and University of Oslo, Norway; [8]Institute of Molecular Medicine, Lisbon, Portugal; [9]Medical University of Warsaw, Poland; [10]Palacky University, Olomouc, Czech Republic; [11]Institute of Neurology CCS, School of Medicine, University of Belgrade, Serbia; [12]Katholieke Universiteit Leuven, Belgium; [13]Central Hospital Bremerhaven, Germany, and University Hospital, Lund, Sweden; [14]Innsbruck Medical University, Austria; [15]University Hospital and University of Toulouse, Toulouse, France; [16]Laboratório de Farmacologia Clinica e Terapeutica e Instituto de Medicina Molecular, Faculdade de Medicina de Lisboa, Portugal; [17]INSERM CIC-9503, Hôpital Pitié-Salpétrière, Paris, France, and Bern University Hospital and University of Bern, Switzerland; [18]Universitat de Barcelona, Spain; [19]Paracelsus-Elena Hospital, Kassel, and University of Goettingen, Germany

Background

In the initial stages of disease, levodopa is the most effective therapy for improving motor symptoms in Parkinson's disease (PD). However, long-term treatment is accompanied by the development of fluctuations in motor performance, dyskinesias, and neuropsychiatric complications. Furthermore, as PD progresses, patients develop features that do not respond well to levodopa therapy, such as freezing episodes, autonomic dysfunction, postural instability, falling, dementia, and symptoms related to the administration of other drugs. The increasingly diverse possibilities in the therapy of PD, and the many side effects and complications of therapy, require reliable standards for patient care that are based on current scientific knowledge.

This chapter provides these scientifically supported treatment recommendations.

If the level of available evidence is only Level IV, i.e if the evidence is based on expert opinion and scientific evidence is lacking and therefore the rating of recommendation is below C, best practice is recommended (GPP).

Methods

Search strategy

Searches were made in MEDLINE, the full database of the Cochrane Library, and the International Network of Agencies for Health Technology Assessment (INAHTA). The databases were also searched for existing guidelines and management reports, and requests were made to EFNS societies for their National Guidelines. For the 2010 update, the Movement Disorder Society's Evidence Based Medicine Task Force conducted systematic checking of reference lists published in review articles and other clinical reports, and provided the results of a literature search for articles published until September 2009.

Method for reaching consensus

Classification of scientific evidence and the rating of recommendations are made according to the EFNS guidance [1]. This report focuses on the highest levels of evidence available. If the level of available evidence is only Level IV, i.e if the evidence is based on the experience of

European Handbook of Neurological Management: Volume 1, 2nd edition. Edited by N. E. Gilhus, M. P. Barnes and M. Brainin.
© 2011 Blackwell Publishing Ltd.

the guidelines development group (expert opinion) and/or scientific evidence is lacking and therefore the rating of recommendation is below C, best practice is recommended (GPP).

Meetings of the original author group were held in Chicago in June 2008 and in Paris in May 2009 to agree the strategy for revision of the original review, and additional members were invited to join the author group. Two authors were assigned to review the recent publications relating to each section of the original document, grade the evidence, and make any necessary revisions.

For recommendations concerning drug dosage, method and route of administration, and contraindications, the reader is referred to the local formulary or manufacturer's instruction, except when provided within the guidelines' recommendation itself.

Interventions for the management of early (uncomplicated) Parkinson's disease

This section discusses drug classes used in the pharmacological treatment of PD. Following this, there is consideration of the non-pharmacological interventions in early (uncomplicated) PD.

Neuroprotection and disease modification

To date, no adequate clinical trial has provided unequivocal evidence for pharmacological neuroprotection. While many agents appear to be promising based on laboratory studies, selecting clinical endpoints for clinical trials that are not confounded by symptomatic effects of the study intervention has been difficult. As matters stand at present, neuroprotective trials of riluzole (Class II: [2], coenzyme Q10 (CoQ) (Class II: [3], and glial-derived neurotrophic factor (GDNF) (Class II: [4] do not support the use of any of these drugs for neuroprotection in routine practice. Although a meta-analysis of seven observational studies suggested that dietary intake of vitamin E protects against PD (Class III: [5], vitamin E did not have a neuroprotective effect in patients with PD (Class I: [6]).

Likewise, no adequate clinical trial has provided unequivocal evidence for a disease-modifying effect of any available pharmacotherapy. The sections below describe the investigations on the neuroprotective and disease-modifying effect of drugs primarily known for their symptomatic effect.

MAO-B inhibitors

Studies in early PD (Class I and II: [6–10] showed that selegiline postpones the need for dopaminergic treatment by >6 months, suggesting a delay in disability progression. However, the initial advantages of selegiline were not sustained [11]. Rasagiline had been shown to have symptomatic effect in early *de novo* PD patients in the TEMPO study (Class I: [12]. These patients were followed in a so-called delayed-start design[1] with 1 mg or 2 mg rasagiline for 12 months. They showed less functional decline (UPDRS-score) than subjects whose treatment with rasagiline was delayed for 6 months, suggesting that a disease modification may be present (Class I: [13]. In the ADAGIO study (Class I: [14]; delayed start design) rasagiline was studied in less affected patients under randomized double-blind placebo-controlled conditions for 18 months. The combined primary endpoint was reached for 1 mg, but not for 2 mg. The authors themselves advise caution in the interpretation of the results, given they were not replicated in the 2 mg/day arm. The long-lasting beneficial effect of the 1 mg dose may be interpreted as being due to a potential 'disease-modifying effect', or a symptomatic effect combined with other confounding factors [14]. A disease modifying effect of 1 mg rasagiline can be hypothesized, but is currently not proven.

In summary, the delayed-start results are compatible with the concept that 1 mg/day rasagiline is possibly efficacious for disease modification. However, in the absence of long-term follow-up, such trials do not provide sufficient evidence to conclude on any potential disease-modifying – as opposed to the symptomatic – effect of rasagiline in PD in respect to its usefulness in the practical management of early PD.

Levodopa

The only available placebo-controlled study of levodopa in relation to neuroprotection is inconclusive about any neuroprotective, as opposed to symptomatic, effect

---

[1]The introduction of the 'delayed start design' for studying a potential disease-modifying effect has not resolved the issues that: (1) the primary endpoint(s) are not confounded by a symptomatic effect of the intervention under study; (2) the study duration may not be long enough; and (3) the enrolled group of PD patients may already be too far in the course of the disease to address the issue of disease modification.

(Class I: [15]. Mortality studies suggest improved survival with levodopa therapy (Class III: [16]; review: [17]).

Dopamine agonists

Class I randomized, controlled trials with bromocriptine, pergolide, pramipexole, and ropinirole produced no convincing evidence of neuroprotection or disease modification [9, 18–20].

Starting treatment of PD patients with bromocriptine, rather than with levodopa, is not effective in improving mortality (Class II: [21, 22]).

Anticholinergics, amantadine, COMT inhibitors

For these medications, either clinical studies are not available or the agents are unable to prevent the progression of PD.

Symptomatic pharmacotherapy of parkinsonism

Anticholinergics

Mechanism of action

Anticholinergics are believed to act by correcting the disequilibrium between striatal dopamine and acetylcholine neurotransmission. Some anticholinergics, e.g. benzotropine, can also block dopamine uptake in central dopaminergic neurons. The anticholinergics used to treat PD specifically block muscarinic receptors.

Symptomatic treatment of parkinsonism (monotherapy)

Three Class II trials found anticholinergic monotherapy more effective than placebo in improving motor function in PD (bornaprine [23], benzhexol [24, 25]). Biperiden is as effective as apomorphine in patients with parkinsonian tremor (Class III: [26]). However, data conflict over whether anticholinergic drugs have a better effect on tremor than on other outcome measures or a better effect on tremor than other antiparkinsonian agents. These results are consistent with reviews concluding that anticholinergics have only a small effect on PD symptoms, and that evidence for a special effect on tremor is inconclusive [27, 28].

Adjunctive therapy of parkinsonism

Class II studies of trihexyphenidyl [29], benzotropine [30], and bornaprine [31] in levodopa-treated patients,

and two reviews, indicate that adjunctive anticholinergics have only a minor effect on PD symptoms in patients on levodopa therapy, and that the tremor-specific data are inconclusive [27, 28].

Prevention of motor complications

No studies available.

Symptomatic treatment of non-motor problems

Because of the risk of side effects (see below), centrally acting anticholinergics are usually not advised for the therapy of non-motor, i.e. autonomic, dysfunctions (see Part II of the review).

Safety

The clinical use of anticholinergics has been limited by their side-effect profiles and contraindications. The most commonly reported side effects are blurred vision, urinary retention, nausea, constipation (rarely leading to paralytic ileus), and dry mouth. The incidence of reduced sweating, particularly in those patients on neuroleptics, can lead to fatal heat stroke. Anticholinergics are contraindicated in patients with narrow-angle glaucoma, tachycardia, hypertrophy of the prostate, gastrointestinal obstruction, and megacolon.

Impaired mental function (mainly immediate memory and memory acquisition) and acute confusional state are a well-documented central side effect that resolves after drug withdrawal (Class IV: [32]. Therefore, if dementia is present, the use of anticholinergics is contraindicated.

The abrupt withdrawal of anticholinergics may lead to a rebound effect with marked deterioration of parkinsonism. Consequently, anticholinergics should be discontinued gradually and with caution [33, 34].

Amantadine

Mechanism of action

Amantadine's mechanism of action appears to be multiple. A blockade of NMDA glutamate receptors and an anticholinergic effect are proposed, whereas other evidence suggests an amphetamine-like action to release presynaptic dopamine stores.

Symptomatic treatment of parkinsonism (monotherapy)

Class II studies [24, 35–37] and reviews [28, 38] show that amantadine induces symptomatic improvement.

Adjunctive therapy of parkinsonism

The addition of amantadine to anticholinergic agents is superior to placebo, with the improvement more pronounced in severely affected patients (Class II: [39, 40].

Over 9 weeks, amantadine was beneficial as an adjunctive treatment to levodopa (Class II: [41]), with a more noticeable improvement in patients on low levodopa doses (Class II: [42]. Together with the results of low class evidence studies (reviews: [28, 38]), data suggest that amantadine is probably effective as adjunct therapy, with an unproven long-term duration of effect.

Prevention of motor complications

No studies available.

Symptomatic treatment of non-motor problems

Not applicable.

Safety

Side effects are generally mild, most frequently including dizziness, anxiety, impaired co-ordination and insomnia (>5%), nausea and vomiting (5–10%), peripheral distal oedema (unresponsive to diuretics), and headache, nightmares, ataxia, confusion/agitation, drowsiness, constipation/diarrhoea, anorexia, xerostomia, and livedo reticularis (<5%). Less common side effects include psychosis, abnormal thinking, amnesia, slurred speech, hyperkinesia, epileptic seizures (rarely, and at higher doses), hypertension, urinary retention, decreased libido, dyspnoea, rash, and orthostatic hypotension (during chronic administration) [28].

MAO-B inhibitors

Mechanism of action

Selegiline and rasagiline inhibit the action of monoamine oxidase isoenzyme type B (MAO-B). MAO-B inhibition prevents the breakdown of dopamine, producing greater dopamine availability. Mechanisms besides MAO-B inhibition may also contribute to the clinical effects [43]. Unlike selegiline, rasagiline is not metabolized to amphetamine, and has no sympathomimetic activity.

Symptomatic treatment of parkinsonism (monotherapy)

Five of six studies with a typical follow-up period of 3–12 months (Class I and II: [6, 8, 10, 44–46], and a meta-analysis [47], demonstrated a small symptomatic effect of selegiline monotherapy (Class I).

Two large scale placebo-controlled trials with rasagiline monotherapy in early PD with a follow-up of 6–9 months (Class I: TEMPO-study [12, 13]; ADAGIO-study [14]) provided consistent and significant results for a modest symptomatic benefit of early use of 1 mg and 2 mg/daily to early *de novo* PD patients.

Adjunctive therapy of parkinsonism

In clinical studies (Class I: [48–52]) and a meta-analysis [47] investigating the addition of selegiline to other antiparkinsonian therapies (mainly levodopa), no consistent beneficial effect was demonstrated on the core symptoms of PD in non-fluctuating patients. Rasagiline has not been studied in this context.

Prevention of motor complications

Selegiline has shown no effect in preventing motor fluctuations including wearing-off, ON–OFF fluctuations and dyskinesia (Class I: [53]; Class II: [54, 55]). Rasagiline has not been studied in this context.

Symptomatic treatment of non-motor problems

A Class II study detected no effect of selegiline on depression in PD [56]. MAO-B inhibitors have not been investigated for the treatment of other non-motor problems.

Safety

As with any dopaminergic drug, MAO-B inhibitors can induce a variety of dopaminergic adverse reactions. At the daily doses of selegiline currently recommended, the risk of tyramine-induced hypertension (the 'cheese effect') is low [57]. The tyramine-effect does not need to be taken into consideration when using rasagiline. Concerns that the selegiline/levodopa combination increased mortality rates [58] have been allayed [59].

COMT inhibitors

Mechanism of action

Catechol-O-methyltransferase (COMT) inhibitors reduce the metabolism of levodopa, extending its plasma half-life and prolonging the action of each levodopa dose. Therapeutic doses of entacapone only act peripherally and do not alter cerebral COMT activity. Entacapone is administered together with each dose of levodopa. Entacapone is not approved for use in early (uncomplicated) and non-fluctuating PD patients (see Part II).

Tolcapone (a second-line drug – see safety in Part II) also acts peripherally; in addition a small central effect is discussed. Due to its stronger and longer action, tolcapone is recommended to be taken three times a day. Tolcapone is not approved for use in early (uncomplicated) and non-fluctuating PD patients (see Part II).

Symptomatic treatment of parkinsonism (monotherapy)

Not applicable (COMT inhibitors should always be given with levodopa).

Adjunctive therapy of parkinsonism

There are six published studies (Class I and II) where the issue of efficacy in non-fluctuating patients is addressed. Two of these tested tolcapone [60, 61] and the further two examined entacapone [62, 63]. All trials showed a small benefit in the control of the symptoms of parkinsonism, mostly reflected in UPDRS part II (activities of daily living), but the results were not consistent across all endpoints.

In two recent trials, levodopa/cerbidopa/entacapone showed only borderline significance when compared to levodopa/carbidopa alone in the UPDRS parts II and III in patients with no or minimal fluctuations in the QUEST-AP study [64]. In the FIRST STEP STUDY [65], a 39-week, randomized, double-blind, multicentre study, the efficacy, safety, and tolerability of levodopa/carbidopa/entacapone (LCE, Stalevo®) was compared with levodopa/carbidopa (LC, Sinemet IR) in patients with early, *de novo* PD. A significant difference was present in the combined UPDRS II and III, but not in the UPDRS part III between the two treatment arms (Class I: [65]).

Prevention of motor complications

In addition the FIRST STEP study assessed as secondary endpoints the occurrence of motor fluctuations and dyskinesias. When the initiation of treatment with levodopa/carbidopa/entacapone was compared to that with levodopa/carbidopa, no difference was found between the two treatment arms [65].

Symptomatic treatment of non-motor problems

No studies available.

Safety

COMT inhibitors increase levodopa bioavailability, so they can increase the incidence of dopaminergic adverse reactions, including nausea, and cardiovascular and neuropsychiatric complications. Diarrhoea and urine discolouration are the most frequently reported non-dopaminergic adverse reactions.

The combination with selective MAO-B inhibitors (selegiline) is allowed if the dose of MAO-B inhibitor does not exceed the recommended dose.

For tolcapone including safety see Part II.

Levodopa

(a) Standard levodopa formulation

Mechanism of action

Levodopa exerts its symptomatic benefits through conversion to dopamine, and is routinely administered in combination with a decarboxylase inhibitor (benserazide, carbidopa) to prevent its peripheral conversion to dopamine with the resultant nausea and vomiting. Levodopa passes the blood–brain barrier – in contrast to dopamine. Levodopa has a short half-life, which eventually results in short-duration responses with a wearing-off (end-of-dose) effect.

Symptomatic treatment of parkinsonism (monotherapy)

The efficacy of levodopa is firmly established from more than 30 years of use in clinical practice [28, 66]. A recent Class I trial confirmed a dose-dependent significant reduction in UPDRS scores with levodopa versus placebo [15].

In terms of symptomatic effects, levodopa proved to be better than the dopamine agonists. Levodopa was better than bromocriptine, at least during the first year (Class II: [21]), and a Cochrane review found comparable effects of bromocriptine and levodopa on impairment and disability [67]. Levodopa's symptomatic effect also proved better than ropinirole (Class I: [19]), pramipexole (Class I: [68]), pergolide (Class I: [20, 69]; Class I: [20]), lisuride (Class III: [70]), and cabergoline (Class I: [71]). The results of these individual studies are confirmed by systematic reviews showing that levodopa monotherapy – in general – produced lower UPDRS scores than cabergoline, pramipexole, and ropinirole [28, 66], and bromocriptine, lisuride, and pergolide [66].

Adjunctive therapy of parkinsonism

Supplementation of levodopa to other antiparkinsonian medications in stable PD is common clinical practice to improve symptomatic control (Class IV).

Prevention of motor complications (risk reduction)

The prevention of motor complications (i.e. fluctuations and dyskinesia) by levodopa seems contradictory because these complications are actually caused by levodopa. Usually, levodopa is started three times daily, which offers symptomatic control throughout the day, but after several months or years of chronic treatment, motor complications may arise (see safety section, below). However, by carefully shortening the dose interval to compensate for shortening of the duration of effect of each levodopa dose (wearing-off), and by reducing the dose of each levodopa intake to reduce the magnitude of the effect (peak dose dyskinesia), the clinical emergence of these motor problems may be postponed.

For a comment on non-disabling and disabling dyskinesia in studies with initial levodopa monotherapy versus initial dopamine agonist therapy, see below 'Dopamine agonist, Prevention of motor complications'.

Symptomatic treatment of non-motor problems

Whether or not levodopa improves mood in PD is a matter of debate [72–74], as is the influence of levodopa on cognition (reviews: [75–77]). Off-period psychiatric symptoms (anxiety, panic attacks, depression) and other non-motor symptoms (drenching sweats, pain, fatigue, and akathisia) may be alleviated by modifying the treatment schedule of levodopa (Class IV: [78–81]).

Safety

Most studies in animal models and humans failed to show accelerated dopaminergic neuronal loss with long-term levodopa therapy at usual clinical doses (reviews: [28, 82, 83]). A meta-analysis reported no treatment-related deaths or life-threatening events [66]. Peripheral side effects include gastrointestinal and cardiovascular dysfunction (reviews: [28, 66, 80, 84, 85]).

Central adverse effects include levodopa motor problems such as fluctuations, dyskinesia, and dystonia, and psychiatric side effects such as confusion, hallucinations, and sleep disorders (reviews: [66, 80, 84]. A meta-analysis found ~40% likelihood of motor fluctuations and dyskinesias after 4–6 years of levodopa therapy [86]. Risk factors are younger age, longer disease duration, and levodopa [15, 87–92]; reviews: [66, 80, 84]. In individual studies, the percentage of fluctuations and dyskinesia may range from 10 to 60% of patients at 5 years, and up to 80–90% in later years [66, 80]. Neuropsychiatric complications occur in less than 5% of *de novo* patients on levodopa monotherapy (reviews: [66, 80]).

(b) Controlled-release (CR) levodopa formulations

Mechanism of action

Levodopa has a short half-life, which eventually results in short-duration responses with a wearing-off (end-of-dose) effect. Controlled-release (CR) formulations aim to prolong the effect of a single dose of levodopa, and reduce the number of daily doses.

Symptomatic treatment of parkinsonism (monotherapy)

Standard and CR levodopa maintain a similar level of control in *de novo* PD after 5 years (Class I: [93]), and also in more advanced PD with a duration of about 10 years and without motor fluctuations (Class I: [94]).

Prevention of motor complications

CR levodopa has no significant preventive effect on the incidence of motor fluctuations or dyskinesia, as compared with standard levodopa (Class I: [93, 95, 96].

(c) Intrajejunal application of Levodopa

Not applicable; only approved for very advanced PD patients.

Dopamine agonists

Mechanism of action

Of the 10 dopamine agonists presently marketed for the treatment of PD, five are ergot derivatives (bromocriptine, cabergoline, dihydroergocryptine, lisuride, and pergolide) and five are non-ergot derivatives (apomorphine, piribedil, pramipexole, ropinirole, and rotigotine).

It is generally accepted that the shared D_2-like receptor agonistic activity produces the symptomatic antiparkinsonian effect. This D_2 effect also explains peripheral (gastrointestinal – nausea and vomiting), cardiovascular (orthostatic hypotension), and neuropsychiatric (somnolence, psychosis, and hallucinations) side effects. In addition, dopamine agonists have other properties (e.g. anti-apoptotic effect) that have prompted their testing as putative neuroprotective agents.

Apart from apomorphine or rotigotine, which are used via the subcutaneous (penject and pumps) or transdermal (patch) routes respectively [97, 98], all dopamine agonists are used orally. A once-daily controlled-release formulation of ropinirole has recently became available

[99], while one such formulation for pramipexole is currently under development [100].

Symptomatic treatment of parkinsonism (monotherapy)

Agonists versus placebo Dihydroergocryptine [101], pergolide [102], pramipexole [103], ropinirole [104], piribedil [105], and rotigotine [106–108] are effective in early PD (Class I). Bromocriptine and cabergoline are probably effective as monotherapy in early PD (Class II and III: [71, 109–111]. Lisuride is possibly effective [70] (Class IV).

Agonists versus levodopa Levodopa is more efficacious than any orally active dopamine agonist monotherapy (see section on levodopa). The proportion of patients able to remain on agonist monotherapy falls progressively over time to <20% after 5 years of treatment (Class I: bromocriptine [55, 110, 112]), cabergoline [111], pergolide [20], pramipexole [113, 114]), and ropinirole ([18a, 115]). For this reason, after a few years of treatment, most patients who start on an agonist will receive levodopa as a replacement or adjunct treatment to keep control of motor Parkinsonian signs. Over the past decade, a commonly tested strategy has been to start with an agonist and to add levodopa later if worsening of symptoms cannot be controlled with the agonist alone. However, previously, it was common practice to combine an agonist like bromocriptine or lisuride with levodopa within the first months of treatment ('early combination strategy') (Class II: bromocriptine [116] and lisuride [117]). There are no studies assessing whether one strategy is better than the other.

Agonists versus agonists From the limited data available (Class II: bromocriptine versus ropinirole [118, 119]; Class III: bromocriptine versus pergolide [120]), the clinical relevance of the reported difference between agonists, if any, remains questionable. On the other hand, ropinirole controlled-release was shown to be non-inferior to ropinirole immediate-release [99], while this was not demonstrated for rotigotine in comparison to ropinirole immediate release, possibly because of methodological issues [106] (Class I evidence).

Agonists versus other antiparkinsonian medications There are no published head-to-head comparisons between agonist monotherapy and any other antiparkinsonian medication in early PD. Changes in UPDRS scores reported for most agonists are usually larger than those reported with MAO-B inhibitors, suggesting a greater symptomatic effect with the agonists.

Adjunctive therapy of parkinsonism

Agonists versus placebo Based on Class I evidence, most agonists have been shown to be effective in improving the cardinal motor signs of parkinsonism in patients already treated with levodopa. This is true for apomorphine [121], bromocriptine [122, 123], cabergoline [124], pergolide [125], piribedil [126], pramipexole [127–129], and ropinirole [130]. The available evidence is less convincing (Class II) for dihydroergocryptine [131] and lisuride [117].

Agonists versus agonists Several Class I and II studies have compared the symptomatic effect of two different dopamine agonists on parkinsonism when given as adjunct to levodopa – with bromocriptine as the reference comparator. Such data cannot have a strong impact on clinical practice because of methodological problems in the reported studies (cabergoline [132], lisuride [133, 134], pergolide [120, 135–137], pramipexole [123], piribedil [138], rotigotine [139], and ropinirole [140]). Switching from one agonist to another for reasons of efficacy or safety is sometimes considered in clinical practice. Most of the available data are based on open-label Class IV trials with an overnight switch [141–150]). An empirical conversion chart of dose equivalence is usually proposed, with 10 mg bromocriptine = 1 mg pergolide = 1 mg pramipexole = 2 mg cabergoline = 5 mg ropinirole. There is Class I evidence that ropinirole can be switched overnight at the same dose from immediate- to controlled-release formulation [99].

Agonists versus other antiparkinsonian medications Bromocriptine [151] and pergolide [152] have been compared with the COMT inhibitor tolcapone (Class II), and no significant difference was reported in terms of efficacy on parkinsonian cardinal signs.

Prevention of motor complications

Agonists versus levodopa Class I randomized, controlled trials demonstrate how early use of an agonist can reduce the incidence of motor complications versus levodopa (cabergoline [111, 153], pramipexole [113], pergolide [20], and ropinirole ([18a, 19]). Similar conclusions were reported with bromocriptine (Class II: [55, 110, 154]. Conflicting results have been reported with lisuride [70, 117]. The risk of dyskinesia reappears once levodopa is adjunct to initial agonist monotherapy. From that time-point, the incidence of dyskinesia does not differ, after adjusting for disease duration and levodopa daily dose, among subjects initially randomized to levodopa or an agonist [155, 156]. Long follow-up (6–15 years) of patients initially randomized early to an agonist (bromocriptine, pramipexole, ropinirole) or levodopa are available [112, 114, 115, 157].

Overall, the risk of motor complications remains lower for those starting on an agonist, but the importance of this observation is controversial in such advanced cases because of: (1) methodological issues including high drop-out rate, (2) greater incidence of daytime somnolence, peripheral oedema, and psychiatric/behavioural changes on agonists (see below); and (3) greater impact of other symptoms than dyskinesia (falls, dementia) on patients' disability.

Finally it should be mentioned, that the frequency of disabling dyskinesias – as opposed to non-disabling dyskinesias – was found not to differ in the above listed Class I studies in early PD, which directly compared the effect of initial levodopa monotherapy versus initial dopamine agonist monotherapy on the latency to dyskinesia and the occurrence of dyskinesia over the course of 2–6 years.

Agonists versus agonists There is no available indication that one agonist might be more efficacious than another in preventing or delaying 'time to motor complications'. The only published Class II comparison (ropinirole versus bromocriptine: [119] did not show any difference in dyskinesia incidence at 3 years.

Agonists versus other antiparkinsonian medications No studies available.

Symptomatic treatment of non-motor problems

Dopamine agonists may improve depression, as indicated by clinical trials conducted in non-parkinsonian subjects with major or bipolar depression pramipexole, which showed to be superior to placebo [158, 159]. However, only uncontrolled or low-quality clinical trails of pergolide, pramipexole, and ropinirole have addressed this issue in PD patients [160–163].

The effect of dopamine agonists over Health-related Quality of Life (HRQuOL) has been explored in several clinical trials as secondary outcomes [164]. Rotigotine improved HRQuOL versus placebo at 6 months in early PD [107]. Pramipexole had a similar impact than levodopa on HRQuOL over 6 years of follow-up [114, 165, 166].

There is no indication that symptoms such as anxiety, sleep disturbance, or pain are responsive to dopamine agonists. It is conceivable that such symptoms, if partly 'dopa-responsive' and occurring or worsening during OFF episodes, might be improved by dopamine agonists, as with any dopaminergic medication, but no convincing data are available. Conversely, dysautonomic parkinsonian symptoms such as orthostatic hypotension can be aggravated by dopaminergic medication, including agonists, probably through sympatholytic mechanisms (see also the management recommendations section on neuropsychiatric complications and autonomic dysfunction in Part II of the guidelines).

Safety

Dopamine agonists and all other active dopamine-mimetic medications share a common safety profile reflecting dopamine stimulation. Accordingly, side effects such as nausea, vomiting, orthostatic hypotension, confusion, psychosis, and somnolence may occur with administration of any of these agents. Peripheral leg oedema is also commonly observed with most agonists.

Hallucinations and somnolence are more frequent with some agonists than with levodopa, (Class I: [167, 168] even in healthy subjects, in the case of somnolence [169]. Similarly, leg oedemas appear to be more frequent on agonists than levodopa [18a, 153, 165]). Though there is no convincing evidence that any agonist is better tolerated than bromocriptine, a recent meta-analysis suggested that while frequencies of somnolence, hallucination, or anxiety cases were higher with non-ergot DAs, incidence of vomiting, arterial hypotension, or depression was higher with ergots [170]. The rare but severe risk of pleuropulmonary/retroperitoneal fibrosis is greater with ergot agonists than with non-ergot agonists. The same is true for valvular heart disorders [171–173]). As pergolide and cabergoline have been the most frequently reported drugs at the present time, they are only used as a second-line alternative option, when other agonists have not provided an adequate response. If employed, regular monitoring of heart valves by ultrasound is mandatory.

Impulse-control disorders have recently been identified as a common adverse drug reaction to dopamine agonists. Prevalence ranges between 5 and 15% depending on the author [174]. The principal risk factor is treatment with dopamine agonists, although they can occur on levodopa as well [174]. Personal traits, disturbed decision-making abilities, and younger age have also been implicated [174, 175]. Comorbidities, cognitive impairment, disease severity, and polytherapy are sometimes also mentioned [176]. Up to the present there is no evidence about between-agonists difference in the frequency of these events.

Neurosurgical management of early stage PD

There are no studies available on deep brain stimulation or lesional neurosurgery in patients with uncomplicated PD before the appearance of motor complications.

Non-pharmacological/non-neurosurgical management of early stage PD

In addition to medical management, many patients with PD receive one or more forms of non-pharmacological treatment during the course of their disease. This includes a broad range of disciplines, among others rehabilitation specialists, allied health professionals (physiotherapy, occupational therapy, speech-language therapy), PD nurse specialists, social workers, and sex therapists. These disciplines can be engaged either as monotherapy, or as part of a team approach (interdisciplinary or multi-disciplinary rehabilitation [198]). Non-pharmacological management can be engaged both as an adjunctive treatment for symptoms that also respond to dopaminergic therapy and as the mainstay treatment for symptoms that are otherwise treatment-resistant.

Physiotherapy is the only allied health discipline that explicitly distinguishes the management of early-versus late-stage PD as documented in an evidence-based guideline [177, 178]. The guideline recommends that standard medical care should be complemented with early referral to physiotherapy services (GPP). The guideline also stresses that any physiotherapy interventions should be aimed at clear goals and outcomes, based on a thorough interview and physical assessment. Non-pharmacological management supports patients and their families in coping with the disability and in teaching them how to compensate for their motor and non-motor deficits caused by PD. In the early to middle stages of PD, physiotherapy is aimed mainly at increasing levels of physical activity to preserve or improve physical capacity and physical functioning. This requires expert decisions and adapted exercise programmes to ensure that those aspects of physical capacity that best increase safety and independence in the later stages are targeted.

The weight of the evidence points at positive effects of exercise-based interventions, particularly on motor signs and gait (Class II). A recent meta-analysis recommends exercise therapy as an effective approach to enhance general physical functioning and quality of life in PD (Class II) [179]. Evidence of effectiveness (Class II–III) has now emerged in the following areas.
• There is evidence that cueing strategies improve the quality of gait and increase the confidence to carry out functional activities (Class II) [180]. Cueing does not increase the risk of falling. However, effects are not retained at 6 weeks follow-up without cues. Cued training is likely to improve gait during performance of a secondary motor task (Class III) [181].
• Increases of muscle power can be achieved through resistance exercise (several Class III studies [182]).
• Aerobic training with an appropriate duration (7 weeks) and intensity (50–60% of maximum heart rate reserve) induces significant changes in several cardiorespiratory measures of endurance (Class II) [183].
• Treadmill training for patients with PD results in sustained gains in gait speed (Class II) [184, 197]. Alternative forms of exercise such as Tai Chi (Class II) [185] or Qijong (Class II) [186] have beneficial effects on balance and gait measures, and Unified Parkinson Disease Rating Scale scores.
Other disciplines may also be used in the non-pharmacological management of early stage PD. Similar to physiotherapy, early referral is felt to be useful for occupational therapy and speech-language therapy (Expert opinion), but this is not yet grounded in international guidelines (see also Part II).

Recommendations

Early untreated patients

The optimal time frame for onset of therapy has not been clearly defined. Once parkinsonian signs start to have an impact on the patient's life, initiation of treatment is recommended. For each patient, the choice between the numerous effective drugs available is based on a subtle combination of subjective and objective factors. These factors include considerations related to the drug (efficacy for symptomatic control of parkinsonism/prevention of motor complications, safety, practicality, costs, etc.), to the patient (symptoms, age, needs, expectations, experience, comorbidity, socioeconomic level, etc.), and to their environment (drug availability according to national markets in the European Union, variability in economic and health insurance systems, etc.). However, based on the available level of evidence alone, two main issues are usually considered when initiating a symptomatic therapy for early PD: the symptomatic control of parkinsonism, and the prevention of motor complications (see table 14.1).

Currently, there is no uniform proposal across Europe on initiating symptomatic medication for PD. Options include starting treatment with:

- *MAO-B inhibitor*, like selegiline or rasagiline (Level A). The symptomatic effect is more modest than that of levodopa and (probably) dopamine agonists, but they are easy to administer (one dose, once daily, no titration),and well tolerated (especially rasagiline)

- *amantadine or an anticholinergic* (Level B). The impact on symptoms is smaller than that of levodopa. Anticholinergics are poorly tolerated in the elderly and their use is mainly restricted to young patients

- *levodopa*, the most effective symptomatic antiparkinsonian drug (Level A). After a few years of treatment, levodopa is frequently associated with the development of motor complications. As older patients are more sensitive to neuropsychiatric adverse reactions and are less prone to developing motor complications, the early use of levodopa is recommended in the older population (GPP). The early use of controlled-release levodopa formulations is not effective in the prevention of motor complications (Level A)

- orally active dopamine agonist. Pramipexole, piribedil, and ropinirole immediate- or controlled-release are effective as monotherapy in early PD (Level A), with a lower risk of motor complications than levodopa for pramipexole or ropinirole (Level A). Older drugs like bromocriptine are supported by lower class evidence, giving a Level B recommendation. However, there is no convincing evidence that they are less effective in managing patients with early PD. The benefit of agonists in preventing motor complications (Level A, with data up to 5 years only) must be balanced with the smaller effect on symptoms and the greater incidence of hallucinations, impulse-control disorders, somnolence, and leg oedema, as compared with levodopa. Patients must be informed of these risks, e.g. excessive daytime somnolence is especially relevant to drivers. Younger patients are more prone to developing levodopa-induced motor complications, and therefore initial treatment with an agonist can be recommended in this population (GPP). Ergot derivatives such as pergolide, bromocriptine, and cabergoline are not recommended as first-line medication because of the risk of fibrotic reactions. Rotigotine is administered transdermally using a patch and ropinirole CR once daily orally, as opposed to the other agonists that are administered orally three times a day. Subcutaneous apomorphine is not appropriate at this stage of the disease. The early combination of low doses of a dopamine agonist with low doses of levodopa is another option, although the benefits of such a combination have not been properly documented

- *rehabilitation*. Due to the lack of evidence of the efficacy of physical therapy and speech therapy in the early stage of the disease, a recommendation cannot be made.

Adjustment of initial monotherapy in patients without motor complications
Patients not on dopaminergic therapy

If a patient has started on an MAO-B inhibitor, anticholinergic, amantadine, or a combination of these drugs, a stage will come when, because of worsening motor symptoms, there is a requirement for:

- *addition of levodopa or a dopamine agonist* (GPP). Just like in *de novo* patients, at this stage, the choice between levodopa and an agonist again mainly depends on the impact of improving motor disability (better with

levodopa) compared with the risk of motor complications (less with agonists in the first 3–5 years) and neuropsychiatric complications (greater with agonists). In addition, there is the effect of age on the occurrence of motor complications (more frequent in younger patients) and neuropsychiatric/behavioural complications (more frequent in older and cognitively impaired patients). In general, dopaminergic therapy may/could be started with agonists in younger patients, whereas levodopa may be preferred in older patients (GPP, see previous section) and in multimorbid patients of any age.

Table 14.1 Recommendations for the treatment of early PD.

Therapeutic interventions	Recommendation level	
	Symptomatic control of parkinsonism	Prevention of motor complications
Levodopa	effective (Level A)	not applicable
Levodopa CR	effective (Level A)	ineffective (Level A)
Apomorphine	not used[a]	not used[a]
Bromocriptine[b]	effective (Level B)	effective (Level B)
Cabergoline[b]	effective (Level B)	effective (Level A)
Dihydroergocryptine[b]	effective (Level A)	no recommendation[c]
Lisuride[b]	effective (Level B)	effective (Level C)
Pergolide[b]	effective (Level A)	effective (Level B)
Piribedil	effective (Level C)	no recommendation[c]
Pramipexole	effective (Level A)	effective (Level A)
Pramipexole CR[e]	not available	not available
Ropinirole	effective (Level A)	effective (Level A)
Ropinirole CR[e]	effective (Level A)	no recommendation[c]
Rotigotine[f]	effective (Level A)	no recommendation[c]
Selegiline	effective (Level A)	ineffective (Level A)
Rasagiline	effective (Level A)	no recommendation[c]
Entacapone[d]	no recommendation[c]	no recommendation[c]
Tolcapone[d]	no recommendation[c]	no recommendation[c]
Amantadine	effective (Level B)	no recommendation[c]
Anticholinergics	effective (Level B)	no recommendation[c]
Rehabilitation	no recommendation[c]	no recommendation[c]
Surgery	not used	not used

[a]Subcutaneous apomorphine is not used in early PD.
[b]Pergolide, bromocriptine, cabergoline and, precautionarily, other ergot derivates, cannot be recommended as a first-line treatment for early PD because of the risk of valvular heart disorder [187, 188].
[c]No recommendation can be made due to insufficient data.
[d]As COMT inhibitors, entacapone and tolcapone should always be given with levodopa. Due to hepatic toxicity, tolcapone is not recommended in early PD.
[e]Controlled-release.
[f]Transdermal patch delivery system.

Patients on dopaminergic therapy

Once receiving therapy with a dopamine agonist or levodopa, adjustments of these drugs will also become necessary over time because of worsening motor symptoms.

Recommendations

If on dopamine agonist therapy:

- *increase the dopamine agonist dose* (GPP). However, even when the dopamine agonist dose is increased over time, it cannot control parkinsonian symptoms for more than about 3–5 years of follow-up in most patients
- *switch between dopamine agonists* (Level C)
- *add levodopa* (GPP).

If on levodopa:

- *increase the levodopa dose* (GPP)
- *add a dopamine agonist* (GPP), although the efficacy of adding an agonist has been insufficiently evaluated
- *add a COMT-inhibitor* to levodopa at the transition of a non-fluctuating to a fluctuating status, i.e. if motor fluctuations evolve (GPP) – preferably in older patients and multimorbid patients of any age.

Patients with persistent, or emerging disabling, tremor

If a significant tremor persists despite usual therapy with dopaminergic agents or amantadine, the following treatment options exist for tremor at rest.

Recommendations

- *Anticholinergics* (GPP: possibly useful, although no full consensus could be made). Cave: anticholinergic side effects, particularly cognitive dysfunction in older patients (see section on anticholinergics).
- *Clozapine* (Level B: [189–191]). Due to safety concerns (see Part II of the guidelines on the treatment of psychosis), clozapine is not advised for routine use, but it is considered as an experimental approach for exceptionally disabled patients requiring specialised monitoring (GPP).
- *Beta-blockers (propanolol)*. Beta-blockers can be effective in both resting and postural tremor (Level C: [192–195]). However, due to methodological problems, a Cochrane review found it impossible to determine whether beta-blocker therapy is effective for tremor in PD [196]. Further studies are needed to judge the efficacy of beta-blockers in the treatment of tremor in PD (no recommendation can be made).
- *Consider deep brain stimulation*. Usually subthalamic nucleus stimulation, rarely thalamic stimulation (GPP, see Part II of the guidelines).

Statement of the likely time when the guidelines will need to be updated

No later than 2013.

Funding sources supporting the work

Financial support from MDS-ES, EFNS and Stichting De Regenboog (the Netherlands – review 2006) and Competence Network Parkinson (Germany – review 2010).

Conflicts of interest

A. Berardelli has received speaker honoraria from Allergan and Boehringer Ingelheim.

U. Bonuccelli has acted as scientific advisor for, or obtained speaker honoraria from, Boehringer Ingelheim, Chiesi, GlaxoSmithKline, Novartis, Pfizer, and Schwarz-Pharma. He has received departmental grants and performed clinical studies for Boehringer Ingelheim, Chiesi, Eisai, GlaxoSmithKline, Novartis, Schwarz-Pharma, and Teva.

D. Burn has served on medical advisory boards for Teva, Boehringer-Ingelheim, Archimedes, and Merck Serono. He has received honoraria to speak at meetings from Teva-Lundbeck, Orion, Boehringer-Ingelheim, GlaxoSmithKline, Novartis, Eisai, UCB, and GE Healthcare.

G. Deuschl has acted as scientific advisor for, or obtained speaker honoraria from, Orion, Novartis, Boehringer Ingelheim, and Medtronic.

E. Dietrichs has received honoraria for lecturing and/or travelling grants from GlaxoSmithKline, Lundbeck, Medtronic, Orion, Solvay, and UCB.

G. Fabbrini has received honoraria for lectures from Boehringer Ingelheim, Glaxo Pharmaceuticals, and Novartis Pharmaceuticals, and is member of an advisory board for Boehringer Ingelheim.

J. Ferreira has received honoraria for lecturing and/or consultancy from GlaxoSmithKline, Novartis, TEVA, Lundbeck, Solvay, and BIAL.

Andrzej Friedman received honoraria for presentations at educational conferences from Roche Poland, MSD Poland, and Allergan Poland.

P. Kanovsky has received honoraria for lectures from Ipsen and GSK, and received a research grant from Novartis.

V. Kostić has received honoraria for lecturing from Novartis, Boehringer Ingelheim, Merck, Lundbeck, and Glaxo-Smith-Kline, and is a member of the Regional South-Eastern European Pramipexole Advisory Board of Boehringer Ingelheim.

P. Odin has received honoraria for lectures from Boehringer Ingelheim, UCB, GSK, Solvay, and Cephalon, and participated in advisory boards for Boehringer Ingelheim, Cephalon, and Solvay.

W.H. Oertel has received honoraria for consultancy and presentations from Bayer-Schering, Boehringer Ingelheim, Cephalon, Desitin, GlaxoSmithKline, Medtronic, Merck-Serono, Neurosearch, Novartis, Orion Pharma, Schwarz-Pharma Neuroscience, Servier, Synosia, Teva, UCB, and Vifor Pharma.

W. Poewe has received honoraria for lecturing and advisory board membership from Novartis, GlaxoSmithKline, Teva, Boehringer Ingelheim, Schwarz-Pharma, and Orion.

O. Rascol has received scientific grants and consulting fees from GlaxoSmithKline, Novartis, Boehringer Ingelheim, Teva Neuroscience, Eisai, Schering, Solvay,

XenoPort, Oxford BioMedica, Movement Disorder Society, UCB, Lundbeck, Schwarz-Pharma, and Servier.

C. Sampaio has received departmental research grants from Novartis Portugal. Her department has also charged consultancy fees to Servier and Lundbeck, and she has received honoraria for lectures from Boehringer Ingelheim.

M. Schüpbach has received speaker's honoraria and travel reimbursement from Medtronic.

E. Tolosa has received honoraria for lectures from Boehringer Ingelheim, Novartis, UCB, GlaxoSmithKline, Solvay, Teva, and Lundbeck, and participated in advisory boards for Boehringer Ingelheim, Novartis, Teva, and Solvay.

C. Trenkwalder has received honoraria for lectures from Boehringer Ingelheim, UCB, Glaxo Pharmaceuticals, and Astra Zeneca, and is member of advisory boards for Boehringer Ingelheim, UCB, Cephalon, Solvay, Novartis, and TEVA/Lundbeck.

Disclosure statement

The reader's attention should be drawn to the fact that the opinions and views expressed in the paper are those of the authors and not necessarily those of the MDS or the MDS Scientific Issues Committee (SIC).

Acknowledgements

The authors acknowledge the contribution of the late Martin Horstink as first author of the original publication. We are grateful to Susan Fox who provided the Movement Disorder Society's Evidence-based Medicine Task Force 2009 literature review. Niall Quinn is thanked for reviewing the manuscript. The authors would like to thank Karen Henley for co-ordinating the manuscript revision and Heidi Schudrowitz for technical assistance.

References

1. Brainin M, Barnes M, Baron JC, Gilhus NE, Hughes R, Selmaj K, Waldemar G. Guidance for the preparation of neurological management guidelines by EFNS scientific task forces – revised recommendations 2004. *Eur J Neurol* 2004;**11**:577–81.

2. Jankovic J, Hunter C. A double-blind, placebo-controlled and longitudinal study of riluzole in early Parkinson's disease. *Parkinsonism Relat Disord* 2002;**8**:271–6.

3. Shults CW, Oakes D, Kieburtz K, *et al.* Effects of coenzyme Q10 in early Parkinson disease: evidence of slowing of the functional decline. *Arch Neurol* 2002;**59**: 1541–50.

4. Nutt JG, Burchiel KJ, Comella CL, *et al.* Randomized, double-blind trial of glial cell line-derived neurotrophic factor (GDNF) in PD. *Neurology* 2003;**60**:69–73.

5. Etminan M, Gill SS, Samii A. Intake of vitamin E, vitamin C, and carotenoids and the risk of Parkinson's disease: a meta-analysis. *Lancet Neurol* 2005;**4**:362–5.

6. Parkinson Study Group. Effect of deprenyl on the progression of disability in early Parkinson's disease. *N Engl J Med* 1989;**321**:1364–71.

7. Tetrud JW, Langston JW. The effect of deprenyl (selegiline) on the natural history of Parkinson's disease. *Science* 1989;**245**:519–22.

8. Myllyla VV, Sotaniemi KA, Vuorinen JA, Heinonen EH. Selegiline as initial treatment in de novo parkinsonian patients. *Neurology* 1992;**42**:339–43.

9. Olanow CW, Hauser RA, Gauger L, *et al.* The effect of deprenyl and levodopa on the progression of Parkinson's disease. *Ann Neurol* 1995;**38**:771–7.

10. Palhagen S, Heinonen EH, Hagglund J, *et al.* Selegiline delays the onset of disability in de novo parkinsonian patients. Swedish Parkinson Study Group. *Neurology* 1998;**51**:520–5.

11. Parkinson Study Group. Impact of deprenyl and tocopherol treatment on Parkinson's disease in DATATOP patients requiring levodopa. *Ann Neurol* 1996;**39**:37–45.

12. Parkinson Study Group. A controlled trial of rasagiline in early Parkinson disease. The TEMPO study. *Arch Neurol* 2002;**59**:1937–43.

13. Parkinson Study Group. A controlled, randomized, delayed-start study of rasagiline in early Parkinson disease. *Arch Neurol* 2004;**61**:561–6.

14. Olanow CW, Rascol O, Hauser R, *et al.*, Adagio Study Investigators. A double-blind, delayed start trial of rasagiline in Parkinson's disease. *N Engl J Med* 2009;**361**: 1268–78.

15. Parkinson Study Group. Levodopa and the progression of Parkinson's disease. *N Engl J Med* 2004;**351**:2498–508.

16. Rajput AH. Levodopa prolongs life expectancy and is non-toxic to substantia nigra. *Parkinsonism Relat Disord* 2001;**8**:95–100.

17. Clarke CE. Does levodopa therapy delay death in Parkinson's disease? A review of the evidence. *Mov Disord* 1995;**10**:250–6.

18. Parkinson Study Group. Dopamine transporter brain imaging to assess the effects of pramipexole vs levodopa on Parkinson disease progression. *JAMA* 2002;**287**:1653–61.

18a. Rascol O, Brooks DJ, Korczyn AD, De Deyn PP, Clarke CE, Lang AE. A five-year study of the incidence of dyskinesia in patients with early Parkinson's disease who were treated with ropinirole or levodopa. 056 Study Group. *N Engl J Med.* 2000 May 18;**342**(20):1484–91.

19. Whone AL, Watts RL, Stoess AJ, *et al.* Slower progression of Parkinson's disease with ropinirole versus levodopa: the REAL-PET study. *Ann Neurol* 2003;**54**:93–101.

20. Oertel WH, Wolters E, Sampaio C, *et al.* Pergolide versus levodopa monotherapy in early Parkinson's disease patients: the PELMOPET study. *Mov Disord* 2006;**21**: 343–53.

21. Lees AJ, Katzenschlager R, Head J, Ben-Shlomo Y. Ten-year follow-up of three different initial treatments in de-novo PD. A randomized trial. *Neurology* 2001;**57**: 1687–94.

22. Montastruc JL, Desboeuf K, Lapeyre-Mestre M, Senard JM, Rascol O, Brefel-Courbon C. Long-term mortality results on the randomized controlled study comparing bromocriptine to which levodopa was later added with levodopa alone in previously untreated patients with Parkinson's disease. *Mov Disord* 2001;**16**:511–4.

23. Iivanainen M. KR 339 in the treatment of Parkinsonian tremor. *Acta Neurol Scand* 1974;**50**:469–70.

24. Parkes JD, Baxter RC, Marsden CD, Rees J. Comparative trial of benzhexol, amantadine, and levodopa in the treatment of Parkinson's disease. *J Neurol Neurosurg Psychiatry* 1974;**37**:422–6.

25. Cooper JA, Sagar HJ, Doherty SM, Jordan N, Tidswell P, Sullivan EV. Different effects of dopaminergic and anticholinergic therapies on cognitive and motor function in Parkinson's disease. *Brain* 1992;**115**:1701–25.

26. Schrag A, Schelosky L, Scholz U, Poewe W. Reduction of parkinsonian signs in patients with Parkinson's disease by dopaminergic versus anticholinergic single-dose challenges. *Mov Disord* 1999;**14**:252–5.

27. Katzenschlager R, Sampaio C, Costa J, Lees A. Anticholinergics for symptomatic management of Parkinson's disease. *Cochrane Database Syst Rev* 2002;(3):CD003735.

28. Management of Parkinson's disease: an evidence-based review. *Mov Disord* 2002;**17**:S1–166.

29. Martin WE, Loewenson RB, Resch JA, Baker AB. A controlled study comparing trihexyphenidyl hydrochloride plus levodopa with placebo plus levodopa in patients with Parkinson's disease. *Neurology* 1974;**24**:912–9.

30. Tourtellotte WW, Potvin AR, Syndulko K, *et al.* Parkinson's disease: cogentin with Sinemet, a better response. *Prog Neuropsychopharmacol Biol Psychiatry* 1982;**6**:51–5.

31. Cantello R, Riccio A, Gilli M, *et al.* Bornaprine vs placebo in Parkinson disease: double-blind controlled cross-over trial in 30 patients. *Ital J Neurol Sci* 1986;**7**:139–43.

32. van Herwaarden G, Berger HJ, Horstink MW. Short-term memory in Parkinson's disease after withdrawal of long-term anticholinergic therapy. *Clin Neuropharmacol* 1993;**16**:438–43.

33. Hughes RC, Polgar JG, Weightman D, Walton JN. Levodopa in Parkinsonism: the effects of withdrawal of anticholinergic drugs. *Br Med J* 1971;**2**:487–91.

34. Horrocks PM, Vicary DJ, Rees JE, Parkes JD, Marsden CD. Anticholinergic withdrawal and benzhexol treatment in Parkinson's disease. *J Neurol Neurosurg Psychiatry* 1973; **36**:936–41.

35. Cox B, Danta G, Schnieden H, Yuill GM. Interactions of levodopa and amantadine in patients with parkinsonism. *J Neurol Neurosurg Psychiatry* 1973;**36**:354–61.

36. Butzer JF, Silver DE, Sans AL. Amantadine in Parkinson's disease. A double-blind, placebo-controlled, crossover study with long-term follow-up. *Neurology* 1975;**25**: 603–6.

37. Fahn S, Isgreen WP. Long-term evaluation of amantadine and levodopa combination by double-blind crossover analyses. *Neurology* 1975;**25**:695–700.

38. Crosby NJ, Deane KH, Clarke CE. Amantadine for dyskinesia in Parkinson's disease. *Cochrane Database Syst Rev* 2003;(2):CD003467.

39. Appleton DB, Eadie MJ, Sutherland JM. Amantadine hydrochloride in the treatment of parkinsonism. A controlled study. *Med J Aust* 1970;**2**:626–9.

40. Jorgensen PB, Bergin JD, Haas L, *et al.* Controlled trial of amantadine hydrochloride in Parkinson's disease. *N Z Med J* 1971;**73**:263–7.

41. Savery F. Amantadine and a fixed combination of levodopa and carbidopa in the treatment of Parkinson's disease. *Dis Nerv Syst* 1971;**38**:605–8.

42. Fehling C. The effect of adding amantadine to optimum levodopa dosage in Parkinson's syndrome. *Acta Neurol Scand* 1973;**49**:245–51.

43. Olanow CW, Riederer P. Selegiline and neuroprotection in Parkinson's disease. *Neurology* 1996;**47C**(Suppl. 3):51.

44. Teravainen H. Selegiline in Parkinson's disease. *Acta Neurol Scand* 1990;**81**:333–6.

45. Allain H, Pollak P, Neukirch HC. Symptomatic effect of selegiline in de novo Parkinsonian patients. The French Selegiline Multicenter Trial. *Mov Disord* 1993;**8**(Suppl. 1):S36–40.

46. Mally J, Kovacs AB, Stone TW. Delayed development of symptomatic improvement by (−)-deprenyl in Parkinson's disease. *J Neurol Sci* 1995;**134**:143–5.

47. Ives NJ, Stowe RL, Marro J, *et al.* Monoamine oxidase type B inhibitors in early Parkinson's disease: meta-analysis of 17 randomised trials involving 3525 patients. *BMJ* 2004;**329**:593.

48. Przuntek H, Kuhn W. The effect of R-(-)-deprenyl in de novo Parkinson patients on combination therapy with levodopa and decarboxylase inhibitor. *J Neural Transm Suppl* 1987;**25**:97–104.

49. Sivertsen B, Dupont E, Mikkelsen B, *et al.* Selegiline and levodopa in early or moderately advanced Parkinson's disease: a double-blind controlled short- and long-term study. *Acta Neurol Scand Suppl* 1989;**126**: 147–52.

50. Nappi G, Martignoni E, Horowski R, *et al.* Lisuride plus selegiline in the treatment of early Parkinson's disease. *Acta Neurol Scand* 1991;**83**:407–10.

51. Lees AJ. Comparison of therapeutic effects and mortality data of levodopa and levodopa combined with selegiline in patients with early, mild Parkinson's disease. Parkinson's Disease Research Group of the United Kingdom. *BMJ* 1995;**311**:1602–7.

52. Larsen JP, Boas J. The effects of early selegiline therapy on long-term levodopa treatment and parkinsonian disability: an interim analysis of a Norwegian–Danish 5-year study. Norwegian-Danish Study Group. *Mov Disord* 1997;**12**: 175–82.

53. Larsen JP, Boas J, Erdal JE. Does selegiline modify the progression of early Parkinson's disease? Results from a five-year study. The Norwegian-Danish Study Group. *Eur J Neurol* 1999;**6**:539–47.

54. Shoulson I, Oakes D, Fahn S, *et al.* Parkinson Study Group. Impact of sustained deprenyl (selegiline) in levodopa-treated Parkinson's disease: a randomized placebo-controlled extension of the deprenyl and tocopherol antioxidative therapy of parkinsonism trial. *Ann Neurol* 2002;**51**:604–12.

55. Parkinson's Disease Research Group in the United Kingdom. Comparisons of therapeutic effects of levodopa, levodopa and selegiline, and bromocriptine in patients with early, mild Parkinson's disease: three year interim report. *BMJ* 1993;**307**:469–72.

56. Lees AJ, Shaw KM, Kohout LJ, Stern GM. Deprenyl in Parkinson's disease. *Lancet* 1977;**15**:791–5.

57. Heinonen EH, Myllyla V. Safety of selegiline (deprenyl) in the treatment of Parkinson's disease. *Drug Saf* 1998;**19**: 11–22.

58. Ben-Shlomo Y, Churchyard A, Head J, *et al.* Investigation by Parkinson's Disease Research Group of United Kingdom into excess mortality seen with combined levodopa and selegiline treatment in patients with early, mild Parkinson's disease: further results of randomised trial and confidential inquiry. *BMJ* 1998;**316**:1191–6.

59. Olanow CW, Myllyla VV, Sotaniemi KA, *et al.* Effect of selegiline on mortality in patients with Parkinson's disease: a meta-analysis. *Neurology* 1998;**51**:825–30.

60. Waters CH, Kurth M, Bailey P, *et al.* Tolcapone in stable Parkinson's disease: efficacy and safety of long-term treatment. The Tolcapone Stable Study Group. *Neurology* 1997;**49**:665–71.

61. Dupont E, Burgunder JM, Findley LJ, Olsson JE, Dorflinger E. Tolcapone added to levodopa in stable parkinsonian patients: a double-blind placebo-controlled study. Tolcapone in Parkinson's Disease Study Group II (TIPS II). *Mov Disord* 1997;**12**:928–34.

62. Myllyla VV, Kultalahti ER, Haapaniemi H, Leinonen M, FILOMEN Study Group. Twelve-month safety of entacapone in patients with Parkinson's disease. *Eur J Neurol* 2001;**8**:53–60.

63. Brooks DJ, Sagar H, UK-Irish Entacapone Study Group. Entacapone is beneficial in both fluctuating and non-fluctuating patients with Parkinson's disease: a randomised, placebo controlled, double blind, six month study. *J Neurol Neurosurg Psychiatry* 2003;**74**:1071–9.

64. Fung VS, Herawati L, Wan Y, Movement Disorder Society of Australia Clinical Research and Trials Group; QUEST-AP Study Group. Quality of life in early Parkinson's disease treated with levodopa/carbidopa/entacapone. *Mov Disord* 2009;**24**:25–31.

65. Hauser RA, Panisset M, Abbruzzese G, Mancione L, Dronamraju N, Kakarieka A, FIRST STEP Study Group. Double-blind trial of levodopa/carbidopa /entacapone versus levodopa/carbidopa in early Parkinson's disease. *Mov Disord* 2009;**24**:541–50.

66. Levine CB, Fahrbach KR, Siderowf AD, Estok RP, Ludensky VM, Ross SD. Diagnosis and treatment of Parkinson's disease: a systematic review of the literature. *Evid Rep Technol Assess* 2003;**57**:1–306.

67. Ramaker C, van Hilten JJ. Bromocriptine versus levodopa in early Parkinson's disease. *Cochrane Database Syst Rev* 2000;(2):CD002258.

68. Parkinson Study Group. Pramipexole vs levodopa as initial treatment for Parkinson disease: a 4-year randomized controlled trial. *Arch Neurol* 2004;**61**:1044–53.

69. Kulisevsky J, Lopez-Villegas D, Garcia-Sanchez C, Barbanoj M, Gironell A, Pascual-Sedano B. A six-month study of pergolide and levodopa in de novo Parkinson's disease patients. *Clin Neuropharmacol* 1998;**21**: 358–62.

70. Rinne UK. Lisuride, a dopamine agonist in the treatment of early Parkinson's disease. *Neurology* 1989;**39**: 336–9.

71. Rinne UK, Bracco F, Chouza C, *et al.* Cabergoline in the treatment of early Parkinson's disease: results of the first year of treatment in a double-blind comparison of cabergoline and levodopa. The PKDS009 Collaborative Study Group. *Neurology* 1997;**48**:363–8.

72. Marsh GG, Markham CH. Does levodopa alter depression and psychopathology in Parkinsonism patients? *J Neurol Neurosurg Psychiatry* 1973;**36**:925–35.

73. Maricle RA, Nutt JG, Carter JH. Mood and anxiety fluctuation in Parkinson's disease associated with levodopa infusion: preliminary findings. *Mov Disord* 1995;**10**: 329–32.

74. Morrison CE, Borod JC, Brin MF, Halbig TD, Olanow CW. Effects of levodopa on cognitive functioning in moderate-to-severe Parkinson's disease (MSPD). *J Neural Transm* 2004;**111**:1333–41.

75. Nieoullon A. Dopamine and the regulation of cognition and attention. *Prog Neurobiol* 2002;**67**:53–83.

76. Pillon B, Czernecki V, Dubois B. Dopamine and cognitive function. *Curr Opin Neurol* 2003;**16**(Suppl. 2):S17–22.

77. Bosboom JL, Stoffers D, Wolters EC. Cognitive dysfunction and dementia in Parkinson's disease. *J Neural Transm* 2004;**111**:1303–15.

78. Nissenbaum H, Quinn NP, Brown RG, Toone B, Gotham AM, Marsden CD. Mood swings associated with the 'on-off' phenomenon in Parkinson's disease. *Psychol Med* 1987;**17**:899–904.

79. Raudino F. Non motor off in Parkinson's disease. *Acta Neurol Scand* 2001;**104**:312–5.

80. Olanow CW, Watts RL, Koller WC. An algorithm (decision tree) for the management of Parkinson's disease: treatment guidelines. *Neurology* 2001;**56**(Suppl. 5):S1–88.

81. Witjas T, Kaphan E, Azulay JP, et al. Nonmotor fluctuations in Parkinson's disease: frequent and disabling. *Neurology* 2002;**59**:408–13.

82. Katzenschlager R, Lees AJ. Treatment of Parkinson's disease: levodopa as the first choice. *J Neurol* 2002;**249** (Suppl. 2):II19–24.

83. Olanow CW, Agid Y, Mizuno Y, et al. Levodopa in the treatment of Parkinson's disease: current controversies. *Mov Disord* 2004;**19**:997–1005.

84. Jankovic J. Motor fluctuations and dyskinesias in Parkinson's disease: clinical manifestations. *Mov Disord* 2005;**20**(Suppl. 11):S11–6.

85. Adler CH. Nonmotor complications in Parkinson's disease. *Mov Disord* 2005;**20**(Suppl. 11):S23–9.

86. Ahlskog JE, Muenter MD. Frequency of levodopa-related dyskinesias and motor fluctuations as estimated from the cumulative literature. *Mov Disord* 2001;**16**:448–58.

87. Poewe WH, Lees AJ, Stern GM. Low-dose L-dopa therapy in Parkinson's disease: a 6-year follow-up study. *Neurology* 1986;**36**:1528–30.

88. Kostic V, Przedborski S, Flaster E, Sternic N. Early development of levodopa-induced dyskinesias and response fluctuations in young-onset Parkinson's disease. *Neurology* 1991;**41**:202–5.

89. Blanchet PJ, Allard P, Gregoire L, Tardif F, Bedard PJ. Risk factors for peak dose dyskinesia in 100 levodopa-treated parkinsonian patients. *Can J Neurol Sci* 1996;**23**: 189–93.

90. Grandas F, Galiano ML, Tabernero C. Risk factors for levodopa-induced dyskinesias in Parkinson's disease. *J Neurol* 1999;**246**:1127–33.

91. Denny AP, Behari M. Motor fluctuations in Parkinson's disease. *J Neurol Sci* 1999;**165**:18–23.

92. Kumar N, Van Gerpen JA, Bower JH, Ahlskog JE. Levodopa-dyskinesia incidence by age of Parkinson's disease onset. *Mov Disord* 2005;**20**:342–4.

93. Koller WC, Hutton JT, Tolosa E, Capilldeo R. Immediate-release and controlled-release carbidopa/levodopa in PD: a 5-year randomized multicenter study. Carbidopa/Levodopa Study Group. *Neurology* 1999;**53**: 1012–9.

94. Goetz CG, Tanner CM, Shannon KM, et al. Controlled-release carbidopa/levodopa (CR4-Sinemet) in Parkinson's disease patients with and without motor fluctuations. *Neurology* 1988;**38**:1143–6.

95. Dupont E, Andersen A, Boas J, et al. Sustained-release Madopar HBS compared with standard Madopar in the long-term treatment of de novo parkinsonian patients. *Acta Neurol Scand* 1996;**93**:14–20.

96. Block G, Liss C, Reines S, Irr J, Nibbelink D. Comparison of immediate-release and controlled release carbidopa/levodopa in Parkinson's disease. A multicenter 5-year study. The CR First Study Group. *Eur Neurol* 1997;**37**: 23–7.

97. Katzenschlager R, Hughes A, Evans A, et al. Continuous subcutaneous apomorphine therapy improves dyskinesias in Parkinson's disease: a prospective study using single-dose challenges. *Mov Disord* 2005;**20**:151–7.

98. Rascol O, Perez-Lloret S. Rotigotine transdermal delivery for the treatment of Parkinson's disease. *Expert Opin Pharmacother* 2009;**10**:677–91.

99. Stocchi F, Hersh BP, Scott BL, Nausieda PA, Giorgi L. Ropinirole 24-hour prolonged release and ropinirole immediate release in early Parkinson's disease: a randomized, double-blind, non-inferiority crossover study. *Curr Med Res Opin* 2008;**24**:2883–95.

100. Jenner P, Könen-Bergman M, Schepers C, Haertter S. Pharmacokinetics of a once-daily extended-release formulation of pramipexole in healthy male volunteers: three studies. *Clin Therap* 2009;**31**:2698–711.

101. Bergamasco B, Frattola L, Muratorio A, Piccoli F, Mailland F, Parnetti L. Alpha-dihydroergocryptine in the treatment of de novo parkinsonian patients: results of a multicentre, randomized, double-blind, placebo-controlled study. *Acta Neurol Scand* 2000;**101**:372–80.

102. Barone P, Bravi D, Bermejo-Pareja F, *et al.* and the Pergolide Monotherapy Study Group. Pergolide monotherapy in the treatment of early PD. A randomized controlled study. *Neurology* 1999;**53**:573–9.

103. Shannon KM, Bennett JP, Friedman JH. Efficacy of pramipexole, a novel dopamine agonist, as monotherapy in mild to moderate Parkinson's disease. The Pramipexole Study Group. *Neurology* 1997;**49**:724–8.

104. Adler CH, Sethi KD, Hauser RA, *et al.* for the Ropinirole Study Group. Ropinirole for the treatment of early Parkinson's disease. *Neurology* 1997;**49**:393–9.

105. Rascol O, Dubois B, Caldas AC, Senn S, Del SS, Lees A. Early piribedil monotherapy of Parkinson's disease: a planned seven-month report of the REGAIN study. *Mov Disord* 2006;**21**:2110–5.

106. Giladi N, Boroojerdi B, Korczyn AD, Burn DJ, Clarke CE, Schapira AH. Rotigotine transdermal patch in early Parkinson's disease: a randomized, double-blind, controlled study versus placebo and ropinirole. *Mov Disord* 2007;**22**:2398–404.

107. Jankovic J, Watts RL, Martin W, Boroojerdi B. Transdermal rotigotine: double-blind, placebo-controlled trial in Parkinson disease. *Arch Neurol* 2007;**64**:676–82.

108. Parkinson Study Group. A controlled trial of rotigotine monotherapy in early Parkinson's disease. *Arch Neurol* 2003;**60**:1721–8.

109. Riopelle RJ. Bromocriptine and the clinical spectrum of Parkinson's disease. *Can J Neurol Sci* 1987;**14**:455–9.

110. Montastruc JL, Rascol O, Senard JM, Rascol A. A randomized controlled study comparing bromocriptine to which levodopa was later added, with levodopa alone in previously untreated patients with Parkinson's disease: a five year follow-up. *J Neurol Neurosurg Psychiatry* 1994;**57**:1034–8.

111. Rinne UK, Bracco F, Chouza C, *et al.* Early treatment of Parkinson's disease with cabergoline delays the onset of motor complications. The PKDS009 Study Group. *Drugs* 1998;**55**(Suppl. 1):23–30.

112. Katzenschlager R, Head J, Schrag A, Ben-Shlomo Y, Evans A, Lees AJ. Fourteen-year final report of the randomized PDRG-UK trial comparing three initial treatments in PD. *Neurology* 2008;**71**:474–80.

113. Parkinson Study Group. Pramipexole vs levodopa as initial treatment for Parkinson disease: a randomized controlled trial. *JAMA* 2000;**284**:1931–8.

114. Parkinson's Disease Study Group. Long-term effect of initiating pramipexole vs levodopa in early Parkinson disease. *Arch Neurol* 2009;**66**:563–70.

115. Hauser RA, Rascol O, Korczyn AD, *et al.* Ten-year follow-up of Parkinson's disease patients randomized to initial therapy with ropinirole or levodopa. *Mov Disord* 2007;**22**:2409–17.

116. Przuntek H, Welzel D, Gerlach M, *et al.* Early institution of bromocriptine in Parkinson's disease inhibits the emergence of levodopa-associated motor side effects. Long-term results of the PRADO study. *J Neural Transm* 1996;**103**:699–715.

117. Allain H, Destée A, Petit H, *et al.* Five-year follow-up of early lisuride and levodopa combination therapy versus levodopa monotherapy in de novo Parkinson's disease. The French Lisuride Study Group. *Eur Neurol* 2000;**44**:22–30.

118. Korczyn AD, Brooks DJ, Brunt ER, Poewe WH, Rascol O, Stocchi F. Ropinirole versus bromocriptine in the treatment of early Parkinson's disease: a 6-month interim report of a 3-year study. 053 Study Group. *Mov Disord* 1998;**13**:46–51.

119. Korczyn AD, Brunt ER, Larsen JP, Nagy Z, Poewe WH, Ruggieri S. A 3-year randomized trial of ropinirole and bromocriptine in early Parkinson's disease. The 053 Study Group. *Neurology* 1999;**53**:364–70.

120. Mizuno Y, Kondo T, Narabayashi H. Pergolide in the treatment of Parkinson's disease. *Neurology* 1995;**45**(Suppl. 31):S13–21.

121. Dewey RB Jr, Hutton JT, LeWitt PA, Factor SA. A randomized, double-blind, placebo-controlled trial on subcutaneously injected apomorphine for parkinisonian off-state events. *Arch Neurol* 2001;**58**:1385–92.

122. Guttman M. Double-blind randomized, placebo controlled study to compare safety, tolerance and efficacy of pramipexole and bromocriptine in advanced Parkinson's disease. International Pramipexole-Bromocriptine Study Group. *Neurology* 1997;**49**:1060–5.

123. Mizuno Y, Yanagisawa N, Kuno S, *et al.* Japanese Pramipexole Study Group. Randomized double-blind study of pramipexole with placebo and bromocriptine in advanced Parkinson's disease. *Mov Disord* 2003;**18**:1149–56.

124. Hutton JT, Koller WC, Ahlskog JE, *et al.* Multicenter, placebo-controlled trial of cabergoline taken once daily in the treatment of Parkinson's disease. *Neurology* 1996;**46**:1062–5.

125. Olanow CW, Fahn S, Muenter M, *et al.* A multicenter double-bind placebo-controlled trial of pergolide as an adjunct to Sinemet in Parkinson's disease. *Mov Disord* 1994;**9**:40–7.

126. Ziegler M, Castro-Caldas A, Del Signore S, Rascol O. Efficacy of piribedil as early combination to levodopa in patients with stable Parkinson's disease: a 6-month, randomized placebo-controlled study. *Mov Disord* 2003;**18**:418–25.

127. Pinter MM, Pogarell O, Oertel WH. Efficacy, safety, and tolerance of the non-ergoline dopamine agonist pramipexole in the treatment of advanced Parkinson's disease: a

double-blind, placebo controlled, randomized, multicentre study. *J Neurol Neurosurg Psychiatry* 1999;**66**:436–41.

128. Pogarell O, Gasser T, van Hilten JJ, *et al.* Pramipexole in patients with Parkinson's disease and marked drug resistant tremor: a randomized, double-blind, placebo-controlled multicentre trial. *J Neurol Neurosurg Psychiatry* 2002;**72**:713–20.

129. Moller JC, Oertel WH, Koster J, Pezzoli G, Provinciali L. Long-term efficacy and safety of pramipexole in advanced Parkinson's disease: results from a European multicenter trial. *Mov Disord* 2005;**20**:602–10.

130. Mizuno Y, Abe T, Hasegawa K, *et al.* Ropinirole is effective on motor function when used as an adjunct to levodopa in Parkinson's disease: STRONG study. *Mov Disord* 2007;**22**:1860–5.

131. Martignoni E, Pacchetti C, Sibilla L, Bruggi P, Pedevilla M, Nappi G. Dihydroergocryptine in the treatment of Parkinson's disease: a six month's double-blind clinical trial. *Clin Neuropharmacol* 1991;**14**:78–83.

132. Inzelberg R, Nisipeanu P, Rabey JM, *et al.* Double-blind comparison of cabergoline and bromocriptine in Parkinson's disease patients with motor fluctuations. *Neurology* 1996;**47**:785–8.

133. Le Witt PA, Gopinathan G, Ward CD, *et al.* Lisuride versus bromocriptine treatment in Parkinson disease: a double-blind study. *Neurology* 1982;**32**:69–72.

134. Laihinen A, Rinne UK, Suchy I. Comparison of lisuride and bromocriptine in the treatment of advanced Parkinson's disease. *Acta Neurol Scand* 1992;**86**:593–5.

135. Le Witt PA, Ward CD, Larsen TA, *et al.* Comparison of pergolide and bromocriptine therapy in parkinsonism. *Neurology* 1983;**33**:1009–14.

136. Pezzoli G, Martignoni E, Pacchetti C, *et al.* A cross-over, controlled study comparing pergolide with bromocriptine as an adjunct to levodopa for the treatment of Parkinson's disease. *Neurology* 1995;**45**(Suppl. 3):S22–7.

137. Boas J, Worm-Petersen J, Dupont E, Mikkelsen B, Wermuth L. The levodopa dose-sparing capacity of pergolide compared with that of bromocriptine in an open-label, cross-over study. *Eur J Neurol* 1996;**3**:44–9.

138. Castro-Caldas A, Delwaide P, Jost W, *et al.* The Parkinson-Control study: a 1-year randomized, double-blind trial comparing piribedil (150 mg/day) with bromocriptine (25 mg/day) in early combination with levodopa in Parkinson's disease. *Mov Disord* 2006;**21**:500–9.

139. Poewe WH, Rascol O, Quinn N, *et al.* Efficacy of pramipexole and transdermal rotigotine in advanced Parkinson's disease: a double-blind, double-dummy, randomised controlled trial. *Lancet Neurol* 2007;**6**:513–20.

140. Brunt ER, Brooks DJ, Korczyn AD, Montastruc JL, Stocchi F, 043 study group. A six-month multicentre, double-blind, bromocriptine-controlled study of the safety and efficacy of ropinirole in the treatment of patients with Parkinson's disease not optimally controlled by L-dopa. *J Neural Transm* 2002;**109**:489–502.

141. Goetz CG, Shannon KM, Tanner CM, Carroll VS, Klawans HL. Agonist substitution in advanced Parkinson's disease. *Neurology* 1989;**39**:1121–2.

142. Goetz CG, Blasucci L, Stebbins GT. Switching dopamine agonists in advanced Parkinson's disease: is rapid titration preferable to slow? *Neurology* 1999;**52**:1227–9.

143. Canesi M, Antonini A, Mariani CB, *et al.* An overnight switch to ropinirole therapy in patients with Parkinson's disease. Short communication. *J Neural Transm* 1999;**106**:925–9.

144. Gimenez-Roldan S, Esteban EM, Mateo D. Switching from bromocriptine to ropinirole in patients with advanced Parkinson's disease: open label pilot responses to three different dose-ratios. *Clin Neuropharmacol* 2001;**24**:346–51.

145. Hanna PA, Ratkos L, Ondo WG, Jankovic J. Switching from pergolide to pramipexole in patients with Parkinson's disease. *J Neural Transm* 2001;**108**:63–70.

146. Reichmann H, Herting B, Miller A, Sommer U. Switching and combining dopamine agonists. *J Neural Transm* 2003;**110**:1393–400.

147. Grosset K, Needleman F, Macphee G, Grosset D. Switching from ergot to nonergot dopamine agonists in Parkinson's disease: a clinical series and five-drug dose conversion table. *Mov Disord* 2004;**19**:1370–4.

148. LeWitt PA, Boroojerdi B, MacMahon D, Patton J, Jankovic J. Overnight switch from oral dopaminergic agonists to transdermal rotigotine patch in subjects with Parkinson disease. *Clin Neuropharmacol* 2007;**30**:256–65.

149. Takahashi H, Nogawa S, Tachibana H, *et al.* Pramipexole safely replaces ergot dopamine agonists with either rapid or slow switching. *J Int Med Res* 2008;**36**:106–14.

150. Linazasoro G, Spanish Dopamine Agonists Study Group. Conversion from dopamine agonists to pramipexole. An open-label trial in 227 patients with advanced Parkinson's disease. *J Neurol* 2004;**251**:335–9.

151. Tolcapone Study Group. Efficacy and tolerability of tolcapone compared with bromocriptine in levodopa-treated parkinsonian patients. *Mov Disord* 1999;**14**:38–44.

152. Koller W, Lees A, Doder M, Hely M, Tolcapone/Pergolide Study Group. Randomised trial of tolcapone versus pergolide as add-on to levodopa therapy in Parkinson's disease patients with motor fluctuations. *Mov Disord* 2001;**16**:858–66.

153. Bracco F, Battaglia A, Chouza C, *et al.* The long-acting dopamine receptor agonist cabergoline in early

Parkinson's disease: final results of a 5-year, double-blind, levodopa-controlled study. *CNS Drugs* 2004;**18**:733–46.

154. Hely MA, Morris JGL, Reid WGJ. The Sydney multicentre study of Parkinson's disease: a randomized, prospective five year study comparing low dose bromocriptine with low dose levodopa-carbidopa. *J Neurol Neurosurg Psychiatry* 1994;**57**:903–10.

155. Rascol O, Brooks DJ, Korczyn AD, *et al.* Development of dyskinesias in a 5-year trial of ropinirole and L-dopa. *Mov Disord* 2006;**21**:1844–50.

156. Constantinescu R, Romer M, McDermott MP, Kamp C, Kieburtz, CALM-PD Investigators of the Parkinson Study Group. Impact of pramipexole on the onset of levodopa-related dyskinesias. *Mov Disord* 2007;**22**(9):1317–9.

157. Hely MA, Morris JG, Reid WG, Trafficante R. Sydney Multicenter Study of Parkinson's disease: non-L-dopa-responsive problems dominate at 15 years. *Mov Disord* 2005;**20**:190–9.

158. Corrigan MH, Denahan AQ, Wright CE, Ragual RJ, Evans DL. Comparison of pramipexole, fluoxetine, and placebo in patients with major depression. *Depress Anxiety* 2000;**11**: 58–65.

159. Zarate CA, Jr, Payne JL, Singh J, *et al.* Pramipexole for bipolar II depression: a placebo-controlled proof of concept study. *Biol Psychiatry* 2004;**56**:54–60.

160. Barone P, Scarzella L, Marconi R, *et al.* Pramipexole versus sertraline in the treatment of depression in Parkinson's disease: a national multicenter parallel-group randomized study. *J Neurol* 2006;**253**:601–7.

161. Izumi T, Inoue T, Kitagawa N, *et al.* Open pergolide treatment of tricyclic and heterocyclic antidepressant-resistant depression. *J Affect Disord* 2000;**61**:127–32.

162. Rektorova I, Balaz M, Svatova J, *et al.* Effects of ropinirole on nonmotor symptoms of Parkinson disease: a prospective multicenter study. *Clin Neuropharmacol* 2008;**31**: 261–6.

163. Rektorova I, Rektor I, Bares M, *et al.* Pramipexole and pergolide in the treatment of depression in Parkinson's disease: a national multicentre prospective randomized study. *Eur J Neurol* 2003;**10**:399–406.

164. Gallagher DA, Schrag A. Impact of newer pharmacological treatments on quality of life in patients with Parkinson's disease. *CNS Drugs* 2008;**22**:563–86.

165. Holloway RG, Shoulson I, Fahn S, *et al.* Pramipexole vs levodopa as initial treatment for Parkinson disease: a 4-year randomized controlled trial. *Arch Neurol* 2004;**61**: 1044–53.

166. Noyes K, Dick AW, Holloway RG. Pramipexole versus levodopa in patients with early Parkinson's disease: effect on generic and disease-specific quality of life. *Value Health* 2006;**9**:28–38.

167. Etminan M, Samii A, Takkouche B, Rochon P. Increased risk of somnolence with the new dopamine agonists in patients with Parkinson's disease. A meta-analysis of randomised controlled trials. *Drug Saf* 2001;**24**:863–8.

168. Avorn J, Schneeweiss S, Sudarsky LR, *et al.* Sudden uncontrollable somnolence and medication use in Parkinson disease. *Arch Neurol* 2005;**62**:1242–8.

169. Micallef J, Rey M, Eusebio A, *et al.* Antiparkinsonian drug-induced sleepiness: a double-blind placebo-controlled study of L-dopa, bromocriptine and pramipexole in healthy subjects. *Br J Clin Pharmacol* 2009;**67**: 333–40.

170. Stowe RL, Ives NJ, Clarke C, *et al.* Dopamine agonist therapy in early Parkinson's disease. *Cochrane Database Syst Rev* 2008;(16):CD006564.

171. Van Camp G, Flamez A, Cosyns B, *et al.* Treatment of Parkinson's disease with pergolide and relation to restrictive valvular heart disease. *Lancet* 2004;**363**:1179–83.

172. Steiger M, Jost W, Grandas F, Van CG. Risk of valvular heart disease associated with the use of dopamine agonists in Parkinson's disease: a systematic review. *J Neural Transm* 2009;**116**:179–91.

173. Antonini A, Poewe W. Fibrotic heart-valve reactions to dopamine-agonist treatment in Parkinson's disease. *Lancet Neurol* 2007;**6**:826–9.

174. Antonini A, Cilia R. Behavioural adverse effects of dopaminergic treatments in Parkinson's disease: incidence, neurobiological basis, management and prevention. *Drug Saf* 2009;**32**:475–88.

175. Rossi M, Gerschcovich ER, de Achaval D, Perez-Lloret S, Cerquetti D, Cammarota A, Inés Nouzeilles M, Fahrer R, Merello M, Leiguarda R. Decision-making in Parkinson's disease patients with and without pathological gambling. *Eur J Neurol.* 2010 Jan;**17**(1):97–102.

176. Voon V, Fox SH. Medication-related impulse control and repetitive behaviors in Parkinson disease. *Arch Neurol* 2007;**64**:1089–96.

177. Keus SH, Munneke M, Nijkrake MJ, Kwakkel G, Bloem BR. Physical therapy in Parkinson's disease: evolution and future challenges. *Mov Disord* 2009;**24**:1–14.

178. Keus SH, Bloem BR, Hendriks EJ, Bredero-Cohen AB, Munneke M. Evidence-based analysis of physical therapy in Parkinson's disease with recommendations for practice and research. *Mov Disord* 2007;**22**:451–60.

179. Goodwin VA, Richards SH, Taylor RS, Taylor AH, Campbell JL. The effectiveness of exercise interventions for people with Parkinson's disease: a systematic review and meta-analysis. *Mov Disord* 2008;**23**:631–40.

180. Nieuwboer A, Kwakkel G, Rochester L, *et al.* Cueing training in the home improves gait-related mobility in

Parkinson's disease: the RESCUE trial. *J Neurol Neurosurg Psychiatry* 2007;**78**:134–40.

181. Rochester L, Nieuwboer A, Baker K, *et al.* The attentional cost of external rhythmical cues and their impact on gait in Parkinson's disease: effect of cue modality and task complexity. *J Neural Transm* 2007;**114**(10):1243–8.

182. Falvo MJ, Schilling BK, Earhart GM. Parkinson's disease and resistive exercise: rationale, review, and recommendations. *Mov Disord* 2008;**23**:1–11.

183. Burini D, Farabollini B, Iacucci S, *et al.* A randomised controlled cross-over trial of aerobic training versus Qigong in advanced Parkinson's disease. *Eura Medicophys* 2006;**42**:231–8.

184. Herman T, Giladi N, Hausdorff JM. Treadmill training for the treatment of gait disturbances in people with Parkinson's disease: a mini-review. *J Neural Transm* 2009;**116**:307–18.

185. Hackney ME, Earhart GM. Tai Chi improves balance and mobility in people with Parkinson disease. *Gait Posture* 2008;**28**:456–60.

186. Schmitz-Hubsch T, Pyfer D, Kielwein K, Fimmers R, Klockgether T, Wullner U. Qigong exercise for the symptoms of Parkinson's disease: a randomized, controlled pilot study. *Mov Disord* 2006;**21**:543–8.

187. Rascol O, Pathak A, Bagheri H, Montastruc J.-L. New concerns about old drugs: valvular heart disease on ergot derivative dopamine agonists as an exemplary situation of pharmacovigilance. *Mov Disord* 2004;**19**:611–3.

188. Rascol O, Pathak A, Bagheri H, Montastruc J.-L. Dopamine agonists and fibrotic valvular heart disease: further considerations. *Mov Disord* 2004;**19**:1524–5.

189. Bonuccelli U, Ceravolo R, Salvetti S, *et al.* Clozapine in Parkinson's disease tremor. Effects of acute and chronic administration. *Neurology* 1997;**49**:1587–90.

190. Friedman JH, Koller WC, Lannon MC, Busenbark K, Swanson-Hyland E, Smith D. Benztropine versus clozapine for the treatment of tremor in Parkinson's disease. *Neurology* 1997;**48**:1077–81.

191. Parkinson Study Group. Low-dose clozapine for the treatment of drug-induced psychosis in Parkinson's disease. The Parkinson Study Group. *N Engl J Med* 1999;**340**:757–63.

192. Marsden CD, Parkes JD, Rees JE. Propranolol in Parkinson's disease. *Lancet* 1974;**2**:410.

193. Foster NL, Newman RP, LeWitt PA, Gillespie MM, Larsen TA, Chase TN. Peripheral beta-adrenergic blockade treatment of parkinsonian tremor. *Ann Neurol* 1984;**16**:505–8.

194. Koller WC, Herbster G. Adjuvant therapy of parkinsonian tremor. *Arch Neurol* 1987;**44**:921–3.

195. Henderson JM, Yiannikas C, Morris JG, Einstein R, Jackson D, Byth K. Postural tremor of Parkinson's disease. *Clin Neuropharmacol* 1994;**17**:277–85.

196. Crosby NJ, Deane KHO, Clarke CE. Beta-blocker therapy for tremor in Parkinson's disease. *Cochrane Database Syst Rev* 2003;(1):CD003361.

197. Mehrholz J, Friis R, Kugler J, Twork S, Storch A, Pohl M. Treadmill training for patients with Parkinson's disease. *Cochrane Database Syst Rev* 2010 Jan 20;(1):CD007830.

198. Munneke M, Nijkrake MJ, Keus SH, *et al.* Efficacy of community-based physiotherapy networks for patients with Parkinson's disease: a cluster-randomised trial. *Lancet Neurol* 2010;**9**:46–54.

CHAPTER 15

Late (complicated) Parkinson's disease

W. H. Oertel,[1] A. Berardelli,[2] B. R. Bloem,[3] U. Bonuccelli,[4] D. Burn,[5] G. Deuschl,[6] E. Dietrichs,[7] G. Fabbrini,[2] J. J. Ferreira,[8] A. Friedman,[9] P. Kanovsky,[10] V. Kostic,[11] A. Nieuwboer,[12] P. Odin,[13] W. Poewe,[14] O. Rascol,[15] C. Sampaio,[16] M. Schüpbach,[17] E. Tolosa,[18] C. Trenkwalder[19]

[1]Philipps-University of Marburg, Centre of Nervous Diseases, Germany; [2]Sapienza, Università di Roma, Italy; [3]Donders Institute for Brain, Cognition and Behavior, Radboud University Nijmegen Medical Center, The Netherlands; [4]University of Pisa, Italy; [5]Institute for Ageing and Health, Newcastle University, Newcastle upon Tyne, UK; [6]Christian-Albrechts-University Kiel, Germany; [7]Oslo University Hospital and University of Oslo, Norway; [8]Institute of Molecular Medicine, Lisbon, Portugal; [9]Medical University of Warsaw, Poland; [10]Palacky University, Olomouc, Czech Republic; [11]Institute of Neurology CCS, School of Medicine, University of Belgrade, Serbia; [12]Katholieke Universiteit Leuven, Leuven, Belgium; [13]Central Hospital Bremerhaven, Germany, and University Hospital, Lund, Sweden; [14]Innsbruck Medical University, Austria; [15]University Hospital and University of Toulouse, Toulouse, France; [16]Laboratório de Farmacologia Clínica e Terapeutica e Instituto de Medicina Molecular, Faculdade de Medicina de Lisboa, Portugal; [17]INSERM CIC-9503, Hôpital Pitié-Salpétrière, Paris, France, and Bern University Hospital and University of Bern, Switzerland; [18]Universitat de Barcelona, Spain; [19]Paracelsus-Elena Hospital, Kassel, and University of Goettingen, Germany

Methods

For background, search strategy, and method for reaching consensus, see Part I of these guidelines (Chapter 14).

Patients with advanced Parkinson's disease (PD) may suffer from any combination of motor and non-motor problems. Doctors and patients must make choices and decide which therapeutic strategies should prevail for each particular instance.

Interventions for the symptomatic control of motor complications

Motor complications are divided into motor fluctuations and dyskinesia. With advancing PD, patients may begin to fluctuate in motor performance, i.e. they experience a wearing-off (end-of-dose) effect because the motor improvement after a dose of levodopa becomes reduced in duration and Parkinsonism reappears. However, wearing-off can also manifest in symptoms such as

depression, anxiety, akathisia, unpleasant sensations, and excessive sweating. Besides fluctuations, dyskinesias may occur, which are involuntary movements in response to levodopa and/or dopamine agonist intake. Most dyskinesias emerge at peak-dose levels and are typically choreatic, but may involve dystonia or – rarely – myoclonus. A minority of patients may experience diphasic dyskinesia, in which they exhibit dyskinesia at the beginning of turning ON and/or at the beginning of turning OFF, but have different and less severe or absent dyskinesias at the time of peak levodopa effect. Eventually, patients may begin to experience rapid and unpredictable fluctuations between ON and OFF periods, known as the ON–OFF phenomenon.

The diagnosis and therapeutic management of motor complications depends on detecting the type of movement involved and the time of day when they occur in relation to the timing of levodopa and the resulting ON–OFF cycle. Diaries may be helpful in assessing this course over time. It must be noted that many patients prefer being ON with dyskinesia rather than OFF without dyskinesia.

Pharmacological interventions

Mechanisms of action: if not mentioned, see Part I of the guidelines.

European Handbook of Neurological Management: Volume 1, 2nd edition. Edited by N. E. Gilhus, M. P. Barnes and M. Brainin.
© 2011 Blackwell Publishing Ltd.

Amantadine

Using patient diaries, one study found that oral amantadine significantly decreased the duration of daily OFF time (Class I: [1];), whereas a second study found no significant differences in ON or OFF duration (Class I: [2], oral amantadine).

In patients on chronic levodopa, oral amantadine significantly reduced the dyskinetic effect of an orally administered acute levodopa/decarboxylase inhibitor challenge of 1.5 times their usual dose (Class I: [3]. Similar results were found by Luginger *et al.* [2] (Class I). During 3 weeks of stable oral amantadine, levodopa-dyskinesia was reduced by 60%, with a similar effect observed under long-term oral amantadine therapy at 1-year follow-up [4]. According to another study (Class I: [5] the antidyskinetic effect of oral amantadine may only last for 3–8 months, although several subjects experienced a rebound in dyskinesia severity after discontinuation.

Intravenous infusion of amantadine was employed for the treatment of levodopa-induced dyskinesias in one double-blind placebo-controlled [6] and two open-label trials [7], [8]. When in the later study amantadine was intravenously infused continuously for 3 days to bridge an oral levodopa 3 days withdrawal ('levodopa drug holidays'), a significant improvement of motor complications (motor fluctuations and dyskinesias) was observed for up to 4 months under reinstalled oral levodopa treatment without concomitant oral or i.v. amantadine.

MAO-B inhibitors

Short-duration studies (<3 months) showed no consistent effect of selegiline in the reduction of OFF time, although an improvement in PD symptoms was observed (Class I and II: [9–11]). Zydis selegiline, which dissolves on contact with saliva, reduces daily OFF time when used as adjunctive therapy with levodopa (Class I: [12]).

Rasagiline produced a significant reduction in OFF time in patients on levodopa (Class I: rasagiline 1 mg, −0.94 h/day [13] and rasagiline 1 mg, −0.78 h/day [14]). In the latter study, rasagiline achieved a similar magnitude of effect to the active comparator, entacapone, which reduced OFF time by 0.80 h/day (Class I: [14]).

Selegiline might increase or provoke dyskinesia in levodopa-treated patients, but this was not the primary outcome measure in the studies referred to (Class I: [9, 15]). Golbe *et al.* noted that dyskinesia lessened after levodopa was reduced (Class I: [11]). Rasagiline increased

dyskinesia in one study [13], whereas it had no significant impact in another [14]. The reason for this difference remains unknown, since levodopa dose adjustment was allowed equally in both trials.

COMT inhibitors

Due to their mechanism of action, COMT inhibitors should always be given with levodopa.

With entacapone the overall conclusion from four studies was a reduction in OFF time of 41 min/day (95% CI: 13 min, 1 h 8 min) as compared with placebo (Class I: [16]). Entacapone reduces mean daily OFF time in levodopa-treated patients by a similar extent to rasagiline (Class I: [14]). Entacapone also demonstrated long-term efficacy as shown in the meta-analysis of Class I studies and their open-label extensions [17] and was efficacious in terms of activities of daily living (ADL) in fluctuating patients (Class I: [18]). In the trials cited above, dyskinesias were more frequent with entacapone adjunct therapy than with placebo. In the majority of the trials, entacapone produced an improvement in Unified PD Rating Scale (UPDRS) motor scores.

Class I studies with tolcapone demonstrated that it was efficacious in reducing OFF time [19–22]. The effect size of tolcapone and dopamine agonists (bromocriptine, pergolide) may be similar (Class II: [23–25]), but these studies lacked the power to be fully conclusive [26].

In a double-blind 'switch study' PD patients with motor fluctuations on optimized 'levodopa plus entacapone therapy' were switched to 'levodopa plus tolcapone'. There was a tendency of tolcapone to offer enhanced efficacy, especially in PD patients with marked fluctuations [27].

Safety issue of tolcapone

Tolcapone rarely can elevate liver transaminases, and few fatal cases of liver injury have been reported. The European Agency for the Evaluation of Medicinal Products (EMEA) lifted the suspension of tolcapone for use in patients with motor fluctuations on levodopa who fail to respond to other COMT inhibitors, but imposed strict safety restrictions [26a]. Tolcapone can only be prescribed by physicians experienced in the management of advanced PD, with a recommended daily dose of 100 mg three times daily. Patients must have fortnightly blood tests for liver function in the first year, at four-weekly intervals for the next 6 months and, subsequently, every 8 weeks. Patients with abnormal liver function or a history of neuroleptic malignant syndrome, rhabdomyolysis or hyperthermia have to be excluded.

For adverse events and further safety issues of COMT-inhibitors see Part I.

Levodopa

Immediate release (standard) levodopa is the most important component of pharmacotherapy in advanced PD. Based on its short half-life, dosing schedules may consist of up to eight, or even more, individual doses with additional dosing of immediate- or slow-release levodopa. The action of levodopa can be prolonged and enhanced when combined with a COMT-inhibitor and/or MAO-B-inhibitor. Due to its lower – compared with dopamine agonists – potency to induce hallucinations, levodopa is the drug of choice in advanced PD patients with cognitive impairment and dementia (see 'Non-motor problems, Dementia' section).

It is common practice to reduce the size of individual doses of levodopa in cases of peak-dose dyskinesia, whereas the dose interval is shortened in wearing-off ([28, 29]).

To reduce the occurrence of delayed ON, no ON, or reduced symptomatic effect due to gastrointestinal absorption failure, methods are being developed to improve levodopa absorption. Fluctuations and wearing-off could be reduced by methods providing more constant gastrointestinal delivery (reviews: [28, 30]).

(a) Controlled-release (CR) levodopa formulations

Controlled-release (CR) levodopa has been shown to have a significant beneficial effect on daily ON time in a minority of studies, but the improvement is often only minor and transient. No Class I study shows long-lasting (>6 months) daily improvement of >1 h ON, or a reduction in hours with dyskinesia as measured by diaries, although some studies found an improvement using 1–4 ratings similar to the UPDRS-Complications scale [28, 31–33]. Levodopa CR is preferably administered at bedtime or during the night to ease nocturnal akinesia (GPP).

(b) Alternative levodopa formulations and delivery routes

In fluctuating PD, oral dispersible levodopa/benserazide significantly shortened time to peak plasma levels compared with the standard formulation (Class III: [34].

A 4 weeks, double-blind, double-dummy study comparing levodopa methylester/carbidopa (melevodopa) with standard levodopa/carbidopa for the treatment of the afternoon OFF periods showed that melevodopa induced a faster ON than standard levodopa/carbidopa (Class II: [35]). Melevodopa had a similar safety profile to standard levodopa/carbidopa. A large double-blind study on 327 fluctuating patients demonstrated that eti-levodopa/carbidopa, another form of soluble levodopa, did not differ from standard levodopa/carbidopa in total daily time to ON after levodopa dosing, in reducing response failures, or in decreasing total off time (Class I: [36]).

Continuous duodenal infusions of levodopa/carbidopa resulted in statistically significant increases in ON time (Class III: [37]). Continuous intrajejunal infusion of levodopa/carbidopa enteral gel resulted in a significant improvement in motor function during ON time, accompanied by a significant decrease in OFF time, and no increase, or even a decrease, in dyskinesia. Median total UPDRS score also decreased (short-term, single randomised comparison to oral levodopa, Class III: [38]). Open-label trials have confirmed the beneficial effect of this therapy in very advanced PD patients in respect to reduced OFF time and – after several months – decreasing dyskinesia, but also have detailed the technical problems encountered in its long-term use in a substantial number of patients (Class III: [39]; [40]; [41]).

Dopamine agonists

Several dopamine agonists have been shown to reduce the duration of OFF episodes. There is Class I evidence for pergolide [42], pramipexole [43, 44], ropinirole [45, 46], ropinirole controlled-release [47], rotigotine transdermal patch [48, 49], and for apomorphine as intermittent subcutaneous injection (Class I: [50, 51]) or continuous infusion (Class IV: [52–54]. There is Class II evidence for bromocriptine [43, 55, 56] and cabergoline [57], and Class IV evidence for other agonists such as lisuride or piribedil ([28]).

The available comparative Class II–III trials showed no major differences between bromocriptine and other agonists such as cabergoline [58], lisuride [59], pergolide [60], and pramipexole [43]. The same was true when comparing bromocriptine [24] and pergolide [25], to the COMT inhibitor tolcapone (Class II), or cabergoline to entacapone (Class I: [61]).

When levodopa-treated patients with advanced PD receive an agonist to reduce OFF episodes, dyskinesia may occur or, if already present, worsen. In clinical practice, when an agonist is given as adjunct in patients with dyskinesias, the levodopa dose is usually reduced to minimize this problem.

Dopamine agonists can deliver more continuous dopamine stimulation than levodopa, due to their longer plasma elimination half-life and receptor occupancy. Therefore, high doses of dopamine agonists might allow a reduction in levodopa daily dose and, consequently, lessen the duration and severity of levodopa-induced dyskinesias. There are only a few open-label reports to support this practice (Class IV), involving small cohorts of patients with continuous subcutaneous infusions of apomorphine [53, 62–64] or oral administration of high doses of pergolide [65] or ropinirole [66].

The continuous subcutaneous infusion of apomorphine and the intrajejunal infusion of levodopa are – as is deep brain stimulation – expensive and, to a different degree, invasive therapeutical options. Studies on a direct comparison on the efficacy and safety of apomorphine infusion, levodopa infusion, and deep brain stimulation are lacking.

For use of dopamine agonists in PD patients with dementia, see 'Non-motor problems, Dementia' section.

Functional neurosurgery

Pallidotomy and deep brain stimulation (DBS) are discussed in detail here, as they are the only surgical treatments frequently used to treat PD symptoms. Other treatments are covered only briefly and the reader is referred to special reviews [67].

All surgical interventions for PD involve lesioning or stimulating nuclei or fibre connections of the basal ganglia loops (direct or indirect loop) [68]. Lesioning of these nuclei destroys the circuit, and continuous electrical stimulation is likely to reversibly block the neuronal activity in the loop.

In general the level I-evidence definition of the EFNS with blinded outcome assessments is difficult to achieve for surgical studies as blinding of the investigators remains often a fiction. Therefore, randomisation and adequate power of the studies are more imporant criteria.

Pallidotomy

This section focuses on unilateral pallidotomy. Bilateral pallidotomy is only rarely performed and there are insuf-

ficient studies to allow a conclusion on the safety of the technique.

Adjunctive therapy of parkinsonism

Unilateral pallidotomy has been tested in prospective studies with control groups receiving best medical treatment or subthalamic nucleus (STN) stimulation (Class II: [69–72]) and was found to be efficacious for the treatment of PD. According to one study (Class I: [73]) parkinsonian motor signs are more improved after 1 year with bilateral STN stimulation than with unilateral pallidotomy.

Symptomatic control of motor complications

The improvement of dyskinesia on the body side contralateral to pallidotomy is usually 50–80% (Class III: [69, 72, 74–78]).

Safety

Side effects with unilateral pallidotomy are generally limited, but the potential for severe complications due to haemorrhage or peri-operative complications is common to all stereotactic procedures. Symptomatic infarction was found in 3.9% of patients, and the mortality rate was 1.2%. Speech problems were found in 11.1% of patients and facial paresis in 8.4% (reviews: [70, 75]). Neuropsychological functioning is usually unaffected [79, 80], but frontal lobe functions and depression may show a modest deterioration (Class III: [81, 82]). Visual field defects were common in earlier series, but have decreased to <5% with modification of the surgical technique [83].

Deep brain stimulation (DBS)

Stimulation of the STN (reviews: [29, 84–87]; Class II: [88]) has become the most frequently applied surgical procedure for PD (at least in Europe), because treating neurologists and neurosurgeons consider it more efficient than pallidal stimulation. However, this is not scientifically proven. Deep brain stimulation of the STN has been found to be superior to medical treatment in patients with advanced disease and motor fluctuations which can no longer be sufficiently treated medically in a large randomized study (Class II: [88]). STN-stimulation showed an improvement of 24% of quality of life, an improvement of motor fluctuations, and a 41% improvement of the motor score. In comparisons of STN- or GPi-DBS versus best medical treatment, DBS was found to be equally superior to medical treatment

(Class I: [89]). Both large studies compared 6 months' data. Data on long-term outcome show a slow deterioration of axial and akinesia scores with stable improvement of tremor and rigidity [90]. One small study found only a non-significant trend towards better efficacy of stimulation of STN over GPi. The trial was, however, underpowered [91]. Manual dexterity was equivalently improved by GPi and STN stimulation in a subgroup of patients of a prospective randomized trial [92]. The question wether STN or GPi-stimulation is superior is still open.

Stimulation of the posteroventral pallidum

Adjunctive therapy of parkinsonism Pallidal DBS may improve the symptoms of advanced PD, as assessed by the UPDRS-Motor score, by 33% for study periods of up to 6 and 12 months (Class II: [93]). Over time, deterioration occurs in some patients who are subsequently successfully reoperated on, with implantation of electrodes into the STN (Class III: [84]).

Symptomatic control of motor complications One of the most consistent effects of DBS on the pallidum is reduction of dyskinesias and of OFF time. In Class II and III studies, the reduction in OFF time was 35–60% ([84, 93]). The few long-term observations available show no loss of effect on dyskinesias [86].

Symptomatic control of non-motor problems Under stimulation, there is a mild but significant improvement in mood [94], but the symptomatic control of non-motor complications has not been primarily studied.

Safety The general surgical risks for pallidal stimulation are the same as for STN DBS (see next section). However, stimulation-specific side effects are less frequent. The incidence and severity of the neuropsychological and psychiatric effects of this technique are understudied [84, 95–98]. A randomized comparison between stimulation of the GPi or the STN showed similar mild reductions in neuropsychological test performance for both targets, mainly for verbal fluency and working memory after unilateral and bilateral stimulation [99]. A review found neuropsychiatric complications in 2.7% of patients, speech and swallowing disturbances in 2.6%, sensory disturbances in 0.9%, and oculomotor disturbances in 1.8% of patients [86].

Stimulation of the subthalamic nucleus (STN)

Adjunctive therapy of parkinsonism In two large randomized trials of DBS versus medical treatment, the UPDRS-Motor score improved by 54% for STN stimulation [88] and 28% for STN- or GPi-stimulation [89], thereby confirming ealier uncontrolled data [93]. This is consistent with a meta-analysis of 20 studies, showing an average improvement of 53% [84]. Smaller controlled studies found similar results [72, 100, 101]. At the same time, the levodopa equivalence dosage could be reduced by 50–60%. UPDRS-Motor scores during stimulation were still improved by 54% after 5 years, although slightly deteriorated compared with 1 year after the operation (Class III: [90, 102]).

Quality of life is significantly better in patients undergoing DBS than medical treatment in advanced stages of the disease [89, 103].

Symptomatic control of motor complications Two Class I studies found an improvement of dyskinesias by 54% and likewise OFF-time improved from 6.2 to 2 h or 5.7 to 3.4 h respectively versus no change compared with the medically treated group [88, 89]. Similar results were obtained in uncontrolled studies [93]. Dyskinesias have been reduced by 54–75% [88, 89, 93, 104].

Two open randomized controlled studies (Class I and II: [88, 89]) have shown the superiority of STN stimulation over medical treatment for parkinsonian motor scores OFF medication. The UPDRS OFF-score was reduced by 41% or 35 %. OFF time and time in troublesome dyskinesia was reduced and sleep and ON time without troublesome dyskinesia was increased with STN stimulation after 6 months. Dyskinesia was still improved after 5 years (Class III: [90, 102]). Thus, STN stimulation is as effective in reducing dyskinesia as pallidotomy or pallidal stimulation.

A pilot study in 20 patients with earlier disease (mean disease duration 7 years) comparing STN-DBS and best medical treatment showed similar results as in the two large randomized studies [105].

Symptomatic control of non-motor problems Depression and anxiety scores improve at 6 and 12 months after the operation in a controlled study against medical treatment [106] as well as in open studies [90, 107–110]. However, verbal fluency and the Stroop test were found to be significantly worse in the DBS group versus the medically treated group [106]. See also safety section, below.

Disease-related quality of life was the primary or secondary outcome in large studies on advanced complicated PD over 6 months (Class I: [88, 89]) and in a small pilot trial on early complicated PD over 18 months (Class I: [105]). In all these studies quality of life was improved by 20–24% by stimulation and remained unchanged in the medical control group.

Safety In general, reviews [29, 104] and those studies referred to below, show that adverse effects of DBS may occur in about 50% of patients, but are permanent only in about 20%. However, the severity of adverse events seldom warrants suspension of DBS. The occurrence of adverse effects related to the procedure, i.e. acute confusion, intracerebral bleeding, stroke, and seizures, or to device dysfunction, i.e. infection or stimulator repositioning, causing permanent severe morbidity or death, reaches up to about 4% (review: [104]). In a large observational study of more than 1,100 patients the mortality was found to be 0.4% and the permanent morbidity was 1% [111]. The major risk factor is age.

However, most adverse effects are related to the treatment (either stimulatory or stimulatory in combination with pharmacological). Neuropsychological tests were not worsened or showed only slight deterioration in various areas of cognition particularly verbal fluency and stroop test [80, 106, 108, 112–119]. Older patients or patients with moderate cognitive impairment prior to surgery may be at greater risk of cognitive deterioration [97, 114–116, 120]. Apathy, hypomania, psychosis, depression, anxiety, and emotional lability occur in up to 10% of patients [84, 90, 118, 121, 122], although many of these might instead be caused by a reduction in dopaminergic therapy.

Suicide has been reported in 0.45%, and suicide attempts in 0.9% of patients with STN stimulation. The risk of suicide is over 15-fold increased in the first postoperative year after STN surgery and tapers down to the risk in the general population within 3 years [123]. Weight gain is reported in 13% of patients, speech and swallowing disturbances in 7.1%, sensory disturbances in 0.4%, and oculomotor disturbances (apraxia of eyelid opening) in 1.5% [103]. However, a number of these stimulation-associated side effects can be corrected. Gait disorder, speech and swallowing difficulties, and disequilibrium are probably not related to the stimulation itself [90, 122], but could in part result from disease progression or a reduction in levodopa dose.

Surgical treatments that are now rarely used in the treatment of PD

Thalamotomy

Thalamotomy has been performed for many years in patients with tremor insufficiently controlled by oral medications. It improves tremor, and rigidity is also reduced in 70% of patients, but it has no consistent effect on akinesia (Class IV: [124]). Unilateral thalamotomy, as assessed in historical case series, has a permanent morbidity rate of 4–47%, and bilateral thalamotomy is associated with a 30% chance of developing serious dysarthria [125].

Stimulation of the thalamus

Stimulation of the thalamus is frequently used for the treatment of tremors, especially essential tremor [126, 127] and, unlike thalamotomy, can be relatively safely applied bilaterally. Stimulation of the thalamus improves tremor (and rigidity) in PD, but not akinesia [127, 128], and is therefore rarely employed. Thalamotomy and stimulation of the thalamus were found to be equally efficient after 6 months, but DBS had fewer side effects (Class I: [129]). An open-label 5-year follow-up suggests that thalamic stimulation may be preferable over unilateral thalamotomy to improve functional abilities (Class III: [130]).

Lesioning of the subthalamic nucleus

Lesioning of the STN has only been used in experimental protocols in small patient series with a high incidence of persistent dyskinesias after surgery (Class III: [131, 132]). Therefore, presently, this technique is not recommended if STN DBS is an available option.

Fetal mesencephalic grafts

Two Class I studies found that the symptoms of parkinsonism were not improved by fetal mesencephalic grafts, and some patients developed serious dyskinesias [133, 134]. However, in the study by Freed *et al.*, the younger group, but not the older, showed an improvement of UPDRS-Motor OFF scores of 34%, and of Schwab and England OFF scores of 31%, while sham surgery patients did not improve. Subsequent analysis showed that it was not patient age, but the preoperative response to levodopa that predicted the magnitude of neurological change after transplant. Some patients in open studies (Class IV) have also shown major improvement [135–137]. Therefore, although transplantation of mesencephalic cells has, at the moment, to be considered ineffective as routine treatment for PD (Level A), further investigation is probably warranted.

Non-pharmacological, non-surgical management of motor symptoms

Despite optimal medical and/or neurosurgical treatment, the clinical picture of PD becomes progressively complicated by an increased risk of falling, marked mobility problems (e.g. freezing of gait or difficulty rising from a chair), disabling communication and swallowing problems, and a variety of non-motor symptoms. These motor symptoms and signs generally respond poorly to dopaminergic treatment, and this underscores the importance of non-pharmacological treatment approaches. As in early stage PD, this includes a broad range of disciplines, among others rehabilitation specialists, allied health professionals (physiotherapy, occupational therapy, speech-language therapy), PD nurse specialists, and social workers.

Sufficient PD-specific expertise is required to strike a balance between promoting mobility and maintaining optimal levels of physical activity on the one hand, versus the need for safety and prevention of falls and injuries on the other hand [138, 139].

Specifically, the evidence-based guideline of physiotherapy in PD recommends training of transfer difficulties using compensatory cognitive strategies and cueing.
• The effectiveness of cued training of sitting to standing transfers is supported by recent evidence (Class II: [140]).
• Cognitive movement strategy training for ADL functions and transfer movements probably improves functional performance and quality of life, when embedded in a 2-week inpatient rehabilitation period (Class II: [141]). However, effects of strategy training were similar to musculoskeletal exercises of the same duration and intensity. Benefits of training declined after 3 months follow-up without training.
Recent evidence has emerged that physiotherapy intervention improves freezing of gait and balance.
• Cued gait training in the home is probably effective in reducing the severity of freezing of gait (Class II: [142]). The combination of 4 weeks of treadmill training and cueing induces even greater benefits for freezing of gait than cueing alone (Class II: [143, 332]).
• Physical activity and exercise are probably effective in improving postural instability and balance task performance (Class II: [144]). Also, treadmill training is beneficial for balance measures (Class II: [145]). Furthermore, physical activity likely reduces the risk of sustaining near-

falls (Class II: [146]) and possibly the risk of actual falls (some Class III studies, in a systematic review [144]).

Three reviews found insufficient evidence for the efficacy of speech and language therapy for dysarthria [147–149]. Lee Silverman Voice Therapy (LSVT) improves vocal intensity and phonation (Class II: [150–152]). The Pitch Limiting Voice Treatment (PLVT) produces the same increase in loudness, but limits an increase in vocal pitch and prevents a strained voicing (Class IV) [153]. No scientific evidence supports or refutes the efficacy of non-pharmacological swallowing therapy for dysphagia in PD [154, 155].

One Cochrane review concluded that there is insufficient evidence to support or refute the efficacy of occupational therapy for PD, in light of the substantial methodological drawbacks in the studies, the small number of patients examined, and the possibility of publication bias [156].

Clinical experience suggests that PD nurse specialists are beneficial for patients with PD, for example by providing information to patients and their families, or by acting as a liaison within a multidisciplinary team, or by enabling the application of complex treatments such as apomorphine, intrajejunal levodopa-carbidopa, and DBS. However, a systematic review did not support the clinical and cost effectiveness of specialized PD nurses in the management of PD [157].

Recommendations for the symptomatic control of motor complications

Recommendations
Motor fluctuations
Wearing-off (end of dose akinesia, predictable ON-OFF)
• *Adjust levodopa dosing.* In an early phase, when motor fluctuations are just becoming apparent, adjustments in the frequency of levodopa dosing during the day, tending to achieve 4–6 daily doses, may attenuate wearing-off (GPP).

• *Add COMT inhibitors or MAO-B inhibitors.* No recommendations can be made on which treatment should be chosen first – on average, all reduce OFF time by about 1–1.5 h/day. The only published direct comparison (Level A) showed no difference between entacapone and rasagiline. Tolcapone, although more effective than entacapone, is potentially hepatotoxic, and is only recommended in patients failing on all other available medications (see Part I of the guidelines). Rasagiline should not be added to selegiline (Level C) because of cardiovascular safety issues.

- *Add dopamine agonists.* Non-ergot dopamine agonists are first-line compounds. Pergolide and other ergot agonists are reserved for second-line treatment, due to their association with lung, retroperitoneal, and heart valve fibrosis. Oral dopamine agonists are efficacious in reducing OFF time in patients experiencing wearing-off. Currently, no dopamine agonist has proven better than another, but switching from one agonist to another can be helpful in some patients (Level B/C).

- *Switch from standard levodopa to CR formulation.* CR formulations of levodopa can also improve wearing-off (Level C). This formulation is useful for the treatment of night-time akinesia (nocturnal end of dose akinesia) (GPP).

- *Add amantadine or an anticholinergic.* In patients with disabling recurrent OFF symptoms that fail to improve further with the above-mentioned strategies, the addition of an anticholinergic (in younger patients), or amantadine, may improve symptoms in some cases (GPP).

Most patients will eventually receive a combination of several of these treatments because a single treatment fails to provide adequate control of fluctuations. There is insufficient evidence on the combination of more than two strategies, and the choice of drugs is mainly based on safety, tolerability, ease of use, experience of the treating physician, and patient preference. All the above options may provoke or increase dyskinesias, but usually this can be managed by decreasing the levodopa dose.

Note: reduction or redistribution of total daily dietary proteins may reduce wearing-off effects in some patients. Restricting protein intake mainly to one meal a day may facilitate better motor responses to levodopa following other meals during the day. A more practical approach could be to take levodopa on an empty stomach about 1 h before, or at least 1 h after, each meal (Class IV: [158, 159]).

Oral dispersible levodopa can be useful for delayed ON (Level B).

Severe motor fluctuations

Try oral therapy, as outlined above. If oral therapy fails to improve (marked to) severe predictable motor fluctuations, the following strategies can be recommended.

- *Deep brain stimulation of the STN* is effective against motor fluctuations and dyskinesia (Level A), but because of risk for adverse events the procedure is only recommended for patients below the age of 70 without major psychiatric problems or cognitive decline. Stimulation of other targets may also be effective, but results are less well documented.

- *Subcutaneous apomorphine* as penject (Level A) or pump (Level C).

- *Intrajejunal levodopa/carbidopa enteric gel* administered through percutaneous gastrostomy (PEG) can also help to stabilize patients with refractory motor fluctuations and dyskinesia (Level C).

Unpredictable ON–OFF

Deep brain stimulation of the STN is effective for unpredictable ON-OFF fluctuations (Level A). In the large studies of oral medical treatment for wearing-off, patients with unpredictable ON–OFF were either not included or constituted <5% of the total population Therefore, insufficient evidence exists to conclude whether the results that are valid for wearing-off are also valid for unpredictable ON–OFF. There are only a few small studies specifically including only patients suffering from unpredictable ON–OFF, although studies evaluating continuous dopaminergic stimulation also include patients suffering concomitantly from wearing-off and unpredictable ON–OFF. The same is true for concomitant dyskinesia, which frequently occurs during the ON phase of ON–OFF. Thus, there is insufficient evidence to conclude on specific oral medical strategies for ON–OFF, although the strategies described for dyskinesia and for wearing-off should be considered for unpredictable ON–OFF (GPP).

Unpredictable ON–OFF can have several components, one of which is delayed ON and, for which, oral dispersible levodopa formulations could have some value (Level C).

Note: by shortening the interval between levodopa doses to prevent wearing-off, and reducing the size of individual doses, the relation between the moment of intake of each dose and the subsequent motor effect can become difficult to disclose, especially when inadequate absorption also occurs. The resulting pattern of fluctuation and dyskinesia may falsely suggest unpredictable ON–OFF. In such patients, the actual mechanism of wearing-off and peak-dose dyskinesia may reappear by increasing the levodopa intake interval to about 4 h. However, in some patients, the benefit may wane after weeks or months.

Recommendations

Dyskinesias

Peak-dose dyskinesia

- *Reduce individual levodopa dose size*, at the risk of increasing OFF time. The latter can be compensated for by increasing the number of daily doses of levodopa or increasing the doses of a dopamine agonist (Level C).

- *Discontinue or reduce dose of MAO-B inhibitors or COMT inhibitors* (GPP), at the risk of worsening wearing-off.

- Add amantadine (Level A) – most studies use oral 200–400 mg/day. The benefit may last <8 months. The use of other antiglutamatergic drugs is investigational. In some cases discontinuation of oral levodopa for a short period of time (3 days) with simultaneous continuous intravenous infusion of amantadine may temporarily improve dyskinesia (GPP).

- *Deep brain stimulation of the STN*, which allows reduction of dopaminergic treatment (Level A). Effective inhibition of severe dyskinesia may also be obtained by GPi stimulation (Level C).

- *Add atypical antipsychotics*, clozapine (Level C: [160, 161]), in dosages ranging between 12.5–75 mg/day up to 200 mg/day, or quetiapine (Level C: [162, 163]). However, clozapine is associated with potential serious adverse events (agranulocytosis and myocarditis), which limits its use (GPP).

- *Apomorphine continuous subcutaneous infusion*, which allows reduction of levodopa therapy (Level C).

- *Intrajejunal levodopa infusion* in patients with marked peak dose dyskinesia and motor fluctuations (Level C).

Biphasic dyskinesia

Biphasic dyskinesias can be very difficult to treat, and have not been the subject of specific and adequate Class I–III studies. Deep brain stimulation of the STN is effective (Level A) and the strategies described for peak-dose dyskinesias can also be considered for biphasic dyskinesia (GPP). Another option is increasing the size and frequency of levodopa dose, at the risk of inducing or increasing peak-dose dyskinesia. This latter strategy can be helpful, generally transiently, in those cases without peak-dose dyskinesia, or where they are considered less disabling than the biphasic type. A further option could be larger, less frequent doses, to give a more predictable response, which would better enable patients to plan daily activities (GPP). Finally apomorphine- and intrajejunal levodopa-infusion can be tried (Level C).

Recommendations

Off-period and early morning dystonias

- *Usual strategies for wearing-off* can be applied in cases of off-period dystonia (GPP).

- *Additional doses of levodopa or dopamine agonist therapy at night* may be effective for the control of dystonia appearing during the night or early in the morning (GPP).

- *Deep brain stimulation of the STN* (Level A) or GPi (Level C).

- *Botulinum toxin* can be employed in both off-period and early morning dystonia (GPP).

Freezing

Freezing, particularly freezing of gait, often occurs during the OFF phase, and less frequently in both OFF and ON. The latter scenario often does not respond to dopaminergic strategies.

Options for OFF freezing are the same as those described for wearing-off. In addition, the use of visual or auditory cues is empirically useful for facilitating the start of the motor act once freezing has occurred (Level C).

In ON freezing, a reduction in dopaminergic therapy can be tried, although this may result in worsening of wearing-off.

Interventions and recommendations for the symptomatic control of non-motor problems

Neuropsychiatric complications

Dementia

The prevalence of dementia in PD is 30–40% [164], although the cumulative incidence is closer to 80% [165]. Current age, rather than disease duration, is the highest risk factor for development of dementia associated with PD [166]. The pathological and neurochemical substrates underpinning cognitive decline in PD are heterogeneous, although a profound cortical cholinergic deficiency is characteristic [167, 168].

Interventions for the treatment of dementia in PD

Several drugs, particularly anticholinergics, can impair cognitive function and a gradual, graded discontinuation of such drugs is recommended. Other possible interventions are therapy with cholinesterase inhibitors or the N-methly D-aspartate receptor antagonist memantine (see below).

Cholinesterase inhibitors Several reports on cognitive dysfunction in patients with dementia in PD have claimed beneficial treatment effects with donepezil (Class I: [169–171]), rivastigmine (Class I: [172]), galantamine (Class III: [173]), and tacrine (Class IV: [174, 175]). A Cochrane review concluded that cholinesterase inhibitors lead to a clinically significant benefit in 15% of cases, but that further studies were required to better ascertain impact on quality of life, as well as health economic measures [176].

For the effect of cholinesterase inhibitors on neuropsychiatric symptoms (including hallucinations) see below.

Increased tremor is an uncommon reason for discontinuation of cholinesterase inhibitors [177], while nausea and vomiting can also result in discontinuation of therapy in a minority of patients. These drugs may also be associated with a modest increase in risk for syncope, need for pacemaker insertion and hip fracture [178]. They may also worsen urinary frequency, urgency, and urge incontinence.

Memantine Two relatively small randomized trials in patients with either dementia associated with PD (PDD) or the closely related dementia with Lewy bodies (DLB) demonstrated benefit for memantine, although the effects were very modest (Class I: [179, 180]). In both studies the drug was well tolerated.

Recommendations
Treatment of dementia in PD
Most of the recommendations are off-label recommendations.

- *Discontinue potential aggravators.* Anticholinergics (Level B), amantadine (Level C), tricyclic antidepressants (Level C), tolterodine and oxybutynin (Level C), and benzodiazepines (Level C).
- *Add cholinesterase inhibitors.* Rivastigmine (Level A), donepezil (Level A), galantamine (Level C). Given the hepatotoxicity of tacrine, its use is not recommended (GPP). There may be idiosyncrasy in clinical response and side effects with these agents so it may be worth trying an alternative agent before abandoning (GPP).
- *Add or substitute with memantine if cholinesterase inhibitors not tolerated or lacking efficacy* (Level C).

Psychosis
Psychosis is one of the most disabling non-motor complications of PD. Visual hallucinations have been observed in up to 40% of patients with advanced disease in hospital-based series [181].

Interventions for the treatment of psychosis in PD
Due to the prominent role of dopaminergic treatment in inducing psychosis in PD, interventions are primarily based on reduction or withdrawal of the offending drugs, complemented by adjunct treatment with atypical antipsychotics, if necessary. However, infection and metabolic disorders can provoke psychosis and, in such cases, the underlying disorder should be treated.

Visual hallucinations often preceed or accompany cognitive decline and should be considered as a warning sign for developing dementia in PD.

Atypical antipsychotics
Clozapine The efficacy of clozapine was documented in two 4-week trials (Class I: [182, 183]). There was no worsening of UPDRS-Motor scores, and one study [182] found significant improvement of tremor in patients receiving clozapine versus placebo. In an open-label extension of one of these studies, efficacy was maintained over an additional 12 weeks [184]. Leucopenia is a rare (0.4%) but serious adverse event with clozapine as is myocarditis [185]. Consistently reported side effects (even with low-dose clozapine) include sedation, dizziness, increased drooling, orthostatic hypotension, and weight gain.

Olanzapine In two Class I studies, olanzapine failed to show antipsychotic efficacy [186, 187]. Both studies also found significant motor worsening with olanzapine, as did Goetz *et al.* [188] (Class I). Olanzapine is associated with unacceptable worsening of PD, and is no longer recommended because of the risk of cerebrovascular events in the elderly [189]. However, a relationship between olanzapine and stroke has been denied by others [190].

Quetiapine A recent trial found no significant improvement in psychosis rating with quetiapine versus placebo (Class I: [331]). This study contradicts previous encouraging results from several Class III studies [191–197], and a study by Morgante *et al.* [162] (Class II), which found no difference between quetiapine and clozapine.

Risperidone Risperidone improves hallucinations and psychosis in PD (Class IV: [198–201]). However, motor worsening was observed in most of these reports and, therefore, risperidone is not recommended in patients with PD [202].

Cholinesterase inhibitors
Rivastigmine (Class III: [202a, 203] and donepezil (Class IV: [204, 205]) have been reported to improve psychosis in PD patients. In a study of dementia in PD, rivastigmine improved hallucinations (Class III, as hallucination was analysed post hoc in this trial: [172, 206]). Motor worsening was reported in two cases in one study only. A small minority of patients discontinued therapy because of increased tremor, nausea or vomiting.

Recommendations
Treatment of psychosis in PD
- *Control triggering factors* (GPP). Treat infection and metabolic disorders, rectify fluid/electrolyte balance, treat sleep disorder.
- *Reduce polypharmacy* (GPP). Reduce/stop anticholinergic antidepressants, reduce/stop anxiolytics/sedatives.
- *Reduce antiparkinsonian drugs* (GPP). Stop anticholinergics, stop amantadine, reduce/stop dopamine agonists, reduce/stop MAO-B and COMT inhibitors, lastly, reduce levodopa. Stopping antiparkinsonian drugs can be at the cost of worsening motor symptoms. As a rule dopamine agonists have a higher psychosis-inducing potential than levodopa (GPP).
- *Add atypical antipsychotics.* Clozapine (Level A) – although it can be associated with serious haematological adverse events, requiring monitoring. There is insufficient data on quetiapine, and it is possibly useful (GPP). Quetiapine is thought to be relatively safe and does not require blood monitoring. Olanzapine (Level A), risperidone (Level C), and aripripazole (GPP) are not recommended, but can induce – sometimes with a delay – parkinsonism (harmful).
- *Typical antipsychotics* (e.g. phenothiazines, butyrophenones) should not be used because they worsen parkinsonism.
- *Add cholinesterase inhibitors.* Rivastigmine (Level B), donepezil (Level C).

Depression
Depression is one of the most common non-motor symptoms of PD and, overall, available studies suggest that it may be found in about 40% of patients [207, 208].

Depressive episodes and panic attacks may occur before the onset of overt motor symptoms [209, 210] and, in established PD, depression is a major determinant of quality of life [211, 212].

There is consensus that PD-specific neurobiological changes also play a key role [213–215].

Interventions for the treatment of depression in PD
Despite its clinical importance, relatively few pharmacological intervention studies on how to treat PD-associated depression have been reported and ony recently Class I trials have been published and initiated.

Levodopa There are no studies on the effects of chronic levodopa treatment on depressive symptoms in PD.

Dopamine agonists There have been early anecdotal claims of antidepressant effects of the dopamine agonists, initially related to bromocriptine (Class IV: [216]). In addition, a small study has compared the antidepressive efficacy of standard doses of pergolide and pramipexole as adjunct therapy. After 8 months, both treatments were associated with significant improvements in depression scores (Class III: [217]). A meta-analysis of seven randomized controlled trials of the effect of the non-ergot dopamine agonist pramipexole on depression in PD suggests that this compound has a beneficial effect on mood and motivational symptoms in PD patients, who do not suffer from major depressive disorder [218].

MAO inhibitors In a study of the effects of selegiline on motor fluctuations, Lees et al. [9] (Class II) failed to detect any significant changes in depression score in a subgroup analysis. However, depression was not the primary target of this trial.

In another study, after 6 weeks of therapy, Hamilton Depression rating scale (HAM-D) scores showed significantly greater improvement in patients receiving combined MAO-A (moclobemide 600 mg/day) plus MAO-B (selegiline 10 mg/day) inhibition, as compared with treatment with moclobemide alone (Class III: [219]). However, this study was confounded by motor improvement in the combined treatment group.

Tricyclic antidepressants This class of agents features among others an anticholinergic effect and is an established treatment modality in major depression. One randomised placebo-controlled study in 19 patients (all on levodopa 7 of whom also were on anticholinergics) dates back more than 20 years and is related to nortriptyline (titrated from 25 mg/day to a maximum of 150 mg/day) (Class II: [220]), which showed a significant improvement over placebo, on a depression rating scale designed by the author. Although evidence-based reviews ([28, 221]) found little evidence supporting the use of tricyclic antidepressants in PD, a randomized controlled trial of paroxetine CR versus nortriptyline versus placebo in 52 patients with PD and depression showed that nortriptyline was efficacious but paroxetine CR was not. The primary endpoint in this study was the Hamilton Depression Scale and the percentage of depression responders at 8 weeks [222, 223].

Selective serotonin reuptake inhibitors (SSRIs) The use of SSRIs in PD-associated depression has been reported as beneficial in numerous small, open-label studies covering a variety of agents (fluoxetine, sertraline, paroxetine; Class II–IV: see [224] for review). One small double-blind placebo-controlled study of sertraline has assessed this approach. No statistically significant differences in the change of Montgomery Asberg Depression Rating Scale (MADRS) scores was detected between treatment arms (Class II: [225]).

The two largest uncontrolled trials of SSRIs in the treatment of depression in PD investigated the use of paroxetine in 33 and 65 patients over a period of 3–6 months (Class III: [226, 227]). In both studies, paroxetine was titrated to 20 mg/day and produced statistically significant improvements over baseline in HAM-D rating scores. There were no changes in UPDRS-Motor scores in either study. Avila *et al.* [228] (Class II) compared nefazodone with fluoxetine. Significant improvements in BDI scores were observed with both treatments. However, according to a recent review, large effect sizes have been seen with both active and placebo treatments in PD, but with no difference between the active and placebo groups [224]. The controlled, although small study by Menza *et al.* [222] also failed to demonstrate a beneficial effect of an SSRI, i.e. paroxetine CR, on depression in PD (see above) – in contrast to nortriptyline.

When added to dopaminergic therapy, SSRIs have the potential to induce a 'serotonin syndrome', which is a rare but serious adverse event.

'New' antidepressants Reboxetine (Class III: [229]) and venlafaxine (Class III: [230]) have been reported beneficial in PD-associated depression. However, these studies have been small and of short duration.

Non-pharmacological interventions A recent review identified 21 articles, covering a total of 71 patients with PD receiving electroconvulsive therapy (ECT) to treat concomitant depression [28]. These data are insufficient to conclude on the efficacy and safety of ECT to treat depression in PD.

Two double-blind studies have assessed repetitive transcranial magnetic stimulation (rTMS) in PD depression. There was no difference between sham and effective stimulation with respect to depression and PD measures (Class I: [231]. A Class I study [232] found rTMS as effective as fluoxetine in improving depression at week 2 – an effect maintained to week 8. However, interpretation of this study is hampered by lack of a placebo.

Recommendations
Treatment of depression in PD
- *Optimize antiparkinsonian therapy* (GPP).
- *Tricyclic antidepressants* (Level B).
- *SSRIs* (GPP). SSRIs are less likely to produce adverse effects than tricyclic antidepressants (GPP).
- *'New' antidepressants (mirtazapine, reboxetine, venlafaxine).* No recommendation can be made.

Autonomic dysfunction

Autonomic dysfunction is a common complication of PD. However, it may also occur as a side effect of standard medical therapy in PD. A significant minority of parkinsonian patients experience severe and disabling autonomic impairment.

Orthostatic hypotension

Interventions for the treatment of orthostatic hypotension in PD

Midodrine Midodrine is a peripheral alpha-adrenergic agonist without adverse effects on cardiac function. Two Class II studies of midodrine that included PD and other causes of neurogenic orthostatic hypotension revealed a significant increase in standing blood pressure [233,

234]. Such effect lasts only a few hours, which may be an advantage in some cases since patients can take it only when the effects are needed. The main side effects are supine hypertension (4% of patients) [234], paresthesias, and goose bumps.

Fludrocortisone Fludrocortisone (also called fluorohydrocortisone) enhances sodium reabsorption and potassium excretion in the kidney. The rise in blood pressure is assumed to be due to an increase in blood volume and cardiac output. Only one study (Class IV) evaluated PD patients and showed an increase in systolic pressure upon standing, as well as disappearance of orthostatic symptoms [235]. In a more recent, small (17 patients with PD) crossover clinical trial (Class III; [236]*) with four dropouts, both fludrocortisone and domperidone improved scores on two clinical scales used as outcome measures (CGI and COMPASS-OD), with only a trend towards reduced blood pressure drop on tilt table testing (domperidone > fludrocortisone). Hypertension, hypokalaemia, and ankle oedema [237] are the main side effects of fludrocortisone. Other studies have found fludrocortisone effective in various other causes of orthostatic hypotension. At least 4-5 days of treatment are necessary before therapeutic response is observed and full benefit requires a high dietary salt and adequate fluid intake.

Dihydroergotamine, etilefrine hydrochloride, indomethacin, yohimbine, L-DOPS (L-threo-3,4-dihydroxyphenylserine), desmopressin acetate, pyridostigmine and EPO (erythropoietin) Insufficient evidence is available in PD and in other disorders causing neurogenic orthostatic hypotension.

Recommendations
Treatment of orthostatic hypotension in PD
General measures
- *Avoid aggravating factors* such as large meals, alcohol, caffeine at night, exposure to a warm environment, volume depletion, and drugs known to cause orthostatic hypotension, such as diuretics or antihypertensive drugs, tricyclic antidepressants, nitrates, alpha-blockers used to treat urinary disturbances related to prostatic hypertrophy. Levodopa, dopamine agonists, and MAO-B inhibitors may also induce orthostatic hypotension.

- *Increase salt intake (1g per meal)* in symptomatic orthostatic hypotension.
- *Head-up tilt of the bed at night (30–40°)*, which may be helpful.
- *Wear waist-high elastic stockings and/or abdominal binders.*
- *Exercise as tolerated.*
- *Introduce counter-manoeuvres to prolong the time for which the patient can be upright* (leg crossing, toe raising, thigh contraction, bending at the waist).
- *Highlight postprandial effects.* In some patients, hypotension occurs only postprandially. Warning the patient about this effect and taking frequent small meals may be helpful.

Drug therapy
- *Add midodrine* (Level A).
- *Add fludrocortisone* (GPP: possibly effective, but note side effects).

Urinary disturbance

Interventions for the treatment of urinary disturbance in PD

Dopaminergic drugs There are indications that dopaminergic therapy (apomorphine, L-dopa) can improve storage urodynamic properties in patients with PD, at least in *de novo* patients (Class IV: [238]). In non-*de novo* patients the results of different studies are partly conflicting and variable concerning effects of dopaminergic therapy (Class III: [239–246]). With subcutaneous apomorphine a reduction of bladder outflow resistance and improved voiding was demonstrated (Class III: [242]).

Peripherally acting anticholinergics Neurogenic bladder problems with overactive bladder in general improve with anticholinergics [247, 248] but there are no placebo-controlled double-blind/randomized studies on this treatment in patients with PD. It is important to balance the therapeutic benefits with the adverse effects of these drugs. Dry mouth, constipation, and cognitive adverse events are a concern. It has been suggested that anticholinergic drugs that do not pass the blood–brain barrier so readily should have priority because of their lower risk of cognitive side effects, but there are no studies addressing this issue.

Intranasal desmopressin spray Intranasal desmopressin spray showed a good response in PD patients with nocturia (Class IV: [249]).

Deep brain stimulation Deep brain stimulation might have benefitial effects with improved bladder capacity, and increased voiding volumes, but does not influence bladder emptying (Class III: [250, 251]).

Recommendations
Treatment of urinary disturbance in PD
Most PD patients develop bladder problems. The symptoms include urgency, frequency, nocturia, and sometimes urge incontinence. The most common bladder disturbance is detrusor hyperactivity. Detrusor hypoactivity is uncommon, and usually caused by anticholinergic and tricyclic antidepressive drugs. Pronounced incontinence is relatively uncommon and when it occurs it mostly relates to late stage disease or akinesia. PD patients with bladder problems should be referred to a urologist, at least if response to anticholinergic therapy is insufficient or if incontinence is present. Further management includes the following.

- *When symptoms appear suddenly*: exclude urinary tract infection.

- *When frequency and polyuria dominate*: exclude diabetes mellitus.

- *Nocturia*: reduce intake of fluid after 6pm. Sleep with head-up tilt of bed to reduce urine production.

- *Night-time dopaminergic therapy should be optimized* (GPP). Apomorphine injections can be considered if outflow obstruction is the dominating problem (GPP).

- *Use anticholinergic drugs* (GPP): drugs that do not pass the blood–brain barrier should have priority (since those that pass the blood–brain barrier tend to cause cognitive side effects in this patient category (GPP)). Substances: trospium chloride (10–20 mg two to three times per day), tolterodine (2 mg twice per day), oxybutynin (2.5–5 mg twice per day). Compared to other alternatives trospium is less apt to penetrate the blood–brain barrier. In case of cognitive side effects the advantage of better control of the urine must be balanced against the cognitive drawbacks. Postmicturation residual urine should be measured before and especially after start of anticholinergic therapy.

- A recent pilot study showed that botulinum toxin type A injected in the detrusor muscle under cystostopic guidance ameliorated clinical symptoms and urodynamic variables in a small sample of PD patients with overactive bladder. [252].

Gastrointestinal motility problems

Dysphagia: therapeutic interventions
The literature on treatment of dysphagia in Parkinson's disease is limited. Several studies have methodological problems and results are difficult to compare because of heterogeneous methods and outcome measures. Levodopa and apomorphine can improve the early phases (oral and pharyngeal) of swallowing, resulting in a shorter swallowing time, but do not affect all patients and might reduce swallowing efficiency (Class III: [253–259]). Percutaneous injection of botulinum toxin can be considered in selected patients (Class III: [260]). The effects of cricopharyngeal myotomy have not been fully evaluated (Class IV: [261, 262]). The effect of different rehabilitative treatments and modification of food/drink could be effective in some patients (Class III: [263–267]).

Recommendations
Dysphagia
Dysphagia difficulties in PD usually relate to disease severity and are rare in early PD. They are connected to a risk for asphyxia, aspiration pneumonia, malnutrition, and dehydration. There is a high risk of silent aspiration in PD. Pneumonia is a leading cause of death in later disease stages. The following recommendations can be given (GPP).

- Optimization of motor symptom control should be given priority3. Levodopa and apomorphine can improve dysphagia at least in some patients.

- Early referral to speech therapist for assessment, swallowing advice, and further instrumental investigations if needed.

- Videofluoroscopy in selected cases to exclude silent aspiration.

- Enteral feeding options may need to be considered (short-term nasogastric tube feeding or longer-term feeding systems (percutaneous endoscopic gastrostomy)).

Concerning surgical therapies, rehabilitative treatments, and botulinum toxin therapies there is still very limited experience and these treatments can not be generally recommended.

Gastric dysfunction: therapeutic interventions
Domperidone has been reported to accelerate gastric emptying and reduces dopaminergic drug-related gastrointestinal symptoms in patients with PD (Class II–IV: [268–271]). Mosapride, a selective 5-hydroxytryptamine

type 4 (5HT4) agonist drug, improved gastric emptying in PD patients with motor fluctuations (Class III: [272]*)

Metoclopramide also blocks peripheral dopamine receptors and reduces nausea and vomiting [269] by blocking dopamine receptors in the area postrema. However, in contrast to domperidone, it also crosses the blood–brain barrier, thus can also worsen or induce parkinsonism [273–275], which is considered an unacceptable risk in patients with PD.

Recommendations
Gastric dysfunction

- Gastric emptying is often delayed in PD, both in early and advanced patients. In addition to nausea and vomiting, symptoms may include early satiety, postprandial fullness, and abdominal pain. Through delayed absorption of medication motor fluctuations such as 'delayed on' can result. Domperidone can be considered to accelerate gastric emptying (GPP).

- Parenteral treatment such as transdermal patches can be considered for patients with severe fluctuations due to erratic gastric emptying (GPP). In cases with gastroparesis a PEG often becomes necessary.

Nausea and vomiting: therapeutic interventions

These symptoms often occur as adverse events in the initiation of dopaminergic therapy (see Part I) or when dopaminergic therapy is increased. To block or reduce nausea (and vomiting) and improve compliance to the symptomatic therapy, antiemetics can be used as concomitant therapy.

Recommendations
Nausea and vomiting

Domperidone (30–60 mg/daily) reduces dopaminergic drug-related gastrointestinal symptoms in patients with PD (Class II–IV: [268–271]). Ondansetron may be used as second-line drug. No other antiemetic is recommended. In fact, metoclopramide, cinnarizine, and prochlorperazine must be avoided (GPP) (see above).

Constipation: therapeutic interventions

Psyllium was reported to increase stool frequency (Class II: [276]). A placebo-controlled study showed Macrogol to be effective in the treatment of chronic constipation

in 57 patients with PD (Class I: [277]). Also tagaserode (a 5-HT4 partial agonist) has proven to be an efficacious and safe therapy (Class II: [278]).

Recommendations
Constipation

- Constipation is the most commonly reported gastrointestinal symptom in PD patients. It can occur in both clinical and preclinical stages of the disease and worsens with disease progression. Anticholinergic drugs can worsen constipation and should be removed (GPP).

- Among non-pharmacological therapies, increased intake of fluid and fibre are recommended (GPP).

- Increased physical activity can be beneficial (GPP).

- As medication polyethylene glycol solution (Macrogol) is recommended (Level A).

- Alternative treatments are fibre supplements such as psyllium (Level B) or methylcellulose and osmotic laxatives (e.g. lactulose) (GPP).

- Irritant laxatives should be reserved for selected patients and short treatment duration.

Erectile dysfunction

Interventions for the treatment of erectile dysfunction in PD

Sildenafil On the basis of trials using validated questionnaires, sildenafil was found to be efficacious in the treatment of erectile dysfunction (Class I: [279]; Class IV: [280, 281]). Side effects of this drug include a group of mild and transitory adverse reactions (headache, transient visual effects, flushing) and, occasionally, severe reactions (hypotension, priapism, cardiac arrest).

Alprostadil Insufficient evidence.

Dopamine agonists Apomorphine, administered 30 min before sexual activity, may improve erectile function (Class IV: [282, 283]).

Nausea, headache, yawning, and orthostatic hypotension are the most common side effects of apomorphine. Pergolide may improve sexual function in younger male patients (Class IV: [284]).

Recommendations

Treatment of erectile dysfunction in PD

Erectile dysfunction is more common in PD patients compared with age matched controls. Urological investigation should be considered. Comorbidities, such as endocrine abnormalities (e.g. hypothyroidism, hyperprolactinemia, low testosterone) and depression should be considered and treated. Drugs associated with erectile dysfunction (e.g. alpha-blockers) or anorgasmia (e.g. SSRIs) should be discontinued. Dopaminergic therapy can have both negative and positive effects on this symptom. Sildenafil (50–100 mg, 1 h before sex) can be tried in PD patients with these problems (Level B). Other drugs of this class, like tadalafil (10 mg, 30 min–12 h before sex) or vardenafil (10 mg, 1 h before sex) can be alternative choices (GPP; no published experience in PD). In some patients apomorphine injections (5–10 min before sex) can also be an alternative treatment (GPP). Intracavernous injections of papaverine or alprostadil can be considered in selected patients (GPP; no published experience in PD).

Sleep disorders

Clinically significant sleep disorders are common in PD. It is estimated that 60–90% of patients complain of difficulties associated with sleep [285]. These disorders can be classified into those that involve nocturnal sleep (insomnia), daytime manifestations such as excessive daytime sleepiness, and those that involve specific nocturnal motor problems such as akinesia, dystonia, periodic limb movements, and restless legs syndrome. The causes of sleep disorders are related to the disease itself, to comorbidity or ageing, or linked to the effects of medications. There are a limited number of controlled clinical trials specifically on sleep problems associated with PD. There are also data on sleep outcomes generated in trials that selected patients who were not specifically recruited because of their sleep problems.

Daytime somnolence

There is huge variability in the frequency of daytime sleepiness depending on the population investigated and the tools used [286, 287]. Using the Epworth Sleepiness Scale (ESS) to define daytime somnolence, the frequency reaches 33% of patients as compared to 11–16% in a population of non-PD controls [288–290].

Interventions for the treatment of daytime somnolence in PD

Modafinil Modafinil is an orally administered wake-promoting agent, indicated to improve wakefulness in adults with excessive sleepiness associated with obstructive sleep apnoea, shift work disorder, and narcolepsy. Three small Class II, short-term, placebo-controlled, randomized, double-blinded trials evaluated the effect of oral modafinil on daytime sleepiness in PD [291, 292, 293]. The two trials with a crossover design [291, 292] found a small improvement in the ESS, while in the parallel trial [293] modafinil failed to significantly improve ESS. There was no benefit documented in other secondary sleep related outcomes [291–293].

Other pharmacological treatments An open-label study (Class III: [294]) on STN-stimulated patients with advanced PD with severe gait disorders, treated with high doses of methylphenidate, reported an improvement in the ESS.

Recommendations

Treatment of daytime somnolence in PD

General measures

- Assessment of nocturnal sleep disturbances (GPP).
- Optimize improvement of nocturnal sleep by reducing disturbing factors, such as akinesia, tremor, urinary frequency, etc. (GPP).
- Recommendation to stop driving (GPP).

Drug therapy

- Decrease dose or discontinue sedative drugs prescribed for another medical condition (GPP).
- Decrease dose of dopaminergic drugs (mainly dopamine agonists; GPP). All dopaminergic drugs may induce daytime somnolence.
- Switch to other dopamine agonist (GPP).
- Add modafinil (Level B).
- Add other wake-promoting agents like methylphenidate (GPP).

Sudden-onset sleep episodes

Sudden-onset sleep episodes ('sleep attacks') were originally described as 'sudden, irresistible, and overwhelming sleepiness without awareness of falling asleep'. The percentage of PD patients complaining of sleep episodes varies greatly in different reports between 3.8 and 20.8% [288, 295–300].

Nocturnal sleep problems

Nocturnal sleep disorders may not be a major clinical problem in the early stages of the disease, although changes of motor events, REM sleep behaviour disorder (RBD), and sleep fragmentation are recognized in untreated PD [301]. However, with disease progression there are specific symptoms of PD that may interfere with global sleep quality. The most frequent sleep problems include sleep fragmentation and nocturia. Other problems include difficulty in turning over in bed, a restless legs-like syndrome, vivid dreams, hallucinations, dyskinesias, pain, dystonia, and others [302]. All these phenomena result in worse quality of sleep when compared with a control group without PD [290]. Another frequent sleep disorder both in early and late stage PD is RBD.

REM sleep behaviour disorder

REM sleep behaviour disorder is a parasomnia characterized by the occurrence of muscle activity enabling dream enactment during REM sleep [303]. Patients may present complex, vigorous, and sometimes violent behaviours [304]. RBD is present in 25–50% of PD patients [304, 305] and may precede the onset of clinical symptoms of parkinsonism by many years [306].

Interventions for the treatment of RBD

There are no controlled trials that specifically addressed the treatment of RBD in Parkinson's disease or any parkinsonian syndrome.

Clonazepam Two case series (Class IV: [307, 308]) that have included patients with PD concluded that small doses of clonazepam (0.5–2 mg) are efficacious for the treatment of RBD. Clonazepam may induce daytime sedation and exacerbate underlying obstructive breathing in sleep and increase the risk of nocturnal falling in the elderly.

Dopamine agonists Three small open-label studies (Class III: [309–311] reported contradictory results on the effi-

cacy of pramipexole for the treatment of RBD in PD patients.

Antidepressants Most antidepressants, especially serotonin reuptake inhibitors and mirtazapine, may carry a risk of worsening pre-existing RLS, periodic leg movements and RBD (Class IV: [312]).

Other sleep disorders

In the available studies, the translation of the concept of night-time sleep disorders to the inclusion criteria of the different trials is very heterogeneous. The applied criteria varied from sleep fragmentation (frequency of nocturnal awakenings) to subjective complaint of unsatisfactory night-time sleep with nocturnal akinesia as a frequent and clinically relevant complaint.

Interventions for the treatment of other night-time sleep disorders in PD

Levodopa Two randomized, crossover placebo controlled trials (Class II: [313]; [314]) suggested that a bedtime intake of a standard or slow release dose of L-dopa may improve nocturnal and early morning disabilities. A small trial (Class II: [313]) comparing three different night-time doses (100 mg levodopa/25 mg carbidopa) found an increased sleep quality, decreased number of spontaneous moves in bed, and improved walking time in the morning. A placebo-controlled trial (Class II: [314]) reported an improvement in nocturnal akinesia and sleeping time with a bedtime single dose of slow-release levodopa/carbidopa. In a crossover double-blind trial, both levodopa/benserazide formulations (controlled release vs standard release) reduced nocturnal and early-morning disability scores (compared with baseline) [315].

Dopamine agonists A Class II [316] randomized, double-blind, placebo-controlled trial demonstrated that a night-time dose of 1 mg pergolide worsened sleep (sleep efficiency, movement, and fragmentation index) in PD patients with fragmented sleep. A small open-label trial that evaluated the effect of nocturnal continuous subcutaneous overnight apomorphine infusion (Class III: [317]) documented a reduction of nocturnal awakenings and off periods and improvement of nocturia and nocturnal and early-morning akinesia in PD patients with nocturnal disabilities.

Nocturnal disturbances were measured with the Parkinson's Disease Sleep Scale (PDSS) – as secondary outcome criteria and not as an eligibility criteria in two Class I trials [47, 49]. It was concluded that transdermal rotigotine, pramipexole, and ropinirole prolonged release improved most aspects of sleep and night quality (PDSS) in advanced PD.

Two small open-label studies (Class III: [318, 319]) evaluated the benefit of a single evening intake of cabergoline. In the first trial, cabergoline improved early morning motor function, did not change sleep efficiency, and aggravated fragmented sleep. In the second trial, there was significant increase of sleep efficiency and sleep quality (PDSS).

Melatonin An improvement in night sleep outcomes was reported in two randomized placebo-controlled studies (Class II: [320, 321]) with two completely different doses of melatonin (50 mg and 3 mg). There were no reports of relevant adverse events.

Other pharmacological treatments Two case series with zolpidem (Class IV: [322]), an imidazopyrimidine short-acting hypnotic, and quetiapine (Class IV: [323]), an atypical antipsychotic with sedative properties, suggested an improvement of insomnia. Low doses of clozapine (mean dose 26 mg at bedtime) were reported to improve nocturnal akathisia and rest tremor with no serious side effects observed (Class IV: [324]).

An open-label study (Class III: [249]) showed a reduction in the frequency of nocturnal voids with bedtime desmopressin (nasal spray) in PD patients with nocturia. However, desmopressin treatment is not advised in the elderly.

Deep brain surgery Several open-label studies (Class III: [325–330]) concluded that subthalamic nucleus stimulation consistently improves sleep duration and reduces nigh time akinesia, sleep fragmentation, and early morning dystonia. There were also consistent reports of no improvement on periodic leg movements, restless legs symptoms, RBD. and excessive daytime sleepiness.

Recommendations
Treatment of sleep problems in PD
- Add a bed-time intake of a standard or slow-release dose of levodopa (Level B).
- Transdermal rotigotine, pramipexole, and prolonged-release ropinirole improve sleep quality in advanced PD patients with motor fluctuations (Level A).
- Subthalamic nucleus deep brain stimulation improves sleep quality in advanced PD patients except for nocturnal motor phenomena of sleep disorders (Level B).

Need of update
No later than 2013.

Funding sources supporting the work
Financial support from MDS-ES, EFNS and Stichting De Regenboog (the Netherlands – review 2006) and Competence Network Parkinson (Germany – review 2010).

Conflicts of interest
A. Berardelli has received speaker honoraria from Allergan and Boehringer Ingelheim.

U. Bonuccelli has acted as scientific advisor for, or obtained speaker honoraria from, Boehringer Ingelheim, Chiesi, GlaxoSmithKline, Novartis, Pfizer, and Schwarz-Pharma. He has received departmental grants and performed clinical studies for Boehringer Ingelheim, Chiesi, Eisai, GlaxoSmithKline, Novartis, Schwarz-Pharma, and Teva.

D. Burn has served on medical advisory boards for Teva, Boehringer-Ingelheim, Archimedes, and Merck Serono. He has received honoraria to speak at meetings from Teva-Lundbeck, Orion, Boehringer-Ingelheim, GlaxoSmithKline, Novartis, Eisai, UCB, and GE Healthcare.

G. Deuschl has acted as scientific advisor for, or obtained speaker honoraria from, Orion, Novartis, Boehringer Ingelheim, and Medtronic.

E. Dietrichs has received honoraria for lecturing and/or travelling grants from GlaxoSmithKline, Lundbeck, Medtronic, Orion, Solvay, and UCB.

G. Fabbrini has received honoraria for lectures from Boehringer Ingelheim, Glaxo Pharmaceuticals, and Novartis Pharmaceuticals, and is member of an advisory board for Boehringer Ingelheim.

J. Ferreira has received honoraria for lecturing and/or consultancy from GlaxoSmithKline, Novartis, TEVA, Lundbeck, Solvay, and BIAL.

Andrzej Friedman received honoraria for presentations at educational conferences from Roche Poland, MSD Poland, and Allergan Poland.

P. Kanovsky has received honoraria for lectures from Ipsen and GSK, and received a research grant from Novartis.

V. Kostić has received honoraria for lecturing from Novartis, Boehringer Ingelheim, Merck, Lundbeck, and Glaxo-Smith-Kline, and is a member of the Regional South-Eastern European Pramipexole Advisory Board of Boehringer Ingelheim.

P. Odin has received honoraria for lectures from Boehringer Ingelheim, UCB, GSK, Solvay, and Cephalon, and participated in advisory boards for Boehringer Ingelheim, Cephalon, and Solvay.

W.H. Oertel has received honoraria for consultancy and presentations from Bayer-Schering, Boehringer Ingelheim, Cephalon, Desitin, GlaxoSmithKline, Medtronic, Merck-Serono, Neurosearch, Novartis, Orion Pharma, Schwarz-Pharma Neuroscience, Servier, Synosia, Teva, UCB, and Vifor Pharma.

W. Poewe has received honoraria for lecturing and advisory board membership from Novartis, GlaxoSmith-Kline, Teva, Boehringer Ingelheim, Schwarz-Pharma, and Orion.

O. Rascol has received scientific grants and consulting fees from GlaxoSmithKline, Novartis, Boehringer Ingelheim, Teva Neuroscience, Eisai, Schering, Solvay, Xeno-Port, Oxford BioMedica, Movement Disorder Society, UCB, Lundbeck, Schwarz-Pharma, and Servier.

C. Sampaio has received departmental research grants from Novartis Portugal. Her department has also charged consultancy fees to Servier and Lundbeck, and she has received honoraria for lectures from Boehringer Ingelheim.

M. Schüpbach has received speaker's honoraria and travel reimbursement from Medtronic.

E. Tolosa has received honoraria for lectures from Boehringer Ingelheim, Novartis, UCB, GlaxoSmithKline, Solvay, Teva, and Lundbeck, and participated in advisory boards for Boehringer Ingelheim, Novartis, Teva, and Solvay.

C. Trenkwalder has received honoraria for lectures from Boehringer Ingelheim, UCB, Glaxo Pharmaceuticals, and Astra Zeneca, and is member of advisory boards for Boehringer Ingelheim, UCB, Cephalon, Solvay, Novartis, and TEVA/Lundbeck.

Disclosure statement

The reader's attention should be drawn to the fact that the opinions and views expressed in the paper are those of the authors and not necessarily those of the MDS or the MDS Scientific Issues Committee (SIC).

Acknowledgements

The authors acknowledge the contribution of the late Martin Horstink as first author of the original publication. We are grateful to Susan Fox who provided the Movement Disorder Society's Evidence-based Medicine Task Force 2009 literature review. Niall Quinn is thanked for reviewing the manuscript. The authors would like to thank Karen Henley for co-ordinating the manuscript revision and Heidi Schudrowitz for technical assistance.

References

1. Verhagen Metman L, Del Dotto P, van den Munckhof P, Fang J, Mouradian MM, Chase TN. Amantadine as treatment for dyskinesias and motor fluctuations in Parkinson's disease. *Neurology* 1998;**50**:1323–6.
2. Luginger E, Wenning GK, Bosch S, Poewe W. Beneficial effects of amantadine on levodopa-induced dyskinesias in Parkinson's disease. *Mov Disord* 2000;**15**:873–8.
3. Snow BJ, Macdonald L, Mcauley D, Wallis W. The effect of amantadine on levodopa-induced dyskinesias in Parkinson's disease: a double-blind, placebo-controlled study. *Clin Neuropharmacol* 2000;**23**:82–5.
4. Verhagen Metman L, Del Dotto P, LePoole K, Konitsiotis S, Fang J, Chase TN. Amantadine for levodopa-induced dyskinesias. A 1-year follow-up. *Arch Neurol* 1999;**56**:1383–6.
5. Thomas A, Iacono D, Luciano AL, Armellino K, Di Iorio A, Onofrj M. Duration of amantadine benefit on dyskinesia of severe Parkinson's disease. *J Neurol Neurosurg Psychiatry* 2004;**75**:141–3.
6. Del Dotto P, Pavese N, Gambaccini G, *et al.* Intravenous amantadine improves levodopa-induced dyskinesias: an

acute double-blind placebo-controlled study. *Mov Disord* 2001;**16**:515–20.

7. Růžicka E, Streitová H, Jech R, *et al*. Amantadine infusion in treatment of motor fluctuations and dyskinesias in Parkinson's disease. *J Neural Transm* 2000;**107**:1297–306.

8. Koziorowski D, Friedman A. Levodopa 'drug holiday' with amantadine infusions as a treatment of complications in Parkinson's disease. *Mov Disord* 2007;**22**:1033–6.

9. Lees AJ, Shaw KM, Kohout LJ, Stern GM. Deprenyl in Parkinson's disease. *Lancet* 1977;**15**:791–5.

10. Lieberman AN, Gopinathan G, Neophytides A, Foo SH. Deprenyl versus placebo in Parkinson disease: a double-blind study. *N Y State J Med* 1987;**87**:646–9.

11. Golbe LI, Lieberman AN, Muenter MD, *et al*. Deprenyl in the treatment of symptom fluctuations in advanced Parkinson's disease. *Clin Neuropharmacol* 1988;**11**:45–55.

12. Waters CH, Sethi KD, Hauser RA, Molho E, Bertoni JM, Zydis Selegiline Study Group. Zydis selegiline reduces off time in Parkinson's disease patients with motor fluctuations: a 3-month, randomized, placebo-controlled study. *Mov Disord* 2004;**19**:426–32.

13. Parkinson Study Group. A randomized placebo-controlled trial of rasagiline in levodopa-treated patients with Parkinson disease and motor fluctuations. The PRESTO study. *Arch Neurol* 2005;**62**:241–8.

14. Rascol O, Brooks DJ, Melamed E, *et al*., LARGO study group. Rasagiline as an adjunct to levodopa in patients with Parkinson's disease and motor fluctuations (LARGO, Lasting effect in Adjunct therapy with Rasagiline Given Once daily, study): a randomised, double-blind, parallel-group trial. *Lancet* 2005;**365**:947–54.

15. Shoulson I, Oakes D, Fahn S, *et al*. Parkinson Study Group. Impact of sustained deprenyl (selegiline) in levodopa-treated Parkinson's disease: a randomized placebo-controlled extension of the deprenyl and tocopherol antioxidative therapy of parkinsonism trial. *Ann Neurol* 2002;**51**:604–12.

16. Deane KHO, Spieker S, Clarke CE. Catechol-O-methyltransferase inhibitors for levodopa-induced complications in Parkinson's disease. *Cochrane Database Syst Rev* 2004;(4):CD004554.

17. Brooks DJ, Leinonen M, Kuoppamäki M, Nissinen H. Five-year efficacy and safety of levodopa/DDCI and entacapone in patients with Parkinson's disease. *J Neural Transm* 2008;**115**:843–9.

18. Reichmann H, Boas J, Macmahon D, Myllyla V, Hakala A, Reinikainen K, ComQol Study Group. Efficacy of combining levodopa with entacapone on quality of life and activities of daily living in patients experiencing wearing-off type fluctuations. *Acta Neurol Scand* 2005;**111**:21–8.

19. Rajput AH, Martin W, Saint-Hilaire MH, Dorflinger E, Pedder S. Tolcapone improves motor function in parkinsonian patients with the 'wearing-off' phenomenon: a double-blind, placebo-controlled, multicenter trial. *Neurology* 1997;**49**:1066–71.

20. Kurth MC, Adler CH, Hilaire MS, *et al*. Tolcapone improves motor function and reduces levodopa requirement in patients with Parkinson's disease experiencing motor fluctuations: a multicenter, double-blind, randomized, placebo-controlled trial. Tolcapone Fluctuator Study Group I. *Neurology* 1997;**48**:81–7.

21. Baas H, Beiske AG, Ghika J, *et al*. Catechol-O-methyltransferase inhibition with tolcapone reduces the 'wearing off' phenomenon and levodopa requirements in fluctuating parkinsonian patients. *J Neurol Neurosurg Psychiatry* 1997;**63**:421–8.

22. Adler CH, Singer C, O'Brien C. Randomized, placebo-controlled study of tolcapone in patients with fluctuating Parkinson disease treated with levodopa-carbidopa. Tolcapone Fluctuator Study Group III. *Arch Neurol* 1998;**55**:1089–95.

23. Agid Y, Destee A, Durif F, Montastruc J-L, Pollak P. Tolcapone, bromocriptine, and Parkinson's disease. French Tolcapone Study Group. *Lancet* 1997;**350**:712–3.

24. Tolcapone Study Group. Efficacy and tolerability of tolcapone compared with bromocriptine in levodopa-treated parkinsonian patients. *Mov Disord* 1999;**14**:38–44.

25. Koller W, Lees A, Doder M, Hely M, Tolcapone/Pergolide Study Group. Randomised trial of tolcapone versus pergolide as add-on to levodopa therapy in Parkinson's disease patients with motor fluctuations. *Mov Disord* 2001;**16**:858–66.

26. Deane KHO, Spieker S, Clarke CE. Catechol-O-methyltransferase inhibitors versus active comparators for levodopa-induced complications in Parkinson's disease. *Cochrane Database Syst Rev* 2004;(4):CD004553.

26a. European Agency for the Evaluation of Medicinal Products (EMEA). (2004). EMEA public statement on the lifting of the suspension of the marketing authorisation for tolcapone (Tasmar). London, 29 April 2004 (http://www.emea.eu.int/pdfs/human/press/pus/1185404en.pdf, date accessed 10 January 2006).

27. The Entacapone to Tolcapone switch study investigators. Entacapone to tolcapone: multicenter double-blind, randomised, active controlled trial in advanced Parkinson's disease. *Mov Disord* 2007;**22**:14–9.

28. Management of Parkinson's disease: an evidence-based review. *Mov Disord* 2002;**17**:S1–166.

29. Levine CB, Fahrbach KR, Siderowf AD, Estok RP, Ludensky VM, Ross SD. Diagnosis and treatment of Parkinson's

disease: a systematic review of the literature. *Evid Rep Technol Assess* 2003;**57**:1–306.

30. Nyholm D, Aquilonius SM. Levodopa infusion therapy in Parkinson disease: state of the art in 2004. *Clin Neuropharmacol* 2004;**27**:245–56.

31. Ahlskog JE, Muenter MD, McManis PG, Bell GN, Bailey PA. Controlled-release Sinemet (CR-4): a double-blind crossover study in patients with fluctuating Parkinson's disease. *Mayo Clin Proc* 1988;**63**:876–86.

32. Jankovic J, Schwartz K, Vander LC. Comparison of Sinemet CR4 and standard Sinemet: double blind and long-term open trial in parkinsonian patients with fluctuations. *Mov Disord* 1989;**4**:303–9.

33. Lieberman A, Gopinathan G, Miller E, Neophytides A, Baumann G, Chin L. Randomized double-blind cross-over study of Sinemet-controlled release (CR4 50/200) versus Sinemet 25/100 in Parkinson's disease. *Eur Neurol* 1990;**30**:75–8.

34. Contin M, Riva R, Martinelli P, Cortelli P, Albani F, Baruzzi A. Concentration-effect relationship of levodopa-benserazide dispersible formulation versus standard form in the treatment of complicated motor response fluctuations in Parkinson's disease. *Clin Neuropharmacol* 1999;**22**: 351–5.

35. Stocchi F, Fabbri L, Vecsei L, Krygowska-Wajs A, Monici Preti PA, Ruggieri SA. Clinical efficay of a single afternoon dose of effervescent levodopa-carbidopa preparation (CHF 1512) in fluctuating Parkinson disease. *Clin Neuropharmacol* 2007;**30**(1):18–24.

36. Blindauer K, Shoulson I, Oakes D, *et al.* A randomized controlled trial of etilevodopa in patients with Parkinson disease who have motor fluctuations. *Arch Neurol* 2006; **63**(2):210–6.

37. Kurth MC, Tetrud JW, Tanner CM, *et al.* Double-blind, placebo-controlled, crossover study of duodenal infusion of levodopa/carbidopa in Parkinson's disease patients with 'on-off' fluctuations. *Neurology* 1993;**43**:1698–703.

38. Nyholm D, Nilsson Remahl AI, Dizdar N, *et al.* Duodenal levodopa infusion monotherapy vs oral polypharmacy in advanced Parkinson disease. *Neurology* 2005;**64**:216–23.

39. Antonini A, Isaias IU, Canesi M, *et al.* Duodenal levodopa infusion for advanced Parkinson's disease: 12-month treatment outcome. *Mov Disord* 2007;**22**(8):1145–9.

40. Eggert K, Schrader C, Hahn M, *et al.* Continuous jejunal Levodopa infusion in patients with advanced Parkinson's disease: practical aspects and outcome of motor and non-motor complications. *Clin Neuropharmacol* 2008;**31**: 151–66.

41. Devos D, French DUODOPA Study Group. Patient profile, indications, efficacy and safety of duodenal levodopa infusion in advanced Parkinson's disease. *Mov Disord* 2009;**24**(7):993–1000.

42. Olanow CW, Fahn S, Muenter M, *et al.* A multicenter double-blind placebo-controlled trial of pergolide as an adjunct to Sinemet in Parkinson's disease. *Mov Disord* 1994;**9**:40–7.

43. Guttman M. Double-blind randomized, placebo controlled study to compare safety, tolerance and efficacy of pramipezole and bromocriptine in advanced Parkinson's disease. International Pramipexole-Bromocriptine Study Group. *Neurology* 1997;**49**:1060–5.

44. Mizuno Y, Yanagisawa N, Kuno S, *et al.*, Japanese Pramipexole Study Group. Randomized double-blind study of pramipexole with placebo and bromocriptine in advanced Parkinson's disease. *Mov Disord* 2003;**18**:1149–56.

45. Rascol O, Lees AJ, Senard JM, Pirtosek Z, Montastruc JL, Fuell D. Ropinirole in the treatment of levodopa-induced motor fluctuations in patents with Parkinson's disease. *Clin Neuropharmacol* 1996;**19**:234–45.

46. Lieberman A, Olanow CW, Sethi K, *et al.* A multicenter trial of ropinirole as adjunct treatment for Parkinson's disease. Ropinirole Study Group. *Neurology* 1998;**51**:1057–62.

47. Pahwa R, Stacy MA, Factor SA, *et al.* Ropinirole 24-hour prolonged release: randomized, controlled study in advanced Parkinson disease. *Neurology* 2007;**68**: 1108–15.

48. LeWitt PA, Lyons KE, Pahwa R. Advanced Parkinson disease treated with rotigotine transdermal system: PREFER Study. *Neurology* 2007;**68**:1262–7.

49. Poewe WH, Rascol O, Quinn N, *et al.* Efficacy of pramipexole and transdermal rotigotine in advanced Parkinson's disease: a double-blind, double-dummy, randomised controlled trial. *Lancet Neurol* 2007;**6**:513–20.

50. Ostergaard L, Werdelin L, Odin P. Pen injected apomorphine against off phenomena in late Parkinson's disease: a double blind, placebo controlled study. *J Neurol Neurosurg Psychiatry* 1995;**58**:681–7.

51. Dewey RB Jr, Hutton JT, LeWitt PA, Factor SA. A randomized, double-blind, placebo-controlled trial on subcutaneously injected apomorphine for parkinsonian off-state events. *Arch Neurol* 2001;**58**:1385–92.

52. Manson AJ, Turner K, Lees AJ. Apomorphine monotherapy in the treatment of refractory motor complications of Parkinson's disease: long-term follow-up study of 64 patients. *Mov Disord* 2002;**17**:1235–41.

53. Katzenschlager R, Hughes A, Evans A, *et al.* Continuous subcutaneous apomorphine therapy improves dyskinesias in Parkinson's disease: a prospective study using single-dose challenges. *Mov Disord* 2005;**20**:151–7.

54. Garcia Ruiz PJ, Sesar IA, Ares PB, *et al.* Efficacy of long-term continuous subcutaneous apomorphine infusion in advanced Parkinson's disease with motor fluctuations: a multicenter study. *Mov Disord* 2008;**23**:1130–6.

55. Hoehn MMM, Elton RL. Low dosages of bromocriptine added to levodopa in Parkinson's disease. *Neurology* 1985;**35**:199–206.

56. Toyokura Y, Mizuno Y, Kase M, *et al.* Effects of bromocriptine on parkinsonism. A nation-wide collaborative double-blind study. *Acta Neurol Scand* 1985;**72**:157–70.

57. Hutton JT, Koller WC, Ahlskog JE, *et al.* Multicenter, placebo-controlled trial of cabergoline taken once daily in the treatment of Parkinson's disease. *Neurology* 1996;**46**:1062–5.

58. Inzelberg R, Nisipeanu P, Rabey JM, *et al.* Double-blind comparison of cabergoline and bromocriptine in Parkinson's disease patients with motor fluctuations. *Neurology* 1996;**47**:785–8.

59. Laihinen A, Rinne UK, Suchy I. Comparison of lisuride and bromocriptine in the treatment of advanced Parkinson's disease. *Acta Neurol Scand* 1992;**86**:593–5.

60. Mizuno Y, Kondo T, Narabayashi H. Pergolide in the treatment of Parkinson's disease. *Neurology* 1995;**45** (Suppl. 31):S13–21.

61. Deuschl G, Vaitkus A, Fox GC, Roscher T, Schremmer D, Gordin A. Efficacy and tolerability of Entacapone versus Cabergoline in parkinsonian patients suffering from wearing-off. *Mov Disord* 2007;**22**:1550–5.

62. Colzi A, Turner K, Lees AJ. Continuous subcutaneous waking day apomorphine in the long term treatment of levodopa induced interdose dyskinesias in Parkinson's disease. *J Neurol Neurosurg Psychiatry* 1998;**64**:573–6.

63. Stocchi F, Vacca L, De Pandis MF, Barbato L, Valente M, Ruggieri S. Subcutaneous continuous apomorphine infusion in fluctuating patients with Parkinson's disease: long-term results. *Neurol Sci* 2001;**22**:93–4.

64. Kanovsky P, Kubova D, Bares M, *et al.* Levodopa-induced dyskinesias and continuous subcutaneous infusions of apomorphine: results of a two-year, prospective follow-up. *Mov Disord* 2002;**17**:188–91.

65. Facca A, Sanchez-Ramos J. High-dose pergolide monotherapy in the treatment of severe levodopa-induced dyskinesias. *Mov Disord* 1996;**11**:327–9.

66. Cristina S, Zangaglia R, Mancini F, Martignoni E, Nappi G, Pacchetti C. High-dose ropinirole in advanced Parkinson's disease with severe dyskinesias. *Clin Neuropharmacol* 2003;**26**:146–50.

67. Deuschl G, Volkmann J, Krack P. Deep brain stimulation for movement disorders. *Mov Disord* 2002;**17**:S1.

68. Alexander GE, Crutcher MD, DeLong MR. Basal ganglia-thalamocortical circuits: parallel substrates for motor, oculomotor, 'prefrontal' and 'limbic' functions. *Prog Brain Res* 1990;**85**:119–46.

69. de Bie RM, de Haan RJ, Nijssen PC, *et al.* Unilateral pallidotomy in Parkinson's disease: a randomised, single-blind, multicentre trial. *Lancet* 1999;**354**:1665–9.

70. de Bie RM, de Haan RJ, Schuurman PR, Esselink RA, Bosch DA, Speelman JD. Morbidity and mortality following pallidotomy in Parkinson's disease: a systematic review. *Neurology* 2002;**58**:1008–12.

71. Vitek JL, Bakay RA, Freeman A, *et al.* Randomized trial of pallidotomy versus medical therapy for Parkinson's disease. *Ann Neurol* 2003;**53**:558–69.

72. Esselink RA, de Bie RM, de Haan RJ, *et al.* Unilateral pallidotomy versus bilateral subthalamic nucleus stimulation in PD: a randomized trial. *Neurology* 2004;**62**:201–7.

73. Esselink RA, de Bie RM, de Haan RJ, *et al.* Unilateral pallidotomy versus bilateral subthalamic nucleus stimulation in Parkinson's disease: one year follow-up of a randomised observer-blind multicentre trial. *Acta Neurochir (Wien)* 2006;**148**(12):1247–55.

74. Baron MS, Vitek JL, Bakay RA, *et al.* Treatment of advanced Parkinson's disease by posterior GPi pallidotomy: 1-year results of a pilot study. *Ann Neurol* 1996;**40**:355–66.

75. Hariz MI, De Salles AA. The side-effects and complications of posteroventral pallidotomy. *Acta Neurochir Suppl* 1997;**68**:42–8.

76. Kumar R, Lozano AM, Montgomery E, Lang AE. Pallidotomy and deep brain stimulation of the pallidum and subthalamic nucleus in advanced Parkinson's disease. *Mov Disord* 1998;**13**:73–82.

77. Kondziolka D, Bonaroti E, Baser S, Brandt F, Kim YS, Lunsford LD. Outcomes after stereotactically guided pallidotomy for advanced Parkinson's disease. *J Neurosurg* 1999;**90**:197–202.

78. de Bie RM, Schuurman PR, Bosch DA, de Haan RJ, Schmand B, Speelman JD. Outcome of unilateral pallidotomy in advanced Parkinson's disease: cohort study of 32 patients. *J Neurol Neurosurg Psychiatry* 2001;**71**:375–82.

79. Green J, McDonald WM, Vitek JL, *et al.* Neuropsychological and psychiatric sequelae of pallidotomy for PD: clinical trial findings. *Neurology* 2002;**58**:858–65.

80. Gironell A, Kulisevsky J, Rami L, Fortuny N, Garcia-Sanchez C, Pascual-Sedano B. Effects of pallidotomy and bilateral subthalamic stimulation on cognitive function in Parkinson disease. A controlled comparative study. *J Neurol* 2003;**250**:917–23.

81. Perrine K, Dogali M, Fazzini E, *et al.* Cognitive functioning after pallidotomy for refractory Parkinson's disease. *J Neurol Neurosurg Psychiatry* 1998;**65**:150–4.

82. Trepanier LL, Saint-Cyr JA, Lozano AM, Lang AE. Neuro-psychological consequences of posteroventral pallidotomy for the treatment of Parkinson's disease. *Neurology* 1998; **51**:207–15.

83. Biousse V, Newman NJ, Carroll C, *et al.* Visual fields in patients with posterior GPi pallidotomy. *Neurology* 1998; **50**:258–65.

84. Volkmann J, Allert N, Voges J, Sturm V, Schnitzler A, Freund HJ. Long-term results of bilateral pallidal stimulation in Parkinson's disease. *Ann Neurol* 2004;**55**:871–5.

85. Verhagen Metman L, O'Leary ST. Role of surgery in the treatment of motor complications. *Mov Disord* 2005;**20** (Suppl. 11):S45–56.

86. Lang AE, Houeto J-L, Krack P, *et al.* Deep brain stimulation: preoperative issues. *Mov Disord* 2006;**21**(Suppl. 14):S171–96.

87. Rezai AR, Kopell BH, Gross R, *et al.* Deep brain stimulation for Parkinson's disease: surgical issues. *Mov Disord* 2006;**21**(Suppl. 14):S197–218.

88. Deuschl G, Schade-Brittinger C, Krack P, *et al.* (on behalf of the German Parkinson Study Group). A randomized trial of deep-brain stimulation for Parkinson's disease. *N Engl J Med* 2006;**355**(9):896–908.

89. Weaver FM, Follett K, Stern M, *et al.* Bilateral deep brain stimulation vs best medical therapy for patients with advanced Parkinson disease: a randomized controlled trial. *JAMA* 2009;**301**(1):63–73.

90. Krack P, Batir A, Van Blercom N, *et al.* Five-year follow-up of bilateral stimulation of the subthalamic nucleus in advanced Parkinson's disease. *N Engl J Med* 2003;**349**: 1925–34.

91. Anderson VC, Burchiel KJ, Hogarth P, Favre J, Hammerstad JP. Pallidal vs subthalamic nucleus deep brain stimulation in Parkinson disease. *Arch Neurol* 2005;**62**(4):554–60.

92. Nakamura K, Christine CW, Starr PA, Marks WJ Jr. Effects of unilateral subthalamic and pallidal deep brain stimulation on fine motor functions in Parkinson's disease. *Mov Disord* 2007;**22**(5):619–26.

93. Deep Brain Stimulation for Parkinson's Disease Study Group. Deep-brain stimulation of the subthalamic nucleus or the pars interna of the globus pallidus in Parkinson's disease. *N Engl J Med* 2001;**345**:956–63.

94. Ardouin C, Pillon B, Peiffer E, *et al.* Bilateral subthalamic or pallidal stimulation for Parkinson's disease affects neither memory nor executive functions: a consecutive series of 62 patients. *Ann Neurol* 1999;**46**:217–23.

95. Vingerhoets G, van der Linden C, Lannoo E, *et al.* Cognitive outcome after unilateral pallidal stimulation in Parkinson's disease. *J Neurol Neurosurg Psychiatry* 1999;**66**: 297–304.

96. Fields JA, Troster AI. Cognitive outcomes after deep brain stimulation for Parkinson's disease: a review of initial studies and recommendations for future research. *Brain Cogn* 2000;**42**:268–93.

97. Trepanier LL, Kumar R, Lozano AM, Lang AE, Saint-Cyr JA. Neuropsychological outcome of GPi pallidotomy and GPi or STN deep brain stimulation in Parkinson's disease. *Brain Cogn* 2000;**42**:324–47.

98. Troster AI, Woods SP, Fields JA, Hanisch C, Beatty WW. Declines in switching underlie verbal fluency changes after unilateral pallidal surgery in Parkinson's disease. *Brain Cogn* 2002;**50**:207–17.

99. Rothlind JC, Cockshott RW, Starr PA, Marks WJ Jr. Neuropsychological performance following staged bilateral pallidal or subthalamic nucleus deep brain stimulation for Parkinson's disease. *J Int Neuropsychol Soc* 2007;**13**(1): 68–79.

100. Katayama Y, Kasai M, Oshima H, *et al.* Subthalamic nucleus stimulation for Parkinson disease: benefits observed in levodopa-intolerant patients. *J Neurosurg* 2001;**95**:213–21.

101. Ostergaard K, Sunde N, Dupont E. Effects of bilateral stimulation of the subthalamic nucleus in patients with severe Parkinson's disease and motor fluctuations. *Mov Disord* 2002;**17**:693–700.

102. Schüpbach WM, Chastan N, Welter ML, *et al.* Stimulation of the subthalamic nucleus in Parkinson's disease: a 5 year follow-up. *J Neurol Neurosurg Psychiatry* 2005;**76**(12): 1640–4.

103. Deuschl G, Herzog J, Kleiner-Fisman G, *et al.* Deep brain stimulation: postoperative issues. *Mov Disord* 2006;**21**(Suppl. 14):S219–37.

104. Kleiner-Fisman G, Herzog J, Fisman DN, *et al.* Subthalamic nucleus deep brain stimulation: summary and meta-analysis of outcomes. *Mov Disord* 2006;**21**(Suppl. 14): S290–304.

105. Schüpbach WM, Maltête D, Houeto JL, *et al.* Neurosurgery at an earlier stage of Parkinson disease: a randomized, controlled trial. *Neurology* 2007;**68**(4):267–71.

106. Witt K, Daniels C, Reiff J, *et al.* Neuropsychological and psychiatric changes after deep brain stimulation for Parkinson's disease: a randomised, multicentre study. *Lancet Neurol* 2008;**7**(7):605–14.

107. Romito LM, Scerrati M, Contarino MF, Bentivoglio AR, Tonali P, Albanese A. Long-term follow up of subthalamic nucleus stimulation in Parkinson's disease. *Neurology* 2002;**58**:1546–50.

108. Daniele A, Albanese A, Contarino MF, *et al.* Cognitive and behavioural effects of chronic stimulation of the subthalamic nucleus in patients with Parkinson's disease. *J Neurol Neurosurg Psychiatry* 2003;**74**:175–82.

109. Herzog J, Volkmann J, Krack P, *et al*. Two-year follow-up of subthalamic deep brain stimulation in Parkinson's disease. *Mov Disord* 2003;**18**:1332–7.

110. Houeto JL, Mallet L, Mesnage V, *et al*. Subthalamic stimulation in Parkinson disease: behavior and social adaptation. *Arch Neurol* 2006;**63**(8):1090–5.

111. Voges J, Hilker R, Botzel K, *et al*. Thirty days complication rate following surgery performed for deep-brain-stimulation. *Mov Disord* 2007;**22**:1486–9.

112. Burchiel KJ, Anderson VC, Favre J, Hammerstad JP. Comparison of pallidal and subthalamic nucleus deep brain stimulation for advanced Parkinson's disease: results of a randomized, blinded pilot study. *Neurosurgery* 1999;**45**:1375–84.

113. Morrison CE, Borod JC, Brin MF, *et al*. A program for neuropsychological investigation of deep brain stimulation (PNIDBS) in movement disorder patients: development, feasibility, and preliminary data. *Neuropsychiatry Neuropsychol Behav Neurol* 2000;**13**:204–19.

114. Saint-Cyr JA, Trepanier LL, Kumar R, Lozano AM, Lang AE. Neuropsychological consequences of chronic bilateral stimulation of the subthalamic nucleus in Parkinson's disease. *Brain* 2000;**123**:2091–108.

115. Alegret M, Junque C, Valldeoriola F, *et al*. Effects of bilateral subthalamic stimulation on cognitive function in Parkinson disease. *Arch Neurol* 2001;**58**:1223–7.

116. Dujardin K, Defebvre L, Krystkowiak P, Blond S, Destee A. Influence of chronic bilateral stimulation of the subthalamic nucleus on cognitive function in Parkinson's disease. *J Neurol* 2001;**248**:603–11.

117. Berney A, Vingerhoets F, Perrin A, *et al*. Effect on mood of subthalamic DBS for Parkinson's disease: a consecutive series of 24 patients. *Neurology* 2002;**59**:1427–9.

118. Funkiewiez A, Ardouin C, Caputo E, *et al*. Long term effects of bilateral subthalamic nucleus stimulation on cognitive function, mood, and behaviour in Parkinson's disease. *J Neurol Neurosurg Psychiatry* 2004;**75**:834–9.

119. Smeding HM, Speelman JD, Koning-Haanstra M, *et al*. Neuropsychological effects of bilateral STN stimulation in Parkinson disease: a controlled study. *Neurology* 2006;**66**(12):1830–6.

120. Kleiner-Fisman G, Fisman DN, Sime E, Saint-Cyr JA, Lozano AM, Lang AE. Long-term follow-up of bilateral deep brain stimulation of the subthalamic nucleus in patients with advanced Parkinson disease. *J Neurosurg* 2003;**99**:489–95.

121. Houeto JL, Mesnage V, Mallet L, *et al*. Behavioural disorders, Parkinson's disease and subthalamic stimulation. *J Neurol Neurosurg Psychiatry* 2002;**72**:701–7.

122. Rodriguez-Oroz MC, Obeso JA, Lang AE, *et al*. Bilateral deep brain stimulation in Parkinson's disease: a multicentre study with 4 years follow-up. *Brain* 2005;**128**:2240–9.

123. Voon V, Krack P, Lang AE, *et al*. A multicentre study on suicide outcomes following subthalamic stimulation for Parkinson's disease. *Brain* 2008:**131**;2720–8.

124. Speelman JD, Schuurman R, de Bie RM, Esselink RA, Bosch DA. Stereotactic neurosurgery for tremor. *Mov Disord* 2002;**17**(Suppl. 3):S84–8.

125. Tasker RR. Deep brain stimulation is preferable to thalamotomy for tremor suppression. *Surg Neurol* 1998;**49**:145–54.

126. Koller WC, Lyons KE, Wilkinson SB, Pahwa R. Efficacy of unilateral deep brain stimulation of the VIM nucleus of the thalamus for essential head tremor. *Mov Disord* 1999;**14**:847–50.

127. Limousin P, Speelman JD, Gielen F, Janssens M. Multicentre European study of thalamic stimulation in parkinsonian and essential tremor. *J Neurol Neurosurg Psychiatry* 1999;**66**:289–96.

128. Koller W, Pahwa R, Busenbark K, *et al*. High-frequency unilateral thalamic stimulation in the treatment of essential and parkinsonian tremor. *Ann Neurol* 1997;**42**:292–9.

129. Schuurman PR, Bosch DA, Bossuyt PM, *et al*. A comparison of continuous thalamic stimulation and thalamotomy for suppression of severe tremor. *N Engl J Med* 2000;**342**:461–8.

130. Schuurman PR, Bosch DA, Merkus MP, Speelman JD. Long-term follow-up of thalamic stimulation versus thalamotomy for tremor suppression. *Mov Disord* 2008;**23**(8):1146–53.

131. Alvarez L, Macias R, Guridi J, *et al*. Dorsal subthalamotomy for Parkinson's disease. *Mov Disord* 2001;**16**:72–8.

132. Alvarez L, Macias R, Lopez G, *et al*. Bilateral subthalamotomy in Parkinson's disease: initial and long-term response. *Brain* 2005;**128**:570–83.

133. Freed CR, Greene PE, Breeze RE, *et al*. Transplantation of embryonic dopamine neurons for severe Parkinson's disease. *N Engl J Med* 2001;**344**:710–9.

134. Olanow CW, Goetz CG, Kordower JH, *et al*. A double-blind controlled trial of bilateral fetal nigral transplantation in Parkinson's disease. *Ann Neurol* 2003;**54**:403–14.

135. Lopez-Lozano JJ, Bravo G, Brera B, *et al*. Long-term improvement in patients with severe Parkinson's disease after implantation of fetal ventral mesencephalic tissue in a cavity of the caudate nucleus: 5-year follow up in 10 patients. Clinica Puerta de Hierro Neural Transplantation Group. *J Neurosurg* 1997;**86**:931–42.

136. Brundin P, Pogarell O, Hagell P, *et al*. Bilateral caudate and putamen grafts of embryonic mesencephalic tissue treated with lazaroids in Parkinson's disease. *Brain* 2000;**123**:1380–90.

137. Schumacher JM, Ellias SA, Palmer EP, *et al*. Transplantation of embryonic porcine mesencephalic tissue in patients with PD. *Neurology* 2000;**54**:1042–50.

138. Keus SH, Bloem BR, Hendriks EJ, Bredero-Cohen AB, Munneke M. Evidence-based analysis of physical therapy in Parkinson's disease with recommendations for practice and research. *Mov Disord* 2007;**22**:451–60.

139. Keus SH, Munneke M, Nijkrake MJ, Kwakkel G, Bloem BR. Physical therapy in Parkinson's disease: evolution and future challenges. *Mov Disord* 2009;**24**(1):1–14. Review.

140. Mak MK, Hui-Chan CW. Cued task-specific training is better than exercise in improving sit-to-stand in patients with Parkinson's disease: a randomized controlled trial. *Mov Disord* 2008;**23**:501–9.

141. Morris ME, Iansek R, Kirkwood B. A randomized controlled trial of movement strategies compared with exercise for people with Parkinson's disease. *Mov Disord* 2009;**24**:64–71.

142. Nieuwboer A, Kwakkel G, Rochester L, *et al.* Cueing training in the home improves gait-related mobility in Parkinson's disease: the RESCUE trial. *J Neurol Neurosurg Psychiatry* 2007;**78**:134–40.

143. Frazzitta G, Maestri R, Uccellini D, Bertotti G, Abelli P. Rehabilitation treatment of gait in patients with Parkinson's disease with freezing: a comparison between two physical therapy protocols using visual and auditory cues with or without treadmill training. *Mov Disord* 2009;**24**: 1139–43.

144. Dibble LE, Addison O, Papa E. The effects of exercise on balance in persons with Parkinson's disease: a systematic review across the disability spectrum. *J Neurol Phys Ther* 2009;**33**:14–26.

145. Herman T, Giladi N, Hausdorff JM. Treadmill training for the treatment of gait disturbances in people with Parkinson's disease: a mini-review. *J Neural Transm* 2009;**116**: 307–18.

146. Ashburn A, Fazakarley L, Ballinger C, Pickering R, McLellan LD, Fitton C. A randomised controlled trial of a home based exercise programme to reduce the risk of falling among people with Parkinson's disease. *J Neurol Neurosurg Psychiatry* 2007;**78**:678–84.

147. Deane KH, Whurr R, Playford ED, Ben-Shlomo Y, Clarke CE. A comparison of speech and language therapy techniques for dysarthria in Parkinson's disease. *Cochrane Database Syst Rev* 2001;(2):CD002814. Review.

148. Rascol O, Goetz CG, Koller W, Poewe W, Sampaio C. Treatment interventions for Parkinson's disease: an evidence based assessment. *Lancet* 2002;**359**:1589–98.

149. Pinto S, Ozsancak C, Tripoliti E, Thobois S, Limousin-Dowsey P, Auzou P. Treatments for dysarthria in Parkinson's disease. *Lancet Neurol* 2004;**3**:547–56.

150. Ramig LO, Countryman S, O'Brien C, Hoehn M, Thompson L. Intensive speech treatment for patients with Parkinson's disease: short-and long-term comparison of two techniques. *Neurology* 1996;**47**:1496–504.

151. Ramig LO, Sapir S, Countryman S, *et al.* Intensive voice treatment (LSVT) for patients with Parkinson's disease: a 2 year follow up. *J Neurol Neurosurg Psychiatry* 2001;**71**: 493–8.

152. Ramig LO, Sapir S, Fox C, Countryman S. Changes in vocal loudness following intensive voice treatment (LSVT) in individuals with Parkinson's disease: a comparison with untreated patients and normal age-matched controls. *Mov Disord* 2001;**16**:79–83.

153. de Swart BJ, Willemse SC, Maassen BA, Horstink MW. Improvement of voicing in patients with Parkinson's disease by speech therapy. *Neurology* 2003;**60**:498–500.

154. Deane KH, Whurr R, Clarke CE, Playford ED, Ben-Shlomo Y. Non-Pharmacological Therapies for Dysphagia in Parkinson's Disease (Cochrane Review). *Cochrane Database Syst Rev* 2001;(1):CD002816. Review.

155. Deane KH, Ellis-Hill C, Jones D, *et al.* Systematic review of paramedical therapies for Parkinson's disease. *Mov Disord* 2002;**17**:984–91.

156. Deane KH, Ellis-Hill C, Playford ED, Ben-Shlomo Y, Clarke CE. Occupational therapy for patients with Parkinson's disease. *Cochrane Database Syst Rev* 2001;(3): CD002813. Review. Update in: *Cochrane Database Syst Rev.* 2007;(3):CD002813.

157. Hagell P. Nursing and multidisciplinary interventions for Parkinson's disease: what is the evidence? *Parkinsonism Relat Disord* 2007;**13**(Suppl. 3):S501–8.

158. Bracco F, Malesani R, Saladini M, Battistin L. Protein redistribution diet and antiparkinsonian response to levodopa. *Eur Neurol* 1991;**31**:68–71.

159. Karstaedt PJ, Pincus JH. Protein redistribution diet remains effective in patients with fluctuating parkinsonism. *Arch Neurol* 1992;**49**:149–51.

160. Pierelli F, Adipietro A, Soldati G, Fattapposta F, Pozzessere G, Scoppetta C. Low dosage clozapine effects on L-dopa induced dyskinesias in parkinsonian patients. *Acta Neurol Scand* 1998;**97**:295–9.

161. Durif F, Debilly B, Galitzky M. Clozapine improves dyskinesias in Parkinson disease: a double-blind, placebo-controlled study. *Neurology* 2004;**62**:381–8.

162. Morgante L, Epifanio A, Spina E, *et al.* Quetiapine and clozapine in parkinsonian patients with dopaminergic psychosis. *Clin Neuropharmacol* 2004;**27**:153–6.

163. Katzenschlager R, Manson AJ, Evans A, Watt H, Lees AJ. Low dose quetiapine for drug induced dyskinesias in Parkinson's disease: a double blind cross over study. *J Neurol Neurosurg Psychiatry* 2004;**75**:295–7.

164. Aarsland D, Zaccai J, Brayne C. A systematic review of prevalence studies of dementia in Parkinson's disease. *Mov Disord* 2005;**10**:1255–63.

165. Aarsland D, Andersen K, Larsen JP, Lolk A, Kragh-Sorensen P. Prevalence and characteristics of dementia in

Parkinson disease: an 8-year prospective study. *Arch Neurol* 2003;**60**:387–92.

166. Buter TC, van den Hout A, Matthews FE, Larsen JP, Brayne C, Aarsland D. Dementia and survival in Parkinson disease: a 12-year population study. *Neurology* 2008;**70**: 1017–22.

167. Tiraboschi P, Hansen LA, Alford M, *et al*. Corey-Bloom J. Cholinergic dysfunction in diseases with Lewy bodies. *Neurology* 2000;**54**:407–10.

168. Bohnen NI, Kaufer DI, Ivanco LS, *et al*. Cortical cholinergic function is more severely affected in parkinsonian dementia than in Alzheimer disease. *Arch Neurol* 2003;**60**: 1745–8.

169. Aarsland D, Laake K, Larsen JP, Janvin C. Donepezil for cognitive impairment in Parkinson's disease: a randomised controlled study. *J Neurol Neurosurg Psychiatry* 2002;**72**:708–12.

170. Leroi I, Brandt J, Reich SG, *et al*. Randomized placebo-controlled trial of donepezil in cognitive impairment in Parkinson's disease. *Int J Geriatr Psychiatry* 2004;**19**: 1–8.

171. Ravina B, Putt M, Siderowf A, *et al*. Donepezil for dementia in Parkinson's disease: a randomised, double blind, placebo controlled, crossover study. *J Neurol Neurosurg Psychiatry* 2005;**76**:934–9.

172. Emre M, Aarsland D, Albanese A, *et al*. Rivastigmine in Parkinson's disease patients with dementia: a randomized, double-blind, placebo-controlled study. *N Engl J Med* 2004;**351**:2509–18.

173. Litvinenko IV, Odinak MM, Mogil'naya VI, Emelin AY. Efficacy and safety of galantamine (reminyl) for dementia in patients with Parkinson's disease (an open controlled trial). *Neurosci Behav Physiol* 2008;**38**:937–45.

174. Hutchinson M, Fazzini E. Cholinesterase inhibition in Parkinson's disease. *J Neurol Neurosurg Psychiatry* 1996;**61**: 324–5.

175. Werber E, Rabey J. The beneficial effect of cholinesterase inhibitors on patients suffering from Parkinson's disease and dementia. *J Neural Transm* 2001;**108**:1319–25.

176. Maidment I, Fox C, Boustani M. Cholinesterase inhibitors for Parkinson's disease dementia. *Cochrane Database Syst Rev* 2006; (1):CD004747. Review.

177. Oertel W, Poewe W, Wolters E, *et al*. Effects of rivastigmine on tremor and other motor symptoms in patients with Parkinson's disease dementia: a retrospective analysis of a double-blind trial and an open-label extension. *Drug Saf* 2008;**31**:79–94.

178. Gill SS, Anderson GM, Fischer HD, *et al*. Syncope and its consequences in patients with dementia receiving cholinesterase inhibitors: a population-based cohort study. *Arch Intern Med* 2009;**169**:867–73.

179. Leroi I, Overshott R, Byrne EJ, Daniel E, Burns A. Randomized controlled trial of memantine in dementia associated with Parkinson's disease. *Mov Disord* 2009;**24**: 1217–21.

180. Aarsland D, Ballard C, Walker Z, *et al*. Memantine in patients with Parkinson's disease dementia or dementia with Lewy bodies: a double-blind, placebo-controlled, multicentre trial. *Lancet Neurol* 2009;**8**:613–8.

181. Fenelon G, Mahieux F, Huon R, Ziegler M. Hallucinations in Parkinson's disease. Prevalence, phenomenology and risk factors. *Brain* 2000;**123**:733–45.

182. Parkinson Study Group. Low-dose clozapine for the treatment of drug-induced psychosis in Parkinson's disease. *N Engl J Med* 1999;**340**:757–63.

183. French Clozapine Parkinson Study Group. Clozapine in drug-induced psychosis in Parkinson's disease. *Lancet* 1999;**353**:2041.

184. Factor SA, Friedman JH, Lannon MC, Oakes D, Bourgeois K, Parkinson Study Group. Clozapine for the treatment of drug-induced psychosis in Parkinson's disease: results of the 12 week open label extension in the PSYCLOPS trial. *Mov Disord* 2001;**16**:135–9.

185. Honigfeld G, Arellano F, Sethi J, Bianchini A, Schein J. Reducing clozapine-related morbidity and mortality: 5 years of experience with the Clozaril National Registry. *J Clin Psychiatry* 1998;**59**:3–7.

186. Ondo W, Levy J, Vuong K, Hunter C, Jankovic J. Olanzapine treatment for dopaminergic-induced hallucinations. *Mov Disord* 2002;**17**:1031–5.

187. Breier A, Sutton VK, Feldman PD, *et al*. Olanzapine in the treatment of dopaminetic-induced psychosis in patients with Parkinson's disease. *Biol Psychiatry* 2002;**52**: 438–45.

188. Goetz C, Blasucci L, Leurgans S, Pappert E. Olanzapine and clozapine: comparative effects on motor function in hallucinating PD patients. *Neurology* 2000;**55**: 748–9.

189. Bullock R. Treatment of behavioural and psychiatric symptoms in dementia: implications of recent safety warnings. *Curr Med Res Opin* 2005;**21**:1–10.

190. Herrmann N, Lanctot KL. Do atypical antipsychotics cause stroke? *CNS Drugs* 2005;**19**:91–103.

191. Fernandez H, Friedman J, Jacques C, Rosenfeld M. Quetiapine for the treatment of drug-induced psychosis in Parkinson's disease. *Mov Disord* 1999;**14**:484–7.

192. Dewey RB Jr, O'Suilleabhain PE. Treatment of drug-induced psychosis with quetiapine and clozapine in Parkinson's disease. *Neurology* 2000;**55**:1753–4.

193. Brandstaedter D, Oertel WH. Treatment of drug-induced psychosis with quetiapine and clozapine in Parkinson's disease. *Neurology* 2002;**58**:160–1.

194. Fernandez H, Trieschmann ME, Burke MA, Friedmann JH. Quetiapine for psychosis in Parkinson's disease versus dementia with Lewy bodies. *J Clin Psychiatry* 2002;**63**: 513–5.

195. Reddy S, Factor SA, Molho ES, Feustel PJ. The effect of quetiapine on psychosis and motor function in parkinsonian patients with and without dementia. *Mov Disord* 2002;**17**:676–81.

196. Fernandez HH, Trieschmann ME, Burke MA, Jacques C, Friedman JH. Long-term outcome of quetiapine use for psychosis among Parkinsonian patients. *Mov Disord* 2003;**18**:510–4.

197. Juncos JL, Roberts VJ, Evatt ML, *et al.* Quetiapine improves psychotic symptoms and cognition in Parkinson's disease. *Mov Disord* 2004;**19**:29–35.

198. Mohr E, Mendis T, Hildebrand K, De Deyn PP. Risperidone in the treatment of dopamine-induced psychosis in Parkinson's disease: an open pilot trial. *Mov Disord* 2000;**15**:1230–7.

199. Ellis T, Cudkowicz ME, Sexton PM, Growdon JH. Clozapine and risperidone treatment of psychosis in Parkinson's disease. *J Neuropsychiatry Clin Neurosci* 2000;**12**:364–9.

200. Leopold NA. Risperidone treatment of drug-related psychosis in patients with parkinsonism. *Mov Disord* 2000;**15**:301–4.

201. Meco G, Alessandria A, Bonifati V, Giustini P. Risperidone for hallucinations in levodopa-treated Parkinson's disease patients. *Lancet* 1994;**343**:1370–1.

202. Friedman JH, Factor SA. Atypical antipsychotics in the treatment of drug-induced psychosis in Parkinson's disease. *Mov Disord* 2000;**15**:201–11.

202a. Reading PJ, Luce AK, McKeith IG. Rivastigmine in the treatment of parkinsonian psychosis and cognitive impairment: preliminary findings from an open trial. *Mov Disord* 2001 Nov;**16**(6):1171–4.

203. Bullock R, Cameron A. Rivastigmine for the treatment of dementia and visual hallucinations associated with Parkinson's disease: a case series. *Curr Med Res Opin* 2002;**18**:258–64.

204. Fabbrini G, Barbanti P, Aurilia C, Pauletti C, Lenzi GL, Meco G. Donepezil in the treatment of hallucinations and delusions in Parkinson's disease. *Neurol Sci* 2002;**23**:41–3.

205. Bergmann J, Lerner V. Successful use of donepezil for the treatment of psychotic symptoms in patients with Parkinson's disease. *Clin Neuropharmacol* 2002;**25**:107–10.

206. Burn D, Emre M, McKeith I, *et al.* Effects of rivastigmine in patients with and without visual hallucinations in dementia associated with Parkinson's disease. *Mov Disord* 2006;**21**(11):1899–907.

207. Cummings JL. Depression and Parkinson's disease: a review. *Am J Psychiatry* 1992;**149**:443–54.

208. Burn DJ. Beyond the iron mask: towards better recognition and treatment of depression associated with Parkinson's disease. *Mov Disord* 2002;**17**:445–54.

209. Santamaria J, Tolosa E, Valles A. Parkinson's disease with depression: a possible subgroup of idiopathic parkinsonism. *Neurology* 1986;**36**:1130–3.

210. Gonera EG, van't Hof M, Berger HJC, van Weel C, Horstink MWIM. Prodromal symptoms in Parkinson's disease. *Mov Disord* 1997;**12**:871–6.

211. Findley LJ. Quality of life in Parkinson's disease. *Int J Clin Pract* 1999;**53**:404–5.

212. Schrag A, Jahanshahi M, Quinn N. What contributes to quality of life in patients with Parkinson's disease? *J Neurol Neurosurg Psychiatry* 2000;**69**:308–12.

213. Hornykiewicz O. Imbalance of brain monoamines and clinical disorders. *Prog Brain Res* 1982;**55**:419–29.

214. Mayeux R, Stern Y, Cote L, Williams JBW. Altered serotonin metabolism in depressed patients with Parkinson's disease. *Neurology* 1984;**34**:642–6.

215. Zgaljardic DJ, Foldi NS, Borod JC. Cognitive and behavioral dysfunction in Parkinson's disease: neurochemical and clinicopathological contributions. *J Neural Transm* 2004;**111**:1287–301.

216. Agid Y, Ruberg M, Dubois B, *et al.* Parkinson's disease and dementia. *Clin Neuropharmacol* 1986;**9**(Suppl. 2):22–36.

217. Rektorová I, Rektor I, Bares M, *et al.* Pramipexole and pergolide in the treatment of depression in Parkinson's disease: a national multicentre prospective randomized study. *Eur J Neurol* 2003;**10**:399–406.

218. Leentjens AF, Koester J, Fruh B, Shephard DT, Barone P, Houben JJ. The effect of pramipexole on mood and motivational symptoms in Parkinson's disease: a metaanalysis of placebo-controlled studies. *Clin Ther* 2009;**31**(1):89–98.

219. Steur EN, Ballering LA. Moclobemide and selegeline in the treatment of depression in Parkinson's disease. *J Neurol Neurosurg Psychiatry* 1997;**63**:547.

220. Andersen J, Aabro E, Gulmann N, Hjelmsted A, Pedersen HE. Antidepressive treatment in Parkinson's disease: a controlled trial of the effect of nortriptyline in patients with Parkinson's disease treated with L-dopa. *Acta Neurol Scand* 1980;**62**:210–9.

221. Ghazi-Noori S, Chung TH, Deane KHO, Rickards H, Clarke CE. Therapies for depression in Parkinson's disease. *Cochrane Database Syst Rev* 2003;(2):CD003465.

222. Menza M, Dobkin RD, Marin H, *et al.* The impact of treatment of depression on quality of life, disability and relapse in patients with Parkinson's disease. *Mov Disord* 2009;**24**(9):1325–32.

223. Menza M, Dobkin R, Marin H, *et al.* A controlled trial of antidepressants in patients with Parkinson Disease and depression. *Neurology* 2009;**72**(10):886–92.

224. Weintraub D, Morales KH, Moberg PJ, *et al.* Antidepressant studies in Parkinson's disease: a review and meta-analysis. *Mov Disord* 2005;**20**:1161–9.

225. Leentjens AF, Vreeling FW, Luijeckx GJ, Verhey FR. SSRIs in the treatment of depression in Parkinson's disease. *Int J Geriatr Psychiatry* 2003;**18**:552–4.

226. Ceravolo R, Nuti A, Piccinni A, *et al.* Paroxetine in Parkinson's disease: effects on motor and depressive symptoms. *Neurology* 2000;**55**:1216–8.

227. Tesei S, Antonini A, Canesi M, Zecchinelli A, Mariani CB, Pezzoli G. Tolerability of paroxetine in Parkinson's disease: a prospective study. *Mov Disord* 2000;**15**:986–9.

228. Avila A, Cardona X, Martin-Baranera M, Maho P, Sastre F, Bello J. Does nefazodone improve both depression and Parkinson disease? A pilot randomized trial. *J Clin Psychopharmacol* 2003;**23**:509–13.

229. Lemke MR. Effect of reboxetine on depression in Parkinson's disease patients. *J Clin Psychiatry* 2002;**63**:300–4.

230. Bayulkem K, Torun F. Therapeutic efficiency of venlafaxin in depressive patients with Parkinson's disease. *Mov Disord* 2002;**17**(Suppl. 5):P204.

231. Okabe S, Ugawa Y, Kanazawa I, Effectiveness of rTMS on Parkinson's Disease Study Group. 0.2-Hz repetitive transcranial magnetic stimulation has no add-on effects as compared to a realistic sham stimulation in Parkinson's disease. *Mov Disord* 2003;**18**:382–8.

232. Fregni F, Santos CM, Myczkowski ML, *et al.* Repetitive transcranial magnetic stimulation is as effective as fluoxetine in the treatment of depression in patients with Parkinson's disease. *J Neurol Neurosurg Psychiatry* 2004;**75**:1171–4.

233. Jankovic J, Gilden JL, Hiner BC, *et al.* Neurogenic orthostatic hypotension: a double-blind placebo-controlled study with midodrine. *Am J Med* 1993;**95**:38–48.

234. Low PA, Gilden FL, Freeman R, Sheng KN, McElligott MA. Efficacy of midodrine vs placebo in neuogenic orthostatic hypotension. A randomized double-blind multicenter study. Midodrine study group. *JAMA* 1997;**277**:1046–51.

235. Hoehn MM. Levodopa induced postural hypotension. Treatment with fludrocortisone. *Arch Neurol* 1975;**32**:50–1.

236. Schoffer KL, Henderson RD, O'Maley K, O'Sullivan JD. Nonpharmacological treatment, fludrocortisone, and domperidone for orthostatic hypotension in Parkinson's disease. *Mov Disord* 2007;**22**(11):1543–9.

237. Riley DE. Orthostatic hypotension in multiple system atrophy. *Curr Treat Options Neurol* 2000;**2**:225–30.

238. Aranda B, Cramer P. Effect of apomorphine and l-dopa on the parkinsonian bladder. *Neurourol Urodyn* 1993;**12**:203–9.

239. Kuno S, Mizuta E, Yamasaki S, Araki I. Effects of pergolide on nocturia in Parkinson's disease: three female cases selected from over 400 patients. *Parkinsonism Relat Disord* 2004;**10**:181–7.

240. Yamamoto M. Pergolide improves neurogenic bladder in patients with Parkinson's disease. *Mov Disord* 1997;**12**:328.

241. Benson GS, Raezer DM, Anderson JR, Saunders CD, Corrierie JN Jr. Effect of levodopa on urinary bladder. *Urology* 1976;**7**:24–8.

242. Christmas TJ, Kempster PA, Chapple CR, *et al.* Role of subcutaneous apomorphine in parkinsonian voiding dysfunction. *Lancet* 1988;**2**:1451–3.

243. Fitzmaurice H, Fowler CJ, Rickards D, *et al.* Micturition disturbance in Parkinson's disease. *Br J Urol* 1985;**57**:652–6.

244. Winge K, Werdelin LM, Nielsen KK, Stimpel H. Effects of dopaminergic treatment on bladder function in Parkinson's disease. *Neurourol Urodyn* 2004;**23**:689–96.

245. Brusa L, Petta F, Pisani A, *et al.* Central acute D2 stimulation worsens bladder function in patients with mild Parkinson's disease. *J Urol* 2006;**175**:202–6.

246. Uchiyama T, Sakakibara R, Hattori T, Yamanishi T. Short-term effect of a single levodopa dose on micturition disturbance in Parkinson's disease patients with the wearing-off phenomenon. *Mov Disord* 2003;**18**:573–8.

247. Andersson KE. Treatment of overactive bladder: other drug mechanisms. *Urology* 2000;**55**:51–7.

248. Appell RA. Clinical efficacy and safety of tolterodine in the treatment of overactive bladder: a pooled analysis. *Urology* 1997;**50**:90–6.

249. Suchowersky O, Furtado S, Rohs G. Beneficial effect of intranasal desmopressin for nocturnal polyuria in Parkinson's disease. *Mov Disord* 1995;**10**:337–40.

250. Finazzi-Agro E, Peppe A, d'Amico A, *et al.* Effects of subthalamic nucleus stimulation on urodynamic findings in patients with Parkinson's disease. *J Urol* 2003;**169**:1388–91.

251. Seif C, Herzog J, van der HC, *et al.* Effect of subthalamic deep brain stimulation on the function of the urinary bladder. *Ann Neurol* 2004;**55**:118–20.

252. Giannantoni A, Rossi A, Mearini E, Del Zingaro M, Porena M, Berardelli A. Botulinum toxin a for overactive bladder and detrusor muscle overactivity in patients with parkinson's disease and multiple system atrophy. *J Urol* 2009;**182**(4):1453–57.

253. Bushmann M, Dobmeyer SM, Leeker L, Perlmutter JS. Swallowing abnormalities and their response to treatment in Parkinson's disease. *Neurology* 1989;**39**:1309–14.

254. Fuh JL, Lee RC, Wang SJ, *et al.* Swallowing difficulty in Parkinson's disease. *Clin Neurol Neurosurg* 1997;**99**:106–12.

255. Hunter PC, Crameri J, Austin S, Woodward MC, Hughes AJ. Response of parkinsonian swallowing dysfunction to dopaminergic stimulation. *J Neurol Neurosurg Psychiatry* 1997;**63**:579–83.

256. Ciucci MR, Barkmeier-Kraemer JM, Sherman SJ. Subthalamic nucleus deep brain stimulation improves deglutition in Parkinson's disease. *Mov Disord* 2008;**23**:676–83.

257. Tison F, Wiart L, Guatterie M, *et al*. Effects of central dopaminergic stimulation by apomorphine on swallowing disorders in Parkinson's disease. *Mov Disord* 1996;**11**: 729–32.

258. Calne DB, Shaw DG, Spiers AS, Stern GM. Swallowing in Parkinsonism. *Br J Radiol* 1970;**43**:456–7.

259. Lim A, Leow L, Huckabee ML, Frampton C, Anderson T. A pilot study of respiration and swallowing integration in Parkinson's disease: 'on' and 'off' levodopa. *Dysphagia* 2008;**23**:76–81.

260. Restivo DA, Palmeri A, Marchese-Ragona R. Botulinum toxin for cricopharyngeal dysfunction in Parkinson's disease. *N Engl J Med* 2002;**346**:1174–5.

261. Born LJ, Harned RH, Rikkers LF, Pfeiffer RF, Quigley EM. Cricopharyngeal dysfunction in Parkinson's disease: role in dysphagia and response to myotomy. *Mov Disord* 1996;**11**:53–8.

262. Byrne KG, Pfeiffer R, Quigley EM. Gastrointestinal dysfunction in Parkinson's disease. A report of clinical experience at a single center. *J Clin Gastroenterol* 1994;**19**:11–6.

263. Logemann JA, Gensler G, Robbins J, *et al*. A randomized study of three interventions for aspiration of thin liquids in patients with dementia or Parkinson's disease. *J Speech Lang Hear Res* 2008;**51**:173–83.

264. El Sharkawi A, Ramig L, Logemann JA, *et al*. Swallowing and voice effects of Lee Silverman Voice Treatment (LSVT): a pilot study. *J Neurol Neurosurg Psychiatry* 2002;**72**:31–6.

265. Nagaya M, Kachi T, Yamada T. Effect of swallowing training on swallowing disorders in Parkinson's disease. *Scand J Rehabil Med* 2000;**32**:11–5.

266. Pinnington LL, Muhiddin KA, Ellis RE, Playford ED. Non-invasive assessment of swallowing and respiration in Parkinson's disease. *J Neurol* 2000;**247**:773–7.

267. Troche MS, Sapienza CM, Rosenbek JC. Effects of bolus consistency on timing and safety of swallow in patients with Parkinson's disease. *Dysphagia* 2008;**23**:26–32.

268. Agid Y, Pollak P, Bonnet AM, Signoret JL, Lhermitte F. Bromocriptine associated with a peripheral dopamine blocking agent in treatment of Parkinson's disease. *Lancet* 1979;**1**:570–2.

269. Quinn N, Illas A, Lhermitte F, Agid Y. Bromocriptine and domperidone in the treatment of Parkinson's disease. *Neurology* 1981;**31**:662–7.

270. Day JP, Pruitt RE. Diabetic gastroparesis in a patient with Parkinson's disease: effective treatment with domperidone. *Am J Gastroenterol* 1989;**84**:837–8.

271. Soykan I, Sarosiek I, Shifflett J, Wooten GF, McCallum RW. Effect of chronic oral domperidone therapy on gastrointestinal symptoms and gastric emptying in patients with Parkinson's disease. *Mov Disord* 1997;**12**:952–7.

272. Asai H, Udaka F, Hirano M, *et al*. Increased gastric motility during 5-HT4 agonist therapy reduces response fluctuations in Parkinson's disease. *Parkinsonism Relat Disord* 2005;**11**:499–502.

273. Bateman DN, Rawlins MD, Simpson JM. Extrapyramidal reactions with metoclopramide. *Br Med J* 1985;**291**: 930–2.

274. Miller LG, Jankovic J. Metoclopramide-induced movement disorders. Clinical findings with a review of the literature. *Arch Intern Med* 1989;**149**:2486–92.

275. Ganzini L, Casey DE, Hoffman WF, McCall AL. The prevalence of metoclopramide-induced tardive dyskinesia and acute extrapyramidal movement disorders. *Arch Intern Med* 1993;**153**:1469–75.

276. Ashraf W, Pfeiffer RF, Park F, Lof J, Quigley EM. Constipation in Parkinson's disease: objective assessment and response to psyllium. *Mov Disord* 1997;**12**:946–51.

277. Zangaglia R, Martignoni E, Glorioso M, *et al*. Macrogol for the treatment of constipation in Parkinson's disease. A randomized placebo-controlled study. *Mov Disord* 2007; **22**:1239–344.

278. Sullivan KL, Staffetti JF, Hauser RA, Dunne PB, Zesiewicz TA. Tegaserod (Zelnorm) for the treatment of constipation in Parkinson's disease. *Mov Disord* 2006;**21**: 115–6.

279. Hussain IF, Brady CM, Swinn MJ, Mathias CJ, Fowler CJ. Treatment of erectile dysfunction with sildenafil citrate in parkinsonism due to Parkinson's disease and multiple system atrophy with observations on orthostatic hypotension. *J Neurol Neurosurg Psychiatry* 2001;**71**:371–4.

280. Zesiewicz TA, Helal M, Hauser RA. Sildenafil citrate (Viagra) for the treatment of erectile dysfunction in men with Parkinson's disease. *Mov Disord* 2000;**15**:305–8.

281. Raffaele R, Vecchio I, Giammusso B, Morgia G, Brunetto MB, Rampello L. Efficacy and safety of fixed-dose oral sildenafil in the treatment of sexual dysfunction in depressed patients with idiopathic Parkinson's disease. *Eur Urol* 2002;**41**:382–6.

282. O'Sullivan JD. Apomorphine as an alternative to sildenafil in Parkinson's disease. *J Neurol Neurosurg Psychiatry* 2002;**72**(5):681.

283. O'Sullivan JD, Hughes AJ. Apomorphine-induced penile erections in Parkinson's disease. *Mov Disord* 1998;**13**: 536–9.

284. Pohanka M, Kanovsky P, Bares M, Pulkrabek J, Rektor I. Pergolide mesylate can improve sexual dysfunction in patients with Parkinson's disease: the results of an open, prospective, 6-month follow-up. *Eur J Neurol* 2004;**11**: 483–8.

285. Factor SA, McAlarney T, Sanchez-Ramos JR, Weiner WJ. Sleep disorders and sleep effect in Parkinson's disease. *Mov Disord* 1990;**5**:280–5.

286. van Hilten JJ, Weggeman M, van der Velde EA, Kerkhof GA, van Dijk JG, Roos RA. Sleep, excessive daytime sleepiness and fatigue in Parkinson's disease. *J Neural Transm Park Dis Dement Sect* 1993;**5**:235–44.

287. Tandberg E, Larsen JP, Karlsen K. Excessive daytime sleepiness and sleep benefit in Parkinson's disease: a community-based study. *Mov Disord* 1999;**14**:922–9227.

288. Tan EK, Lum SY, Fook-Chong SM, *et al*. Evaluation of somnolence in Parkinson's disease: comparison with age- and sex-matched controls. *Neurology* 2002;**58**: 465–8.

289. Högl B, Rothdach A, Wetter TC, Trenkwalder C. The effect of cabergoline on sleep, periodic leg movements in sleep, and early morning motor function in patients with Parkinson's disease. *Neuropsychopharmacology* 2003;**28**: 866–70.

290. Ferreira JJ, Desboeuf K, Galitzky M, *et al*. Sleep disruption, daytime somnolence and 'sleep attacks' in Parkinson's disease: a clinical survey in PD patients and age matched healthy volunteers. *Eur J Neurol* 2006;**13**:209–14.

291. Högl B, Saletu M, Brandauer E, *et al*. Modafinil for the treatment of daytime sleepiness in Parkinson's disease: a double-blind, randomized, crossover, placebo-controlled polygraphic trial. *Sleep* 2002;**25**:905–9.

292. Adler CH, Caviness JN, Hentz JG, Lind M, Tiede J. Randomized trial of modafinil for treating subjective daytime sleepiness in patients with Parkinson's disease. *Mov Disord* 2003;**18**:287–93.

293. Ondo WG, Fayle R, Atassi F, Jankovic J. Modafinil for daytime somnolence in Parkinson's disease: double blind, placebo controlled parallel trial. *J Neurol Neurosurg Psychiatry* 2005;**76**(12):1636–9.

294. Devos D, Krystkowiak P, Clement F, *et al*. Improvement of gait by chronic, high doses of methylphenidate in patients with advanced Parkinson's disease. *J Neurol Neurosurg Psychiatry* 2007;**78**:470–5.

295. Stove NP, Okun MS, Watts RL. 'Sleep attacks' and excessive daytime sleepiness in Parkinson's disease: a survey of 200 consecutive patients. *Neurology* 2001;**56**: P03.140.

296. Montastruc JL, Brefel-Courbon C, Senard JM, *et al*. Sleep attacks and antiparkinsonian drugs: a pilot prospective pharmacoepidemiologic study. *Clin Neuropharmacol* 2001;**24**:181–3.

297. Hobson DE, Lang AE, Martin WR, Razmy A, Rivest J, Fleming J. Excessive daytime sleepiness and sudden-onset sleep in Parkinson disease: a survey by the Canadian Movement Disorders Group. *JAMA* 2002;**287**:455–63.

298. Paus S, Brecht HM, Koster J, Seeger G, Klockgether T, Wullner U. Sleep attacks, daytime sleepiness, and dopamine agonists in Parkinson's disease. *Mov Disord* 2003;**18**: 659–67.

299. Brodsky MA, Godbold J, Roth T, Olanow CW. Sleepiness in Parkinson's disease: a controlled study. *Mov Disord* 2003;**18**:668–72.

300. Körner Y, Meindorfner C, Moeller JC, *et al*. Predictors of sudden onset of sleep in Parkinson's disease. *Mov Disord* 2004;**19**:1298–305.

301. Wetter TC, Collado-Seidel V, Pollmacher T, Yassouridis A, Trenkwalder C. Sleep and periodic leg movement patterns in drug-free patients with Parkinson's disease and multiple system atrophy. *Sleep* 2000;**23**:361–7.

302. Lees AJ, Blackburn NA, Campbell VL. The nighttime problems of Parkinson's disease. *Clin Neuropharmacol* 1988;**11**:512–9.

303. Schenck CH, Bundlie SR, Ettinger MG, Mahowald MW. Chronic behavioral disorders of human REM sleep: a new category of parasomnia. *Sleep* 1986;**9**:293–308.

304. Comella CL, Nardine TM, Diederich NJ, Stebbins GT. Sleep related violence, injury, and REM sleep behavior disorder in Parkinson's disease. *Neurology* 1998;**51**:526–9.

305. Gagnon JF, Bedard MA, Fantini ML, *et al*. REM sleep behavior disorder and REM sleep without atonia in Parkinson's disease. *Neurology* 2002;**59**:585–9.

306. Iranzo A, Molinuevo JL, Santamaria J, *et al*. Rapid-eye-movement sleep behaviour disorder as an early marker for a neurodegenerative disorder: a descriptive study. *Lancet Neurol* 2006;**5**:572–7.

307. Iranzo A, Santamaria J, Rye DB, *et al*. Characteristics of idiopathic REM sleep behavior disorder and that associated with MSA and PD. *Neurology* 2005;**65**:247–52.

308. Olson EJ, Boeve BF, Silber MH. Rapid eye movement sleep behaviour disorder: demographic, clinical and laboratory findings in 93 cases. *Brain* 2000;**123**:331–9.

309. Fantini ML, Gagnon JF, Filipini D, Montplaisir J. The effects of pramipexole in REM sleep behavior disorder. *Neurology* 2003;**61**:1418–20.

310. Schmidt MH, Koshal VB, Schmidt HS. Use of pramipexole in REM sleep behavior disorder: results from a case series. *Sleep Med* 2006;**7**:418–23.

311. Kumru H, Iranzo A, Carrasco E, *et al*. Lack of effects of pramipexole on REM sleep behavior disorder in Parkinson disease. *Sleep* 2008;**31**:1418–21.

312. Winkelman JW, James L. Serotonergic antidepressants are associated with REM sleep without atonia. *Sleep* 2004;**27**: 317–21.

313. Leeman AL, O'Neill CJ, Nicholson PW, *et al.* Parkinson's disease in the elderly: response to and optimal spacing of night time dosing with levodopa. *Br J Clin Pharmacol* 1987;**24**:637–43.

314. Stocchi F, Barbato L, Nordera G, Berardelli A, Ruggieri S. Sleep disorders in Parkinson's disease. *J Neurol* 1998;**245** (Suppl. 1):S15–8.

315. The U.K. Madopar CR Study Group. A comparison of Madopar CR and standard Madopar in the treatment of nocturnal and early-morning disability in Parkinson's disease. *Clin Neuropharmacol* 1989;**12**(6):498–505.

316. Comella CL, Morrissey M, Janko K. Nocturnal activity with nighttime pergolide in Parkinson disease: a controlled study using actigraphy. *Neurology* 2005;**64**:1450–1.

317. Reuter I, Ellis CM, Ray Chaudhuri K. Nocturnal subcutaneous apomorphine infusion in Parkinson's disease and restless legs syndrome. *Acta Neurol Scand* 1999;**100**:163–7.

318. Romigi A, Stanzione P, Marciani MG, *et al.* Effect of cabergoline added to levodopa treatment on sleep-wake cycle in idiopathic Parkinson's disease: an open label 24-hour polysomnographic study. *J Neural Transm* 2006;**113**: 1909–13.

319. Högl B, Seppi K, Brandauer E, *et al.* Increased daytime sleepiness in Parkinson's disease: a questionnaire survey. *Mov Disord* 2003;**18**:319–23.

320. Dowling GA, Mastick J, Colling E, Carter JH, Singer CM, Aminoff MJ. Melatonin for sleep disturbances in Parkinson's disease. *Sleep Med* 2005;**6**:459–66.

321. Medeiros CA, Carvalhedo de Bruin PF, Lopes LA, Magalhaes MC, de Lourdes Seabra M, de Bruin VM. Effect of exogenous melatonin on sleep and motor dysfunction in Parkinson's disease. A randomized, double blind, placebo-controlled study. *J Neurol* 2007;**254**: 459–64.

322. Abe K, Hikita T, Sakoda S. A hypnotic drug for sleep disturbances in patients with Parkinson's disease. *No To Shinkei* 2005;**57**:301–5.

323. Juri C, Chana P, Tapia J, Kunstmann C, Parrao T. Quetiapine for insomnia in Parkinson disease: results from an open-label trial. *Clin Neuropharmacol* 2005;**28**:185–7.

324. Linazasoro G, Marti Masso JF, Suarez JA. Nocturnal akathisia in Parkinson's disease: treatment with clozapine. *Mov Disord* 1993;**8**:171–4.

325. Arnulf I, Bejjani BP, Garma L, *et al.* Improvement of sleep architecture in PD with subthalamic nucleus stimulation. *Neurology* 2000;**55**:1732–4.

326. Iranzo A, Valldeoriola F, Santamaria J, Tolosa E, Rumia J. Sleep symptoms and polysomnographic architecture in advanced Parkinson's disease after chronic bilateral subthalamic stimulation. *J Neurol Neurosurg Psychiatry* 2002;**72**:661–4.

327. Hjort N, Ostergaard K, Dupont E. Improvement of sleep quality in patients with advanced Parkinson's disease treated with deep brain stimulation of the subthalamic nucleus. *Mov Disord* 2004;**19**:196–9.

328. Monaca C, Ozsancak C, Jacquesson JM, *et al.* Effects of bilateral subthalamic stimulation on sleep in Parkinson's disease. *J Neurol* 2004;**251**:214–8.

329. Lyons KE, Pahwa R. Effects of bilateral subthalamic nucleus stimulation on sleep, daytime sleepiness, and early morning dystonia in patients with Parkinson disease. *J Neurosurg* 2006;**104**:502–5.

330. Zibetti M, Torre E, Cinquepalmi A, *et al.* Motor and non-motor symptom follow-up in parkinsonian patients after deep brain stimulation of the subthalamic nucleus. *Eur Neurol* 2007;**58**:218–23.

331. Ondo WG, Tintner R, Voung KD, Lai D, Ringholz G. Double-blind, placebo-controlled, unforced titration parallel trial of quetiapine for dopaminergic-induced hallucinations in Parkinson's disease. *Mov Disord* 2005;**20**: 958–63.

332. Mehrholz J, Friis R, Kugler J, Twork S, Storch A, Pohl M. Treadmill training for patients with Parkinson's disease. *Cochrane Database Syst Rev* 2010;(1):CD007830.

CHAPTER 16

Alzheimer's disease

J. Hort,[1] J. T. O'Brien,[2] G. Gainotti,[3] T. Pirttila,[4] B. O. Popescu,[5] I. Rektorova,[6] S. Sorbi,[7] P. Scheltens[8]

[1]Charles University in Prague, Second Faculty of Medicine and Motol Hospital, Czech Republic; [2]Institute for Ageing and Health, Newcastle University, UK; [3]Policlinico Gemelli/Catholic University, Rome, Italy; [4]Kuopio University Hospital, Finland; [5]University Hospital, 'Carol Davila' University of Medicine and Pharmacy, Bucharest, Romania; [6]Masaryk University and St Anne's Hospital, Brno, Czech Republic; [7]University of Florence, Italy; [8]VU University Medical Center, Amsterdam, The Netherlands

Objectives

The objective of the task force set up in 2008 was to revise previous European Federation of Neurological Societies (EFNS) recommendations on the diagnosis and management of Alzheimer's disease (AD) [1]. The previous guideline reflected Diagnostic and Statistical Manual, 4th edition (DSM IV) and National Institute of Neurological, Communicative Disorders and Stroke – Alzheimer's Disease and Related Disorders Association (NINCDS-ADRDA) criteria for dementia syndrome and AD. In the revised guideline special attention was given to whether further evidence had become available for bio-markers of disease, such as magnetic resonance imaging (MRI), positron emission tomography (PET) and cere-brospinal fluid (CSF), that have been proposed to increase the confidence of the clinical diagnosis [2]. Special attention was given to results of recent clinical trials in AD, both for cognitive and behavioural aspects of the disease. Because AD is the focus of this guideline, non-Alzheimer's dementias such as vascular (VaD), frontotemporal (FTLD), Parkinson's disease dementia (PDD), dementia with Lewy bodies (DLB), corticobasal degeneration (CBD), progressive supranuclear palsy (PSP), Creutzfeldt-Jacob (CJD), and others will be dealt with separately. This guideline represents desirable standards to guide practice, but may not be appropriate in all

circumstances as clinical presentation of the individual patient and available resources should be taken into account. Cost-effectiveness is not discussed, as heterogeneity across Europe will result in different, country-specific, conclusions.

Background

Dementia affects 5.4% of the over-65s and its prevalence further increases with age [3]. AD is responsible for the majority of cases. The European Collaboration on Dementia, co-ordinated by Alzheimer Europe, found there were currently 8.45 million people in Europe with AD. Dementia causes a significant financial burden to society, estimated at €141 billion of annual cost for the whole of Europe, of which 56% are the costs of informal care. The costs per person with dementia was about €21 000 per year, while disability caused by the illness is estimated at 350 disability-adjusted life years (DALYs) per 100 000 persons, compared to 247 caused by diabetes [4]. With increasing longevity, numbers of people with dementia are set to double in the next 30 years [3]. AD with early onset (<65 years) merits special consideration because of its greater genetic predisposition, and its differing clinical and cognitive profile and course, which is characteristically more aggressive than in late-onset cases. In addition subjects may still be working and of childbearing age. Early-onset AD, therefore, poses particular management issues.

Clinical AD is often preceded by a phase called mild cognitive impairment (MCI) in which there are

European Handbook of Neurological Management: Volume 1, 2nd edition. Edited by N. E. Gilhus, M. P. Barnes and M. Brainin.

complaints and objective impairments in one or more cognitive domains, but with preserved activities of daily living (ADL) ([5]. The panel decided not to review MCI syndrome extensively since discussions around the nosological status of MCI and its relationship to AD are ongoing.

Search strategy

The evidence for this guideline was collected from Cochrane Library reviews, meta-analyses and systematic reviews, and original scientific papers published in peer-reviewed journals before May 2009 accessed using the MEDLINE database. The scientific evidence was evaluated according to pre-specified levels of certainty (classes of evidence I, II, III, and IV) by the expert group members, and the recommendations were graded according to the strength of evidence (Level A, B, or C), using the definitions given in the EFNS guidance [6]. In addressing important clinical questions, for which no evidence was available, Good Practice Points were recommended based on the experience and consensus of the expert task force group.

Reaching of the consensus

A proposed guideline with specific recommendation was drafted for circulation to task force members and displayed on EFNS web pages for comments from all panel members. Consensus was reached at three task force meetings during 2009.

Results

Clinical diagnosis: medical history, laboratory, neurological and physical examination

The history, from the patient and a close informant, should focus on the affected cognitive domains, the course of the illness, and the impact on ADL and any associated non-cognitive symptoms. Past medical history, comorbidities, family and educational history are important. The neurological and general physical examination is particularly important in distinguishing AD from other

primary degenerative and secondary dementias and comorbidities [1]. There exist no evidence-based data to support the usefulness of specific routine blood tests for evaluation of those with dementia but these are useful in excluding comorbidities. Most expert opinion advises to screen for vitamin B12, folate, thyroid-stimulating hormone, calcium, glucose, complete blood cell count, renal and liver function abnormalities. Serological tests for syphilis, Borrelia, and HIV should be considered in individual cases at high risk or where there are suggestive clinical features.

Assessment of cognitive functions

There are two main reasons for neuropsychological assessment in AD: (1) the diagnosis of dementia requires evidence of multiple cognitive defects; (2) initial stages of all principal forms of dementia have a selective anatomical localization reflected by typical patterns of neuropsychological impairment. Screening tests are used to assess cognitive functions globally to identify patients who require more detailed investigation. This is then undertaken with a battery of neuropsychological tests which should evaluate memory, executive functions, language, praxis and visual-spatial abilities. The most widely used *screening test* (Class I) is the Mini-Mental State Examination (MMSE), in which standard cut-off score (24) should be increased to 27 in highly educated individuals [7] and lowered in patients whose native tongue is another language or with low education. Patients with early AD fail mainly in orientation and memory tasks, whereas FTLD individuals exhibit early impairment in speech, and DLB patients may be affected in visuospatial components (pentagons) [8]. Other neuropsychological or clinical screening instruments reported in Table 16.1 provide an equal or greater accuracy in the diagnosis of AD (Class III).

Memory functions Memory, especially episodic memory, should be systematically assessed (Class I), because it is the function most commonly impaired early in AD as consequence of mesial temporal lobe atrophy (entorhinal cortex, hippocampus) which disables consolidation. Retrieval, which depends on frontal lobe and subcortical structures, is less affected. This can be clarified by cuing as applied in California Verbal Learning Test (CVLT) [9] or Buschke Free and Cued Selective Reminding test (FCSRT), to distinguish patients at an early stage of AD

Table 16.1 Neuropsychological instruments

Screening test	Sensitivity	Specificity	[Ref]
MMSE	80–85%	76–80% (Demented vs non-demented very old patients)	[24]
7 Minutes	93%	93% (AD vs various forms of depression and dementia)	[25]
ACE	94%	89% (AD vs NC and other forms of dementia)	[26]
MOCA	90%	90% (Mild AD vs MCI and NC)	[27]
Mattis D.R.S.	85%	85% (AD vs FTD)	[28]
Clock Drawing	67%	97% (Very mild AD vs NC)	[29]
CERAD Battery	80%	81% (Mild AD vs MCI and NC)	[30]
5 Words test	91%	87% (AD vs functional memory disorders)	[15]
Assessment of specific cognitive domains			
Episodic memory			
Logical memory	89% (free recall)	87% (very mild AD vs NC)	[14]
FCSRT	80% (free and cued recall)	90% (MCI converters vs non-converters)	[10]
CVLT	50% (free and cued recall)	98% (Mild AD vs MCI and NC)	[9]
Category Cued Recall	88%	89% (Very mild AD vs NC)	[12]
RAVLT	50% (0 score)	97% (AD vs other forms of dementia)	[11]
Semantic memory (category fluency)			
Language (Naming)			[16]
Graded Naming			[21]
Boston Naming	Overall accuracy: 77% (AD vs NC)		[20]
Visual-spatial abilities			
BVRT			[22]
Executive functions			
Verbal fluency tests			[16]
WCST			[17]
TMT			[18]
Stroop test			[19]

MMSE = Mini-Mental State Examination; ACE = Addenbrooke's Cognitive Examination; MOCA = Montreal Cognitive Assessment; FCSRT = Free and Cued Selective Reminding test; CVLT = California Verbal Learning Test; RAVLT = Rey Auditory Verbal Learning Test; BVRT = Benton Visual Retention Test; CST = Wisconsin Card Sorting test; TMT = Trail Making test; AD = Alzheimer's disease; MCI = mild cognitive impairment; FTD = fronto-temporal dementia; NC = normal controls.

from other subjects [10]. The Rey Auditory Verbal Learning Test (RAVLT) can distinguish between patients with AD and those without dementia, or between AD and other forms of dementia with a diagnostic accuracy of 83–86% [11]. In particular, a very severe impairment (0 score) on RAVLT delayed free recall has a very high (97%) specificity for AD (Class I) [11]. A less severe score can raise diagnostic problems, since it can be due to defective encoding resulting from depression, anxiety, or attentional deficit. A comparison between free recall and cued recall revealed different results in mild AD patients. Vogel *et al.* found that cued and free recall had the same values of sensitivity and specificity [12], whereas Ivanoiu

et al. found that cued recall test was the best predictor of mild AD [13]. High values of sensitivity and specificity have also been obtained by Salmon *et al.* [14] with the delayed recall from the 'Logical Memory' test or in the '5-word' test [15].

Semantic memory (category fluency test, pictures naming task, word and picture definition) testing may confirm deficits in AD or more prominently in semantic dementia [16].

Executive functions A predominance of executive dysfunction over episodic memory impairment is typical for

FTLD and VaD (Class III) and is more frequent in early onset AD. Decreased fluency on verbal fluency tests, perseverations on the Wisconsin card sorting test (WCST) [17], reduced speed of processing on the Trail Making test (TMT) [18], and defects in inhibiting automatic responses on the Stroop test [19] may be caused by subcortical or frontal lesions [18, 19].

Language (speech comprehension and production, reading, and writing) *praxis and visual-spatial abilities* can be variably affected according to type and stage of dementia suggesting for prominent cortical involvement. Boston Naming test [20] or the Graded Naming test [21] are frequently impaired in the earliest stages of AD. High number of errors on the Benton Visual Retention Test (BVRT) can predict the development of AD more than a decade before diagnosis [22].

Studies of apraxia are remarkably few in AD, but a significant relationship has been found between apraxia severity and dependency in ADL [23].

The ADAS cog is an 11-item cognitive test battery that has been particularly useful for detecting changes in severity of AD, mainly in clinical trials, but it is not useful for diagnostic purposes.

Assessment of activities of daily living

Functional decline is required for the diagnosis of dementia. It also allows evaluation of the need for personal and institutional care. ADL are divided into basic (e.g. bathing, toileting) and instrumental (e.g. shopping, handling finances), the latter being more vulnerable to cognitive decline early in the course of the disease. There is no 'gold standard' available for ADL assessment. Out of 12 systematically reviewed scales the informant-based questionnaires the Disability Assessment for Dementia (DAD) and the Bristol ADL are among the most useful, though their overall psychometric properties were still only of moderate quality [31]. ADL are reflected in the Clinical Dementia Rating (CDR) scale which is widely used for rating of dementia severity. The Blessed Roth Dementia Scale and the Informant Questionnaire on Cognitive Decline in the Elderly are also helpful in detection of dementia [1]. The AD8 is a brief, sensitive, informant-based questionnaire that reliably differentiates between non-demented and demented individuals. The respondent rates change (yes versus no) in memory, problem-solving abilities, orientation, and ADL [32].

Assessment of behavioural and psychological symptoms

The term 'behavioural and psychological symptoms of dementia' (BPSD) is used to describe the spectrum of non-cognitive symptoms of dementia (apathy, psychosis, affective and hyperactive behaviours) [33]. Identification of neuropsychiatric symptoms is essential since BPSD occur in the majority of persons with dementia over the course of the disease, and in 35–75% of MCI patients [34] (Class I). BPSD are associated with declining cognitive and functional ability [34], decreased quality of life, and increased institutionalization. Somatic comorbidity and environmental triggers should be ruled out as a possible cause. Several global reliable and validated scales are used to assess BPSD and their change as a result of treatment [35]. They rely on the report of an informant and include the Neuropsychiatric Inventory (NPI), and the Behaviour Rating Scale for Dementia of the CERAD (CERAD–BRSD) [36]. For assessing treatment effects the change in scales representing a clinically meaningful improvement has not been established. More focused scales evaluating agitation or depression in dementia are also available [36]. The Cornell Scale for Depression in Dementia (CSDD) is based on combined caregiver and patient interviews. The 15-item Geriatric Depression Scale (GDS-15) has also been validated for use in AD, but the CSDD appears to be a more sensitive and specific tool for detecting depression independently of the severity of dementia [37].

Assessment of comorbidity

AD patients commonly have comorbid medical conditions such as depression, cardiovascular and pulmonary diseases, infections, arthritis, other neurological disorders, sleep disturbances, falls and incontinence, and drug-related adverse effects, especially in older patients. There is a strong association between medical conditions and impaired cognitive status in AD and the prompt identification and treatment of the associated medical illnesses at the time of diagnosis and throughout the disease evolution may improve cognition in AD patients [38].

Neuroimaging

Structural imaging in the diagnostic work-up of AD serves two purposes: it excludes other, potentially surgically treatable diseases and includes specific findings for AD.

For the former, computed tomography (CT) and magnetic resonance imaging (MRI) perform as well and most current guidelines agree that such an imaging procedure should be carried out once in every patient. However, MRI is more sensitive to subtle vascular changes (strategic infarcts for instance) and to changes that may indicate specific conditions such as multiple sclerosis, PSP, multiple-system atrophy, CBD, prion disease, FTLD (for review see [39]). For practice purposes a standard MR protocol involving at least coronal T1 and axial T2 or FLAIR sequences should be used. Contrast is not indicated. Of note, vascular changes seen on CT or MRI need not preclude a diagnosis of AD, especially in older age, but should prompt adequate evaluation and treatment of cardiovascular risk factors.

Hippocampal atrophy is best seen on MRI but may also be visualized on the more modern type CT scanner [40] and yields sensitivity and specificity values between 80 and 90 % in most studies [39–41] (Class II). Since the previous guideline only one prospective study has been performed examining the added value of hippocampal atrophy on MRI in the diagnosis of AD with postmortem verification [42]. However, being a single-centre, small study in a selected population it just fails Class I evidence.

AD patients with early age of onset often present with complaints and cognitive deficits other than memory impairment [43]. Several structural MRI studies localize the pattern of the atrophy in early-onset AD to more posterior regions, with prominent involvement of the precuneus and posterior cingulate cortex [44].

In addition, MRI may be useful to monitor changes over time and may aid the clinician in following the disease process and explaining it to the patient (GPP).

Functional neuroimaging (i.e. fluorodeoxy-glucose-[FDG-] PET and single photon emission computed tomography [SPECT]) may increase diagnostic confidence in the evaluation of dementia. In a clinical-pathological study, a positive perfusion SPECT scan raised the likelihood of AD to 92%, whereas a negative SPECT scan lowered the likelihood to 70%. SPECT was more useful when the clinical diagnosis was 'possible' AD, with the likelihood of 84% with a positive SPECT, and 52% with a negative SPECT [45]. Dopaminergic SPECT imaging (FP-CIT or DATScan) is useful to differentiate AD from DLB with sensitivity and specificity around 85% (Class I). Care should be taken that stan-

dardized acquisition and analysis methods are used since results and interpretation of DAT scans may otherwise vary [46]. FDG-PET has become a practically applicable tool since the wide distribution of PET CT machines. It may reveal specific abnormalities in AD by showing reduced glucose metabolism in the parietal and superior/posterior temporal regions, posterior cingulate cortex, and precuneus. In advanced stages of AD, frontal lobe defects are also seen. [18]FDG-PET has been reported to have a sensitivity of 93% and a specificity of 63% in predicting a pathological diagnosis of AD (Class II) [47]. FDG-PET is particularly useful in the differential diagnosis of AD towards other dementias with specificity higher than 95% in early-onset cases [48]. Based on the study by Foster et al. [49] FDG-PET is reimbursed in the USA for the distinction between AD and FTD only. A very promising development is the possibility of imaging amyloid with new PET ligands. As of yet these are not available for routine use.

Electroencephalography (EEG)

The EEG may help to differentiate between AD, subjective complains, and psychiatric diagnoses. EEG is recommended in differential diagnosis of atypical clinical presentations of AD. It can also provide early evidence for CJD or suggest the possibility of a toxic-metabolic disorder, transient epileptic amnesia, or other previously unrecognized seizure disorder. Even though reduced alpha power, increased theta power, and lower mean frequency are characteristic for AD patients, EEG can be normal early in the course of the disease in up to 14% of cases. In different studies, the diagnosis accuracy of EEG for AD patients versus healthy control subjects with similar demographic characteristics varied widely, with diagnosis odds ratios between 7 and 219 [50]. EEG with only diffuse abnormalities argues for AD, EEG with both diffuse and focal changes suggests AD or other forms of dementia [51].

CSF analysis

Routine CSF cell count, protein, glucose, and protein electrophoresis assessment is mandatory when vasculitis, inflammatory, haematologic, or demyelinating disease is suspected and in cases of suspected CJD in differentiation with AD.

The elevation of the 14-3-3 protein reflects acute neuronal loss and supports diagnosis of CJD [52] (Class II), while high to very high levels of total tau yield high specificity for CJD [53, 54]. In AD, decreased levels of beta-amyloid 42 (Aβ42) and increased total-tau or phospho-tau in CSF are frequently found. The pooled sensitivity and specificity for Aβ42 in AD versus controls from 13 studies involving 600 patients and 450 controls were 86% and 90% [55]. For total-tau, the sensitivity was 81% and the specificity 90%, pooled from 36 studies with 2,500 patients and 1,400 controls. Across 11 studies with a total of 800 patients and 370 controls, phospho-tau had a mean sensitivity of 80% and specificity was set at 92%, but sensitivities varied widely among studies using different methods. Combined assessment of Aβ42 and total-tau revealed sensitivities (85–94%) and specificities (83–100%) in AD versus controls [55] (Class I).

Specificity of these markers for AD has been lower (39–90%) in differential to the other dementias in clinic-based series [56], which may relate to the presence of comorbid AD pathology [57] (Class III).

There are considerable differences in absolute concentrations of these markers between laboratories, even when the same kit is used [58, 59]. Before CSF can be widely accepted as a reliable tool a consensus for processing and handling of the samples is needed [58].

Genetic testing

The genetics of dementia is complex and genetic testing is associated with many ethical concerns. APP, PS1, and PS2 gene mutations explain 50% of the familial form of early-onset AD [60]. The ApoE ε4 allele is the only genetic factor consistently implicated in late-onset AD, but it is neither necessary nor sufficient for development of the disease [61]. Hence, there is no evidence to suggest ApoE testing is useful in a diagnostic setting. Autopsy diagnosis in familial dementias can be valuable for subsequent diagnosis and counselling. Testing of patients with familial dementia and of unaffected at-risk relatives should be accompanied by neurogenetic counselling and undertaken only after full consent and by specialist centres. Pre-symptomatic testing may be performed in at-risk member of family-carrying mutation. It is recommended that the Huntington's disease protocol is followed for pre-symptomatic testing [62].

Other investigations

A number of non-nervous tissue specimens (mostly fibroblasts, platelets, olfactory and vascular epithelium)

have been investigated in AD, including analysis of DNA damage and repair, autophagy, proteomic analysis, oxidative processes, ionic channels and transduction, APP levels, and intracellular calcium regulation. However, these studies, while potentially informative about the disease process, are presently not of clinical use. Skin and muscle biopsy are used in cerebral autosomal dominant arteriopathy with subcortical infarcts and leukoencephalopathy (CADASIL) diagnosis. Brain biopsy may have a role in the diagnosis of dementia where a treatable disease cannot be excluded by other means. However, it has been shown that information obtained at biopsy affected treatment in only 11% of cases biopsied for the suspicion of an infectious or inflammatory aetiology, though the role of brain biopsy may increase as disease-modifying therapies become available [63].

Recommendations

Diagnosis

- Clinical history should be supplemented by an informant (Level A). A neurological and physical examination should be performed in all patients with dementia (GPP). ADL impairment due to cognitive decline is an essential part of the diagnostic criteria for dementia and should be assessed in the diagnostic evaluation (Level A).

- Several informant-based questionnaires are available and should be used where possible (GPP).

- Cognitive assessment should be performed in all patients (Level A). Quantitative neuropsychological testing should be made in patients with questionable or very early AD (Level B). The assessment of cognitive functions should include a general cognitive measure and more detailed testing of the main cognitive domains, and in particular an assessment of delayed recall (Level A). In patients with moderate memory impairment cued recall could be more appropriate than free recall (Level B).

- Assessment of BPSD should be performed in each patient (Level A). Information should be gathered from an informant using an appropriate rating scale (GPP).

- Assessment of comorbidity is important in AD patients, both at the time of diagnosis and throughout the course of the illness (GPP) and should always be considered as a possible cause of BPSD (Level C). Blood levels of folate, vitamin B12, thyroid-stimulating hormone, calcium, glucose, complete blood cell count, renal and liver function tests should be evaluated at the time of diagnosis and serological tests for syphilis, Borelia, and HIV might also be needed in cases with atypical presentation or clinical features suggestive of these disorders (GPP).

- CT and MRI may be used to exclude treatable causes of dementia. Multislice CT and coronal MRI may be used to assess hippocampal atrophy to support a clinical diagnosis of AD (Level B). FDG-PET and perfusion SPECT are useful adjuncts when diagnosis remains in doubt (Level B). Dopaminergic SPECT is useful to differentiate AD from DLB (Level A). Follow up with serial MRI is useful in a clinical setting to document disease progression (GPP).

- EEG is recommended in differential diagnosis of atypical clinical presentations of AD (GPP) and when CJD or transient epileptic amnesia is suspected (Level B).

- Routine CSF analysis is recommended in differential diagnosis for atypical clinical presentations of AD (GPP). CSF 14-3-3 or total tau measurement are recommended for the identification of CJD in patients with rapidly progressive dementia (Level B). Alterations in CSF total tau, phospho-tau, and Aβ42 support diagnosis of AD (Level B).

- Screening for known pathogenic mutations can be undertaken in patients with appropriate phenotype or a family history of an autosomal dominant dementia. Routine Apo E genotyping is not recommended.

Management of Alzheimer's disease

The first step in AD management is accurate recognition and diagnosis of the disorder, and then disclosing that diagnosis in a sensitive and timely way to the patient and others as appropriate. Disclosure of diagnosis is not harmful, and actually decreases depression and anxiety in patients and their caregivers [64] (Class II). The vast majority of patients with mild dementia wish to be fully informed and 75% of caregivers wish their relative to be informed [65]. Differences among ethnic, cultural, and religious groups may influence how and what disclosure occurs. It offers the patient opportunity to pursue desired activities and maximizes individual autonomy and choice by providing information necessary for decision making and advance planning, including the decision to give informed consent to research projects and autopsy. At time of diagnosis several issues need to be addressed, including the provision of high-quality, understandable information about the illness and its course to patient and caregiver, a careful assessment for any comorbidities, and consideration given to other services that may be required, including social services, mental stimulation, occupational therapy, physiotherapy, speech and language therapy (Class IV). Occupational therapy can

benefit patients' daily functioning and reduce the need for informal care [66] (Class II). Medico-legal issues need to be addressed, with driving often needing prompt attention and action taken according to the legal framework operating in that particular country. Caregiver support should consist of education about AD, and attending peer support groups may be helpful. Caregiver stress and depression are common and, if present, more intensive caregiver support and counselling and/or specific treatment for depression may be needed. The provision of a standard education and support package to caregivers has been shown in randomized controlled trials (RCT) to decrease psychiatric symptoms in caregivers and lead to delays in institutionalization for patients [67, 68] (Class I). Management should include clear arrangements for follow-up, as regular monitoring of medication response and adverse effects, as well as changes in the severity of dementia (using scales like the MMSE), should be undertaken. Reassessment for development of comorbidity (including carer stress) should be an integral part of management.

Primary prevention of AD

This refers to the prevention of subsequent dementia in cognitively normal subjects and is the ultimate goal for AD management. Several risk factors have been well established for AD, though some (such as age, sex, and genotype) are not modifiable. Potentially modifiable risk factors that have been established through several epidemiological studies include vascular risk factors (hypertension, smoking, diabetes, atrial fibrillation, and obesity) and head injury, while protective factors described include use of antihypertensives, non-steroidal anti-inflammatories, statins and hormone replacement therapy, high education, diet, physical activity, and engagement in social and intellectual activities. However, whether modifying these factors will reduce risk of dementia is not yet known. A meta-analysis concluded that there is no good evidence to recommend statins for reducing the risk of AD [69], while results of the large, prospective, placebo-controlled 'Women's Health Initiative Memory Study' showed that the use of oestrogen plus progestin in post-menopausal women was actually associated with a significantly increased risk of dementia [70] (I).

Treatment of hypertension for prevention of dementia, including AD, has been the best-studied risk factor to date. However, most RCTs have been stopped early because cardiovascular endpoints were reached, meaning they were underpowered to detect differences in rates of dementia. A study of treating hypertension in the very old (HYVET) reached similar conclusions, and contained a meta-analysis of all studies supporting a significant risk reduction [71] (I). However, the period over which treatment needs to be given is not known, nor has it been established whether treating vascular risk factors, including hypertension, in those with established AD affects disease progression. Currently, no clear recommendations about dementia prevention can be made.

Secondary prevention of AD

This refers to the prevention of development of AD in non-demented subjects with some evidence of cognitive impairment. The groups most often studied in this regard are those with MCI, and several RCTs of cholinesterase inhibitors (ChEIs) have been undertaken in MCI, most using 'conversion' to dementia as the primary outcome. A meta-analysis included eight studies involving all three ChEIs, with duration of treatment ranging from 16 weeks to 3 years [72]. There were no differences in rate of conversion to AD between active and placebo groups, and most secondary outcomes were also negative (Class I). There have also been negative studies of aspirin in primary prevention of cognitive decline and of anti-inflammatories and vitamin E in MCI (Class I). A large study showed no effect of Ginkgo on preventing AD [73] (Class I). Therefore, no treatments have demonstrated efficacy for preventing or delaying development of AD in MCI subjects until now, while evidence exists that ChEIs, Vitamin E, Ginkgo biloba, and anti-inflammatories are not substantively helpful.

Treatment of established AD

Cholinesterase inhibitors

There have been several well-conducted, placebo-controlled, large-scale RCTs with the three ChEIs, donepezil, rivastigmine, and galantamine, which have shown efficacy on cognitive function, global outcome, and ADL in patients with mild to moderate AD (Class I), usually defined as MMSE between 16 and 26. Mean global improvement over placebo is 3–4 points on the ADAS-Cog, a level of improvement roughly equivalent to the naturalistic decline expected over a 6-month period. Most studies have been of relatively short duration (6

months), though 1- and 3-year studies have been reported with donepezil, which suggest the benefits of ChEIs continue in the longer term (Class I). Retrospective analysis and some long-term open studies suggest a possible effect of ChEIs on disease modification, but more data are needed before this can be confirmed [74]. RCTs of ChEIs in more severe AD (MMSE < 10) have also shown positive results [75, 76] and a Cochrane review concluded that trials supported evidence of benefit in mild, moderate, and severe AD [77]. In light of current evidence, limiting prescribing of ChEIs to only some AD subjects according to certain cut-offs on a measure such as the MMSE, as operated in many countries, does not seem justified. Although a point will be reached in severe AD when ChEIs are unlikely to continue to have benefit, it is currently unclear at what point in the disease process ChEIs should be withdrawn.

ChEIs are generally well tolerated, although common gastrointestinal adverse effects such as nausea, diarrhoea, and vomiting may sometimes lead to discontinuation of treatment in some patients. There have been few direct comparisons between ChEIs, and those which have been undertaken have been small in size and have not produced consistent evidence of better efficacy of one drug over another (Class II). There is some evidence from open-label studies that patients who do not tolerate or do not seem to benefit from one ChEI may tolerate or draw benefit from the other (Class III). One of the ChEIs, rivastigmine, is now available in a transdermal (patch) formulation which appears to have lower incidence of side effects than oral administration but equal efficacy [78] (Class I).

A disease-modifying effect of ChEIs has been proposed, and has some basic scientific support, but no convincing clinical data, either from trials of clinical endpoints or of those using biomarkers, has yet been forthcoming to support these claims (Class IV).

Effects on non-cognitive behavioural and psychological symptoms of dementia (BPSD) have also been shown, though as with cognition effect sizes are modest (Class I). There remains uncertainty as to which particular non-cognitive symptoms may respond best, though effects on psychosis and apathy are consistently reported (Class II). Effects on agitation are less clear, and a large placebo-controlled RCT in moderate to severe AD failed to show an effect of donepezil on patients with clinically significant agitation [79] (Class I).

Memantine

Memantine, a non-competitive N-Methyl-D-Aspartate (NMDA) receptor antagonist, also has been subject to several RCTs in AD. Studies in moderate to severe AD have been more consistently positive than those in mild to moderate AD; previous reviews of the literature have concluded that while there is a significant effect in cognition at all severities, but effects on global outcome, ADL and behaviour were only apparent in the moderate to severe studies [80] (Class I). Once-daily dosing has been shown to be as effective as the original recommendation of administration twice daily (Class I) [81]. Modest effects on behaviour were also found in a pooled analysis of six studies which included all those with MMSE<20, with delusions, agitation/aggression, and irritability being the most responsive symptoms [82] (Class II), though studies of subjects primarily selected for the presence of these behavioural features have not yet been reported.

The benefits of adding memantine to ChEIs are not clear; an early study of adding memantine to donepezil was positive, but a recent study of more than 400 subjects which added the drug or placebo to those stable on any of the three ChEIs showed no evidence of benefit in either cognitive or non-cognitive symptoms [83] (Class I). Further studies are needed before clear recommendations can be made about the benefits of adding memantine to ChEIs.

Other drugs and interventions

Several other treatments have been suggested as potentially beneficial for AD, including non-steroidal anti-inflammatory drugs (NSAIDs), oestrogens, and statins. A large, placebo-controlled RCT of vitamin E (1000 IU, twice a day over 2 years) in moderate AD was found to significantly delay the time to a composite outcome of primary outcome measures, but a study in MCI has been negative and the conclusion of a Cochrane review is that there is insufficient evidence for the efficacy of vitamin E in the treatment of AD or MCI [84] (Class I). Studies of steroidal, non-steroidal, and cyclo-oxygenase-2 inhibitors in AD and MCI have been negative, yet have had potentially serious side effects (Class I). Evidence-based data report studies of Ginkgo biloba extract (explicitly EGb 761), but there remains controversy about the role of the EGb 761 as studies to date have included mixed populations and have not been consistent in results. A

meta-analysis concluded that the evidence that Ginkgo biloba has predictable and clinically significant benefit for people with dementia or cognitive impairment is inconsistent and unreliable [85] (Class I). However two Class I studies [86, 87] demonstrating positive effects were omitted because of significant heterogeneity between the trials. Further evidence is needed before efficacy for Ginkgo can be clearly established.

Many other compounds, such as piracetam, nicergoline, selegiline, vinpocetine, pentoxyphylins, and Cerebrolysin are prescribed in some countries as treatments for AD. For example, a recent Cochrane review of piracetam, one of the most widely studied drugs to date, found poor study design, possible publication bias, and that overall the evidence from trials did not support the use of piracetam in people with dementia or cognitive impairment [88]. A review of six Cerebrolysin trials [89] found an effect on global outcome but no consistent effect on other scales. Further evidence is therefore required before its use can be recommended. Similarly, a Cochrane review of selegiline found no evidence for its efficacy in AD [90]. At present, therefore, there is no convincing evidence for efficacy of any of these drugs for AD.

There is much interest in the use of cognitive therapies in AD. Preliminary studies seem to suggest a beneficial effect of cognitive stimulation, also known as Reality Orientation (see www.nice.org.uk, dementia guideline (no. 42) for comprehensive review). More studies are needed before it can be classified as Class I evidence, but in individual cases the clinician may decide to try this form of therapy (GPP).

There are many ongoing clinical studies aimed at modifying the underlying disease process, including international trials of passive and active amyloid immunisation [91] and of the drug Dimebon [92]. However, recommendations about the usefulness of these and other agents must await final results from rigorous Phase III studies.

Treatment of behavioural and psychological symptoms (BPSD)

Management of BPSD begins with a careful search for trigger and/or exacerbating factors, including environmental cues, physical problems (infections, constipation), medication, and depression or psychosis. As studies of BPSD indicate a high placebo response, safe non-pharmacological management (education, exercise, aromatherapy, sensory stimulation, personalized music) should be tried wherever possible in the first instance, as symptoms may naturally resolve within a short time. The beneficial effects of ChEIs and memantine for mild BPSD have been described above, but a recent RCT found donepezil did not help clinically significant agitation in those with moderate to severe AD [79]. Both conventional and atypical antipsychotics reduce BPSD, with particular effects demonstrated for risperidone for agitation/aggression and psychosis [93, 94] (Class I). However, antipsychotics have important and potentially serious side effects, most especially increased stroke risk, increased mortality, parkinsonism, and cognitive impairment [95]. They should be used with caution, at low dose, and for the shortest period needed only for those with moderate to severe symptoms causing distress, and after careful assessment of risk and benefit and after dis-

cussion with the caregiver and, where possible, the patient. There is no evidence that conventional agents are any safer in regard to risk of stroke or mortality than atypical agents [96] and they have a less established evidence base and greater side effects. Low doses of antipsychotics should be used with careful monitoring, and drugs prescribed for the minimum period required. When BPSD have settled, antipsychotics can be withdrawn in most cases without re-emergence of BPSD, unless behavioural disturbance is still present [97]. Evidence for other drugs is limited; carbamazepine may help aggression [98] (Class II), though most studies of valproate have been negative [99] (Class II). Antidepressants, especially selective serotonin reuptake inhibitors (SSRIs), may be useful for depression in dementia and do not have the adverse anticholinergic effects of older tricyclics [100] (Class II).

Recommendations
Management

- Diagnosis of AD should be disclosed to the patient (and caregivers as appropriate) (Level B). Disclosure of diagnosis should be individually tailored. It should be accompanied by information and counselling, as well as useful contacts such as Alzheimer's patient organizations. Patients and caregivers should be provided with education and support (Level A). Driving, medico-legal issues, and the need for other support services should be considered (GPP). If possible, physicians may encourage patients to draw up advance directives containing future treatment and care preferences (GPP).

- There is insufficient evidence to support the use of any drugs purely for the primary prevention of dementia. ChEIs, vitamin E, ginkgo, and oestrogens should not be used as treatments for those with MCI (Level A).

- In patients with AD, treatment with ChEIs (donepezil, galantamine, or rivastigmine) should be considered at the time of diagnosis, taking into account expected therapeutic benefits and potential safety issues (Level A). Benefits on cognitive and non-cognitive symptoms have been demonstrated in those with mild, moderate, and severe disease (Level A). Realistic expectations for treatment effects and potential side effects should be discussed with the patient and caregivers (GPP).

- In patients with moderate to severe AD, treatment with memantine should be considered, taking into account expected therapeutic benefits and potential safety issues (Level A). Benefits on cognitive and non-cognitive symptoms are apparent, some non-cognitive symptoms (agitation,

delusions) may respond better than others (Level B). Realistic expectations for treatment effects and potential side effects should be discussed with the patient and caregivers (GPP).

- Regular patient follow-up, which should include scales like the MMSE to monitor response to treatment and disease progression, should be an integral part of management (GPP).

- Aspirin should not be used as a treatment for AD (Level A), though it can be used in those with AD who also have other indications for its use (e.g. to prevent cardiovascular events). Vitamin E should not be used as a treatment for AD (Level A).

- Currently, there is insufficient evidence to support the use of other agents, including anti-inflammatory drugs, nootropics (including piracetam, nicergoline), selegiline, oestrogens, pentoxyphylin, or statins, and inconsistent evidence for EGb 761 and Cerebrolysin in the treatment or prevention of AD (Level A).

- Cognitive stimulation or rehabilitation may be considered in patients with mild to moderate AD (GPP). Occupational therapy can improve patients' functioning and reduce need for informal care (Level B).

- Management of BPSD should begin with a careful search for triggers and causative factors (i.e. physical illness). Where possible, initial treatment should be non-pharmacological (Level C).

- Antipsychotics should only be used for moderate or severe BPSD symptoms causing significant distress, which have either not responded to other treatments (like non-pharmacological measures or cholinesterase inhibitors) or when other treatments are not appropriate (Level A). Low dose of atypical agents should be used only after assessment of risk benefit and full discussion with the patient (when capacity allows) and caregiver (GPP).

• Atypical agents have fewer side effects and do not confer a greater risk of stroke or mortality than conventional drugs (Level B).

• Selective serotonin reuptake inhibitors rather than tricyclic antidepressants should be used to treat depression in AD (Level B).

Scheduled update

2012.

Conflicts of interest

The authors have received speaker's and/or consultancy honoraria from Eisai, GE Healthcare, Janssen-Cilag, Lundbeck, Mertz, Shire, Novartis, Elan, Zentiva, Pfizer, Wyeth, and Elan. For the conception and writing of this guideline no honoraria or any other compensation were received by any of the authors.

References

1. Waldemar G, Dubois B, Emre M, *et al.*, EFNS. Recommendations for the diagnosis and management of Alzheimer's disease and other disorders associated with dementia: EFNS guideline. *Eur J Neurol* 2007;14.

2. Dubois B, Feldman HH, Jacova C, *et al.* Research criteria for the diagnosis of Alzheimer's disease: revising the NINCDS-ADRDA criteria. *Lancet Neurol* 2007;**6**:734–46.

3. Ferri CP, Prince M, Brayne C, *et al.*, Alzheimer's Disease International. Global prevalence of dementia: a Delphi consensus study. *Lancet* 2005;**366**:2112–7.

4. Packo I. *Dementia in Europe Yearbook 2008.* Luxembourg: Alzheimer Europe, 2008.

5. Petersen RC, Stevens JC, Ganguli M, Tangalos EG, Cummings JL, DeKosky ST. Practice parameter: Early detection of dementia: mild cognitive impairment (an evidence-based review). Report of the quality standards subcommittee of the Amerian Academy of Neurology. *Neurology* 2001;**56**:1133–42.

6. Brainin M, Barnes M, Gilhus NE, Selmaj K, Waldemar G. Guidance for the preparation of neurological management guidelines by EFNS scientific task forces – revised recommendations. *Eur J Neurol* 2004;**11**:577–81.

7. O'Bryant SE, Humphreys JD, Smith GE, *et al.* Detecting dementia with the mini-mental state examination in highly educated individuals. *Arch Neurol* 2008;**65**:963–7.

8. Ala TA, Hughes LF, Kyrouac GA, Ghobrial MW, Elble RJ. Pentagon copying is more impaired in dementia with Lewy

bodies than in Alzheimer's disease. *J Neurol Neurosurg Psychiatry* 2001;**70**:483–8.

9. Lange KL, Bondi MW, Salmon DP, *et al.* Decline in verbal memory during preclinical Alzheimer's disease: examination of the effect of APOE genotype. *J Int Neuropsychol Soc* 2002;**8**:943–55.

10. Sarazin M, Berr C, De Rotrou J, *et al.* Amnestic syndrome of the medial temporal type identifies prodromal AD: a longitudinal study. *Neurology* 2007;**69**:1859–67.

11. Gainotti G, Marra C, Villa G, Parlato V, Chiarotti F. Sensitivity and specificity of some neuropsychological markers of Alzheimer dementia. *Alzheimer Dis Assoc Disord* 1998;**12**:152–62.

12. Vogel A, Mortensen EL, Gade A, Waldemar G. The Category Cued Recall test in very mild Alzheimer's disease: discriminative validity and correlation with semantic memory functions. *Eur J Neurol* 2007;**14**:102–8.

13. Ivanoiu A, Adam S, Van der Linden M, *et al.* Memory evaluation with a new cued recall test in patients with mild cognitive impairment and Alzheimer's disease. *J Neurol* 2005;**252**:47–55.

14. Salmon DP, Thomas RG, Pay MM, *et al.* Alzheimer's disease can be accurately diagnosed in very mildly impaired individuals. *Neurology* 2002;**59**:1022–8.

15. Dubois B, Touchon J, Portet F, Ousset PJ, Vellas B, Michel B. 'The 5 words': a simple and sensitive test for the diagnosis of Alzheimer's disease. *Presse Med* 2002;**31**:1696–9.

16. Nestor PJ, Fryer TD, Hodges JR. Declarative memory impairments in Alzheimer's disease and semantic dementia. *Neuroimage* 2006;**30**:1010–20.

17. Nagahama Y, Okina T, Suzuki N, Nabatame H, Matsuda M. The cerebral correlates of different types of perseveration in the Wisconsin Card Sorting Test. *J Neurol Neurosurg Psychiatry* 2005;**76**:169–75.

18. Zakzanis KK, Mraz R, Graham SJ. An fMRI study of the Trail Making Test. *Neuropsychologia* 2005;**43**:1878–86.

19. Kramer JH, Reed BR, Mungas D, Weiner MW, Chui HC. Executive dysfunction in subcortical ischaemic vascular disease. *J Neurol Neurosurg Psychiatry* 2002;**72**:217–20.

20. Coen RF, Kirby M, Swanwick GR, *et al.* The utility of naming tests in the diagnosis of Alzheimer's disease. *Ir J Psychol Med* 1999;**16**:43–6.

21. Ahmed S, Arnold R, Thompson SA, Graham KS, Hodges JR. Naming of objects, faces and buildings in mild cognitive impairment. *Cortex* 2008;**44**:746–52.

22. Kawas CH, Corrada MM, Brookmeyer R, *et al*. Visual memory predicts Alzheimer's disease more than a decade before diagnosis. *Neurology* 2003;**60**:1089–93.

23. Hanna-Pladdy B, Heilman KM, Foundas AL. Ecological implications of ideomotor apraxia: evidence from physical activities of daily living. *Neurology* 2003;**60**:487–90.

24. Kahle-Wrobleski K, Corrada MM, Li B, Kawas CH. Sensitivity and specificity of the mini-mental state examination for identifying dementia in the oldest-old: the 90+ study. *J Am Geriatr Soc* 2007;**55**:284–9.

25. Meulen EF, Schmand B, van Campen JP, *et al*. The seven minute screen: a neurocognitive screening test highly sensitive to various types of dementia. *J Neurol Neurosurg Psychiatry* 2004;**75**:700–5.

26. Mioshi E, Dawson K, Mitchell J, Arnold R, Hodges JR. The Addenbrooke's Cognitive Examination Revised (ACE-R): a brief cognitive test battery for dementia screening. *Int J Geriatr Psychiatry* 2006;**21**:1078–85.

27. Nasreddine ZS, Phillips NA, Bédirian V, *et al*. The Montreal Cognitive Assessment, MoCA: a brief screening tool for mild cognitive impairment. *J Am Geriatr Soc* 2005;**53**:695–9.

28. Rascovsky K, Salmon DP, Hansen LA, Galasko D. Distinct cognitive profiles and rates of decline on the Mattis Dementia Rating Scale in autopsy-confirmed frontotemporal dementia and Alzheimer's disease. *J Int Neuropsychol Soc* 2008;**14**:373–83.

29. Lee H, Swanwick GR, Coen RF, Lawlor BA. Use of the clock drawing task in the diagnosis of mild and very mild Alzheimer's disease. *Int Psychogeriatr* 1996;**8**(3):469–76.

30. Chandler MJ, Lacritz LH, Hynan LS, *et al*. A total score for the CERAD neuropsychological battery. *Neurology* 2005;**65**:102–6.

31. Sikkes SAM, de Lange-de Klerk ESM, Pijnenburg YAL, Scheltens P, Uitdehaag BMJ. A systematic review of instrumental activities of daily living scales in dementia: room for improvement. *J Neurol Neurosurg Psychiatry* 2009;**80**: 7–12.

32. Galvin JE, Roe CM, Powlishta KK, *et al*. The AD8: a brief informant interview to detect dementia. *Neurology* 2005;**65**:559–64.

33. Aalten P, Verhey FRJ, Boziki M, *et al*. Consistency of neuropsychiatric syndromes across dementias: results from the European Alzheimer Disease Consortium. *Dement Geriatr Cogn Disord* 2008;**25**:1–8.

34. Apostolova LG, Cummings JL. Neuropsychiatric manifestations in mild cognitive impairment: A systematic review of the literature. *Dement Geriatr Cogn Disord* 2008;**25**: 115–26.

35. Perrault A, Oremus M, Demers L, Vida S, Wolfson C. Review of outcome measurement instruments in Alzheimer's disease drug trials: psychometric properties of behavior and mood scales. *J Geriatr Psychiatry Neurol* 2000;**13**:181–96.

36. Conn D, Thorpe L. Assessment of behavioural and psychological symptoms associated with dementia. *Can J Neurol Sci* 2007;**34**:S67–71.

37. Müller-Thomsen T, Arlt S, Mann U, *et al*. Detecting depression in Alzheimer's disease: evaluation of four different scales. *Arch Clin Neuropsychol* 2005;**20**:271–6.

38. Doraiswamy PM, Leon J, Cummings JL, Marin D, Neumann PJ. Prevalence and impact of medical comorbidity in Alzheimer's disease. *J Gerontol A Biol Sci Med Sci* 2002;**57**:M173–7.

39. Scheltens P. Imaging in Alzheimer's disease. *Dialogues Clin Neurosci* 2009;**11**:191–9.

40. Wattjes MP, Henneman WJ, van der Flier WM, *et al*. Diagnostic imaging of patients in a memory clinic: comparison of MR imaging and 64-detector row CT. *Radiology* 2009;[Epub ahead of print].

41. Scheltens P, Fox N, Barkhof F, De Carli C. Structural magnetic resonance imaging in the practical assessment of dementia: beyond exclusion. *Lancet Neurol* 2002;**1**:13–21.

42. Burton EJ, Barber R, Mukaetova-Ladinska EB, *et al*. Medial temporal lobe atrophy on MRI differentiates Alzheimer's disease from dementia with Lewy bodies and vascular cognitive impairment: a prospective study with pathological verification of diagnosis. *Brain* 2009;**132**(Pt 1):195–203.

43. Hodges JR. Alzheimer's centennial legacy: origins, landmarks and the current status of knowledge concerning cognitive aspects. *Brain* 2006;**129**:2811–22.

44. Karas G, Scheltens P, Rombouts S, *et al*. Precuneus atrophy in early-onset Alzheimer's disease: a morphometric structural MRI study. *Neuroradiology* 2007;**49**:967–76.

45. Jagust W, Thisted R, Devous MD Sr, *et al*. SPECT perfusion imaging in the diagnosis of Alzheimer's disease: a clinical-pathologic study. *Neurology* 2001;**56**:950–6.

46. McKeith I, O'Brien J, Walker Z, *et al*., DLB Study Group. Sensitivity and specificity of dopamine transporter imaging with 123I-FP-CIT SPECT in dementia with Lewy bodies: a phase III, multicentre study. *Lancet Neurol* 2007;**6**: 305–13.

47. Silverman DH, Alavi A. PET imaging in the assessment of normal and impaired cognitive function. *Radiol Clin North Am* 2005;**43**:67–77.

48. Panegyres PK, Rogers JM, McCarthy M, Campbell A, Wu JS. Fluorodeoxyglucose-positron emission tomography in the differential diagnosis of early-onset dementia: a prospective, community-based study. *BMC Neurol* 2009;**9**: 41–50.

49. Foster NL, Heidebrink JL, Clark CM, *et al.* FDG-PET improves accuracy in distinguishing frontotemporal dementia and Alzheimer's disease. *Brain* 2007;**130**(Pt 10): 2616–35.

50. Jelic V, Kowalski J. Evidence-based evaluation of diagnostic accuracy of resting EEG in dementia and mild cognitive impairment. *Clin EEG Neurosci* 2009;**40**:129–42.

51. Liedorp M, van der Flier WM, Hoogervorst EL, Scheltens P, Stam CJ. Associations between patterns of EEG abnormalities and diagnosis in a large memory clinic cohort. *Dement Geriatr Cogn Disord* 2009;**27**:18–23.

52. WHO. WHO Manual for Surveillance of Human Transmissible Spongiform Encephalopathies. 2003.

53. Otto M, Wiltfang J, Cepek L, *et al.* Tau protein and 14-3-3 protein in the differential diagnosis of Creutzfeldt-Jakob disease. *Neurology* 2002;**58**:192–7.

54. Sanchez-Juan P, Green A, Ladogana A, *et al.* CSF tests in the differential diagnosis of Creutzfeldt-Jakob disease. *Neurology* 2006;**67**:637–43.

55. Blennow K, Hampel H. CSF markers for incipient Alzheimer's disease. *Lancet Neurol* 2003;**2**:605–13.

56. Mattsson N, Zetterberg H, Hansson O, *et al.* CSF biomarkers and incipient Alzheimer disease in patients with mild cognitive impairment. *JAMA* 2009;**302**:385–93.

57. Tapiola T, Alafuzoff I, Herukka SK, *et al.* CSF beta-amyloid42 and Tau proteins are markers of Alzheimer-type pathology in the brain. *Arch Neurol* 2009;**66**: 382–9.

58. Hort J, Bartos A, Pirttilä T, Scheltens P. Use of cerebrospinal fluid biomarkers in diagnosis of dementia across Europe. *Eur J Neurol* 2009.

59. Verwey NA, van der Flier WM, Blennow K, *et al.* A worldwide multicentre comparison of assays for cerebrospinal fluid biomarkers in Alzheimer's disease. *Ann Clin Biochem* 2009;**46**:235–40.

60. Chen Q, Schubert D. Presenilin interacting proteins. *Expert Rev Mol Med* 2002;**22**(4):1–18.

61. Brouwers N, Sleegers K, Van Broeckhoven C. Molecular genetics of Alzheimer's disease: an update. *Ann Med* 2008;**40**:562–83.

62. Tibben A. Predictive testing for Huntington's disease. *Brain Res Bull* 2007;**72**:165–71.

63. Warren JD, Schott JM, Fox NC, *et al.* Brain biopsy in dementia. *Brain* 2005;**128**:2016–25.

64. Carpenter BD, Xiong C, Porensky EK, *et al.* Reaction to a dementia diagnosis in individuals with Alzheimer's disease and mild cognitive impairment. *J Am Geriatr Soc* 2008;**56**: 405–12.

65. Pinner G, Bouman WP. Attitudes of patients with mild dementia and their carers towards disclosure of the diagnosis. *Int Psychogeriatr* 2003;**15**:279–88.

66. Graff MJ, Adang EM, Vernooij-Dassen MJ, *et al.* Community occupational therapy for older patients with dementia and their care givers: cost effectiveness study. *BMJ* 2008;**336**(7636):134–8.

67. Mittelman MS, Haley WE, Clay OJ, Roth DL. Improving caregiver well-being delays nursing home placement of patients with Alzheimer disease. *Neurology* **67**:1592–9.

68. Mittelman MS, Brodaty H, Wallen AS, Burns A. A three-country randomized controlled trial of a psychosocial intervention for caregivers combined with pharmacological treatment for patients with Alzheimer disease: effects on caregiver depression. *Am J Geriatr Psychiatry* 2008;**16**: 893–904.

69. McGuinness B, Craig D, Bullock R, Passmore P. Statins for the prevention of dementia. *Cochrane Database Syst Rev* 2009;(2):CD003160.

70. Shumaker SA, Legault C, Kuller L, *et al.*, Women's Health Initiative Memory Study. Conjugated equine estrogens and incidence of probable dementia and mild cognitive impairment in postmenopausal women: Women's Health Initiative Memory Study. *JAMA* 2004;**291**:2947–58.

71. Peters R, Beckett N, Forette F, *et al.*, HYVET investigators. Incident dementia and blood pressure lowering in the Hypertension in the Very Elderly Trial cognitive function assessment (HYVET-COG): a double-blind, placebo controlled trial. *Lancet Neurol* 2008;**7**:683–9.

72. Raschetti R, Albanese E, Vanacore N, Maggini M. Cholinesterase inhibitors in mild cognitive impairment: a systematic review of randomised trials. *Plos Med* 2007;**4**: e338.

73. DeKosky ST, Williamson JD, Fitzpatrick AL, *et al.* Ginkgo Evaluation of Memory (GEM) Study Investigators. Ginkgo biloba for prevention of dementia: a randomized controlled trial. *JAMA* 2008;**300**:2253–62.

74. Farlow MR. The search for disease modification in moderate to severe Alzheimer's disease. *Neurology* 2005; **65**(Suppl. 3):S25- 30.

75. Black SE, Doody R, Li H, *et al.* Donepezil preserves cognition and global function in patients with severe Alzheimer disease. *Neurology* 2007;**69**:459–69.

76. Burns A, Bernabei R, Bullock R, *et al.* Safety and efficacy of galantamine (Reminyl) in severe Alzheimer's disease (the SERAD study): a randomised, placebo-controlled, double-blind trial. *Lancet Neurol* 2009;**8**:39–47.

77. Birks J, Harvey RJ. Donepezil for dementia due to Alzheimer's disease. *Cochrane Database Syst Rev* 2006;(1): CD001190.

78. Birks J, Grimley Evans J, Iakovidou V, Tsolaki M, Holt FE. Rivastigmine for Alzheimer's disease. *Cochrane Database Syst Rev* 2009;(2):CD001191.

79. Howard RJ, Juszczak E, Ballard CG, *et al.*, CALM-AD Trial Group. Donepezil for the treatment of agitation in Alzheimer's disease. *N Engl J Med* 2007;**357**:1382–92.

80. Burns A, O'Brien J, BAP Dementia Consensus group, Auriacombe S, Ballard C, Broich K, Bullock R, Feldman H, Ford G, Knapp M, McCaddon A, Iliffe S, Jacova C, Jones R, Lennon S, McKeith I, Orgogozo JM, Purandare N, Richardson M, Ritchie C, Thomas A, Warner J, Wilcock G, Wilkinson D, British Association for Psychopharmacology. Clinical practice with anti-dementia drugs: a consensus statement from British Association for Psychopharmacology. *J Psychopharmacol* 2006;**20**:732–55.

81. Jones RW, Bayer A, Inglis F, Barker A, Phul R. Safety and tolerability of once-daily versus twice-daily memantine: a randomised, double-blind study in moderate to severe Alzheimer's disease. *Int J Geriatr Psychiatry* 2007;**22**(3):258–62.

82. Gauthier S, Loft H, Cummings J. Improvement in behavioural symptoms in patients with moderate to severe Alzheimer's disease by memantine: a pooled data analysis. *Int J Geriatr Psychiatry* 2008;**23**:537–45.

83. Porsteinsson AP, Grossberg GT, Mintzer J, Olin JT, Memantine MEM-MD-12 Study Group. Memantine treatment in patients with mild to moderate Alzheimer's disease already receiving a cholinesterase inhibitor: a randomized, double-blind, placebo-controlled trial. *Curr Alzheimer Res* 2008;**5**:83–9.

84. Isaac MG, Quinn R, Tabet N. Vitamin E for Alzheimer's disease and mild cognitive impairment. *Cochrane Database Syst Rev* 2008;(3):CD002854.

85. Birks J, Grimley Evans J. Ginkgo biloba for cognitive impairment and dementia. *Cochrane Database Syst Rev* 2009;(1):CD003120.

86. Mazza M, Capuano A, Bria P, Mazza S. Ginkgo biloba and donepezil: a comparison in the treatment of Alzheimer's dementia in randomized placebo controlled double blind study. *Eur J Neurol* 2006;**13**:981–5.

87. Napryeyenko O, Borzenko I, GINDEM-NP Study Group. Ginkgo biloba special extract in dementia with neuropsychiatric features. *Drug Res* 2007;**57**(1):4–11.

88. Flicker L, Grimley Evans G. Piracetam for dementia or cognitive impairment. *Cochrane Database Syst Rev* 2001;(2):CD001011.

89. Wei ZH, He QB, Wang H, Su BH, Chen HZ. Meta-analysis: the efficacy of nootropic agent Cerebrolysin in the treatment of Alzheimer's disease. *J Neural Transm* 2007;**114**:629–34.

90. Birks J, Flicker L. Selegiline for Alzheimer's disease. *Cochrane Database Syst Rev* 2003;(1):CD000442.

91. Wisniewski T, Konietzko U. Amyloid-beta immunisation for Alzheimer's disease. *Lancet Neurol* 2008;**7**:805–11.

92. Doody RS, Gavrilova SI, Sano M, *et al.*, dimebon investigators. Effect of dimebon on cognition, activities of daily living, behaviour, and global function in patients with mild-to-moderate Alzheimer's disease: a randomised, double-blind, placebo-controlled study. *Lancet* 2008;**372**:207–15.

93. De Deyn PP, Katz IR, Brodaty H, Lyons B, Greenspan A, Burns A. Management of agitation, aggression, and psychosis associated with dementia: a pooled analysis including three randomized, placebo-controlled double-blind trials in nursing home residents treated with risperidone. *Clin Neurol Neurosurg* 2005;**107**:497–508.

94. Katz I, de Deyn PP, Mintzer J, Greenspan A, Zhu Y, Brodaty H. The efficacy and safety of risperidone in the treatment of psychosis of Alzheimer's disease and mixed dementia: a meta-analysis of 4 placebo-controlled clinical trials. *Int J Geriatr Psychiatry* 2007;**22**:475–84.

95. Schneider LS, Dagerman KS, Insel P. Risk of death with atypical antipsychotic drug treatment for dementia: meta-analysis of randomized placebo-controlled trials. *JAMA* 2005;**294**:1934–43.

96. Gill SS, Bronskill SE, Normand SL, *et al.* Antipsychotic drug use and mortality in older adults with dementia. *Ann Intern Med* 2007;**146**:775–86.

97. Ballard CG, Thomas A, Fossey J, *et al.* A 3-month, randomized, placebo-controlled, neuroleptic discontinuation study in 100 people with dementia: the neuropsychiatric inventory median cutoff is a predictor of clinical outcome. *J Clin Psychiatry* 2004;**65**:114–9.

98. Tariot PN, Erb R, Podgorski CA, *et al.* Efficacy and tolerability of carbamazepine for agitation and aggression in dementia. *Am J Psychiatry* 1998;**155**:54–61.

99. Konovalov S, Muralee S, Tampi RR. Anticonvulsants for the treatment of behavioral and psychological symptoms of dementia: a literature review. *Int Psychogeriatr* 2008;**20**:293–308.

100. Bains J, Birks JS, Dening TR. Antidepressants for treating depression in dementia. *Cochrane Database Syst Rev* 2009;(4):CD003944.

CHAPTER 17

Management of amyotrophic lateral sclerosis

The EFNS Task Force on Diagnosis and Management of Amyotrophic Lateral Sclerosis:
P. M. Andersen (chairman),[1] S. Abrahams,[2] G. D. Borasio,[3] M. de Carvalho,[4] A. Chio,[5]
P. Van Damme,[6] O. Hardiman,[7] K. Kollewe,[8] K. E. Morrison,[9] S. Petri,[8] P.-F. Pradat,[10]
V. Silani,[11] B. Tomik,[12] M. Wasner,[3] M. Weber[13]

[1]Umeå University Hospital, Sweden; [2]University of Edinburgh, UK; [3]Munich University Hospital, Germany; [4]Hospital de Santa Maria, Lisbon, Portugal; [5]University of Turin and San Giovanni Hospital, Turin, Italy; [6]University of Leuven, Belgium; [7]Trinity College and Beaumont Hospital, Dublin, Ireland; [8]Medizinische Hochschule Hannover, Germany; [9]Queen Elizabeth Hospital and School of Clinical and Experimental Medicine, University of Birmingham, UK; [10]Hôpital de la Salpêtrière, Paris, France; [11]University of Milan Medical School, Italy; [12]Jagiellonian University Medical College, Krakow, Poland; [13]Kantonsspital St. Gallen, Switzerland

Introduction

Amyotrophic lateral sclerosis (ALS; also known as motor neuron disease, or MND) is characterized by symptoms and signs of degeneration of the upper and lower motor neurons, leading to progressive weakness of the bulbar, limb, thoracic and abdominal muscles. Other brain functions, including oculomotor and sphincter function, are relatively spared, although these may be involved in some patients. Cognitive dysfunction occurs in 20–50% of cases, and 5–15% develop dementia that is usually of frontotemporal type. Death due to respiratory failure follows on average 2–4 years after symptom onset, but a subgroup (approximately 10%) of patients may survive for a decade or more [1]. The mean age of onset is 47–52 years in familial and 58–63 years in sporadic cases of ALS [2]. The life-time risk of developing ALS is about 1 in 400–800, with male sex, increasing age, and hereditary disposition being the main risk factors [2, 3]. When diagnosing and managing a patient with ALS, it is important to recognize that ALS is a heterogeneous syndrome that overlaps with a number of other conditions, and that

misdiagnoses are not infrequent [4, 5]. This systematic review is an objective appraisal of the evidence regarding the diagnosis and clinical management of patients with ALS. The primary aim has been to establish evidence-based and patient- and carer-centred guidelines, with the secondary aim of identifying areas where further research is needed.

Search strategy

From 2008 through September 2009, two investigators screened potentially relevant citations independently. We searched the Cochrane Central Register of Controlled Trials (CENTRAL) (The Cochrane Library to date); MEDLINE-OVID (January 1966 on); MEDLINE-ProQuest; MEDLINE-EIFL; EMBASE-OVID (January 1990 on); the Science Citation Index (ISI); the National Research Register; the Oxford Centre for Evidence-based Medicine; the American Speech Language Hearing Association (ASHA); the World Federation of Neurology ALS page of reviews of published research; the Oxford Textbook of Palliative Medicine; and the UK Department of Health National Research Register (http://www.update-software.com/). We also searched national neurological databases (e.g. http://www.alsa.org and http://alsod.org) and personal collections of references and reference lists

European Handbook of Neurological Management: Volume 1,
2nd edition. Edited by N. E. Gilhus, M. P. Barnes and M. Brainin.
© 2011 Blackwell Publishing Ltd.

of articles. There were no constraints based on language or publication status. Any differences at any stage of the review were resolved by discussion. An earlier version of this report has already been published [6].

Results

Thirteen central issues in the management of ALS were addressed by the task force. The guidelines were prepared following the European Federation of Neurological Societies criteria [7], and the level of evidence and grade of recommendation are expressed in accordance with Brainen *et al.* [7]. Where there is a lack of evidence but consensus is clear, we have stated our opinion as Good Practice Points (GPP).

Diagnosing ALS/MND

Diagnosing ALS is usually straightforward if the patient has progressive, generalized symptoms in the bulbar and limb regions (table 17.1) [8]. Diagnosing the disease *early* in the disease course when the patient has limited symptoms in one or two regions (bulbar, upper limb, trunk, lower limb) may be difficult and depends on the presence

---

Table 17.1 Diagnostic criteria for ALS.

The diagnosis of ALS requires the presence of:
(positive criteria)
Lower motor neuron signs (including EMG features in clinically
   unaffected muscles)
Upper motor neuron signs
Progression of symptoms and signs

The diagnosis of ALS requires the absence of
(diagnosis by exclusion):
Sensory signs
Sphincter disturbances
Visual disturbances
Autonomic features
Basal ganglion dysfunction
Alzheimer-type dementia
ALS 'mimic' syndromes (Table 17.3)

The diagnosis of ALS is supported by:
Fasciculations in one or more regions
Neurogenic changes in EMG results
Normal motor and sensory nerve conduction
Absence of conduction block

ALS, amyotrophic lateral sclerosis; EMG, electromyography.

---

of signs in other affected regions and supportive findings in ancilliary investigations [9, 10]. The mean time from the onset of symptoms to confirmation of the diagnosis of ALS is 13–18 months [11, 12]. Delays tend to arise due to early or intermittent symptoms being unrecognized or denied by the patient or because of inefficient referral pathways to a neurologist. There are cogent reasons for making the diagnosis as early as possible. Psychologically, the lack of diagnosis, even of a disorder carrying a poor prognosis, causes distress and anxiety. Early diagnosis may save patients from undertaking onerous, unnecessary, and often expensive, tours of the healthcare system and allows them to better plan their future. Another motivator for early diagnosis is that it would give the chance of instigating neuroprotective therapies at an earlier stage in the disease process, when fewer neuronal cells are irreversibly compromised. Although no hard evidence exists on the kinetics of cell loss in ALS, it is reasonable to assume that the earlier neuroprotective medication is started, the greater its effect will be [13]. Studies in experimental animal models and humans with *SOD1* gene mutations indicate that the loss of motor neurons is preceded by a period of cellular dysfunction [14]. In both patients and animal models, the life-prolonging effect of riluzole is greater the earlier medication is initiated. The early administration of potential disease-modifying drugs can have a profound positive psychological effect [15].

The objective here is to present guidelines for making the correct diagnosis *and* to do this as early as possible. Since no single investigation is specific for ALS, and there is still no sensitive surrogate disease biomarker, diagnosis is based on symptoms, clinical examination findings, and the results of electrodiagnostic, neuroimaging, and laboratory studies (tables 17.1 and 17.2) [16]. Great care should be taken to rule out diseases that can masquerade as ALS (table 17.3) [17, 18]. In specialist practice, 5–8% of apparent ALS patients have an alternative diagnosis, which may be treatable in about half the cases [18–20]. An evolution of atypical symptoms and a lack of progression of typical symptoms are the most important 'red flags' suggesting an incorrect diagnosis of ALS [18]. The diagnosis should be regularly reviewed at different stages of the disease [21]. The revised El Escorial criteria (table 17.4, adapted from [22]) are too restrictive for use in routine clinical practice and are not suitable if the objective is to establish the diagnosis as early as possible [23]. The new Awaji algorithm may improve diagnostic

Table 17.2 Diagnosing amyotrophic lateral sclerosis/motor neuron disease: recommended investigations.

Test	Evidence class	Recommended mandatory tests	Recommended additional tests in selected cases
Clinical chemistry			
Blood			
Erythrocyte sedimentation rate	IV	x	–
C-reactive protein	IV	x	–
Haematological screen	IV	x	–
Aspartate aminotransferase, alanine aminotransferase, lactate dehydrogenase	IV	x	–
Thyroid-stimulating hormone, free T_4, free T_3 hormone assays	IV	x	–
Vitamin B_{12} and folate	IV	x	–
Serum protein electrophoresis	IV	x	–
Serum immunoelectrophoresis	IV	x	–
Creatine kinase	IV	x	–
Creatinine	IV	x	–
Electroclytes (Na^+, K^+, Cl^-, Ca^{2+}, HPO_4^{2-})	IV	x	–
Glucose	IV	x	–
Angiotensin-converting enzyme	IV	–	x
Lactate	IV	–	x
Hexoaminidase A and B assay	IV	–	x
Ganglioside GM-1 antibodies	IV	–	x
Anti-Hu, anti-MAG	IV	–	x
RA, antinuclear antibodies, anti-DNA	IV	–	x
Anti-acetylcholine receptor and anti-muscle-specific receptor tyrosine kinase antibodies	IV	–	x
Serology (*Borrelia*, virus including HIV)	IV	–	x
DNA analysis (for SOD1, SMN1/2, SBMA)	IV	–	x
CSF			
Cell count	IV	–	x
Cytology	IV	–	x
Total protein concentration	IV	–	x
Glucose, lactate	IV	–	x
Protein electrophoresis including IgG index	IV	–	x
Serology (*Borrelia*, virus)	IV	–	x
Ganglioside antibodies	IV	–	x
Urine			
Cadmium	IV	–	x
Lead (24-h secretion)	IV	–	x
Mercury	IV	–	x
Manganese	IV	–	x
Urine immunoelectrophoresis	IV	–	x
Neurophysiology		–	–
Electromyography	III	x	–
Nerve conduction velocity	III	x	–
Motor evoked potential	IV	–	x
Radiology			
Magnetic resonance imaging/computed tomography (cranial/cervical, thoracic, lumbar)	IV	x	–
Chest X-ray	IV	x	–
Mammography	IV	–	x
Biopsy			
Muscle	III	–	x
Nerve	IV	–	x
Bone marrow	IV	–	x
Lymph node	IV	–	x

Table 17.3 Diseases that can masquerade as ALS/MND.

Anatomical abnormalities/compression syndromes
Arnold–Chiari type 1 and other hindbrain malformations
Cervical, foramen magnum, or posterior fossa region tumours
Cervical disc herniation with osteochondrosis
Cervical meningeoma
Retropharyngeal tumour
Spinal epidural cyst
Spondylotic myelopathy and/or motor radiculopathy
Syringomyelia

Acquired enzyme defects
Adult GM_2 gangliosidosis (hexosaminidase A or B deficiency)
Polyglucosan body disease
Pompe's Disease (Glycogen Storage Disease type II)

Autoimmune syndromes
Monoclonal gammopathy with motor neuropathy
Multifocal motor neuropathy with/without conduction block
Dysimmune lower motor neuron syndromes (with GM_1, GD_{1b}, and asialo-GM_1 antibodies)
Other dysimmune lower motor neuron syndromes, including chronic inflammatory demyelinating polyneuropathy
Multiple sclerosis
Myasthenia gravis (in particular the anti-muscle-specific receptor tyrosine kinase positive variant)

Endocrine abnormalities
Allgrove syndrome
Diabetic 'amyotrophy'
Insulinoma causing neuropathy
Hyperthyroidism with myopathy
Hypothyroidism with myopathy
Hyperparathyroidism (primary)
Hyperparathyroidism (secondary due to vitamin D deficiency)
Hypokalemia (Conn's syndrome)

Exogenous toxins
Lead (?), mercury (?), cadmium, aluminium, arsenic, thallium, manganese, organic pesticides; neurolathyrism, konzo

Infections
Acute poliomyelitis
Post-poliomyelitis progressive muscular atrophy syndrome
HIV-1 (with vacuolar myelopathy)
HTLV-1-associated myelopathy (tropical spastic paraplegia)
Neuroborreliosis
Syphilitic hypertrophic pachymeningitis
Spinal encephalitis lethargica, varicella-zoster
Trichinosis
Brucellosis, cat-scratch disease
Prion disorders

Myopathies
Cachectic myopathy
Carcinoid myopathy
Dystrophin-deficient myopathy
Inclusion body myositis
Inflammatory myopathies

Nemaline myopathy
Polymyositis
Sarcoid myositis

Neoplastic syndromes
Chronic lymphocytic leukemia
Intramedullary glioma
Lymphoproliferative disorders with paraproteinemia and/or oligoclonal bands in the cerebrospinal fluid
Pancoast tumour syndrome
Paraneoplastic encephalomyelitis with anterior horn cell involvement
'Stiff person plus' syndromes

Physical injury
Electric shock neuronopathy
Radiation-induced radiculo-plexopathies and/or myelopathy

Vascular disorders
Arterioveneous malformation
Dejerine's anterior bulbar artery syndrome
Stroke
Vasculitis

Other neurological conditions
Western Pacific atypical forms of MND/ALS (Guam, New Guinea, Kii Peninsula of Japan)
Carribean atypical forms of MND–dementia–PSP (Guadeloupe)
Madras-form of juvenile onset MND/ALS (South India)
Frontotemporal dementia with MND/ALS (including Pick's disease with amyotrophy)
Multiple system atrophy
Olivo-ponto cerebellar atrophy syndromes
Primary lateral sclerosis (some subtypes not related to ALS)
Progressive encephalomyelitis with rigidity
PSP
Hereditary spastic paraplegia (many variants, some subtypes with distal amyotrophy)
Progressive spinal muscular atrophy (some subtypes not related to ALS)
Spinobulbar muscular atrophy with/without dynactin or androgen receptormutation
Spinal muscular atrophy I–IV
Brown–Vialetto–van Laere syndrome (early-onset bulbar and spinal ALS with sensorineural deafness)
Fazio–Londe syndrome (infantile progressive bulbar palsy)
Harper–Young syndrome (laryngeal and distal spinal muscular atrophy)
Monomelic sporadic spinal muscular atrophy (benign focal amyotrophy, including Hirayama syndrome)
Polyneuropathies with dominating motor symptoms (like hereditary motor and sensory neuropathy type 2, hereditary motor neuropathy type 5)
Familial amyloid polyneuropathy
Benign fasciculations
Myokymia

ALS, amyotrophic lateral sclerosis; MDN, motor neuron disease; PSP, Progressive supranuclear palsy.

Table 17.4 Revised El Escorial research diagnostic criteria for ALS – a summary.

Clinically definite ALS
UMN and LMN signs in three regions

Clinically definite ALS – laboratory supported
UMN and/or LMN signs in one region *and* the patient is a carrier of a pathogenic gene mutation

Clinically probable ALS
UMN and LMN signs in two regions with some UMN signs rostral to the LMN signs

Clinically probable ALS – laboratory supported
UMN signs in one or more regions *and* LMN signs defined by EMG in at least two regions

Clinically possible ALS
UMN and LMN signs in one region, or
UMN signs in at least two regions, or
UMN and LMN signs in two regions with no UMN signs rostral to LMN signs

ALS, amyotrophic lateral sclerosis; EMG, electromyography; LMN, lower motor neuron; UMN, upper motor neuron.

sensitivity with no loss in specificity as reported in a recent study [24, 32]. We do not recommend that patients are told they have 'definite, probable, or possible' ALS. Experience suggests that pursuing an early diagnosis of ALS outweighs the potential increase in risk of misdiagnosis (GPP). The clinician must decide, on the balance of probability, whether or not the patient has ALS, even in the absence of unequivocal upper and lower motor neuron signs [25] (GPP).

Good Practice Points

1. The diagnosis should be pursued as early as possible. Patients in whom ALS is suspected should be referred with high priority to an experienced neurologist.

2. All suspected new cases should undergo prompt detailed clinical and paraclinical examinations (see tables 17.1 and 17.2).

3. In some cases, additional investigations may be needed (see table 17.2).

4. Repetition of the investigations may be needed if initial tests do not result in a diagnosis.

5. Review of the diagnosis is advisable if there is no evidence of typical progression or if the patient develops atypical features (see table 17.1).

Breaking the news: communicating the diagnosis

Telling the patient and the family that the diagnosis is ALS is a daunting task for the physician. If not performed appropriately, the effect can be devastating, leaving the patient with a sense of abandonment and destroying the patient–physician relationship [26]. Surveys of patients and caregivers have demonstrated that the way the diagnosis is communicated is less than satisfactory in half of all cases [27, 28]. Studies of other fatal illnesses [29–31] clearly demonstrate the advantages of using specific techniques, such as those outlined in table 17.5. Better patient/caregiver satisfaction has been shown if effective communication strategies are used and more time is spent discussing the diagnosis [28]. A survey has shown that physicians in 44% of ALS centres routinely spend 30 min or less discussing the diagnosis [33]. Callous delivery of the diagnosis may affect the families'/carers' psychological adjustment to bereavement later [34].

Good Practice Points

1. The diagnosis should be communicated by a consultant with a good knowledge of the patient.

2. The physician should start the consultation by asking what the patient already knows or suspects.

3. The physician should give the diagnosis and discuss its implications in a *stepwise fashion*, checking that the patient understands what is being communicated. The diagnosis should be given in person, ensuring that enough time is available for an unhurried discussion (suggest at least 45–60 min). Provide printed materials about the disease, about support and advocacy organizations, and about informative websites if appropriate. A copy letter or audiotape summarising the discussion can be helpful for patients and their families.

4. Assure patients that they and their families will not be 'abandoned' by healthcare services but will be supported by a professional ALS care team (where available) and with regular follow-up visits to a neurologist. Before the end of the consultation, make arrangements for a follow-up visit (ideally within 2–4 weeks).

5. Avoid the following: withholding the diagnosis, providing insufficient information, imposing unwanted information, delivering information callously, and taking away or not providing hope.

Table 17.5 How should a physician tell patients that they have ALS?

Task	Recommendations
Location	Quiet, comfortable, and private
Structure	In person, face-to-face Convenient time (at least 45–60 minutes) Enough time to ensure there is no rushing or interruptions Make eye contact and sit close to the patient
Participants	Know the patient *before* the meeting, including the family, emotional, and social situation, case history, and all relevant test results. Have all the facts at hand Have the patient's support network present (relatives). Have a clinical nurse specialist or equivalent present or available
What is said	Find out what the patient already knows about the condition Ascertain how much the patient wants to know about ALS and tailor your information accordingly Give a warning comment that bad news is coming. The whole truth may need to come by instalments Use the correct ALS-term, not 'wear and tear of the motor nerves' Explain the anatomy of the disease (make a simple drawing) If the patient indicates that they want to know the course of the disease, be honest about the likely progression and prognosis, but give a broad time frame and recognise the limitations of any predictions There is no cure, symptoms tend to steadily worsen, and prognosis is highly variable Some patients survive 5, 10, or more years Acknowledge and explore the patient's reaction and allow for emotional expression Summarise the discussion verbally, in writing, and/or on an audiotape Allow plenty of time for questions
Reassurance	Acknowledge that this is devastating news, but discuss reasons for hope such as research, drug trials, and the variability of the disease Explain that the complications of ALS are treatable Reassure that every attempt will be made to maintain the patient's function and that the patient's treatment decisions will be respected Reassure that the patient will continue to be cared for and will not be abandoned Inform about patient support groups (offer contact details and leaflets) Inform about neuroprotective treatment (i.e. riluzole) and ongoing research Discuss opportunities to participate in research treatment protocols (if available) Acknowledge a willingness to get a second opinion if the patient wishes
How it is said	Emotional manner: warmth, caring, empathy, respect Be honest and sympathetic but not sentimental Give news at the person's pace; allow the patient to dictate what he or she is told
Language	Simple and careful word choice, yet direct; no euphemisms or medical jargon

ALS, amyotrophic lateral sclerosis.
Modified from Miller *et al.* [32].

Multidisciplinary care

Ideally, patients with ALS should be followed in specialist multidisciplinary clinics. These tertiary centres can provide both diagnostic and management services [25, 35, 36] with the emphasis on patient autonomy and choice. Comparisons between clinic-based cohorts and population-based cohorts of patients have confirmed a referral bias: patients attending multidisciplinary clinics tend to be younger and to have had symptoms for longer than those who do not [35, 37]. An independent survival benefit has been identified in two studies [36, 38], more relevant in bulbar patients, while another study has shown no effect [39]. Importantly, patients attending multidisciplinary clinics have fewer hospital admissions and shorter inpatient stays than those who attend general clinics [36]. Tertiary centres can also increase the sense of patient well-being, perhaps [40] related to a greater provision of appropriate aids and appliances [41]. The increased use of riluzole and non-invasive ventilation, attention to nutrition, and earlier referral to palliative care services are likely to contribute to the increased survival of those attending multidisciplinary clinics [35, 42]. Effective multidisciplinary clinics can be developed at modest cost using existing healthcare structures [43]. Excellent communication and cooperation between specialized clinics and the primary health care sector is crucial.

Good Practice Points

1. Multidisciplinary care should be available for people affected by ALS as attendance at multidisciplinary clinics improves care, promotes a sense of well-being, and may extend survival.

2. The following specialists should be part of or readily available to the multidisciplinary clinic team: a neurologist, respiratory physician, gastroenterologist, rehabilitation medicine physician, social counsellor, occupational therapist, speech therapist, respiratory therapist, specialized nurse, physical therapist, dietitian, psychologist, dentist, and palliative care physician.

3. Patients should generally be reviewed every 2–3 months, although they may require more frequent review in the first half-year following diagnosis or in the later stages of disease, and less frequent review if their disease is only slowly progressive. The patient support team should maintain regular contact with the patient and relatives between visits.

4. Ideally, the patient should from the outset be followed by one neurologist or palliative care specialist liaising closely with the patient's primary care physician (family general practitioner).

5. Effective channels of communication and co-ordination are essential between the hospital-based multidisciplinary clinic team, the primary care team, the palliative care team, and the community services.

ALS caregivers and strains

ALS causes a progressive loss of independence and an increased need for help with activities of everyday life. Carers therefore have to progressively increase the time they devote to caring [44], with resultant effects on their physical, psychological, and emotional well-being. The caregivers' burden relates to personal and social restrictions and psychological and emotional problems [45, 46]. Caregivers frequently search for information about ALS, and many actively participate in interactions between the patient and physician, from the time of diagnosis through to decision-making regarding advance directives and end of life care.

Certain ALS symptoms cause particular strain in carers. If the patient loses effective communication, carers can become intellectually and emotionally isolated. The use of augmentative alternative communication devices can help to restore communication. Several studies have shown that respiratory problems, in particular the provision of mechanical ventilation for patients, causes particular strain on caregivers, reducing their quality of life and raising their responsibilities related to managing the ventilator and providing for the increasing caring costs [47–49]. Although only rarely studied, data indicate that sexuality is an important and problematic issue for several ALS patient–caregiver couples. The problems reported were mainly decreased libido, passivity of the partner, and the carer's own passivity. The most frequent reasons cited were the physical weakness and the body image changes due to ALS [50].

Around 50% of patients with ALS in a cohort from the UK and Germany died at home [51]. The anticipation of patients' imminent deaths may increase caregiver distress and anxiety. However, Neudert *et al.* [51] report that most patients with ALS died peacefully and no patient 'choked to death' if good palliative care measures were in place. The likelihood of a peaceful death process should be communicated to patients and their caregivers/relatives (GPP).

Some caregivers go through the grieving process starting from the time that diagnosis is given. [52, 53]. It seems that the anticipation of future loss is as important as the loss itself in leading to psychological difficulties. Issues for the caregiver in particular are a feeling of being burned out from providing care, repercussions from forced changes in living arrangements to accommodate the patient's progressive weakness, and financial hardships [54].

Good Practice Points

1. Caregivers should be acknowledged in their double role in the disease process: they are one of the most important resources for the patient, yet they are affected themselves, and their needs as carers need to be addressed.

2. Ideally, caregivers should be involved when the diagnosis is given and in all clinical decisions, while preserving patients' autonomy.

3. Carers' own health needs should be considered. Physical, psychological, and spiritual support should be provided if appropriate.

4. Maintaining communication between patients and caregivers is of utmost importance.

5. Detailed information about the usual death process in patients with ALS should be given to caregivers if they ask for this.

6. Bereavement counselling and support should be offered to all caregivers.

Neuroprotective treatment/ disease-modifying treatment

To date, riluzole is the only drug that has been shown to slow the course of ALS in four Class I studies, possibly due to its anti-glutamatergic properties [55, 56]; a Cochrane review has also been published [57]. These studies did not include patients with early disease (i.e. with suspected or possible ALS according to the El Escorial criteria). Oral administration of 100 mg riluzole daily improved the 1-year survival by 15% and prolonged survival by about 3 months after 18 months' treatment. There was a clear dose effect. In clinical practice, retrospective Phase IV studies from four large clinical databases indicate that the overall gain in survival (i.e. over the whole extent of the disease course), may extend from around 6 to 20 months, although these estimates are almost certainly subject to various statistical biases [58–61]. The drug is safe, with few serious side effects. Guidelines for monitoring have been published by the National Institute for Health and Clinical Excellence. Although patients with progressive spinal muscular atrophy or primary lateral sclerosis were not included in the riluzole trials, pathological and genetic studies show that some patients with progressive spinal muscular atrophy and primary lateral sclerosis fall within the ALS syndrome, so may benefit from the drug [5, 62]. Riluzole may have little effect in late-stage ALS, and it is not clear if and when treatment should be terminated. A large number of other drugs have been tested in ALS, unfortunately with negative results (table 17.6).

Good Practice Points

1. Patients with ALS should be offered treatment with riluzole 50 mg twice daily (Class IA).

2. Patients treated with riluzole should be monitored regularly for safety (Class IA).

3. Treatment should be initiated as early as possible after diagnosis, taking into account expected therapeutic benefits and potential safety issues (Class IA). Realistic expectations for treatment effects and potential side effects should be discussed with the patient and caregivers.

4. Treatment with riluzole should be considered in patients with progressive spinal muscular atrophy and primary lateral sclerosis who have a first-degree relative with ALS.

5. Patients with slowly progressive sporadic progressive spinal muscular atrophy, sporadic primary lateral sclerosis or hereditary spastic paraplegia should as a rule not be treated with riluzole, but treatment should be considered in 'ALS-like' patients with clinical progressive spinal muscular atrophy or primary lateral sclerosis.

6. Irrespective of familial disposition, all patients with a symptomatic progressive MND and carrying a *SOD1* gene mutation should be offered treatment with riluzole.

7. Currently, there is insufficient evidence to recommend treatment with vitamins, testosterone, antioxidants such as co-enzyme Q-10 and gingko biloba, intravenous immunoglobulin therapy, cyclosporin, interferons, Copaxone, KDI tripeptide, neurotrophic factors (including vascular endothelial growth factor, insulin-like growth factor-1, and mecasermin rinfabate), ceftriaxone, creatine, gabapentin, minocycline, stem cells, or lithium.

Symptomatic treatment

Symptomatic treatment aims to improve the quality of life of patients and caregivers. Symptoms should be treated as they become prominent and incapacitating in individual patients.

Sialorrhoea

Sialorrhoea (drooling or excessive salivation) is a common symptom and may be socially disabling. It can result from impaired swallowing and may be treatable.

Amitriptyline is most commonly used, with reasonable efficacy at low cost [63]. Oral doses of not more than 25–50 mg two or three times a day are usually sufficient. Benefit can also be obtained using atropine drops, 0.5% or 1%, administered three or four times a day sublin-

Table 17.6 Summary of the most important controlled therapeutic studies in amyotrophic lateral sclerosis (ALS).

Completed trials	
N-Acetylcysteine*	Vitamin E* (two trials)
Brain-derived neurotrophic factor*	Xaliproden*
Branched-chain amino acids*	**Ongoing Phase II/III trials (2006–2010)**
Buspirone*	Arimoclomol
Celecoxib*	Ceftriaxone
Ciclosporin*	Cistanche total glycosides
Ciliary neurotrophic factor* (two trials)	Combination therapy (celecoxib, creatine, minocycline)
Co-enzyme Q10*	Copaxone
Creatine* (three trials)	Edaravone
Dextromethorphan*	Granulocyte colony-stimulating factor
Gabapentin*	Growth hormone
Glial-derived neurotrophic factor*	Lithium
IGF-1*(three trials)	Mecobalamin
Indinavir*	Olanzapine
Interferon-beta-1a*	Olesoxime
Lamotrigine* (two trials)	Pioglitazone
Lymphoid irradiation*	Pyrimethamine
Memantine*	SOD1 DNA antisense oligonucleotides
Minocyclin*	Talampanel
Nimodipine*	Tauroursodeoxycholic acid
ONO-2506*	**Phase III trials being planned or considered**
Oxandrolone*	AEOL 10150
Pentoxifylline*	Celastrol
Riluzole†	IGF-1 – viral delivery
Selegiline*	KNS-760704
TCH346*	NAALADase inhibitors
Thalidomide*	Nimesulide
Topiramate*	Ritonavir and hydroxyurea
Valproic acid*	Sodium phenylbutyrate
Verapamil*	Scriptaid
	VEGF

IGF-1, Insulin-like growth factor.
*No therapeutic benefit was observed.
†Riluzole is the only one of the drugs tested that has been shown to have an effect against ALS.

gually, which has the advantage of having a fairly short duration of action – valuable in patients who suffer from sialorrhoea alternating with an uncomfortably dry mouth. Glycopyrrolate (in nebulized or i.v. form) has been shown to be effective in patients with cerebral palsy or developmental disabilities in a Class I study [64], but no studies in ALS are known. Hyoscine (scopolamine) can also be effective, given orally or applied as a dermal patch. Two Class IV studies [65, 66] showed a reduction of salivary flow with transdermal scopolamine (1.5 mg every third day). Care is needed in elderly patients, due to the not infrequent side effect of confusion. Patients with severe drooling may need two patches (GPP). Injection of botulinum toxin (type A and type B) into the salivary glands may be beneficial [67–69]. The injections are generally well tolerated and may improve quality of life, but caution is recommended in patients with significant bulbar palsy as increased dysphagia may occur (GPP). In rare instances, serious side effects have been reported [70]. Another option is external irradiation of the salivary glands, with four Class IV studies showing satisfactory results [71–74].

Surgical interventions, such as transtympanic neurectomy, parotid duct ligation and relocation, and submandibular gland excision, have been reported to yield effective long-term results in children with drooling [75, 76]. However, case reports suggest that such procedures are less satisfactory in patients with ALS and may lead to problematic effects such as increased secretion of thick mucus; thus, they are not recommended [77].

Good Practice Points

1. Treat sialorrhoea in ALS with amitriptyline, oral or transdermal hyoscine, glycopyrrolate, or sublingual atropine drops.

2. Botulinum toxin injections into the parotid and/or submandibular gland may be effective and are generally well tolerated.

3. Irradiation of the salivary glands may be tried when pharmacological treatment fails.

4. Provide a portable mechanical home suction device.

5. Surgical interventions are not recommended.

Bronchial secretions

Patients with bulbar or respiratory insufficiency commonly report difficulties in effectively clearing tenacious sputum, and indeed mucus accumulation is a negative prognostic factor in ALS patients treated with non-invasive ventilation [78]. The mucosa of the nasal cavity, larynx, trachea, bronchial airways, and lungs contribute a constant flow of serous and mucoid fluids. Although no studies exist, it is likely that dehydration increases the viscosity of mucus. A portable home suction device may be useful for clearing the upper airways (and excess saliva in the mouth). However, secretions in the lower airways can be difficult to reach, and repeated use of a catheter may stimulate secretions. Medication with mucolytics like guaifenesin or N-acetylcysteine, a beta-receptor antagonist (such as metoprolol or propranolol), and/or an anticholinergic bronchodilator like ipratropium and/or theophylline, or even furosemide, can be of value, but no controlled studies in ALS exist [79]. In a Class I study in critically ill patients with chronic obstructive pulmonary disease, sublingual potassium dichromate signifi-

cantly decreased the amount of stringy tracheal secretions [80]. Mechanical cough-assist devices (insufflator–exsufflator) via a face mask have been reported to be effective in ALS patients in uncontrolled trials [81,82].

Good Practice Points

1. Consider using a mucolytic like N-acetylcysteine, 200–400 mg three times daily.

2. Try a nebulizer with saline and a beta-receptor antagonist and/or an anticholinergic bronchodilator and/or a mucolytic and/or furosemide in combination. Mucolytics should only be used if sufficient cough flow is present.

3. Sublingual potassium dichromate may be helpful.

4. Teach the patient and carers the technique of assisting expiratory movements using a manual assisted cough (can also be performed by a physical therapist).

5. The use of a mechanical insufflator–exsufflator may be helpful, particularly in the setting of an acute respiratory infection.

6. Provide a portable home suction device and a room humidifier.

7. Cricopharyngeal myotomy may be helpful in rare cases with frequent episodes of cricopharyngeal spasm and severe bronchial secretions.

Pseudobulbar emotional lability

Emotional lability occurs in at least 50% of ALS patients irrespective of the presence or absence of bulbar motor signs [83]. Emotional lability does not correlate with cognitive impairment [84]. Prominent pseudobulbar features such as pathological weeping, laughing, or yawning can be socially disabling and affect patients' quality of life. Currently, there are no approved treatments for pseudobulbar emotional lability. The most commonly used agents are tricyclic antidepressants and selective serotonin reuptake inhibitors (SSRIs), which have been found to be effective in small placebo-controlled studies or case series [85]. Dopamine and lithium have been tested with good effect in other neurological diseases [86, 87]. A randomized controlled trial of a combination of dextrometorphan and quinidine showed efficacy in improving emotional lability and quality of life [88]. Side effects were experienced by 89% of patients, and 24% discontinued treatment.

Cramps

Cramps may be an early and troublesome symptom, particularly at night. Class I studies using quinine sulphate or vitamin E in non-ALS patients with leg cramps showed a positive effect only for quinine [89, 90]. Treatments such as massage, physical exercise, hydrotherapy in heated pools, carbamazepine, diazepam, phenytoin, and verapamil have be tried, but evidence of efficacy is lacking.

Spasticity

Physical therapy is the mainstay of treatment of spasticity in ALS, and has been shown to be effective in a Class IIB study [91]. Other interventions such as hydrotherapy, heat, cold, ultrasound, electrical stimulation, chemodenervation, and in rare cases surgery can be used, although no controlled studies in ALS exist. In a Class III study of 20 patients with spinal cord injury, the use of hydrotherapy in heated pools three times per week produced a significant decrease in spasm severity and a reduction of oral baclofen medication [92]. Cryotherapy of the facial muscles reduced spasticity to facilitate dental care in 24 patients with cerebral palsy [93]. Intrathecal baclofen in patients with ALS, intractable spasticity, and associated pain was more effective than oral medication and greatly improved patients' quality of life [94, 95]. Other drugs

have not been tested formally in ALS, but in clinical practice gabapentin (900–2400 mg daily), tizanidine (6–24 mg daily), memantine (10–60 mg daily), dantrolene (25–100 mg daily), tetrazepam (100–200 mg daily), and diazepam (10–30 mg daily) have been used. Botulinum toxin A has successfully been used to treat trismus and stridor in single cases [96].

Depression and anxiety

Depression and anxiety occur frequently in ALS patients and their caregivers [97, 98]. Anxiety seems to be particularly prevalent during the diagnostic and terminal phases [97, 99]. No formal studies with antidepressants have been conducted in patients with ALS, but empirically tricyclic antidepressants (e.g. amitriptyline) and SSRIs such as escitalopram are effective. A new alternative is mirtazapine, which is well tolerated in the later stages when SSRIs and amitriptyline may not be. The choice may be guided by additional symptoms (e.g. sialorrhoea, insomnia, apathy, appetite loss), which are differently affected by the various antidepressants. There are no systematic studies on anxiolytics in ALS. Some antidepressants, such as escitalopram, exert anxiolytic effects, but oral diazepam or sublingual lorazepam may be necessary.

Insomnia and fatigue

Insomnia is common in the final months of life in patients with ALS [100]. There are likely to be several causes, including depression, cramps, pain, and respiratory distress, which if identified should be treated first. For insomnia in ALS, amitriptyline and zolpidem are the most commonly used medications [63]. Fatigue is a frequent and potentially debilitating symptom. It is multifactorial and may be of central and/or peripheral origin [101]. One open-label study and one Class I study with modafinil revealed a significant reduction of fatigue with a number-needed-to-treat of 1.6 [102, 103]. However, its long-term effects in ALS have not yet been studied.

Good Practice Points

1. Treat insomnia with amitriptyline, mirtazapine, or appropriate hypnotics (e.g. zolpidem).
2. For debilitating, fatigue modafinil may be considered.

Pain

Pain occurs frequently in ALS, more often in the advanced stages of the disease, and is mainly due to immobility [51, 104] or respiratory insufficiency with morning headache. Treatment is unspecific and should follow accepted principles. Opioids can be used, following the 1990 World Health Organization analgesic ladder guidelines, when non-narcotics fail [105]: begin treatment with non-steroidal anti-inflammatory drugs, followed by weak opioids such as tramadol, followed by strong opioids such as morphine or ketobemidone. A liberal use of opioids may be appropriate when non-narcotics fail, and these have the secondary advantages of alleviating dyspnoea and anxiety.

Good Practice Points

Treat pain in ALS following accepted guidelines.

Venous thrombosis

Patients with ALS have an increased risk of deep venous thrombosis (DVT), with an annual incidence rate of 2.7% [106, 107]. The increased risk correlates with greater immobility and impaired respiratory function,

but is independent of the patient's age. Since DVTs may be asymptomatic, the incidence of venous thrombosis is probably underestimated. There are no studies regarding the management of DVT in patients with ALS.

Good Practice Points

1. DVT should be treated with anticoagulants.
2. The optimum management of risk factors for venous thrombosis should be pursued. Physiotherapy, limb elevation, and/or compression stockings are recommended.
3. There is currently insufficient evidence to recommend prophylactic treatment with anticoagulants.

Unproven therapies

The use of complementary and alternative medicine (CAM) is frequent in ALS. Wasner *et al.* found that 54% of 350 patients reported the use of CAM, in most cases (60%) performed by a physician [108]. In a survey in 53 ALS patients, the most frequently used types of CAM were vitamins, herbal supplements, or alternative therapies such as homeopathy and acupuncture [109].

Stem cell therapy is still in the early experimental development in ALS. However, the nature of the disease may induce patients to seek transplantation procedures. The intravenous, intrathecal, or intraparenchymal administration of haematopoietic stem cells derived from peripheral blood or bone marrow has been tested in small series of patients [110–114]. In these uncontrolled studies, even if safety and lack of side effects were claimed, the majority of these studies did not exhibit good scientific evidence for the procedure before translation to clinical application [115, 116]. Clinical efficacy is unproven, and long-term safety needs to be demonstrated.

A number of patients with ALS have been reported having received intracerebral transplantation of olfactory ensheathing cells [117, 118], sometimes with serious side effects [119]. No sham operations have been documented, and the scientific basis for the use of such cells for treating ALS is meager. Frequently, these studies have not been performed in accordance with good scientific practice in well-designed clinical trials.

The intrathecal application of neuroprotective agents has been tried in order to circumvent the blood–brain barrier. Pilot trials have used thyrotropin-releasing hormone [120], interferon-alfa [121], human recombinant SOD1 [122], ciliary neurotrophic factor, and brain-derived neurotrophic factor [123–125], all without evidence of clinical benefit. Recently, insulin-like growth factor-1 has been injected intrathecally in nine ALS patients safely and with a reported modest clinical effect [126].

In randomized, controlled, and open studies, liquor-pheresis (filtration of cerebrospinal fluid) has been performed in one familial ALS and 10 sporadic ALS patients, without clinical effect [127, 128].

A Phase 1 safety study of hyperbaric oxygen therapy in five patients with ALS reported some efficacy on fatigue in four patients [129].

Repetitive transcranial magnetic stimulation of the motor cortex reportedly had a beneficial effect in a pilot trial, but a double-blind study is recommended [130].

3. Patients with ALS must be carefully informed about existing reliable data related to cell therapies. It should be emphasized to the patient that all treatments with cell transplantation are experimental and that there is no proven scientific effect on disease outcome. If they then decide to undergo transplantation, thorough examination before and after the stem cell treatment should be performed and documented to improve our knowledge of benefits and/or side effects.

4. Adequate and updated unbiased information related to cell therapies and other unproven/alternative therapies need to be delivered to the patient community.

5. All studies, including transplantation of stem cells in ALS, should be performed in full accordance with the Declaration of Helsinki (WMA, 1964).

6. Larger surveys are needed to evaluate the use of alternative/complementary therapies by ALS patients.

Good Practice Points

1. For cellular therapies to become a reality, a more thorough preclinical evaluation and elucidation of several open questions is mandatory.

2. Even if cell transplantation might be a possible approach for the future, no well-designed clinical trials testing cellular therapies have been completed demonstrating safety and clinical efficacy supported by pathological evidence in a sufficient number of patients.

Genetic testing and counselling

In different populations, the frequency of familial ALS is reportedly 5–10% of all ALS cases (table 17.7) but may be underestimated for a number of reasons (table 17.8). Presently, mutations in eight genes – *SOD1*, *VAPB*, *SETX*, *ALSIN*, *ANG*, *FUS*, *OPTN*, and TDP43 – have been found to cause ALS. At present, mutations in the latter seven genes appear to be very rare, and analysis is only performed in a research setting. A few patients (often

Table 17.7 Frequency of familial ALS in some epidemiological studies.

Study area:	% Familial ALS	*n*	Year	Reference
British Columbia, Canada	18.5	254	2008	Eisen *et al.* [131]
Germany	13.5	251	1959	Haberlandt [132]
Central Finland	11.6	36	1983	Murros, Fogelholm [133]
USA	9.5	1200	1995	Haverkamp *et al.* [2]
Belgium	8.6	140	2000	Thijs *et al.* [134]
Nova Scotia, Canada	5.8	52	1974	Murray *et al.* [135]
Wärmland, Sweden	5.6	89	1984	Gunnarsson, Palm [136]
England	5.0	580	1988	Li *et al.* [137]
USA	4.9	668	1978	Rosen AD [11]
Northern Sweden	4.7	128	1983	Forsgren *et al.* [1]
Sardinia, Italy	4.4	182	1983	Giagheddu *et al.* [138]
Jutland, Denmark	2.7	186	1989	Højer-Pedersen *et al.* [139]
Hong Kong	1.2	84	1996	Fong *et al.* [140]
Finland	0.8	255	1977	Jokelainen [141]

ALS, amyotrophic lateral sclerosis.

Table 17.8 Factors that may lead to underrepresentation of familial ALS cases.

1. Different diagnostic ALS-criteria have been used
2. Inadequate recording of a pertinent family history in patients' charts
3. The ALS disease expresses itself with different subtypes of ALS (e.g. progressive bulbar palsy, progressive spinal muscular atrophy) in different members of the family and os therefore not recognized as being one disease entity
4. Reluctance of the patient to report a hereditary disease
5. Loss of contact between different members of a family
6. Early death to other causes of individuals in the family who transmits the gene defect
7. The child develops ALS before the parent who transmitted the gene defect
8. Incomplete disease penetrance
9. Family members with ALS were misdiagnosed
10. Illegitimacy
11. Genealogical investigations were not performed

ALS, amyotrophic lateral sclerosis.

Table 17.9 Disease penetrance in amyotrophic lateral sclerosis associated with a *SOD1* gene mutation.

Complete penetrance (symptomatic disease in over 90% by age 70 years)
A4V, G37R, L38V, G41S, H43R, H46R, D76V, L84F, L84V, N86K, D90A homozygous, E100G, D101H, I104F, G108V, C111Y, I112M, G114A, L126GQRWKX, G127GGQRWKX, G141E, L144F, V148G, V148I

Incomplete penetrance
A4T, L8Q, N19S, E21G, N65S, G72S, D76Y, N86S, A89V, D90A heterozygous, G93D, A95T, G93S, S105L, D109Y, I113T, L117V, L126S, N139H

Table 17.10 *SOD1* gene mutations reported in patients with apparently sporadic amyotrophic lateral sclerosis.

A4V, L8V, G12R, V14G, G16S, N19S, E21K, V29A, H48Q, C57R, N65S, G72S, D76Y, H80R (only *de novo* mutation confirmed), L84F, N86I, N86S, N86D, A89V, D90A,G93S, A95T, V97L, I99V, D101N, S105delSL, L106P, D109Y, I113T, T116R, L117V, V118L, V118KTGPX, D124G, G127R, E133ΔE, K136X, L144F

Table 17.11 Disease survival time in amyotrophic lateral sclerosis associated with *SOD1* gene mutations (without artificial ventilation).

Short (<3 years)	Intermediate (3–10 years)	Long (>10 years)	Variable
A4T	G12R	G41D	E21G
A4V	G93V	H46R	G37R
C6F	E100G	N65S	L38V
C6G	D101G	D76V	D76Y
V7E	D101N	A89V	L84F
L8Q	S105L	D90A hom	L84V
G10V	G108V	G93C	N86S
G41S	C111Y	G93D	D90A het
H43R	N139H	G93S	G93R
H48Q	G141E	E100K	I104F
D90V		I113F	I113I
G93A			L144F
D101H			L144S
D101Y			
L106V			
I112M			
I112T			
R115G			
L126X			
G127X			
A145T			
V148G			
V148I			

het, heterozygous; hom, homozygous.

diagnosed as sporadic ALS) with private DNA mutations in the *NF-H, EAAT2, NAIP*, peripherin, *HFE, PON1, PON2, SPG4*, chromogranin, and dynactin genes have also been reported, but causation remains to be proved.

Since 1993, 155 mutations have been reported in the *SOD1* gene [62]. The most frequent mutation is D90A, which in many European countries is inherited as a recessive trait with a characteristic slowly progressing phenotype, although pedigrees with dominantly (heterozygous) inherited D90A-*SOD1* and an aggressive phenotype have also been reported [62, 142]. Around 12–23% of patients diagnosed with familial ALS carry a *SOD1* mutation. *SOD1* mutations have also been described in 2–7%

of apparently sporadic ALS patients, suggesting that some *SOD1* mutations are frequently non-penetrant (tables 17.9 and 17.10) [143]. A DNA *SOD1* diagnostic test speeds up the diagnostic process and can be of help in diagnosing patients with atypical features [62], as well as providing some prognostic information (tables 17.11 and 17.12) [142] (GPP). There is no specific therapy for patients with *SOD1* gene mutations, but clinical trials targeting *SOD1* specifically are currently underway. Pre-

Table 17.12 *SOD1* gene mutations associated with atypical features of amyotrophic lateral sclerosis (such as neuralgic pain syndrome, heat sensations, bladder disturbance, severe cognitive dysfunction).

A4V, V14G, E21G, G41S, H46R, H48Q, L84F, D90A, G93S, E100G, D101Y, I104F, I113T, L117V, V118L, L144F, I151T.

symptomatic (predictive) genetic testing should only be performed in first-degree adult blood-relatives of patients with a known *SOD1* gene mutation (GPP). Testing should only be performed on a strictly voluntary basis as outlined (table 17.13). Special consideration should be taken before presymptomatic testing is performed in familial ALS families where the mutation is associated with reduced disease penetrance (see table 17.9) or with a variable prognosis (see table 17.11) (GPP).

Good Practice Points

1. In all patients suspected of suffering from ALS, progressive spinal muscular atrophy, primary lateral sclerosis, or frontotemporal dementia, a detailed medical history of the patient, siblings, parents, *and* grandparents *and* their siblings should be obtained to disclose a familial disease with reduced disease penetrance.

2. Clinical DNA analysis for *SOD1* gene mutation should only be performed in cases with a known family history of ALS, and in sporadic ALS cases with the characteristic phenotype of the D90A mutation.

3. Clinical DNA analysis for *SOD1* gene mutations should *not* be performed in cases with sporadic ALS with a typical classical ALS phenotype.

4. In familial or sporadic cases where the diagnosis is uncertain, a SMN, androgen receptor, or *SOD1* DNA analysis may accelerate the diagnostic process.

5. Before blood is drawn for DNA analysis, the patient should receive genetic counselling. Give the patient time for consideration. DNA analysis should be performed only with the patient's informed consent.

6. Presymptomatic genetic testing should *only* be performed in first-degree adult blood-relatives of patients with a known *SOD1* gene mutation. Testing should only be performed on a strictly voluntary basis and should follow accepted ethical principles (table 17.13).

7. Results of DNA analysis performed on patients and their relatives as part of a research project should not be used in clinical practice or disclosed to the unaffected relative. The research results should be kept in a separate file and not in the patient's standard medical chart.

Respiratory management in patients with ALS

Respiratory complications are the main cause of death in ALS. They predominantly derive from diaphragmatic weakness but can be precipitated by aspiration and infection [144]. Forced vital capacity and vital capacity are the most widely used tests to evaluate respiratory function and should be performed regularly, along with an assessment of symptoms suggestive of respiratory insufficiency (table 17.14). Sniff nasal pressure (SNP) may be more accurate in patients with weak lips, but neither forced vital capacity nor SNP is a sensitive predictor of respiratory insufficiency in patients with severe bulbar involvement [145]. Percutaneous nocturnal oximetry is an easy tool to screen patients with and can be useful to determine the need for non-invasive positive-pressure ventilation (NIPPV) [146]. Phrenic nerve responses can predict hypoventilation in ALS [147]. Blood gas abnormalities are generally a late finding. Peak cough flow can access cough effectiveness [148].

NIPPV and, less frequently, invasive mechanical ventilation (IMV), is used to alleviate symptoms of respiratory insufficiency and prolong survival. There is no clear evidence regarding the timing and criteria for use of NIPPV and IMV in patients with ALS (table 17.15). The use of mechanical ventilation varies between countries, reflecting economic and cultural differences [32, 149]. Ideally, the patient's advance directives and a plan for management of respiratory insufficiency should be established before respiratory complications occur [25, 32, 149].

NIPPV increases survival and overall improves patient quality of life (Class I evidence), and is the preferred therapy to alleviate respiratory insufficiency [49, 151–154]. It is usually initially used only at night to alleviate symptoms of nocturnal hypoventilation (see table 17.14). NIPPV has not been shown to prolong survival in bulbar-onset patients, but even so, it improves quality of life in this subgroup too [152]. Bulbar-onset patients tend to be less compliant with NIPPV, due in part to increased secretions [78]. NIPPV also prolongs survival in patients presenting with respiratory insufficiency, who represent about 3% of all patients with ALS [155]. The use of diaphragmatic pacing or respiratory exercise in ALS is not established [156, 157].

IMV can prolong survival in ALS, in some cases for many years. However, it is not documented that quality

Table 17.13 Guidelines for presymptomatic genetic testing in amyotrophic lateral sclerosis.

1. The test subject should belong to a family with a known *SOD1* gene mutation
2. The test subject should be a first-degree relative of an affected blood relative, or a second-degree relative of an affected case if the first-degree relative is deceased from other causes
3. The test subject should be 18 years or older
4. The test subject should be mentally and physically healthy
5. The test subject should not be under emotional stress (e.g. recently married or divorced, has become unemployed, pregnant, etc.)
6. The test subject should participate as a volunteer without influence from a third party
7. The test subject should receive a minimum of two genetic counselling sessions before the blood is drawn
8. The test subject can request more than two genetic counselling sessions
9. Genetic counselling should be given by professionals with a specific knowledge about amyotrophic lateral sclerosis and genetics
10. After the blood sample has been drawn, the mutation analysis should be performed as quickly as possible to minimise the emotional discomfort of the procedure
11. The test subject should be informed of the test result at a personal meeting with a genetic counsellor. The test result should never be given by letter or electronic communication
12. It is advisable that the test subject be accompanied by a close friend at the genetic counselling sessions and when the test result is announced
13. The test subject can at any time demand that the blood sample and test records be destroyed
14. The test subject can at any time and without explanation withdraw from the test procedure and choose not to be informed of the test result
15. Professional and community resources should be available to deal with the impact of the test result on the test subject and relatives
16. The test result is private and should be kept in a separate file in the medical chart
17. The test result is private, and no third party can request taking part in the result (unless regulated otherwise by national legislation)

Table 17.14 Symptoms and signs of respiratory insufficiency in amyotrophic lateral sclerosis.

Symptoms	Signs
Dyspnoea on minor exertion or talking	Tachypnoea
Orthopnoea	Use of auxiliary respiratory muscles
Frequent nocturnal awakenings	Paradoxical movement of the abdomen
Excessive daytime sleepiness	Decreased chest wall movement
Daytime fatigue	Weak cough
Morning headache	Sweating
Difficulty clearing secretions	Tachycardia
Apathy	Morning confusion, hallucinations
Poor appetite	Weight loss
Poor concentration and/or memory	Mouth dryness

Modified from Leigh *et al.* [25].

of life is improved by IMV, and there is a risk that some patients will become totally unable to communicate and develop a 'locked-in' state. The availability and cultural acceptability of IMV in ALS patients varies greatly between different countries and cultures. It is costly and has significant emotional and social impact on patients and caregivers (table 17.16) [32, 48, 158].

A difficult issue is that of when to terminate ventilatory support. Parenteral morphine, a benzodiazepine, and an antiemetic are used when the patient decides that ventilatory support should be withdrawn [32]. There is good evidence for the use of opioids and/or oxygen to treat dyspnoea in patients with terminal cancer or chronic obstructive pulmonary disease (Class I) [159, 160], but no controlled studies in ALS exist.

Improving the clearance of bronchial secretions is important in patients with ALS to promote quality of life, improve NIPPV tolerance, and decrease the risk of infection. Techniques such as the provision of cough-assist devices and chest wall oscillation may be of value (see above) [82, 161, 162].

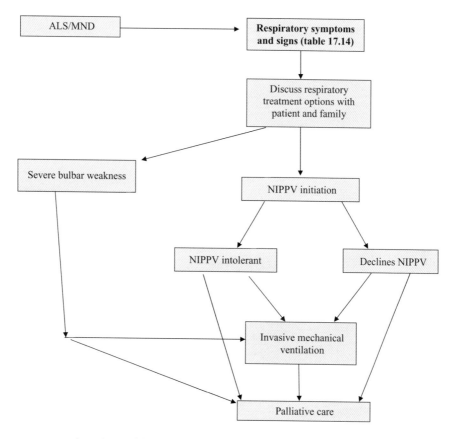

NIPPV, non-invasive positive-pressure ventilation.

Figure 17.1. Flowchart for the management of respiratory dysfunction in amyotrophic lateral sclerosis (ALS)/motor neuron disease (MND).

Good Practice Points

1. Symptoms or signs of respiratory insufficiency (including symptoms of nocturnal hypoventilation) should be checked at each visit.

2. Forced vital capacity and vital capacity are the most available and practical tests for the regular monitoring of respiratory function.

3. SNP may be used for monitoring, particularly in bulbar patients with weak lips.

4. Percutaneous nocturnal oximetry is recommended as a screening test and for monitoring respiratory function.

5. Symptoms or signs of respiratory insufficiency should prompt discussions with the patient and caregivers about treatment options and the terminal phase. Early discussions are needed to allow advance planning and directives.

6. NIPPV should be considered in preference to IMV in patients with symptoms or signs of respiratory insufficiency.

7. Active management of secretions and provision of cough assist devices can increase the effectiveness of assisted ventilation in ALS.

8. NIPPV can prolong survival for many months and can improve the patient's quality of life.

9. NIPPV and IMV have a major impact upon caregivers, and should be initiated only after informed discussion.

10. Unplanned (emergency) IMV should be avoided through an early discussion of end of life issues, co-ordination with palliative care teams, and appropriate advance directives.

11. Oxygen therapy alone should be avoided as it may exacerbate carbon dioxide retention and oral dryness. Use oxygen only if symptomatic hypoxia is present.

12. The medical treatment of intermittent dyspnoea should involve:

– for short dyspnoeic bouts: relieve anxiety and give lorazepam 0.5–2.5 mg sublingually;

– for longer phases of dyspnoea (>30 minutes): give morphine 2.5 mg orally or s.c.

13. For the medical treatment of chronic dyspnoea, start with morphine 2.5 mg orally four to six times daily. For severe dyspnoea, give morphine s.c. or as an i.v. infusion. Start with 0.5 mg/h and titrate. If needed, add midazolam (2.5–5 mg) or diazepam for nocturnal symptom control and to relieve anxiety (figure 17.1).

Table 17.15 Proposed criteria for NIPPV [25,146, 150].

Symptoms/signs related to respiratory muscle weakness. At least one of the following:
Dyspnoea
Tachypnoea
Orthopnoea
Disturbed sleep due to nocturnal desaturation/arousals
Morning headache
Use of auxiliary respiratory muscles at rest
Paradoxical respiration
Daytime fatigue
Excessive daytime sleepiness (ESS > 9)

and

Abnormal respiratory function tests. At least one of the following:
Forced vital capacity <80% of predicted value
Sniff nasal pressure <40 cmH$_2$O
PI max <60 mmH2O
Significant nocturnal desaturation on overnight oximetry
Morning blood gas pCO$_2$ > 45 mmHg

ESS, Epworth Sleepiness Score.

Table 17.16 The advantages and drawbacks of invasive mechanical ventilation.

Advantages
Prevents aspiration
Ability to provide more effective ventilator pressures and better gas exchange

Drawbacks
Generates more bronchial secretions
Increases risk of infection
Introduces risk of tracheo-oesophageal fistula, tracheal stenosis, or tracheomalacia
Greatly increased costs
Increased family and carer burden, including 24-h nursing requirement
Ethical issues regarding discontinuation

Enteral nutrition in patients with ALS

Weight loss and body impedance analysis changes [163] are independent prognostic factors of survival in ALS. Data are appearing indicating that ALS patients have an increased resting energy expenditure [164, 165]. The initial management of dysphagia in patients with ALS is based on dietary counselling, modification of food and fluid consistency (blending food, adding thickeners to liquids), prescription of high-protein and high-caloric supplements, and education of the patient and carers in feeding and swallowing techniques such as supraglottic swallowing and postural changes [166, 167]. Flexing the neck forward on swallowing to protect the airway ('chin-tuck manoeuvre') may be helpful. Some patients with difficulty swallowing tap water can drink fluids containing carbonate and/or citrate, and/or ice-cold fluids. As dysphagia progresses, these measures become insufficient, and tube feeding is needed. Three procedures obviate the need for major surgery and general anaesthesia: percutaneous endoscopic gastrostomy (PEG), percutaneous radiologic gastrostomy (PRG, or radiologically inserted gastrostomy), and nasogastric tube (NGT) feeding.

PEG is the standard procedure for enteral nutrition in ALS and is widely available [166, 167]. PEG improves nutrition, but there is no convincing evidence that it prevents aspiration or improves quality of life or survival [167]. The procedure requires mild sedation and is therefore more hazardous in patients with respiratory impairment and/or at an advanced stage of the disease [166, 167]. Non-invasive ventilation during the PEG procedure may be feasible in ALS patients with respiratory impairment. The timing of PEG is mainly based on symptoms, nutritional status, and respiratory function [167]. To minimize risks, PEG should be performed before vital capacity falls below 50% of predicted [168, 169].

PRG is a newer alternative to PEG and has the major advantage that it does not require patient sedation for insertion [167, 170, 171]. The rate of successful PRG insertion is reportedly higher than that for PEG [170, 172], but PRG is not widely available. NGT insertion is a minor procedure that can be performed on all patients, but it has several disadvantages [167, 173]. NGT placement increases oropharyngeal secretions and is associated with nasopharyngeal discomfort, pain, or even ulceration.

A recent observational study suggested that home parenteral nutrition is possible in patients with advanced ALS and poor respiratory function as an alternative to enteral feeding [174]. However, further studies are needed to evaluate the safety and efficacy of this method.

Good Practice Points

1. Bulbar dysfunction and nutritional status, including at least weight, should be checked at each visit. Difficulty drinking tap water is frequently the first sign of significant dysphagia.

2. Patients should be referred to a dietitian as soon as dysphagia appears. A speech and language therapist can give valuable advice on swallowing techniques.

3. The timing of PEG/PRG is based on an individual approach taking into account bulbar symptoms, malnutrition (weight loss of over 10 %), respiratory function, and the patient's general condition. Early insertion of a feeding tube is highly recommended.

4. When PEG is indicated, patient and carers should be informed: (1) of the benefits and risks of the procedure; (2) that it is possible to continue to take food orally as long as it is possible; and (3) that deferring PEG to a late disease stage may increase the risk of the procedure.

5. PRG is a suitable alternative to PEG. This procedure can be used as the procedure of choice or when PEG is deemed hazardous.

6. Tubes with relatively large diameter (e.g. 18–22 Charrière) are recommended for both PEG and PRG in order to prevent tube obstruction.

7. Prophylactic medication with antibiotics on the day of the operation may reduce the risk of infections.

8. NGT may be used for short-term feeding and when PEG or PRG is not suitable.

Cognition in ALS

ALS is associated with a frontotemporal syndrome in a significant proportion of cases, and these patients have a shorter survival [175]. Suggested risk factors include old age, male sex, poor education, family history of dementia, low forced vital capacity, pseudobulbar palsy, and a bulbar site of onset, although the data are not conclusive [176].

Between 5% and 15% of patients with ALS meet the diagnostic criteria for frontotemporal dementia, typically a frontal variant with marked executive dysfunction and behaviour change [177]. Progressive non-fluent aphasia and semantic dementia have also been reported [178]. Another 25–50% show mild cognitive (ALSci) and/or behavioural (ALSbi) impairment [179]. ALSci is associated with early deficits in verbal fluency and a mild dysexecutive syndrome [180]. ALSbi presents with behaviour change that partially meets the criteria for frontotemporal dementia, including disinhibition, loss of insight, lack of volition/apathy, and stereotyped and ritualistic behaviour [181, 182]. Impairment in emotional processing and social cognition has also been described [183, 184].

Carers may be unaware of mild impairment as increasing physical disability results in a loss of autonomy and a greater reliance on others for daily tasks. Executive dysfunction may manifest as difficulties in managing affairs/finances, planning for the future, making decisions, and learning new tasks, including the use of equipment associated with symptomatic treatment for ALS (e.g. gastrostomy, NIPPV). Language changes may manifest as reduced verbal output (see the next section).

Assessing predictors of frontotemporal dysfunction in ALS is an important research area. Atrophy on magnetic resonance imaging, or ocular fixation instabilities, may be biomarkers of behavioural and cognitive abnormalities [185–187].

A number of screening batteries have been proposed for diagnosing cognitive impairment [176, 188, 189]. Verbal fluency deficits are a sensitive measure of cognitive dysfunction if testing is appropriately modified to account for physical deficits and results standardized to educational attainment and premorbid IQ [176]. More extensive full neuropsychological assessment is warranted where cognitive impairment has been suspected. Considering the progression of cognitive impairment in the disease, a careful prospective population-based cohort study is required to determine prevalence and incidence of cognitive impairment in ALSci and ALSbi, the rate of progression, and the degree of clinical overlap between the subgroups.

Communication in ALS patients

The majority of clinically apparent communication difficulties in ALS result from dysarthria. However, subtle changes in language function may also occur, as evidenced by reduced verbal output, reduced spelling ability, increased word-finding difficulties, and impaired auditory comprehension of specific classes of language (e.g. verbs more than nouns) and more complex language constructs [190–192]. Deficits may be subtle and only identifiable with formal neuropsychological testing [176, 193]. Language impairment can have a deleterious effect on the quality of life of both patients and carers, and can render clinical management more difficult [193].

Communication should be routinely assessed by a speech and language therapist. Formal neuropsychological evaluation and support may be required in patients with concomitant evolving language deficits (see the previous section). The overall goal should be to optimize the effectiveness of communication, concentrating on meaningful interpersonal communication with the primary carer and family. This should include strategies for effec-

tive conversation, and the introduction of alternative communication devices where appropriate. Augmentive and alternative communication systems can substantially improve the quality of life for both patients and carers

Prosthetic treatments (palatal lift and/or a palatal augmentation prosthesis) can be useful in the reduction of hypernasality and improvement of articulation. For those requiring full mechanical ventilation, eye-pointing, eye-gaze or head-tracking augmentive high-tech communication devices may be useful. Brain–computer interfaces and electroencephalogram and evoked potential methods may prove useful in the future.

Palliative and end of life care

A palliative care approach should be incorporated into the care plan for patients and carers from the time of diagnosis [194] (Class III recommendation). Early referral to a specialist palliative care team is often appropriate. Palliative care based in the community or through hospice contacts (e.g. home care teams) can proceed in partnership with clinic-based neurological multidisciplinary care. The aim of palliative care is to maximize the quality of life of patients and families by relieving symptoms, providing emotional, psychological, and spiritual support as needed, removing obstacles to a peaceful death, and supporting the family in bereavement [104, 195]. A small proportion of ALS patients express interest in assisted suicide [196] and may choose euthanasia where it is legalized [197]. Various other aspects of terminal care have been covered in previous sections.

Good Practice Points

1. Whenever possible, offer input from a palliative care team early in the course of the disease.

2. Initiate discussions on end of life decisions when the patient asks or provides an opportunity for a discussion on the provision of end of life information and/or interventions.

3. Discuss the options for respiratory support and end of life issues if the patient has dyspnoea, other symptoms of hypoventilation (see table 17.15), or a forced vital capacity below 50%.

4. Inform the patient of the legal situation regarding advance directives and the naming of a healthcare proxy. Offer assistance in formulating an advance directive.

5. Re-discuss the patient's preferences for life-sustaining treatments every 6 months.

6. Initiate early referral to hospice or homecare teams well in advance of the terminal phase of ALS.

7. Be aware of the importance of spiritual issues for the quality of life and treatment choices. Establish a liaison with local pastoral care workers in order to be able to address the needs of the patient and relatives.

8. For the symptomatic treatment of dyspnoea and/or pain of intractable cause use opioids alone or in combination with benzodiazepines if anxiety is present. Titrating the dosages against the clinical symptoms will rarely if ever result in a life-threatening respiratory depression ([198], Class I A recommendation; [195]).

9. For treating terminal restlessness and confusion due to hypercapnia, neuroleptics may be used (e.g. chlorpromazine 12.5 mg every 4–12 h p.o., i.v., or p.r.).

10. Use oxygen only if symptomatic hypoxia is present.

Future developments

Being a syndrome with low incidence and short survival, most recommendations are GPPs based on consensus of experts from the field of ALS. Further randomized and double-blinded clinical trials are urgently needed to improve the management of ALS.

Research Recommendations

1. Further studies of biomarkers (imaging, blood and cerebrospinal fluid proteomics and metabolomics, neurophysiological markers) to aid earlier specific ALS diagnosis and to monitor possible effects in clinical trials.

2. Further studies of the impact of specialist MD clinics on clinical outcomes, quality of life, and carer burden.

3. Further studies to optimize the symptomatic treatment of muscle cramps, drooling, and bronchial secretions in ALS patients.

4. Better criteria for defining the use of PEG, PRG, NIPPV, and IMV.

5. Further studies to evaluate the effects of PEG/PRG, cough-assisting devices, and ventilation support on quality of life and survival.

6. Further studies to evaluate language dysfunction and its treatment in ALS.

7. Systematic studies to assess the cognitive impairment and the frequency of frontal lobe dysfunction in ALS and to standardize clinical, neuropsychological, and neuroradiological methods in this field. Future ALS diagnostic criteria should include parameters regarding cognitive dysfunction and dementia.

8. Studies of the medico-economical impact of more expensive procedures (NIPPV, IMV, cough-assist devices, advanced communication equipment).

9. Further studies to harmonize the patient databases of ALS centres.

10. Further studies on the psychosocial and spiritual determinants of quality of life in patients and their family caregivers are needed, as well as studies on the prevalence of and determinants for wishes for a hastened death.

Conflicts of interest

The present guidelines were prepared without external financial support. None of the authors reports conflicting interests.

References

1. Forsgren L, Almay BG, Holmgren G, Wall S. Epidemiology of motor neuron disease in northern Sweden. *Acta Neurol Scand* 1983;**68**:20–9.

2. Haverkamp LJ, Appel V, Appel SH. Natural history of amyotrophic lateral sclerosis in a database population. Validation of a scoring system and a model for survival prediction. *Brain* 1995;**118**:707–19.

3. Scott KM, Abhinav K, Stanton BR, *et al.* Geographical clustering of amyotrophic lateral sclerosis in South-East England: a population study. *Neuroepidemiology* 2009;**32**: 81–8.

4. Ince PG, Lowe J, Shaw PJ. Amyotrophic lateral sclerosis: current issues in classification, pathogenesis and molecular pathology. *Neuropathol Appl Neurobiol* 1998;**24**:104–17.

5. Brugman F, Wokke JH, Vianney de Jong JM, Franssen H, Faber CG, Van den Berg LH. Primary lateral sclerosis as a phenotypic manifestation of familial ALS. *Neurology* 2005;**64**:1778–9.

6. Andersen PM, Borasio GD, Dengler R, *et al.* EFNS Task Force on Management of Amyotrophic Lateral Sclerosis. Guidelines for diagnosing and clinical care of patients and relatives. An evidence-based review with Good Practice Points. *Eur J Neurol* 2005;**12**:921–38.

7. Brainin M, Barnes M, Baron J-C, *et al.* Guidance for the preparation of neurological management guidelines by EFNS scientific task forces – revised recommendations 2004. *Eur J Neurol* 2004;**11**:577–81.

8. Li TM, Day SJ, Alberman E, Swash M. Differential diagnosis of motoneurone disease from other neurological conditions. *Lancet* 1986;**2**:731–3.

9. Wilbourn AJ. Clinical neurophysiology in the diagnosis of amyotrophic lateral sclerosis: the Lambert and the El Escorial criteria. *J Neurol Sci* 1998;**160**(Suppl. 1):S25–9.

10. Meininger V. Getting the diagnosis right: beyond El Escorial. *J Neurol* 1999;**246**(Suppl. 3):III10–5.

11. Rosen AD. Amyotrophic lateral sclerosis. Clinical features and prognosis. *Arch Neurol* 1978;**35**:638–42.

12. Chio A, Mora G, Calvo A, Mazzini L, Bottacchi E, Mutani R, PARALS. Epidemiology of ALS in Italy: a 10-year prospective population-based study. *Neurology* 2009;**72**:725–31.

13. Bromberg M. Accelerating the diagnosis of amyotrophic lateral sclerosis. *Neurologist* 1999;**5**:63–74.

14. Aggarwal A, Nicholson G. Detection of preclinical motor neurone loss in SOD1 mutation carriers using motor unit number estimation. *J Neurol Neurosurg Psychiatry* 2002;**73**:199–201.

15. Dengler R, Tröger M. Impact of riluzole on the relationship between patient and physician. *J Neurol* 2001;**244**(Suppl. 2):S30–2.

16. Lima A, Evangelista T, de Carvalho M. Increased creatine kinase and spontaneous activity on electromyography, in amyotrophic lateral sclerosis. *Electromyogr Clin Neurophysiol* 2003;**43**:189–92.

17. Evangelista T, Carvalho M, Conceicao I, Pinto A, de Lurdes M, Luis ML. Motor neuropathies mimicking amyotrophic lateral sclerosis/motor neuron disease. *J Neurol Sci* 1996;**139**(Suppl.):95–8.

18. Traynor BJ, Codd MB, Corr B, Forde C, Frost E, Hardiman O. Amyotrophic lateral sclerosis mimic syndromes. *Arch Neurol* 2000;**57**:109–13.

19. Belsh JM, Schiffman PL. The amyotrophic lateral sclerosis (ALS) patient perspective on misdiagnosis and

its repercussions. *J Neurol Sci* 1996;**139**(Suppl.):110–16.

20. Davenport RJ, Swingler RJ, Chancellor AM, Warlow CP. Avoiding false positive diagnoses of motor neuron disease: lessons from the Scottish Motor Neuron Disease Register. *J Neurol Neurosurg Psychiatry* 1996;**60**:147–51.

21. Brooks BR. Earlier is better: the benefits of early diagnosis. *Neurology* 1999;**53**(Suppl. 5):S53–4.

22. Brooks BR, Miller RG, Swash M, *et al.* El Escorial revisited: revised criteria for the diagnosis of amyotrophic lateral sclerosis. *Amyotroph Lateral Scler Other Motor Neuron Disord* 2000;**1**:293–9.

23. Ross MA, Miller RG, Berchert L, *et al.* Towards earlier diagnosis of ALS. Revised criteria. *Neurology* 1998;**50**:768–72.

24. Carvalho M, Dengler R, Eisen A, *et al.* Electrodiagnostic criteria for diagnosis of ALS. *Clin Neurophysiol* 2008;**110**:497–503.

25. Leigh PN, Abrahams S, Al-Chalabi A, *et al.* The management of motor neuron disease. *J Neurol Neurosurg Psychiatry* 2003;**70**(Suppl. IV):iv32–47.

26. Lind SE, Good MD, Seidel S, Csordas T, Good BJ. Telling the diagnosis in cancer. *J Clin Oncol* 1989;**7**:583–9.

27. Borasio GD, Sloan R, Pongratz DE. Breaking the news in amyotrophic lateral sclerosis. *J Neurol Sci* 1998;**160**(Suppl. 1):S127–33.

28. McCluskey L, Casarett D, Siderowf A. Breaking the news: a survey of ALS patients and their caregivers. *Amyotroph Lateral Scler Other Motor Neuron Disord* 2004;**5**:131–5.

29. Damian D, Tattersall MHN. Letters to patients: improving communication in cancer care. *Lancet* 1991;**338**:923–5.

30. Doyle D. Breaking bad news. *J Royal Soc Med* 1996;**89**:590–1.

31. Davies E, Hopkins A. Good practice in the management of adults with malignant cerebral glioma: clinical guidelines. Working Group. *Br J Neurosurg* 1997;**11**:318–30.

32. Douglass CP, Kandler RH, Shaw PJ, McDermott CJ. An evaluation of neurophysiological criteria used in the diagnosis of Motor Neurone Disease. *J Neurol, Neurosurg Psychiatry*, in press, 2010.

33. Borasio GD, Shaw PJ, Hardiman O, Ludolph AC, Sales Luis ML, Silani V, for the European ALS Study Group. Standards of palliative care for patients with amyotrophic lateral sclerosis: results of a European survey. *Amyotroph Lateral Scler Other Motor Neuron Disord* 2001a;**2**:159–64.

34. Ackerman GM, Oliver D. Psychosocial support in an outpatient clinic. *Palliat Med* 1997;**11**:167–8.

35. Howard RS, Orrell RW. Management of motor neurone disease. *Postgrad Med J* 2002;**78**:736–41.

36. Chio A, Bottacchi E, Buffa C, Mutani R, Mora G. Positive effects of tertiary centres for amyotrophic lateral sclerosis on outcome and use of hospital facilities. *J Neurol Neurosurg Psychiatry* 2006;**77**:948–50.

37. Sorenson EJ, Mandrekar J, Crum B, Stevens JC. Effect of referral bias on assessing survival in ALS. *Neurology* 2007;**68**:600–2.

38. Traynor BJ, Alexander M, Corr B, *et al*. Effects of a multidisciplinary ALS clinic on survival. *J Neurol Neurosurg Psychiatry* 2003a;**74**:1258–61.

39. Zoccolella S, Beghi E, Palagano G, *et al*. ALS multidisciplinary clinic and survival. Results from a population-based study in Southern Italy. *J Neurol* 2007;**254**:1107–12.

40. Van den Berg JP, Kalmijn S, Lindeman E, *et al*. Multidisciplinary ALS care improves quality of life in patients with ALS. *Neurology* 2005;**65**:1264–7.

41. Mayadev AS, Weiss MD, Distad BJ, Krivickas LS, Carter GT. The amyotrophic lateral sclerosis center: a model of multidiciplinary management. *Phys Med Rehabil Clin N Am* 2008;**19**:619–31.

42. Kareus SA, Kagebein S, Rudnicki SA. The importance of a respiratory therapist in the ALS clinic. *Amyotroph Lateral Scler* 2008;**9**:173–6.

43. Corr B, Frost E, Traynor BJ, Hardiman O. Service provision for patients with ALS/MND: a cost-effective multidisciplinary approach. *J Neurol Sci* 2008;**160**(Suppl. 1):S141–5.

44. Chiò A, Gauthier A, Vignola A, *et al*. Caregiver time use in ALS. *Neurology* 2006;**67**:902–4.

45. Hecht MJ, Graesel E, Tigges S, *et al*. Burden of care in amyotrophic lateral sclerosis. *Palliat Med* 2003;**17**:327–33.

46. Gauthier A, Vignola A, Calvo A, *et al*. A longitudinal study on quality of life and depression in ALS patient-caregiver couples. *Neurology* 2007;**68**:923–6.

47. Gelinas DF, O'Connor P, Miller RG. Quality of life for ventilator-dependent ALS patients and their caregivers. *J Neurol Sci* 1998;**160**(Suppl. 1):S134–6.

48. Kaub-Wittemer D, Steinbüchel N, Wasner M, Laier-Groeneveld G, Borasio GD. Quality of life and psychosocial issues in ventilated patients with amyotrophic lateral sclerosis and their caregivers. *J Pain Symptom Manage* 2003;**26**:890–6.

49. Mustfa N, Walsh E, Bryant V, *et al*. The effect of noninvasive ventilation on ALS patients and their caregivers. *Neurology* 2006;**66**:1211–17.

50. Wasner M, Bold U, Vollmer TC, Borasio GD. Sexuality in patients with amyotrophic lateral sclerosis and their partners. *J Neurol* 2004;**251**:445–8.

51. Neudert C, Oliver D, Wasner M, Borasio GD. The course of the terminal phase in patients with amyotrophic lateral sclerosis. *J Neurol* 2001;**248**:612–16.

52. Hebert RS, Lacomis D, Easter C, Frick V, Shear MK. Grief support for informal caregivers of patients with ALS: a national survey. *Neurology* 2005;**64**:137–8.

53. Paz-Rodriguez F, Andrade-Palos P, Llanos-Del Pilar AM. Emotional consequences of providing care to amyotrophic lateral sclerosis patients. *Rev Neurol* 2005;**40**: 459–64.

54. Martin J, Turnbull J. Lasting impact in families after death from ALS. *Amyotroph Lateral Scler Other Motor Neuron Disord* 2001;**2**:181–7.

55. Bensimon G, Lacomblez L, Meininger V, *et al*. A controlled trial of riluzole in amyotrophic lateral sclerosis. ALS/ Riluzole Study Group. *N Engl J Med* 1994;**330**:585–91.

56. Lacomblez L, Bensimon G, Leigh PN, *et al*. Dose-ranging study of riluzole in amyotrophic lateral sclerosis. Amyotrophic Lateral Sclerosis/Riluzole Study Group II. *Lancet* 1996;**347**:1425–31.

57. Miller RG, Mitchell JD, Lyon M, Moore DH. Riluzole for amyotrophic lateral sclerosis (ALS)/motor neuron disease (MND). *Cochrane Database Syst Rev* 2007;(2): CD001447.

58. Riviere M, Meininger V, Zeisser P, Munsat T. An analysis of extended survival in patients with ALS treated with riluzole. *Arch Neurol* 1998;**55**:526–8.

59. Brooks BR, Belden DS, Roelke K, *et al*. Survival in non-riluzole treated ALS patients is identical before and since 1996: a clinic-based epidemiological study. *Amyotroph Lateral Scler Other Motor Neuron Disord* 2001;**2**(Suppl. 2):60–1. (Abstract #P15).

60. Turner MR, Bakker M, Sham P, Shaw CE, Leigh PN, Al-Chalabi A. Prognostic modelling of therapeutic interventions in amyotrophic lateral sclerosis. *Amyotroph Lateral Scler Other Motor Neuron Disord* 2002;**3**:15–21.

61. Traynor BJ, Alexander M, Corr B, Frost E, Hardiman O. An outcome study of riluzole in amyotrophic lateral sclerosis – a population-based study in Ireland, 1996–2000. *J Neurol* 2003b;**250**:473–9.

62. Andersen PM, Sims KB, Xin WW, *et al*. Sixteen novel mutations in the gene encoding CuZn-superoxide dismutase in ALS. *Amyotroph Lateral Scler Other Motor Neuron Disord* 2003;**2**:62–73.

63. Forshew DA, Bromberg MB. A survey of clinicans' practice in the symptomatic treatment of ALS. *Amyotrophic Lateral Scler Other Motor Neuron Disord* 2003;**4**:258–63.

64. Mier RJ, Bachrach SJ, Lakin RC, Barker T, Childs J, Moran M. Treatment of sialorrhea with glycopyrrolate: a double-blind, dose-ranging study. *Arch Pediatr Adolesc Med* 2000;**154**:1214–18.

65. Talmi YP, Finkelstein Y, Zohar Y. Reduction of salivary flow in amyotrophic lateral sclerosis with scopoderm TTS. *Head Neck* 1989;**11**:565.

66. Talmi YP, Finkelstein Y, Zohar Y. Reduction of salivary flow with transdermal scopolamine: a four-year experience. *Otolaryngol Head Neck Surg* 1990;**103**:615–18.

67. Giess R, Naumann M, Werner E, *et al.* Injections of botulinum toxin A into the salivary glands improve sialorrhoea in amyotrophic lateral sclerosis. *J Neurol Neurosurg Psychiatry* 2000;**69**:121–3.

68. Lipp A, Trottenberg T, Schink T, Kupsch A, Arnold G. A randomized trial of botulinum toxin A for treatment of drooling. *Neurology* 2003;**61**:1279–81.

69. Jackson CE, Gronseth G, Rosenfeld J, *et al.* Randomized double-blind study of botulinum toxin type B for sialorrhea in ALS patients. *Muscle Nerve* 2009;**39**:137–43.

70. Winterholler MG, Erbguth FJ, Wolf S, Kat S. Botulinum toxin for the treatment of sialorrhoea in ALS: serious side effects of a transductal approach. *J Neurol Neurosurg Psychiatry* 2001;**70**:417–18.

71. Andersen PM, Grönberg H, Funegård U, Franzen L. X-ray radiation of the parotid glands significantly reduces drooling in patients with progressive bulbar palsy. *J Neurol Sci* 2001;**191**:111–14.

72. Harriman M, Morrison M, Hay J, *et al.* Use of radiotherapy for control of sialorrhea in patients with amyotrophic lateral sclerosis. *J Otolaryngol* 2001;**30**:242–5.

73. Stalpers LJ, Moser EC. Results of radiotherapy for drooling in amyotrophic lateral sclerosis. *Neurology* 2002;**58**:1308.

74. Neppelberg E, Haugen DF, Thorsen L, Tysnes OB. Radiotherapy reduces sialorrhea in amyotrophic lateral sclerosis. *Eur J Neurol* 2007;**14**:1373–7.

75. Burton MJ. The surgical management of drooling. *Dev Med Child Neurol* 1991;**33**:1110–6.

76. Hockstein NG, Samadi DS, Gendron K, Handler SD. Sialorrhea: a management challenge. *Am Fam Physician* 2004;**69**:2628–34.

77. Janzen VD, Rae RE, Hudson AJ. Otolaryngologic manifestations of ALS. *J Otolaryngol* 1988;**17**:41–2.

78. Peysson S, Vandenberghe N, Phillit F, *et al.* Factors predicting survival following noninvasive ventilation in amyotrophic lateral sclerosis. *Eur Neurol* 2008;**59**: 164–71.

79. Newall AR, Orser R, Hunt M. The control of oral secretions in bulbar ALS/MND. *J Neurol Sci* 1996;**139** (Suppl.):43–4.

80. Frass M, Dielacher C, Linkesch M, *et al.* Influence of potassium dichromate on tracheal secretions in critically ill patients. *Chest* 2005;**127**:936–41.

81. Hanayama K, Ishikawa Y, Bach JR. Amyotrophic lateral sclerosis: successful treatment of of mucous plugging by mechanical insufflation-exsufflation. *Am J Phys Med Rehabil* 1997;**76**:338–9.

82. Sancho J, Servera E, Diaz J, Marin J. Efficacy of mechanical insufflation-exsufflation in medically stable patients with amyotrophic lateral sclerosis. *Chest* 2004;**125**:1400–5.

83. Gallagher JP. Pathologic laughter and crying in ALS: a search for their origin. *Acta Neurol Scand* 1989;**80**: 114–17.

84. Palmieri A, Abrahams S, Sorarù G, *et al.* Emotional lability in MND: relationship to cognition and psychopathology and impact on caregiver. *J Neurol Sci* 2009;**278**:16–20.

85. Rosen H. Dextromethorphan/quinidine sulfate for pseudobulbar affect. *Drugs Today* 2008;**44**:661–8.

86. Schiffer RB, Herndon RM, Rudick RA. Treatment of pathological laughing and weeping with amitriptyline. *N Engl J Med* 1985;**312**:1480–2.

87. Andersen G, Vestergaard K, Riis JO. Citalopram for post-stroke pathological crying. *Lancet* 1993;**342**:837–9.

88. Brooks BR, Thisted RA, Appel SH, *et al.* Treatment of pseudobulbar affect in ALS with dextromethorphan/ quinidine: a randomized trial. The AVP-923 ALS Study Group. *Neurology* 2004;**63**:1364–70.

89. Connolly PS, Shirley EA, Wasson JH, Nierenberg DW. Treatment of nocturnal leg cramps. A crossover trial of quinine vs vitamin E. *Arch Intern Med* 1992;**152**: 1877–80.

90. Diener HC, Dethlefsen U, Dethlefsen-Gruber S, Verbeek P. Effectiveness of quinine in treating muscle cramps: a double-blind, placebo-controlled, parallel-group, multicentre trial. *Int J Clin Pract* 2002;**56**:243–6.

91. Drory VW, Goltsman E, Renik JG, *et al.* The value of muscle exercise in patients with amyotrophic lateral sclerosis. *J Neurol Sci* 2001;**191**:133–7.

92. Kesiktas N, Paker N, Erdogan N, Gulsen G, Bicki D, Yilmaz H. The use of hydrotherapy for the management of spasticity. *Neurorehabil Neural Repair* 2004;**18**:268–73.

93. dos Santos MT, de Oliveira LM. Use of cryotherapy to enhance mouth opening in patients with cerebral palsy. *Spec Care Dentist* 2004;**24**:232–4.

94. Marquardt G, Seifert V. Use of intrathecal baclofen for treatment of spasticity in amyotrophic lateral sclerosis. *J Neurol Neurosurg Psychiatry* 2002;**72**:275–6.

95. McClelland S 3rd, Bethoux FA, Boulis NM, *et al.* Intrathecal baclofen for spasticity-related pain in amyotrophic lateral sclerosis: efficacy and factors associated with pain relief. *Muscle Nerve* 2008;**37**:396–8.

96. Winterholler MG, Heckmann JG, Hecht M, Erbguth FJ. Recurrent trismus and stridor in an ALS patient: successful treatment with botulinum toxin. *Neurology* 2002;**58**: 502–3.

97. Vignola A, Guzzo A, Calvo A, *et al.* Anxiety undermines quality of life in ALS patients and caregivers. *Eur J Neurol* 2008;**15**:1231–6.

98. Wicks P, Abrahams S, Masi D, Hejda-Forde S, Leigh PN, Goldstein LH. Prevalence of depression in a 12-month consecutive sample of patients with ALS. *Eur J Neurol* 2007;**14**:993–1001.

99. Mandler RN, Anderson FA Jr, Miller RG, *et al.* The ALS Patient Care Database: insights into end-of-life care in ALS. *Amyotrophic Lateral Scler Other Motor Neuron Disord* 2001;**2**:203–8.

100. Ganzini L, Johnston WS, Silveira MJ. The final month of life in patients with ALS. *Neurology* 2002;**59**:428–31.

101. Lou JS. Fatigue in amyotrophic lateral sclerosis. *Phys Med Rehabil Clin N Am* 2008;**19**:533–43.

102. Carter GT, Weiss MD, Lou JS, *et al.* Modafinil to treat fatigue in amyotrophic lateral sclerosis: an open label pilot study. *Am J Hosp Palliat Care* 2005;**22**:55–9.

103. Rabkin JG, Gordon PH, McElhiney M, Rabkin R, Chew S, Mitsumoto H. Modafinil treatment of fatigue in patients with ALS: a placebo-controlled study. *Muscle Nerve* 2009;**39**:297–303.

104. Oliver D, Borasio GD, Walsh D. *Palliative Care in Amyotrophic Lateral Sclerosis*, 2nd edn. Oxford: Oxford University Press, 2006.

105. Brettscheneider J, Kurent J, Ludolph A, Mitchell JD. Drug therapy for pain in amyotrophic lateral sclerosis or motor neuron disease. *Cochrane Database Syst Rev* 2008;**3**: CD005226.

106. Elman LB, Siderowf A, Houseman G, Kelley M, McCluskey LF. *Amyotroph Lateral Scler Other Motor Neuron Disord* 2005;**6**:246–9.

107. Qureshi MM, Cudkowicz ME, Zhang H, Raynor E. Increased incidense of deep venous thrombosis in ALS. *Neurology* 2007;**68**:76–7.

108. Wasner M, Klier H, Borasio GD. The use of alternative medicine by patients with amyotrophic lateral sclerosis. *J Neurol Sci* 2001;**191**:151–4.

109. Vardeny O, Bromberg MB. The use of herbal supplements and alternative therapies by patients with amyotrophic lateral sclerosis (ALS). *J Herb Pharmacother* 2005;**5**:23–31.

110. Janson CG, Ramesh TM, During MJ, Leone P, Heywood J. Human intrathecal transplantation of peripheral blood stem cells in amyotrophic lateral sclerosis. *J Hematother Stem Cell Res* 2001;**10**:913–15.

111. Mazzini L, Mareschi K, Ferrero I, *et al.* Stem cell treatment in amyotrophic lateral sclerosis. *J Neurol Sci* 2008;**265**: 78–83.

112. Appel SH, Engelhardt JI, Henkel JS, *et al.* Hematopoietic stem cell transplantation in patients with sporadic amyotrophic lateral sclerosis. *Neurology* 2008;**71**:1326–34.

113. Deda H, Inci MC, Kürekçi AE, *et al.* Treatment of amyotrophic lateral sclerosis patients by autologous bone marrow-derived hematopoietic stem cell transplantation: a 1-year follow-up. *Cytotherapy* 2009;**11**:18–25.

114. Martinez HR, Gonzalez-Garza MT, Moreno-Cuevas JE, Caro E, Gutierrez-Jimenez E, Segura JJ. Stem-cell transplantation into the frontal motor cortex in amyotrophic lateral sclerosis patients. *Cytotherapy* 2009;**11**:26–34.

115. Silani V, Cova L, Corbo M, Ciammola A, Polli E. Stem-cell therapy for amyotrophic lateral sclerosis. *Lancet* 2004;**364**: 200–2.

116. Badayan I, Cudkowicz ME. Is it too soon for mesenchymal stem cell trials in people with ALS? *Amyotroph Lateral Scler* 2009;**10**:123–4.

117. Huang H, Chen L, Xi H, *et al.* Fetal olfactory ensheathing cells transplantation in amyotrophic lateral sclerosis patients: a controlled pilot study. *Clin Transplant* 2008;**22**: 710–18.

118. Huang H, Chen L, Xi H, *et al.* Olfactory ensheathing cells transplantation for central nervous system diseases in 1,255 patients. *Zhongguo Xiu Fu Chong Jian Wai Ke Za Zhi* 2009;**23**:14–20.

119. Chen L, Huang H, Zhang J, *et al.* Short-term outcome of olfactory ensheathing cells transplantation for treatment of amyotrophic lateral sclerosis. *Zhongguo Xiu Fu Chong Jian Wai Ke Za Zhi* 2007;**21**:961–6.

120. Stober T, Schimrigk K, Dietzsch S, Thielen T. Intrathecal thyrotropin-releasing hormone therapy of amyotrophic lateral sclerosis. *J Neurol* 1985;**232**:13–14.

121. Mora JS, Munsat TL, Kao KP, *et al.* Intrathecal administration of natural human interferon alpha in amyotrophic lateral sclerosis. *Neurology* 1986;**36**:1137–40.

122. Cudkowicz ME, Warren L, Francis JW, *et al.* Intrathecal administration of recombinant human superoxide dismutase 1 in amyotrophic lateral sclerosis: a preliminary safety and pharmacokinetic study. *Neurology* 1997;**49**: 213–22.

123. Aebischer P, Schluep M, Déglon N, *et al.* Intrathecal delivery of CNTF using encapsulated genetically modified xenogeneic cells in amyotrophic lateral sclerosis patients. *Nat Med* 1996;**2**:696–9.

124. Penn RD, Kroin JS, York MM, Cedarbaum JM. Intrathecal ciliary neurotrophic factor delivery for treatment of amyotrophic lateral sclerosis (phase I trial). *Neurosurgery* 1997;**40**:94–9.

125. Ochs G, Penn RD, York M, *et al.* A phase I/II trial of recombinant methionyl human brain derived neurotrophic factor administered by intrathecal infusion to patients with amyotrophic lateral sclerosis. *Amyotroph Lateral Scler Other Motor Neuron Disord* 2000;**1**:201–6.

126. Nagano I, Shiote M, Murakami T, *et al.* Beneficial effects of intrathecal IGF-1 administration in patients with amyotrophic lateral sclerosis. *Neurol Res* 2005;**27**:768–72.

127. Finsterer J, Mamoli B. Liquorpheresis (CSF filtration) in familial amyotrophic lateral sclerosis. *Spinal Cord* 1999;**37**:592–3.

128. Finsterer J, Mamoli B. Cerebrospinal fuid filtration in amyotrophic lateral sclerosis. *Eur J Neurol* 1999;**6**:597–600.

129. Steele J, Matos LA, Lopez EA, *et al.* A phase I safety study of hyperbaric oxygen therapy for amyotrophic lateral sclerosis. *Amyotroph Lateral Scler Other Motor Neuron Disord* 2004;**5**:250–4.

130. Zanette G, Forgione A, Manganotti P, Fiaschi A, Tamburin S. The effect of repetitive transcranial magnetic stimulation on motor performance, fatigue and quality of life in amyotrophic lateral sclerosis. *J Neurol Sci* 2008;**270**: 18–22.

131. Eisen A, Mezei MM, Stewart HG, Fabros M, Gibson G, Andersen PM. SOD1 gene mutations in ALS patients from British Columbia, Canada: clinical features, neurophysiology and ethical issues in management. *Amyotroph Lateral Scler* 2008;**9**:108–19.

132. Haberlandt WF. Genetic aspects of amyotrphic lateral sclerosis and progressive bulbar paralysis. *Acta Genet Med Gemell* 1959;**8**:369–73.

133. Murros K, Fogelholm R. Amyotrophic lateral sclerosis in middle-Finland: an epidemiological study. *Acta Neurol Scand* 1983;**67**:41–7.

134. Thijs V, Peeters E, Theys P, Matthijs G, Robberecht W. Demographic characteristics and prognosis in a Flemish amyotrophic lateral sclerosis population. *Acta Neurol Belg* 2000;**100**:84–90.

135. Murray TJ, Pride S, Haley G. Motor neuron disease in Nova Scotia. *CMAJ* 1974;**110**:814–17.

136. Gunnarsson L-G, Palm R. Motor neuron disease and heavy labour: an epidemiological survey of Värmland county, Sweden. *Neuroepidemiology* 1984;**3**:195–206.

137. Li T-M, Alberman E, Swash M. Comparison of sporadic and familial disease amongst 580 cases of motor neuron disease. *J Neurol Neurosurg Psychiatry* 1988;**51**:778–84.

138. Giagheddu M, Puggioni G, Masala C, *et al.* Epidemiologic study of amyotrophic lateral sclerosis in Sardinia, Italy. *Acta Neurol Scand* 1983;**68**:394–404.

139. Højer-Pedersen E, Christensen PB, Jensen NB. Incidence and prevalence of motor neuron disease in two Danish counties. *Neuroepidemiology* 1989;**8**:151–9.

140. Fong KY, Yu YL, Chan YW, *et al.* Motor neuron disease in Hong Kong Chinese: epidemiology and clinical picture. *Neuroepidemiology* 1996;**15**:239–45.

141. Jokelainen M. Amyotrophic lateral sclerosis in Finland. II: clinical characteristics. *Acta Neurol Scand* 1977;**56**: 194–204.

142. Andersen PM, Forsgren L, Binzer M, *et al.* Autosomal recessive adult-onset ALS associated with homozygosity for Asp90Ala CuZn-superoxide dismutase mutation. A clinical and genealogical study of 36 patients. *Brain* 1996;**119**:1153–72.

143. Jones CT, Swingler RJ, Simpson SA, Brock DJ. Superoxide dismutase mutations in an unselected cohort of Scottish amyotrophic lateral sclerosis patients. *J Med Genet* 1995;**32**:290–2.

144. Gil J, Funalot B, Verschueren A. Causes of death amongst French patients with amyotrophic lateral sclerosis: a prospective study. *Eur J Neurol* 2008;**15**:1245–51.

145. Lyall RA, Donaldson N, Polkey MI, Leigh PN, Moxham J. Respiratory muscle strength and ventilatory failure in amyotrophic lateral sclerosis. *Brain* 2001;**124**:2000–13.

146. Pinto A, de Carvalho M, Evangelista T, Lopes A, Sales-Luis L. Nocturnal pulse oxymetry: a new approach to establish the appropriate time for non-invasive ventilation. *Amyotroph Lateral Scler* 2003;**4**:31–5.

147. Pinto S, Turkman A, Pinto A, Swash M, de Carvalho M. Predicting respiratory insufficiency in amyotrophic lateral sclerosis: the role of phrenic nerve studies. *Clin Neurophysiol* 2009;**120**:941–6.

148. Sancho J, Servera E, Dias J, Marin J. Prediction of ineffective cough during a chest infection in patients with stable amyotrophic lateral sclerosis. *Am J Respir Crit Care Med* 2007;**175**:1266–71.

149. Bourke SC, Gibson GJ. Non-invasive ventilation in ALS: current practice and future role. *Amyotroph Lateral Scler Other Motor Neuron Disord* 2004;**5**:67–71.

150. Mendoza M, Gelinas DF, Moore DH, Miller RG. A comparison of maximal inspiratory pressure and forced vital capacity as potential criteria for initiating non-invasive ventilation in ALS. *Amyotroph Lateral Scler* 2007;**8**: 106–11.

151. Pinto A, Evangelista T, de Carvalho M, Alves MA, Sales-Luis ML. Respiratory assistance with a non-invasive ventilator (BiPAP) in MND/ALS patients: survival rates in a controlled trial. *J Neurol Sci* 1995;**129**(Suppl.):19–26.

152. Bourke SC, Tomlinson M, Williams TL, Bullock RE, Shaw PJ, Gibson GJ. Effects of non-invasive ventilation on survival and quality of life in patients with amyotrophic lateral sclerosis: a randomised controlled trial. *Lancet Neurol* 2006;**5**:140–7.

153. Lo Cocco D, Marchese S, Pesco MC, La Bella V, Piccoli F, Lo Cocco A. The amyotrophic lateral sclerosis functional rating scale predicts survival time in amyotrophic lateral sclerosis patients on invasive mechanical ventilation. *Chest* 2007;**132**:64–9.

154. Lechtzin N, Scott Y, Busse AM, Clawson LL, Kimball R, Wiener CM. Early use of non-invasive ventilation prolongs survival in subjects with ALS. *Amyotr Lat Scler* 2007;**8**: 185–8.

155. Shoesmith CL, Findlater K, Rowe A, Strong MJ. Prognosis of amyotrophic lateral sclerosis with respiratory onset. *J Neurol Neurosurg Psychiatry* 2007;**78**:629–31.

156. Onders RP, Carlin AM, Elmo M, Sivashankaran S, Katirii B, Schilz R. Amyotrophic lateral sclerosis: the Midwestern surgical experience with diaphragm pacing stimulation system shows that general anesthesia can be safely performed. *Am J Surg* 2009;**197**:386–90.

157. Nardin R, O'Donnell C, Loring SH, *et al.* Diaphragm training in amyotrophic lateral sclerosis. *J Clin Neuromusc Dis* 2008;**10**:56–60.

158. Cazzolli PA, Oppenheimer EA. Home mechanical ventilation for amyotrophic lateral sclerosis: nasal compared to tracheostomy-intermittent positive pressure ventilation. *J Neurol Sci* 1996;**139**(Suppl.):123–8.

159. Jennings AL, Davies AN, Higgins JP, Gibbs JS, Broadley KE. A systematic review of the use of opioids in the management of dyspnoea. *Thorax* 2002;**57**:939–44.

160. Bruera E, Sweeney C, Willey J, *et al.* A randomized controlled trial of supplemental oxygen versus air in cancer patients with dyspnea. *Palliat Med* 2003;**17**:659–63.

161. Winck JC, Gonçalves MR, Lourenço C, Viana P, Almeida J, Bach JR. Effects of mechanical insufflation-exsufflation on respiratory parameters for patients with chronic airway secretion encumbrance. *Chest* 2004;**126**:774–80.

162. Lange DJ, Lechtzin N, Davey C, *et al.* High-frequency chest wall oscillation in ALS: an exploratory randomized, controlled trial. *Neurology* 2006;**67**:991–7.

163. Desport JC, Marin B, Funalot B, Preux PM, Curatirer P. Phase angle is a prognostic factor for survival in amyotrophic lateral sclerosis. *Amyotroph Lateral Scler* 2008;**9**:273–8.

164. Desport JC, Torny F, Lacoste M, Preux PM, Couratier P. Hypermetabolism in ALS: correlations with clinical and paraclinical parameters. *Neurodegener Dis* 2005;**2**:202–7.

165. Vaisman N, Lusaus M, Nefussy B, *et al.* Do patients with amyotrophic lateral sclerosis (ALS) have increased energy needs? *J Neurol Sci* 2009;**279**:26–9.

166. Desport JC, Preux PM, Truong CT, Courat L, Vallat JM, Couratier P. Nutritional assessment and survival in ALS patients. *Amyotroph Lateral Scler Other Motor Neuron Disord* 2000;**1**:91–6.

167. Heffernan C, Jenkinson C, Holmes T, *et al.* Nutritional management in MND/ALS patients: an evidence based review. *Amyotroph Lateral Scler Other Motor Neuron Disord* 2004;**5**:72–83.

168. Shaw AS, Ampong MA, Rio A, *et al.* Survival of patients with ALS following institution of enteral feeding is related to pre-procedure oximetry: a retrospective review of 98 patients in a single centre. *Amyotroph Lateral Scler* 2006;**7**:16–21.

169. Mathus-Vliegen LM, Louwerse LS, Merkus MP, Tytgat GN, Vianney de Jong JM. Percutaneous endoscopic gastrostomy in patients with amyotrophic lateral sclerosis and impaired pulmonary function. *Gastrointest Endosc* 1994;**40**:463–9.

170. Chio A, Galletti R, Finocchiaro C, *et al.* Percutaneous radiological gastrostomy: a safe and effective method of nutritional tube placement in advanced ALS. *J Neurol Neurosurg Psychiatry* 2004;**75**:645–7.

171. Shaw AS, Ampong MA, Rio A, McClure J, Leigh PN, Sidhu PS. Entristar skin-level gastrostomy tube: primary placement with radiologic guidance in patients with amyotrophic lateral sclerosis. *Radiology* 2004;**233**:392–9.

172. Thornton FJ, Fotheringham T, Alexander M, Hardiman O, McGrath FP, Lee MJ. Amyotrophic lateral sclerosis: enteral nutrition provision – endoscopic or radiologic gastrostomy? *Radiology* 2002;**224**:713–17.

173. Scott AG, Austin HE. Nasogastric feeding in the management of severe dysphagia in motor neurone disease. *Palliat Med* 1994;**8**:45–9.

174. Verschueren A, Monnier A, Attarian S, Lardillier D, Pouget J. Enteral and parenteral nutrition in the later stages of ALS: an observational study. *Amyotroph Lateral Scler* 2009;**10**:42–6.

175. Olney RK, Murphy J, Forshew D, *et al.* The effects of executive and behavioral dysfunction on the course of ALS. *Neurology* 2005;**65**:1774–7.

176. Phukan J, Pender N, Hardiman O. Cognitive impairment in ALS. *Lancet Neurol* 2007;**6**:994–1003.

177. Neary D, Snowden JS, Mann DM. Classification and description of frontotemporal dementias. *Ann N Y Acad Sci* 2000;**920**:46–51.

178. Lomen-Hoerth C, Murphy J, Langmore S, Kramer JH, Olney RK, Miller B. Are amyotrophic lateral sclerosis patients cognitively normal? *Neurology* 2003;**60**:1094–7.

179. Strong MJ, Grace GM, Freedman M, *et al.* Consensus criteria for the diagnosis of frontotemporal cognitive and behavioural syndromes in amyotrophic lateral sclerosis. *Amyotroph Lateral Scler* 2009;**10**:3–131.

180. Abrahams S, Leigh PN, Goldstein LH. Cognitive change in ALS: a prospective study. *Neurology* 2005;**64**:1222–6.

181. Grossman AB, Woolley-Levine S, Bradley WG, Miller RG. Detecting neurobehavioral changes in amyotrophic lateral sclerosis. *Amyotroph Lateral Scler* 2007;**8**:56–61.

182. Gibbons ZC, Richardson A, Neary D, Snowden JS. Behaviour in amyotrophic lateral sclerosis. *Amyotroph Lateral Scler* 2008;**9**:67–74.

183. Papps B, Abrahams S, Wicks P, Leigh PN, Goldstein LH. Changes in memory for emotional material in amyotrophic lateral sclerosis (ALS). *Neuropsychologia* 2005;**43**: 1107–14.

184. Gibbons ZC, Snowden JS, Thompson JC, Happe F, Richardson A, Neary D. Inferring thought and action in motor neurone disease. *Neuropsychologia* 2007;**45**: 1196–207.

185. Abrahams S, Goldstein LH, Suckling J, *et al*. Frontotemporal white matter changes in amyotrophic lateral sclerosis. *J Neurol* 2005;**252**:321–31.

186. Murphy JM, Henry RG, Langmore S, Kramer JH, Miller BL, Lomen-Hoerth C. Continuum of frontal lobe impairment in amyotrophic lateral sclerosis. *Arch Neurol* 2007;**64**: 53053–4.

187. Donaghy C, Pinnock R, Abrahams S. Ocular fixation instabilities in motor neurone disease. A marker of frontal lobe dysfunction? *J Neurol* 2009;**256**:420–6.

188. Flaherty-Craig C, Eslinger P, Stephens B, Simmons Z. A rapid screening battery to identify frontal dysfunction in patients with ALS. *Neurology* 2006;**67**:2070–2.

189. Gordon PH, Wang Y, Doorish C, *et al*. A screening assessment of cognitive impairment in patients with ALS. *Amyotroph Lateral Scler* 2007;**8**:362–5.

190. Grossman M, Anderson C, Khan A, *et al*. Impaired action knowledge in amyotrophic lateral sclerosis. *Neurology* 2008;**71**:1396–401.

191. Raaphorst J, De Visser M, Linssen WH, *et al*. The cognitive profile of amyotrophic lateral sclerosis: a meta-analysis. *Amyotroph Lateral Scler* 2010;**11**:27–37.

192. Bak TH, Hodges JR. Motor neurone disease, dementia and aphasia. Coincidence, co-occurrence or continuum. *J Neurol* 2001;**248**:260–70.

193. Cobble M. Language impairment in motor neurone disease. *J Neurol Sci* 1998;**160**(Suppl. 1):S47–52.

194. Borasio GD, Voltz R, Miller RG. Palliative care in amyotrophic lateral sclerosis. *Neurol Clin* 2001;**19**:829–47.

195. Mitsumoto H, Bromberg M, Johnston W, *et al*. Promoting excellence in end-of-life care in ALS. *Amyotroph Lateral Scler Other Motor Neuron Disord* 2005;**6**:145–54.

196. Ganzini L, Johnston WS, McFarland BH, Tolle SW, Lee MA. Attitudes of patients with amyotrophic lateral sclerosis and their care givers toward assisted suicide. *N Engl J Med* 1998;**339**:967–73.

197. Veldink JH, Wokke JH, van der Wal G, Vianney de Jong JM, van den Berg LH. Euthanasia and physician-assisted suicide among patients with amyotrophic lateral sclerosis in the Netherlands. *N Engl J Med* 2002;**346**: 1638–44.

198. Sykes N, Thorns A. Sedative use in the last week of life and the implications for end-of-life decision making. *Arch Intern Med* 2003;**163**:341–4.

CHAPTER 18

Post-polio syndrome

E. Farbu,[1] N. E. Gilhus,[2] M. P. Barnes,[3] K. Borg,[4] M. de Visser,[6] R. Howard,[7] F. Nollet,[6] J. Opara,[8] E. Stalberg[9]

[1]Stavanger University Hospital, Norway; [2]University of Bergen, and Haukeland University Hospital, Bergen, Norway; [3]Hunters Moor Hospital, Newcastle upon Tyne, UK; [4]Karolinska Intitutet/Karolinska Hospital, Stochkholm, Sweden; [6]University of Amsterdam, 1100 DD Amsterdam, The Netherlands; [7]St Thomas' Hospital, London, UK; [8]Repty Rehab Centre. ul. Sniadeckio 1, PL 42-604 Tarnowskie Góry, Poland; [9]University Hospital, S-75185 Uppsala, Sweden

Objectives

The aim was to revise the existing EFNS task force document, with regard to a common definition of PPS, and evaluation of the existing evidence for the effectiveness and safety of therapeutic interventions. By this revision, clinical guidelines for management of PPS are provided.

Background

Many previous polio patients experience new muscle weakness, fatigue, myalgia and joint pain, and cold intolerance, and develop new atrophy several years after acute paralytic poliomyelitis. The first case of new atrophy and weakness many years after acute paralytic polio was first described in 1875 by Raymond [1, 2].

The term post-polio syndrome (PPS) was introduced by Halstead in 1985 [3]. In general, PPS has been interpreted as a condition with new muscle weakness or fatigability in persons with a confirmed history of acute paralytic polio, usually occurring several decades after the acute illness.

As PPS is reckoned to be a chronic disease, the EFNS task force on post-polio syndrome recommends that the criteria published by March of Dimes (MoD) in 2000 [4] should be regarded as universal criteria for PPS.

European Handbook of Neurological Management: Volume 1, 2nd edition. Edited by N. E. Gilhus, M. P. Barnes and M. Brainin. © 2011 Blackwell Publishing Ltd.

1 Prior paralytic poliomyelitis with evidence of motor neuron loss, as confirmed by history of the acute paralytic illness, signs of residual weakness, and atrophy of muscles on neurological examination, and signs of denervation on electromyography (EMG).

2 A period of partial or complete functional recovery after acute paralytic poliomyelitis, followed by an interval (usually 15 years or more) of stable neurologic function.

3 Gradual or sudden onset of progressive and persistent muscle weakness or abnormal muscle fatigability (decreased endurance), with or without generalized fatigue, muscle atrophy, or muscle and joint pain. (Sudden onset may follow a period of inactivity, or trauma, or surgery.) Less commonly, symptoms attributed to PPS include new problems with swallowing or breathing.

4 Symptoms persist for at least 1 year.

5 Exclusion of other neurologic, medical, and orthopaedic problems as causes of symptoms.

The symptoms reported for PPS are the same from all parts of the world. Muscle weakness, atrophy, generalized fatigue, post-exercise fatigue, muscle pain, fasciculations, cramps, cold intolerance, and joint pain dominate[3, 5–12]. A history of previous paralytic polio seems to increase long-term mortality [13].

Deterioration of the neuromuscular function, overuse of motor units, the general ageing process, and inflammatory changes in the central nervous system and serum, have all been proposed as possible explanations for the new symptoms [14–17]. However, the underlying mechanisms are not fully elucidated, and we cannot conclude which underlying factors are causing PPS. Regarding the clinical course, there is increasing evidence that the decline in muscle strength is slow with modest effect on functional tasks [18, 19]. Generalized fatigue is a common complaint among PPS patients, and not well understood, although both neuromuscular decline and increased levels of inflammatory cytokines indicate that fatigue in PPS should be reckoned as a physical entity [16, 20]. From a clinical point of view it should be emphasized that comorbidity could cause PPS- mimicking conditions, requiring other investigations and treatments [10, 21–23].

The prevalence of PPS has been reported from 15 to 80% of all patients with previous polio, depending on the criteria applied and population studied [5, 10, 24–28]. In many population-based studies, terms such as 'late-onset polio symptoms' have been used instead of PPS. Hospital-based studies use the term PPS, but in these studies it is always debatable whether the patient material is representative. Exact prevalence of PPS is therefore difficult to establish. For European populations, one Dutch study reported a prevalence of late-onset polio symptoms of 46%, one study from Edinburgh reported a prevalence of more than 60%, in Estonia a prevalence of 52% has been reported, Norway 60%, and Denmark 63% [5, 29–31].

With regard to symptomatic treatment and clinical purposes, the difference between stable muscle weakness after polio and PPS seems as yet rather irrelevant. Still, it would be of great benefit to have a consensus on the term PPS for research and when evidence-based therapeutic interventions have become available. The MoD criteria are based on the principle of exclusion of other causes for new deterioration, where PPS is characterized with new muscle weakness or abnormal muscle fatigability, and persistence of symptoms for at least 1 year. The diagnosis of PPS is an exclusion diagnosis with no test or analysis specific for PPS, and the role of the investigation is to rule out every other possible cause for the new symptoms and clinical deterioration.

Many patients report a sense of weakening in the muscles before it is detectable by clinical examination, although dynamometric muscle strength evaluation and computed tomography (CT) imaging may be helpful [32, 33]. Atrophy is the end stage of new neuromuscular deterioration and by using this as a necessary criterion, patients in an earlier stage of neuromuscular deterioration will be excluded.

Role of clinical neurophysiology

Clinical neurophysiology is used for four main reasons. First, to establish typical lower motor neuron involvement (neurogenic EMG findings, normal findings of the sensory and motor nerves except for parameters reflecting muscle atrophy). Second, to exclude other causes. This is part of the PPS definition, and it is not uncommon to find patients in whom the initial diagnosis of polio must be revised. Third, to find concomitant nerve or muscle disorders, such as entrapments and radiculopathies. Fourth, to assess the degree of motor neuron loss. This cannot be quantified clinically, since loss of neurones may be completely masked by compensatory nerve sprouting and muscle fibre hypertrophy. Macro EMG studies have shown that loss of up to 50% of neurons may be compatible with a normal clinical picture [15].

In longitudinal studies with macro EMG, a continuous loss of neurons is demonstrated with exaggerated speed compared to normal age-dependent degeneration [34]. New weakness appears when the compensatory mechanisms are no longer sufficient, and occurs when macro motor unit potential (MUP) exceeds 20 times the normal size [34].

Search strategy

MEDLINE via Pubmed, EMBASE, ISI, and Cochrane were searched with time limits 1966 until 2004. Search terms were post-polio syndrome, postpoliomyelitis, PPMA, PPMD, poliomyelitis, in combination with management, therapy, treatment, medicaments, physiotherapy, and intervention.

In the present revised document, the database search was supplied with the years 2004–2009.

No meta-analyses of intervention for PPS were found when searching the databases, but one Cochrane review is being prepared [35]. Data were classified according to their scientific level of evidence as Class I–IV [36]. Recommendations are given as Level A–C according to the scheme for EFNS guidelines. When only Class IV evidence was available but consensus could be reached the task force gives our recommendations as Good Practice Points (GPP)[36]. Consensus was reached mainly through email correspondence.

A questionnaire about diagnosis, management, and care of post-polio patients was answered by the group members from The Netherlands, Norway, Poland, Sweden, and the United Kingdom in the first version; this has not been repeated in this revision.

Results

Therapeutic interventions

Acetylcholinesterase inhibitors, steroids, amantadine, modafinil, lamotrigine, coenzyme Q10, intravenous immunoglobulin (IVIg)

The effect of acetylcholinesterase inhibitors in PPS has been investigated in four studies with particular emphasis on fatigue, muscular strength, and quality of life. One open pilot study indicated a positive effect on fatigue [37, 38], but this was not confirmed in two double-blinded randomized controlled trials using a daily dose of 180 mg pyridostigmine [39, 40]. Horemans et al. reported a significant improvement in walking performance, but the difference in quadriceps strength was not significant as reported by Trojan et al. Hence, there is evidence at Class I that pyridostigmine is not effective in the management of fatigue and muscular strength in PPS. One randomized study explored the effect on fatigue of 400 mg modafinil daily in PPS [41]. Modafinil was not superior to placebo, and there is Class I evidence that modafinil is not effective on fatigue in PPS. There are two randomized placebo-controlled studies investigating the effect of high-dose prednisolone (80 mg daily) and amantandine (200 mg daily) on muscular weakness and fatigue (prednisone), and fatigue (amantadine) [42, 43]. They included a small number of patients, 17 and 23 respectively, and only Stein et al. included statistical power calculations. There was no significant effect on muscular strength or fatigue in any of these Class I studies.

Lamotrigine has been tried in an open study (15 patients treated with 50–100 mg lamotrigine daily), where a positive effect on quality of life (Nottingham Health Profile), pain (VAS), and fatigue (FSS) was found after 2 and 4 weeks [44]. A double-blinded randomized study is needed to confirm this finding. In a randomized double-blinded pilot study of coenzyme Q10 (200 mg daily) including 14 patients, no additional effect to resistance muscle training was found [45].

Several reports of increased levels of inflammatory markers in serum and CSF in PPS have raised the question whether immunological changes could be a part of the pathophysiology in PPS [16, 17, 46]. These findings have also presented a rationale for investigating immune-modulating therapies in PPS. Intravenous immunoglobulin (IVIg) has been tried in three therapeutic intervention studies. Gonzalez et al. performed a multicentre double-blinded randomized study including 135 patients where the primary endpoints were muscle strength in a pre-selected muscle group and quality of life measured with the SF-36 scale. The patients were treated with either placebo or 90 g IvIg, repeated after 3 months. A significant difference on muscle strength was found, but no significant effect on the SF-36 on pain, balance, or sleep quality[47]. Farbu et al. performed a double-blinded randomized study with 20 patients with the primary endpoints muscle strength (isometric), pain (VAS), and fatigue (FSS) after 3 months [48]. The patients were treated with one dose of IvIg (2 g/kg body weight). A significant effect was found on pain, but not on muscle strength or fatigue. One open study with 14 patients explored the effect of 90 mg IvIg on muscle strength, physical ability measured by walking test, and quality of life (SF-36) [49]. There was a positive effect on quality of life, but not on muscle strength or physical ability. These studies indicate that IvIg could have a modest therapeutic benefit in PPS, but they include a small number of patients, the results are diverging according to which symptoms improving after treatment, and the IvIg has not been compared with other therapies like specific training programmes. There is also a remaining question about the appropriate dose of IvIg and therapeutic interval. Hence, IvIg can at present not be recommended as standard treatment in PPS, despite two Class 1 studies [50].

Muscular training

It has been claimed that muscular overuse and training may worsen the symptoms in patients with residual weakness after paralytic polio, and even provoke a further loss of muscular strength.[51]. Many post-polio patients have been advised to avoid muscular overuse and intensive training [4, 52]. Studies of morphology and oxidative capacity in the tibialis anterior muscle indicate a high muscular activity due to gait and weight bearing [53, 54]. When followed prospectively, the macro EMG motor unit potential amplitude (MUP) in the tibialis anterior muscle was found to be increased after 5 years, whereas there was no change in the macro MUP amplitude in the biceps brachii muscle [55]. This indicates a more pronounced denervation-reinnervation process in the tibialis muscle, which may be due to daily use and higher muscle activities in the leg muscles. However, there are no prospective studies, which show that increased muscle activity or training lead to loss of muscular strength compared to absence of training or less muscular activity. On the contrary, patients who reported regular physical activity had fewer symptoms and a higher functional level than physically inactive patients [11, 56]. One randomized controlled trial reported significant improvement in muscular strength after a 12-week training programme with isometric contraction of hand muscles [57]. Non-randomized trials with training programmes lasting from 6 weeks to 6 months involving both isokinetic, isometric, and endurance muscular training have shown a significant increase in both isokinetic and isometric muscle strength [58–61]. Oncu et al. found that both time-limited hospital and home exercise programmes improved fatigue and quality of life in the short term [62]. No complications or side effects were reported. Hence, there is evidence at Class II and III that supervised training programmes increase muscle strength and can improve quality of life and relieve fatigue in patients with post-polio syndrome. Two follow-up open studies of multidisciplinary rehabilitation report a positive effect on fatigue and physical capacity up to 1 year after the intervention [63, 64]. This is promising, but long-term effects (several years) of training are not documented and deserve prospective studies. For patients without cardiovascular disease, one randomized controlled study reported improved cardiovascular fitness after supervised exercise programmes using ergometer cycle [65] (Class I). Aerobic training in upper extremities had a beneficial effect on oxygen consumption, minute ventilation, power, and exercise time [66] (Class II). Aerobic walking exercises can help to economize movements and increase endurance without improvement in cardiovascular fitness [67]. Ernstoff et al. reported an increase in work performance by reduction of heart rate during exercises; hence endurance training seems to improve cardiovascular conditioning (Class IV). It is important to emphasize that most exercise studies have been executed with supervision, sub-maximal work load, intermittent breaks, and rest periods between exercise sessions to prevent the likelihood of overuse effects. This is an important aspect for PPS patients in general. Most of the participating patients in these studies younger than 60 years, and the effect of exercise programmes older patients is therefore less documented.

One randomized controlled study of post-polio patients with pain, weakness, and fatigue in their shoulder muscles compared the effect of exercise only, exercise in combination with lifestyle modification, and lifestyle modification only [68]. Significant improvement was found only for the two groups with exercise (Class II). The endpoints in this study were combinations of several symptoms. Further studies are needed to identify improvement on particular symptoms before conclusions are drawn regarding lifestyle modifications.

Treatment in a warm climate and training in water

Anecdotal reports from post-polio patients indicate a positive effect of a warm climate and of training in warm water with respect to pain and fatigue. One randomized controlled study reported a significant reduction in pain, health-related problems, and depression for both groups after completing identical training programmes in either Norway or Tenerife [69]. No significant difference in walking tests was seen. Both groups improved their walking skills, reduced their level of fatigue, depression, and health-related problems. However, the effect remained significantly longer in the Tenerife group (Class I).

Dynamic non-swimming water exercises for post-polio patients have been reported to reduce pain, improve cardiovascular conditioning, and increase subjective wellbeing in a controlled but not randomized study (Class III) [70]. A qualitative interview study (Class IV) indicated a positive effect on the self-confidence when performing group training in water [71].

Respiratory aid

Reduced pulmonary function due to weak respiratory muscles and/or chest deformities may occur in patients with previous polio [22, 72]. Patients with chest deformities have an increased risk of nocturnal hypoventilation and sleep-disordered breathing [22, 73, 74]. The prevalence of respiratory impairment is highest among patients who were treated with artificial ventilation in the acute phase [22]. Shortness of breath is a common complaint in many post-polio patients, but is not necessarily related to respiratory impairment, but rather to orthopaedic and general medication problems. Two hospital-based studies showed that respiratory function was normal in the majority of patients reporting shortness of breath, and cardiovascular deconditioning and being overweight were the most common cause for this symptom [10, 75]. Respiratory impairment can occur without shortness of breath and can present with daytime somnolence, morning headache, and fatigue [67]. There are no randomized trials evaluating the effect of respiratory aids. Reports indicate that early introduction of non-invasive respiratory aids like intermittent positive pressure ventilation (IPPV) or biphasic positive pressure (BIPAP) ventilators via mouthpiece or nasal application can stabilize the situation and prevent complications such as chest infections, further respiratory decline, and invasive ventilatory aid (tracheostomy) [73, 76], and also improve exercise capacity [77] (Class IV). If invasive ventilatory aid is needed, PPS patients with a tracheostomy and mechanical home ventilation are reported to have good perceived health despite severe physical disability [78] (Class III). For patients already using intermittent respiratory aids, respiratory muscle training is useful [79] (Class IV). General precautions such as stopping smoking, mobilization of secretions, and cough assistance are beneficial [73].

Bulbar symptoms

Weakening of bulbar muscles causing dysphagia, weakness of voice, and vocal changes have been reported among patients with PPS [80–83]. Case reports indicate that speech therapy and laryngeal muscle training are useful for these patients (Class IV) [83].

Weight control, assistive devices, and lifestyle modifications

The importance of reducing weight, adaptation to assistive devices, and modification of activities of daily living has been emphasized [4, 6, 84, 85]. The scientific evidence for these recommendations is limited, but there was consensus in our group that an individual with weak muscles benefits from losing excess weight, and that

proper orthoses, walking sticks, and wheelchairs facilitate daily life activities (GPPs). Participating in muscle-training programmes and endurance training will, in many cases, also lead to weight loss, but there is no evidence that weight reduction alone can ameliorate symptoms. Patients with BMI (body mass index) > 25, which is defined as overweight, did not report more symptoms than those of normal weight [10]. On the other hand, a recent weight gain was found to be a predictive factor for PPS [86]. Sleep disorders are common among PPS patients [10], and can be a mix of obstructive sleep apnoea, frequency of tiredness on waking up and during the day, headache on waking up, daytime sleepiness, restless legs, and hypoventilation [87–89]. It is widely accepted that obesity is related to obstructive sleep apnoea, and weight control is crucial for this disorder [90]. The number of patients receiving mechanical home ventilation because of obesity-induced hypoventilation has increased [91]. From this perspective, there is a rationale for reducing excess weight in PPS patients (Class IV).

One pilot study reported that a change from metal braces to lightweight carbon orthoses can be useful and increase walking ability in polio patients with new pareses [92]. This has been confirmed in two other open uncontrolled studies [93, 94], and there is Class III evidence that lightweight orthoses should be preferred compared to metal braces. Biomechanical analysis of the walking pattern can lead to optimal design of orthoses and improve function in the lower limbs (Class IV) [94, 95].

Frequent periods of rest, energy conservation, and work simplification skills are thought to be useful for patients with fatigue [96].

Coming to terms with new disabilities, educational interventions

New loss of function, increase in disability, and handicap are common in post-polio patients [5, 10, 97]. This can lead to reduced wellbeing and emotional stress. Group training with other post-polio patients, participation, and regular follow-up at post-polio clinics can prevent a decline in mental status and give a more positive experience of the 'self' [71, 98] (Class III). Acceptance of assistive devices, environmental support, and spending more time on daily tasks can facilitate coping with home and occupational life (Class III) [99].

Recommendations

Level A

- Some controlled studies of potential specific medical treatments for PPS have been completed, and no definitive therapeutic effect has been reported for the agents pyridostigmine, steroids, amantadine, modafinil, and coenzyme Q10.

Level B

- Supervised muscular training, both isokinetic and isometric, is a safe and effective way to prevent further decline of muscle strength in slightly or moderately weak muscle groups and can even reduce symptoms of muscular fatigue, muscle weakness, and pain in selected post-polio patients. A prolonged effect up to one year after well-defined training programmes has been reported.
- There are no studies evaluating the effect of muscular training in patients with severe weakness and the long-term effect of such training is not yet explored.
- Precautions to avoid muscular overuse should be taken with intermittent breaks, periods of rest between series of exercises, and submaximal work load.
- Training in a warm climate and non-swimming water exercises are particularly useful.

Level C

- Recognition of respiratory impairment and early introduction of non-invasive ventilatory aids prevent or delay further respiratory decline and the need of invasive respiratory aids.
- Respiratory muscle training can improve pulmonary function.
- Group training, regular follow-ups, and patient education are useful for the patients' mental status and wellbeing.
- Lightweight carbon orthoses can be more proper than metal orthoses.

Good Practice Points

- Weight loss, and adjustment and introduction of properly fitted assistive devices is helpful, but lack significant scientific evidence.

New revision of guidelines

Prospective follow-up studies evaluating muscle strength and function during the natural course of the disorder are welcomed. Studies evaluating the effects of muscular training in patients with severe muscular weakness are needed, in addition to prospective studies evaluating the long-term effects of muscular training. A potential positive effect of IvIg in PPS has been claimed in three recent studies, and follow-up studies to investigate whether IvIg could be a therapeutic option are needed.

Conflicts of interest

The authors have reported no conflicts of interests.

References

1. Nollet F, de Visser M. Postpolio syndrome. *Arch Neurol* 2004;**61**(7):1142–4.
2. Raymond M. Paralysie essentielle de l'enfance, atrophie musculaire con,cutive. *C R Soc Biol* 1875;**27**:158.
3. Halstead LS, Rossi CD. New problems in old polio patients: results of a survey of 539 polio survivors. *Orthopedics* 1985;**8**(7):845–50.
4. MarchofDimes. March of Dimes International Conference on Post Polio Syndrome. Identifying best practices in diagnosis and care. www.marchofdimes.com/files/PPSreport.pdf *March of Dimes*, NY, USA: White Plains, 2000; pp. 9–11.
5. Ivanyi B, Nollet F, Redekop WK, *et al.* Late onset polio sequelae: disabilities and handicaps in a population- based cohort of the 1956 poliomyelitis outbreak in the Netherlands. *Arch Phys Med Rehabil* 1999;**80**(6):687–90.
6. Jubelt B, Agre JC. Characteristics and management of post-polio syndrome. *JAMA* 2000;**284**(4):412–4.
7. Chang CW, Huang SF. Varied clinical patterns, physical activities, muscle enzymes, electromyographic and histologic findings in patients with post-polio syndrome in Taiwan. *Spinal Cord* 2001;**39**(10):526–31.
8. Farbu E, Gilhus NE. Former poliomyelitis as a health and socioeconomic factor. A paired sibling study. *J Neurol* 2002;**249**(4):404–9.
9. Farbu E, Gilhus NE. Education, occupation, and perception of health amongst previous polio patients compared to their siblings. *Eur J Neurol* 2002;**9**(3):233–41.
10. Farbu E, Rekand T, Gilhus NE. Post polio syndrome and total health status in a prospective hospital study. *Eur J Neurol* 2003;**10**(4):407–13.
11. Rekand T, Korv J, Farbu E, *et al.* Lifestyle and late effects after poliomyelitis. A risk factor study of two populations. *Acta Neurologica Scandinavica* 2004;**109**(2):120–5.
12. Takemura J, Saeki S, Hachisuka K, Aritome K. Prevalence of post-polio syndrome based on a cross-sectional survey in Kitakyushu, Japan. *J Rehab Med* 2004;**36**(1):1–3.

13. Nielsen NM, Rostgaard K, Juel K, Askgaard D, Aaby P. Long-term mortality after poliomyelitis. *Epidemiology* 2003;**14**(3):355–60.

14. Dalakas MC. Pathogenetic mechanisms of post-polio syndrome: morphological, electrophysiological, virological, and immunological correlations. *Ann N Y Acad Sci* 1995;**753**: 167–85.

15. Stalberg E, Grimby G. Dynamic electromyography and muscle biopsy changes in a 4-year follow-up: study of patients with a history of polio. *Muscle Nerve* 1995;**18**(7): 699–707.

16. Gonzalez H, Khademi M, Andersson M, Wallstrom E, Borg K, Olsson T. Prior poliomyelitis-evidence of cytokine production in the central nervous system. *J Neurol Sci* 2002;**205**(1):9–13.

17. Fordyce CB, Gagne D, Jalili F, *et al*. Elevated serum inflammatory markers in post-poliomyelitis syndrome. *J Neurol Sci* 2008;**271**(1–2):80–6.

18. Sorenson EJ, Daube JR, Windebank AJ. A 15-year follow-up of neuromuscular function in patients with prior poliomyelitis. *Neurology* 2005;**64**(6):1070–2.

19. Stolwijk-Swuste JM, Beelen A, Lankhorst GJ, Nollet F. The course of functional status and muscle strength in patients with late-onset sequelae of poliomyelitis: a systematic review. *Arch Phys Med Rehabil* 2005;**86**(8):1693–701.

20. Sunnerhagen KS, Grimby G. Muscular effects in late polio. *Acta Physiol Scand* 2001;**171**(3):335–40.

21. Howard RS. Poliomyelitis and the postpolio syndrome. *BMJ* 2005;**330**(7503):1314–8.

22. Howard RS, Wiles CM, Spencer GT. The late sequelae of poliomyelitis. *Q J Med* 1988;**66**(251):219–32.

23. Stolwijk-Swuste JM, Beelen A, Lankhorst G, Nollet F. Impact of age and co-morbidity on the functioning of patients with sequelae of poliomyelitis: a cross-sectional study. *J Rehabil Med* 2007;**39**(1):56–62.

24. Burger H, Marincek C. The influence of post-polio syndrome on independence and life satisfaction. *Disabil Rehabil* 2000;**22**(7):318–22.

25. Dalakas MC. The post-polio syndrome as an evolved clinical entity. Definition and clinical description. *Ann N Y Acad Sci* 1995;**753**:68–80.

26. Halstead LS. Post-polio syndrome. *Sci Am* 1998;**278**(4):42–7.

27. Halstead LS, Rossi CD. Post-polio syndrome: clinical experience with 132 consecutive outpatients. *Birth Defects Orig Artic Ser* 1987;**23**(4):13–26.

28. Ramlow J, Alexander M, LaPorte R, Kaufmann C, Kuller L. Epidemiology of the post-polio syndrome. *Am J Epidemiol* 1992;**136**(7):769–86.

29. Lonnberg F. Late onset polio sequelae in Denmark. Results of a nationwide survey of 3,607 polio survivors. *Scand J Rehabil Med Suppl* 1993;**28**:1–32.

30. Pentland B, Hellawell D, Benjamin J, Prasad R, Ainslie A. Survey of the late consequences of polio in Edinburgh and the Lothians. *Health Bull* 2000;**58**(4):267–75.

31. Rekand T, Korv J, Farbu E, *et al*. Long term outcome after poliomyelitis in different health and social conditions. *J Epidemiol Community Health* 2003;**57**(5):368–72.

32. Ivanyi B, Redekop W, De Jongh R, De Visser M. Computed tomographic study of the skeletal musculature of the lower body in 45 postpolio patients. *Muscle Nerve* 1998;**21**(4): 540–2.

33. Hildegunn L, Jones K, Grenstad T, Dreyer V, Farbu E, Rekand T. Perceived disability, fatigue, pain and measured isometric muscle strength in patients with post-polio symptoms. *Physiother Res Int* 2007;**12**(1):39–49.

34. Grimby G, Stalberg E, Sandberg A, Sunnerhagen KS. An 8-year longitudinal study of muscle strength, muscle fiber size, and dynamic electromyogram in individuals with late polio. *Muscle Nerve* 1998;**21**(11):1428–37.

35. Koopman FS, Uegaki K, Gilhus NE, Beelen A, De Visser M, Nollet F. Treatment for postpolio syndrome (Protocol). *Cochrane Database Syst Rev* 2009;(2):CD 007818.

36. Brainin M, Barnes M, Baron JC, *et al*. Guidance for the preparation of neurological managment guidelines by EFNS scientific task forces – revised recommendations 2004. *Eur J Neurol* 2004;**11**:1–6.

37. Trojan DA, Cashman NR. An open trial of pyridostigmine in post-poliomyelitis syndrome. *Can J Neurol Sci* 1995;**22**(3): 223–7.

38. Trojan DA, Gendron D, Cashman NR. Anticholinesterase-responsive neuromuscular junction transmission defects in post-poliomyelitis fatigue. *J Neurol Sci* 1993;**114**(2): 170–7.

39. Trojan DA, Collet JP, Shapiro S, *et al*. A multicenter, randomized, double-blinded trial of pyridostigmine in postpolio syndrome. *Neurology* 1999;**53**(6):1225–33.

40. Horemans HLD, Nollet F, Beelen A, *et al*. Pyridostigmine in postpolio syndrome: no decline in fatigue and limited functional improvement. *J Neurol, Neurosurg Psych* 2003;**74**(12): 1655–61.

41. Vasconcelos OM, Prokhorenko OA, Salajegheh MK, *et al*. Modafinil for treatment of fatigue in post-polio syndrome: a randomized controlled trial. *Neurology* 2007;**68**(20): 1680–6.

42. Dinsmore S, Dambrosia J, Dalakas MC. A double-blind, placebo-controlled trial of high-dose prednisone for the treatment of post-poliomyelitis syndrome. *Ann N Y Acad Sci* 1995;**753**:303–13.

43. Stein DP, Dambrosia JM, Dalakas MC. A double-blind, placebo-controlled trial of amantadine for the treatment of fatigue in patients with the post-polio syndrome. *Ann N Y Acad Sci* 1995;**753**:296–302.

44. On AY, Oncu J, Uludag B, Ertekin C. Effects of lamotrigine on the symptoms and life qualities of patients with post polio syndrome: a randomized, controlled study. *Neuro Rehabil* 2005;**20**(4):245–51.

45. Skough K, Krossen C, Heiwe S, Theorell H, Borg K. Effects of resistance training in combination with coenzyme Q10 supplementation in patients with post-polio: a pilot study. *J Rehabil Med* 2008;**40**(9):773–5.

46. Gonzalez H, Khademi M, Andersson M, *et al*. Prior polio-myelitis-IVIg treatment reduces proinflammatory cytokine production. *J Neuroimmunol* 2004;**150**(1–2):139–44.

47. Gonzalez H, Sunnerhagen KS, Sjoberg I, Kaponides G, Olsson T, Borg K. Intravenous immunoglobulin for post-polio syndrome: a randomised controlled trial. *Lancet Neurol* 2006;**5**(6):493–500.

48. Farbu E, Rekand T, Vik-Mo E, Lygren H, Gilhus NE, Aarli JA. Post-polio syndrome patients treated with intravenous immunoglobulin: a double-blinded randomized controlled pilot study. *Eur J Neurol* 2007;**14**(1):60–5.

49. Kaponides G, Gonzalez H, Olsson T, Borg K. Effect of intravenous immunoglobulin in patients with post-polio syndrome–an uncontrolled pilot study. *J Rehabil Med* 2006;**38**(2):138–40.

50. Elovaara I, Apostolski S, van Doorn P, *et al*. EFNS guidelines for the use of intravenous immunoglobulin in treatment of neurological diseases: EFNS task force on the use of intra-venous immunoglobulin in treatment of neurological dis-eases. *Eur J Neurol* 2008;**15**(9):893–908.

51. Bennett RL, Knowlton GC. Overwork weakness in partially denervated skeletal muscle. *Clin Orthop* 1958;**15**(12):22–9.

52. Halstead LS, Gawne AC. NRH proposal for limb classifica-tion and exercise prescription. *Disabil Rehabil* 1996;**18**(6):311–6.

53. Borg K, Henriksson J. Prior poliomyelitis-reduced capillary supply and metabolic enzyme content in hypertrophic slow-twitch (type I) muscle fibres. *J Neurol, Neurosurg Psych* 1991;**54**(3):236–40.

54. Grimby L, Tollback A, Muller U, Larsson L. Fatigue of chronically overused motor units in prior polio patients. *Muscle Nerve* 1996;**19**(6):728–37.

55. Sandberg A, Stalberg E. Changes in macro electromyogra-phy over time in patients with a history of polio: a compari-son of 2 muscles. *Arch Phys Med Rehabil* 2004;**85**(7):1174–82.

56. Veicsteinas A, Sarchi P, Mattiotti S, Bignotto M, Belleri M. Cardiorespiratory and metabolic adjustments during sub-maximal and maximal exercise in polio athletes. *Medicina Dello Sport* 1998;**51**(4):361–73.

57. Chan KM, Amirjani N, Sumrain M, Clarke A, Strohschein FJ. Randomized controlled trial of strength training in post-polio patients. *Muscle Nerve* 2003;**27**(3):332–8.

58. Einarsson G. Muscle conditioning in late poliomyelitis. *Arch Phys Med Rehabil* 1991;**72**(1):11–4.

59. Ernstoff B, Wetterqvist H, Kvist H, Grimby G. Endurance training effect on individuals with postpoliomyelitis. *Arch Phys Med Rehabil* 1996;**77**(9):843–8.

60. Spector SA, Gordon PL, Feuerstein IM, Sivakumar K, Hurley BF, Dalakas MC. Strength gains without muscle injury after strength training in patients with postpolio muscular atrophy. *Muscle Nerve* 1996;**19**(10):1282–90.

61. Agre JC, Rodriquez AA, Franke TM. Strength, endurance, and work capacity after muscle strengthening exercise in postpolio subjects. *Arch Phys Med Rehabil* 1997;**78**(7):681–6.

62. Oncu J, Durmaz B, Karapolat H. Short-term effects of aerobic exercise on functional capacity, fatigue, and quality of life in patients with post-polio syndrome. *Clin Rehabil* 2009;**23**(2):155–63.

63. Bertelsen M, Broberg S, Madsen E. Outcome of phy-siotherapy as part of a multidisciplinary rehabilitation in an unselected polio population with one-year follow-up: an uncontrolled study. *J Rehabil Med* 2009;**41**(1):85–7.

64. Davidson AC, Auyeung V, Luff R, Holland M, Hodgkiss A, Weinman J. Prolonged benefit in post-polio syndrome from comprehensive rehabilitation: a pilot study. *Disabil Rehabil* 2009;**31**(4):309–17.

65. Jones DR, Speier J, Canine K, Owen R, Stull A. Car-diorespiratory responses to aeroic training by patients with postpoliomyelitis sequelae. *JAMA* 1989;**261**(22):3255–8.

66. Kriz JL, Jones DR, Speier JL, Canine JK, Owen RR, Serfass RC. Cardiorespiratory responses to upper extremity aerobic training by postpolio subjects. *Arch Phys Med Rehabil* 1992;**73**:49–54.

67. Dean E, Ross J. Effect of modified aerobic training on move-ment energetics in polio survivors. *Orthopedics* 1991;**14**(11):1243–6.

68. Klein MG, Whyte J, Esquenazi A, Keenan MA, Costello R. A comparison of the effects of exercise and lifestyle modifi-cation on the resolution of overuse symptoms of the shoul-der in polio survivors: a preliminary study. *Arch Phys Med Rehabil* 2002;**83**(5):708–13.

69. Strumse YAS, Stanghelle JK, Utne L, Ahlvin P, Svendsby EK. Treatment of patients with postpolio syndrome in a warm climate. *Disabil Rehabil* 2003;**25**(2):77–84.

70. Willen C, Sunnerhagen KS, Grimby G. Dynamic water exer-cise in individuals with late poliomyelitis. *Arch Phys Med Rehabil* 2001;**82**(1):66–72.

71. Willen C, Scherman MH. Group training in a pool causes ripples on the water: experiences by persons with late effects of polio. *J Rehabil Med* 2002;**34**(4):191–7.

72. Kidd D, Howard RS, Williams AJ, Heatley FW, Panayiotopoulos CP, Spencer GT. Late functional deterioration following paralytic poliomyelitis. *QJM* 1997;**90**(3): 189–96.

73. Bergholtz B, Mollestad SO, Refsum H. Post-polio respiratory failure. New manifestations of a forgotten disease. *Tidsskr Nor Laegeforen* 1988;**108**(29):2474–5.

74. Howard R. Late post-polio functional deterioration. *Pract Neurol* 2003;**3**(2):66–77.

75. Stanghelle JK, Festvag L, Aksnes AK. Pulmonary function and symptom-limited exercise stress testing in subjects with late sequelae of poliomyelitis. *Scand J Rehabil Med* 1993;**25**(3):125–9.

76. Bach JR. Management of post-polio respiratory sequelae. *Ann N Y Acad Sci* 1995;**753**:96–102.

77. Vaz Fragoso CA, Kacmarek RM, Systrom DM. Improvement in exercise capacity after nocturnal positive pressure ventilation and tracheostomy in a postpoliomyelitis patient. *Chest* 1992;**101**(1):254–7.

78. Markstrom A, Sundell K, Lysdahl M, Andersson G, Schedin U, Klang B. Quality-of-life evaluation of patients with neuromuscular and skeletal diseases treated with noninvasive and invasive home mechanical ventilation. *Chest* 2002;**122**(5):1695–700.

79. Klefbeck B, Lagerstrand L, Mattsson E. Inspiratory muscle training in patients with prior polio who use part-time assisted ventilation. *Arch Phys Med Rehabil* 2000;**81**(8): 1065–71.

80. Sonies BC, Dalakas MC. Dysphagia in patients with the post-polio syndrome. *N Eng J Med* 1991;**324**(17):1162–7.

81. Ivanyi B, Phoa SS, de Visser VM. Dysphagia in postpolio patients: a videofluorographic follow-up study. *Dysphagia* 1994;**9**(2):96–8.

82. Driscoll BP, Gracco C, Coelho C, *et al.* Laryngeal function in postpolio patients. *Laryngoscope* 1995;**105**(1):35–41.

83. Abaza MM, Sataloff RT, Hawkshaw MJ, Mandel S. Laryngeal manifestations of postpoliomyelitis syndrome. *J Voice* 2001;**15**(2):291–4.

84. Halstead LS, Gawne AC, Pham BT. National rehabilitation hospital limb classification for exercise, research, and clinical trials in post-polio patients. *Ann N Y Acad Sci* 1995;**753**: 343–53.

85. Thorsteinsson G. Management of postpolio syndrome. *Mayo Clin Proc* 1997;**72**(7):627–38.

86. Trojan DA, Cashman NR, Shapiro S, Tansey CM, Esdaile JM. Predictive factors for post-poliomyelitis syndrome. *Arch Phys Med Rehabil* 1994;**75**(7):770–7.

87. Steljes DG, Kryger MH, Kirk BW, Millar TW. Sleep in post-polio syndrome. *Chest* 1990;**98**(1):133–40.

88. Van Kralingen KW, Ivanyi B, Van Keimpema ARJ, Venmans BJW, De Visser M, Postmus PE. Sleep complaints in post-polio syndrome. *Arch Phys Med Rehabil* 1996;**77**(6): 609–11.

89. Hsu AA, Staats BA. 'Postpolio' sequelae and sleep-related disordered breathing. *Mayo Clin Proc* 1998;**73**(3):216–24.

90. Gami AS, Caples SM, Somers VK. Obesity and obstructive sleep apnea. *Endocrinol Metab Clin North Am* 2003;**32**(4): 869–94.

91. Janssens JP, Derivaz S, Breitenstein E, *et al.* Changing patterns in long-term noninvasive ventilation: a 7-year prospective study in the Geneva Lake Area. *Chest* 2003;**123**(1): 67–79.

92. Heim M, Yaacobi E, Azaria M. A pilot study to determine the efficiency of lightweight carbon fibre orthoses in the management of patients suffering from post-poliomyelitis syndrome. *Clin Rehabil* 1997;**11**(4):302–5.

93. Hachisuka K, Makino K, Wada F, Saeki S, Yoshimoto N, Arai M. Clinical application of carbon fibre reinforced plastic leg orthosis for polio survivors and its advantages and disadvantages. *Prosthet Orthot Int* 2006;**30**(2):129–35.

94. Brehm MA, Beelen A, Doorenbosch CA, Harlaar J, Nollet F. Effect of carbon-composite knee-ankle-foot orthoses on walking efficiency and gait in former polio patients. *J Rehabil Med* 2007;**39**(8):651–7.

95. Perry J, Clark D. Biomechanical abnormalities of post-polio patients and the implications for orthotic management. *Neurorehabilitation* 1997;**8**(2):119–38.

96. Packer TL, Martins I, Krefting L, Brouwer B. Activity and post-polio fatigue. *Orthopedics* 1991;**14**(11):1223–6.

97. Nollet F, Beelen A, Prins MH, *et al.* Disability and functional assessment in former polio patients with and without post-polio syndrome. *Arch Phys Med Rehabil* 1999;**80**(2): 136–43.

98. Stanghelle JK, Festvag LV. Postpolio syndrome: a 5 year follow-up. *Spinal Cord* 1997;**35**(8):503–8.

99. Thoren-Jonsson AL. Coming to terms with the shift in one's capabilities: a study of the adaptive process in persons with poliomyelitis sequelae. *Disabil Rehabil* 2001;**23**(8):341–51.

CHAPTER 19

Autoimmune neuromuscular transmission disorders

G. O. Skeie,[1] S. Apostolski,[2] A. Evoli,[3] N. E. Gilhus,[1] I. Illa,[4] L. Harms,[5] D. Hilton-Jones,[6] A. Melms,[7] J. Verschuuren,[8] H. Westgaard Horge[9]

[1]University of Bergen, Norway; [2]Institute of Neurology, School of Medicine, University of Belgrade, Serbia and Montenegro; [3]Catholic University, Rome, Italy; [4]Hospital Sta Creu i Sant Pau, Barcelona, Spain; [5]Universitätsmedizin Berlin Charité, Neurologische Klinik Berlin, Germany; [6]Radcliffe Infirmary, Oxford, UK; [7]Neurologische Klinik, Universität Tübingen, Germany; [8]LUMC, Leiden, The Netherlands; [9]The Norwegian Muscular Disorders Association, Norway

Background and objectives

Autoimmune neuromuscular transmission (NMT) disorders are relatively rare, but often debilitating diseases. Myasthenia gravis (MG) is caused by autoantibodies against components of the postsynaptic neuromuscular junction. The autoimmune attack at the muscle endplate leads to NMT failure and muscle weakness. Lambert–Eaton myasthenic syndrome (LEMS) is caused by antibodies against the voltage-gated calcium channels (VGCC) at the presynaptic side of the muscle endplate. The antibodies inhibit acetylcholine release and cause NMT failure and muscle weakness. Neuromyotonia (peripheral nerve hyperexcitability; Isaacs' syndrome) is caused by antibodies to nerve voltage-gated potassium channels (VGKC) that produce nerve hyperexcitability and spontaneous and continuous skeletal muscle overactivity, presenting as twitching and painful cramps and stiffness.

Our increased understanding of the basic mechanisms of neuromuscular transmission and autoimmunity has led to the development of novel treatment strategies. NMT disorders are now amenable to treatment and their prognoses are good. Treatment developed for other and more common antibody-mediated autoimmune disor-

ders with similar pathogenetic processes have also been applied for NMT disorders. Although present treatment strategies are increasingly underpinned by scientific evidence, they are still based partly on clinical experience. In this paper, we have evaluated the available literature and give evidence-based treatment guidelines.

Materials and methods

Search strategy

MEDLINE 1966–2009 and EMBASE 1966–2004 were examined with appropriate MESH and free subject terms: 1 Myasthenia, 2 Myasthenia gravis, 3 Lambert Eaton, 4 Lambert Eaton myasthenic syndrome/LEMS, 5 Neuromyotonia, 6 Isaacs' syndrome.

1–6 was combined with the terms: 7 Treatment, 8 Medication, 9 Therapy, 10 Controlled clinical trial, 11 Randomized controlled trial, 12 Clinical trial, 13 Multicentre study, 14 Meta-analysis, 15 Crossover studies, 16 Thymectomy, 17 Immunosuppression

The Cochrane Central Register of Controlled Trials (CENTRAL) was also sought.

Articles in English that contained data which could be rated according to the guidance statement for neurological management guidelines of EFNS were included [1].

Information from patient and other voluntary organizations and existing guidelines including those from the American Academy of Neurology was reviewed and validated according to the above criteria. Finished and ongoing Cochrane data-based projects on LEMS treatment, immunosuppressive MG treatment, IVIg for MG, plasmapheresis for MG, and corticosteroids for MG in addition to thymectomy for MG were reviewed.

Methods for reaching consensus

Four members of the task force prepared parts of the manuscript and draft statements about the treatment of MG, LEMS, and neuromyotonia. Evidence was classified as Class I–IV and recommendations as Level A–C according to the scheme agreed for EFNS guidelines [1]. When only Class IV evidence was available but consensus could be reached the task force has offered advice as Good Practice Points (GPP) [1]. The statements were revised and collated into a single document, which was then revised iteratively until consensus was reached.

Myasthenia gravis (MG)

MG is characterized by a fluctuating weakness of skeletal muscle with remissions and exacerbations [2]. In 85% of MG patients, the disease is caused by antibodies against the AChR at the postsynaptic side of the neuromuscular junction which cause transmission failure and produce destruction of the endplate. Of the 15% of generalized MG patients without AChR antibodies, 20–50% have antibodies against another synaptic antigen, muscle-specific tyrosine kinase [MuSK] [3]. The remaining patients probably have antibodies against unknown antigens at the neuromuscular junction or low level/affinity antibodies against AChR or MuSK that are not detectable by standard assays. MG is closely associated with thymic pathology. Fifteen per cent of MG patients have a thymoma and often have antibodies against additional striated muscle antigens such as titin [4] and ryanodine receptors [5]. These antibodies are more common in thymoma and severe MG and are considered as useful markers [6, 7]. A hypertrophic thymus is found in 60% of MG patients, typically young females, while most patients with debut after 50 years of age, have a normal or atrophic thymus.

MG often used to cause chronic, severe disability and had a high mortality. However, improved treatment allied with advances in critical care have transformed the long-term prognosis and life expectancy is now near normal [8–11].

Symptomatic treatment

Acetylcholine esterase inhibitors (of which pyridostigmine is the most widely used) inhibit the breakdown of ACh at the neuromuscular junction. This increases the availability of ACh to stimulate AChR and facilitates muscle activation and contraction. These drugs are most helpful as initial therapy in newly diagnosed MG patients, and as sole long-term treatment of milder disease.

These drugs are usually well tolerated at standard doses of up to 60 mg five times per day. Adverse effects are caused by the increased concentration of ACh at both nicotinic and muscarinic synapses. The common muscarinic effects are gut hypermotility (stomach cramps, diarrhoea), increased sweathing, excessive respiratory and gastrointestinal secretions [12, 13], and bradycardia. The main nicotinic adverse effects are muscle fasciculations and cramps.

There are no placebo-controlled randomized studies of these drugs, but case reports, case series, and daily clinical experience demonstrate an objective and marked clinical effect (Class IV evidence). Although there is inadequate evidence for a formal recommendation, the task force agreed that an anticholinesterase drug should be the first-line treatment for all forms of MG (Class IV evidence, GPP). However, its use should be cautious in patients with anti-MuSK antibodies who often show Ach hypersensitivity [14].

The optimal dose is determined by the balance between clinical improvement and adverse effects, and can vary over time and with concomitant treatment. There is one report of additional effect of intranasally administered pyridostigmine, although this is not commercially available [15] (Class III evidence).

3,4-diaminopyridine releases ACh from nerve terminals. In a double-blind, placebo-controlled trial the drug seemed effective in congenital (hereditary and non-immune) myasthenia patients. Juvenile MG patients did not respond [16](Class III evidence). The drug is not recommended in autoimmune MG, although it may prove useful in some forms of congenital myasthenia (Level C recommendation).

Ephedrine, increases ACh release. It has probably less effect and more severe side effects including sudden death and myocardial infarction, compared with pyridostigmine [17] (Class III evidence). Terbutalin, a B2-adrenergic agonist, has also been tried and seems promising as an adjunct for a subgroup of MG patients [18]. Pyridostigmine should be preferred to ephedrine in the symptomatic treatment of MG (Level C recommendation).

Immune-directed treatment

Definitive MG treatments target the autoimmune response by suppressing the production of pathogenic antibodies or the damage induced by the antibodies. The aim of immunotherapy is to induce and then maintain remission. MG patients with a thymoma and other patients with anti-titin and anti-RyR antibodies usually have a severe disease [6, 19](Class III evidence), thus, suggesting that more aggressive treatment strategies should be considered in these patients (Level C recommendation).

Most MG treatment studies are insufficient. There is no consideration of whether patients have had thymectomy. In non-operated patients, it is unknown how many of them had thymoma. In studies conducted before 1980, the percentage of patients with and without AChR antibodies is not known, and the MuSK antibodies were detected recently. There are no controlled and prospective trials of immunosuppressive treatment in children and adolescents. Evidence suggests that each immunological subtype of MG may be associated with a different spectrum of clinical phenotypes and thymus pathologies that should be considered when designing optimum treatment strategies [20].

Plasma exchange

Antibodies are removed from patient sera by membrane filtration or centrifugation. The onset of improvement is within the first week and the effect lasts for 1–3 months. From unrandomized reports, semi-selective immunoadsorption to tryptophan-linked polyvinylalcohol gels or protein-A-columns appears to be as effective as plasmapheresis, with the advantage that protein substitution is not required.

Short-term benefits of plasma exchange have been reviewed by Gajdos *et al.* (Cochrane review)[21], who conclude: 'There are no adequate randomized controlled trials, but many case series report short-term benefit from plasma exchange in myasthenia gravis, especially in myasthenic crisis.' The NIH consensus of 1986 states: 'the panel is persuaded that plasma exchange can be useful in strengthening patients with myasthenia gravis before thymectomy and during the postoperative period. It can

also be valuable in lessening symptoms during initiation of immunosuppressive drug therapy and during an acute crisis.' (Class IV evidence). Plasma exchange is recommended as a short-term treatment in MG, especially in severe cases to induce remission and in preparation for surgery (Level B recommendation).

There is one report on the use of repeated plasma exchange over a long period in refractory MG. It failed to show any cumulative long-term benefit in combination with immunosuppressive drugs [22](Class II evidence), [21] (Class I evidence). Repeated plasma exchange is not recommended as a treatment to obtain a continuous and lasting immunosuppression in MG (Level B recommendation).

Intravenous immunoglobulin (IVIg)

IVIg had a positive effect in several open studies, especially in the acute phase of MG [23, 24] (Class IV evidence). It has been used for the same indications as plasma exchange; rapidly progressive disease, preparation of weak patients for surgery including thymectomy, and as an adjuvant to minimize long-term side effects of oral immunosuppressive therapy [25]. A recent Cochrane review compared the efficacy of IVIg compared to plasma exchange, other treatments, or placebo. It concluded: 'the only randomised controlled trial examining early treatment effects did not show a significant difference between IVIg and plasma exchange for the treatment of myasthenia gravis exacerbations.' Non-randomized evidence consistently favours the interpretation that they are equally effective in this situation [26, 27](Class I evidence) (Level A recommendation). Two multicentre randomized controlled studies suggest that, although efficacy is equal, side effects of IVIg may be fewer and less severe. Thus, IVIg may be the preferred option [28] (Class I evidence). However, the controlled study by Gajdos *et al.* (1997) used a lower volume of plasma exchange than usual for the treatment of MG crisis, and the endpoint was improvement at a time point set too late to allow proper assessment of whether one therapy worked quicker than the other. There are published abstracts but no papers suggesting that plasma exchange work faster in MG crisis.

In mild or moderate MG, no significant difference in efficacy of IVIg and placebo was found after 6 weeks. In moderate exacerbations of MG no statistically significant difference in efficacy was found between IVIg and methylprednisolone. Randomized controlled trials have not shown evidence of improved functional outcome or steroid-sparing effect with the repeated use of IVIg in moderate or severe stable MG [26, 27] (Class I evidence). However, a randomized, placebo-controlled study showed a significant response in patients treated with IVIg, the greatest improvement occurring in subjects with more severe disease [29].

Thymectomy (TE)

There are several surgical approaches to TE: full or partial sternotomy, transcervical, and thoracoscopic. There are no randomized controlled studies for TE in MG.

It is difficult to compare the outcomes of the different operative techniques (confounding factors influenced both the controlled and the uncontrolled studies) but outcomes are probably similar [30] (Class III evidence).

Despite the absence of randomized, well-controlled studies, TE in MG patients with and without thymoma is widely practised. Postoperative improvement can take months or years to appear, making it difficult to distinguish TE effects from those of immunosuppressive drugs, which are often used concomitantly. In a controlled study, a 34% remission and a 32% improvement rate were achieved after TE, compared with 8% and 16% for matched patients without the operation [31] (Class III evidence). The patient should be in a clinically stable condition before this elective intervention. The perioperative morbidity is very low and consists of wound-healing disorders, bronchopneumonia, phrenic nerve damage, and sternum instability.

The Quality Standard Subcommittee of the American Academy of Neurology [32, 33] analysed 28 articles written between 1953 and 1998 describing outcomes in 21 MG cohorts with or without TE (Class II evidence). Most series used the trans-sternal approach and the follow-up ranged from 3 to 28 years. There are a number of methodological problems in the studies, including the definition of remission, the selection criteria, the medical therapy applied in both groups, and data on antibody status. However, 18 of the 21 cohorts showed improvement in MG patients who underwent TE. MG patients undergoing TE were twice as likely to attain medication-free remission, 1.6 times as likely to become asymptomatic, and 1.7 times as likely to improve. No study found a significant negative influence of TE. Patients with purely ocular manifestations did not benefit from TE.

The outcome for younger TE patients was not significantly different from the total MG group. Mild MG (Ossermann grade 1–2) did not profit from surgery, while more severe cases (Ossermann grade 2b–4) were 3.7 times as likely to achieve remission after TE than those without surgery (p < 0.0077).

Gronseth *et al.* asserted unequivocally that 'for patients with nonthymomatous autoimmune MG, thymectomy is recommended as an option to increase the probability of remission or improvement'. Their recommendation is supported by this task force with the specification that patients with generalized MG and AChR antibodies are the group most likely to benefit (Level B recommendation).

The widespread opinion that an early TE in the course of MG improves the chance of a quick remission is based on observations that lack detailed information and cannot be verified by meta-analysis. However, from pathogenic considerations it is tempting to assume that early TE should be preferred to TE after many years.

The indication for TE in AChR antibody-negative MG patients is controversial. This group is heterogenic. Some patients are false-negative as they have low-affinity AChR antibodies not detected by standard assays [34], while others have MuSK antibodies and possible other still-undetected antibodies. A retrospective cohort study displayed a similar postoperative course in AChR antibody-negative and AChR antibody-positive patients with a follow-up of at least 3 years [35]. Remission or improvement after TE occurred in 57% of AChR antibody-negative patients and in 51% of AChR antibody-positive patients. One study [36] could not prove any effect of TE in 15 MuSK antibody-positive patients, while MuSK antibodies predicted a poor outcome of TE in another study [37]. Available evidence suggests that TE should not be recommended in MuSK antibody-positive patients. Early-onset generalized MG without AChR and MuSK antibodies should have TE in the same way as MG with AChR antibodies.

In MG patients with a thymoma, the main aim of TE is to treat the tumour rather than for any effect on the MG. Once thymoma is diagnosed, TE is indicated irrespective of the severity of MG (GPP). Thymoma is a slow-growing tumour and TE should be performed only after stabilization of the MG. After TE, the AChR-antibody titre usually falls less in patients with thymoma than in those with thymic hyperplasia [38].

The prognosis depends on early and complete tumour resection [39].

Corticosteroids

In observational studies, remission or marked improvement is seen in 70–80 % of MG patients treated with oral corticosteroids, usually prednisolone [40] (Class IV evidence), but the efficacy has not been studied in double-blind, placebo-controlled trials. Steroids have side effects including weight gain, fluid retention, hypertension, diabetes, anxiety/depression/insomnia/ psychosis, glaucoma, cataract, gastrointestinal haemorrhage and perforations, myopathy, increased susceptibility to infections, and avascular joint necrosis. The risk of osteoporosis is reduced by giving bisphosphonate [41] (Class IV evidence), and antacids may prevent gastrointestinal complications. The task force agreed that oral prednosolone should be a first-choice drug when immunosuppressive drugs are necessary in MG (GPP). Some patients have a temporary worsening of MG if prednisolone is started at high dose. This steroid dip occurs after 4–10 days and sometimes can precipitate a MG crisis. Thus, we recommend starting treatment at low dose, 10–25 mg on alternate days increasing the dose gradually (10 mg per dose) to 60–80 mg on alternate days. If the patient is critically ill, one should start on a high dose every day and use additional short-time treatments to overcome the temporary worsening. When remission occurs, usually after 4–16 weeks, the dose should be slowly reduced to the minimum effective dose given on alternate days (GPP).

Azathioprine

Azathioprine is in extensive use as an immunosuppressant. It is metabolized to 6-mercaptopurine, which inhibits DNA and RNA synthesis and interferes with T-cell function. The onset of therapeutic response may be delayed for 4–12 months, and maximal effect is obtained after 6–24 months. Azathioprine is usually well tolerated, but idiosyncratic flu-like symptoms or gastrointestinal disturbances including pancreatitis occur in 10%, usually within the first few days of treatment. Some patients develop hepatitis with elevations of liver enzymes. Leucopenia, anemia, thrombocytopenia, or pancytopenia usually respond to drug withdrawal. Blood cell effects and hepatitis often do not recur after cautious reintroduction of the drug. Careful monitoring of full blood cell count and liver enzymes is mandatory and the dosage should be adjusted according to the results. About 11% of the population are heterozygous and 0.3% homozygous for mutations of the thiopurine methyltransferase gene (which can be monitored in blood) and have an increased risk of azathioprine-induced myelosuppression.

One large double-blind randomized study has demonstrated the efficacy of azathioprine as a steroid-sparing agent with a better outcome in patients on a combination of azathioprine and steroids than in patients treated with steroids alone [42] (Class I evidence). It has an immunosuppressive effect when used alone without steroids [43] (Class III evidence). In a small randomized study, prednisone was associated with better and more predictable early improvement in muscle strength than azathioprine [44] (Class III evidence). In patients where long-term immunosuppression is necessary, we recommend starting azathioprine together with steroids to allow tapering of the steroids to the lowest dose possible, while maintaining azathioprine (Level A recommendation).

Methotrexate

Methotrexate should be used in selected MG patients who do not respond to first-choice immunosuppressive drugs (GPP). It is well studied in other autoimmune disorders, but there is no evidence of sufficient quality published for MG.

Cyclophosphamide

Cyclophosphamide is an alkylating agent with immunosuppressive properties. It is a strong suppressor of B-lymphocyte activity and antibody synthesis and at high doses it also affects T-cells. In a randomized, double-blind, placebo-controlled study including 23 MG patients, those on treatment had significantly improved muscle strength and a lower steroid dose compared with the placebo group. Intravenous pulses of cyclophosphamide allowed reduction of systemic steroids without deterioration of muscle strength or serious side effects [45] (Class II evidence). However, the relatively high risk of toxicity, including bone marrow suppression, opportunistic infections, bladder toxicity, sterility, and neoplasms, limits the use of this medication to MG patients intolerant or unresponsive to steroids plus azathioprine, methotrexate, ciclosporin, or mycophenolate mofetil (Level B recommendation).

Ciclosporin

Ciclosporin has an immunosuppressive effect in both organ transplantation and autoimmune disorders. It is an inhibitor of T-cell function through inhibition of calcineurin signalling [46]. Tindall *et al.* conducted a placebo-controlled, double-blind, randomized study in 20 patients for 6 months with an open extension [47] (Class II evidence) [48, 49] (Class III evidence). The ciclosporin group had significantly improved strength and reduction in AChR antibody titre compared with the placebo group. Two open trials of 1 and 2 years' treatment and one retrospective study all support the beneficial effect of ciclosporin [10, 50–52] (Class III evidence). Cyclosporin is effective in MG, has significant side effects of nephrotoxicity and hypertension, and should be considered only in patients intolerant or unresponsive to azathioprine (Level B recommendation).

Mycophenolate mofetil

Mycophenolate mofetil's active metabolite, mycophenolic acid, is an inhibitor of purine nucleotide synthesis and impares lymphocyte proliferation selectively. A few studies including a small double-blind, placebo-controlled study of 14 patients have shown that mycophenolate mofetil is effective in patients with poorly controlled MG and as a steroid-sparing medication [53–59] (Class III, Class IV evidence). These findings could not be reproduced in a recent placebo-controlled study over 9 months [60] (Class II evidence). The effect of mycophenolate mofetil in MG is therefore not unequivocally documented, but it may be tried in patients intolerant or unresponsive to azathioprine (Level B recommendation).

FK506 (tacrolimus)

Tacrolimus (FK506) is a macrolide molecule of the same immunosuppressant class as ciclosporin. It inhibits the proliferation of activated T-cells via the calcium-calcineurin pathway. FK506 also acts on ryanodine receptor-mediated calcium release from sarcoplasmic reticulum to potentiate excitation–contraction coupling in skeletal muscle [61]. Case reports and a small open trial all showed a useful improvement of MG with minor side effects [9, 62–66] (Class III evidence). Interestingly, patients with anti-RyR antibodies (and potential excitation–contraction coupling dysfunction) had a rapid response to treatment indicating a symptomatic effect on muscle strength in addition to the immunosuppression (53). FK506 should be tried in MG patients with poorly controlled disease, especially in RyR antibody positive patients (Level C recommendation).

Antibodies against leucocyte antigens

There are case reports of improvement of refractory MG with monoclonal antibodies against different lymphocyte subsets such as anti-CD20 (rituximab) (B-cell inhibitor) [67–70] (Class IV evidence), and anti-CD4 (T-cell inhibitor) [71] (Class IV evidence), both reporting good clinical outcome. These treatment strategies are promising, but more evidence is needed before any recommendations can be given.

Training, weight control and lifestyle modifications

The importance of reducing weight and modification of activities of daily living has been suggested, but there is no hard scientific evidence to this. There are reports that show some benefit of respiratory muscle training in MG [72, 73] (Class III evidence) and strength training in mild MG [74] (Class III evidence). Physical training can be carried out safely in mild MG and produces some improvement of muscle force (Level C recommendation). Seasonal flu vaccination should be recommended in MG patients (GPP).

MG is associated with a slightly increased rate of complications during birth and more frequent need of operative interventions [75, 76] (Class II evidence). Transient neonatal MG occurs in 10–20% of children born to MG mothers. Maternal MG is also a rare cause of arthrogryphosis congenita and of recurrent miscarriages [77]. Acetylcholine esterase inhibitors and immunosuppressive drugs should be continued during pregnancy when necessary for the MG, except for methotrexate, which is damaging to ova and sperm and should be stopped at least 3 months before attempting conception. Mycophenolate mofetil and other new drugs where no safety data are available should also be stopped 3 months before conception [78] (GPP). Effective immunosuppression can improve severe fetal MG-related conditions (Class III evidence). Women with MG should not be discouraged from conceiving, and pregnancy does not worsen the long-term outcome of MG [79] (Class II evidence).

Recommendations

Myasthenia gravis

After the diagnosis of MG is established an acetylcholine esterase inhibitor should be introduced. Thymoma patients should have thymectomy. AChR antibody-positive early-onset patients with generalized MG and insufficient response to pyridostigmine therapy should be considered for thymectomy, ideally within 1 year of disease onset. Immunosuppressive medication should be considered in all patients with progressive MG symptoms. We recommend starting with prednisolone covered by bisphosphonate and antacid, and azathioprine. Non-responders or patients intolerant to this regime should be considered for treatment with one of the other recommended immunosupressive drugs. Recommendation levels are B, C or Good Practice Points.

Lambert-Eaton myasthenic syndrome (LEMS)

Antibodies to peripheral nerve P/Q-type VGCC antibodies are present in the serum of at least 85% of LEMS patients [80]. The disease is characterized by ascending muscle weakness that usually starts in the proximal lower-limb muscles and is associated with autonomic dysfunction. Ptosis and ophthalmoplegia tend to be milder than in MG [81]. LEMS rarely causes respiratory failure [81]. In half of the patients LEMS is a paraneoplastic disease and a small cell lung carcinoma (SCLC) will be found [82].

Symptomatic and immune-directed treatment

Evidence from small randomised controlled trials showed that both 3,4-diaminopyridine and IVIg improved muscle strength scores and compound muscle action potential amplitudes in LEMS patients [83] (Cochrane Review) (Class I evidence).

First-line treatment is 3,4-diaminopyridine [84]. An additional therapeutic effect may be obtained if combined with pyridostigmine. If symptomatic treatment is insufficient, immunosuppressive therapy should be started, usually with a combination of prednisone and azathioprine. Other drugs such as ciclosporin or mycophenolate can be used, although evidence of benefit is limited to case series reports (Class IV evidence) (Level C recommendation).

For patients with a paraneoplastic LEMS it is essential to treat the tumour. Chemotherapy is the first choice in SCLC and this will have an additional immunosuppressive effect. In LEMS patients with a possible underlying SCLC, corticosteroids, when required for the disease treatment, can be used; immunosuppressants should be avoided before the tumour is ruled out. This does not apply to thymoma, which has a slow growth.

The presence of LEMS in a patient with SCLC improves tumour survival [85]. For a more detailed description of LEMS consult the Guidelines for the management of paraneoplastic disorders [86].

Neuromyotonia (peripheral nerve hyperexcitability)/Isaacs' syndrome

This commonest acquired form of generalized peripheral nerve hyperexcitability is autoimmune and caused by antibodies to nerve voltage-gated potassium channels (VGKC). [87], although the only generally available assay detects these antibodies in only 30–50% of all patients [87]. Neuromyotonia is paraneoplastic in up to 25% of patients and can predate the detection of neoplasia, usually thymus or lung, by up to 4 years [88]. The clinical hallmark is spontaneous and continuous skeletal muscle overactivity presenting as twitching and painful cramps and often accompanied by stiffness, pseudomyotonia, pseudotetany, and weakness [89]. One-third of patients also have sensory features and up to 50% have hyperhidrosis suggesting autonomic involvement. Central nervous system features can occur (Morvan's syndrome) [88, 90].

Symptomatic and immune-directed treatment

Neuromyotonia usually improves with symptomatic treatment [89], although evidence is case reports and case series (Class IV evidence). Carbamazepine, phenytoin, lamotrigine, and sodium valproate can be used, if necessary in combination.

Neuromyotonia often improves and can remit after treatment of an underlying cancer [89]. In patients whose symptoms are debilitating or refractory to symptomatic therapy, immunomodulatory therapies should be tried [89, 91]. Plasma exchange often produces useful clinical improvement lasting about 6 weeks accompanied by a reduction in EMG activity [89] and a fall in VGKC antibody titres [92]. Single case studies suggest that IVIg can also help [93]. There are no good trials of long-term oral immunosuppression. However, prednisolone, with or without azathioprine or methotrexate, has been useful in selected patients 86[94] (Class IV evidence) (GPP).

Conflicts of interest

The following author has reported conflicts of interest.

I. Illa has received speaker honoraria from Talecris and an educational grant from Grifols.

The other authors have nothing to declare.

References

1. Brainin M, Barnes M, Baron JC, *et al.* Guidance for the preparation of neurological management guidelines by EFNS scientific task forces–revised recommendations. *Eur J Neurol* 2004;**2004**(11):577–81.

2. Vincent A. Unravelling the pathogenesis of myasthenia gravis. *Nat Rev Immunol* 2002;**2**:797–804.

3. Hoch W, McConville J, Helms S, Newsom-Davis J, Melms A, Vincent A. Auto-antibodies to the receptor tyrosine kinase MuSK in patients with myasthenia gravis without acetylcholine receptor antibodies. *Nat Med* 2001;**7**:365–8.

4. Aarli JA, Stefansson K, Marton LS, Wollmann RL. Patients with myasthenia gravis and thymoma have in their sera IgG autoantibodies against titin. *Clin Exp Immunol* 1990;**82**:284–8.

5. Mygland A, Tysnes OB, Matre R, Volpe P, Aarli JA, Gilhus NE. Ryanodine receptor autoantibodies in myasthenia gravis patients with a thymoma. *Ann Neurol* 1992;**32**:589–91.

6. Skeie GO, Mygland A, Aarli JA, Gilhus NE. Titin antibodies in patients with late onset myasthenia gravis: clinical correlations. *Autoimmunity* 1995;**20**:99–104.

7. Somnier FE, Skeie GO, Aarli JA, Trojaborg W. EMG evidence of myopathy and the occurrence of titin autoantibodies in patients with myasthenia gravis. *Eur J Neurol* 1999;**6**:555–63.

8. Gerber NL, Steinberg AD. Clinical use of immunosuppressive drugs: part II. *Drugs* 1976;**11**:90–112.

9. Evoli A, Di Schino C, Marsili F, Punzi C. Successful treatment of myasthenia gravis with tacrolimus. *Muscle Nerve* 2002;**25**:111–4.

10. Goulon M, Elkharrat D, Gajdos P. Treatment of severe myasthenia gravis with cyclosporin. A 12-month open trial. *Presse Med* 1989;**18**:341–6.

11. Owe JF, Daltveit AK, Gilhus NE. Causes of death among patients with myasthenia gravis in Norway between 1951 and 2001. *J Neurol Neurosurg Psychiatry* 2006;**77**:203–7.

12. Szathmary I, Magyar P, Szobor A. Air-flow limitation in myasthenia gravis. The effect of acetylcholinesterase inhibitor therapy on air-flow limitation. *Am Rev Respir Dis* 1984;**130**:145.

13. Shale DJ, Lane DJ, Davis CJ. Air-flow limitation in myasthenia gravis. The effect of acetylcholinesterase inhibitor therapy on air-flow limitation. *Am Rev Respir Dis* 1983;**128**:618–21.

14. Punga AR, Flink R, Askmark H, Stalberg EV. Cholinergic neuromuscular hyperactivity in patients with myasthenia gravis seropositive for MuSK antibody. *Muscle Nerve* 2006;**34**:111–5.

15. Sghirlanzoni A, Pareyson D, Benvenuti C, *et al.* Efficacy of intranasal administration of neostigmine in myasthenic patients. *J Neurol* 1992;**239**:165–9.

16. Anlar B, Varli K, Ozdirim E, Ertan M. 3,4-diaminopyridine in childhood myasthenia: double-blind, placebo-controlled trial. *J Child Neurol* 1996;**11**:458–61.

17. Sieb JP, Engel AG. Ephedrine: effects on neuromuscular transmission. *Brain Res* 1993;**623**:167–71.

18. Soliven B, Rezania K, Gundogdu B, Harding-Clay B, Oger J, Arnason BG. Terbutaline in myasthenia gravis: a pilot study. *J Neurol Sci* 2009;**277**:150–4.

19. Romi F, Skeie GO, Aarli JA, Gilhus NE. The severity of myasthenia gravis correlates with the serum concentration of titin and ryanodine receptor antibodies. *Arch Neurol* 2000;**57**:1596–600.

20. Meriggioli MN, Sanders DB. Autoimmune myasthenia gravis: emerging clinical and biological heterogeneity. *Lancet Neurol* 2009;**8**:475–90.

21. Gajdos P, Chevret S, Toyka K. Plasma exchange for myasthenia gravis. *Cochrane Database Syst Rev* 2002;CD002275.

22. Gajdos P, Simon N, de Rohan-Chabot P, Raphael JC, Goulon M. Long-term effects of plasma exchange in myasthenia. Results of a randomized study. *Presse Med* 1983;**12**:939–42.

23. Fateh-Moghadam A, Wick M, Besinger U, Geursen RG. High-dose intravenous gammaglobulin for myasthenia gravis. *Lancet* 1984;**1**:848–9.

24. Elovaara I, Apostolski S, van Doorn P, *et al.* EFNS guidelines for the use of intravenous immunoglobulin in treatment of neurological diseases: EFNS task force on the use of intravenous immunoglobulin in treatment of neurological diseases. *Eur J Neurol* 2008;**15**:893–908.

25. Dalakas MC. Intravenous immunoglobulin in the treatment of autoimmune neuromuscular diseases: present status and practical therapeutic guidelines. *Muscle Nerve* 1999;**22**:1479–97.

26. Gajdos P, Chevret S, Toyka K. Intravenous immunoglobulin for myasthenia gravis. *Cochrane Database Syst Rev* 2008;CD002277.

27. Gajdos P, Chevret S, Toyka K. Intravenous immunoglobulin for myasthenia gravis. *Cochrane Database Syst Rev* 2003;CD002277.

28. Gajdos P, Chevret S, Clair B, Tranchant C, Chastang C. Clinical trial of plasma exchange and high-dose intravenous immunoglobulin in myasthenia gravis. Myasthenia Gravis Clinical Study Group. *Ann Neurol* 1997;**41**:789–96.

29. Zinman L, Ng E, Bril V. IV immunoglobulin in patients with myasthenia gravis: a randomized controlled trial. *Neurology* 2007;**68**:837–41.

30. Meyer DM, Herbert MA, Sobhani NC, *et al.* Comparative clinical outcomes of thymectomy for myasthenia gravis performed by extended transsternal and minimally invasive approaches. *Ann Thorac Surg* 2009;**87**:385–90; discussion 390–81.

31. Buckingham JM, Howard FM, Jr, Bernatz PE, *et al.* The value of thymectomy in myasthenia gravis: a computer-assisted matched study. *Ann Surg* 1976;**184**:453–8.

32. Gronseth GS, Barohn RJ. Thymectomy for Myasthenia Gravis. *Curr Treat Options Neurol* 2002;**4**:203–9.

33. Gronseth GS, Barohn RJ. Practice parameter: thymectomy for autoimmune myasthenia gravis (an evidence-based review): report of the Quality Standards Subcommittee of the American Academy of Neurology. *Neurology* 2000;**55**: 7–15.

34. Leite MI, Jacob S, Viegas S, *et al.* IgG1 antibodies to acetylcholine receptors in "seronegative" myasthenia gravis. *Brain* 2008;**131**:1940–52.

35. Guillermo GR, Tellez-Zenteno JF, Weder-Cisneros N, *et al.* Response of thymectomy: clinical and pathological characteristics among seronegative and seropositive myasthenia gravis patients. *Acta Neurol Scand* 2004;**109**:217–21.

36. Evoli A, Tonali PA, Padua L, *et al.* Clinical correlates with anti-MuSK antibodies in generalized seronegative myasthenia gravis. *Brain* 2003;**126**:2304–11.

37. Pompeo E, Tacconi F, Massa R, Mineo D, Nahmias S, Mineo TC. Long-term outcome of thoracoscopic extended thymectomy for nonthymomatous myasthenia gravis. *Eur J Cardiothorac Surg* 2009;**36**:164–9.

38. Reinhardt C, Melms A. Normalization of elevated CD4-/CD8- (double-negative) T cells after thymectomy parallels clinical remission in myasthenia gravis associated with thymic hyperplasia but not thymoma. *Ann Neurol* 2000;**48**: 603–8.

39. Chen G, Marx A, Wen-Hu C, *et al.* New WHO histologic classification predicts prognosis of thymic epithelial tumors: a clinicopathologic study of 200 thymoma cases from China. *Cancer* 2002;**95**:420–9.

40. Pascuzzi RM, Coslett HB, Johns TR. Long-term corticosteroid treatment of myasthenia gravis: report of 116 patients. *Ann Neurol* 1984;**15**:291–8.

41. Saag KG. Prevention of glucocorticoid-induced osteoporosis. *South Med J* 2004;**97**:555–8.

42. Palace J, Newsom-Davis J, Lecky B. A randomized double-blind trial of prednisolone alone or with azathioprine in myasthenia gravis. Myasthenia Gravis Study Group. *Neurology* 1998;**50**:1778–83.

43. Witte AS, Cornblath DR, Parry GJ, Lisak RP, Schatz NJ. Azathioprine in the treatment of myasthenia gravis. *Ann Neurol* 1984;**15**:602–5.

44. Bromberg MB, Wald JJ, Forshew DA, Feldman EL, Albers JW. Randomized trial of azathioprine or prednisone for initial immunosuppressive treatment of myasthenia gravis. *J Neurol Sci* 1997;**150**:59–62.

45. De Feo LG, Schottlender J, Martelli NA, Molfino NA. Use of intravenous pulsed cyclophosphamide in severe, generalized myasthenia gravis. *Muscle Nerve* 2002;**26**: 31–6.

46. Matsuda S, Koyasu S. Mechanisms of action of cyclosporine. *Immunopharmacology* 2000;**47**:119–25.

47. Tindall RS, Rollins JA, Phillips JT, Greenlee RG, Wells L, Belendiuk G. Preliminary results of a double-blind, randomized, placebo-controlled trial of cyclosporine in myasthenia gravis. *N Engl J Med* 1987;**316**:719–24.

48. Tindall RS. Immunointervention with cyclosporin A in autoimmune neurological disorders. *J Autoimmun* 1992;5(Suppl. A):301–13.

49. Tindall RS, Phillips JT, Rollins JA, Wells L, Hall K. A clinical therapeutic trial of cyclosporine in myasthenia gravis. *Ann N Y Acad Sci* 1993;**681**:539–51.

50. Goulon M, Elkharrat D, Lokiec F, Gajdos P. Results of a one-year open trial of cyclosporine in ten patients with severe myasthenia gravis. *Transplant Proc* 1988;**20**:211–7.

51. Bonifati DM, Angelini C. Long-term cyclosporine treatment in a group of severe myasthenia gravis patients. *J Neurol* 1997;**244**:542–7.

52. Ciafaloni E, Nikhar NK, Massey JM, Sanders DB. Retrospective analysis of the use of cyclosporine in myasthenia gravis. *Neurology* 2000;**55**:448–50.

53. Ciafaloni E, Massey JM, Tucker-Lipscomb B, Sanders DB. Mycophenolate mofetil for myasthenia gravis: an open-label pilot study. *Neurology* 2001;**56**:97–9.

54. Chaudhry V, Cornblath DR, Griffin JW, O'Brien R, Drachman DB. Mycophenolate mofetil: a safe and promising immunosuppressant in neuromuscular diseases. *Neurology* 2001;**56**:94–6.

55. Schneider C, Gold R, Reiners K, Toyka KV. Mycophenolate mofetil in the therapy of severe myasthenia gravis. *Eur Neurol* 2001;**46**:79–82.

56. Hauser RA, Malek AR, Rosen R. Successful treatment of a patient with severe refractory myasthenia gravis using mycophenolate mofetil. *Neurology* 1998;**51**:912–3.

57. Meriggioli MN, Rowin J. Single fiber EMG as an outcome measure in myasthenia gravis: results from a double-blind, placebo-controlled trial. *J Clin Neurophysiol* 2003;**20**: 382–5.

58. Meriggioli MN, Rowin J. Treatment of myasthenia gravis with mycophenolate mofetil: a case report. *Muscle Nerve* 2000;**23**:1287–9.

59. Meriggioli MN, Ciafaloni E, Al-Hayk KA, *et al.* Mycophenolate mofetil for myasthenia gravis: an analysis of efficacy, safety, and tolerability. *Neurology* 2003;**61**:1438–40.

60. Sanders DB, Hart IK, Mantegazza R, *et al.* An international, phase III, randomized trial of mycophenolate mofetil in myasthenia gravis. *Neurology* 2008;**71**:400–6.

61. Timerman AP, Ogunbumni E, Freund E, Wiederrecht G, Marks AR, Fleischer S. The calcium release channel of sarcoplasmic reticulum is modulated by FK-506-binding protein. Dissociation and reconstitution of FKBP-12 to the calcium release channel of skeletal muscle sarcoplasmic reticulum. *J Biol Chem* 1993;**268**:22992–9.

62. Takamori M, Motomura M, Kawaguchi N, *et al.* Anti-ryanodine receptor antibodies and FK506 in myasthenia gravis. *Neurology* 2004;**62**:1894–6.

63. Konishi T, Yoshiyama Y, Takamori M, Yagi K, Mukai E, Saida T. Clinical study of FK506 in patients with myasthenia gravis. *Muscle Nerve* 2003;**28**:570–4.

64. Yoshikawa H, Mabuchi K, Yasukawa Y, Takamori M, Yamada M. Low-dose tacrolimus for intractable myasthenia gravis. *J Clin Neurosci* 2002;**9**:627–8.

65. Tada M, Shimohata T, Oyake M, *et al.* Long-term therapeutic efficacy and safety of low-dose tacrolimus (FK506) for myasthenia gravis. *J Neurol Sci* 2006;**247**:17–20.

66. Nagaishi A, Yukitake M, Kuroda Y. Long-term treatment of steroid-dependent myasthenia gravis patients with low-dose tacrolimus. *Intern Med* 2008;**47**:731–6.

67. Wylam ME, Anderson PM, Kuntz NL, Rodriguez V. Successful treatment of refractory myasthenia gravis using rituximab: a pediatric case report. *J Pediatr* 2003;**143**: 674–7.

68. Illa I, Diaz-Manera J, Rojas-Garcia R, *et al.* Sustained response to Rituximab in anti-AChR and anti-MuSK positive Myasthenia Gravis patients. *J Neuroimmunol* 2008;**201–202**:90–4.

69. Lebrun C, Bourg V, Tieulie N, Thomas P. Successful treatment of refractory generalized myasthenia gravis with rituximab. *Eur J Neurol* 2009;**16**:246–50.

70. Stieglbauer K, Topakian R, Schaffer V, Aichner FT. Rituximab for myasthenia gravis: three case reports and review of the literature. *J Neurol Sci* 2009;**280**:120–2.

71. Ahlberg R, Yi Q, Pirskanen R, *et al.* Treatment of myasthenia gravis with anti-CD4 antibody: improvement correlates to decreased T-cell autoreactivity. *Neurology* 1994;**44**:1732–7.

72. Weiner P, Gross D, Meiner Z, *et al.* Respiratory muscle training in patients with moderate to severe myasthenia gravis. *Can J Neurol Sci* 1998;**25**:236–41.

73. Rassler B, Hallebach G, Kalischewski P, Baumann I, Schauer J, Spengler CM. The effect of respiratory muscle endurance training in patients with myasthenia gravis. *Neuromuscul Disord* 2007;**17**:385–91.

74. Lohi EL, Lindberg C, Andersen O. Physical training effects in myasthenia gravis. *Arch Phys Med Rehabil* 1993;**74**: 1178–80.

75. Hoff JM, Daltveit AK, Gilhus NE. Myasthenia gravis: consequences for pregnancy, delivery, and the newborn. *Neurology* 2003;**61**:1362–6.

76. Wen JC, Liu TC, Chen YH, Chen SF, Lin HC, Tsai WC. No increased risk of adverse pregnancy outcomes for women with myasthenia gravis: a nationwide population-based study. *Eur J Neurol* 2009;**16**:889–94.

77. Vincent A, Newland C, Brueton L, *et al.* Arthrogryposis multiplex congenita with maternal autoantibodies specific for a fetal antigen. *Lancet* 1995;**346**:24–5.

78. Ferrero S, Pretta S, Nicoletti A, Petrera P, Ragni N. Myasthenia gravis: management issues during pregnancy. *Eur J Obstet Gynecol Reprod Biol* 2005;**121**:129–38.

79. Batocchi AP, Majolini L, Evoli A, Lino MM, Minisci C, Tonali P. Course and treatment of myasthenia gravis during pregnancy. *Neurology* 1999;**52**:447–52.

80. Motomura M, Johnston I, Lang B, Vincent A, Newsom-Davis J. An improved diagnostic assay for Lambert-Eaton myasthenic syndrome. *J Neurol Neurosurg Psychiatry* 1995;**58**:85–7.

81. Wirtz PW, Sotodeh M, Nijnuis M, *et al.* Difference in distribution of muscle weakness between myasthenia gravis and the Lambert-Eaton myasthenic syndrome. *J Neurol Neurosurg Psychiatry* 2002;**73**:766–8.

82. Wirtz PW, Willcox N, van der Slik AR, *et al.* HLA and smoking in prediction and prognosis of small cell lung cancer in autoimmune Lambert-Eaton myasthenic syndrome. *J Neuroimmunol* 2005;**159**:230–7.

83. Maddison P, Newsom-Davis J. Treatment for Lambert-Eaton myasthenic syndrome. *Cochrane Database Syst Rev* 2003;CD003279.

84. McEvoy KM, Windebank AJ, Daube JR, Low PA. 3,4-Diaminopyridine in the treatment of Lambert-Eaton myasthenic syndrome. *N Engl J Med* 1989;**321**:1567–71.

85. Maddison P, Newsom-Davis J, Mills KR, Souhami RL. Favourable prognosis in Lambert-Eaton myasthenic syndrome and small-cell lung carcinoma. *Lancet* 1999;**353**: 117–8.

86. Vedeler CA, Antoine JC, Giometto B, *et al.* Management of paraneoplastic neurological syndromes: report of an EFNS Task Force. *Eur J Neurol* 2006;**13**:682–90.

87. Hart IK, Maddison P, Newsom-Davis J, Vincent A, Mills KR. Phenotypic variants of autoimmune peripheral nerve hyperexcitability. *Brain* 2002;**125**:1887–95.

88. Hart IK, Waters C, Vincent A, *et al.* Autoantibodies detected to expressed K+ channels are implicated in neuromyotonia. *Ann Neurol* 1997;**41**:238–46.

89. Newsom-Davis J, Mills KR. Immunological associations of acquired neuromyotonia (Isaacs' syndrome). Report of five cases and literature review. *Brain* 1993;**116**(Pt 2): 453–69.

90. Liguori R, Vincent A, Clover L, *et al.* Morvan's syndrome: peripheral and central nervous system and cardiac involve-ment with antibodies to voltage-gated potassium channels. *Brain* 2001;**124**:2417–26.

91. Hayat GR, Kulkantrakorn K, Campbell WW, Giuliani MJ. Neuromyotonia: autoimmune pathogenesis and response to immune modulating therapy. *J Neurol Sci* 2000;**181**: 38–43.

92. Shillito P, Molenaar PC, Vincent A, *et al.* Acquired neuro-myotonia: evidence for autoantibodies directed against K+ channels of peripheral nerves. *Ann Neurol* 1995;**38**:714–22.

93. Alessi G, De Reuck J, De Bleecker J, Vancayzeele S. Success-ful immunoglobulin treatment in a patient with neuromyo-tonia. *Clin Neurol Neurosurg* 2000;**102**:173–5.

94. Nakatsuji Y, Kaido M, Sugai F, *et al.* Isaacs' syndrome suc-cessfully treated by immunoadsorption plasmapheresis. *Acta Neurol Scand* 2000;**102**:271–3.

CHAPTER 20

Chronic inflammatory demyelinating polyradiculoneuropathy

P. Y. K. Van den Bergh,[1] R. D. M. Hadden,[2] Pierre Bouche,[3] D. R. Cornblath,[4] A. Hahn,[5] I. Illa,[6] C. L. Koski,[7] J.-M. Léger,[3] E. Nobile-Orazio,[8] J. Pollard,[9] C. Sommer,[10] P. A. van Doorn,[11] I. N. van Schaik[12]

[1]Centre de Référence Neuromusculaire, Cliniques universitaires St-Luc, Brussels, Belgium; [2]King's College London School of Medicine, London, UK; [3]Consultation de Pathologie Neuromusculaire Groupe Hospitalier, Pitié Salpêtriére, Paris, France; [4]Johns Hopkins University, Baltimore, MD, USA; [5]London Health Sciences Centre, London, ON, Canada; [6]Hospital Universitari de la Sta Creu i Sant Pau, Barcelona, Spain; [7]University of Maryland, School of Medicine, Baltimore, MD, USA; [8]University of Milan IRCCS Humanitas Clinical Institute, Italy; [9]University of Sydney, Australia; [10]University of Würzburg, Germany; [11]Erasmus Medical Centre, Rotterdam, The Netherlands; [12]Academic Medical Center, University of Amsterdam, The Netherlands

Objectives

The aim is to update the EFNS/PNS guideline on management of CIDP (2005), based on newly available evidence and, where adequate evidence was not available, consensus.

Background

Several different sets of diagnostic criteria for CIDP have been created, but sensitivity and specificity vary [2]. Patients who meet AAN research criteria [3] certainly have CIDP, but many patients who are diagnosed with CIDP by clinicians do not meet these criteria. The EFNS/PNS consensus guideline [1] was designed to offer diagnostic criteria to balance more evenly specificity, which needs to be higher in research than clinical practice, and sensitivity which might miss disease if set too high.

Since the first treatment trial of prednisone in CIDP by Dyck *et al.* [4], a small but growing body of evidence from randomized trials has accumulated to allow evidence-based statements about treatments. These trials have been the subject of Cochrane reviews on which our recommendations are based.

Search strategy

We searched MEDLINE and the Cochrane Library from August 2004 to July 2009 for articles on CIDP and 'diagnosis' or 'treatment' or 'guideline'.

Methods for reaching consensus

Task force members prepared draft statements about definition, diagnosis, and treatment. Evidence and recommendations were classified according to the scheme agreed for EFNS guidelines [5]. When only Class IV evidence was available but consensus could be reached, the task force offered advice as Good Practice Points [5]. The statements were revised and collated into a single document, which was then revised iteratively until consensus was reached.

European Handbook of Neurological Management: Volume 1, 2nd edition. Edited by N. E. Gilhus, M. P. Barnes and M. Brainin.
© 2011 Blackwell Publishing Ltd.

Results

Diagnostic criteria for CIDP

In almost all diagnostic criterion sets for CIDP, the diagnosis rests on a combination of clinical, electrodiagnostic, and laboratory features with exclusions to eliminate other disorders that may appear as CIDP. In practice, criteria for CIDP have been most closely linked to criteria for detection of peripheral nerve demyelination. At least 12 sets of electrodiagnostic criteria for primary demyelination have been published to identify CIDP (for review, see [2]). The EFNS/PNS criteria [1], which included clinical and electrodiagnostic criteria, proposed new electrodiagnostic criteria which have been successfully used in subsequent clinical trials [6]. Additionally, Rajabally *et al.* [7] applied the EFNS/PNS criteria to 151 CIDP patients from four European centres and reported 81% sensitivity and 96% specificity.

Koski and coworkers recently derived another set of diagnostic criteria [8]. Experts reviewed the case notes, including longitudinal follow-up of each other's patients diagnosed with CIDP, excluding those with paraproteins and genetic neuropathy, chronic acquired demyelinating polyneuropathy including those with paraproteins, and other chronic neuropathies. Using classification and regression tree analysis, two sets of criteria were developed: one that included electrodiagnostic criteria (recordable compound muscle action potential in ≥75% of nerves and either abnormal distal latency or abnormal motor conduction velocity or abnormal F-wave latency in >50% of studied nerves) and one that relied on clinical criteria alone (symmetric onset or examination, weakness of four limbs, and proximal weakness in ≥ one limb). The diagnostic criteria were validated and shown to distinguish CIDP from Lewis-Sumner syndrome, multifocal motor neuropathy, and other chronic neuropathy types. The authors reported 83% sensitivity and 97% specificity. Although the Koski and coworker's criteria have the advantage of diagnosing CIDP when electrodiagnostic criteria are not fulfilled, all prior criteria sets included electrodiagnostic criteria. Thus, the task force was uncertain whether to adopt these criteria at this time.

While the majority of those with CIDP have a chronic onset of a progressive or relapsing phase of more than 8 weeks, there are patients eventually diagnosed with CIDP who have an acute onset resembling Guillain-Barré syndrome (GBS). This may occur in up to 16% of all CIDP patients. 'Acute-onset CIDP' in a patient initially diagnosed as GBS is likely if deterioration continues >2 months from onset or if ≥ three treatment-related fluctuations occur [9]. 'Acute-onset CIDP' should be suspected in GBS patients with prominent sensory symptoms and signs at presentation [10]. Different clinical presentations have been associated with CIDP with pure motor or sensory impairment or with distal, multifocal, or focal distributions. The task force considered these as atypical CIDP. Both typical and atypical CIDP are rarely associated with multifocal central nervous system demyelination, resembling multiple sclerosis [11, 12].

Based on case reports, numerous diseases have been associated with CIDP. These include diabetes mellitus, IgG or IgA monoclonal gammopathy of undetermined significance (MGUS), IgM monoclonal gammopathy without antibodies to myelin-associated glycoprotein (MAG), HIV infection, chronic active hepatitis, systemic lupus erythematosus or other connective tissue diseases, sarcoidosis, thyroid disease, inflammatory bowel disease [13], membranous glomerulonephritis [14], bone marrow or solid organ transplantation [15]. There is insufficient evidence to consider CIDP associated with these diseases different from idiopathic CIDP.

Recommended strategy for investigation to confirm the diagnosis of CIDP

Based on consensus expert opinion, CIDP should be considered in any patient with a progressive symmetrical or asymmetrical polyradiculoneuropathy in whom the clinical course is relapsing and remitting or progresses for more than 2 months, especially if there are positive sensory symptoms, proximal weakness, areflexia without wasting, or preferential loss of vibration or joint position sense. Electrodiagnostic tests are mandatory and the major features suggesting a diagnosis of CIDP are listed in table 20.1. The sensitivity of electrodiagnostic criteria for motor nerves may be improved by examining more than four nerves, by including proximal stimulation in the upper limbs [16, 17], and by examining sensory nerves [18, 19]. Somatosensory evoked potentials (SSEP) can be useful to demonstrate abnormal proximal sensory conduction, particularly in sensory CIDP [20, 21] (Good Practice Point[GPP]). If electrodiagnostic criteria for definite CIDP are not met initially, repeat study at a later date should be considered. CSF examination, gadolinium-

Table 20.1 Electrodiagnostic criteria.

I *Definite: at least one of the following*

   A Motor distal latency prolongation at least 50% above ULN in two nerves (excluding median neuropathy at the wrist from carpal tunnel syndrome), or

   B Reduction of motor conduction velocity at least 30% below LLN in two nerves, or

   C Prolongation of F-wave latency at least 30% above ULN in two nerves (at least 50% if amplitude of distal negative peak CMAP <80% of LLN values), or

   D Absence of F-waves in two nerves if these nerves have distal negative peak CMAP amplitudes at least 20% of LLN + at least one other demyelinating parameter* in at least one other nerve, or

   E Partial motor conduction block: at least 50% amplitude reduction of the proximal negative peak CMAP relative to distal, if distal negative peak CMAP at least 20% of LLN, in two nerves, or in one nerve + at least one other demyelinating parameter* in at least one other nerve, or

   F Abnormal temporal dispersion (>30% duration increase between the proximal and distal negative peak CMAP) in at least two nerves, or

   G Distal CMAP duration (interval between onset of the first negative peak and return to baseline of the last negative peak) increase in at least one nerve (median ≥6.6 ms, ulnar ≥6.7 ms, peroneal ≥7.6 ms, tibial ≥8.8 ms)** + at least one other demyelinating parameter* in at least one other nerve

II *Probable*

   At least 30% amplitude reduction of the proximal negative peak CMAP relative to distal, excluding the posterior tibial nerve, if distal negative peak CMAP at least 20% of LLN, in two nerves, or in one nerve + at least one other demyelinating parameter* in at least one other nerve

III *Possible*

   As in I but in only one nerve

To apply these criteria, the median, ulnar (stimulated below the elbow), peroneal (stimulated below the fibular head), and tibial nerves on one side are tested. If criteria are not fulfilled, the same nerves are tested at the other side, and/or the ulnar and median nerves are stimulated bilaterally at the axilla and at Erb's point. Motor conduction block is not considered in the ulnar nerve across the elbow and at least 50% amplitude reduction between Erb's point and the wrist is required for probable conduction block. Temperatures should be maintained to at least 33°C at the palm and 30°C at the external malleolus (GPP)

*Any nerve meeting any of the criteria (A–G)

**Isose *et al.*, in press [47]

CMAP, compound muscle action potential; ULN, upper limit of normal values; LLN, lower limit of normal values

---

enhanced MRI of spinal roots, brachial or lumbar plexus, and trial of immunotherapy with objective assessment of endpoints [22] may assist the diagnosis. Nerve biopsy, usually of the sural nerve, can provide supportive evidence for the diagnosis of CIDP, but positive findings are not specific and negative findings do not exclude the diagnosis. The nerve selected for biopsy should be clinically and electrophysiologically affected and is usually the sural, but occasionally the superficial peroneal, superficial radial, or gracilis motor nerve. Supportive features for the diagnosis of CIDP are macrophage-associated demyelination, onion bulb formation, demyelinated and to a lesser extent remyelinated nerve fibres, endoneurial oedema, endoneurial mononuclear cell infiltration, and variation between fascicles. There is only Class IV evidence concerning all these matters. Investigations to dis-

cover possible concomitant diseases should also be considered (GPP, table 20.2).

Treatment of CIDP

Corticosteroids

In one unblinded RCT with 28 participants, prednisone was superior to no treatment [4, 23] (Class II evidence). Six weeks of oral prednisolone starting at 60 mg daily produced benefit that was not significantly different from that produced by a single course of IVIg 2.0 g/kg [24, 25] (Class II evidence). In addition, many observational studies report a beneficial effect from corticosteroids except in pure motor CIDP, where they can be harmful [26, 27]. Consequently, a trial of corticosteroids may be considered in all patients with significant disability (Level

Table 20.2 Investigations to be considered.

To diagnose CIDP
- Electrodiagnostic studies including sensory and motor nerve conduction studies, which may be repeated, done bilaterally, or use proximal stimulation for motor nerves
- CSF examination including cells and protein
- MRI spinal roots, brachial plexus, and lumbosacral plexus
- Nerve biopsy

To detect concomitant diseases
A Recommended studies
- *Serum and urine paraprotein detection by immunofixation
- Fasting blood glucose
- Complete blood count
- Renal function
- Liver function
- Antinuclear factor
- Thyroid function
B Studies to be performed if clinically indicated
- *Skeletal survey
- Oral glucose tolerance test
- Borrelia burgdorferi serology
- C-reactive protein
- Extractable nuclear antigen antibodies
- Chest radiograph
- Angiotensin-converting enzyme
- HIV antibody

To detect hereditary neuropathy
- Examination of parents and siblings
- Appropriate gene testing (especially PMP22 duplication and connexin 32 mutations)
- Nerve biopsy

*repeating these should be considered in patients who are or become unresponsive to treatment

C recommendation). There is no evidence and no consensus about whether to use daily or alternate-day prednisolone or prednisone, or intermittent high-dose monthly intravenous or oral regimens. The generally accepted dosage for prednisolone is 60 mg/d (1–1.5 mg/kg in children) as induction with maintenance therapy slowly tapering over months to years [28].

Plasma exchange (PE)

Two small double-blind, randomized controlled trials (RCTs) with altogether 47 participants showed that PE provides significant short-term benefit in about two-thirds of patients, but rapid deterioration may occur afterwards [29–31] (Class I evidence). Plasma exchange might be considered as an initial treatment as neurological disability may improve rapidly (Level A recommendation). For stabilization of CIDP, PE needs to be combined with other treatments. Because adverse events related to difficulty with venous access, use of citrate, and haemodynamic changes are not uncommon, either corticosteroids or IVIg should be considered first (GPP).

Intravenous immunoglobulin

Meta-analysis of four double-blind RCTs with altogether 235 participants showed that IVIg 2.0 g/kg produces significant improvement in disability lasting 2–6 weeks [25, 32–36] (Class I evidence, Level A recommendation). A recent international study of 117 patients from 33 countries showed that the efficacy of IVIg (2.0 g/kg baseline loading dose divided over 2–4 days followed by maintenance infusions of 1.0 g/kg over 1–2 days every 3 weeks) was maintained over 24 weeks and possibly over 48 weeks with greater improvement of disability and fewer relapses as compared with placebo [37]. Because the benefit from IVIg is short-lived, treatment needs to be repeated at intervals and doses that need to be judged on an individual basis [28]. Crossover trials have shown no significant short-term difference between IVIg and PE [38] or between IVIg and prednisolone [24], but the samples were too small to establish equivalence (both Class II evidence).

Immunosuppressive agents

RCTs have been reported only for azathioprine and methotrexate. Azathioprine (2 mg/kg) showed no benefit when added to prednisone in 14 patients for 9 months [39, 40], but the trial was likely too short and the dose too low to be able to show a benefit. No significant benefit was observed when methotrexate 15 mg daily for 24 weeks was compared with placebo in 62 patients treated with IVIg or corticosteroids [6]. Immunosuppressive agents (table 20.3) are often used together with corticosteroids to reduce the need for IVIg or PE, or to treat patients who have not responded to any of these treatments but there is only Class IV evidence on which to base this practice [28, 40]. More research is needed before any recommendation can be made. In the meantime immunosuppressant treatment may be considered when the response to corticosteroids, IVIg, or PE is inadequate (GPP).

Table 20.3 Immunosuppressant and immunomodulatory drugs that have been reported to be beneficial in CIDP (Class IV evidence [28, 40]).

Alemtuzemab
Azathioprine
Cyclophosphamide
Ciclosporin
Etanercept
Interferon-α
Interferon-β1a
Mycophenolate mofetil
Methotrexate
Rituximab
Stem cell transplantation (hematopoietic)

Interferons

One crossover trial of interferon beta 1a for 12 weeks did not detect significant benefit [41], but the trial only included 10 patients. In a more recent non-randomized open study of intramuscular beta interferon 1a 30 μg weekly, seven of 20 patients treated showed clinical improvement, 10 remained stable, and three worsened [42]. An open study of interferon alpha showed benefit in nine of 14 treatment-resistant patients [43] and there have been other favourable smaller reports. In the absence of evidence interferon treatment may be considered when the response to corticosteroids, IVIg, or PE is inadequate (GPP).

Initial management (Good Practice Points)

Patients with very mild symptoms that do not or only slightly interfere with activities of daily living may be monitored without treatment. Treatment with corticosteroids or IVIg should be offered to patients with moderate or severe disability. Plasma exchange is similarly effective but may be less tolerated. IVIg is often the first choice as improvement can be fast. The usual first dose of IVIg is 2.0 g/kg given as 2 g/kg over 2–5 consecutive days. Contraindications to corticosteroids will influence the choice towards IVIg and vice versa. For pure motor CIDP, IVIg treatment should be the first choice and if corticosteroids are used, patients should be monitored closely for deterioration.

Therapy of CIDP patients requires individualized assessment of the treatment response. For patients starting on corticosteroids, a course of up to 12 weeks on their starting dose should be considered before deciding whether there is no treatment response. If there is a response, tapering the dose slowly to a low maintenance level over 1 or 2 years and eventual withdrawal should be considered. Patients starting on IVIg should be closely monitored to objectify occurrence and duration of response to the first course before embarking on further treatment. Between 15 and 30% of patients require only a single course of IVIg.

Long-term management (Good Practice Points)

No evidence-based guideline can be given as none of the trials systematically assessed long-term management. IVIg given in a dose of 1 g/kg over 1–2 days every 3 weeks has been shown to be efficacious over 24 (and possibly 48) weeks with improvement of grip strength, disability, and health-related quality of life [37, 44], but the appropriate dose needs to be individualized (usually 0.4–1.2 g/kg every 2–6 weeks) [28]. If a patient becomes stable on a regime of intermittent IVIg, the dose (or, perhaps, frequency) of IVIg should be reduced periodically to establish the need for ongoing therapy because patients may need less IVIg than they receive or in fact none at all. In a recent international study, the IVIg dose could be reduced by over 20% without deterioration in almost half of the patients [6]. If frequent high-dose IVIg is required, addition of corticosteroids or an immunosuppressive agent should be considered, but there is not sufficient evidence to recommend a particular drug. Patients benefiting from long-term IVIg treatment who become refractory to IVIg may respond again after a short course of PE [45]. Approximately 15% of patients fail to respond to any of the proposed treatments.

General treatment

There is a dearth of evidence concerning general aspects of treatment for symptoms of CIDP such as pain and fatigue. There is also a lack of research into the value of exercise and occupational and physical therapy in the management of CIDP. Evidence is limited concerning immunizations. International and national support groups offer information and support to patients (www.gbs-cidp.org) (GPP).

Recommendations

Good Practice Points for defining diagnostic criteria for CIDP:

1 Clinical: typical and atypical CIDP (table 20.4)

2 Electrodiagnostic: definite, probable and possible CIDP (table 20.1)

3 Supportive: including CSF, MRI, nerve biopsy, and treatment response (table 20.5)

4 Categories: definite, probable, and possible CIDP (table 20.6)

Recommendations for treatment

For induction of treatment

1 IVIg (Level A recommendation) or corticosteroids (Level C recommendation) should be considered in sensory and motor CIDP in the presence of disabling symptoms. Plasma exchange is similarly effective (Level A recommendation) but may be less tolerated. The presence of relative contraindications to any of these treatments should influence the choice (GPP). The advantages and disadvantages should be explained to the patient who should be involved in the decision making (GPP).

2 The advantages and disadvantages should be explained to the patient, who should be involved in the decision making (GPP).

3 In pure motor CIDP, IVIg should be considered as the initial treatment (GPP).

For maintenance treatment

1 If the first-line treatment is effective, continuation should be considered until the maximum benefit has been achieved and then the dose reduced to find the lowest effective maintenance dose (GPP).

2 If the response is inadequate or the maintenance doses of the initial treatment (IVIg, steroids, or PE) result in adverse effects, the other first-line treatment alternatives should be tried before considering combination treatments or adding an immunosuppressant or immunomodulatory drug may be considered but there is no sufficient evidence to recommend any particular drug (table 20.3) (GPP).

3 Advice about foot care, exercise, diet, driving, and lifestyle management should be considered. Neuropathic pain should be treated with drugs according to the EFNS guideline on treatment of neuropathic pain [46]. Depending on the needs of the patient, orthoses, physiotherapy, occupational therapy, psychological support, and referral to a rehabilitation specialist should be considered (GPP).

4 Information about patient support groups should be offered (GPP).

Table 20.4 Clinical diagnostic criteria.

I *Inclusion criteria*
　A Typical CIDP
　　• Chronically progressive, stepwise, or recurrent symmetric proximal and distal weakness and sensory dysfunction of all extremities, developing over at least 2 months; cranial nerves may be affected; and
　　• Absent or reduced tendon reflexes in all extremities
　B Atypical CIDP (still considered CIDP but with different features)
　　One of the following, but otherwise as in A (tendon reflexes may be normal in unaffected limbs)
　　• Predominantly distal (distal acquired demyelinating symmetric, DADS)
　　• Asymmetric (multifocal acquired demyelinating sensory and motor neuropathy [MADSAM], Lewis–Sumner syndrome)
　　• Focal (e.g. involvement of the brachial or lumbosacral plexus or of one or more peripheral nerves in one upper or lower limb)
　　• Pure motor
　　• Pure sensory (including chronic immune sensory polyradiculopathy affecting the central process of the primary sensory neuron)

II *Exclusion criteria*
　• Borrelia burgdorferi infection (Lyme disease), diphtheria, drug, or toxin exposure likely to have caused the neuropathy
　• Hereditary demyelinating neuropathy
　• Prominent sphincter disturbance
　• Diagnosis of multifocal motor neuropathy (MMN)
　• IgM monoclonal gammopathy with high titre antibodies to myelin-associated glycoprotein (MAG)
　• Other causes for a demyelinating neuropathy including POEMS syndrome, osteosclerotic myeloma, diabetic and non-diabetic lumbosacral radiculoplexus neuropathy. PNS lymphoma and amyloidosis may occasionally have demyelinating features

Table 20.5 Supportive criteria.

1 Elevated CSF protein with leukocyte count <10/mm^3 (Level A recommendation)
2 MRI showing gadolinium enhancement and/or hypertrophy of the cauda equina, lumbosacral or cervical nerve roots, or the brachial or lumbosacral plexuses (Level C recommendation)
3 Abnormal sensory electrophysiology in at least one nerve (GPP):
  a normal sural with abnormal median (excluding median neuropathy at the wrist from carpal tunnel syndrome) or radial sensory nerve action potential (SNAP) amplitudes, or
  b conduction velocity <80% of lower limit of normal (<70% if SNAP amplitude <80% of lower limit of normal), or
  c delayed somatosensory evoked potentials (SSEP) without central nervous system disease
4 Objective clinical improvement following immunomodulatory treatment (Level A recommendation)
5 Nerve biopsy showing unequivocal evidence of demyelination and/or remyelination by electron microscopy or teased fibre analysis (GPP)

Table 20.6 Diagnostic categories.

Definite CIDP
Clinical criteria I (A or B) and II with electrodiagnostic criterion I; or
Probable CIDP + at least one supportive criterion; or
Possible CIDP + at least two supportive criteria

Probable CIDP
Clinical criteria I (A or B) and II with electrodiagnostic criterion II; or
Possible CIDP + at least one supportive criterion

Possible CIDP
Clinical criteria I (A or B) and II with electrodiagnostic criterion III
CIDP (definite, probable, possible) associated with concomitant diseases

Conflicts of interest

The following authors have reported conflicts of interest.

D. Cornblath, personal honoraria from Merck, Pfizer, Mitsubishi Pharma, Sangamo, Bristol-Myers Squibb, Eisai, Octapharma, Sun Pharma, Acorda, DP Clinical, Geron, Exelixis, Johnson&Johnson, Genzyme, Cebix, Abbott, CSL Behring, Pfizer, Schwartz Biosciences, Avigen, FoldRx.

R. D. M. Hadden, personal honoraria from Janssen-Cilag and Talecris.

A. Hahn, personal honoraria from Baxter, Bayer, and Biogen-Idec, Talecris.

I. Illa, personal none, departmental research grant from Grifols.

C. Koski, personal honoraria from Baxter, CSL, and Talecris.

J.-M. Léger, personal none, departmental research grants or honoraria from Biogen-Idec, Baxter, LFB, Octapharma.

E. Nobile-Orazio, personal honoraria from Kedrion, Grifols, Baxter, and LFB (and he has been commissioned by Kedrion and Baxter to give expert opinions to the Italian Ministry of Health on the use of IVIg in dysimmune neuropathies).

J. Pollard, personal none, departmental research grants from Biogen-Idec, Schering.

P. van Doorn, personal none, departmental research grants or honoraria from Baxter, Talecris, and Bayer.

The other authors have nothing to declare.

References

1. European Federation of Neurological Societies, Peripheral Nerve Society. Guideline on management of chronic inflammatory demyelinating polyradiculoneuropathy. Report of a joint task force of the European Federation of Neurological Societies and the Peripheral Nerve Society. *J Peripher Nerv Syst* 2005;**10**:220–8.
2. Van den Bergh PYK, Piéret F. Electrodiagnostic criteria for acute and chronic inflammatory demyelinating polyradiculoneuropathy. *Muscle Nerve* 2004;**29**:565–74.
3. Ad Hoc Subcommittee of the American Academy of Neurology AIDS Task Force. Research criteria for the diagnosis of

chronic inflammatory demyelinating polyradiculoneuropathy (CIDP). *Neurology* 1991;**41**:617–8.

4. Dyck PJ, O'Brien PC, Oviatt KF, *et al.* Prednisone improves chronic inflammatory demyelinating polyradiculoneuropathy more than no treatment. *Ann Neurol* 1982;**11**:136–41.

5. Brainin M, Barnes M, Baron J-C, *et al.* Guidance for the preparation of neurological management guidelines by EFNS scientific task forces – revised recommendations 2004. *Eur J Neurol* 2004;**11**:577–81.

6. RMC Trial Group. Randomised controlled trial of methotrexate for chronic inflammatory demyelinating polyradiculoneuropathy (RMC trial): a pilot, multicentre study. *Lancet Neurol* 2009;**8**:158–64.

7. Rajabally YA, Nicolas G, Piéret F, Bouche P, Van den Bergh PYK. Validity of diagnostic criteria for chronic inflammatory demyelinating polyneuropathy: a multicentre European study. *J Neurol Neurosurg Psychiatry* 2009; Online First 19 August 2009.

8. Koski CL, Baumgarten M, Magder LS, *et al.* Derivation and validation of diagnostic criteria for chronic inflammatory demyelinating polyneuropathy. *J Neurol Sci* 2009; **277**:1–8.

9. Ruts L, van Koningsveld R, van Doorn PA. Distinguishing acute-onset CIDP from Guillain-Barré syndrome with treatment-related fluctuations. *Neurology* 2005;**65**:138–40.

10. Dionne A, Nicolle MW, Hahn AF. Clinical and electrophysiological parameters distinguishing acute-onset CIDP from acute inflammatory demyelinating polyneuropathy. *Muscle Nerve* 2009; Oct 30 (Epub ahead of print).

11. Thomas PK, Walker RW, Rudge P, *et al.* Chronic demyelinating peripheral neuropathy associated with multifocal central nervous system demyelination. *Brain* 1987;**110**:53–76.

12. Zéphir H, Stojkovic T, Latour P, *et al.* Relapsing demyelinating disease affecting both the central and peripheral nervous systems. *J Neurol Neurosurg Psychiatry* 2008;**79**:1032–9.

13. Gondim FA, Brannagan TH 3rd, Sander HW, *et al.* Peripheral neuropathy in patients with inflammatory bowel disease. *Brain* 2005;**128**:867–79.

14. Smyth S, Menkes DL. Coincident membranous glomerulonephritis and chronic inflammatory demyelinating polyradiculoneuropathy: questioning the autoimmunity hypothesis. *Muscle Nerve* 2008;**37**:130–5.

15. Echaniz-Laguna A, Anheim M, Wolf P, *et al.* Chronic inflammatory demyelinating polyradiculoneuropathy (CIDP) in patients with solid organ transplantation: a clinical, neurophysiological and neuropathological study of 4 cases. *Rev Neurol* 2005;**161**:1213–20.

16. Rajabally YA, Jacob S, Hbahbih M. Optimizing the use of electrophysiology in the diagnosis of chronic inflammatory demyelinating polyneuropathy: a study of 20 cases. *J Peripher Nerv Syst* 2005;**10**:282–92.

17. Rajabally YA, Jacob S. Proximal nerve conduction studies in of chronic inflammatory demyelinating polyradiculoneuropathy. *Clin Neurophysiol* 2006;**117**:2079–84.

18. Rajabally YA, Narasimhan M. The value of sensory electrophysiology in of chronic inflammatory demyelinating polyradiculoneuropathy. *Clin Neurophysiol* 2007;**118**:1999–2004.

19. Bragg JA, Benatar MG. Sensory nerve conduction slowing is a specific marker for CIDP. *Muscle Nerve* 2008;**38**:1599–603.

20. Sinnreich M, Klein CJ, Daube JR, Engelstad J, Spinner RJ, Dyck PJB. Chronic immune sensory polyradiculopathy: a possibly treatable sensory ataxia. *Neurology* 2004;**63**:1662–9.

21. Yiannikas C, Vucic S. Utility of somatosensory evoked potentials in chronic acquired demyelinating neuropathy. *Muscle Nerve* 2008;**38**:1447–54.

22. French CIDP Study Group. Recommendations on diagnostic strategies for chronic inflammatory demyelinating polyradiculoneuropathy. *J Neurol Neurosurg Psychiatry* 2008;**79**:115–8.

23. Mehndiratta MM, Hughes RAC. Corticosteroids for chronic inflammatory demyelinating polyradiculoneuropathy. *Cochrane Database Syst Rev* 2002;(3):CD002062.

24. Hughes RAC, Bensa S, Willison HJ, *et al.,* the Inflammatory Neuropathy Cause and Treatment Group. Randomized controlled trial of intravenous immunoglobulin versus oral prednisolone in chronic inflammatory demyelinating polyradiculoneuropathy. *Ann Neurol* 2001;**50**:195–201.

25. Eftimov F, Winer JB, Vermeulen M, de Haan R, van Schaik IN. Intravenous immunoglobulin for chronic inflammatory demyelinating polyradiculoneuropathy. *Cochrane Database Syst Rev* 2009;CD001797.

26. Sabatelli M, Madia F, Mignogna T, Lippi L, Quaranta L, Tonali P. Pure motor chronic inflammatory demyelinating polyneuropathy. *J Neurol* 2001;**248**:772–7.

27. Molenaar DS, van Doorn PA, Vermeulen M. Pulsed high dose dexamethasone treatment in chronic inflammatory demyelinating polyneuropathy: a pilot study. *J Neurol Neurosurg Psychiatry* 1997;**62**:388–90.

28. Kuitwaard K, van Doorn PA. Newer therapeutic options for chronic inflammatory demyelinating polyradiculoneuropathy. *Drugs* 2009;**69**:987–1001.

29. Dyck PJ, Daube J, O'Brien P, *et al.* Plasma exchange in chronic inflammatory demyelinating polyradiculoneuropathy. *N Engl J Med* 1986;**314**:461–5.

30. Hahn AF, Bolton CF, Pillay N, *et al.* Plasma-exchange therapy in chronic inflammatory demyelinating polyneuropathy (CIDP): a double-blind, sham-controlled, cross-over study. *Brain* 1996a;**119**:1055–66.

31. Mehndiratta MM, Hughes RAC, Agarwal P. Plasma exchange for chronic inflammatory demyelinating polyradiculoneuropathy (Cochrane Review). *Cochrane Database Syst Rev* 2004;(3):CD003906.

32. van Doorn PA, Brand A, Strengers PF, Meulstee J, Vermeulen M. High-dose intravenous immunoglobulin treatment in chronic inflammatory demyelinating polyneuropathy: a double-blind, placebo-controlled, crossover study. *Neurology* 1990;**40**:209–12.

33. Vermeulen M, van Doorn PA, Brand A, Strengers PFW, Jennekens FGI, Busch HFM. Intravenous immunoglobulin treatment in patients with chronic inflammatory demyelinating polyneuropathy: a double blind, placebo controlled study. *J Neurol Neurosurg Psychiatry* 1993; **56**:36–9.

34. Hahn AF, Bolton CF, Zochodne D, Feasby TE. Intravenous immunoglobulin treatment (IVIg) in chronic inflammatory demyelinating polyneuropathy (CIDP): a double-blind placebo-controlled cross-over study. *Brain* 1996b;**119**: 1067–78.

35. Mendell JR, Barohn RJ, Freimer ML, *et al.* Randomized controlled trial of IVIg in untreated chronic inflammatory demyelinating polyradiculoneuropathy. *Neurology* 2001;**56**: 445–9.

36. Elovaara I, Apostolski S, van Doorn P, *et al.* EFNS guidelines for the use of intravenous immunoglobulin in treatment of neurological diseases: EFNS task force on the use of intravenous immunoglobulin in treatment of neurological diseases. *Eur J Neurol* 2008;**15**:893–908.

37. Hughes RA, Donofrio P, Bril V, *et al.*, ICE Study Group. Intravenous immune globulin (10% caprylate-chromatography purified) for the treatment of of chronic inflammatory demyelinating polyradiculoneuropathy (ICE study): a randomised placebo-controlled trial. *Lancet Neurol* 2008; **7**:136–44.

38. Dyck PJ, Litchy WJ, Kratz KM, *et al.* A plasma exchange versus immune globulin infusion trial in chronic inflammatory demyelinating polyradiculoneuropathy. *Ann Neurol* 1994;**36**:838–45.

39. Dyck PJ, O'Brien P, Swanson C, Low P, Daube J. Combined azathioprine and prednisone in chronic inflammatory-demyelinating polyneuropathy. *Neurology* 1985;**35**:1173–6.

40. Hughes RAC, Swan AV, van Doorn PA. Cytotoxic drugs and interferons for chronic inflammatory demyelinating polyradiculoneuropathy (Update). *Cochrane Database Syst Rev* 2004;(4):CD003280.

41. Hadden RD, Sharrack B, Bensa S, Soudain SE, Hughes RAC. Randomized trial of interferon beta-1a in chronic inflammatory demyelinating polyradiculoneuropathy. *Neurology* 1999;**53**:57–61.

42. Vallat JM, Hahn AF, Leger JM, *et al.* Interferon beta-1a as an investigational treatment for CIDP. *Neurology* 2003;**60**: S23–S28.

43. Gorson KC, Ropper AH, Clark BD, Dew RB III, Simovic D, Allam G. Treatment of chronic inflammatory demyelinating polyneuropathy with interferon-alpha 2a. *Neurology* 1998; **50**:84–7.

44. Merkies IS, Bril V, Dalakas MC, *et al.*, ICE Study Group. Health-related quality-of-life improvements in CIDP with immune globulin IV 10%: the ICE Study. *Neurology* 2009; **72**:1337–44.

45. Berger AR, Herskovitz S, Scelsa S. The restoration of IVIg efficacy by plasma exchange in CIDP. *Neurology* 1995;**45**: 1628–9.

46. Cruccu G, Anand P, Attal N, Garcia-Larrea L, *et al.* EFNS guidelines on neuropathic pain assessment. *Eur J Neurol* 2004;**11**:153–62.

47. Isose S, Kuwabara S, Kokubun N, *et al.*, the Tokyo Metropolitan Neuromuscular Electrodiagnosis Study Group. *J Periph Nerv Syst* 2009;**14**:151–58.

CHAPTER 21

Multifocal motor neuropathy

I. N. van Schaik,[1] J.-M. Léger,[2] E. Nobile-Orazio,[3] D. R. Cornblath,[4] R. D. M. Hadden,[5] C. L. Koski,[6] J. Pollard,[7] C. Sommer,[8] I. Illa,[9] P. Van den Bergh,[10] P. A. van Doorn[11]

[1]Academic Medical Center, University of Amsterdam, The Netherlands; [2]Hôpital de la Salpêtrière, Paris, France; [3]University of Milan IRCCS Humanitas Clinical Institute, Italy; [4]Johns Hopkins University School of Medicine, Baltimore, MD, USA; [5]King's College Hospital, London, UK; [6]University of Maryland, Baltimore, MD, USA; [7]University of Sydney, Australia; [8]University of Wurzburg, Germany; [9]Hospital Sta Creu i Sant Pau, Universitat Autonoma de Barcelona, Spain; [10]Centre de Référence Neuromusculaire, Cliniques universitaires St-Luc, Brussels, Belgium; [11]Erasmus Medical Center, Rotterdam, The Netherlands

Objectives

The aim is to update the EFNS/PNS guideline for the definition, diagnosis, and treatment of multifocal motor neuropathy (MMN) based on available evidence and, where adequate evidence was not available, consensus.

Background

Patients with a pure motor, asymmetric neuropathy with multifocal conduction blocks (CB) have been reported from 1986 onwards [1–3]. Pestronk and colleagues first introduced the term multifocal motor neuropathy and highlighted the association with IgM anti-ganglioside GM1 antibodies and the response to immune-modulating therapies [4]. The diagnosis of MMN is based on clinical, laboratory, and electrophysiological characteristics [5–8]. Several diagnostic criteria for this neuropathy have been proposed [9–11]. These criteria share the following clinical features: slowly progressive, asymmetric, predominantly distal weakness without objective loss of sensation in the distribution of two or more individual peripheral nerves, and absence of upper motor neuron signs. The hallmark of the disease is the presence of mul-

tifocal conduction block on electrophysiological testing outside the usual sites of nerve compression [5, 12–15]. Conduction block is a reduction in the amplitude and area of the compound muscle action potential (CMAP) obtained by proximal versus distal stimulation of motor nerves in the absence of abnormal temporal dispersion [7, 12, 16]. The extent of reduction of the CMAP amplitude and/or area necessary to classify a reduction as a true conduction block is still a matter of debate. For this guideline, we present clinical and electrophysiological diagnostic criteria based on published criteria and consensus agreed upon by the task force.

MMN is a treatable disorder. A beneficial effect of various immunomodulatory drugs has been suggested in several uncontrolled studies [4, 17–25], and reviewed in a Cochrane systematic review [26]. Four trials have shown intravenous immunoglobulin (IVIg) therapy to be effective in MMN in the short term, and this treatment currently is considered the standard treatment for MMN [27–30]. These trials have also been reviewed in a Cochrane systematic review [31] This small body of evidence has allowed evidence-based statements about treatment.

Search strategy

We searched MEDLINE from August 2004 to July 2009 for articles on 'multifocal motor neuropathy' and 'diagnosis' or 'treatment' or 'guideline'. We also searched the Cochrane Library in July 2009.

European Handbook of Neurological Management: Volume 1, 2nd edition. Edited by N. E. Gilhus, M. P. Barnes and M. Brainin.
© 2011 Blackwell Publishing Ltd.

Methods for reaching consensus

Task force members prepared draft statements about definition, diagnosis, and treatment. Evidence and recommendations were classified according to the scheme agreed for EFNS guidelines [32]. When only Class IV evidence was available but consensus could be reached, the task force offered advice as Good Practice Points (GPP). The statements were revised and collated into a single document that was then revised iteratively until consensus was reached.

Results

Diagnostic criteria for MMN

The task force developed its own diagnostic criteria based on the published criteria [5–11]. The clinical criteria are listed in table 21.1. The main clinical features are weakness without objective sensory loss, slowly progressive or stepwise progressive course, asymmetric involvement of two or more nerves, and absence of upper motor neuron signs. Recently, the extent of sensory signs and symptoms in MMN has been reconsidered and development of elec-

trophysiological sensory changes with or without sensory signs and symptoms over the course of MMN has been described [33, 34].

The presence of conduction block (CB) in motor nerve fibres is the hallmark of the disease. However, some patients with otherwise typical MMN have no detectable CB, probably because these blocks are activity dependent [35] or are located in nerve segments that cannot be assessed by routine electrophysiological examination [36, 37]. More recently, other techniques with restricted availability, such as transcranial magnetic stimulation, triple-stimulation technique, and transcutaneous cervical root stimulation, have been used to identify conduction blocks with greater sensitivity. These techniques may be useful, especially where CBs are proximally situated. The value of these techniques in routine clinical use has yet to be determined. The first papers defined CB as a 20–30% amplitude or area reduction if the distal CMAP duration did not exceed 15% greater than normal. Computer modelling of CB and temporal dispersion in an animal model has demonstrated that up to 50% area reduction of the proximal to distal CMAP can be due entirely to interphase cancellation [38]. Similar studies in man have shown that distal CMAP duration and proximal CMAP duration

Table 21.1 Clinical criteria for MMN.

Core criteria (both must be present)
  1 Slowly progressive or stepwise progressive, focal, asymmetric[a] limb weakness, i.e. motor involvement in the motor nerve distribution of at least two nerves, for more than one month[b]. If symptoms and signs are present only in the distribution of one nerve only a possible diagnosis can be made (see table 21.4).
  2 No objective sensory abnormalities except for minor vibration sense abnormalities in the lower limbs[c]
Supportive clinical criteria
  3 Predominant upper limb involvement[d]
  4 Decreased or absent tendon reflexes in the affected limb[e]
  5 Absence of cranial nerve involvement[f]
  6 Cramps and fasciculations in the affected limb
  7 Response in terms of disability or muscle strength to immunomodulatory treatment
Exclusion criteria
  8 Upper motor neuron signs
  9 Marked bulbar involvement
 10 Sensory impairment more marked than minor vibration loss in the lower limbs
 11 Diffuse symmetric weakness during the initial weeks

[a]asymmetric = a difference of 1 MRC grade if strength is MRC >3 and 2 MRC grades if strength is MRC ≤3;
[b]usually more than 6 months;
[c]sensory signs and symptoms may develop over the course of MMN;
[d]at onset, predominantly lower limb involvement account for nearly 10% of the cases;
[e]slightly increased tendon reflexes, in particular in the affected arm have been reported and do not exclude the diagnosis of MMN provided criterion 8 is met;
[f]12th nerve palsy has been reported.

prolongation are important factors for the definition of CB in the median nerve segment over the forearm: the shorter the distal duration and proximal duration prolongation the less CMAP amplitude reduction is needed to diagnose a conduction block [39]. In one of the main papers concerning the diagnostic criteria of MMN, grading of CB was defined as definite or probable, and in the other as definite, probable, and possible [9–11]. There is only Class IV evidence concerning all these matters. Nevertheless, the task force agreed on Good Practice Points to define clinical and electrophysiological diagnostic criteria for MMN (tables 20.1 and 20.2).

Investigation of MMN

Based on consensus expert opinion, consideration of MMN should enter the differential diagnosis of any patient with a slowly or stepwise progressive asymmetrical limb weakness without objective sensory abnormalities, upper motor neuron, or bulbar signs or symptoms. MMN should be differentiated from motor neuron disease, entrapment neuropathies, hereditary neuropathy with liability to pressure palsies, Lewis–Sumner syndrome, and chronic inflammatory demyelinating polyradiculoneuropathy, in particular its purely motor variant [1, 3, 9, 40–51].

Clinical examination and electrodiagnostic tests are mandatory and the features suggesting a diagnosis of MMN are listed under diagnostic criteria. A family history should be obtained. The association between MMN and IgM anti-ganglioside GM1 (anti-GM1) antibodies was already suggested in the first report recognizing MMN as a distinct disease entity [4]. However, the diagnostic accuracy of anti-GM1 testing in diagnosing MMN is unclear. The literature reports the presence of anti-GM1 IgM antibodies in between 30 and 80% of MMN patients [52, 53]. Furthermore, anti-GM1 antibodies don't seem to be specific for MMN. Anti-GM1 antibodies have been reported to occur in other dysimmune neuropathies and in patients with motor neuron disease, which may mimic MMN, albeit infrequently and in lower titres. Other tests that can support the diagnosis of MMN are CSF protein <1 g/l [54], and increased signal intensity on T2-weighted MRI scans of the brachial plexus associated with a diffuse nerve swelling [6, 9, 22].

Cerebrospinal fluid (CSF), anti-ganglioside GM1 antibodies, and magnetic resonance imaging (MRI) scans of the brachial plexus are not normally needed for patients fulfilling the clinical and electrodiagnostic criteria of MMN. Nerve biopsies are not routinely performed in MMN but can be useful in detecting an alternative cause [55, 56]. Needle EMG, serum and urine paraprotein detection by immunofixation [57], thyroid function [58], creatine kinase [6, 20], CSF cells, and protein [6, 59] are investigations that can be helpful to discover concomitant disease or exclude other possible causes. This list is not complete and additional investigations should be guided by the clinical findings.

Treatment of MMN

The treatment options for people with MMN are limited. In contrast to the response in CIDP, MMN does not usually respond to steroids or plasma exchange (PE), and patients may worsen when they receive these treatments [7, 51, 60–63].

Table 21.2 Electrophysiological criteria for conduction block.[a]

1 Definite motor CB[a]

Negative peak CMAP area reduction on proximal versus distal stimulation of at least 50% whatever the nerve segment length (median, ulnar, and peroneal). Negative peak CMAP amplitude on stimulation of the distal part of the segment with motor CB must be >20% of the lower limit of normal and >1 mV and increase of proximal to distal negative peak CMAP duration must be ≤30%.

2 Probable motor CB[a]

Negative peak CMAP area reduction of at least 30% over a long segment (e.g. wrist to elbow, or elbow to axilla) of an upper limb nerve with increase of proximal to distal negative peak CMAP duration ≤30%;

OR

Negative peak CMAP area reduction of at least 50% (same as definite) with an increase of proximal to distal negative peak CMAP duration >30%;

3 Normal sensory nerve conduction in upper limb segments with CB (see exclusion criteria).

[a]Evidence for CB must be found at sites distinct from common entrapment or compression syndromes.

The efficacy of IVIg has been suggested by many open, uncontrolled studies. Four randomized controlled, double-blind trials of IVIg for treating MMN have been done [27–30]. These four RCTs included a total of 45 patients with MMN and have been summarized in a Cochrane systematic review [31]. IVIg treatment was superior to placebo in inducing an improvement in muscle strength in patients with MMN (NNT 1.4, 95% CI 1.1–1.8). As weakness is the only determinant of disability in patients with MMN, it is to be expected that in patients whose muscle strength improves after IVIg treatment, disability will improve as well. Elevated anti-ganglioside GM1 antibodies and definite CB were significantly correlated with a favourable response to IVIg in one large retrospective study [6], but in a more recent retrospective study no factors associated with treatment response were found [25]. In this series, approximately 20% of patients achieved prolonged remission (>12 months) after IVIg alone; approximately 70% of patients needed repeated long term IVIg infusions and, of them, half needed additional immunosuppressive treatment [25]. Maintenance IVIg therapy should be tailored to the need of individual patients [64]. During long-term IVIg treatment effectiveness declines as muscle strength decreases, even when dosage is increased [65–69]. This process is due to ongoing axonal degeneration [66,67,69]. In one retrospective study, treatment with higher than normal maintenance doses of IVIg (1.6–2.0 g/kg given over 4–5 days) promoted reinnervation, decreased the number of CBs, and prevented axonal degeneration in 10 MMN patients for up to 12 years [68]. However, further long-term studies are needed to determine whether disease progression can be prevented by high-dose IVIg.

One randomized, single-blinded trial and one open pilot study suggest that short-term subcutaneous administered Ig is feasible, safe, and as effective as IVIg [70, 71]. Mycophenolate mofetil added to IVIg has no additional beneficial effect and no IVIg-sparing effect [72]. Uncontrolled studies suggest a beneficial effect in some patients of cyclophosphamide [4, 17, 18, 20–22, 73], interferon beta1a [23, 24], cyclosporine [74], methotrexate [75], and azathioprine [19]. There is conflicting evidence for rituximab [76–80]. Cyclophosphamide was not recommended by one group of experts because concern exists about its short- and long-term toxicity and lack of evidence of efficacy in MMN [10].

Recommendations

Diagnostic criteria
1 Clinical: the two core criteria and all exclusion criteria should be met (see infront of table 21.1) (GPP).

2 Electrodiagnostic: definite or probable conduction block in at least one nerve (table 21.2) (GPP).

3 Supportive: anti-GM1 antibodies, MRI, CSF, and treatment response (table 21.3) (GPP).

4 Categories: definite and probable MMN (table 21.4) (GPP).

Diagnostic tests
1 Clinical examination and electrodiagnostic tests should be done in all patients (GPP).

2 Anti-ganglioside GM1 antibody testing, MRI of the brachial plexus, and CSF examination should be considered in selected patients (GPP).

3 Investigations to discover concomitant disease or exclude other possible causes should be considered but the choice of tests will depend on the individual circumstances (GPP).

Treatment
1 IVIg (2 g/kg (total cumulative dose) given over 2–5 days) should be the first-line treatment (Level A) when disability is sufficiently severe to warrant treatment.

2 Corticosteroids are not recommended (GPP).

3 If an initial treatment with IVIg is effective, repeated IVIg treatment should be considered in selected patients (Level C). The frequency of IVIg maintenance therapy should be guided by the response (GPP). Typical treatment regimens are 1 g/kg every 2–4 weeks, or 2 g/kg every 1–2 months (GPP).

4 If IVIg is not or not sufficiently effective then immunosuppressive treatment may be considered. However, no agent has shown to be beneficial in a clinical trial and data from case series are conflicting (GPP).

5 Toxicity makes cyclophosphamide a less desirable option (GPP).

Table 21.3 Supportive criteria.

1 Elevated IgM anti-ganglioside GM1 antibodies.
2 Laboratory: increased CSF protein (<1 g/l)
3 Magnetic resonance imaging showing increased signal intensity on T2-weighted imaging associated with a diffuse nerve swelling of the brachial plexus.
4 Objective clinical improvement following IVIg treatment.

Table 21.4 Diagnostic categories.

Definite MMN
• Clinical criteria 1, 2 and 8–11 (table 21.1) AND electrophysiological criteria 1 and 3 in one nerve (table 21.2)

Probable MMN
• Clinical criteria 1, 2 and 8–11 AND electrophysiological criteria 2 and 3 in two nerves
• Clinical criteria 1, 2 and 8–11 AND electrophysiological criteria 2 and 3 in one nerve AND at least two supportive criteria 1–4 (table 21.3)

Possible MMN
• Clinical criteria 1, 2 and 8–11 AND normal sensory nerve conduction studies AND supportive criteria 4
• Clinical criteria 1 with clinical signs present in only one nerve, 2 and 8–11 AND electrophysiological criteria 1 or 2 and 3 in one nerve

Conflicts of interest

The following authors have reported conflicts of interest.

I. N. van Schaik: personal none, unrestricted departmental research grant from Sanquin blood supply foundation.

D. Cornblath: personal honoraria from Merck, Pfizer, Mitshubishi Pharma, Sangamo, Sanofi-Aventis, Bristol-Myers Squibb, Eisai, Octapharma, Sun Pharma, Acorda, DP Clinical, Exelixis, Geron, Johnson & Johnson, Genyzme, Cebix, Abbott, CSL Behring, Bionevia, Schwarz Biosciences, Avigen, FoldRx, GlaxoSmithKline.

R. D. M. Hadden personal honoraria from Janssen-Cilag and Talecris.

C. Koski: personal honoraria from Baxter and Talecris.

J.-M. Léger: personal none, departmental research grants or honoraria from Biogen-Idec, Baxter, Laboratoire Français du Biofractionnement (LFB), Octapharma.

E. Nobile-Orazio: personal from Kedrion, Baxter, LFB (and he has been commissioned by Kedrion and Baxter to give expert opinions to the Italian Ministry of Health on the use of IVIg in dysimmune neuropathies).

J. Pollard: departmental research grants from Biogen-Idec and Schering.

P. van Doorn: personal none, departmental research grants or honoraria from Baxter, Bayer. and Talecris.

The other authors have nothing to declare.

References

1. Chad DA, Hammer K, Sargent J. Slow resolution of multifocal weakness and fasciculation: a reversible motor neuron syndrome. *Neurology* 1986;**36**:1260–3.
2. Roth G, Rohr J, Magistris MR, Ochsner F. Motor neuropathy with proximal multifocal persistent conduction block, fasciculations and myokymia. Evolution to tetraplegia. *Eur Neurol* 1986;**25**:416–23.
3. Parry GJ, Clarke S. Multifocal acquired demyelinating neuropathy masquerading as motor neuron disease. *Muscle Nerve* 1988;**11**:103–7.
4. Pestronk A, Cornblath DR, Ilyas AA, *et al*. A treatable multifocal motor neuropathy with antibodies to GM1 ganglioside. *Ann Neurol* 1988;**24**:73–8.
5. Parry GJ, Sumner AJ. Multifocal motor neuropathy. In: Dyck PJ, Thomas PK, Griffin JW (eds) *Neurologic Clinics. Peripheral Neuropathy: New Concepts and Treatments*, 1 edn. Philadelphia: WB Saunders company, 1992; pp. 671–84.
6. Van den Berg-Vos RM, Franssen H, Wokke JHJ, Van Es HW, Van den Berg LH. Multifocal motor neuropathy: diagnostic criteria that predict the response to immunoglobulin treatment. *Ann Neurol* 2000;**48**(6):919–26.
7. Nobile-Orazio E. Multifocal motor neuropathy. *J Neuroimmunol* 2001;**115**(1–2):4–18.
8. Nobile-Orazio E, Cappellari A, Priori A. Multifocal motor neuropathy: current concepts and controversies. *Muscle Nerve* 2005;**31**(6):663–80.
9. Van den Berg-Vos RM, Van den Berg LH, Franssen H, *et al*. Multifocal inflammatory demyelinating neuropathy: a distinct clinical entity? *Neurology* 2000;**54**(1):26–32.
10. Hughes RAC. 79th ENMC international workshop: multifocal motor neuropathy: 14–15 April 2000, Hilversum, The Netherlands. *Neuromuscul Disord* 2001;**11**(3):309–14.

11. Olney RK, Lewis RA, Putnam TD, Campellone JVJ. Consensus criteria for the diagnosis of multifocal motor neuropathy. *Muscle Nerve* 2003;**27**:117–21.

12. Cornblath DR, Sumner AJ, Daube J, *et al.* Conduction block in clinical practice. *Muscle Nerve* 1991;**14**:869–71.

13. Kaji R, Kimura J. Nerve conduction block. *Curr Opin Neurology Neurosurgery* 1991;**4**:744–8.

14. Parry GJ. Motor neuropathy with multifocal conduction block. *Sem Neurol* 1993;**13**:269–75.

15. Van Asseldonk JTH, Van den Berg LH, Van den Berg-Vos RM, Wieneke GH, Wokke JHJ, Franssen H. Demyelination and axonal loss in multifocal motor neuropathy: distribution and relation to weakness. *Brain* 2003;**126**(1):186–98.

16. Kaji R. Physiology of conduction block in multifocal motor neuropathy and other demyelinating neuropathies. *Muscle Nerve* 2003;**27**:285–96.

17. Krarup C, Stewart JD, Sumner AJ, Pestronk A, Lipton SA. A syndrome of asymmetric limb weakness with motor conduction block. *Neurology* 1990;**40**:118–27.

18. Feldman EL, Bromberg MB, Albers JW, Pestronk A. Immunosuppressive treatment in multifocal motor neuropathy. *Ann Neurol* 1991;**30**:397–401.

19. Hausmanowa-Petrusewicz I, Rowinska-Marcinska K, Kopec A. Chronic acquired demyelinating motor neuropathy. *Acta Neurol Scand* 1991;**84**(1):40–5.

20. Chaudhry V, Corse AM, Cornblath DR, *et al.* Multifocal motor neuropathy: response to human immune globulin. *Ann Neurol* 1993;**33**:237–42.

21. Meucci N, Cappellari A, Barbieri S, Scarlato G, Nobile-Orazio E. Long term effect of intravenous immunoglobulins and oral cyclophosphamide in multifocal motor neuropathy. *J Neurol Neurosurg Psychiatry* 1997;**63**(6):765–9.

22. Van Es HW, Van den Berg LH, Franssen H, *et al.* Magnetic resonance imaging of the brachial plexus in patients with multifocal motor neuropathy. *Neurology* 1997;**48**(5):1218–24.

23. Martina ISJ, Van Doorn PA, Schmitz PIM, Meulstee J, Van der Meché FGA. Chronic motor neuropathies: response to interferon-β1a after failure of conventional therapies. *J Neurol Neurosurg Psychiatry* 1999;**66**:197–201.

24. Van den Berg-Vos RM, Van den Berg LH, Franssen H, Van Doorn PA, Merkies ISJ, Wokke JHJ. Treatment of multifocal motor neuropathy with interferon-β1A. *Neurology* 2000;**54**(7):1518–21.

25. Léger JM, Viala K, Cancalon F, *et al.* Intravenous immunoglobulin as short- and long-term therapy of multifocal motor neuropathy: a retrospective study of response to IVIg and of its predictive criteria in 40 patients. *J Neurol Neurosurg Psychiatry* 2008;**79**(1):93–6.

26. Umapathi T, Hughes RAC, Nobile-Orazio E, Léger JM. Immunosuppressant and immunomodulatory treatments for multifocal motor neuropathy (review). *Cochrane Database Syst Rev* 2009;(1):CD003217.

27. Azulay J-P, Blin O, Pouget J, *et al.* Intravenous immunoglobulin treatment in patients with motor neuron syndromes associated with anti-GM1 antibodies: a double-blind, placebo-controlled study. *Neurology* 1994;**44**:429–32.

28. Van den Berg LH, Kerkhoff H, Oey PL, *et al.* Treatment of multifocal motor neuropathy with high dose intravenous immunoglobulins: a double blind, placebo controlled study. *J Neurol Neurosurg Psychiatry* 1995;**59**(3):248–52.

29. Federico P, Zochodne DW, Hahn AF, Brown WF, Feasby TE. Multifocal motor neuropathy improved by IVIg: randomized, double-blind, placebo-controlled study. *Neurology* 2000;**55**(9):1256–62.

30. Léger JM, Chassande B, Musset L, Meininger V, Bouche P, Baumann N. Intravenous immunoglobulin therapy in multifocal motor neuropathy: a double-blind, placebo-controlled study. *Brain* 2001;**124**(1):145–53.

31. van Schaik IN, Van den Berg LH, de Haan R, Vermeulen M. Intravenous immunoglobuline for multifocal motor neuropathy. *Cochrane Database Syst Rev* 2005;(2):CD004429.

32. Brainin M, Barnes M, Baron J-C, *et al.* Guidance for the preparation of neurological management guidelines by EFNS scientific task forces – revised recommendations 2004. *Eur J Neurol* 2004;**11**(9):577–81.

33. Lambrecq V, Krim E, Rouanet-Larrivière M, Lagueny A. Sensory loss in multifocal motor neuropathy: a clinical and electrophysiological study. *Muscle Nerve* 2009;**39**(2):131–6.

34. Lievens I, Fournier E, Viala K, Maisonobe T, Bouche P, Léger JM. Multifocal motor neuropathy: a retrospective study of sensory nerve conduction velocities in long-term follow-up of 21 patients. *Rev Neurol* 2009;**165**(3):243–8.

35. Nodera H, Bostock H, Izumi Y, *et al.* Activity-dependent conduction block in multifocal motor neuropathy: magnetic fatigue test. *Neurology* 2006;**67**(2):280–7.

36. Pakiam AS, Parry GJ. Multifocal motor neuropathy without overt conduction block. *Muscle Nerve* 1998;**21**(2):243–5.

37. Delmont E, Azulay JP, Giorgi R, *et al.* Multifocal motor neuropathy with and without conduction block: a single entity? *Neurology* 2006;**67**(4):592–6.

38. Rhee EK, England JD, Sumner AJ. A computer simulation of conduction block: effects produced by actual conduction block versus interphase cancellation. *Ann Neurol* 1990;**28**:146–56.

39. Van Asseldonk JTH, Van den Berg LH, Wieneke GH, Wokke JH, Franssen H. Criteria for conduction block based on computer simulation studies of nerve conduction with human data obtained in the forearm segment of the median nerve. *Brain* 2006;**129**:2447–60.

40. Pestronk A, Chaudhry V, Feldman EL, *et al.* Lower motor neuron syndromes defined by patterns of weakness, nerve conduction abnormalities, and high titer of antiglycolipid antibodies. *Ann Neurol* 1990;**27**:316–26.

41. Veugelers B, Theys P, Lammens M, Van Hees J, Robberecht W. Pathological findings in a patient with amyotrophic lateral sclerosis and multifocal motor neuropathy with conduction block. *J Neurol Sci* 1996;**136**(1–2):64–70.

42. Beydoun SR. Multifocal motor neuropathy with conduction block misdiagnosed as multiple entrapment neuropathies. *Muscle Nerve* 1998;**21**(6):813–5.

43. Saperstein DS, Amato AA, Wolfe GI, *et al.* Multifocal acquired demyelinating sensory and motor neuropathy: the Lewis-Sumner syndrome. *Muscle Nerve* 1999;**22**: 560–6.

44. Parry GJ. Are multifocal motor neuropathy and Lewis-Sumner syndrome distinct nosologic entities? *Muscle Nerve* 1999;**22**:557–9.

45. Ellis CM, Leary S, Payan J, *et al.* Use of human intravenous immunoglobulin in lower motor neuron syndromes. *J Neurol Neurosurg Psychiatry* 1999;**67**(1):15–9.

46. Lewis RA. Multifocal motor neuropathy and Lewis Sumner syndrome: two distinct entities. [comment]. *Muscle Nerve* 1999;**22**(12):1738–9.

47. Molinuevo JL, Cruz-Martinez A, Graus F, Serra J, Ribalta T, Valls-Sole J. Central motor conduction time in patients with multifocal motor conduction block. *Muscle Nerve* 1999; **22**(7):926–32.

48. Mezaki T, Kaji R, Kimura J. Multifocal motor neuropathy and Lewis Sumner syndrome: a clinical spectrum. [comment]. *Muscle Nerve* 1999;**22**(12):1739–40.

49. Visser J, Van den Berg-Vos RM, Franssen H, *et al.* Mimic syndromes in sporadic cases of progressive spinal muscular atrophy. *Neurology* 2002;**58**(11):1593–6.

50. Oh SJ, Claussen GC, Kim DS. Motor and sensory demyelinating mononeuropathy multiplex (multifocal motor and sensory demyelinating neuropathy): a separate entity or a variant of chronic inflammatory demyelinating polyneuropathy? *J Periph Nerv Syst* 2005;**2**:362–9.

51. Slee M, Selvan A, Donaghy M. Multifocal motor neuropathy. The diagnsotic spectrum and response to treatment. *Neurology* 2007;**69**(1680):1687.

52. van Schaik IN, Bossuyt PMM, Brand A, Vermeulen M. The diagnostic value of GM1 antibodies in motor neuron disorders and neuropathies: a meta-analysis. *Neurology* 1995; **45**(8):1570–7.

53. Willison HJ, Yuki N. Peripheral neuropathies and antiglycolipid antibodies. *Brain* 2002;**125**(12):2591–625.

54. Taylor BV, Gross L, Windebank AJ. The sensitivity and specificity of anti-GM1 antibody testing. *Neurology* 1996; **47**(4):951–5.

55. Bouche P, Moulonguet A, Younes-Chennoufi AB, *et al.* Multifocal motor neuropathy with conduction block: a study of 24 patients. *J Neurol Neurosurg Psychiatry* 1995; **59**(1):38–44.

56. Corse AM, Chaudhry V, Crawford TO, Cornblath DR, Kuncl RW, Griffin JW. Sural nerve pathology in multifocal motor neuropathy. *Ann Neurol* 1996;**39**:319–25.

57. Noguchi M, Mori K, Yamazaki S, Suda K, Sato N, Oshimi K. Multifocal motor neuropathy caused by a B-cell lymphoma producing a monoclonal IgM autoantibody against peripheral nerve myelin glycolipids GM1 and GD1b. *Br J Haematol* 2003;**123**(4):600–5.

58. Toscano A, Rodolico C, Benvenga S, *et al.* Multifocal motor neuropathy and asymptomatic Hashimoto's thyroiditis: first report of an association. *Neuromuscul Disord* 2002;**12**(6): 566–8.

59. Taylor BV, Wright RA, Harper CM, Dyck PJ. Natural history of 46 patients with multifocal motor neuropathy with conduction block. *Muscle Nerve* 2000;**23**:900–8.

60. Van den Berg LH, Lokhorst H, Wokke JH. Pulsed high-dose dexamethasone is not effective in patients with multifocal motor neuropathy. [comment]. *Neurology* 1997;**48**(4):1135.

61. Carpo M, Cappellari A, Mora G, *et al.* Deterioration of multifocal motor neuropathy after plasma exchange. *Neurology* 1998;**50**(5):1480–2.

62. Claus D, Specht S, Zieschang M. Plasmapheresis in multifocal motor neuropathy: a case report. *J Neurol Neurosurg Psychiatry* 2000;**68**(4):533–5.

63. Lehmann HC, Hoffmann FR, Fusshoeller A, *et al.* The clinical value of therapeutic plasma exchange in multifocal motor neuropathy. *J Neurol Sci* 2008;**271**(1–2):34–9.

64. Baumann A, Hess CW, Sturzenegger M. IVIg dose increase in multifocal motor neuropathy: a prospective six months follow-up. *J Neurol* 2009;**256**(4):608–14.

65. Azulay JP, Rihet P, Pouget J, *et al.* Long term follow up of multifocal motor neuropathy with conduction block under treatment. *J Neurol Neurosurg Psychiatry* 1997;**62**(4): 391–4.

66. Van den Berg LH, Franssen H, Wokke JHJ. The long-term effect of intravenous immunoglobulin treatment in multifocal motor neuropathy. *Brain* 1998;**121**(3):421–8.

67. Terenghi F, Cappellari A, Bersano A, Carpo M, Barbieri S, Nobile-Orazio E. How long is IVIg effective in multifocal motor neuropathy? *Neurology* 2004;**62**(4):666–8.

68. Vucic S, Black KR, Chong PST, Cros D. Multifocal motor neuropathy. Decrease in conduction blocks and reinnervation with long-term IVIg. *Neurology* 2004;**63**:1264–9.

69. Van Asseldonk JTH, Van den Berg LH, Kalmijn S, *et al.* Axonal loss is an important determinant of weakness in multifocal motor neuropathy. *J Neurol Neurosurg Psychiatry* 2006;**77**:743–7.

70. Harbo T, Andersen H, Hess A, Hansen K, Sindrup SH, Jakobsen J. Subcutaneous versus intravenous immunoglobulin in multifocal motor neuropathy: a randomised, single-blinded cross-over trial. *Eur J Neurol* 2009;**16**:631–8.

71. Eftimov F, Vermeulen M, de Haan RJ, Van den Berg LH, van Schaik IN. Subcutaneous immunoglobulin therapy for multifocal motor neuropathy. *J Periph Nerv Syst* 2009;**14**:93–100.

72. Piepers S, Van den Berg-Vos RM, van der Pol WL, Franssen H, Wokke JH, Van den Berg LH. Mycophenolate mofetil as adjunctive therapy for MMN patients: a randomized, controlled trial. *Brain* 2007;**130**:2004–10.

73. Brannagan TH, III, Pradhan A, Heiman-Patterson T, *et al.* High-dose cyclophosphamide without stem-cell rescue for refractory CIDP. *Neurology* 2002;**58**(12):1856–8.

74. Nemni R, Santuccio G, Calabrese E, Galardi G, Canal N. Efficacy of cyclosporine treatment in multifocal motor neuropathy. *J Neurol* 2003;**250**(9):1118–20.

75. Nobile-Orazio E, Terenghi F, Cocito D, Gallia F, Casellato C. Oral Methotrexate as adjunctive therapy in patients with Multifocal Motor Neuropathy on chronic IVIg therapy. *J Periph Nerv Syst* 2009;**14**(3):203–5.

76. Rojas-Garcia R, Gallardo E, de Andres I, Juarez C, Sanchez P, Illa I. Chronic neuropathy with IgM anti-ganglioside antibodies: lack of long term response to rituximab. *Neurology* 2003;**61**(12):1814–6.

77. Rüegg SJ, Fuhr P, Steck AJ. Rituximab stabilizes multifocal motor neuropathy increasingly less responsive to IVIg. *Neurology* 2004;**63**:2178–9.

78. Gorson KC, Natarajan N, Ropper AH, Weinstein R. Rituximab treatment in patients with IVIg-dependent immune polyneuropathy: a prospective pilot trial. *Muscle Nerve* 2007;**35**:66–9.

79. Stieglbauer K, Topakian R, Hinterberger G, Aichner FT. Beneficial effect of rituximab monotherapy in multifocal motor neuropathy. *Neuromuscul Disord* 2009;**19**(7):473–5.

80. Chaudhry V, Cornblath DR. An open-label trial of rituximab (Rituxan) in multifocal motor neuropathy (MMN). *J Periph Nerv Syst* 2008;**13**:164–5.

CHAPTER 22

Paraproteinaemic demyelinating neuropathies

R. D. M. Hadden,[1] E. Nobile-Orazio,[2] C. Sommer,[3] A. F. Hahn,[4] I. Illa,[5] E. Morra,[6] J. Pollard,[7] M. P. T. Lunn,[8] P. Bouche,[9] D. R. Cornblath,[10] E. Evers,[11] C. L. Koski,[12] J.-M. Léger,[13] P. Van den Bergh,[14] P. van Doorn,[15] I. N. van Schaik[16]

[1]King's College Hospital, London, UK; [2]IRCCS Humanitas Clinical Institute, University of Milan, Italy; [3]University of Würzburg, Germany; [4]University of Western Ontario, London, Canada; [5]Hospital Sta. Creu i Sant Pau, Barcelona, Spain; [6]Niguarda Hospital, Milan, Italy; [7]University of Sydney, Australia; [8]National Hospital for Neurology and Neurosurgery, Queen Square, London, UK; [9]CHU Pitié-Salpêtrière, Paris, France; [10]Johns Hopkins University, Baltimore, MD, USA; [11]Guillain-Barré Syndrome Support Group of the UK; [12]University of Maryland, Baltimore, USA; [13]Faculté de Médecine Pitié-Salpêtrière, Paris, France; [14]Cliniques St.-Luc, Université Catholique de Louvain, Brussels, Belgium; [15]Erasmus Medical Centre, Rotterdam, The Netherlands; [16]Academic Medical Centre, Amsterdam, The Netherlands

Objectives

To construct clinically useful guidelines for the diagnosis, investigation, and treatment of patients with both a demyelinating neuropathy and a paraprotein (paraproteinaemic demyelinating neuropathy, PDN), based on the available evidence and, where evidence was not available, consensus. This is the first revision of the original 2006 guideline [1].

Background

The neuropathies associated with paraproteins are complex and difficult to classify, because of heterogeneity in the clinical and electrophysiological features of the neuropathy, the class, immunoreactivity, and pathogenicity of the paraprotein, and the malignancy of the underlying plasma cell dyscrasia [2, 3]. In the absence of an agreed

diagnostic classification, specific diagnostic criteria are available for only a few of these disorders, and treatment trials are therefore difficult to interpret.

Both demyelinating and axonal neuropathies may be associated with paraproteins, but this guideline concentrates on the demyelinating neuropathies. Many patients with PDN have a neuropathy that is indistinguishable from chronic inflammatory demyelinating polyradiculoneuropathy (CIDP), and there is no consensus as to whether these should be considered the same or different diseases. Paraproteinaemic axonal neuropathies are mentioned briefly in the section 'Other neuropathy syndromes associated with paraproteinaemia'. As both paraproteins and neuropathies are common, it often remains uncertain whether the paraprotein is causing the neuropathy or is coincidental.

Search strategy

We searched MEDLINE and the Cochrane Library on 1 May 2009 for articles on ('paraprotein(a)emic demyelinating neuropathy' AND ('diagnosis' OR 'treatment' OR 'guideline')) and used the personal databases of task force members.

European Handbook of Neurological Management: Volume 1, 2nd edition. Edited by N. E. Gilhus, M. P. Barnes and M. Brainin.
© 2011 Blackwell Publishing Ltd.

Methods for reaching consensus

Evidence was classified as Class I–IV and recommendations as Level A–C [4]. When only Class IV evidence was available but consensus could be reached the task force has offered advice as Good Practice Points (GPP). The original 2006 guideline [1] was revised iteratively until unanimous consensus was reached.

Results

Any diagnostic classification of PDN must take account of the dimensions of clinical phenotype, immunoglobulin (Ig) class, presence of malignancy, antibodies to myelin-associated glycoprotein (MAG), electrophysiological phenotype, and causal relationship of the paraprotein to the neuropathy. There is no consensus as to which should take precedence in classification. This guideline distinguishes IgM from IgG and IgA PDN, because IgM PDN tends to have a typical clinical phenotype, pathogenic antibodies, a causal relationship between paraprotein and neuropathy, and a different response to treatment. Nevertheless, there is significant overlap between the clinical and electrophysiological features of the neuropathy with different types of paraprotein.

Investigation and classification of the paraprotein

Background

While some paraproteins (monoclonal gammopathy, monoclonal immunoglobulin) are detected by standard serum protein electrophoresis (SPEP), both serum immunoelectrophoresis (SIEP) and serum immunofixation electrophoresis (SIFE) are more sensitive techniques that detect lower paraprotein concentrations [5, 6]. Heavy (IgM, IgG, or IgA) and light chain (kappa or lambda) classes should be identified. A paraprotein indicates an underlying clonal B cell expansion, usually in bone marrow, which may be malignant (and may itself require treatment), or a monoclonal gammopathy of uncertain significance (MGUS) (table 22.1) [7].

Most bone lesions causing neuropathy are sclerotic or mixed lytic-sclerotic, most commonly in the vertebral bones or pelvis. Although there is limited evidence on

Table 22.1 Classification of haematological conditions with a paraprotein.

1 Malignant monoclonal gammopathies
  (a) Multiple myeloma (*overt, asymptomatic (smouldering), non-secretory, or osteosclerotic*)
  (b) Plasmacytoma (*solitary, extramedullary, multiple solitary*)
  (c) Malignant lymphoproliferative disease:
    1 Waldenström's macroglobulinaemia
    2 Malignant lymphoma
    3 Chronic lymphocytic leukaemia
  (d) Heavy chain disease
  (e) Primary amyloidosis (AL) (*with or without myeloma*)
2 Monoclonal gammopathy of undetermined significance

imaging of sclerotic lesions, skeletal survey (or computed tomography (CT)), magnetic resonance imaging (MRI), and positron emission tomography (PET)/CT are complementary imaging modalities and more than one may be needed if the index of suspicion is high [8].

Recommended investigations

Table 22.2 suggests investigations to be considered in patients with a paraprotein. SIFE should be performed in patients with a known paraprotein to define the heavy and light chain type, in patients with acquired demyelinating neuropathies, and in patients in whom a paraprotein is suspected but not detected by SPEP.

Definition of MGUS

The definition of IgM MGUS is different to that for IgG and IgA MGUS (table 22.3). Patients with IgM MGUS have alternatively been classified as either 'IgM-related disorders' if they have clinical features attributable to the paraprotein (such as neuropathy), or 'asymptomatic IgM monoclonal gammopathy' if not [9].

Typical syndromes of paraproteinaemic demyelinating neuropathy (PDN)

The most common types of PDN are those with demyelinating neuropathy and MGUS without non-neurological symptoms. The neuropathy is defined as

Table 22.2 Investigation of a paraprotein.

The following should be considered in patients with a paraprotein.

(a) Serum immunofixation electrophoresis

(b) Physical examination for peripheral lymphadenopathy, hepatosplenomegaly, macroglossia, and signs of POEMS syndrome (see page 354)

(c) Full blood count, renal and liver function, calcium, phosphate, erythrocyte sedimentation rate, C-reactive protein, uric acid, beta 2-microglobulin, lactate dehydrogenase, rheumatoid factor, serum cryoglobulins

(d) Total immunoglobulin (Ig)G, IgA, IgM concentrations

(e) Serum free light chains

(f) Random urine collection for the detection of Bence-Jones protein (free light chains), and, if positive, 24-h urine collection for protein quantification

(g) Radiographic X-ray skeletal survey (including skull, pelvis, spine, ribs, long bones) to look for lytic or sclerotic lesions. Part or all of this may be replaced by CT, which is more sensitive but involves greater radiation exposure except where low-dose whole body CT is available. If the index of suspicion is high, CT and/or MRI of the spine, pelvis or whole body, and perhaps whole body FDG-PET/CT, may be considered

(h) Ultrasound or CT of chest, abdomen, and pelvis (to detect lymphadenopathy, hepatosplenomegaly, or malignancy)

(i) Serum VEGF levels if POEMS syndrome suspected

(j) Consultation with a haematologist and consideration of bone marrow examination

Table 22.3 Definition of monoclonal gammopathy of undetermined significance (MGUS).

A IgM-MGUS is defined by the presence of both of the following:

  (a) No lymphoplasmacytic infiltration on bone marrow biopsy, or equivocal infiltration with negative phenotypic studies

  (b) No signs or symptoms suggesting tumour infiltration (e.g. constitutional symptoms, hyperviscosity syndrome, organomegaly)

B IgG or IgA-MGUS is defined by the presence of all of the following:

  1 Serum monoclonal component ≤30 g/L

  2 Bence-Jones proteinuria ≤1 g/24h

  3 No lytic or sclerotic lesions in bone

  4 No anaemia, hypercalcaemia, or chronic renal insufficiency

  5 Bone marrow plasma cell infiltration <10%

IgM Paraproteinaemic Demyelinating Neuropathy

Clinical phenotype

Most patients with IgM PDN have predominantly distal, chronic (duration over 6 months), slowly progressive, symmetric, predominantly sensory impairment, with ataxia, relatively mild or no weakness, and often tremor (Class IV evidence) [2, 11–15]. This phenotype is most strongly associated with IgM anti-MAG antibodies. Some patients have more prominent ataxia with impairment predominantly of vibration and joint position sense. However, the clinical features do not correlate exactly with the paraprotein type: a few patients with IgM PDN have proximal weakness more typical of IgG/IgA PDN, and some CIDP patients have distal weakness without a paraprotein [16].

Electrophysiology

Patients with IgM PDN may meet the definite electrophysiological criteria for CIDP [10]. They may also have additional specific electrophysiological features in one or more nerves which help to distinguish from CIDP, typically uniform symmetrical and predominantly distal reduced conduction velocity (terminal latency index <0.25) without conduction block (table 22.4, adapted from [12, 17, 18]).

demyelinating if it satisfies electrophysiological criteria for CIDP [10]. If there are subtle features of demyelination not meeting these criteria, further investigations should be considered to clarify the possible pathogenic link between the paraprotein and the neuropathy (see section on 'Cerebrospinal fluid and nerve biopsy').

Table 22.4 Electrophysiological features associated with IgM PDN.

(a) Uniform symmetrical reduction of conduction velocities; more severe sensory than motor involvement

(b) Disproportionately prolonged distal motor latency (DML). This may be quantified as terminal latency index (defined as distal distance/[motor conduction velocity x DML]; i.e. 'distal velocity'/'intermediate segment velocity') ≤0.25

(c) Absent sural potential (i.e. less likely to have the 'abnormal median, normal sural' sensory action potential pattern)

(d) Partial motor conduction block (i.e. proximal/distal CMAP amplitude ratio <0.5) and marked distal CMAP dispersion are very rare

Antibodies to myelin-associated glycoprotein (MAG) and other neural antigens

Almost 50% of patients with IgM PDN have high titres of anti-MAG IgM antibodies [19], more commonly associated with kappa than lambda light chains, and this is the best-defined syndrome of PDN [20]. Weakly positive anti-MAG antibodies are less specific and may occur in the absence of neuropathy.

Testing for antibodies to MAG should be considered in all patients with IgM PDN [21]. If negative, then testing for IgM antibodies against other neural antigens, including gangliosides GQ1b, GM1, GD1a and GD1b, and SGPG, may be considered. The presence of these antibodies increases the probability of, but does not prove, a pathogenetic link between the paraprotein and the neuropathy. Their diagnostic relevance is not defined.

IgG or IgA Paraproteinaemic Demyelinating Neuropathy

Patients with IgG or IgA PDN usually have both proximal and distal weakness, with motor and sensory impairment, indistinguishable clinically and electrophysiologically from typical CIDP [10]. They usually have more rapid progression than IgM PDN [14, 15, 22]. However, a minority of patients with IgG or IgA PDN have the clinical and electrophysiological phenotype typical of IgM PDN.

In patients with IgG or IgA paraprotein, no specific antibody has been consistently associated with demyelinating neuropathy, and therefore there is no need to test for serum antibodies to known neural epitopes in routine practice.

Other neuropathy syndromes associated with paraproteinaemia

This section briefly discusses other types of neuropathy associated with a paraprotein, including those with haematological malignancy, systemic symptoms, or axonal electrophysiology, although these are not part of the main guidelines and not discussed in detail.

POEMS

POEMS (Polyneuropathy, Organomegaly, Endocrinopathy, Monoclonal gammopathy, and Skin changes) syndrome usually has an underlying osteosclerotic myeloma, with IgA or IgG lambda paraprotein, or is sometimes associated with Castleman's disease. POEMS neuropathy has similar clinical features to severe CIDP. Many patients are initially thought to have CIDP or ordinary PDN, until POEMS is suggested by the presence of systemic features. Major diagnostic criteria are polyneuropathy; monoclonal plasma cell proliferative disorder (almost always lambda); and sclerotic bone lesions or Castleman disease or raised vascular endothelial growth factor (VEGF) levels [23]. Minor diagnostic criteria are organomegaly (hepatosplenomegaly or lymphadenopathy), extravascular volume overload (oedema, pleural effusion or ascites), endocrinopathy, skin changes (hypertrichosis, hyperpigmentation, plethora, acrocyanosis, flushing, dermal glomeruloid haemangiomata, white nails), papilloedema, or thrombocytosis/polycythaemia [23].

There is no specific diagnostic test for POEMS, so if it is suspected then the diagnostic criteria should be sought by detailed clinical examination and appropriate investigations (table 22.2). Serum or plasma VEGF levels are usually markedly raised in POEMS, and normal or only slightly raised in CIDP or PDN [24], so are a useful supportive diagnostic test. Nerve biopsy may show uncompacted myelin lamellae [25].

Electrophysiology often shows a mixed demyelinating and axonal picture [26]. Features that may help to distinguish POEMS from CIDP include: reduced motor nerve conduction velocities more marked in intermediate than distal nerve segments (increased terminal latency index 0.35–0.6, the opposite of IgM PDN), rarity of conduction block, and severe length-dependent axonal loss [27, 28].

Waldenström's macroglobulinaemia

Waldenström's macroglobulinaemia is defined by the presence of an IgM (usually kappa) paraprotein (irrespective of concentration) and a bone marrow biopsy showing infiltration by lymphoplasmacytic lymphoma with a predominantly intertrabecular pattern, supported by appropriate immunophenotypic studies [9]. The associated neuropathy is clinically heterogeneous, but patients with indolent or asymptomatic Waldenström's macroglobulinaemia may have anti-MAG reactivity and clinical features of IgM anti-MAG neuropathy [29].

CANOMAD

The syndrome of Chronic Ataxic Neuropathy with Ophthalmoplegia, IgM Monoclonal gammopathy, cold Agglutinins and Disialoganglioside (IgM anti-ganglioside GD1b/GQ1b) antibodies (CANOMAD) is a rare neuropathy similar to chronic Fisher syndrome, with mixed demyelinating and axonal electrophysiology [30].

Other neuropathies with a paraprotein

Axonal neuropathy is often present in patients with MGUS, but the pathogenesis and causal relationships vary, and this will not be considered further in these guidelines.

A few patients with cryoglobulinaemia [31] or primary (AL) amyloidosis [32] have demyelinating neuropathy, although far more have axonal neuropathy. AL amyloidosis should be suspected in the presence of prominent neuropathic pain or dysautonomia, and may be demonstrated by biopsy of nerve or other tissues. Chronic axonal polyneuropathy with IgG MGUS, without symptoms or signs of amyloidosis, is usually indistinguishable from chronic idiopathic axonal polyneuropathy.

In patients with lytic multiple myeloma (usually associated with IgA or IgG kappa or lambda paraprotein) neuropathy may be caused by heterogeneous mechanisms, including amyloidosis, metabolic and drug-induced insults, and cord or root compression due to vertebral collapse from lytic lesions [33]. Subacute weakness similar to Guillain-Barré syndrome may be caused by extensive infiltration of nerves or roots by lymphoma or leukaemia [34].

Multifocal motor neuropathy is occasionally associated with an IgM MGUS, which does not seem to affect the behaviour of the disease [35].

Is the paraprotein causing the neuropathy?

A causal relationship of the paraprotein to the neuropathy is more likely with an IgM than an IgG or IgA MGUS. There is still no expert consensus as to whether IgG or IgA PDN may merely be CIDP with a co-incidental paraprotein. The only published criteria of causality were in a study in which all patients had predominantly distal sensory neuropathy, demyelinating physiology, and MGUS (IgM or IgG) [18]. We extensively modified these criteria, and propose factors which suggest whether or not the paraprotein is likely to be causing the neuropathy (table 22.5).

Table 22.5 Causal relationship between paraprotein and demyelinating neuropathy.

1 *Highly probable* if IgM paraprotein (monoclonal gammopathy of uncertain significance (MGUS) or Waldenstrom's) and:
   (a) high titres of IgM anti-MAG or anti-GQ1b antibodies, or
   (b) nerve biopsy shows IgM or complement deposits on myelin, or widely-spaced myelin on electron microscopy
2 *Probable* if either:
   (a) IgM paraprotein (MGUS or Waldenstrom's) with high titres of IgM antibodies to other neural antigens (GM1, GD1a, GD1b, GM2, sulphatide, etc.), and slowly progressive predominantly distal symmetrical sensory neuropathy, or
   (b) IgG or IgA paraprotein and nerve biopsy evidence (as in 1(b) but with IgG or IgA deposits)
3 *Less likely* when any of the following are present in a patient with MGUS and without anti-MAG antibodies (diagnosis may be described as 'CIDP with coincidental paraprotein'):
   (a) time to peak of neuropathy <6 months
   (b) relapsing/remitting or monophasic course
   (c) cranial nerves involved (except CANOMAD)
   (d) asymmetry
   (e) history of preceding infection
   (f) abnormal median with normal sural sensory action potential
   (g) IgG or IgA paraprotein without biopsy features in 2(b)

Table 22.6 Cerebrospinal fluid (CSF) examination and nerve biopsy.

1 **CSF examination** is most likely to be helpful in the following situations
  (a) In patients with borderline demyelinating or axonal electrophysiology or atypical phenotype, where the presence of raised CSF protein would help to suggest that the neuropathy is immune-mediated
  (b) The presence of malignant cells would confirm lymphoproliferative infiltration
2 **Nerve biopsy** (usually sural nerve) is most likely to be helpful when the following conditions are being considered
  (a) amyloidosis.
  (b) vasculitis (e.g. due to cryoglobulinaemia).
  (c) malignant lymphoproliferative infiltration of nerves, or
  (d) IgM PDN with negative anti-MAG antibodies, or IgG or IgA PDN with a chronic progressive course, where the discovery of widely-spaced myelin on electron microscopy or deposits of immunoglobulin and/or complement bound to myelin would support a causal relationship between paraprotein and neuropathy.
However, clinical decisions on treatment are often made without a biopsy.

Cerebrospinal fluid and nerve biopsy

Cerebrospinal fluid (CSF) examination and nerve biopsy may be helpful in selected circumstances (table 22.6, GPP), but are usually not necessary if there is clearly demyelinating physiology with MGUS. The CSF protein is elevated in 75–86% of patients with PDN [12, 18]. The presence of widely spaced myelin outer lamellae on electron microscopy is highly sensitive and specific for anti-MAG neuropathy. Immunoglobulin deposits may be identified on nerve structures [36].

Treatment of paraproteinaemic demyelinating neuropathies

Monitoring of haematological disease

Patients with MGUS or asymptomatic Waldenström's macroglobulinaemia may not need treatment, unless required specifically because of neuropathy or other IgM-related conditions [37]. Whether they have a neuropathy or not, they should have regular haematological evaluation for early detection of malignant transformation, which occurs at approximately 1.3% per year. The following should be measured: paraprotein concentration, Bence Jones protein in the urine, serum immunoglobulin concentrations, ESR, creatinine, calcium, beta 2-microglobulin, and full blood count, at a frequency of once a year for MGUS, every 6 months for asymptomatic Waldenström's macroglobulinaemia, or every 3 months if there is a higher risk of malignant transformation [38, 39] (GPP).

Treatment of IgM Paraproteinaemic Demyelinating Neuropathy

The 2006 Cochrane review of anti-MAG paraproteinaemic neuropathy concluded that there was inadequate evidence to recommend any particular immunotherapy [40]. The same conclusion may be extended to IgM PDN without anti-MAG antibodies. Based on evidence regarding the pathogenicity of anti-MAG antibodies, therapy has been directed at reducing circulating IgM or anti-MAG antibodies by removal (plasma exchange, PE), inhibition (intravenous immunoglobulin, IVIg), or reduction of synthesis (corticosteroids, immunosuppressive or cytotoxic agents, or interferon alpha). Only seven controlled studies on a total of 145 patients have been performed [40], two new studies being added since our first guidelines [41, 42].

Plasma exchange

In a review of uncontrolled studies or case reports [43], PE was temporarily effective in approximately half of the patients, both alone and in combination with other therapies (Class IV evidence). However, this was not confirmed in two controlled studies. In one, a randomized comparative open trial on 44 patients with neuropathy associated with IgM monoclonal gammopathy, 33 of whom had anti-MAG IgM, the combination of PE with chlorambucil was no more effective than chlorambucil alone [44] (Class III). In a double-blind, sham-controlled trial on 39 patients with neuropathy (axonal and demyelinating) associated with all classes of MGUS, PE was significantly effective overall, and in subgroups with IgG and IgA, but not in the 21 patients with IgM MGUS [45] (Class II). In this study anti-MAG reactivity was not examined.

Corticosteroids

In a review of uncontrolled studies or case reports [43], approximately half of the patients responded to corticosteroids given in association with other therapies, but corticosteroids were seldom effective alone (Class IV).

Intravenous immunoglobulin

In one randomized, double-blind, placebo-controlled trial only two of 11 patients improved with IVIg, not significantly better than placebo [46] (Class II). A multicentre double-blind crossover trial of 22 patients with PDN with IgM MGUS, half of whom had anti-MAG IgM, showed significant improvement at 4 weeks with IVIg compared with placebo [47] (Class II). Ten of 22 patients improved with IVIg and four improved with placebo. The short duration of follow-up leaves it unclear whether this was clinically useful. Regular long-term IVIg was not tested. In an open study, 20 participants were randomized to IVIg or interferon alpha and only one of 10 treated with IVIg improved [48] (Class II).

Interferon-alpha

In an open comparative trial against IVIg, eight of 10 patients with PDN and anti-MAG IgM improved with interferon-alpha [48], but the improvement was restricted to sensory symptoms. However, no benefit was shown by the same authors in a randomized, placebo-controlled study on 24 patients with PDN and anti-MAG IgM [49] (Class II).

Immunosuppressive therapies

In a review of uncontrolled studies or case reports [40, 43], *chlorambucil* was effective in one-third of patients when used alone and in a slightly higher proportion in combination with other therapies (Class IV).

A randomized controlled trial (RCT) of pulsed oral *cyclophosphamide* (500 mg daily for 4 days repeated monthly for 6 months) with *prednisolone* (60 mg daily for 5 days) took 8 years to recruit 35 patients, 17 with anti-MAG antibodies [42]. There was no significant difference in the primary outcome measure, the Rivermead Mobility Index (33% improved versus 21% with placebo), although significant improvements were seen in secondary outcomes, including MRC score up to 2 years of follow-up, and sensory, ataxia, quality of life, haematological, and neurophysiological outcomes (Class I evidence). It is unclear whether the risk of malignant

transformation after cyclophosphamide (9% in 5 years in this trial) significantly exceeded the background risk. Cyclophosphamide was effective in 40–100% of patients in two open trials using cyclic high-dose oral or intravenous cyclophosphamide with corticosteroids [50] or PE [51] (Class IV), but was rarely effective when used alone.

In an open study, five of 16 patients treated with *fludarabine* improved with outcomes sustained for at least a year (Class III) [52], complementing previous anecdotal reports [53, 54].

There are anecdotal reports on the efficacy of *cladribine* [55], and *high-dose chemotherapy* followed by *autologous bone marrow transplantation* [56] in IgM PDN. These studies were limited to very small numbers and need to be confirmed in larger series.

Rituximab

Rituximab, the humanized monoclonal antibody against the CD20 antigen, has shown some benefit in several open studies. The usual dose is 375 mg/m^2 intravenously weekly for 4 weeks, with further doses after a longer interval if necessary. In one open prospective study, more than 80% of 21 patients with neuropathy with IgM antibodies to neural antigens (including seven with PDN and anti-MAG IgM) improved in strength, compared with none of 13 untreated patients [57] (Class III). No response to rituximab was observed in another two patients [58]. In an open phase II study of nine patients with chronic polyneuropathy with IgM monoclonal gammopathy and anti-MAG antibodies treated with rituximab, two patients had clinically useful improvement (≥10 points on the Neuropathy Impairment Score), four had marginal improvement (2–5 points), two remained stable and one worsened (Class IV) [59]. Eight (62%) of 13 patients with PDN and anti-MAG IgM improved in the INCAT sensory and MRC scores and seven (54%) also in the INCAT disability score [60]. After a single course of rituximab, improvement lasted 2 years in eight of 10 patients and 3 years in six [61]. Another open study of 17 patients with IgM PDN showed improved disability in two and improved sensory sum score in nine [62]. In non-randomized comparisons, this Dutch group found similar benefits and fewer adverse effects from rituximab as compared with cyclophosphamide/prednisolone or fludarabine [62].

In the only published placebo-controlled RCT, 13 of 26 patients with anti-MAG antibodies were randomized to receive rituximab [41]. The primary outcome measure using the intention-to-treat population of 26 subjects was not significant (Class II). In post hoc, non pre-specified analysis, in which one subject was removed from the treated group, there appeared to be a significant difference between treated and untreated subjects. This method of analysis raises questions about the conclusion of the published paper.

We await the results of another RCT now in progress (RiMAG).

Recommendations

Treatment of IgM PDN

1 In patients without significant disability or haematological reason for treatment, there is no evidence that immunosuppressive or immunomodulatory treatment is beneficial. Patients may be offered symptomatic treatment for tremor and paraesthesiae, and reassurance that symptoms are unlikely to worsen significantly for years.

2 In patients with significant chronic or progressive disability, immunosuppressive or immunomodulatory treatment may be considered, although none is of proven efficacy, and there is no consensus on which treatment to use first. IVIg or PE may be considered, especially in patients with rapid worsening or clinically similar to typical CIDP, although any benefit may be only short term and repeated treatments may be required. In attempts to achieve longer-term benefit (or in patients unresponsive to IVIg or plasma exchange), clinicians have used rituximab, cyclophosphamide with prednisolone, fludarabine, and chlorambucil. All remain unproven and all have risks which must be balanced against any possible benefits.

3 More research on pathogenesis and treatment is needed.

Treatment of IgG and IgA Paraproteinaemic Demyelinating Neuropathy

In a review of uncontrolled studies on small series of patients with an IgG or IgA MGUS, 80% of those with CIDP-like neuropathy responded to the same immuno-therapies used for CIDP (corticosteroids, PE, and IVIg) as compared with 20% of those with axonal neuropathy [63] (Class IV). The only RCT, on 39 patients with neu-ropathy associated with MGUS including 18 with IgG or IgA MGUS and 21 with IgM [45], showed PE was effica-cious compared with sham exchange only in patients with IgG or IgA MGUS (Class II) [64]. No distinction between demyelinating and axonal forms of neuropathy was made in terms of response to therapy.

Recommendations

Treatment of IgG and IgA PDN

In patients with a CIDP-like neuropathy, the detection of IgG or IgA MGUS does not justify a different therapeutic approach from CIDP without a paraprotein.

Treatment of POEMS syndrome

This is a malignant condition which should be managed in consultation with a haemato-oncologist. The 2008 Cochrane Review concluded: 'Despite the absence of evi-dence from randomized trials, the review authors con-sider it clinically logical that the foundation of treatment is radiation for patients with a solitary osteosclerotic lesion …, and high-dose melphalan with autologous peripheral blood stem cell transplantation for patients under 65 years with diffuse disease as demonstrated by multiple bone lesions or documented clonal plasma cells in iliac crest biopsy. Lenalidomide/thalidomide, anti-VEGF monoclonal antibody [bevacizumab], and conven-tional chemotherapy with melphalan or cyclophosphamide may also be treatment options' [65].

Other syndromes

In the neuropathy associated with multiple myeloma, there are no controlled trials and little evidence of response to any treatment in anecdotal reports. There are no controlled treatment trials in the neuropathy associ-ated with Waldenström's macroglobulinaemia. It is beyond the scope of this guideline to discuss the treat-ment of these conditions in general.

Conflicts of interest

The following authors have reported conflicts of interest as follows.

D. Cornblath: personal honoraria from Merck, Pfizer, Mitsubishi Pharma, Sangamo, Sanofi-Aventis, Bristol-Myers Squibb, Eisai, Octapharma, Sun Pharma, Acorda, DP Clinical, Exelixis, Geron, Johnson & Johnson, Genzyme, Cebix, Abbott, CSL Behring, Bionevia, Schwarz Biosciences, Avigen, FoldRx, GlaxoSmithKline.

R. D. M. Hadden: personal honoraria from Janssen-Cilag and Baxter Healthcare.

A. F. Hahn: departmental research grants and personal honoraria from Bayer, Baxter, Biogen-Idec, Talecris.

I. Illa: personal none, departmental research grant from Grifols.

C. Koski: personal honoraria from American Red Cross, Baxter, Bayer, ZLB-Behring.

J.-M. Léger: personal none, departmental research grants or honoraria from Biogen-Idec, Baxter, Laboratoire Français du Biofractionnement (LFB), Octapharma.

M. Lunn: commissioned to give opinions on IVIG and PEx usage by UK Department of Health and received honoraria from Baxter Pharmaceuticals and LFB.

E. Nobile-Orazio: personal from Kedrion, Grifols, Baxter, LFB (and commissioned by Kedrion and Baxter to give expert opinions to the Italian Ministry of Health on IVIg in dysimmune neuropathies).

J. Pollard: departmental research grants from Biogen-Idec, Schering.

C. Sommer: personal honoraria from Biogen Idec and and Baxter International Inc.

P. van Doorn: personal none, departmental research grants or honoraria from Baxter and Bayer.

I. N. van Schaik personal none, unrestricted departmental research grant from Sanquin blood supply foundation.

The other authors have nothing to declare.

References

1. Joint Task Force of the EFNS and the PNS. European Federation of Neurological Societies/Peripheral Nerve Society Guideline on management of paraproteinemic demyelinating neuropathies. Report of a joint task force of the European Federation of Neurological Societies and the Peripheral Nerve Society. *J Periph Nerv Syst* 2006;**11**(1):9–19.

2. Yeung KB, Thomas PK, King RHM, *et al*. The clinical spectrum of peripheral neuropathies associated with benign monoclonal IgM, IgG and IgA paraproteinaemia. Comparative clinical, immunological and nerve biopsy findings. *J Neurol* 1991;**238**:383–91.

3. Ropper AH, Gorson KC. Neuropathies associated with paraproteinemia [Review]. *New Engl J Med* 1998;**338**(22): 1601–7.

4. Brainin M, Barnes M, Baron JC, *et al*. Guidance for the preparation of neurological management guidelines by EFNS scientific task forces – revised recommendations 2004. *Eur J Neurol* 2004;**11**(9):577–81.

5. Keren DF. Procedures for the evaluation of monoclonal immunoglobulins. *Arch Pathol Lab Med* 1999;**123**(2): 126–32.

6. Vrethem M, Larsson B, von Schenck H, Ernerudh J. Immunofixation superior to plasma agarose electrophoresis in detecting small M-components in patients with polyneuropathy. *J Neurol Sci* 1993;**120**:93–8.

7. International Myeloma Working Group. Criteria for the classification of monoclonal gammopathies, multiple myeloma and related disorders: a report of the International Myeloma Working Group. *Br J Haematol* 2003;**121**(5):749–57.

8. Dimopoulos M, Terpos E, Comenzo RL, *et al*. International myeloma working group consensus statement and guidelines regarding the current role of imaging techniques in the diagnosis and monitoring of multiple Myeloma. *Leukemia* 2009;**23**:1545–56.

9. Owen RG, Treon SP, Al-Katib A, *et al*. Clinicopathological definition of Waldenstrom's macroglobulinemia: consensus panel recommendations from the Second International Workshop on Waldenstrom's Macroglobulinemia. *Semin Oncol.* 2003;**30**(2):110–5.

10. Joint Task Force of the EFNS and the PNS. European Federation of Neurological Societies/Peripheral Nerve Society Guideline on management of chronic inflammatory demyelinating polyradiculoneuropathy. Report of a joint task force of the European Federation of Neurological Societies and the Peripheral Nerve Society-First Revision. *J Periph Nerv Syst* 2010;**15**(1):1–9.

11. Chassande B, Leger JM, Younes-Chennoufi AB, *et al*. Peripheral neuropathy associated with IgM monoclonal gammopathy: correlations between M-protein antibody activity and clinical/electrophysiological features in 40 cases. *Muscle Nerve* 1998;**21**(1):55–62.

12. Capasso M, Torrieri F, Di MA, De Angelis MV, Lugaresi A, Uncini A. Can electrophysiology differentiate polyneuropathy with anti-MAG/SGPG antibodies from chronic inflammatory demyelinating polyneuropathy? *Clin Neurophysiol* 2002;**113**(3):346–53.

13. Maisonobe T, Chassande B, Vérin M, Jouni M, Léger JM, Bouche P. Chronic dysimmune demyelinating polyneuropathy: a clinical and electrophysiological study of 93 patients. *J Neurol Neurosurg Psychiatry* 1996;**61**:36–42.

14. Simovic D, Gorson KC, Ropper AH. Comparison of IgM-MGUS and IgG-MGUS polyneuropathy. *Acta Neurol Scand* 1998;**97**(3):194–200.

15. Magy L, Chassande B, Maisonobe T, Bouche P, Vallat JM, Leger JM. Polyneuropathy associated with IgG/IgA monoclonal gammopathy: a clinical and electrophysiological study of 15 cases. *Eur J Neurol* 2003;**10**(6):677–85.

16. Katz JS, Saperstein DS, Gronseth G, Amato AA, Barohn RJ. Distal acquired demyelinating symmetric neuropathy. *Neurology* 2000;**54**(3):615–20.

17. Kaku DA, England JD, Sumner AJ. Distal accentuation of conduction slowing in polyneuropathy associated with

antibodies to myelin-associated glycoprotein and sulphated glucuronyl paragloboside. *Brain* 1994;**117**:941–7.

18. Notermans NC, Franssen H, Eurelings M, Van der Graaf Y, Wokke JH. Diagnostic criteria for demyelinating polyneuropathy associated with monoclonal gammopathy. *Muscle Nerve* 2000;**23**(1):73–9.

19. Nobile-Orazio E, Manfredini E, Carpo M, *et al.* Frequency and clinical correlates of anti-neural IgM antibodies in neuropathy associated with IgM monoclonal gammopathy. *Ann Neurol* 1994;**36**:416–24.

20. Van den Berg LH, Hays AP, Nobile-Orazio E, *et al.* Anti-MAG and anti-SGPG antibodies in neuropathy. *Muscle Nerve* 1996;**19**:637–43.

21. Nobile-Orazio E, Gallia F, Terenghi F, Allaria S, Giannotta C, Carpo M. How useful are anti-neural IgM antibodies in the diagnosis of chronic immune-mediated neuropathies? *J Neurol Sci* 2008;**266**(1–2):156–63.

22. Di Troia A, Carpo M, Meucci N, *et al.* Clinical features and anti-neural reactivity in neuropathy associated with IgG monoclonal gammopathy of undetermined significance. *J Neurol Sci* 1999;**164**(1):64–71.

23. Dispenzieri A. POEMS syndrome. *Blood Rev* 2007;**21**(6):285–99.

24. Watanabe O, Maruyama I, Arimura K, *et al.* Overproduction of vascular endothelial growth factor/vascular permeability factor is causative in Crow-Fukase (POEMS) syndrome. *Muscle Nerve* 1998;**21**(11):1390–7.

25. Vital C, Vital A, Bouillot S, *et al.* Uncompacted myelin lamellae in peripheral nerve biopsy. *Ultrastruct Pathol* 2003;**27**(1):1–5.

26. Kelly JJ. The electrodiagnostic findings in peripheral neuropathy associated with monoclonal gammopathy. *Muscle Nerve* 1983;**6**:504–9.

27. Sung JY, Kuwabara S, Ogawara K, Kanai K, Hattori T. Patterns of nerve conduction abnormalities in POEMS syndrome. *Muscle Nerve* 2002;**26**(2):189–93.

28. Min JH, Hong YH, Lee KW. Electrophysiological features of patients with POEMS syndrome. *Clin Neurophysiol* 2005;**116**(4):965–8.

29. Baldini L, Nobile-Orazio E, Guffanti A, *et al.* Peripheral neuropathy in IgM monoclonal gammopathy and Waldenstrom's macroglobulinemia: a frequent complication in elderly males with low MAG-reactive serum monoclonal component. *Am J Hematol* 1994;**45**(1):25–31.

30. Willison HJ, O'Leary CP, Veitch J, *et al.* The clinical and laboratory features of chronic sensory ataxic neuropathy with anti-disialosyl IgM antibodies. *Brain* 2001;**124**(Pt 10):1968–77.

31. Vital A, Lagueny A, Julien J, *et al.* Chronic inflammatory demyelinating polyneuropathy associated with dysglobu-

linemia: a peripheral nerve biopsy study in 18 cases. *Acta Neuropathol* 2000;**100**(1):63–8.

32. Vital C, Vital A, Bouillot-Eimer S, Brechenmacher C, Ferrer X, Lagueny A. Amyloid neuropathy: a retrospective study of 35 peripheral nerve biopsies. *J Peripher Nerv Syst* 2004;**9**(4):232–41.

33. Kelly JJ, Kyle RA, Miles JM, O'Brien PC, Dyck PJ. The spectrum of peripheral neuropathy in myeloma. *Neurology* 1981;**31**:24–31.

34. Diaz-Arrastia R, Younger DS, Hair L, *et al.* Neurolymphomatosis: a clinicopathologic syndrome re-emerges. *Neurology* 1992;**42**:1136–41.

35. Nobile-Orazio E, Cappellari A, Priori A. Multifocal motor neuropathy: current concepts and controversies. *Muscle Nerve* 2005;**31**(6):663–80.

36. Vallat JM, Tabaraud F, Sindou P, Preux PM, Vandenberghe A, Steck A. Myelin widenings and MGUS-IgA: an immuno-electron microscopic study. *Ann Neurol* 2000;**47**(6):808–11.

37. Kyle RA, Treon SP, Alexanian R, *et al.* Prognostic markers and criteria to initiate therapy in Waldenstrom's macroglobulinemia: consensus panel recommendations from the Second International Workshop on Waldenstrom's Macroglobulinemia. *Semin Oncol* 2003;**30**(2):116–20.

38. Morra E, Cesana C, Klersy C, *et al.* Clinical characteristics and factors predicting evolution of asymptomatic IgM monoclonal gammopathies and IgM-related disorders. *Leukemia* 2004;**18**(9):1512–7.

39. Cesana C, Klersy C, Barbarano L, *et al.* Prognostic factors for malignant transformation in monoclonal gammopathy of undetermined significance and smoldering multiple myeloma. *J Clin Oncol* 2002;**20**(6):1625–34.

40. Lunn MP, Nobile-Orazio E. Immunotherapy for IgM anti-myelin-associated glycoprotein paraprotein-associated peripheral neuropathies. *Cochrane Database Syst Rev* 2006;(2):CD002827.

41. Dalakas MC, Rakocevic G, Salajegheh M, *et al.* Placebo-controlled trial of rituximab in IgM anti-myelin-associated glycoprotein antibody demyelinating neuropathy. *Ann Neurol* 2009;**65**(3):286–93.

42. Niermeijer JM, Eurelings M, van der Linden MW, *et al.* Intermittent cyclophosphamide with prednisone versus placebo for polyneuropathy with IgM monoclonal gammopathy. *Neurology* 2007;**69**(1):50–9.

43. Nobile-Orazio E, Meucci N, Baldini L, Di TA, Scarlato G. Long-term prognosis of neuropathy associated with anti-MAG IgM M-proteins and its relationship to immune therapies. *Brain* 2000;**123**(Pt 4):710–7.

44. Oksenhendler E, Chevret S, Léger JM, Louboutin JP, Bussel A, Brouet JC. Plasma exchange and chlorambucil

in polyneuropathy associated with monoclonal IgM gammopathy. *J Neurol Neurosurg Psychiatry* 1995;**59**: 243–7.

45. Dyck PJ, Low PA, Windebank AJ, *et al*. Plasma exchange in polyneuropathy associated with monoclonal gammopathy of undetermined significance. *New Engl J Med* 1991;**325**: 1482–6.

46. Dalakas MC, Quarles RH, Farrer RG, *et al*. A controlled study of intravenous immunoglobulin in demyelinating neuropathy with IgM gammopathy. *Ann Neurol* 1996; **40**:792–5.

47. Comi G, Roveri L, Swan A, *et al*. A randomised controlled trial of intravenous immunoglobulin in IgM paraprotein associated demyelinating neuropathy. *J Neurol* 2002;**249**(10): 1370–7.

48. Mariette X, Chastang C, Clavelou P, *et al*. A randomised clinical trial comparing interferon-α and intravenous immunoglobulin in polyneuropathy associated with monoclonal IgM. *J Neurol Neurosurg Psychiatry* 1997;**63**: 28–34.

49. Mariette X, Brouet JC, Chevret S, *et al*. A randomised double blind trial versus placebo does not confirm the benefit of alpha-interferon in polyneuropathy associated with monoclonal IgM. *J Neurol Neurosurg Psychiatry* 2000;**69**(2): 279–80.

50. Notermans NC, Lokhorst HM, Franssen H, *et al*. Intermittent cyclophosphamide and prednisone treatment of polyneuropathy associated with monoclonal gammopathy of undetermined significance. *Neurology* 1996;**47**(5): 1227–33.

51. Blume G, Pestronk A, Goodnough LT. Anti-MAG antibody-associated polyneuropathies: improvement following immunotherapy with monthly plasma exchange and IV cyclophosphamide. *Neurology* 1995;**45**:1577–80.

52. Niermeijer JM, Eurelings M, Lokhorst H, *et al*. Neurologic and hematologic response to fludarabine treatment in IgM MGUS polyneuropathy. *Neurology* 2006;**67**(11): 2076–9.

53. Sherman WH, Latov N, Lange DE, Hays RD, Younger DS. Fludarabine for IgM antibody-mediated neuropathies. *Annals Neurology* 1994;**36**:326–7.

54. Wilson HC, Lunn MP, Schey S, Hughes RA. Successful treatment of IgM paraproteinaemic neuropathy with fludarabine. *J Neurol Neurosurg Psychiatry* 1999;**66**(5):575–80.

55. Ghosh A, Littlewood T, Donaghy M. Cladribine in the treatment of IgM paraproteinemic polyneuropathy. *Neurology* 2002;**59**(8):1290–1.

56. Rudnicki SA, Harik SI, Dhodapkar M, Barlogie B, Eidelberg D. Nervous system dysfunction in Waldenstrom's macro-globulinemia: response to treatment. *Neurology* 1998;**51**(4): 1210–3.

57. Pestronk A, Florence J, Miller T, Choksi R, Al-Lozi MT, Levine TD. Treatment of IgM antibody associated polyneu-ropathies using rituximab. *J Neurol Neurosurg Psychiatry* 2003;**74**(4):485–9.

58. Rojas-Garcia R, Gallardo E, de Andres I, *et al*. Chronic neuropathy with IgM anti-ganglioside antibodies: lack of long term response to rituximab. *Neurology* 2003;**61**(12): 1814–6.

59. Renaud S, Gregor M, Fuhr P, *et al*. Rituximab in the treatment of polyneuropathy associated with anti-MAG anti-bodies. *Muscle Nerve* 2003;**27**(5):611–5.

60. Benedetti L, Briani C, Grandis M, *et al*. Predictors of response to rituximab in patients with neuropathy and anti-myelin associated glycoprotein immunoglobulin M. *J Peripher Nerv Syst* 2007;**12**(2):102–7.

61. Benedetti L, Briani C, Franciotta D, *et al*. Long-term effect of rituximab in anti-mag polyneuropathy. *Neurology* 2008;**71**(21):1742–4.

62. Niermeijer JM, Eurelings M, Lokhorst H, *et al*. Rituximab for polyneuropathy with IgM monoclonal gammopathy. *J Neurol Neurosurg Psychiatry* 2009;**80**:1036–9.

63. Nobile-Orazio E, Casellato C, Di Troia A. Neuropathies associated with IgG and IgA monoclonal gammopathy. *Rev Neurol* 2002;**158**(10 Pt 1):979–87.

64. Allen D, Lunn MP, Niermeijer J, Nobile-Orazio E. Treatment for IgG and IgA paraproteinaemic neuropathy. *Cochrane Database Syst Rev* 2007;(1):CD005376.

65. Kuwabara S, Dispenzieri A, Arimura K, Misawa S. Treatment for POEMS (polyneuropathy, organomegaly, endocrinopa-thy, M-protein, and skin changes) syndrome. *Cochrane Database Syst Rev* 2008;(4):CD006828.

CHAPTER 23
Limb girdle muscular dystrophies

F. Norwood,[1,2] M. de Visser,[3] B. Eymard,[4] H. Lochmüller,[5] K. Bushby[1]

[1]Institute of Human Newcastle upon Tyne, UK; [2]King's College Hospital, London, UK; [3]University of Amsterdam, The Netherlands; [4]Hôpital de la Pitié, Salpétriere, Paris, France; [5]Genzentrum, Ludwig-Maximilians-Universität, Munich, Germany

Objectives

To provide guidelines for the best practice management of limb girdle muscular dystrophies (LGMDs) based on the current state of clinical and scientific knowledge in the published literature.

Background

Limb girdle muscular dystrophy was first described as a clinical entity in 1954 by Walton and Natrass [1]. However, it was not until the 1990s that linkage studies and the identification of the group of proteins associated with dystrophin at the sarcolemma began to demonstrate the heterogeneity of LGMDs. Classification of LGMDs was established through workshops held at the European Neuromuscular Centre (ENMC). The most recent classification is shown in table 23.1 (modified from Bushby and Beckmann [2] and updated with the addition of more recently defined entities). LGMDs are grouped into two sections, autosomal dominant (1) or recessive (2), and further subdivided into subtypes, each of which is known by a designated suffix allocated in chronological order of gene identification. As the genes and proteins involved in these disorders are identified, this locus-based approach is being superseded by a classification based on the underlying genetic defect.

With molecular clarification has come the increasing realization that it is possible in some instances to recognize characteristic patterns of disease through thorough clinical assessment. Areas of particular importance are the involvement of the cardiac and respiratory systems, but other features such as the presence of muscle hypertrophy, contractures, and scapular winging may also be of diagnostic help. Prognosis for LGMDs is not uniform and thus timely intervention through early identification of potential complications may improve survival.

An array of diagnostic measures is available but with varying ease of use and availability; mutation analysis for some genes is a huge undertaking and analysis of expressed proteins may be complex. Nevertheless, many causative mutations have been identified and it has been possible to work towards genotype–phenotype correlations. Genetic analysis has also extended the phenotypic range in several of the subtypes, with some genes producing hugely variable clinical features in affected individuals.

Search strategy

The following search protocols were employed with relevant keywords: MEDLINE for original papers and review articles (1985 to 2005); Cochrane database (www.cochrane.org/index0.htm); American Academy of Neurology (AAN) and European Federation of Neurological Sciences (EFNS) practice parameters or management guidelines (www.aan. com/professionals/ practice/guideline/index.cfm;www.efns.org/); EMBASE, patient organizations (www.muscular-dystrophy.org; www.mdausa.org; www.mda.org.au); previous guidelines (www.inahta.org/inahta_web/index.asp; www.york. ac.uk/inst/crd/darehp.htm; www.g-i-n.net/index.cfm? fuseaction=membersarea).

European Handbook of Neurological Management: Volume 1, 2nd edition. Edited by N. E. Gilhus, M. P. Barnes and M. Brainin. © 2011 Blackwell Publishing Ltd.

Table 23.1 105th ENMCworkshop classification (from Bushby and Beckmann [2] and updated with subsequent developments).

Mode of inheritance	Gene location	Gene symbol (gene product)
Limb-girdle MD, dominant		
AD	5q22-q34	LGMD1A (=*TTID*) (myotilin)
AD (AR)	1q11-21	LGMD1B (=*LMNA*) (lamin A/C)
AD (AR)	3p25	LGMD1C (=*CAV3*) (caveolin-3)
AD	7q	LGMD1D (CMD1F)
AD	6q23	LGMD1E
AD	7q32	LGMD1F
AD	4p21	LGMD1G
Limb-girdle MD, recessive		
AR	15q15.1–q21.1	LGMD2A (=*CAPN3*) (calpain 3)
AR	2p13	LGMD2B (=*DYSF*) (dysferlin)
AR	13q12	LGMD2C (=*SGCG*) (γ-sarcoglycan)
AR	17q12–q21.33	LGMD2D (=*SGCA*) (α-sarcoglycan)
AR	4q12	LGMD2E (=*SGCB*) (β-sarcoglycan)
AR	5q33-q34	LGMD2F (=*SGCD*) (δ-sarcoglycan)
AR	17q11-q12	LGMD2G (=*TCAP*) (telethonin)
AR	9q31-q34.1	LGMD2H (=*TRIM32*)
AR	19q13.3	LGMD2I (=*FKRP*) (Fukutin-related protein)
AR	2q	LGMD2J (=*TTN*) (Titin)
AR	9q34	LGMD2K (=*POMT1*)
AR	11p14.3	LGMD2L (=*ANO5*)
AR	9q31	LGMD2M (=*FKTN*) (Fukutin)
AR	14q24	LGMD2N (=*POMT2*)
AR	1p34.1	LGMD2O (=*POMGNT1*)

Method for reaching consensus

The results of the literature review were evaluated by members of the task force; only those studies specific to LGMDs or the subtypes have been included. Older studies pre-1985 include cases of 'limb girdle dystrophy', but without accurate molecular diagnosis it is not possible to extract reliable data from these and so they have been excluded. All the evidence was categorized as class IV [3].

Results

LGMDs are relatively recent in their identification and clarification and efforts are ongoing with further genes and proteins expected to be discovered. In addition, the conditions are individually rare, some with only a few families identified. To date, no substantial randomized controlled trials of management of genetically defined

LGMD have been published. However, as each condition becomes better understood, the phenotypic features of each become apparent through case reports and cohort studies and it is possible to recommend both general and specific Good Practice Points [3] for the management of LGMDs based on this knowledge.

Good Practice Points for management of LGMD

Aspects of care-Diagnosis

Clinical assessment

General principles
Thorough clinical assessment provides the basis for directing further investigation. Neonatal course, timing of developmental motor milestones, and ability to rise

from the floor/presence of Gowers' manoeuvre may all be of relevance. The ability to run, hop, and jump, and sporting ability may be significantly affected in childhood or may be normal until even middle age. The age of onset may vary both between and within subtypes and even between patients with the same mutation.

By definition, LGMDs have in common a predilection for involvement of the proximal musculature in the shoulder and pelvic girdles, but these may be differentially affected, particularly in the early stages, and involvement of distal muscles may also occur. Rate of progression of the muscle weakness may not be linear.

Features such as spinal rigidity, scoliosis, and limb contractures should be sought. Hypertrophy, usually of calf muscles but also of other limb muscles and even the tongue, may be present. Family history may suggest an autosomal dominant inheritance or consanguinity.

Although it is not possible to provide an absolute prediction of the clinical pattern, table 23.2 outlines the presence or absence of typical features in each LGMD to give a guide to the underlying diagnosis [4–6]. Exceptions to the commonly recognized patterns can occur and the table should be seen as a guide only. It is also important to point out that for mutations in some of these genes, there is clinical heterogeneity. Specific examples of this include myotilin mutations (responsible for the rare LGMD1A and myofibrillar myopathy), caveolin 3 mutations (reported with a range of presentations including hyperCKaemia, LGMD1C, and rippling muscle disease), and lamin A/C mutations, which are probably the most clinically variable of all, and have been reported in at least seven distinct diseases, in some of which muscle involvement may be minimal or absent. The variability in presentation for all of these conditions means that different family members, or indeed the same individual, may present with one or more manifestations of mutation in a particular gene.

Specific clinical pointers/indicators

In contrast to the congenital muscular dystrophies and myopathies, the only LGMD that may result in neonatal hypotonia is LGMD1B (lamin A/C). None of the LGMDs has been described in association with neonatal contractures. Those conditions that are most likely to present in early childhood are LGMD1B, 1C (caveolin-3 deficiency), the sarcoglycanopathies, LGMD2A (calpain deficiency),

Table 23.2 Predominant clinical features for the most frequently occurring LGMDs.

Disease	Age of onset[1]	Weakness[2]	CK level[3]	Muscle hypertrophy[4]	Contractures[5]	Special features[6]	Respiratory[7]	Cardiac[8]
LGMD1A	c, d	Proximal/distal	A	No	No	Dysarthria	?	Yes?
LGMD1B	a, b	Proximal/distal	A	No	Yes	–	Yes	Yes A, CM
LGMD1C	a–d	Proximal/distal	B/C	Some cases	No	PIRCs, RMD	No	No
LGMD2A	a–c	Proximal	B/C	Some cases	Yes	–	No	No
LGMD2B	b, c	Proximal/distal	C	No	No	–	No	No
LGMB2C-F	a, b	Proximal	B/C	Yes	Secondary	–	Yes	Yes CM
LGMD2G	a, b	Proximal/distal	A–C	Some cases	No	Brazil	?	No
LGMD2H	b, c	Proximal	B	No	No	Hutterites	?	No
LGMD2I	a–d	Proximal	B/C	Yes	No		Yes	Yes CM
LGMD2J	a, b	Proximal/distal	B	No	No	Finnish	?	No?

[1]Range of age of onset in majority of patients: a = below age 10 years; b = 10–20 years; c = 20–40 years; d = over 40 years.
[2]Pattern of distribution of weakness in limb muscles.
[3]Range of creatine kinase (CK) level at diagnosis: A = normal or mildly elevated at less than 5x upper limit of normal; B = 5–10x upper limit of normal; C = more than 10x upper limit of normal.
[4]Presence of muscle hypertrophy in limb muscles may occur.
[5]Presence of early fixed limb contractures may occur.
[6]Percussion-induced rapid muscle contractions (PIRCs); Rippling muscle disease (RMD).
[7]Presence of frequent respiratory complications.
[8]Presence of frequent cardiac complications: A = arrhythmia, CM = cardiomyopathy.

and some cases of LGMD2I. All of the LGMDs may result in a lifelong decreased sporting ability. This is less likely in LGMD2B (dysferlin deficiency), which in many patients is associated with a normal sporting ability until an abrupt onset of difficulty, occasionally preceded by a transient painful swelling of calf muscles.

Age of onset is relatively well-defined for some conditions: the mean age of onset for LGMD2A is in the early teens and in LGMD2B is 20 +/− 5 years [4]; however, for others a much wider age range is found, such as in LGMD1C where age of onset may be from early childhood to the eighth decade, depending on the phenotype [7]. LGMD2C-F are also variable in their onset and progression; some patients (typically especially β and δ sarcoglycanopathies) may be as severely affected as patients with Duchenne muscular dystrophy (DMD), whereas others are still ambulant into their 40s. Alpha-sarcoglycanopathy (LGMD2D) tends to be the mildest of the sarcoglycanopathies [8].

Most LGMDs by definition involve predominantly proximal musculature, certainly once the full phenotype has evolved, but potential diagnostic difficulty could arise in, for example, the presence of only distal muscle involvement in the early stages of the Miyoshi type of dysferlin deficiency (although the characteristic gastrocnemius weakness is helpful) or in some patients with LGMD1B or 1C. An example of another useful discriminator is the relative preservation of hip abductor muscles in LGMD2A [9, 10] and the striking involvement of the posterior thigh muscles as shown on muscle magnetic resonance imaging (MRI) [11]. Scapular winging is most characteristically seen in LGMD2A and 2C-F.

Associated features such as muscle hypertrophy may be observed quite frequently in LGMD1C, 2C-F, and 2I (Fukutin-related protein, FKRP). Calf hypertrophy is most common but other limb muscles may also be involved, as may the tongue. The calf hypertrophy present in LGMD2I (in addition to the cardiac and respiratory involvement) resembles the Becker phenotype and has led to misdiagnosis of patients in the past. Macroglossia is seen in LGMD2C-F and 2I on occasion. Focal muscle atrophy is most typical of LGMD2A and LGMD2B.

Contractures are most common in LGMD1B, where they may occur in childhood or develop over the course of the condition, representing an overlap with the autosomal dominant Emery–Dreifuss muscular dystrophy (EDMD) phenotype also caused by mutations in lamin A/C. Contractures may also be seen in LGMD2A but tend to be milder. Spinal rigidity is often a feature in LGMD1B and occasionally in LGMD2A [9]. Scoliosis is most often seen in LGMD2C-F, particularly once wheelchair dependence occurs.

Specific indicators include the reported dysarthria in the rare LGMD1A (myotilin) patients [12]. On the other hand, phenotypic variation within the same family as well as overlapping phenotypes are well-recognized; a mutation in a single LGMD gene such as caveolin-3 may produce one or more of a number of manifestations, such as rippling muscles and percussion-induced repetitive contractions. This also occurs in the laminopathies, where some members of the family may have partial lipodystrophy or peripheral neuropathy in addition to their muscle weakness, for example, whereas other members do not, and indeed may have pure cardiac disease.

Intellectual impairment and facial weakness are not characteristically seen. A malignant hyperthermia reaction to general anaesthesia has been reported in two patients from the Hutterite population who have mutations in FKRP (rather than TRIM32).

Geographical location of cases may also be helpful. LGMD2G (telethonin) has so far only been described in Brazilian patients [13]. LGMD2H (TRIM32) is a relatively mild form seen in some areas of Canada with onset in the second or third decade and slow progression; most patients were still ambulant into their 50s [14]. Sarcotubular myopathy is described in patients with the same TRIM 32 mutations [15]. LGMD2J (titin) was described in Finnish patients initially.

Cardiac involvement is very common in LGMD1B, 2C-F, and 2I, whereas significant disease is infrequent in LGMD1C, 2A, and 2B. Cardiac complications may take the form of dysrhythmias or hypertrophic or dilated cardiomyopathy. Isolated familial hypertrophic cardiomyopathy has been described with CAV-3 mutations [16]. Patients may be affected by both a dysrhythmia and cardiomyopathy, especially in LGMD1B. Respiratory muscle weakness does not necessarily accompany cardiac impairment; it is seen most often in LGMD2C-F and in 2I, where diaphragmatic involvement may be seen when patients are still ambulant, but tends to be insignificant in 2A and 2B. Symptoms of nocturnal hypoventilation may herald the development of significant respiratory muscle weakness and need for intervention.

Investigation

Serum *creatine kinase* (CK) is a simple and useful investigation provided that non-muscle conditions are excluded first. The degree of elevation may be helpful in differentiating broadly between diagnoses; typically, it may be normal or only mildly raised in conditions such as LGMD1A and 1B, moderately raised (5–10x upper limit of normal) in LGMD1C, 2A, 2C-F, and 2I, and grossly raised (over 10x) in LGMD2B.

Neurophysiology studies are of little value in refining a diagnosis of LGMD. Nerve conduction studies can exclude a neuropathy if this causes diagnostic doubt in the early stages of presentation. Electromyography (EMG) usually shows myopathic features in patients with any type of LGMD with no ability to further specify the diagnosis. Laminopathy patients may additionally or exclusively have a peripheral neuropathy.

Muscle imaging with computed tomography (CT) or MRI is used increasingly to determine patterns of muscle involvement. No large studies of the LGMDs have been published but case reports and small series suggest characteristic patterns in some conditions. The most consistent examples are LGMD2A, which selectively involves hip extensors and adductors [11], involvement of the glutei in α-sarcoglycanopathy [8], and LGMD2J, where loss of the thigh muscles and involvement of tibialis anterior is present [17].

Muscle biopsy site(s) may be guided by imaging results. They are likely to yield the most useful information if they are undertaken on a clinically affected muscle, but preferably not one that is 'end-stage'. Multiple biopsies may be performed. No studies compare open versus needle biopsies, although with the increasing number of immunohistochemical and immunoblotting procedures possible, it is important to obtain sufficient tissue to allow meaningful interpretation.

Muscle tissue should first be analysed with standard histological techniques. All LGMDs show dystrophic features with variation in fibre size, increased numbers of central nuclei, and endomysial fibrosis. Inflammatory infiltrates are seen most commonly in dysferlin deficiency. Thus, there is the potential for diagnostic confusion and patients may have received a previous diagnosis of polymyositis. Rimmed vacuoles and Z-line streaming may be seen in myotilin mutations as well as with mutations in the other genes causing myofibrillar myopathy. Table 23.3 summarizes typical findings in each condition.

Immunohistochemistry and immunoblotting should be undertaken in a laboratory with sufficient expertise in

Table 23.3 Characteristic muscle biopsy findings in the more common LGMDs.

Disease	Protein	Histological features	Immunoanalysis: primary changes	Secondary changes
LGMD1A*	Myotilin	Dystrophic, inflammatory infiltrate, rimmed vacuoles	Myotilin normal, DGC intact	↓ laminin γ 1
LGMD1B	Lamin A/C	Dystrophic	Lamin A/C usually normal	↓ laminin β1
LGMD1C	Caveolin-3	Myopathic or dystrophic	↓ caveolin-3 labelling	↓ dysferlin
LGMD2A	Calpain-3	Dystrophic	Absent, partial deficiency or normal	Calpain-3 degradation
LGMD2B	Dysferlin	Dystrophic, inflammatory	↓ dysferlin	↓ calpain-3 in half
LGMD2C	γ-sarcoglycan	Dystrophic	↓ γ-sarcoglycan	↓ other SG, dystrophin
LGMD2D	α-sarcoglycan	Dystrophic	↓ α-sarcoglycan	↓ other SG, dystrophin
LGMD2E	β-sarcoglycan	Dystrophic	↓ β-sarcoglycan	Severe ↓ other SG, dystrophin
LGMD2F	δ-sarcoglycan	Dystrophic	↓ δ-sarcoglycan	Severe ↓ other SG, dystrophin
LGMD2G	Telethonin	Dystrophic, rimmed vacuoles	Loss of telethonin labeling	–
LGMD2H	TRIM32	Myopathic, sarcotubular	–	–
LGMD2I	FKRP	Dystrophic	Often normal	↓ laminin α2 and αDG
LGMD2J	Titin	Myopathic, dystrophic, rimmed vacuoles	↓ titin	↓ calpain-3

*EM Z-line streaming.

both the performance and interpretation of these techniques. Immunohistochemical staining with a panel of antibodies ideally including all four anti-sarcoglycan antibodies may show one or more abnormalities. Demonstration of normal dystrophin staining is important (although there may be a mild secondary reduction in sarcoglycan deficiency). Quantitative analysis of proteins by Western blotting may be an additional useful technique for elucidating primary and secondary protein abnormalities [18, 19].

Primary changes on immunoanalysis may be clear and direct analysis specifically towards the underlying genetic defect, such as caveolin-3 reduction in LGMD1C. In other diseases, because of the interdependence of the sarcolemmal and associated proteins, disruption of one member of the complex or pathway may result in the concomitant loss of interacting proteins. This is particularly prominent in disorders of the dystrophin-associated complex, where there may be reduction in all or many of the complex members, and secondary calpain-3 reduction is seen in half of dysferlin deficiency patients and in patients with LGMD2J. These *secondary* changes may lead to diagnostic difficulty, particularly when direct assay for the primary defect is difficult.

In other situations, secondary changes may be the only clue to the underlying disorder. For example, in LGMD1B lamin A/C labelling is usually normal but there is frequently a secondary reduction in laminin-β1 in adult patients. In LGMD2I, secondary reduction of laminin-α2 on immunolabelling was detected in most cases [20] and reduction in α-dystroglycan may also be seen and may correlate with the phenotype [21]. A deficiency of α-dystroglycan is not specific for LGMD2I and may indicate the presence of a mutation in another glycosylation protein such as POMT1, the causative gene in LGMD2K [22]. A summary of commonly observed primary and secondary changes is shown in table 23.3.

Immunoblotting has been the accepted test required for the diagnosis of LGMD2A [23]. However, there is variability in the quantity and function of calpain-3 protein detected on immunoblots, even for those patients in whom a calpain mutation is proven [24] and thus emphasis has shifted to earlier analysis of the calpain-3 gene [25].

One group has developed a blood-based assay for dysferlin expression in monocytes, showing that this correlates with skeletal muscle expression. This potentially avoids the need for muscle biopsy, although it is not in mainstream use at present [26].

DNA analysis directed to provide confirmation of mutation in the affected gene(s) is the gold standard of diagnosis, and necessary to be able to offer carrier or presymptomatic testing to other family members. This is more straightforward in some forms of LGMD than others, depending to a large extent on whether or not there are commonly detected mutations or if mutations in different families tend to be unique. For example, the FKRP 'common mutation' C826A in LGMD2I can be detected readily in a diagnostic laboratory, whereas some of the other causative genes are large, for example dysferlin (55 exons), and screening for mutations is a formidable task. Thus mutation analysis in the lamin A/C, calpain-3, dysferlin, and sarcoglycan genes may be restricted to those exons where most mutations have been detected previously; at present this is available only in selected laboratories. Mutation detection for the rarer types of LGMD may only be available on a research basis.

Recommendations

Careful clinical assessment of factors such as the pattern of muscle involvement, associated features, and family history should suggest the likely diagnosi(e)s in a patient with LGMD. Confirmation of this should be achieved through the selective use of predominantly laboratory-based investigations, some of which are highly specialized and should only be undertaken in a laboratory with appropriate expertise. In some conditions this may be relatively straightforward but in others verification of the underlying mutation presently remains in the realm of the research laboratory. In the UK, patients may be referred for assessment to the centre for limb girdle muscular dystrophy funded by the National Specialised Commissioning Group (NCG).

Assessment and monitoring of adjunctive aspects

Respiratory management

Respiratory muscle weakness resulting in symptomatic hypoventilation and respiratory failure is found in a few of the LGMDs, most frequently in LGMD2I [20] and the sarcoglycanopathies. In LGMD2I and occasionally in the sarcoglycanopathies, respiratory failure may arise while the patient is still ambulant [2, 20].

There are no recommendations specific to the LGMDs but extrapolation from the monitoring and investigation of respiratory involvement in other neuromuscular conditions is helpful. Awareness of symptoms of respiratory insufficiency, such as frequent chest infections, morning headache, and daytime somnolence, is important. Measurements of sitting (and supine if <80%) forced vital capacity (FVC) may be made in the outpatient clinic. Overnight pulse oximetry is recommended if the FVC is <60%. Annual influenza vaccination and prompt treatment of respiratory infections are suggested. Liaison with a respiratory physician with experience in the management of neuromuscular disorders is essential to ensure optimal timing of intervention with nocturnal home ventilation.

Cardiac management

The important issue of cardiac complications in LGMD as well as in other muscle conditions was considered at the 107th ENMC workshop [27]. Cardiac involvement may manifest as a conduction defect and/or cardiomyopathy. In laminopathies, arrhythmias such as atrioventricular block, atrial paralysis, and atrial fibrillation/flutter occur in the majority of patients by age 30 years and permanent pacing is required. However, even with permanent pacing, sudden death may occur in 46% of lamin A/C mutation carriers and therefore an implantable defibrillator is recommended [28]. Dilated cardiomyopathy arises in a third of laminopathy patients and is usually severe. Arrhythmias and hypertrophic or dilated cardiomyopathy are present in approximately 20% of sarcoglycanopathy patients. A third of LGMD2I patients have a cardiomyopathy that is symptomatic. The remaining LGMDs do not characteristically show significant cardiac compromise.

Thus the ability to define precisely the underlying genetic defect allows a tailored approach to monitoring through better anticipation of the onset and progression of cardiac aspects. Monitoring and treatment of LGMD1B, 2C-F, and 2I patients require close cardiological supervision. Electrocardiography and echocardiography are suggested as the standard initial investigations. In the absence of dedicated studies, treatment of heart failure is undertaken on general principles with early use of angiotensin-converting enzyme inhibitors. Anticoagulation may need consideration in patients with atrial fibrillation or standstill. For patients with particularly severe cardiac failure but relatively well-preserved respiratory function, consideration of cardiac transplantation may be appropriate.

Recommendations

Although serial monitoring of basic measurements of respiratory and cardiac function is attainable in the neurology outpatient setting, patients with a LGMD subtype known to place them at additional risk of cardiorespiratory complications ideally should be managed in conjunction with a respiratory physician and/or cardiologist. Intervention in the form of nocturnal ventilatory assistance for respiratory failure and with permanent pacing and/or management of developing cardiomyopathy may be life saving. The need to monitor for and treat complications as appropriate also applies to those patients in whom the underlying diagnosis is unknown as it follows that the attendant risk of cardiorespiratory complications is also unknown, but that general principles of management will apply.

Physical management

There are no papers relating specifically to LGMD and physiotherapy, exercise, or orthotic use. The application of general principles is probably appropriate, as reviewed in Eagle [29]. Prevention of contracture development through stretching and splinting orthoses is important in maximizing functional ability. Release of functionally limiting contractures (especially of the Achilles tendons) may be necessary especially in LGMD1B, LGMD2A, or in childhood-onset sarcoglycanopathy or LGMD2I. Scoliosis in LGMD occurs mainly after wheelchair dependence and attention should be paid to seating. The role of exercise is controversial but basic guidelines as for other types of muscular dystrophy would encourage gentle exercise within comfortable limits and the avoidance of prolonged immobility.

Genetic counselling

Many patients seek medical advice due to concern for themselves, relatives, or descendants. Delineation of the LGMD subtype allows knowledge of its autosomal dominant or recessive inheritance pattern to inform genetic counselling appropriately. Care is required in some conditions such as LGMD1B as, despite the absence of affected members in previous generations, there is a fairly high new dominant mutation rate. Confirmation of the diagnosis in LGMD2I patients in particular has led to altered advice in some, as previously they had been thought to be affected by Becker muscular dystrophy, an X-linked condition.

Drug treatment

There are no established drug treatments for LGMDs. Six patients with sarcoglycan-deficient muscular dystrophy took part in a double-blind, placebo-controlled crossover trial of creatine monohydrate. Thirty patients with other conditions were included. The mean improvement of 3% in muscle strength over the 8-week trial period was found to be significant but modest [30]. There are no relevant studies on the use of co-enzyme Q10 (ubiquinone).

Corticosteroids have an established role in DMD boys [31]; on this basis they have been used empirically in some patients with LGMD2C-F with reported improvement [32, 33]. As these conditions are so much rarer than DMD, it will not be possible to perform adequate treatment trials without collaboration among multiple neuromuscular centres. This is being facilitated by international initiatives such as TREAT-NMD (www.treat-nmd.eu).

Conflict of interests

The authors have reported no conflicts of interest relevant to this manuscript.

References

1. Walton J, Natrass F. On the classification, natural history and treatment of the myopathies. *Brain* 1954;**77**:169–231.
2. Bushby KMD, Beckmann JS. The 105th ENMC sponsored workshop: pathogenesis in the non-sarcoglycan limb-girdle muscular dystrophies, Naarden, April 12–14, 2002. *Neuromusc Disorders* 2003;**13**:80–90.
3. Brainin M, Barnes M, Baron J-C, *et al.* Guidance for the preparation of neurological management guidelines by EFNS scientific task forces – revised recommendations 2004. *Eur J Neurol* 2004;**11**:577–81.
4. Bushby KMD. Making sense of the limb-girdle muscular dystrophies. *Brain* 1999;**122**:1403–20.
5. Beckmann JS, Brown RH, Muntoni F, *et al.* 66th/67th ENMC sponsored international workshop: the limb-girdle muscular dystrophies. *Neuromusc Disorders* 1999;**9**:436–45.
6. Laval SH, Bushby KMD. Limb-girdle muscular dystrophies – from genetics to molecular pathology. *Neuropathol Appl Neurobiol* 2004;**30**:91–105.

7. Woodman SE, Sotgia F, Galbiati F, *et al.* Caveolinopathies. Mutations in caveolin-3 cause four distinct autosomal dominant muscle diseases. *Neurology* 2004;**62**:538–43.
8. Eymard B, Romero NB, Leturcq F, *et al.* Primary adhalinopathy (alpha-sarcoglycanopathy): clinical, pathologic and genetic correlation in 20 patients with autosomal recessive muscular dystrophy. *Neurology* 1997;**48**:1227–34.
9. Pollitt C, Anderson LVB, Pogue R, *et al.* The phenotype of calpainopathy: diagnosis based on a multidisciplinary approach. *Neuromusc Disorders* 2001;**11**:287–96.
10. Saenz A, Leturcq F, Cobo AM, *et al.* LGMD2A: epidemiology and genotype-phenotype correlations based on a large mutational survey on the calpain 3 gene. *Brain* 2005;**128**:732–42.
11. Mercurio E, Bushby K, Ricci E, *et al.* Muscle MRI findings in patients with limb girdle muscular dystrophy with calpain 3 deficiency (LGMD2A) and early contractures. *Neuromusc Disorders* 2005;**15**:164–71.
12. Hauser MA, Horrigan SK, Salmikangas P, *et al.* Myotilin is mutated in limb girdle muscular dystrophy 1A. *Hum Mol Genet* 2000;**9**:2141–7.
13. Moreira ES, Wiltshire TJ, Faulkner G, *et al.* Limb-girdle muscular dystrophy type 2G is caused by mutations in the gene encoding the sarcomeric protein telethonin. *Nat Genet* 2000;**24**:163–6.
14. Frosk P, Weiler T, Nylen E, *et al.* Limb-girdle muscular dystrophy type 2H associated with mutation in TRIM32, a putative E3-ubiquitin-ligase gene. *Am J Hum Genet* 2002;**70**:663–72.
15. Schoser BG, Frosk P, Engel AG, *et al.* Commonality of TRIM32 mutation in causing sarcotubular myopathy and LGMD2H. *Ann Neurol* 2005;**57**:591–5.
16. Hayashi T, Arimura T, Ueda K, *et al.* Identification and functional analysis of a caveolin-3 mutation associated with familial hypertrophic cardiomyopathy. *Biochem Biophys Res Commun* 2004;**313**:178–84.
17. Udd B, Vihola A, Sarparanta J, *et al.* Titinopathies and extension of the M-line mutation phenotype beyond distal myopathy and LGMD2J. *Neurology* 2005;**64**:636–42.
18. Anderson LVB, Davison K. Multiplex Western blotting system for the analysis of muscular dystrophy proteins. *Am J Path* 1999;**154**:1017–22.
19. Cooper ST, Lo HP, North KN. Single section Western blot. Improving the molecular diagnosis of the muscular dystrophies. *Neurology* 2003;**61**:93–7.
20. Poppe M, Cree L, Bourke J, *et al.* The phenotype of limb-girdle muscular dystrophy type 2I. *Neurology* 2003;**60**:1246–51.
21. Brown SC, Torelli S, Brockington M, *et al.* Abnormalities in α-dystroglycan expression in MDC1C and LGMD2I muscular dystrophies. *Am J Path* 2004;**164**:727–37.

22. Balci B, Uyanik G, Dincer P, *et al.* An autosomal recessive limb girdle muscular dystrophy (LGMD2) with mild mental retardation is allelic to Walker-Warburg syndrome (WWS) caused by a mutation in the POMT1 gene. *Neuromuscul Disord* 2005;**15**:271–5.

23. Fanin M, Pegoraro E, Matsuda-Asada C, *et al.* Calpain-3 and dysferlin protein screening in patients with limb-girdle dystrophy and myopathy. *Neurology* 2001;**56**:660–5.

24. Fanin M, Fulizio L, Nascimbeni AC, *et al.* Molecular diagnosis in LGMD2A: mutation analysis or protein testing? *Hum Mutation* 2004;**24**:52–62.

25. Piluso G, Politano L, Aurino S, *et al.* Extensive scanning of the calpain-3 gene broadens the spectrum of LGMD2A phenotypes. *J Med Genet* 2005;**42**:686–93.

26. Ho M, Gallardo E, McKenna-Yasek D, *et al.* A novel, blood-based diagnostic assay for limb girdle muscular dystrophy 2B and Miyoshi myopathy. *Ann Neurol* 2002;**51**:129–33.

27. Bushby K, Muntoni F, Bourke JP. 107th ENMC international workshop: the management of cardiac involvement in muscular dystrophy and myotonic dystrophy. *Neuromusc Disorders* 2003;**13**:166–72.

28. van Berlo JH, de Voogt WG, van der Kooi AJ, *et al.* Meta-analysis of clinical characteristics of 299 carriers of LMNA gene mutations: do lamin A/C mutations portend a high risk of sudden death? *J Mol Med* 2005;**83**:79–83.

29. Eagle M. Report on the Muscular Dystrophy Campaign workshop: Exercise in neuromuscular diseases. *Neuromusc Disorders* 2002;**12**:975–83.

30. Walter MC, Lochmuller H, Reilich P, *et al.* Creatine monohydrate in muscular dystrophies: a double-blind, placebo-controlled clinical study. *Neurology* 2000;**54**:1848–50.

31. Moxley RT, Ashwal S, Pandya S, *et al.* Practice parameter: corticosteroid treatment of Duchenne dystrophy. *Neurology* 2005;**64**:13–20.

32. Angelini C, Fanin M, Menegazzo E, *et al.* Homozygous α-sarcoglycan mutation in two siblings: one asymptomatic and one steroid-responsive mild limb-girdle muscular dystrophy patient. *Muscle Nerve* 1998;**21**:769–75.

33. Connolly AM, Pestronk A, Mehta S, *et al.* Primary α-sarcoglycan deficiency responsive to immunosuppression over three years. *Muscle Nerve* 1998;**21**:1549–53.

CHAPTER 24

Neurological complications of HIV infection

P. Portegies,[1] P. Cinque,[2] A. Chaudhuri,[3] J. Begovac,[4] I. Everall,[5] T. Weber,[6] M. Bojar,[7] P. Martinez-Martin,[8] P. G. E. Kennedy[3]

[1]OLVG Hospital Amsterdam, The Netherlands; [2]San Raffaele Hospital, Milano, Italy; [3]University of Glasgow, Scotland, UK; [4]University of Zagreb, Croatia; [5]Institute of Psychiatry, London, UK; [6]Marienkrankenhaus, Hamburg, Germany; [7]Motol Hospital, Prague, Czech Republic; [8]National Center for Epidemiology, Carlos 111 Institute of Health, Spain

Background and objectives

The introduction and widespread use of highly active antiretroviral therapy (HAART) for the treatment of HIV infection has resulted in dramatic reductions in morbidity, mortality, and healthcare utilization [1–3]. Decreasing rates for opportunistic infections, including the neurological infections, have been reported. Diagnostic tools for these neurological complications have been greatly improved in the past 10 years. The therapeutic approach to the neurologic diseases has been influenced by the success of HAART. However, HIV infection has spread in new populations and the neurological complications are still frequent in patients who are not adequately treated and are immunosuppressed. Furthermore, recent studies show that patients who have been infected and/or treated for many years are at risk for developing neurocognitive dysfunction. Alertness, together with neurological knowledge and expertise remain urgently needed. Together, these developments form the main reason for producing these new guidelines.

The objective of the study was to provide neurologists and others with evidence-based guidelines for the diagnosis and treatment of neurological complications of HIV infection.

Neurological complications

These guidelines deal with the most common neurological complications of HIV infection. Although the epidemiology of neurological complications has changed considerably in recent years in the West, the spectrum has remained relatively unchanged. The most frequent opportunistic infections are cerebral toxoplasmosis, cryptococcal meningitis, progressive multifocal leukoencephalopathy (PML), tuberculous meningitis, cytomegalovirus (CMV) encephalitis, and CMV polyradiculomyelitis. Primary central nervous system (CNS) lymphoma has become less frequent, but is still an important cause of focal brain disease. The neurological diseases that are more directly related to HIV itself are HIV dementia, vacuolar myelopathy, and peripheral neuropathy. HIV dementia is rare in patients who take HAART, but with resistance and compliance problems patients may become at risk. More subtle cognitive dysfunction is only recently recognized in long-term infected patients. The epidemiology and pathogenesis are not clear yet. It has been suggested that an ongoing chronic infection and immunoactivation play a role. Peripheral neuropathy is still a frequent complication, not only in severely immunosuppressed patients. The role of antiretroviral drugs in the pathogenesis remains uncertain.

HAART

An increasing number of potent antiretroviral drugs are available [4]. When used in combinations of three or four

European Handbook of Neurological Management: Volume 1, 2nd edition. Edited by N. E. Gilhus, M. P. Barnes and M. Brainin.

drugs, this treatment is called HAART. In most HIV-infected patients, especially treatment-naive patients, HAART is effective in rapidly reducing plasma levels of HIV-RNA, accompanied by a gradual increase in CD4 cell counts, sometimes to normal levels [4]. For many antiretroviral-naive patients, CD4 cell counts increase to levels at which the patients are no longer generally susceptible to serious opportunistic infections. As currently available antiretroviral regimens will not eradicate HIV, the goal of therapy is to durably inhibit viral replication so that the patient can attain and maintain an effective immune response to most potential microbial pathogens [5, 6]. The recently updated recommendations of the Working Group of the Office of AIDS Research Advisory Council (OARAC) [7] advise the start of treatment in patients with symptomatic HIV disease and in patients with CD4 cell counts below 350 cells/μl or viral loads above 50 000–100 000 copies/ml [6]. The most commonly used regimens to start with contain two nucleoside reverse transcriptase (RT) inhibitors with either a non-nucleoside RT inhibitor or a single (or boosted) protease inhibitor. Antiretroviral activity is evaluated by assessing changes in CD4 cell count and viral load in the plasma. The availability of new drugs has widened the options for patients who fail to respond to their antiretroviral regimen. A patient with one of the neurological complications described below has symptomatic HIV disease and HAART is indicated, but the strength of the evidence for this recommendation varies from complication to complication.

The immune restoration itself, i.e. the result of HAART, may have a beneficial effect on the neurological complication. For some of the neurological diseases (PML, HIV dementia), this has been documented in small, uncontrolled studies. Besides HAART, disease-specific therapy for neurological complications is indicated, as discussed below. The duration of these specific treatments is determined by the level of immunosuppression. Before HAART became available, the treatment for acute infection had to be followed by lifelong secondary prophylaxis to prevent relapses (e.g. for toxoplasmosis, cryptococcosis). The recommendation in general now with HAART is that secondary prophylaxis can be discontinued if CD4 cell counts show a significant and sustained increase in both absolute and percentage terms, for example, if they have increased to above 200 cells/μl and have remained at that level for at least 3 months. Primary prophylaxis for neurological complications is not recommended.

Search strategy

A MEDLINE (National Library of Medicine) search of the relevant literature from 1966 to August 2002 was undertaken using various combinations of the following MeSH headings: HIV-1, acquired immunodeficiency syndrome, HIV-infections, toxoplasmosis cerebral, meningitis cryptococcal, leukoencephalopathy progressive multifocal, polyneuropathies, polyradiculopathy, encephalitis, myelitis transverse, lymphoma, central nervous system, cytomegalovirus infection, tuberculosis central nervous system, diagnosis, therapeutics, drug therapy. The following free text words were used: highly active antiretroviral therapy, cerebral toxoplasmosis, PML, CMV encephalitis, CMV polyradiculomyelitis, primary CNS lymphoma, HIV dementia, AIDS dementia, vacuolar myelopathy, HIV myelopathy, and sensory neuropathy. Limitations included meta-analysis, randomized controlled trial, sensitivity and specificity, cohort studies, case control studies.

Grading of recommendations

All members of the task force prepared one or more of the 10 selected neurological complications. The material available from the literature review was integrated and summarized in graded recommendations. The recommendations were approved by all members.

Cerebral toxoplasmosis

Cerebral toxoplasmosis is a frequent cause of focal brain disease in HIV infection. *Toxoplasma gondii* is an obligate intracellular protozoan parasite in human beings. Toxoplasmic encephalitis is almost always caused by reactivation of *Toxoplasma gondii* cysts in brain parenchyma.

Diagnosis

A presumptive diagnosis of cerebral toxoplasmosis in HIV-infected patients is based on: (1) progressive neurological deficits, (2) contrast-enhancing mass lesion(s) on imaging studies [computed tomography/magnetic resonance imaging (CT/MRI)], (3) successful response within 2 weeks to specific treatment (see below) [Class IV]. Absence of one or more of these characteristics makes cerebral toxoplasmosis less likely. Those patients are possible candidates for brain biopsy. In clinical practice, most patients with mass lesion(s) are given 2 weeks of treatment anyway (including patients with negative serology or a single lesion). Cerebrospinal fluid (CSF) studies, including antibody studies and polymerase chain reaction (PCR) studies, have not produced conclusive results [8].

Treatment

Primary therapy for cerebral toxoplasmosis [9–11]: pyrimethamine 200 mg load, then 50 mg/day (oral) with sulfadiazine 1 g four times daily (oral) (or clindamycin intravenous (i.v.) or oral 600 mg four times daily) with folinic acid 10 mg/day (oral) (Class IIa, Level B recommendation).

Other possible combinations include the following.
1 Trimethroprim/sulfamethoxazol oral or i.v. 2.5–5 mg/kg (TMP) q.i.d. (Class IIa) [12].
2 Pyrimethamine (as above) plus clarithromycin 1 g twice daily (Class III).
3 Pyrimethamine (as above) plus azithromycin 600–1800 mg/day (Class III) [13].
4 Pyrimethamine (as above) plus dapsone 100 mg/day (Class III).
5 Atovaquone 750 mg four times daily (oral) (Class IIa) [14].
For secondary prophylaxis [9, 11]: pyrimethamine 50 mg/day with sulfadiazine 500 mg four times daily (Class IIa, Level B recommendation). Alternatives are: atovaquone 750 mg four times daily (oral) (Class IIa) [15] 13] or pyrimethamine 50 mg/day + sulfadiazine 500 mg four times daily, twice a week (Class IIa) [16].

The primary therapy is usually continued for 6 weeks, followed by secondary prophylaxis. Secondary prophylaxis can be stopped according to the recommendations described above.

Cryptococcal meningitis

Infection with the yeast *Cryptococcus neoformans* in HIV-infected individuals most often leads to a subacute meningitis. The initial infection is a pulmonary infection. In the immunosuppressed host, dissemination occurs afterwards to many organ systems, including the CNS.

Diagnosis

A definitive diagnosis of cryptococcal meningitis is made by using any of the following methods.
1 Visualizing the fungus in the CSF using India ink (sensitivity 75–85%) (Class I).
2 Detecting cryptococcal antigen by latex agglutination assay in the CSF (sensitivity 95%) (Class I).
3 Positive CSF culture for *C. neoformans* (Class I).

Treatment

It is important to be alert (especially in the first week after the diagnosis has been made) for high CSF pressures that may lead to blindness, coma, seizures, etc. [17]. Removing 20–30 ml CSF by (repeated) spinal tap or (in severe cases) a lumbar drain for a few days may be necessary. Based on several randomized clinical trials [18–21] the recommendation for treatment is: amphotericin B 0.7 mg/kg/day i.v. (with or without flucytosine 5-FC; 100 mg/kg/day orally) for 2 weeks (Class Ia). This treatment is followed by: fluconazole 400 mg/day (or itraconazole 400 mg/day) (orally) to complete a course of 10 weeks (Class Ia, Level A recommendation). The addition of flucytosine to amphotericin B did not significantly improve the mortality and clinical course in a randomized clinical trial (RCT); however, flucytosine was well tolerated and there was a trend to a better CSF sterilization with its use in this study [21]. CSF examination should be repeated to confirm a therapeutic response (negative CSF culture).

For secondary prophylaxis fluconazole 200 mg/day (oral) (Class Ia, Level A recommendation; [22–24]. Secondary prophylaxis can be stopped according to the recommendations described above.

Progressive multifocal leukoencephalopathy

Progressive multifocal leukoencephalopathy (PML) is a viral opportunistic infection of oligodendrocytes and astrocytes leading to demyelination in the CNS. The causative agent is a polyomavirus named JC virus. JC virus is ubiquitous in human beings and is usually acquired during adolescence (two-thirds have antibodies at age of 14 years).

Diagnosis

Slowly progressive focal neurological deficits with asymmetrical white matter abnormalities on MRI suggest

PML. The lesions are non-enhancing, hyperintense on T2-weighted MRI, without mass effect. The subcortical 'U' fibres are characteristically involved. This diagnosis is strongly supported by positive CSF-PCR for JC virus DNA (sensitivity 72–100%; specificity 92–100%) (Class I) [25]. If the CSF-PCR is negative, it is recommended to repeat CSF-PCR once or twice. Brain biopsy remains the final confirmatory test, but a positive CSF-PCR offers acceptable evidence.

Treatment

In patients who are being treated with HAART, PML arrests or remits in approximately 50%, and survival is prolonged in these patients [5, 26–28].

Studies with cytarabine [29] and cidofovir [30] failed to show any benefit.

CMV encephalitis

Cytomegalovirus belongs to the family of herpes viruses. CMV infection is endemic; the majority of HIV-infected adults have serologic evidence of prior CMV infection. Clinical syndromes in immunosuppressed patients include retinitis, gastrointestinal ulcers, encephalitis, and polyradiculomyelitis.

Diagnosis

CMV encephalitis is suspected in an HIV-infected patient with (usually) a history of CMV disease (e.g. CMV retinitis), a clinically progressive encephalopathy, and periventricular enhancement (ventriculitis) on imaging (CT/MRI) studies. The diagnosis is strongly supported by: (i) positive CSF-PCR for CMV-DNA (sensitivity 62–100%; specificity 89–100%) (Class I) [31] or (ii) positive CSF culture (Class I) [31], but in general CSF viral cultures are highly insensitive.

Brain biopsy is not a realistic option given the brainstem and periventricular localization of the encephalitis. CSF-PCR is the diagnostic test of choice.

Treatment

Induction treatment (for 3 weeks) [32]: ganciclovir 5 mg/kg i.v. twice daily (Class IV) or foscarnet 90 mg/kg i.v. twice daily (Class IV) or cidofovir 5 mg/kg i.v. every week; after two courses every 2 weeks (Class IV) or ganciclovir and foscarnet (dosages as above) (Class IV, Level C recommendation).

Maintenance treatment [32]: ganciclovir 5 mg/kg/day i.v. (Class IV).

CMV polyradiculomyelitis

This is the most common polyradiculomyelitis in AIDS. The most frequent manifestations are pain (low-back, sciatic), paresthesia, sphincter dysfunction, distal sensory loss, and progressive ascending weakness.

Diagnosis

CMV polyradiculomyelitis is suspected in an HIV-infected patient with (usually) a history of CMV disease (e.g. CMV retinitis), clinically a rapidly ascending polyradiculomyelitis and a highly characteristic CSF polymorphonuclear pleocytosis. The diagnosis is strongly supported by: (i) positive CSF-PCR for CMV-DNA (sensitivity 62–100%; specificity 89–100%) (Class I) [31] or (ii) positive CSF culture (Class I) [31], but in general CSF viral cultures are highly insensitive.

Treatment

Induction treatment (for 3 weeks) [32]: ganciclovir 5 mg/kg i.v. b.i.d. (Class IV) or foscarnet 90 mg/kg i.v. b.i.d. (Class IV) or cidofovir 5 mg/kg i.v. every week; after two courses every 2 weeks (Class IV) or ganciclovir and foscarnet (dosages as above) (Class IV, Level C recommendation).

Maintenance treatment [32]: ganciclovir 5 mg/kg/day i.v. (Class IV).

Tuberculous meningitis

Infection with *Mycobacterium tuberculosis* is the leading cause of death worldwide among persons infected with HIV. Tuberculous meningitis and CNS tuberculomas are common complications. CNS tuberculosis in HIV disease is more frequent in developing countries.

Diagnosis

CNS tuberculosis has been described in 10–20% of patients with HIV-related tuberculosis. Lymphocytic pleocytosis, low glucose, and raised protein are the typical features of tuberculous meningitis. Post-contrast brain scans show enhancement of the meninges and the periphery of the tuberculoma and, on occasion, may reveal miliary lesions. Hydrocephalus may appear early. The diagnosis is based on demonstration of *Mycobacterium tuberculosis* in the CSF [33, 34]: (i) culture (sensitivity 25–86%) (Class I); (ii) CSF smear (ZN) (sensitivity 8–86%) (Class IV); or (iii) CSF-PCR (sensitivity 83–100%; specificity 88–100%) (Class II).

Treatment

Isoniazid 5 mg/kg/day, up to 300 mg/day, and rifampicin 10 mg/kg/day, up to 600 mg/day, and pyrazinamide 15–30 mg/kg/day (max 2.5 g/day), and ethambutol 15–25 mg/kg/day, up to 1600 mg/day (Class III, Level A recommendation; [33, 34].

Ethambutol can be substituted with streptomycin (15 mg/kg/day, up to 1 g/day i.m. or i.v.; max 2 months) or amikacin (15 mg/kg/day i.m. or i.v.). The role of steroids in HIV-positive tuberculous meningitis is unclear. The minimum duration of treatment is 6 months. Isoniazid may lead to pyridoxine deficiency and a sensorimotor distal polyneuropathy. Therefore pyridoxine 20 mg/day should be added to the regimen.

Primary CNS lymphoma

Primary CNS lymphoma is a non-Hodgkin's lymphoma that arises within and is confined to the nervous system. It is the second most frequent CNS mass lesion in adults with AIDS in Western countries. Primary CNS lymphoma is associated with Epstein–Barr virus (EBV) infection. The transforming potential of the virus plays a role in the pathogenesis of this tumour. With the introduction of HAART the incidence has declined [35, 36].

Diagnosis

A definitive diagnosis is made by histological examination of brain tissue (obtained by brain biopsy or at autopsy). In an HIV-infected individual with a single or multiple contrast-enhancing brain lesion(s) on CT or MRI not responding to anti-toxoplasmic therapy, a presumptive diagnosis can be supported by: positive CSF EBV-PCR (sensitivity 83–100%, specificity 93–100%) (Class II) [37–40]. Cytological examination of the CSF rarely reveals pathological cells and its value, although not well studied, seems limited. Data on other potential CSF markers of primary CNS lymphoma are inconclusive. SPECT/PET study results are inconclusive, and these investigations cannot be recommended.

Treatment

HAART improves neurological status and prolongs survival in patients with primary CNS lymphoma [41]. Besides HAART three other treatment options exist: (i)

whole-brain irradiation and corticosteroids (Class III) [42–44]; (ii) intravenous methotrexate followed by whole brain radiation (Class III) [45]; and (iii) methotrexate, thiotepa, and procarbazine intravenously in combination with methotrexate intrathecally (Class III, Level B recommendation; [46].

HIV dementia

HIV dementia is a syndrome of cognitive and motor dysfunction that has also been termed: AIDS dementia complex, HIV-associated cognitive-motor complex, HIV-associated dementia, and AIDS dementia. Its paediatric counterpart is called progressive encephalopathy. The cognitive impairment is compatible with a subcortical dementia. Most patients with HIV dementia are severely immunosuppressed.

Diagnosis

The diagnosis is based on: (i) progressive cognitive impairment (with or without motor dysfunction); (ii) exclusion of CNS opportunistic infections and tumours (by CSF and CT/MRI) [47, 48] and is supported by: (1) high levels of HIV RNA in the CSF (above three log copies/ml) (Class III) [49–51] and (2) diffuse, bilateral (often symmetrical) non-enhancing white-matter hyperintensities on MRI (Class III) [52].

Treatment

Class III evidence for HAART [53, 54] leads to a Level B recommendation. Most nucleosides and non-nucleosides (e.g. nevirapine) penetrate relatively well into the CSF; most protease inhibitors do not (with the exception of indinavir). It seems reasonable to include at least two drugs in the regimen that penetrate well [55]. The data are still limited. Most combinations have not been well studied in HIV dementia.

HIV myelopathy

Spinal cord disease is observed in various stages of HIV infection. The most common type is HIV myelopathy (also named HIV-related vacuolar myelopathy). HIV myelopathy is a progressive non-segmental spinal cord disease. The diagnosis is one of exclusion.

Diagnosis

The diagnosis is based on: (i) progressive myelopathy without sensory level; (ii) absence of focal lesion or mass lesion in spinal cord or compression of spinal cord on MRI; (iii) negative human T-cell lymphotropic virus (HTLV-I) serology; (iv) normal serum vitamin B12; (v) negative CSF PCR for herpesviruses; (vi) negative CSF syphilis tests [56, 57]. All diagnostic tests have only Class IV evidence.

Treatment

HAART (Class III) [58, 59].

HIV polyneuropathy

Polyneuropathies do occur frequently in the course of HIV infection. The pathogenesis is poorly understood and treatment is largely restricted to symptomatic pain therapy.

Diagnosis

The most important neuropathy in HIV infection is the distal sensory polyneuropathy. Its pathogenesis is unclear. This neuropathy is indistinguishable from the toxic neuropathy caused by the nucleosides zalcitabine, didanosine, and stavudine. Symptoms of paraesthesiae and pain predominate; disability caused by loss of sensory or motor function is less prominent. Electrodiagnostic studies may be helpful in confirming the diagnosis but may not be necessary in all cases.

Treatment

Symptomatic treatment: (i) amitriptyline 25–100 mg/day (Class I); (ii) tramadol 50 mg three times daily to 100 mg four times daily (Class I); (iii) carbamazepine 200 mg three or four times daily (Class I) [60] and lamotrigine (Class I) [61]. Gabapentin is a promising drug (2400–3600 mg/day), but has not been studied in RCT.

Immune reconstitution inflammatory syndrome (IRIS)

IRIS has been recognized after the introduction of HAART. Due to an enhanced immune response as a result of an improved immunity after starting HAART, a paradoxal progression (clinically and radiologically) of neurological opportunistic infections may occur. IRIS has been described in PML, toxoplasmosis, cryptococcal meningitis, and VZV-infections. Although studies are lacking, some patients do respond to a brief course of corticosteroids [62].

Summary and conclusions

Despite the success of HAART, HIV-infected individuals are at risk for a variety of neurological complications. The risk for those complications increases with an increasing level of immunodeficiency. Those patients with CD4 cell counts below 200×10^6/ml are particularly at risk for opportunistic infections, lymphoma, and HIV dementia. Nucleic acid amplification in the CSF by PCR has greatly improved the diagnostic accuracy in PML, CMV infections, primary CNS lymphoma, and HIV dementia. Besides HAART, specific treatment options are available for the majority of these complications. In general, the task force recommends rapidity in evaluating these patients to limit damage to the nervous system.

Conflicts of interest

The authors have reported no conflicts of interests.

References

1. Kovacs JA, Vogel S, Albert JM, et al. Controlled trial of interleukin-2 infusions in patients infected with the human immunodeficiency virus. N Engl J Med 1996;**335**:1350–6.
2. Hogg RS, Heath KV, Yip B, et al. Improved survival among HIV-infected individuals following initiation of antiretroviral therapy. JAMA 1998;**279**:450–4.
3. Palella FJ Jr, Delaney KM, Moorman AC, et al. Declining morbidity and mortality among patients with advanced human immunodeficiency virus infection. N Engl J Med 1998;**338**:853–60.
4. Richman DD. HIV chemotherapy. Nature 2001;**410**: 995–1001.
5. De Luca A, Giancola ML, Ammassari A, et al. Potent antiretroviral therapy with or without cidofovir for AIDS-associated progressive multifocal leukoencephalopathy: extended follow-up of an observational study. J Neurovirol 2001;7:364–8.
6. Yeni PG, Hammer SM, Carpenter CCJ, et al. Antiretroviral Treatment for Adult HIV Infection in 2002. Updated recommendations of the International AIDS Society-USA Panel. JAMA 2002;**288**:222–35.
7. Bartlett JG, Clifford Lane H, et al. Panel on Antiretroviral Guidelines for Adults and Adolescents. Guidelines for the use of antiretroviral agents in HIV-1-infected adults and adolescents. Department Health Human Services 2008; pp. 1–139. Available at: http://www.aidsinfo.nih.gov (accessed 28.7.10).
8. Franzen C, Altfeld M, Hegener P, et al. Limited value of PCR for detection of Toxoplasma gondii in blood from human

immunodeficiency virus-infected patients. *J Clin Microbiol* 1997;**35**:2639–41.

9. Leport C, Raffi F, Matheron S, *et al.* Treatment of central nervous system toxoplasmosis with pyrimethamine/sulfadiazine combination in 35 patients with the acquired immunodeficiency syndrome. *Am J Med* 1988;**84**:94–100.

10. Danneman B, McCutchan JA, Israelski D, *et al.* Treatment of toxoplasmic encephalitis in patients with AIDS. A randomized trial comparing pyrimethamine plus clindamycin to pyrimethamine plus sulfadiazine. The California Collaborative Treatment Group. *Ann Intern Med* 1992;**116**:33–43.

11. Katlama C, De Wit S, O'Doherty E, *et al.* Pyrimethamine-clindamycin vs. pyrimethamine-sulfadiazine in acute and long-term therapy for toxoplasmic encephalitis in patients with AIDS. *Clin Infect Dis* 1996;**22**:268–75.

12. Torre D, Casari S, Speranza F, *et al.* Randomized trial of trimethoprim-sulfamethoxazole versus pyrimethamine-sulfadiazine for therapy of toxoplasmic encephalitis in patients with AIDS. Italian Collaborative Study Group. *Antimicrob Agents Chemother* 1998;**42**:1346–9.

13. Jacobsen JM, Hafner R, Remington J, *et al.* Dose-escalation, phase I/II study of zathromycin and pyrimethamine for the treatment of toxoplasmic encephalitis in AIDS. *AIDS* 2001;**15**:583–9.

14. Torres RA, Weinberg W, Stansell J, *et al.* Atovaquone for salvage treatment and suppression of toxoplasmic encephalitis in patients with AIDS. Atovaquone/Toxoplasmic Encephalitis Study Group. *Clin Infect Dis* 1997;**24**:422–9.

15. Katlama C, Mouthon B, Gourdon D, Lapierre D, Rousseau F. Atovaquone as long-term suppressive therapy for toxoplasmic encephalitis in patients with AIDS and multiple drug intolerance. Atovaquone Expanded Access Group. *AIDS* 1996;**10**:1107–12.

16. Podzamczer D, Miro JM, Bolao F, *et al.* Twice-weekly maintenance therapy with sulfadiazine-pyrimethamine to prevent recurrent toxoplasmic encephalitis in patients with AIDS. Spanish Toxoplasmosis Study Group. *Ann Intern Med* 1995;**123**:175–80.

17. Bicanic T, Brouwer AE, Meintjes G, *et al.* Relationship of cerebrospinal fluid pressure, fungal burden and outcome in patients with cryptococcal meningitis undergoing serial lumbar punctures. *AIDS* 2009;**23**:701–6.

18. Larsen RA, Leal M, Chan L. Fluconazole compared with amphotericin B plus flucytosine fpr cryptococcal meningitis in AIDS. *Ann Intern Med* 1990;**113**:183–7.

19. De Gans J, Portegies P, Tiessens G, *et al.* Itraconazole compared with amphotericin B plus flucytosine in AIDS patients with cryptococcal meningitis. *AIDS* 1992;**6**:185–90.

20. Saag MS, Powderly WG, Cloud GA, *et al.* Comparison of amphotericin B with fluconazole in the treatment of acute AIDS-associated cryptococcal meningitis. *N Engl J Med* 1992;**326**:83–9.

21. Van der Horst CM, Saag MS, Cloud GA, *et al.* Treatment of cryptococcal meningitis associated with the acquired immunodeficiency syndrome. *N Engl J Med* 1997;**337**:15–21.

22. Bozzette SA, Larsen R, Chiu J, *et al.* A controlled trial of maintenance therapy with fluconazole after treatment of cryptococcal meningitis in the acquired immunodeficiency syndrome. *N Engl J Med* 1991;**324**:580–4.

23. Powderly WG, Saag MS, Cloud GA, *et al.* A controlled trial of fluconazole or amphotericin B to prevent relapse of cryptococcal meningitis in patients with the acquired immunodeficiency syndrome. *N Engl J Med* 1992;**326**:793–8.

24. Saag MS, Cloud GA, Graybill JR, *et al.* A comparison of itraconazole versus fluconazole as maintenance therapy for AIDS-associated cryptococcal meningitis. National Institute of Allergy and Infectious Diseases Mycoses Study Group. *Clin Infect Dis* 1999;**28**:291–6.

25. Cinque P, Scarpellini P, Vago L, Linde A, Lazzarin A. Diagnosis of central nervous system complications in HIV-infected patients: cerebrospinal fluid analysis by the polymerase chain reaction. *AIDS* 1997;**11**:117.

26. Miralles P, Berenguer J, Garcia de Viedma D, *et al.* Treatment of AIDS-associated progressive multifocal leukoencephalopathy with highly active antiretroviral therapy. *AIDS* 1998;**12**:2467–72.

27. Clifford DB, Yiannoutsos C, Glicksman M, *et al.* HAART improves prognosis in HIV-associated progressive multifocal leukoencephalopathy. *Neurology* 1999;**52**:623–5.

28. De Luca A, Giancola ML, Ammassari A, *et al.* The effect of potent antiretroviral therapy and JC Virus load in cerebrospinal fluid on clinical outcome of patients with AIDS-associated Progressive Multifocal Leukoencephalopathy. *J Inf Dis* 2000;**182**:1077–83.

29. Hall C, Dafni U, Simpson D, *et al.* Failure of cytarabine in progressive multifocal leukoencephalopathy associated with HIV-infection. AIDS Clinical Trial Group 243 Team. *N Engl J Med* 1998;**338**:1345–51.

30. Marra CM, Rajijic N, Barker DE, *et al.* A pilot study of cidofovir for progressive multifocal leukoencephalopathy in AIDS. *AIDS* 2002;**16**:1791–7.

31. Cinque P, Cleator GM, Weber T, *et al.* for the European Union Concerted Action on Virus Meningitis and Encephalitis. Diagnosis and clinical management of neurological disorders caused by cytomegalovirus in AIDS patients. *J Neurovirol* 1998;**4**:120–32.

32. Anduze-Faris BM, Fillet AM, Gozlan J, *et al.* Induction and maintenance therapy of cytomegalovirus central nervous system infection in HIV-infected patients. *AIDS* 2000;**14**:517524.

33. Zuger A, Lowy FD. Tuberculosis. In: Scheld WM, Whitley RJ, Durack DT (eds) *Infections of the Central Nervous System*. Philadelphia, PA: Lippincott-Raven, 1997; pp. 417–43.

34. Gordin F. Mycobacterium tuberculosis. In: Dolin R, Masur H, Saag MS (eds) *AIDS Therapy*. New York: Churchill Livingstone, 1999; pp. 359–74.

35. Newell ME, Hoy JF, Cooper S, *et al.* Human immunodeficiency virus-related primary central nervous system lymphoma: factors influencing survival in 111 patients. *Cancer* 2004;**100**:2627–36.

36. Haldorsen IS, Krakenes J, Goplen AK, Dunlop O, Mella O, Espeland A. AIDS-related primary central nervous system lymphoma: a Norwegian national survey 1989–2003. *BMC Cancer* 2008;**8**:225.

37. Cinque P, Vago L, Dahl H, *et al.* Polymerase chain reaction on cerebrospinal fluid for diagnosis of virus-associated opportunistic diseases of the central nervous system in HIV-infected patients. *AIDS* 1996;**10**:951–8.

38. Arribas JR, Clifford DB, Fichtenbaum CJ, Roberts RL, Powderly WG, Storch GA. Detection of Epstein-Barr virus DNA in cerebrospinal fluid for diagnosis of AIDS-related central nervous system lymphoma. *J Clin Microbiol* 1995;**33**: 1580–3.

39. De Luca A, Antinori A, Cingolani A, *et al.* Evaluation of cerebrospinal fluid EBV-DNA and IL-10 as markers for in vivo diagnosis of AIDS-related primary central nervous system lymphoma. *Br J Haematol* 1995;**90**:844–9.

40. Cinque P, Brytting M, Vago L, *et al.* Epstein-Barr virus DNA in cerebrospinal fluid from patients with AIDS-related primary lymphoma of the central nervous system. *Lancet* 1993;**342**:398–401.

41. Hoffman C, Tabrizian S, Wolf E, *et al.* Survival of AIDS patients with primary central nervous system lymphoma is dramatically improved by HAART-induced immune recovery. *AIDS* 2001;**15**:2119–27.

42. Baumgartner JE, Rachlin JR, Beckstead JH, *et al.* Primary central nervous system lymphomas: natural history and response to radiation therapy in 55 patients with acquired immunodeficiency syndrome. *J Neurosurg* 1990; **73**:206–11.

43. Goldstein JD, Dickson DW, Moser FG, *et al.* Primary central nervous system lymphomas in acquired immunodeficiency syndrome: a clinical and pathological study with results of treatment with radiation. *Cancer* 1991;**67**: 2756–65.

44. Donahue BR, Sullivan JW, Cooper JS. Additional experience with empiric radiotherapy for presumed human immunodeficiency virus-associated primary central nervous system lymphoma. *Cancer* 1995;**76**:328–32.

45. Jacomet C, Girard P-M, Lebrette M-G, Leca Farese V, Montfort L, Rozenbaum W. Intravenous methotrexate for primary central nervous system non-Hodgkin's lymphoma in AIDS. *AIDS* 1997;**11**:1725–30.

46. Forsyth PA, Yahalom J, DeAngelis LM. Combined-modality therapy in the treatment of primary central nervous system lymphoma in AIDS. *Neurology* 1994;**44**:1473–9.

47. Price R. Neurological complications of HIV infection. *Lancet* 1996;**348**:445–52.

48. McArthur JC, Selnes OA. Human immunodeficiency virus-associated dementia. In: Berger JR, Levy RM (eds) *AIDS and the Nervous System*, 2nd edn. Philadelphia, PA: Lippincott-Raven, 1997; pp. 527–67.

49. Brew B, Pemberton L, Cunningham P, *et al.* Levels of human immunodeficiency virus type 1 RNA in cerebrospinal fluid correlate with AIDS dementia stage. *J Infect Dis* 1997;**175**: 963–6.

50. Ellis RJ, Hsia K, Spector S, *et al.* Cerebrospinal fluid human immunodeficiency virus type 1 RNA levels are elevated in neurocognitive impaired individuals with acquired immunodeficiency syndrome: HIV Neurobehavioral Research Center Group. *Ann Neurol* 1997;**42**:679.

51. McArthur JC, McClernon DR, Cronin MF, *et al.* Relationship between human immunodeficiency virus-associated dementia and viral load in cerebrospinal fluid and brain. *Ann Neurol* 1997;**42**:689.

52. Levy RM, Rosenbloom S, Perrett LV. Neuroradiologic findings in AIDS: a review of 200 cases. *Am J Roengenol* 1986;**147**: 977–83.

53. Foudraine NA, Hoetelmans RMW, Lange JMA, *et al.* Cerebrospinal fluid HIV-1 RNA and drug concentrations after treatment with lamivudine plus zidovudine or stavudine. *Lancet* 1998;**351**:1547–51.

54. Sacktor N, McDermott MP, Marder K, *et al.* HIV-associated cognitive impairment before and after the advent of combination therapy. *J Neurovirol* 2002;**8**: 136–42.

55. Letendre S, Marquie-Beck J, Caparelli E, *et al.* Validation of the CNS Penetration-effectiveness rank for quantifying antiretroviral penetration into the central nervous system. *Arch Neurol* 2008;**65**:65–70.

56. Di Rocco A. Diseases of the spinal cord in human immunodeficiency virus infection. *Semin Neurol* 1999;**19**: 151–5.

57. Thurnher MM, Post MJ, Jinkins JR. MRI of infections and neoplasms of the spine and spinal cord in 55 patients with AIDS. *Neuroradiology* 2000;**42**:551–63.

58. Di Rocco A, Geraci A, Tagliati M, Staudinger R, Henry K. Remission of HIV myelopathy after highly active antiretroviral therapy. *Neurology* 2000;**55**:456.

59. Staudinger R, Henry K. Remission of HIV myelopathy after highly active antiretroviral therapy. *Neurology* 2000;**54**: 267–8.

60. Sindrup SH, Jensen TS. Efficacy of pharmacological treatments of neuropathic pain: an update and effect related to mechanism of drug action. *Pain* 1999;**83**:389–400.

61. Simpson DM, McArthur JC, Olney R, *et al.* Lamotrigine for HIV-associated for HIV-associated painful sensory neuropathies: a placebo-controlled trial. *Neurology* 2003;**60**: 1508–14.

62. Venkataramana A, Pardo CA, McArthur JC, *et al.* Immune reconstitution inflammatory syndrome in the CNS of HIV-infected patients. *Neurology* 2006;**67**:383–8.

CHAPTER 25

Viral meningo-encephalitis

I. Steiner,[1,2] H. Budka,[2] A. Chaudhuri,[3] M. Koskiniemi,[4] K. Sainio,[5] O. Salonen,[5] P. G. E. Kennedy[6]

[1]Rabin Medical Center, Petach Tiqva, Israel, and Hadassah University Hospital, Jerusalem, Israel; [2]Institute of Neurology, Medical University of Vienna, Austria; [3]Essex Centre for Neurological Sciences, Queen's Hospital, Romford, UK; [4]Haartman institute, University of Helsinki, Finland; [5]University of Helsinki, Finland; [6]Institute of Neurological Sciences, Southern General Hospital, Glasgow, Scotland, UK

Introduction

Clinical involvement of the central nervous system (CNS) is an unusual manifestation of human viral infection. The spectrum of brain involvement and the outcome of the disease are dependent on the specific pathogen, the immunological state of the host, and environmental factors. Although specific therapy is limited to only several viral agents, correct diagnosis and supportive and symptomatic treatment (when no specific therapy is available) are mandatory to ensure the best prognosis (for reviews see [1–7]). This document addresses the optimal clinical approach to CNS infections caused by viruses.

Classification of evidence levels used in these guidelines for therapeutic interventions and diagnostic measures was according to Brainin *et al.* [8] and detailed in tables 25.1–25.4

Methods

We searched MEDLINE (National Library of Medicine) for relevant literature from 1966 to September 2009. The search included reports of research in humans only and in English. The search terms selected were: viral encephalitis, encephalitis, viral meningitis, meningoencephalitis,

and encephalomyelitis. We then limited the search using the terms diagnosis, MR, PET, SPECT, EEG, cerebrospinal fluid, pathology, treatment, and antiviral therapy. Review articles and book chapters were also included if considered to provide comprehensive reviews of the topic. The final choice of literature and the references included was based on our judgement of their relevance to this subject. Recommendations were reached by consensus of all task force participants and were also based on our own awareness and clinical experience. Where there was lack of evidence but consensus was clear we have stated our opinion as Good Practice Points (GPP).

Definitions and scope

Encephalitis is the presence of an inflammatory process in the brain parenchyma associated with clinical evidence of brain dysfunction. It can be due to a non-infective condition such as in acute disseminated encephalomyelitis (ADEM) or to an infective process, which is diffuse and usually viral. Herpes simplex virus type 1 (HSV-1), varicella zoster virus (VZV), Epstein-Barr virus (EBV), mumps, measles, and enteroviruses are responsible for most cases of viral encephalitis in immuno-competent individuals [1]. This, however, is also based on the continent and on environmental factors. Thus, West Nile virus (WNV) has become an important cause of viral encephalitis in the USA [6]. Other non-viral infective causes of encephalitis may include such diseases as tuberculosis, rickettsial disease and trypanosomiasis, and will be discussed in the differential diagnosis section.

European Handbook of Neurological Management: Volume 1, 2nd edition. Edited by N. E. Gilhus, M. P. Barnes and M. Brainin. © 2011 Blackwell Publishing Ltd.

Table 25.1 Evidence classification scheme for a therapeutic intervention.

Class I: An adequately powered prospective, randomized, controlled clinical trial with masked outcome assessment in a representative population *or* an adequately powered systematic review of prospective randomized controlled clinical trials with masked outcome assessment in representative populations. The following are required
(a) Randomization concealment
(b) Primary outcome(s) is/are clearly defined
(c) Exclusion/inclusion criteria are clearly defined
(d) Adequate accounting for dropouts and crossovers with numbers sufficiently low to have minimal potential for bias
(e) Relevant baseline characteristics are presented and substantially equivalent among treatment groups or there is appropriate statistical adjustment for differences
Class II: Prospective matched group cohort study in a representative population with masked outcome assessment that meets (a)–(e) above *or* a randomized, controlled trial in a representative population that lacks one criteria (a)–(e)
Class III: All other controlled trials (including well-defined natural history controls or patients serving as own controls) in a representative population, where outcome assessment is independent of patient treatment
Class IV: Evidence from uncontrolled studies, case series, case reports, or expert opinion

Table 25.2 Evidence classification scheme for the rating of recommendations for a therapeutic intervention.

Level A   rating (established as effective, ineffective, or harmful) requires at least one convincing Class I study or at least two consistent, convincing Class II studies
Level B   rating (probably effective, ineffective, or harmful) requires at least one convincing Class II study or overwhelming Class III evidence
Level C   (possibly effective, ineffective, or harmful) rating requires at least two convincing Class III studies

Table 25.3 Evidence classification scheme for a diagnostic measure.

Class I: A prospective study in a broad spectrum of persons with the suspected condition, using a 'gold standard' for case definition, where the test is applied in a blinded evaluation, and enabling the assessment of appropriate tests of diagnostic accuracy
Class II: A prospective study of a narrow spectrum of persons with the suspected condition, or a well-designed retrospective study of a broad spectrum of persons with an established condition (by 'gold standard') compared to a broad spectrum of controls, where test is applied in a blinded evaluation, and enabling the assessment of appropriate tests of diagnostic accuracy
Class III: Evidence provided by a retrospective study where either persons with the established condition or controls are of a narrow spectrum, and where test is applied in a blinded evaluation
Class IV: Any design where test is not applied in blinded evaluation *or* evidence provided by expert opinion alone or in descriptive case series (without controls)

Table 25.4 Evidence classification scheme for the rating of recommendations for a diagnostic measure.

Level A   rating (established as useful/predictive or not useful/predictive) requires at least one convincing Class I study or at least two consistent, convincing Class II studies
Level B   rating (established as probably useful/predictive or not useful/predictive) requires at least one convincing Class II study or overwhelming Class III evidence
Level C   rating (established as possibly useful/ predictive or not useful/ predictive) requires at least two convincing Class III studies

Encephalitis should be differentiated from encephalopathy defined as a disruption of brain function that is not due to a direct structural or inflammatory process. It is mediated via metabolic processes and can be caused by intoxications, drugs, systemic organ dysfunction (e. g. liver, pancreas), or systemic infection that spares the brain.

The structure of the nervous system dictates a degree of associated inflammatory meningeal involvement in encephalitis, and therefore symptoms that reflect meningitis are invariable concomitants of encephalitis. Moreover, in textbooks and review articles, the term viral meningo-encephalitis is often used to denote a viral infectious process of both the brain/spinal cord and the meninges.

Clinical manifestations and relevant environmental and personal information

The diagnosis of viral encephalitis is suspected in the context of a febrile disease accompanied by headache, altered level of consciousness, and symptoms and signs of cerebral dysfunction. These may consist of abnormalities that can be categorized into four types: cognitive dysfunction (acute memory, speech, and orientation disturbances, etc.); behavioural changes (disorientation, hallucinations, psychosis, personality changes, agitation); focal neurological abnormalities (such as anomia, dysphasia, hemiparesis); and seizures. After the diagnosis is suspected, the approach should consist of obtaining a meticulous history and a careful general and neurological examination.

The history is mandatory in the assessment of the patient with suspected viral encephalitis. It is very important to obtain the relevant information from an accompanying person (relative, friend, etc.) if the patient is in a confused, agitated, or disoriented state. The geographical location as well as the recent travel history could be of relevance in identifying possible causative pathogens that are endemic or prevalent in certain geographic regions (examples from recent outbreaks include acute respiratory syndrome, SARS, Nipah virus, or avian H5N1 influenza A infections). Likewise, seasonal occurrence can be important for other pathogens such as

polio and WNV. Occupation may well be important (as in a case of a forestry worker with Lyme disease). Contact with animals such as farm animals would sometimes point to the cause, as animals serve as reservoirs for certain viruses (e.g. West Nile fever during the 1999 disease outbreak in New York). A history of insect or other animal bites can be relevant for arbovirus infection as well as rabies. Past contact with an individual afflicted by an infective condition is important. The medical status of the individual is of the utmost relevance. Thus, certain viral and non-viral pathogens cause encephalitis only or much more frequently in immune-suppressed individuals.

The mode of disease course up to the appearance of the neurological signs may provide clues to the aetiology. For example, enterovirus infection has a typical biphasic course. An associated abnormality outside the nervous system (e.g. bleeding tendency in haemorrhagic fever) may also point to a specific pathogen.

General examination. Viral infection of the nervous system is almost always part of a generalized systemic infectious disease. Thus, other organs may be involved prior to or in association with the CNS manifestations and evidence should be obtained either from the history or during the examination. Skin rashes are not infrequent concomitants of viral infections, parotitis may be associated with mumps, gastrointestinal signs with enteroviral disease, and upper respiratory findings may accompany influenza virus infection and HSV-1 encephalitis.

Neurological examination. The findings relate to those of meningitis and disruption of brain parenchyma function. Thus, signs of meningeal irritation and somnolence suggest meningitis, while behavioural, cognitive, and focal neurological signs and seizures reflect the disruption of brain function. Additional signs may include autonomic and hypothalamic disturbances, diabetes insipidus, and the syndrome of inappropriate antidiuretic hormone secretion. The symptoms and signs are not a reliable diagnostic instrument to identify the causative virus. Likewise, the evolution of the clinical signs and their severity depend on host and other factors such as immune state and age, and cannot serve as guidelines to identify the pathogen. In general, the very young and the very old have the most extensive and serious signs of encephalitis.

Diagnostic investigations

General

Peripheral blood count and cellular morphology are helpful in separating viral from non-viral infections. Lymphocytosis in the peripheral blood is common in viral encephalitis. The erythrocyte sedimentation rate (ESR) is another non-specific test that is usually within the normal range in non-disseminated viral infections, although a raised ESR might indicate the alternative possibilities of TB or malignancy [9], or that the viral infection may be widely disseminated. Other, general examinations such as chest X-ray and blood cultures belong to the general investigation of a patient with febrile disease.

The auxiliary studies that examine viral infections of the nervous system include studies that characterize the extent and nature of CNS involvement (electroencephalography (EEG) and neuroimaging) and microbiological attempts to identify the pathogen.

EEG

EEG is generally regarded as a non-specific investigation, although it is still sometimes a useful tool in certain situations. Thus, leukoencephalitides show more diffuse slow activity in the EEG and polioencephalitides more rhythmic slow activity [10, 11]). However, in practice this hardly helps in the differential diagnosis. Likewise, the EEG findings in post-infectious encephalitides differ from infectious encephalitis only in the time schedule of the abnormalities. The main benefit of EEG is to demonstrate cerebral involvement during the early state of the disease. It is an indicator of cerebral involvement and usually shows a background abnormality prior to evidence of parenchyma involvement on neuroimaging [12]. Only in rare instances does the EEG show specific features that may give clues as to the diagnosis. Often, focal abnormalities may be observed. During the acute phase, the severity of EEG abnormalities has been shown to correlate with the prognosis [13]: fast-improving EEG indicates a good prognosis and lack of improvement the opposite [11] (Class IV). The EEG abnormalities usually subside more slowly than the clinical symptoms [10].

The EEG is almost always abnormal in **herpes simplex encephalitis** (HSE). In addition to the background slowing, there is a temporary temporal focus showing periodic lateralized epileptiform discharges (PLEDs). It

can be found during days 2–14 from the beginning of the disease [14], but is non-specific. To detect this, EEG finding often requires serial recordings. In newborns it can be faster with a frequency of 2 Hz and may be other than temporal [15].

In **brainstem encephalitis** the EEG mainly reflects the lowered consciousness and the abnormalities can be mild compared to the clinical state of the patient. In **cerebellitis** the EEG is mostly normal [16].

The EEG pattern in **HIV** infection of the brain is very variable [10]. Likewise the findings in **ADEM** are unspecific [17].

The EEG in **subacute sclerosing panencephalitis (SSPE)** shows a typical generalized periodic pattern repeating with intervals between 4 and 15 s and synchronized with myoclonus of the patient [10]

Neuroimaging

Magnetic resonance imaging (MRI) is more sensitive and specific than computed tomography (CT) and should be the treatment of choice for the evaluation of viral encephalitis. [18–21] Class III, Level C). MRI advantages include the use of non-ionizing radiation, multiplanar imaging capability, improved contrast of soft tissue, and high anatomical resolution. In practical terms, however, many patients who are suspected of having encephalitis often undergo CT scanning before neurological consultation.

A typical MRI protocol consists of routine T1 and T2 spin-echo sequences and a FLAIR (fluid-attenuation inversion recovery) sequence, which is considered extremely sensitive in detecting subtle changes in the early stages of an acute condition. Gradient-echo imaging, with its superior magnetic susceptibility, is also useful in detecting small areas of haemorrhage.

Additional imaging techniques that are available and that can increase sensitivity to small yet clinically relevant lesions, but are mainly used for research, may include *diffusion-weighted MRI*, which distinguishes recent from old insult; *low magnetization transfer ratio*, which reflects myelin damage, cell destruction or changes in water content; *magnetic resonance spectroscopy*, which identifies and quantities concentration of various brain metabolites; and *functional MRI*.

Computed tomography is recommended only as a screening examination or when MRI is unavailable [18–20] (Class IV).

Single photon emission tomography (SPECT) is more readily available than positron emission tomography (PET) and can provide information about brain chemistry, cerebral neurotransmitters, and brain function [22].

Imaging of specific disorders

Herpes simplex encephalitis

CT obtained early is often normal or subtly abnormal. Low attenuation, mild mass effect in temporal lobes and insula, haemorrhage, and enhancement are late features. Follow-up scans 1–2 weeks after disease onset demonstrate progressively more widespread abnormalities with the involvement of contra lateral temporal lobe, insula, and cingulate gyri. MRI is much more sensitive in detecting early changes [19, 20, 23] (Class III, Level C). Involvement of cingulate gyrus and contra lateral temporal lobe is highly suggestive of herpes encephalitis. Typical early findings include gyral oedema on T1WI imaging and high signal intensity in the temporal lobe or cingulate gyrus on T2WI, FLAIR, and DWI, and later haemorrhage. Hypointense on T1, hyperintense on T2WI, FLAIR, high signal on DWI are additional findings [24, 25]. The reinstitution of a normal spectrum over time on MRS could potentially be used as a marker of treatment efficacy [26, 27].

Neonatal **HSV-2 infection** often causes more widespread signal abnormalities than HSV-1 encephalitis, with periventricular white matter involvement and sparing of the medial temporal and inferior frontal lobes [28].

HIV-1

CT demonstrates normal/mild atrophy with white matter hypodensity. MRI usually shows atrophy and non-specific white matter changes. MRS detects early decreases in levels of N-Acetyl-aspartate (NAA) and increases in choline-containing phospholipids (Cho) levels, even before abnormalities are detected by MRI and prior to clinical symptoms [29]. Neuroimaging is an important diagnostic tool for opportunistic infections: toxoplasmosis (ring enhancing mass(es) in basal ganglia), cryptococcosis (gelatinous 'pseudocysts'), meningoencephalitis, vasculitis, infarction, CMV-encephalitis (diffuse white matter hyperintensities), ventriculitis (ependymal enhancement), progressive multifocal leukoencephalopathy (PML, white matter hyperintensities which usually do not enhance), and lymphoma (solitary or multifocal solid or ring-enhancing lesions either in deep grey and white matter or less frequent in subcortical areas) [30, 31]. MRS may be able to distinguish between these different space-occupying lesions based on their chemical profiles and can serve to predict and monitor the efficacy of antiretroviral therapy [32].

Varicella zoster virus

CNS complications of VZV infection (usually due to reactivation of latent VZV in spinal and trigeminal ganglia) include myelitis, encephalitis, large- and small-vessel arteritis, ventriculitis, and meningitis [33]. Large-vessel arteritis presents with ischaemic/haemorrhagic infarctions and may be revealed by MRI/MRA [34].

Miscellaneous

In **polio** and **coxsackie** virus infections, T2-weighted MRI may show hyperintensities in the midbrain and anterior horn of the spinal cord [35], in **EBV** infection in the basal ganglia and thalami [36] and in **Japanese encephalitis** in bilateral thalami, brainstem, and cerebellum [37]. **WNV** can be associated with enhancement of leptomeninges, the periventricular areas, or both, on MRI [38] as well as involvement of basal ganglia brain stem, thalamus and cerebellum [39].

Acute disseminated encephalomyelitis

Initial CT scanning may show low-density, asymmetric lesions with mild mass effect and contrast enhancement multifocal punctate or ring-enhancing lesions. However, CT is normal in 40% of cases. MRI is more sensitive and an essential diagnostic tool. T2WI and FLAIR scans present multifocal, usually bilateral, but asymmetric and large hyperintense lesions, involving peripheral white and grey matter. They do not usually involve the callososeptal interface. Contrast-enhanced T1WI may show ring-enhancing lesions. Cranial nerves may enhance. DWI is variable. On MRS, NAA is transiently low and choline is normal. [19, 21, 40]

MRI is also the most sensitive imaging tool for **PML** [41]. T2WI initially show multiple, bilateral, non-enhancing, oval or round subcortical white matter hyperintensities in the parieto-occipital area. Confluent white matter disease with cavitary change is a late manifestation of PML. Less common imaging manifestations of PML are unilateral white matter and thalamic or basal ganglia lesions.

Rasmussen's encephalitis

Rasmussen's encephalitis typically involves only one cerebral hemisphere, which becomes atrophic and so far its aetiology and pathogenesis are unknown. The earliest CT and MRI abnormalities include high signal on T2WI in cortex and white matter, cortical atrophy, usually of the fronto insular region, with mild or severe enlargement of the lateral ventricle, and moderate atrophy of the head of the caudate nucleus. Fluorodeoxyglucose PET has been reported to present hypometabolism; Tc-99m hexamethylpropyleamine oxime SPECT decreased perfusion and proton MRS reduction of NAA in the affected hemisphere. However, PET and SPECT findings are nonspecific. MRI may become a valuable early diagnostic tool by demonstrating focal disease progression [42, 43].

Paraneoplastic limbic encephalitis

In paraneoplastic limbic encephalitis MRI FLAIR and DWI depicted bilateral involvement of the medial temporal lobes and multifocal involvement of the brain [44].

Virological tests in encephalitis

General

The gold standard of diagnosis in encephalitis is virus isolation in cell culture, but this has now been replaced by the detection of specific nucleic acid from CSF or brain [45–48] (Class Ia). Intrathecal antibody production to a specific virus is similarly a strong evidence for aetiology [49, 50] (Class Ib). Virus detection from throat, stool, urine, or blood, as well as systemic serological responses such as seroconversion or a specific IgM detection provides less strong evidence [1, 51] (Class III). The CSF is a convenient specimen and is recommended for neurological viral diagnosis in general [52]. Brain biopsy is invasive and is now seldom used in routine clinical practice. However, in patients with rapidly deteriorating conditions, it has a high diagnostic yield, particularly in HIV-infected patients, but also 65% in non-HIV-infected patients, including viral encephalitis in 14% [53]. At autopsy, brain specimens can be obtained for virus isolation, nucleic acid and antigen detection, as well as for immunohistochemistry and *in situ* hybridization.

Viral culture

Viral cultures from CSF and brain tissue as well as from throat and stool specimens are performed in four different cell lines: African green monkey cells, Vero cells, human amniotic epithelial cells, and human embryonic skin fibroblasts. Cells are evaluated daily for cytopathic effect and the findings are confirmed by a neutralizing or an immunofluoresence antibody test. Viral cultures from CSF are positive in young children with enteroviral meningoencephalitis but only seldom, in less than 5 %, in other cases [54, 55] (Class III).

Nucleic acid detection

For nucleic acid detection, polymerase chain reaction (PCR) technology provides the most convenient test. Assays for HSV-1, HSV-2, VZV, human herpes viruses (HHV) 6 and 7, CMV, EBV, JCV of PML, Dengue virus, enteroviruses, and respiratory viruses, as well as HIV can be performed from CSF samples or brain tissue. The primers are selected from a conserved region of the viral genome and the PCR product is identified by hybridization with specific probes or by gel electrophoresis. Respiratory viruses' nucleic acid can also be detected from throat samples and enterovirus nucleic acid from stool samples. These, however, cannot confirm the aetiology of encephalitis. Detection of specific nucleic acid from the CSF is dependent on the timing of the CSF sample. The highest yield is obtained during the transient appearance of the virus in the CSF compartment during the first week after symptom onset, much less in the second week and only occasionally after that [47, 50] (Class I). In HSE the sensitivity is 96% and the specificity 99% when CSF is studied between 48 h and 10 days from symptoms onset [47, 48]. The issue of whether or not to routinely repeat the CSF PCR in HSE after 14 days of anti-viral treatment has yet to be resolved.

Alternatively to the single PCR tests, the multiplex PCR technique is also available [56–58] as is the real time PCR [59]. The usage of microarrays that enables to look for several microbes' nucleic acid simultaneously is currently expensive, but has the potential to become a useful diagnostic technique.

Serological tests

Antibodies to HSV-1, HSV-2, VZV, CMV, HHV-6, HHV-7, CMV, EBV, RSV, HIV, adeno, influenza A and B, rota, coxsackie B5, non-typed entero, and parainfluenza 1 viruses are measured from serum and CSF by enzyme immunoassay (EIA) tests [1, 49, 60–64] (Class II). These tests are sensitive enough to detect even low amounts of CSF antibodies. Antibody levels in serum and CSF are compared at the same dilution of 1:200. If the ratio of antibody levels is ≤20, it indicates intrathecal antibody production provided that no other antibodies are present in the CSF, i.e. the blood–brain barrier (BBB) is not damaged [51]. The presence of several antibodies in the CSF suggests BBB breakdown, while the presence of specific IgM in the CSF indicates CNS disease [65]. The tests for measles, mumps, and rubella are only occasionally needed in countries with effective vaccination programmes. Tests for arboviruses and zoonooses will be useful in endemic areas [51, 66]. Oligoclonal bands in the CSF may usually suggest an inflammatory aetiology [67].

Antigen detection

Antigens of HSV, VZV and RSV, influenza A and B, parainfluenza 1 and 3, and adenoviruses can be studied from throat specimens with a conventional immunofluorecence (IF) test or with an EIA test and may provide a possible aetiology for encephalitis. In spite of promising initial results these tests are not helpful in diagnosis using CSF samples.

Conclusion

In a patient with suspected encephalitis, obtaining serum and CSF for virological tests is the core diagnostic procedure of choice. Tests should include: PCR test for nucleic acid detection (from CSF) and serological tests for antibodies (from CSF and serum). In undiagnosed severe cases, PCR should be repeated after 3–7 days, and serological tests repeated after 2–4 weeks to show possible seroconversion or diagnostic increase in antibody levels. In children, viral culture from throat and stool samples as well as antigen detection for herpes and respiratory viruses are recommended during the first week. Viral culture from CSF is useful in children with suspected enteroviral or VZV disease if PCR tests are not available.

Histopathology

Encephalitis features a variety of histopathological changes in the brain, mainly depending on the type of infectious agent, the immunologic response by the host, and the stage of the infection. The aetiologic spectrum is strongly influenced by geography. Primary encephalitic processes may secondarily involve the meninges, with inflammatory infiltration resulting in usually mild CSF pleocytosis (lymphocytes with variable degree of activation, eventually plasmocytes). In encephalitis with a prominent necrotizing component, mixed CSF cellular-

ity may also include granulocytes; this is frequently seen in HSV encephalitis and CMV (peri)ventriculitis/myeloradiculitis of HIV patients.

The histopathological basis of encephalitis is the triad of damage to the parenchyma, reactive gliosis, and inflammatory cellular infiltration [68]. This classical substrate is exemplified by (multi)nodular encephalitis, as in the majority of viral encephalitides consisting of nerve cell damage, followed by nerve cell death and neuronophagia, focal/nodular proliferation of astro- and microglia, and focal/nodular infiltration by lymphocytes, eventually macrophages. Thus, the classical encephalitic nodules are composed of the mixture of microglia, astrocytes, and lymphocytes usually around affected neuron(s) [68].

Distribution and spread of these inflammatory changes are important for aetiologic considerations: four types of meningoencephalitis may be distinguished, affecting the meninges, the grey matter, the white matter, or both, in a focal or a diffuse manner [69]. 'Aseptic' meningitis is most commonly due to enteroviruses, HSV-2, mumps, HIV, LCM, arboviruses, measles, parainfluenza, and adenoviruses [69]. The encephalitic patterns include continuous polioencephalitis (e.g. in luetic general paresis) and patchy-nodular polioencephalitis (e.g. in poliomyelitis, rabies, acute encephalitis by flavi-, toga-, and enteroviruses, HSV brainstem encephalitis), leukoencephalitis (e.g. in PML or HIV leukoencephalopathy), and panencephalitis (e.g. in bacterial septicemia with microabscesses, in Whipple's disease, SSPE, HIV encephalitis, and herpes viruses such as HSV, CMV, and VZV infection). In addition to the inflammatory quality and characteristic distribution of tissue lesions, cytological features such as inclusion bodies (intranuclear in HSV, VZV encephalitis, PML and SSPE, cytoplasmic Negri bodies in rabies) or cytomegalic cell change in CMV disease give important diagnostic clues, especially when the involved cell type is considered: every viral infection of the nervous system usually features a fingerprint signature of selective vulnerability in the nervous system [68]. However, immunosuppression and the effects of potent therapies have become notorious for being able to modify, blur, or even wipe out classical features of specific viral lesions. This has become particularly striking in the recent experience with highly active anti-retroviral therapy (HAART) of HIV infection: its efficiency may result in deterioration by a paradoxical activation of an inflammatory response, the immune reconstitution inflammatory syndrome (IRIS). IRIS features brain inflammation by

predominantly CD8+ lymphocytes [70], including a fulminant leukoencephalitis [71] or a particularly severe
and intensely inflammatory form of PML. IRIS may be
responsive to steroid therapy [72]

Alternatively to direct viral damage to CNS tissue, secondary involvement by infarctions may be due to viral
infection of the CNS vasculature, as seen with VZV [34]
or Nipah virus [73].

The role of special techniques: immunocytochemistry, in situ hybridization, PCR

It is in the field of infections where the techniques of
immunocytochemistry (ICC), *in situ* hybridization
(ISH), and PCR have a profound impact on neuropathological diagnosis. When performed appropriately with
adequate controls and tissue selection, they provide an
aetiologic diagnosis with a high sensitivity and specificity
[68, 74]. Nevertheless, there are caveats for situations in
which they may not be diagnostic.

• Production of the infectious agent may have 'burnt out',
or its products may have become masked, resulting in
negative ICC or ISH.

• Tissue preservation might be unsuitable for ICC or
ISH, or nucleic acid amplification from paraffin embedded tissue may be blocked by yet unidentified factors.

• Since PCR and ISH are very sensitive techniques, positive results may reflect presence of genomic information
resulting from dormant or latent infection, and not necessarily productive and pathogenic infection.

Therefore, prerequisites for the use of ICC, ISH, or
PCR for diagnosis of infections include simultaneous use
of known positive and negative control tissues identically
processed as the material to be examined; availability of
reagents (antibodies, probes, primers) with defined specificities; adequate testing of reagents on control tissues
for optimal signal to noise ratio, and experience with
immunocytochemical antigen retrieval techniques [68].

Viruses may exert damage to the nervous system
not only by productive, but also by indirect means, the
best example being the immune-mediated **ADEM** or
post-infectious/perivenous encephalitis, important for
differential diagnosis from productive viral encephalomyelitis: multiple small demyelinated foci are arranged
around small veins of the white matter, featuring cellular
infiltration composed by lymphocytes, macrophages and
microglia [68].

Other infective causes of meningoencephalitis and differential diagnosis

The clinical distinction between viral encephalitis and
non-viral infective meningoencephalitis may be difficult,
and is sometimes impossible. Epidemiological and
demographic features, such as prevalent or emergent
infections in the community, occupation, a history of
travel, and animal contacts may provide helpful clues. In
a non-epidemic setting, the most common cause of focal
encephalopathic findings is HSE; however, among cases
with biopsy-proven HSE, there were no distinguishing
clinical characteristics between HSV-positive and HSV-
negative patients [3].

ADEM, an autoimmune disease, with evidence of cell-
mediated immunity to the myelin basic protein as its
pathogenic basis [75], is characterized by monophasic
focal neurological signs and a rapidly progressive course
usually with a history of febrile illness or immunization
preceding the neurological syndrome by days or weeks.
It may be distinguished from infective encephalitis by the
younger age of the patient, prodromal history of vaccination or infection, absence of fever at the onset of symptoms, and the presence of multifocal neurological signs
affecting optic nerves, brain, spinal cord, and peripheral
nerve roots. The disturbances of consciousness range
from stupor and confusion to coma. Patients have a mild
fever, often with peripheral blood pleocytosis. CSF shows
lymphocytic pleocytosis, with mildly raised protein, and
may appear similar to the CSF in viral encephalitis. The
clinical course of patients with Hashimoto's encephalopathy would fit a less aggressive form of recurrent ADEM
[76, 77].

CNS vasculitis can be part of a systemic disease or be
confined to the nervous system. Systemic symptoms,
aseptic meningitis, and focal neurological deficit may
occasionally simulate viral encephalitis. This is seen in
both systemic vasculitis and primary CNS angiitis. In
systemic vasculitis affecting the CNS it is usually possible
to make a diagnosis based on a combination of systemic
and CSF serologic and immunological tests, and angiographic appearances of CNS vasculitis. In isolated angiitis
the diagnosis may be more challenging and may require
brain and meningeal biopsy to secure the diagnosis.

Pseudomigraine with pleocytosis. Acute confusion,
psychosis, and focal neurological deficit (hemiplegia,

hemianaesthesia, and aphasia) in association with migraine headache occur in familial hemiplegic migraine [78]. Sterile CSF pleocytosis has been reported in migraine patients who may present similarly [79]. It has been proposed that the pleocytosis in some of these cases is due to predisposition to viral meningitis [80]. Pseudomigraine with pleocytosis and migraine coma are likely to represent reversible forms of ADEM [77].

Therapy

Anti-viral therapy

Acyclovir is the treatment of choice for HSE (Class IA). Monophosphorylation of acyclovir is the critical step in this process and is only catalysed by a viral thymidine kinase induced in cells selectively infected by HSV, VZV, or by a phosphotransferase produced by CMV. Host enzymes subsequently phosphorylate the monophosphate to di-and triphosphate. Acyclovir triphosphate inhibits the synthesis of viral DNA by competing with 2′-deoxyguanosine triphosphate as a substrate for viral DNA polymerase. Viral DNA synthesis is arrested once acyclovir (rather than 2′-deoxyguanosine) is inserted into the replicating DNA. The incorporation of acyclovir into viral DNA is an irreversible process and it also inactivates viral DNA polymerase. Acyclovir is most effective when given early in the clinical course of HSE and reduces both mortality and morbidity [3, 81, 82]. The standard dose for HSE is 10 mg/kg given as an intravenous infusion over 1 h three times daily (30 mg/kg/day) for 14 days. The dose for neonatal HSE is 60 mg/kg/day. The duration of treatment is 21 days for immunosuppressed patients.

Treatment with acyclovir for HSE should be commenced on clinical suspicion. Mortality rates in untreated HSE are around 70% and fewer than 3% would return to normal function. Early acyclovir therapy reduces mortality to 20–30% [81, 83]. Among the acyclovir-treated patients in the NINAID-CASG trials, 26 of the 32 (81%) treated patients survived and serious neurological disability was seen in nearly half of the survivors. Older patients with poor level of consciousness (Glasgow Coma Scale of 6 or less) had the worst outcome. Young patients (30 years or less) with good neurological function at the time of initiating therapy did substantially better (100% survival, more than 60% had little or no sequel). Since more than 80% of acyclovir in circulation is excreted

unchanged in urine, renal impairment can precipitate acyclovir toxicity, and high-dose acyclovir in overweight or obese patients may precipitate renal failure. Rarely, acyclovir can induce a toxic encephalopathy and therefore it is important to establish an early diagnosis of HSE to avoid diagnostic confusion.

In an immunocompetent host with acute encephalopathy, MRI evidence of temporal or frontobasal lobes involvement supports the diagnosis of HSE and such a patient must be treated with acyclovir for a minimum of 14 days (Class IV). If acyclovir is started on admission and the MRI of brain is normal, then treatment should continue until CSF-PCR results become available; the treatment should be withdrawn in cases where this test is negative and an alternative diagnosis has been established. If an alternative diagnosis has not been reached and the CFS-PCR is negative for HSV, then the current consensus is to continue acyclovir therapy for at least 10 days (Class IV) [9]. There has been only a single case report of HSE with normal cerebral MRI scan, where the diagnosis of HSE was made by PCR from a CSF sample obtained on the day of admission but a repeat CSF-PCR after 8 days of acyclovir therapy was negative [84]. Recurrence of HSE has been reported weeks to 3 months later when the treatment was given for 10 days or less [85], and relapse after therapy may be as high as 5%, but relapse has not been documented when higher doses were administered for 21 days [86]. Development of acyclovir resistance in HSE is a possibility following the report of acyclovir resistance in mucocutaneous herpes simplex among AIDS patients and isolation of acyclovir-resistant HSV as the cause of encephalitis in organ transplant recipients and HIV patients. Foscarnet, which inhibits viral DNA polymerases by binding to the pyrophosphate binding site, is recommended in acyclovir-resistant HSE (60 mg/kg intravenously infused over 1 h every 8 hours for 3 weeks). However, acyclovir-resistant HSE has not been reported in immunocompetent patients and foscarnet should be used only in patients with clinically suspected HSE who continue to deteriorate despite acyclovir therapy with a reactive CSF, in whom alternative possibilities have been excluded. Foscarnet can also precipitate a dose-related, reversible renal impairment.

Acyclovir is effective against encephalitis due to VZV [81]. VZV can cause both acute and subacute encephalitis. VZV was the most common alpha-herpesvirus detected in CSF samples from patients with CNS symptoms in the Western Gotaland region of Sweden [87]. Doses of acyclovir in VZV encephalitis are similar to HSE and the treatment should be continued for 3 weeks (Class IV).

Response of CMV encephalitis to antiviral drugs (ganciclovir, foscarnet, and cidofovir) is less than satisfactory. Combination of ganciclovir (5 mg/kg intravenously twice daily) with foscarnet (60 mg/kg every 8 h or 90 mg/kg intravenously every 12 h) is advocated as induction therapy in CMV encephalitis (Class IV), followed by maintenance therapy with ganciclovir (5 mg/kg/day) or foscarnet (60--120 mg/kg/day) [88]. The recommended duration of induction therapy is 3 weeks for immunocompetent and 6 weeks for immunosuppressed patients (Class IV). The rationale for using combination treatment in the induction phase is that monotherapy with ganciclovir or foscarnet alone failed to improve survival.

The present treatment recommendation for HHV-6 encephalitis is foscarnet (60 mg/kg every 8 h for both A and B variants). Ganciclovir (5 mg/kg every 12 h) is an alternative option only for B variant of HHV-6 encephalitis [89].

There have been few successes with antiviral therapy for arboviral encephalitis. A study that evaluated high dose dexamethasone in JE found the treatment to be of no benefit [90].

Neurological complications, including encephalitis, have been widely reported in association with respiratory tract infection with seasonal influenza A or B viruses, and recently with novel influenza A (H1N1) virus. Antiviral therapy with oseltamivir (four patients) and rimantadine (three patients) were clinically effective in patients with suspected encephalitis due to H1N1 infection [91].

PML is commonly caused by JC virus and is regarded as an opportunistic infection of the CNS occurring in the setting of immunosuppression. There have been recent reports of subacutely evolving PML following treatment with rituximab, natalizumab, and efalizumab. Many antiviral drugs, including cytosine arabinoside, amantadine, ribavirin, interferon alpha, and vidarabine, have all been used in small case studies but none has shown a lasting impact.

No antiviral therapy is particularly effective in epizootic or enzootic viral encephalitis; however, because of the high mortality rate associated with B virus (cercopithecine herpes virus) encephalitis in humans, it is currently proposed [3] that patients should be treated with intravenous acyclovir or ganciclovir.

Corticosteroids

Large doses of dexamethasone as an adjunct treatment for acute viral encephalitis are not considered to be effective and their use is controversial. Probably the best evidence for steroid therapy in this context is in VZV encephalitis. Primary VZV infection may cause severe encephalitis in immunocompetent children due to cerebral vasculitis [34, 92]. Vasculitis following primary and secondary VZV infection is recognized as resulting in a chronic course in immunocompetent children and adults (granulomatous angiitis). HSE is occasionally complicated by severe, vasogenic cerebral oedema where high-dose steroids may have a role. Steroid pulse therapy with methylprednisolone has been observed to be beneficial in a small number of patients with acute viral encephalitis who had progressive disturbances of consciousness, an important prognostic factor for outcome [93]. The utility of adjunctive corticosteroid therapy in HSE is about to be evaluated in a multicentre, multinational, randomized, double-blind, placebo-controlled trial [94].

Based on available data, combined acyclovir/steroid treatment may be advised in immunocompetent individuals with severe VZV encephalitis, and probably in other cases of acute viral encephalitis where progressive cerebral oedema documented by CT/MRI complicates the course of illness in the early phase (GPP). High-dose dexamethasone or pulse methylprednisolone are both suitable agents. The duration of steroid treatment should be short (between 3 and 5 days) in order to minimize adverse.

The effect of steroids on IRIS has been demonstrated in anecdotal reports [72, 95], and requires confirmation in controlled trials.

Although no randomized controlled trials have been performed, treatment with high-dose steroids (intravenous pulses of methylprednisolone) and/or plasma exchange is usually the recommended treatment in ADEM [76] (Class IV and GPP).

Surgical intervention

Surgical decompression for acute viral encephalitis is indicated for impending herniation or increased intracranial pressure refractory to medical management

(GPP). Such intervention has been shown to improve outcome in HSE in individual cases [96].

General measures

All cases of acute encephalitis must be hospitalized. Like other critically ill patients, cases with acute viral encephalitis should have access to an intensive care unit equipped with mechanical ventilators. Irrespective of the aetiology, supportive therapy for acute viral encephalitis is an important cornerstone of management [2]. Seizures are controlled with intravenous anticonvulsants such as phenytoin. Careful attention must be paid to the maintenance of respiration, cardiac rhythm, fluid balance, prevention of deep vein thrombosis and aspiration pneumonia, and medical management of raised intracranial pressure and secondary bacterial infections. Secondary neurological complications in the course of viral encephalitis are common and include cerebral infarction, cerebral venous thrombosis, syndrome of inappropriate ADH secretion, aspiration pneumonia, upper gastrointestinal bleeding, urinary tract infections, and disseminated intravascular coagulopathy.

Isolation of patients with community-acquired acute infective encephalitis is not required. Consideration of isolation should be given for severely immunosuppressed patients, rabies encephalitis, patients with exanthematous encephalitis, and those with a contagious viral hemorrhagic fever.

Rehabilitation

Survivors of viral encephalitis and myelitis are a heterogenous group. The nature of the infective pathogen, variability in anatomic lesions, and time to treatment may all contribute to outcome. Longitudinally designed case studies reporting cognitive and psychosocial outcome of mainly following HSE were conducted prior to current era of early diagnosis and effective therapy. While there are anecdotal case reports [97, 98] there are too few studies on the outcome of rehabilitation following encephalitis [99] to allow any conclusions to be drawn.

Preventive measures

Currently vaccines are available against a limited number of viruses with a potential to cause encephalitis. Universal immunization is recommended against mumps, measles, rubella, and poliovirus. European travellers to specific geographic destinations (e.g. South East Asia) should receive advice regarding vaccination against rabies and Japanese encephalitis. Preventive measures against exotic forms of emerging paramyxovirus encephalitis (Nipah and Hendra viruses) are entirely environmental (sanitation, vector control, and avoidance).

Recommendations

Diagnostic tests

Viral encephalitis is still an evolving discipline in medicine. The emergence of new pathogens, the re-emergence of old pathogens, and the constant search for specific therapeutic measures, unavailable in most viral encephalitis cases, suggests that the following years will bring new developments in diagnosis and therapy. At present, adherence to a strict protocol of diagnostic investigations is recommended and includes the following.

Study	Findings	Level of recommendation	Class of evidence
LP	Cells – 5–500 white blood cells, mainly lymphocytes; May be xanthochromic with red blood cells. Glucose – normal (rarely reduced). Protein ≥50 mg/dl	A	II
Serology	CSF and Serum	B	II
PCR	Major aid in diagnosis (CSF). May be false negative in the first 2 days of disease.	A	I
EEG	Early and sensitive. Non specific. May identify focal abnormalities	C	III
Imaging	MRI is usually more sensitive than CT, demonstrating high signal intensity lesion on T2-weighted and FLAIR images.	B	II
Viral culture	Only rarely useful		
Brain biopsy	Highly sensitive. Not used routinely	C	III & GPP

Recommendations

Therapeutic interventions

The following are the specific and symptomatic therapeutic measures available for viral encephalitis.

Interventions	Class of evidence	Level of recommendation
Acyclovir for HSE	II	A
Acyclovir for suspected viral encephalitis	IV	(–)
Acyclovir for VZV encephalitis	IV	(–)
Gancylovir and/Foscarnet for CMV encephalitis	IV	(–)
Acyclovir or ganciclovir for B virus encephalitis	IV	(–)
Pleconaril for enterovirus encephalitis	Not available	(–)
Corticosteroids for viral encephalitis	IV	
Corticosteroids for viral encephalitis	IV	
Surgical decompression	IV	

Statement of the likely time when the guidelines will need to be updated

These guidelines should be regularly reviewed in light of new scientific evidence and medical experience, and updated when necessary.

Conflicts of interest

The authors have reported no conflicts of interests.

References

1. Koskiniemi M, Rantalaiho T, Piiparinen H, *et al.* Infections of the central nervous system of suspected viral origin: a collaborative study from Finland. *J Neurovirol* 2001;7: 400–8.

2. Chaudhuri A, Kennedy PG. Diagnosis and treatment of viral encephalitis. *Postgrad Med J* 2002;78:575–83.

3. Whitley RJ, Gnann JW. Viral encephalitis: familiar infections and emerging pathogens. *Lancet* 2002;359:507–13.

4. Kennedy PGE, Chaudhuri A. Herpes simplex virus encephalitis. *J Neurol Neurosurg Psychiat* 2002;73:237–8.

5. Solomon T, Hart IJ, Beeching NJ. Viral encephalitis: a clinician's guide. *Pract Neurol* 2007;7:288–305.

6. Tyler KL. Emerging viral infections of the central nervous system. *Arch Neurol* 2009;66:1065–74 & 939–48.

7. Shankar SK, Mahadevan A, Kovoor JM. Neuropathology of viral infections of the central nervous system. *Neuroimaging Clin N Am* 2008;18:19–39.

8. Brainin M, Barnes M, Baron JC, *et al.* Guidance for the preparation of neurological management guidelines by EFNS scientific task forces – revised recommendations. *Eur J Neurol* 2004;11:577–81.

9. Kennedy PGE. Viral encephalitis-causes, differential diagnosis and management. *J Neurol Neurosurg Psychiat* 2004;75(Suppl.):i10–5.

10. Westmoreland BF. The EEG in cerebral inflammatory processes. In: Niedermeyer E, Lopes Da Silva F (eds) *Electroencephalography*, 4th edn. Baltimore: Williams & Wilkins, 1999; pp. 302–16.

11. Vas GA, Cracco JB. Inflammatory encephalopathies. In: Daly DD, Pedley TA (eds) *Current Practice of Clinical Electroencephalography*, 2nd edn. New York: Raven Press, 1990; pp. 386–9.

12. Fowler A, Stödberg T, Eriksson M, Wickström R. Childhood encephalitis in Sweden: etiology, clinical presentation and outcome. *Eur J Paediatr Neurol* 2008;12: 484–90.

13. Wang IJ, Lee PI, Huang LM, Chen CJ, Chen CL, Lee WT. The correlation between neurological evaluations and neurological outcome in acute encephalitis: a hospital-based study. *Eur J Paediatr Neurol* 2007;11:63–9.

14. Lai CW, Gragasin ME. Electroencephalography in herpes simplex encephalitis. *J Clin Neurophysiol* 1988;5: 87–103.

15. Sainio K, Granström ML, Pettay O, *et al.* EEG in neonatal herpes simplex encephalitis. *Electroenceph Clin Neurophysiol* 1983;56:556–61.

16. Schmahmann JD, Sherman JC. The cerebellar cognitive affective syndrome. *Brain* 1998;121:561–79.

17. Tenembaum S, Chamoles N, Fejerman N. Acute disseminated encephalomyelitis: a long-term follow-up study of 84 pediatric patients. *Neurology* 2002;59:1224–31.

18. Dun V, Bale JF Jr, Zimmerman RA, Perdue Z, Bell WE. MRI in children with postinfectious disseminated encephalomyelitis. *Magn Reson Imaging* 1986;**4**:25–32.

19. Schroth G, Kretzschmar K, Gawehn J, Voigt K. Advantage of magnetic resonance imaging in the diagnosis of cerebral infections. *Neuroradiology* 1987;**29**:120–6.

20. Marchbank ND, Howlett DC, Sallomi DF, Hughes DV. Magnetic resonance imaging is preferred in diagnosing suspected cerebral infections. *BMJ* 2000;**320**: 187–8.

21. Dale RC, de Sousa C, Chong WK, Cox TC, Harding B, Neville BG. Acute disseminated encephalomyelitis, multiphasic disseminated encephalomyelitis and multiple sclerosis in children. *Brain* 2000;**123**:2407–22.

22. Launes J, Nikkinen P, Lindroth L, Brownell AL, Liewendahl K, Iivanainen M. Diagnosis of acute herpes simplex encephalitis by brain perfusion single photon emission computed tomography. *Lancet* 1988;**i**:1188–91.

23. Steiner I, Kennedy PG, Pachner AR. The neurotropic herpes viruses: herpes simplex and varicella-zoster. *Lancet Neurol* 2007;**6**:1015–28.

24. Tsuchiya K, Katase S, Yoshino A, Hachiya J. Diffusion-weighted MR imaging of encephalitis. *AJR Am J Roentgenol* 1999;**173**:1097–9.

25. Ito S, Hirose Y, Mokuno K. The clinical usefulness of MRI diffusion weighted images in herpes simplex encephalitis-like cases. *Rinsho Shinkeigaku* 1999;**39**:1067–70.

26. Salvan AM, Confort-Gouny S, Cozzone PJ, Vion-Dury J. Atlas of brain proton magnetic resonance spectra. Part III: viral infections. *J Neuroradiol* 1999;**26**:154–61.

27. Menon DK, Sargentoni J, Peden CJ, *et al.* Proton MR spectroscopy in herpes simplex encephalitis: assessment of neuronal loss. *J Comput Assist Tomogr* 1990;**14**:449–52.

28. Hinson VK, Tyor WR. Update on viral encephalitis. *Curr Opin Neurol* 2001;**14**:369–74.

29. Rudkin TM, Arnold DL. Proton magnetic resonance spectroscopy for the diagnosis and management of cerebral disorders. *Arch Neurol* 1999;**56**:919–26.

30. Thurnher MM, Rieger A, Kleibl-Popov C, *et al.* Primary central nervous system lymphoma in AIDS: a wider spectrum of CT and MRI findings. *Neuroradiology* 2001; **43**:29–35.

31. Yin EZ, Frush DP, Donnelly LF, Buckley RH. Primary immunodeficiency disorders in pediatric patients: clinical features and imaging findings. *AJR Am J Roentgenol* 2001; **176**:1541–52.

32. Wilkinson ID, Lunn S, Miszkiel KA, *et al.* Proton MRS and quantitative MRI assessment of the short term neurological response to antiretroviral therapy in AIDS. *J Neurol Neurosurg Psychiatry* 1997;**63**:477–82.

33. Gilden DH, Kleinschmidt-DeMasters BK, LaGuardia JJ, Mahalingam R, Cohrs RJ. Neurologic complications of the reactivation of varicella-zoster virus. *N Engl J Med* 2000; **342**:635–45.

34. Gilden D, Cohrs RJ, Mahalingam R, Nagel MA. Varicella zoster virus vasculopathies: diverse clinical manifestations, laboratory features, pathogenesis, and treatment. *Lancet Neurol* 2009;**8**:731–40.

35. Shen WC, Tsai C, Chiu H, Chow K. MRI of Enterovirus 71 myelitis with monoplegia. *Neuroradiology* 2000;**42**: 124–7.

36. Shian WJ, Chi CS. Epstein-Barr virus encephalitis and encephalomyelitis: MR findings. *Pediatr Radiol* 1996;**26**: 690–3.

37. Abe T, Kojima K, Shoji H, *et al.* Japanese encephalitis. *J Magn Reson Imaging* 1998;**8**:755–61.

38. Sejvar JJ, Haddad MB, Tierney BC, *et al.* Neurologic manifestations and outcome of West Nile virus infection. *JAMA* 2003;**290**:511–5.

39. Davis LE, DeBiasi R, Goade DE, *et al.* West Nile virus neuroinvasive disease. *Ann Neurol* 2006;**60**:286–300.

40. Bizzi A, Ulug AM, Crawford TO, *et al.* Quantitative proton MR spectroscopic imaging in acute disseminated encephalomyelitis. *AJNR Am J Neuroradiol* 2001;**22**: 1125–30.

41. Berger JR, Major EO. Progressive multifocal leukoencephalopathy. *Semin Neurol* 1999;**19**:193–200.

42. Korn-Lubetzki I, Bien CG, Bauer J, *et al.* Rasmussen encephalitis with active inflammation and delayed seizures onset. *Neurology* 2004;**62**:984–6.

43. Chiapparini L, Granata T, Farina L, *et al.* Diagnostic imaging in 13 cases of Rasmussen's encephalitis: can early MRI suggest the diagnosis? *Neuroradiology* 2003;**45**: 171–83.

44. Thuerl C, Muller K, Laubenberger J, Volk B, Langer M. MR imaging of autopsy-proved paraneoplastic limbic encephalitis in non-Hodgkin lymphoma. *AJNR Am J Neuroradiol* 2003;**24**:507–11.

45. Rowley AH, Whitley RJ, Lakeman FD, Wolinsky SM. Rapid detection of herpes-simplex-virus DNA in cerebrospinal fluid of patients with herpes simplex encephalitis. *Lancet* 1990;**335**:440–1.

46. Echevarria JM, Casas I, Tenorio A, de Ory F, Martinez-Martin P. Detection of varicella-zoster virus-specific DNA sequences in cerebrospinal fluid from patients with acute aseptic meningitis and no cutaneous lesions. *J Med Virol* 1994;**43**:331–5.

47. Lakeman FD, Whitley RJ. Diagnosis of herpes simplex encephalitis: application of polymerase chain reaction to cerebrospinal fluid from brain-biopsied patients and correlation with disease. National Institute of Allergy and

Infectious Diseases Collaborative Antiviral Study Group. *J Infect Dis* 1995;**171**:857–63.

48. Tebas P, Nease RF, Storch GA. Use of the polymerase chain reaction in the diagnosis of herpes simplex encephalitis: a decision analysis model. *Am J Med* 1998;**105**:287–95.

49. Levine D, Lauter CB, Lerner M. Simultaneous serum and CSF antibodies in herpes simplex virus encephalitis. *JAMA* 1978;**240**:356–60.

50. Koskiniemi M, Piiparinen H, Rantalaiho T, *et al.* Acute central nervous system complications in varicella zoster virus infections. *J Clin Virol* 2002;**25**:293–301.

51. Burke DS, Nisalak A, Ussery MA, Laorakpongse T, Chantavibul S. Kinetics of IgM and IgG responses to Japanese encephalitis virus in human serum and cerebrospinal fluid. *J Infect Dis* 1985;**151**:1093–9.

52. Cinque P, Linde A. CSF Analysis in the diagnosis of viral meningitis and encephalitis. In: Nath A, Berger JR (eds) *Clinical Neurovirology*. New York, Basel: Marcel Dekker, Inc., 2003; pp. 43–107.

53. Josephson SA, Papanastassiou AM, Berger MS, *et al.* The diagnostic utility of brain biopsy procedures in patients with rapidly deteriorating neurological conditions or dementia. *J Neurosurg* 2007;**106**:72–5.

54. Muir P, vanLoon AM. Enterovirus infections of the central nervous system. *Intervirology* 1997;**40**:153–66.

55. Storch AG. Methodological overview. In Storch AG (ed.) *Essentials of Diagnostic Virology*, New York: Churchill Livinstone. 2000; pp. 1–23.

56. Tenorio A, Echevarria JE, Casas I, Echevarria JM, Tabares E. Detection and typing of human herpesviruses by multiplex polymerase chain reaction. *J Virol Methods* 1993;**44**:261–9.

57. Jaaskelainen AJ, Piiparinen H, Lappalainen M, Koskiniemi M, Vaheri A. Multiplex-PCR and oligonucleotide microarray for detection of eight different herpesviruses from clinical specimens. *J Clin Virol* 2006;**37**:83–90.

58. Pozo F, Tenorio A. Detection and typing of lymphotropic herpesviruses by multiplex polymerase chain reaction. *J Virol Methods* 1999;**79**:9–19.

59. Kessler HH, Muhlbauer G, Rinner B, *et al.* Detection of herpes simplex virus DNA by real-time PCR. *J Clin Microbiol* 2000;**38**:2638–42.

60. MacCallum FO, Chinn IJ, Gostling JVT. Antibodies to herpes-simplex virus in the cerebrospinal fluid of patients with herpetic encephalitis. *J Med Microbiol* 1974;**7**:325–31.

61. Julkunen I, Kleemola M, Hovi T. Serological diagnosis of influenza A and B infections by enzyme immuno assay: comparison with the complement fixation test. *J Virol Methods* 1984;**1**:7–14.

62. Socan M, Beovic B, Kese D. *Chlamydia pneumoniae* and meningoencephalitis. *N Engl J Med* 1994;**331**:406.

63. Gilden DH, Bennett JL, Kleinschmidt-DeMasters BK, Song DD, Yee AS, Steiner I. The value of cerebrospinal fluid antiviral antibody in the diagnosis of neurologic disease produced by varicella zoster virus. *J Neurol Sci* 1998;**159**:140–4.

64. Koskiniemi M, Gencay M, Salonen O, *et al.*, the Study Group. *Chlamydia pneumoniae* associated with central nervous system infections. *Eur Neurol* 1996;**36**:160–3.

65. Jacobi C, Lange P, Reiber H. Quantitation of intrathecal antibodies in cerebrospinal fluid of subacute sclerosing panencephalitis, herpes simplex encephalitis and multiple sclerosis: discrimination between microorganism-driven and polyspecific immune response. *J Neuroimmunol* 2007;**187**:139–46.

66. Wahlberg P, Saikku P, Brummer-Korvenkontio M. Tick-borne viral encephalitis in Finland. The clinical features of Kumlinge disease during 1959–1987. *J Intern Med* 1989;**225**:173–7.

67. Franciotta D, Columba-Cabezas S, Andreoni L, *et al.* Oligoclonal IgG band patterns in inflammatory demyelinating human and mouse diseases. *J Neuroimmunol* 2008;**200**:125–8.

68. Budka H. Viral infections. In: Garcia JH, Budka H, McKeever PE, Sarnat HB, Sima AAF (eds) *Neuropathology – The Diagnostic Approach*. St Louis: Mosby, 1997; pp. 353–91.

69. Love S, Wiley CA. Viral infections. In: Love S, Louis DN, Ellison DW (eds) *Greenfield's Neuropathology*, vol. **2**, 8th edn. London: Hodder Arnold, 2008; pp. 1275–389.

70. Rushing EJ, Liappis A, Smirniotopoulos JD, *et al.* Immune reconstitution inflammatory syndrome of the brain: case illustrations of a challenging entity. *J Neuropathol Exp Neurol* 2008;**67**:819–27.

71. Vendrely A, Bienvenu B, Gasnault J, Thiebault JB, Salmon D, Gray F. Fulminant inflammatory leukoencephalopathy associated with HAART-induced immune restoration in AIDS-related progressive multifocal leukoencephalopathy. *Acta Neuropathol* 2005;**109**:449–55.

72. Tan K, Roda R, Ostrow L, McArthur J, Nath A. PML-IRIS in patients with HIV infection: clinical manifestations and treatment with steroids. *Neurology* 2009;**72**:1458–64.

73. Tan CT, Chua KB. Nipah virus encephalitis. *Curr Infect Dis Rep* 2008;**10**:315–20.

74. Johnson RT. *Viral Diseases of the Nervous System*, 2nd edn. Philadelphia: Lippincott Williams & Wilkins, 1998.

75. Behan PO, Geshwind N, Lamarche JB, *et al.* Delayed hypersensitivity to encephalitogenic protein in disseminated encephalitis. *Lancet* 1968;**ii**:1009–12.

76. Cohen O, Steiner-Birmanns B, Biran I, Abramsky O, Honigman S, Steiner I. Recurrent acute disseminated encephalomyelitis tends to relapse at the previously affected brain site. *Arch Neurol* 2001;**58**:797–801.

77. Chaudhuri A, Behan PO. The clinical spectrum, diagnosis, pathogenesis and treatment of Hashimoto's encephalopathy (recurrent acute disseminated encephalomyelitis). *Current Med Chem* 2003;**10**:1645–53.

78. Feely MP, O'Hare J, Veale D, Callaghan N. Episodes of acute confusion or psychosis in familial hemiplegic migraine. *Acta Neurol Scand* 1982;**65**:369–75.

79. Schraeder PL, Burns RA. Hemiplegic migraine associated with an aseptic meningeal reaction. *Arch Neurol* 1980;**37**: 377–9.

80. Casteels-van Daele M, Standaert L, Boel M, Smeets E, Colaert J, Desmyter J. Basilar migraine and viral meningitis. *Lancet* 1981;**i**:1366.

81. Whitley RJ. Viral encephalitis. *N Eng J Med* 1990;**323**: 242–50.

82. Skoldenberg B, Forsgren M, Alestig K, *et al.* Acyclovir versus vidarabine in herpes simplex encephalitis: randomized multicentre study in consecutive Swedish patients. *Lancet* 1984;**2**:707–12.

83. Whitley RJ, Alford CA, Hirsch MS, *et al.* Vidarabine versus acyclovir therapy in herpes simplex encephalitis. *N Eng J Med* 1986;**314**:144–9.

84. Hollinger P, Matter L. Sturzenegger M. Normal MRI findings in herpes simplex virus encephalitis. *J Neurol* 2000; **247**:799–801.

85. Davis LE. Diagnosis and treatment of acute encephalitis. *The Neurologist* 2000;**6**:145–59.

86. Ito Y, Kimura H, Yabuta Y, *et al.* Exacerbation of herpes simplex encephalitis after successful treatment with acyclovir. *Clin Infect Dis* 2000;**30**:185–7.

87. Persson A, Bergström T, Lindh M, Namvar L, Studahl M. Varicella-zoster virus CNS disease-Viral load, clinical manifestations and sequels. *J Clin Virol* (2009) [Epub ahead of print].

88. Griffiths P. Cytomegalovirus infection of the central nervous system. *Herpes* 2004;**11**(Suppl. 2):95A–104A.

89. Soto-Hernandez JL. Human herpesvirus 6 encephalomyelitis. *Emerg Infect Dis* 2004;**10**:1700–2.

90. Hoke CH Jr, Vaughn DW, Nisalak A, *et al.* Effects of high dose dexamethasone on the outcome of acute Japanese encephalitis. *J Infect Dis* 1992;**165**:131–6.

91. Centers for Disease Control and Prevention (CDC). Neurologic complications associated with novel influenza A (H1N1) virus infection in children – Dallas, Texas, May 2009. *MMWR Morb Mortal Wkly Rep* 2009;**58**:773–8.

92. Hausler M, Schaade L, Kemeny S, *et al.* Encephalitis related to primary varicella-zoster virus infection in immunocompetent children. *J Neurol Sci* 2002;**195**:111–6.

93. Nakano A, Yamasaki R, Miyazaki S, *et al.* Beneficial effect of steroid pulse therapy on acute viral encephalitis. *Eur Neurol* 2003;**50**:225–9.

94. Martinez-Torres F, Menon S, Pritsch M, *et al.*, the GACHE Investigators. Protocol for German trial of Acyclovir and corticosteroids in Herpes-simplex-virus-encephalitis (GACHE): a multicenter, multinational, randomized, doubleblind, placebo-controlled German, Austrian and Dutch trial. *BMC Neurol* 2008;**8**:40.

95. Martinez JV, Mazziotti JV, Efron ED, *et al.* Immune reconstitution inflammatory syndrome associated with PML in AIDS: a treatable disorder. *Neurology* 2006;**67**: 1692–4.

96. Yan HJ. Herpes simplex encephalitis: the role of surgical decompression. *Surg Neurol* 2002;**57**:20–4.

97. Wilson BA, Gracey F, Bainbridge K. Cognitive recovery from 'persistent vegetative state': psychological and personal perspectives. *Brain Inj* 2001;**15**:1083–92.

98. Miotto EC. Cognitive rehabilitation of naming deficits following viral meningo-encephalitis. *Arq Neuropsiquiatr* 2002;**60**:21–7.

99. Moorthi S, Schneider WN, Dombovy ML. Rehabilitation outcomes in encephalitis – a retrospective study 1990–1997. *Brain Inj* 1999;**13**:139–46.42.

CHAPTER 26
Treatment of neuropathic pain

N. Attal,[1] G. Cruccu,[2] R. Baron,[3] M. Haanpää,[4] P. Hansson,[5] T. S. Jensen,[6] T. Nurmikko[7]

[1]Hôpital Ambroise Paré, APHP, Boulogne-Billancourt, and Université Versailles-Saint-Quentin,Versailles, France; [2]La Sapienza University, Rome, Italy; [3]Universitatsklinikum Schleswig-Holstein, Kiel, Germany; [4]Helsinki University Hospital, Helsinki, Finland; [5]Karolinska Institutet/University Hospital, Stockholm, Sweden; [6]Aarhus University Hospital, Aarhus, Denmark; [7]University of Liverpool, UK

Background and objectives

Neuropathic pain (NP) may be caused by a lesion or a disease of the somatosensory system [1] and is estimated to afflict as high as 7–8 % of the general population in Europe [2, 3]. The management of NP is challenging because the response to most drugs remains unpredictable [4] despite attempts to develop a more rationale therapeutic approach [5, 6]. In 2006, the European Federation of Neurological Societies (EFNS) produced the first guidelines on pharmacological treatment of NP [7]. Since 2006, new randomized controlled trials (RCTs) have appeared in various NP conditions, justifying an update.

The objectives of our revised task force were: (a) to examine all the RCTs performed in various NP conditions since 2005; (b) to propose recommendations aiming at helping clinicians in their treatment choice for most NP conditions; (c) to propose studies that may clarify unresolved issues.

Methods

We conducted an initial search of the Cochrane Library from 2005. Whenever the Cochrane search failed to identify top-level study for a given NP condition or a potentially effective drug, we expanded the search to MEDLINE and other electronic databases. As in the first guidelines, we produced individual chapters and guidelines based on aetiological conditions. Each chapter was assigned to two or more task force participants. Classification of evidence and recommendation grading adhered to the EFNS standards [8].

Inclusion criteria were: controlled Class I or II trials (lower-class studies were evaluated in conditions in which no higher-level studies were available); trials including patients with probable or definite NP [1] or trigeminal neuralgia; chronic NP (≥3 months); pain considered as the primary outcome (e.g. studies in which dysaesthesia was the primary outcome, as in chemotherapy-induced neuropathy were excluded); minimum sample of 10 patients; treatment duration and follow-up specified; treatment feasible in an outpatient setting; studies evaluating currently used drugs or drugs under clinical phase-III development; full paper citations in English.

Exclusion criteria included duplicated patient series, conditions with no evidence of lesion in the somatosensory system (e.g. CRPS I, fibromyalgia, low back pain), studies using non-validated primary outcome measures, disease-modifying treatments (i.e. alphalipoic acid for diabetes) and pre-emptive treatments.

We extracted information regarding the efficacy on pain, symptoms/signs, quality of life, sleep and mood and side effects (see supplemental web material).

Results

Our search strategy identified 64 RCTs since January 2005 using placebo or active drugs as comparators and three subgroup or post hoc analyses of prior RCTs.

European Handbook of Neurological Management: Volume 1, 2nd edition. Edited by N. E. Gilhus, M. P. Barnes and M. Brainin.
© 2011 Blackwell Publishing Ltd.

Painful polyneuropathy

Painful polyneuropathy (PPN) is a common NP condition. Diabetic and non-diabetic PPN are similar in symptomatology and with respect to treatment response, with the exception of HIV-induced neuropathy.

Antidepressants

The efficacy of tricyclic antidepressants (TCAs) is largely established in PPN (notably diabetic), although mainly based on single-centre Vlass I or II trials [7, 9, 10]. Three RCTs reported the efficacy of venlafaxine ER in PPN, although this seems lower than imipramine on responders and quality of life in a comparative trial [7, 11]. Side effects are mainly gastrointestinal, but elevated blood pressure and clinically significant electrocardiogram (ECG) changes were reported in 5% of patients. The efficacy of duloxetine is established by three large-scale trials in diabetic PPN [12], with similar efficacy to that of gabapentin/pregabalin based on one industry-funded meta-analysis [13], although direct comparisons are lacking; the effect is reported to persist for 1 year [14]. Frequent adverse events are nausea, somnolence, dry mouth, constipation, diarrhoea, hyperhidrosis and dizziness; discontinuation rates are 15–20 % [15, 16]. Duloxetine induces no/little cardiovascular side effects but rare cases of hepatotoxicity have been reported [15]. Selective serotonin reuptake inhibitors (SSRIs) or mianserin provide little or no pain relief [7, 17].

Antiepileptics

Gabapentin and pregabalin are effective in diabetic PPN [18, 19], with dose-dependent effects for pregabalin (several negative studies for 150 mg/day, mainly positive studies for 300–600 mg/day) [19] and similar efficacy between gabapentin and the TCA nortriptyline in a recent Class I study [20]. Side effects include dizziness, somnolence, peripheral oedema, weight gain, aesthenia, headache, and dry mouth. In a recent comparative trial, only two side effects differentiated gabapentin and nortriptyline: dry mouth (more frequent with nortriptyline) and concentration disorders (more frequent with gabapentin) [20]. Discontinuation rates for pregabalin range from 0 (150 mg/day) to 20% (600 mg/day) [19, 21]. All the other trialled antiepileptics show variable and sometimes discrepant results. Smaller Class III trials (carbamazepine) suggest efficacy [7], while larger placebo-controlled studies usually show no or limited benefit

(table 26.1) [7, 22–29]. One reason for this variability could be a large placebo effect [30].

Opioids

Oxycodone, tramadol [31, 32], and tramadol/acetaminophen combination [33] reduce pain in diabetic PPN. Side effects include mainly nausea and constipation, but long-term use of opioids may be associated with misuse (2.6% in a recent 3-year registry study of oxycodone in mainly diabetic NP, although higher rates were also reported) [4, 34]. Tramadol should be used with caution in elderly patients because of risk of confusion and is not recommended with drugs acting on serotonin reuptake such as SSRIs [7, 32]. The tramadol/acetaminophen combination appears better tolerated [33].

Others

Recent studies reported efficacy of botulinum toxin type A [35], nitrate derivatives [36, 37], and a new nicotinic agonist [38]. Of the other drugs trialled in PPN, one reported a positive outcome (levodopa), another showed discrepant results (NMDA antagonists), while the rest had limited or no efficacy (table 26.1) [10, 39].

Combination

Three Class I studies found a superiority of the gabapentin-opioids (morphine, oxycodone) and gapapentin-nortriptyline combinations compared to each drug alone in patients with diabetic PN, including PHN in two studies [20, 40, 41], while a small study suggested superiority of the gabapentin-venlafaxine combination compared with gabapentin and placebo [7].

HIV neuropathy

Most initial trials of HIV neuropathy were negative (table 26.1) [7, 42]. Only lamotrigine was moderately effective in patients receiving antiretroviral treatment [43]. Recent RCTs found efficacy of smoked cannabis (1–8 % tetrahydrocannabinol for 5 days) on pain intensity but not mood or functioning [44, 45]. A one-off application of high-concentration (8%) capsaicin patch applied to the feet for 30, 60 or 90 min was superior to low concentration (0.04%) in the 30- and 90-min group from weeks 2 to 12 without detectable changes in sensory thresholds [46]. However, another study reported in a systematic review [47] was negative on the primary outcome.

Table 26.1 Classification of evidence for drug treatments in commonly studied NP conditions and recommendations for use[a].

Aetiology	Level A rating for efficacy	Level B rating for efficacy	Level C rating for efficacy	Level A/B rating for inefficacy or discrepant results	Recommendations for first line	Recommendations for second or third line
Diabetic NP[1]	Duloxetine Gabapentin-morphine TCA Gabapentin Nicotine agonist** Nitrate derivatives** Oxycodone Pregabalin TCA[2] Tramadol alone or with acetaminophen Venlafaxine ER	Botulinum toxin* Dextrometorphan Gabapentin-venlafaxine* Levodopa*	Carbamazepine Phenytoine	Capsaicin cream Lacosamide Lamotrigine Memantine Mexiletine Mianserin NK1 antagonist** Oxcarbazepine SSRI Topical clonidine Topiramate Valproate Zonisamide	Duloxetine Gabapentin Pregabalin TCA Venlafaxine ER	Opioids Tramadol[3]
PHN	Capsaicin 8% patch** Gabapentin Gabapentin ER** Lidocaine plasters Opioids (morphine, oxycodone, methadone) Pregabalin TCA[2]	Capsaicin cream Valproate*		Benzydamide topical Dextrometorphan Fluphenazine Memantine Lorazepam Mexiletine COX-2 inhibitor** Tramadol	Gabapentin Pregabalin TCA Lidocaine plasters[4]	Capsaicin Opioids
Classical trigeminal neuralgia	Carbamazepine	Oxcarbazepine	Baclofen* Lamotrigine* Pimozide* Tizanidine*		Carbamazepine Oxcarbazepine	Surgery
Central pain[5]	Cannabinoids (oro-mucosal**, oral) (MS) Pregabalin (SCI)	Lamotrigine (CPSP) TCA (SCI, CPSP) Tramadol (SCI)* Opioids		Carbamazepine Gabapentin Lamotrigine (SCI) Levetiracetam Mexiletine S-ketamine iont. Valproate	Gabapentin Pregabalin TCA	Cannabinoids (MS) Lamotrigine Opioids Tramadol (SCI)

[a]Treatments are presented in alphabetical order. Only drugs used at repeated dosages are shown here (with the exception of treatments with long-lasting effects such as capsaicin patches). Drugs marked with an asterisk were found effective in single Class II or III studies and are generally not recommended. Drugs marked with two asterisks are not yet available for use.
[1]Diabetic neuropathy was the most studied. Only TCAs, tramadol and venlafaxine were studied in non-diabetic neuropathies.
[2]Amitriptyline, clomipramine (diabetic neuropathy), nortriptyline, desipramine, imipramine.
[3]Tramadol may be considered first line in patients with acute exacerbations of pain, especially for the tramadol/acetaminophen combination.
[4]Lidocaine is recommended in elderly patients.
[5]Cannabinoids (positive effects in MS) and lamotrigine (positive effects in CPSP but negative results in MS and SCI except in patients with incomplete lesion and brush-induced allodynia in one study based on post-hoc analysis) are proposed for refractory cases.
Abbreviations: iont.: iontophoresis; CPSP: central poststroke pain; ER: extended release; MS: multiple sclerosis; PHN: postherpetic neuralgia; SCI: spinal cord injury; TCA: tricyclic antidepressants.

Postherpetic neuralgia

Postherpetic neuralgia (PHN) is a common aftermath of herpes zoster in the elderly.

Antidepressants

Systematic reviews concur that TCAs are effective in PHN [9, 49] with superiority over SSRI [7, 50]. No studies were found on the efficacy of SNRIs.

Antiepileptics

Gabapentin and pregabalin have established efficacy in PHN with no difference shown between gabapentin and nortriptyline in a further comparative study [20, 49] An extended-release formulation of gabapentin was more effective than placebo [51]. Good efficacy was reported with divalproex sodium in a small RCT but only results from completers were reported [52].

Opioids

Oxycodone, morphine, and methadone are effective in PHN [49] and have similar or slightly better efficacy compared to TCAs in one comparative trial but are associated with more frequent discontinuation due to side effects [7, 49]. Tramadol was negative on the primary outcome in one Class I trial [7].

Topical agents

Lidocaine plasters (5%) are effective based on five Class I or II RCTs in PHN with brush-induced allodynia, but the therapeutic gain is modest against placebo and the level of evidence is lower than for systemic agents [7, 53]. The largest recent trial including patients with or without allodynia (with enriched-enrolment design) was negative on the primary outcome (time-to-exit), but the groups were not balanced at baseline and many patients withdrew prematurely from the study [54]. In an enriched-design open-label trial, lidocaine plaster was better tolerated than pregabalin [55]. Lidocaine plasters are safe due to their low systemic absorption and well tolerated with local adverse effects only (mild skin reactions) [54–56].

RCTs have reported benefit from topical capsaicin 0.075% [7] but due to the burning effect of capsaicin, blinding was probably compromised. An one-off application of high-concentration (8%) capsaicin patch applied to the skin for 60 min was more effective than a low-concentration patch (0.04%) during 12 weeks [57]. Although a post hoc analysis suggests that blinding was successful, patient randomised to the high-concentration patch required more rescue medication immediately after application. Adverse effects were primarily due to local capsaicin-related reactions at the application site (pain, erythema). Efficacy of capsaicin patches was demonstrated in two other studies reported in a systematic review [47].

Others

NMDA antagonists, lorazepam and a selective Cox2 inhibitor do not provide pain relief in PHN (table 26.1) [7, 58].

Trigeminal neuralgia

Trigeminal neuralgia (TN) typically presents with very brief attacks of pain (electric shocks) and is divided into 'classic', when secondary to vascular compression of the trigeminal nerve in the cerebellopontine angle or when no cause is found, or 'symptomatic', when secondary in particular to cerebellopontine-angle masses or multiple sclerosis [59].

Carbamazepine, oxcarbazepine

Carbamazepine is the drug of choice in TN but its efficacy may be compromised by poor tolerability and pharmacokinetic interactions. Two Class II RCTs found similar effects of oxcarbazepine compared to carbamazepine on the number of attacks and global assessment [60, 61].

Others

Several drugs (i.e. lamotrigine, baclofen) have been reported efficacious in TN based on small single trials each [61, 62] (table 26.1), but a Cochrane review [63] concludes that there is insufficient evidence to recommend them in TN. Small open-label studies also suggested therapeutic benefit from botulinum toxin A and some antiepileptics [62–65] (table 26.1).

Symptomatic TN

There are only small open-label Class IV studies in symptomatic TN associated with multiple sclerosis [62].

Recommendation

In agreement with previous guidelines [7, 61, 62], carbamazepine (Level A) and oxcarbazepine (Level B) are confirmed first line for classical TN. Oxcarbazepine may be preferred because of decreased potential for drug interactions. Patients with intolerable side effects may be prescribed lamotrigine (Level C) but should also be considered for a surgical intervention. We deplore the persistent lack of RCTs in symptomatic TN.

Central neuropathic pain

The most frequent central neuropathic pain (CP) states are caused by stroke (central post-stroke pain, CPSP), spinal cord injury (SCI), or multiple sclerosis (MS).

Antidepressants

The beneficial effects of TCAs was suggested in CPSP but one large-scale study was negative in SCI pain probably because of low doses and lack of specific evaluation of NP [7, 66]. A recent RCT in SCI pain showed that high-dose amitriptyline (150 mg/day) relieved pain more than diphenhydramine and gabapentin (3600 mg) in depressed patients [67]. Despite its limitations (small study, high dose of amitriptyline) it suggests that TCAs can justifiably be considered for SCI patients particularly those with depression. No RCT has evaluated the efficacy of SNRIs in CP.

Antiepileptics

The efficacy of pregabalin was demonstrated in a multicentre study of traumatic SCI pain [68] and confirmed in various CP conditions in a single-centre study [20, 69]. Discrepant results were reported with gabapentin and lamotrigine [7, 43, 67, 70]. Negative results were obtained with other antiepileptics (table 26.1) [7, 71].

Opioids

Evidence for efficacy of opioids in CP is based on only one study comparing high and low doses of levorphanol in which patients with peripheral or central NP participated [72]. A recent RCT showed beneficial effect of tramadol on pain intensity but not pain affect, but many side effects were observed and caused attrition in 43% of cases (17% for the placebo) [73].

Cannabinoids

Cannabinoids (tetrahydrocannabinol, oromucosal sprays 2.7 mg delta-9-tetrahydrocannabinol/2.5 mg cannabidiol) were effective in MS-associated pain in two Class I trials [7]. Adverse events (dizziness, dry mouth, sedation, fatigue, gastrointestinal effects, oral discomfort) were reported by 90% of patients in long-term extension study (up to 3 years) but no tolerance was observed [74].

Others

Negative results were obtained with low-dose mexiletine in SCI pain and S-ketamine iontophoretic transdermal in CP [7, 75].

Recommendation

We recommend pregabalin (Level A), amitriptyline (Level B, Level A in other NP conditions) or gabapentin (Level A in other NP conditions) as first line in CP (table 26.1). Tramadol (Level B) may be considered second line. Strong opioids (Level B) are recommended second or third line if chronic treatment is not an issue. Lamotrigine may be considered in CPSP or SCI pain with incomplete cord lesion and brush-induced allodynia (Level B) and cannabinoids in MS (Level A) only if all other treatments fail.

Other NP conditions

The level of evidence for drugs in other NP conditions is reported in table 26.2.

Cancer NP

There is Level A evidence for the efficacy of gabapentin (one study), Level B for TCAs and tramadol and inefficacy of valproate [7, 76, 77].

Table 26.2 Classification of evidence for drug treatments in less commonly studied NP conditions[a].

Aetiology of NP	Level A rating for efficacy	Level B rating for efficacy	Level A/ B rating for inefficacy/ poor efficacy or discrepant results
HIV neuropathy	Capsaicin 8% patch Smoked cannabis	Lamotrigine	Amitriptyline Capsaicin cream Gabapentin Lidocaine plasters Memantine
Post-traumatic or post-surgical NP		Amitriptyline* Botulinum toxin-A*	Cannabinoids Capsaicin Gabapentin Levetiracetam Propranolol Venlafaxine ER
Chronic radiculo-pathy			Morphine* Nortriptyline* Nortriptyline-morphine* Pregabalin Topiramate
Cancer NP	Gabapentin	Amitriptyline* Tramadol*	Valproate
Phantom pain	Morphine Tramadol		Amitriptyline Gabapentin Memantine Mexiletine
Multi-aetiology NP	Bupropion Cannabinoids (oromucosal, synthetic analog) Levorphanol	Methadone TCA (nortriptyline, clomipramine)	Amitriptyline/ketamine topical CCK2 antagonists Dextrometorphan Dihydrocodeine Gabapentin[1] Venlafaxine ER[1] Lidocaine plasters Lamotrigine Lidocaine plasters Mexiletine[1] Nabilone Riluzole

[a]Treatments are presented in alphabetical order. Drugs marked with an asterisk were found effective in single Class II studies.
[1]These drugs were found effective in some spontaneous NP symptoms (gabapentin) or only on brush-induced or static mechanical allodynia (mexiletine, venlafaxine) in single trials.

Traumatic NP

Gabapentin was reported to be ineffective on the primary outcome in a large multicentre trial but improved several secondary outcomes and may be beneficial in a subgroup of patients (Level A), although predictors of the response need to be identified [78]; antidepressants have Level B evidence, good results were reported for botulinum toxin A and discrepant or negative results were obtained with other drugs [79, 80].

Radiculopathy

Pregabalin (Level A), TCAs, and opioids, and their combination (Level B) are ineffective or slightly effective (the combination TCAs–opioids was effective on maximal pain only in one study) [81–83].

Phantom pain

Efficacy of tramadol and morphine was reported (Level A), while gabapentin induced discrepant results [84, 85].

Multi-aetiology NP

Results in multi-aetiology NP are positive mainly for TCAs, opioids and cannabinoids [7, 86–92].

Effects on pain symptoms and signs and predictors of the response

RCTs increasingly assess symptoms and signs [60] and suggest that drugs (gabapentin, oxycodone, topical lidocaine, cannabinoids) have differential effects on the quality of NP (i.e. burning, deep) [7, 93, 94] and that some may alleviate brush-induced and/or static mechanical allodynia based on single trials (TCA, pregabalin, cannabinoids, topical lidocaine, venlafaxine, NMDA antagonists but not lamotrigine) [7, 50, 87, 88, 95]. Although predictors of response to some drugs (e.g. opioids, lidocaine plasters) were identified in post hoc analyses [79, 96, 97], no RCT has yet been designed to detect predictive factors of the response based on baseline phenotypic profile (Level C).

Effects on quality of life, sleep, and mood

Quality of life (QoL), sleep, and mood are frequently impaired in patients with NP [98, 99]. Generally the effects on pain are related to improvement of QoL [100] (see, however, [75]). Beneficial effects of duloxetine, pregabalin, and gabapentin were reported on these outcomes in Class I trials [7, 40, 99, 101]. However, the most con-sistent effects were observed with pregabalin and gabapentin on sleep quality [40, 98] and poor results were reported with pregabalin on QoL or mood in six trials. Three trials reported the efficacy TCA on QoL [40, 99, 102]. Opioids and tramadol improve pain impact on sleep but have discrepant effects on QoL [99], cannabinoids alleviate QoL or sleep [44, 45, 87] but these drugs generally do not improve mood [32, 72, 73, 76, 87].

Final recommendations and issues for future trials

The present revised EFNS guidelines confirm TCAs (25–150 mg/day), gabapentin (1200–3600 mg/day), and pregabalin (150–600 mg/day) as first line for various NP conditions (except for trigeminal neuralgia) and lidocaine plasters (up to three plasters/day) first line in PHN particularly in the elderly. We now are able to recommend SNRIs (duloxetine 60–120 mg/day, venlafaxine 150–225 mg/day) first line in painful polyneuropathies based on their more established efficacy. TCAs raise safety issues at high doses and in the elderly, they are not more effective than gabapentin based on one comparative trial [20], but they are less costly [99]. Pregabalin has pharmacokinetic advantages compared with gabapentin (bid dosing, dose-dependent efficacy) but similar efficacy and tolerability based on meta-analyses. Second line treatments include tramadol (200–400 mg/day), except in select conditions, and capsaicin cream in PHN. Strong opioids are recommended as second/third line despite established efficacy in neuropathic non-cancer pain due to potential risk for abuse on long-term use, as there are still too few long-term safety trials in neuropathic pain [48]. Capsaicin patches are promising for painful neuropathies or PHN (Level A). Cannabinoids (Level A in MS and peripheral NP) are proposed for refractory cases. Combination therapy (Level A for gabapentin combined with opioids or TCAs) is recommended for patients who show partial response to drugs administered alone.

To date, the choice between these different treatments is mainly on their ratio efficacy/safety and on the patient's clinical condition (e.g. comorbidities, contraindications, concomitant treatments). However, in a recent study investigating more than 2000 patients with neuropathic pain due to diabetic neuropathy and postherpetic neuralgia, Baron and colleagues found that patients with these conditions could be subgrouped according to specific sensory profiles [103]. A classification per sensory profiles rather than based merely on aetiology could contribute to minimize pathophysiological heterogeneity within study groups and increase the positive treatment responses [104, 105].

We propose the following strategy for future trials.

1 Efficacy should be based on standardized endpoints [60]; in establishing such efficacy, symptoms/signs and QoL in addition to overall pain should be identified.

2 Identification of responder profiles based on a detailed characterization of symptoms and signs using sensory examination and specific pain questionnaires should contribute to more successful neuropathic pain management.

3 Identical criteria for assessing harmful events should be obtained.

4 Large-scale comparative trials of drugs should be conducted.

5 More large-scale trials are needed to determine the value of combination therapy.

Conflicts of interest

The following authors did trials or have been consultant for the following pharmaceutical companies.

N. Attal: Grunenthal, Novartis, Pfizer, Eli Lilly, Pierre Fabre, Sanofi-Pasteur Mérieux, Astellas.

R. Baron: Pfizer, Genzyme, Grünenthal, Mundipharma, Allergan, Sanofi Pasteur, Medtronic, Eisai, UCB, Lilly.

G. Cruccu: Boeringer Ingelheim, Eli Lilly, Medtronic, Pfizer.

M. Haanpää: Boeringer-Ingelheim, Janssen-Cilag, GlaxoSmithKline, EMEA, Merck, Mundipharma, Orion, Pfizer, Sanof-Pasteur.

P. Hansson: Bioschwartz, GlaxoSmithKline, Eli Lilly/ Boeringer Ingelheim, Grunenthal, Lundbeck, Medtronic, Neurosearch, Pfizer.

T. S. Jensen: Eli Lilly, GlaxoSmithKline, Grunenthal, Pierre Fabre Takeda Pfizer.

T. Nurmikko: Allergan, AstraZeneca, GlaxoSmith-Kline, GWPharma, Napp, Novartis, Pfizer, Renovis, SchwarzPharma.

The authors have no other conflicts to declare.

References

1. Treede RD, Jensen TS, Campbell JN, *et al.* Neuropathic pain: redefinition and a grading system for clinical and research purposes. *Neurology* 2008;**70**:1630–5.

2. Bouhassira D, Lantéri-Minet M, Attal N, Laurent B, Touboul C. Prevalence of chronic pain with neuropathic characteristics in the general population. *Pain* 2008;**136**: 380–7.

3. Torrance N, Smith BH, Bennett MI, Lee AJ. The epidemiology of chronic pain of predominantly neuropathic origin. Results from a general population survey. *J Pain* 2006;**7**: 281–9.

4. Dworkin RH, O'Connor AB, Backonja M, *et al.* Pharmacologic management of neuropathic pain: evidence based recommendations. *Pain* 2007;**132**:237–51 (class I SR).

5. Finnerup NB, Jensen TS. Mechanisms of disease: mechanism-based classification of neuropathic pain-a critical analysis. *Nature Clin Pract Neurol* 2006;**2**:107–15 (class I SR).

6. Baron R. Mechanisms of disease: neuropathic pain: a clinical perspective. *Nature Clin Pract Neurol* 2006;**2**:95–106 (class I SR).

7. Attal N, Cruccu G, Haanpää M, *et al.* EFNS Task Force. EFNS guidelines on pharmacological treatment of neuropathic pain. *Eur J Neurol* 2006;**13**:1153–69 (class I SR).

8. Brainin M, Barnes M, Baron JC, *et al.* Guideline Standards Subcommittee of the EFNS Scientific Committee. Guidance for the preparation of neurological management guidelines by EFNS scientific task forces – revised recommendations. *Eur J Neurol* 2004;**11**:577–81.

9. Saarto T, Wiffen PJ. Antidepressants for neuropathic pain. *Cochrane Database Syst Rev* 2007;(4):CD005454 (class I SR).

10. Finnerup NB, Otto M, McQuay HJ, Jensen TS, Sindrup SH. Algorithm for neuropathic pain treatment: an evidence based proposal. *Pain* 2005;**118**:289–305 (class I SR).

11. Kadiroglu AK, Sit D, Kayabasi H, Tuzcu AK, Tasdemir N, Yilmaz ME. The effect of venlafaxine HCl on painful peripheral diabetic neuropathy in patients with type 2 diabetes mellitus. *J Diabetes Complications* 2008;**22**:241–5 (class II).

12. Kajdasz DK, Iyengar S, Desaiah D, *et al.* Duloxetine for the management of diabetic peripheral neuropathic pain: evidence-based findings from post hoc analysis of three multicenter, randomized, double-blind, placebo-controlled, parallel-group studies. *Clin Ther* 2007;**29** (Suppl.):2536–46 (class I SR).

13. Quilici S, Chancellor J, Löthgren M, *et al.* Meta-analysis of duloxetine versus pregabalin and gabapentin in the treatment of diabetic peripheral neuropathic pain. *BMC Neurology* 2009;**9**:6 (class I SR).

14. Skljarevski V, Desaiah D, Zhang Q, *et al.* Evaluating the maintenance of effect of duloxetine in patients with diabetic peripheral neuropathic pain. *Diab Met Res Rev* 2009;**25**:623–31 (class IV).

15. Gahimer J, Wernicke J, Yalcin I, Ossanna MJ, Wulster-Radcliffe M, Viktrup L. A retrospective pooled analysis of duloxetine safety in 23983 subjects. *Curr Med Res Opin* 2007;**23**:175–84 (class I SR).

16. Sultan A, Gaskell H, Derry S, Moore RA. Duloxetine for painful diabetic neuropathy and fibromyalgia pain: systematic review of randomised trials. *BMC Neurol* 2008;**8**:29 (class I SR).

17. Otto M, Bach FW, Jensen TS, Brøsen K, Sindrup SH. Escitalopram in painful polyneuropathy: a randomized, placebo-controlled, cross-over trial. *Pain* 2008;**139**:275–83 (class I).

18. Wiffen P, McQuay H, Edwards J, Moore RA. Gabapentin for acute and chronic pain. *Cochrane Database Syst Rev* 2005;(20):CD005452 (class I SR).

19. Freeman R, Durso-Decruz E, Emir B. Efficacy, safety and tolerability of pregabalin treatment for painful diabetic peripheral neuropathy; findings from seven randomized controlled trials accross a range of doses. *Diabetes Care* 2008;**31**:1448–54 (class I SR).

20. Gilron I, Baley JM, Tu D, Holdern DR, Jackson AC, Houlden RL. Nortritpyline and gabapentin, alone and in combination for neuropathic pain: a double-blind, randomised controlled crossover trial. *Lancet* 2009;**374**:1252–61.

21. Moore RA, Straube S, Wiffen PJ, Derry S, McQuay HJ. Pregabalin for acute and chronic pain in adults. *Cochrane Database Syst Rev* 2009;(3):CD007076 (class I SR).

22. Rauck RL, Shaibani A, Biton V, Simpson J, Koch B. Lacosamide in painful diabetic peripheral neuropathy: a phase 2 double-blind placebo-controlled study. *Clin J Pain* 2007;**23**:150–8 (class I).

23. Wymer JP, Simpson J, Sen J, Bongardt S. Efficacy and safety of lacosamide in diabetic neuropathic pain: a 18 weeks double blind placebo controlled trial of fixed doses regimens. *Clin J Pain* 2009;**25**:376–85 (class I).

24. Dogra S, Beydoun S, Mazzola J, Hopwood M, Wan Y. Oxcarbazepine in painful diabetic neuropathy: a randomized, placebo-controlled study. *Eur J Pain* 2005;**9**:543–54 (class I).

25. Grosskopf J, Mazzola J, Wan Y, Hopwood M. A randomized, placebo-controlled study of oxcarbazepine in painful diabetic neuropathy. *Acta Neurol Scand* 2006;**114**:177–80 (class I).

26. Beydoun A, Shaibani A, Hopwood M, Wan Y. Oxcarbazepine in painful diabetic neuropathy: results of a dose-ranging study. *Acta Neurol Scand* 2006;**113**:395–404 (class I).

27. Vinik AI, Tuchman M, Safirstein B, *et al.* Lamotrigine for treatment of pain associated with diabetic neuropathy: results of two randomized, double-blind, placebo-controlled studies. *Pain* 2007;**128**:169–79 (class I).

28. Atli A, Dogra S. Zonisamide in the treatment of painful diabetic neuropathy: a randomized, double-blind, placebo-controlled pilot study. *Pain Med* 2005;**6**:225–34 (class II).

29. Shaibani A, Fares S, Selam JL, *et al.* Lacosamide in painful diabetic neuropathy: an 18-week double-blind placebo-controlled trial. *J Pain* 2009;**10**:818–28 (class I).

30. Katz J, Finnerup NB, Dworkin RH. Clinical outcome in neuropathic pain: relationship to study characteristics. *Neurology* 2008;**28**:263–72 (class I SR).

31. Eisenberg E, McNicol ED, Carr DB. Efficacy of mu-opioid agonists in the treatment of evoked neuropathic pain: systematic review of randomized controlled trials. *Eur J Pain* 2006;**10**:667–76 (class I SR).

32. Hollingshead J, Dühmke RM, Cornblath DR. Tramadol for neuropathic pain. *Cochrane Database Syst Rev* 2006;(3):CD003726 (class I SR).

33. Freeman R, Raskin P, Hewitt DJ, *et al.* Randomized study of tramadol/acetaminophen versus placebo in painful diabetic peripheral neuropathy. *Curr Med Res Opin* 2007;**23**:147–61 (class I).

34. Portenoy RK, Farrar JT, Backonja MM, *et al.* Long-term use of controlled-release oxycodone for noncancer pain: results of a 3-year registry study. *Clin J Pain* 2007;**23**:287–99 (class IV).

35. Yuan RY, Sheu JJ, Yu JM, *et al.* Botulinum toxin for diabetic neuropathic pain: a randomized double-blind crossover trial. *Neurology* 2009;**72**:1473–8 (class II).

36. Yuen KC, Baker NR, Rayman G. Treatment of chronic painful diabetic neuropathy with isosorbide dinitrate spray: a double-blind placebo-controlled cross-over study. *Diabetes Care* 2002;**25**:1699–703 (class I).

37. Agrawal RP, Choudhary R, Sharma P, *et al.* Glyceryl trinitrate spray in the management of painful diabetic neuropathy: a randomized double blind placebo controlled cross-over study. *Diabetes Res Clin Pract* 2007;**77**:161–7 (class I).

38. Rowbotham MC, Rachel Duan W, Thomas J, Nothaft W, Backonja MM. A randomized, double-blind, placebo-controlled trial evaluating the efficacy and safety of ABT-594 in patients with diabetic peripheral neuropathic pain. *Pain* 2009;**146**:245–52 (class I).

39. Sindrup SH, Graf A, Sfikas N. The NK1-receptor antagonist TKA731 in painful diabetic neuropathy: a randomised, controlled trial. *Eur J Pain* 2006;**10**:567–71 (class I).

40. Gilron I, Bailey JM, Tu D, Holden RR, Weaver DF, Houlden RL. Morphine, gabapentin, or their combination for neuropathic pain. *N Engl J Med* 2005;**352**:1324–34 (class I).

41. Hanna M, O'Brien C, Wilson MC. Prolonged-release oxycodone enhances the effects of existing gabapentin therapy

in painful diabetic neuropathy patients. *Eur J Pain* 2008;**12**:804–13 (class I).

42. Schifitto G, Yiannoutsos CT, Simpson DM, *et al.* A placebo-controlled study of memantine for the treatment of human immunodeficiency virus-associated sensory neuropathy. *J Neurovirol* 2006;**12**:328–31 (class II).

43. Wiffen PJ, Rees J. Lamotrigine for acute and chronic pain. *Cochrane Database Syst Rev* 2007;(2):CD006044 (class I SR).

44. Abrams DI, Jay CA, Shade SB, *et al.* Cannabis in painful HIV-associated sensory neuropathy: a randomized placebo-controlled trial. *Neurology* 2007;**68**:515–21 (class I).

45. Ellis RJ, Toperoff W, Vaida F, *et al.* Smoked medicinal cannabis for neuropathic pain in HIV: a randomized, crossover clinical trial. *Neuropsychopharmacology* 2009; **34**:672–80 (class II).

46. Simpson DM, Brown S, Tobias J. NGX-4010 C107 Study Group. Controlled trial of high-concentration capsaicin patch for treatment of painful HIV neuropathy. *Neurology* 2008;**70**:2305–13 (class I).

47. Noto C, Pappagallo M, Szallasi A. NGX-4010, a high-concentration capsaicin dermal patch for lasting relief of peripheral neuropathic pain. *Curr Opin Investig Drugs* 2009;**10**:702–10 (class I SR).

48. Eisenberg E, McNicol ED, Carr DB. Efficacy and safety of opioid agonists in the treatment of neuropathic pain of nonmalignant origin: systematic review and meta-analysis of randomized controlled trials. *JAMA* 2005;**293**:3043–52 (class I SR).

49. Hempenstall K, Nurmikko TJ, Johnson RW, A'Hern RP, Rice AS. Analgesic therapy in postherpetic neuralgia: a quantitative systematic review. *PLOS Med* 2005;**2**:e164 (class I SR).

50. Rowbotham MC, Reisner LA, Davies PS, Fields HL. Treatment response in antidepressant-naive postherpetic neuralgia patients: double-blind, randomized trial. *J Pain* 2005;**6**:741–6 (class I).

51. Irving G, Jensen M, Cramer M, *et al.* Efficacy and tolerability of gastric-retentive gabapentin for the treatment of postherpetic neuralgia. *Clin J Pain* 2009;**25**:185–92 (class I).

52. Chandra K, Shafiq N, Pandhi P, Gupta S, Malhotra S. Gabapentin versus nortriptyline in post-herpetic neuralgia patients: a randomized, double-blind clinical trial-the GONIP Trial. *Int J Clin Pharmacol Ther* 2006;**44**:358–63 (class II).

53. Khaliq W, Alam S, Puri N. Topical lidocaine for the treatment of postherpetic neuralgia. *Cochrane Database Syst Rev* 2007;(18):CD004846 (class I SR).

54. Binder A, Bruxelle J, Rogers P, Hans G, Böster I, Baron R. Topical 5% lidocaine (lignocaine) medicated plaster treat-

ment for post-herpetic neuralgia. *Clin Drug Investig* 2009;**29**:393–408 (class II).

55. Baron R, Mayoral V, Leijon G, Binder A, Stergelwald I, Serpell M. 5% lidocaine medicated plaster versus pregabalin in post-herpetic neuralgia and diabetic polyneuropathy: an open-label, non-inferiority two-stage RCT study. *Curr Med Res Op* 2009;**27**:1663–76 (class IV).

56. Hans G, Sabatowski R, Binder A, Boesl I, Rogers P, Baron R. Efficacy and tolerability of a 5% lidocaine medicated plaster for the topical treatment of post-herpetic neuralgia: results of a long-term study. *Curr Med Res Opin* 2009; **25**:1295–305 (class IV).

57. Backonja M, Wallace MS, Blonsky ER, *et al.* NGX-4010, a high concentration capsaicin patch, for the treatment of postherpetic neuralgia: a randomised, double-blind study. *Lancet Neurol* 2009;**7**:1106–2 (class I).

58. Shackelford S, Rauck R, Quessy S, Blum D, Hodge R, Philipson R. A randomized, double-blind, placebo controlled trial of a selective COX2 inhibitor GW406381 in patients with postherpetic neuralgia. *J Pain* 2009;**10**:654–60 (class I).

59. Cruccu G, Truini A. Trigeminal neuralgia and orofacial pains. In: Pappagallo M. (ed.) *The Neurological Basis of Pain*, New York: McGraw Hill, 2005; pp. 401–14.

60. Cruccu G, Sommer C, Anand P, *et al.* EFNS guidelines on neuropathic pain assessment. 2009 revision, *Eur J Neurol* (submitted) 2010; Mar 8; epud ahead of print.

61. Gronseth G, Cruccu G, Alksne J, *et al.* Practice parameter: the diagnostic evaluation and treatment of trigeminal neuralgia (an evidence-based review): report of the Quality Standards Subcommittee of the American Academy of Neurology and the European Federation of Neurological Societies. *Neurology* 2008;**71**:1183–90 (class I SR).

62. Cruccu G, Gronseth G, Alksne J, *et al.* AAN-EFNS guidelines on trigeminal neuralgia management. *Eur J Neurol* 2008;**15**:1013–28 (class I SR).

63. Nurmikko T, Cruccu G. Botulinum toxin for trigeminal neuralgia. *Eur J Neurol* 2009;**16**:e104.

64. Lemos L, Flores S, Oliveira P, Almeida A. Gabapentin supplemented with ropivacain block of trigger points improves pain control and quality of life in trigeminal neuralgia patients when compared with gabapentin alone. *Clin J Pain* 2008;**24**:64–75 (class IV).

65. He L, Wu B, Zhou M. Non-antiepileptic drugs for trigeminal neuralgia. *Cochrane Database Syst Rev* 2006;(3): CD004029 (class I SR).

66. Klit H, Finnerup NB, Jensen TS. Central post-stroke pain: clinical characteristics, pathophysiology, and management. *Lancet Neurol* 2009;**9**:857–68 (class I SR).

67. Siddall PJ, Cousins MJ, Otte A, Griesing T, Chambers R, Murphy TK. Pregabalin in central neuropathic pain associ-

ated with spinal cord injury: a placebo-controlled trial. *Neurology* 2006;**67**:1792–800 (class I).

68. Vranken JH, Dijkgraaf MG, Kruis MR, Van der Vegt MH, Hollmann MW, Heesen M. Pregabalin in patients with central neuropathic pain: a randomized, double-blind, placebo-controlled trial of a flexible-dose regimen. *Pain* 2008;**136**:150–7 (class I).

69. Rintala DH, Holmes SA, Courtade D, Fiess RN, Tastard LV, Loubser PG. Comparison of the effectiveness of amitriptyline and gabapentin on chronic neuropathic pain in persons with spinal cord injury. *Arch Phys Med Rehab* 2007;**88**:1547–60 (class II).

70. Breuer B, Pappagallo M, Knotkova H, Guleyupoglu N, Wallenstein S, Portenoy RK. A randomized, double-blind, placebo-controlled, two-period, crossover, pilot trial of lamotrigine in patients with central pain due to multiple sclerosis. *Clin Ther* 2007;**29**:2022–30 (class II).

71. Finnerup NB, Grydehoj J, Bong J, *et al.* Levetiracetam in spinal cord injury pain: a randomized controlled trial. *Spinal Cord* 2009;**47**:861–7 (class I).

72. Rowbotham MC, Twilling L, Davies PS, Reisner L, Taylor K, Mohr D. Oral opioid therapy for chronic peripheral and central neuropathic pain. *New Engl J Med* 2003;**348**:1223–32 (class I).

73. Norrbrink C, Lundeberg T. Tramadol in neuropathic pain after spinal cord injury: a randomized double blind placebo-controlled trial. *Clin J Pain* 2009;**25**:177–84 (class II).

74. Rog DJ, Nurmikko TJ, Young CA. Oromucosal delta9-tetrahydro cannabinolcannabidiol for neuropathic pain associated with multiple sclerosis: an uncontrolled, open-label, 2-year extension trial. *Clin Ther* 2007;**29**:2068–79 (class IV).

75. Vranken JH, Dijkgraaf MG, Kruis MR, Van Dasselaar NT, Van der Vegt MH. Iontophoretic administration of S(+)-ketamine in patients with intractable central pain: a placebo-controlled trial. *Pain* 2005;**118**:224–31 (class II).

76. Arbaiza D, Vidal O. Tramadol in the treatment of neuropathic cancer pain: a double-blind, placebo-controlled study. *Clin Drug Investig* 2007;**27**:75–83 (class I).

77. Hardy JR, Rees EA, Gwilliam B, Ling J, Broadley K, A'Hern R. A phase II study to establish the efficacy and toxicity of sodium valproate in patients with cancer-related neuropathic pain. *J Pain Symptom Manage* 2001;**21**:204–9 (class II).

78. Gordh TE, Stubhaug A, Jensen TS, *et al.* Gabapentin in traumatic nerve injury pain: a randomized, double-blind, placebo-controlled, cross-over, multi-center study. *Pain* 2008;**138**:255–66 (class I).

79. Ranoux D, Attal N, Morain F, Bouhassira D. Botulinum toxin a induces direct analgesic effects in neuropathic pain: a double blind placebo controlled study. *Ann Neurol* 2008;**64**:274–83 (class I).

80. Vilholm OJ, Cold S, Rasmussen L, Sindrup SH. Effect of levetiracetam on the postmastectomy pain syndrome. *Eur J Neurol* 2008;**15**:851–7 (class I).

81. Khoromi S, Patsalides A, Parada S, Salehi V, Meegan JM, Max MB. Topiramate in chronic lumbar radicular pain. *J Pain* 2005;**6**:829–36 (class II).

82. Khoromi S, Cui L, Nackers L, Max MB. Morphine, nortriptyline and their combination vs. placebo in patients with chronic lumbar root pain. *Pain* 2007;**130**:66–75 (class II).

83. Baron R, Freyhagen R, Tolle TR, Cloutier C, Leon T, Murphy TK, Phillips K. The efficacy and safety of pregabalin in the treatment of neuropathic pain associated with chronic lumbosacral radiculopathy. *Pain* 2010; may 19, epud ahead of print.

84. Wu CL, Agarwal S, Tella PK, *et al.* Morphine versus mexiletine for treatment of postamputation pain: a randomized, placebo-controlled, crossover trial. *Anesthesiology* 2008;**109**:289–96 (class I).

85. Wilder-Smith CH, Hill LT, Laurent S. Postamputation pain and sensory changes in treatment-naive patients: characteristics and responses to treatment with tramadol, amitriptyline, and placebo. *Anesthesiology* 2005;**103**:619–28 (class II).

86. Karst M, Salim K, Burstein S, Conrad I, Hoy L, Schneider U. Analgesic effect of the synthetic cannabinoid CT-3 on chronic neuropathic pain: a randomized controlled trial. *JAMA* 2003;**290**:1757–62 (class I).

87. Nurmikko TJ, Serpell MG, Hoggart B, Toomey PJ, Morlion BJ, Haines D. Sativex successfully treats neuropathic pain characterised by allodynia: a randomised, double-blind, placebo-controlled clinical trial. *Pain* 2007;**133**:210–20 (class I).

88. Yucel A, Ozyalcin S, Koknel Talu G, *et al.* The effect of venlafaxine on ongoing and experimentally induced pain in neuropathic pain patients: a double blind, placebo controlled study. *Eur J Pain* 2005;**9**:407–16 (class II).

89. Frank B, Serpell MG, Hughes J, Matthews JN, Kapur D. Comparison of analgesic effects and patient tolerability of nabilone and dihydrocodeine for chronic neuropathic pain: randomised, crossover, double blind study. *BMJ* 2008;**336**:199–201 (class I).

90. Ho KY, Huh BK, White WD, Yeh CC, Miller EJ. Topical amitriptyline versus lidocaine in the treatment of neuropathic pain. *Clin J Pain* 2008;**24**:51–5 (class II).

91. Silver M, Blum D, Grainger J. Double blind placebo-controlled trial of lamotrigine in combination with other medications for neuropathic pain. *J Pain Symptom Manage* 2007;**34**:446–54 (class I).

92. Yelland MJ, Poulos CJ, Pillans PI, *et al*. N-of-1 randomized trials to assess the efficacy of gabapentin for chronic neuropathic pain. *Pain Med* 2009;**10**:754–61.

93. Jensen MP, Friedman M, Bonzo D, Richards P. The validity of the neuropathic pain scale for assessing diabetic neuropathic pain in a clinical trial. *Clin J Pain* 2006;**22**:97–103 (class II).

94. Jensen MP, Chiang Y-K, Wu J. Assessment of pain quality in a clinical trial of gabapentin extended release for postherpetic neuralgia. *Clin J Pain* 2009;**25**:286–92 (class II).

95. Stacey BR, Barrett JA, Whalen E, Phillips KF, Rowbotham MC. Pregabalin for postherpetic neuralgia: placebo-controlled trial of fixed and flexible dosing regimens on allodynia and time to onset of pain relief. *J Pain* 2008;**9**:1006–17 (class I).

96. Edwards RR, Haythornthwaite JA, Tella P, Max MB, Raja S. Basal heat pain thresholds predict opioid analgesia in patients with postherpetic neuralgia. *Anesthesiology* 2006;**104**:1243–8 (class II).

97. Wasner G, Kleinert A, Binder A, Schattschneider J, Baron R. Postherpetic neuralgia: topical lidocaine is effective in nociceptor deprived skin. *J Neurol* 2005;**252**:677–6 (class II).

98. Jensen MP, Chodroff MJ, Dworkin RH. The impact of neuropathic pain on health-related quality of life: review and implications. *Neurology* 2007;**68**:1178–82 (class I SR).

99. O'Connor AB. Neuropathic pain. Quality-of-life impact, costs and cost effectiveness of therapy. *Pharmacoeconomics* 2009;**27**:95–112 (class I SR).

100. Deshpande MA, Holden RR, Gilron I. The impact of therapy on quality of life and mood in neuropathic pain: what is the effect of pain reduction? *Anesth Analg* 2006;**102**:1473–9.

101. Armstrong DG, Chappell AS, Le TK, *et al*. Duloxetine for the management of diabetic peripheral neuropathic pain: evaluation of functional outcomes. *Pain Med* 2007;**8**:410–8 (class I SR).

102. Otto M, Bach FW, Jensen TS, Sindrup SH. Health-related quality of life and its predictive role for analgesic effect in patients with painful polyneuropathy. *Eur J Pain* 2007;**11**:572–8 (class I SR).

103. Baron R, Tölle TR, Gockel U, Brosz M, Freynhagen R. A cross-sectional cohort survey in 2100 patients with painful diabetic neuropathy and postherpetic neuralgia: differences in demographic data and sensory symptoms. *Pain* 2009;**146**:34–40.

104. Cruccu G, Truini A. Sensory profiles: a new strategy for selecting patients in treatment trials for neuropathic pain. *Pain* 2009;**146**:5–6.

105. Attal N, Fermanian C, Fermanian J, Lanteri-Minet M, Alchaar H, Bouhassira D. Neuropathic pain: are there distinct subtypes depending on the aetiology or anatomical lesion? *Pain* 2008;**138**:343–53.

CHAPTER 27

Acute relapses of multiple sclerosis

F. Sellebjerg,[1] D. Barnes,[2] G. Filippini,[3] R. Midgard,[4] X. Montalban,[5] P. Rieckmann,[6] K. Selmaj,[7] L. H. Visser,[8] P. Soelberg Sørensen[1]

[1]University of Copenhagen and Rigshospitalet, Copenhagen, Denmark; [2]Atkinson Morley's Hospital, Wimbledon, UK; [3]Fondazione Istituto Nazionale Neurologico C. Besta, Milan, Italy; [4]Molde Hospital, Norway; [5]University Hospital Vall d'Hebron, Barcelona, Spain; [6]University of British Columbia and Vancouver Coastal Health, Vancouver, British Columbia, Canada; [7]Medical University of Lodz, Poland; [8]St Elisabeth Hospital, Tilburg, The Netherlands

Background

Attacks or relapses are the dominating feature of relapsing–remitting multiple sclerosis (MS), but are also observed in patients with secondary progressive MS with superimposed relapses. Even patients with primary progressive MS may experience relapses, becoming progressive-relapsing MS [1, 2]. In the McDonald criteria for the diagnosis of MS, a relapse is defined as 'an episode of neurological disturbance of the kind seen in MS, when the clinicopathological studies have established that the causative lesions are inflammatory and demyelinating in nature' [3, 4]. An attack should last for at least 24 h. and, according to the McDonald criteria, there should be expert opinion that the event is not a pseudoattack as might be caused by an increase in body temperature or infection. Although the majority of relapses improve to some extent, incomplete recovery is an important determinant of irreversible, or at least long-lasting, neurological impairment in relapsing–remitting MS [5, 6].

Glucocorticoid treatment is recommended as the first-line treatment of MS relapses in North American guidelines and in the recommendations of a European MS therapy consensus group [7, 8]. The aim of the European Federation of Neurological Societies (EFNS) task force was to review the current literature on relapse treatment. Key issues addressed are whether treatment of MS

relapses: (1) can improve the speed of recovery; (2) can influence long-term recovery; (3) can influence subsequent disease activity; (4) has significant side effects. Furthermore, the task force sought to provide guidelines on whether all relapses should be treated and how relapses during pregnancy should be managed.

Search strategy

We searched literature databases (EMBASE and PubMed), in English, for papers using the search terms 'multiple sclerosis', 'attack', 'relapse', 'exacerbation', and 'treatment' in November 2004 and November 2009. The Cochrane Library and the reference lists of individual papers were searched for studies not identified in the EMBASE and PubMed searches. Studies of various treatments for patients suffering from relapses of MS were considered for the guidelines and were rated as Class I to Class IV studies according to the recommendations for EFNS scientific task forces [9].

Method for reaching consensus

The results of the literature searches were circulated by email to the task force members for comments. The task force chairman prepared a first draft of the manuscript based on the results of the literature review and comments from the task force members. The draft and the recommendations were discussed during telephone conferences until consensus was reached within the task

European Handbook of Neurological Management: Volume 1, 2nd edition. Edited by N. E. Gilhus, M. P. Barnes and M. Brainin. © 2011 Blackwell Publishing Ltd.

force. Recommendations were rated from A to C according to the EFNS guidelines for scientific task forces [9]. Where there was insufficient evidence to support firm recommendations the term 'Good Practice Point' (GPP) was used.

Results

Effect of glucocorticoid and adrenocorticotrophic hormone (ACTH) treatment on MS relapses

Glucocorticoid or ACTH treatment of MS relapses was analysed in a Cochrane review that included results from six randomized, placebo-controlled clinical trials of either ACTH (two trials), intravenous (i.v.) methylprednisolone treatment (three trials) or oral methylprednisolone treatment (one trial) [10–15]. All trials reported a benefit in terms of rate of recovery compared to placebo [16]. A similar conclusion was reached in another meta-analysis, which used less stringent criteria for study inclusion than the Cochrane review [17].

Three trials have compared the efficacy of i.v. methylprednisolone and ACTH treatment in MS relapses [18–20]. One study including 14 patients treated with i.v. methylprednisolone (1 g daily for 7 days) and 11 patients treated with intramuscular (IM) ACTH (80 units, 60 units, 40 units, and 20 units daily, each for 1 week) reported more rapid improvement (after 3 and 28 days) after i.v. methylprednisolone than after ACTH treatment, but there was no significant difference after 3 months [19]. However, the patient blinding and the primary outcome were not clearly defined, for which reason this study should be considered a Class III study. One Class II study compared the administration of 1 g of methylprednisolone once daily for 3 days to ACTH treatment (80 units for 7 days, 40 units for 4 days and 20 units for 3 days) in 61 patients, and found no difference in terms of rate of recovery or final outcome after 12 weeks [20]. A Class III study including 60 patients, treated with either i.v. methylprednisolone (20 mg/kg day 1–3, 10 mg/kg day 4–7, 5 mg/kg day 8–10, and 1 mg/kg day 11–15) or ACTH (1 mg i.v. daily for 15 days), also found no difference in the efficacy of ACTH and methylprednisolone treatment [18]. The studies found no major differences in adverse events between methylprednisolone and ACTH treatment. Thus there is no evidence of any major difference

in the efficacy of ACTH and methylprednisolone treatment from comparative studies, but the clinical trials were too small to rule out some difference in efficacy. Indeed, in the Cochrane review it was suggested that methylprednisolone treatment could still confer greater benefit than treatment with ACTH, and the administration of methylprednisolone is simpler than the more prolonged ACTH treatment regimen [16].

In a separate meta-analysis of three double-blind, randomized, placebo-controlled trials [21], it was concluded that treatment with i.v. methylprednisolone (15 mg/kg day 1–3, 10 mg/kg day 4–6, 5 mg/kg day 7–9, 2.5 mg/kg day 10–12, 1 mg/kg day 13–15 followed by oral prednisone tapered slowly over 120 days [10]), i.v. methylprednisolone without a tapering dose (500 mg once daily for 5 days [13]), or oral methylprednisolone (500 mg once daily for 5 days followed by 400, 300, 200, 100, 64, 48, 32, 16, 8, and 8 mg once daily the subsequent 10 days [15]) resulted in significantly faster recovery than did treatment with placebo (table 27.1). The first two trials provided follow-up data in a placebo-controlled design for 15 days [10] and 28 days [13]. The oral methylprednisolone study found significant differences between the methylprednisolone and the placebo group after 8 weeks and a trend to better improvement in the methylprednisolone group after 1 year [15]. In the latter trial there was no evidence that the 1-year risk of subsequent relapses was influenced by oral high-dose methylprednisolone treatment.

Specific glucocorticoids, dose, and route of administration

The clinical trials of glucocorticoid treatment in relapses of MS have mainly assessed the effect of methylprednisolone treatment. Two trials have compared the effect of methylprednisolone treatment given i.v. or orally. One Class III study compared the effect of methylprednisolone (500 mg once daily for 5 days) given orally or i.v. in 35 patients with an MS relapse, and found no significant difference in recovery between the two treatment arms after 5 and 28 days [22]. Another study (Class I) compared the effect of oral methylprednisolone (48 mg daily for 7 days, 24 mg daily for 7 days, and 12 mg daily for 7 days) to treatment with i.v. methylprednisolone (1 g daily for 3 days) [23]. In this study, recovery from the relapse was similar in the 38 patients in the i.v. treatment group and the 42 patients in the oral treatment group at all time points for

Table 27.1 Summary of three randomized, placebo-controlled trials comparing methylprednisolone (MP) treatment to placebo in patients with relapses of MS (Durelli *et al.* [10]; Milligan *et al.* [12]; Sellebjerg *et al.* [15]). Data are changes in Kurtzke EDSS scores from baseline (mean and standard deviation in brackets) or differences (mean and 95% confidence intervals in brackets) between MP and placebo reported in a meta-analysis (Miller *et al.* [21]).

Study and treatment	Change from baseline	Difference (MP vs placebo)
Day 5–7		
Durelli, placebo (*n* = 8)	0 (0)	
i.v. methylprednisolone (*n* = 12)	−1.00 (0.6)	−1.00 (−1.45 to −0.55)
Milligan, placebo (*n* = 9)	−0.28 (0.51)	
i.v. methylprednisolone (*n* = 13)	−1.46 (1.38)	−1.18 (−2.19 to −0.17)
Sellebjerg, placebo (*n* = 25)	−0.06 (0.44)	
Oral methylprednisolone (*n* = 26)	−0.58 (0.82)	−0.52 (−0.89 to −0.14)
Pooled difference:		−0.76 (standard error 0.14)
Day 21–28		
Durelli, placebo (*n* = 8)	−0.38 (0.52)	
i.v. methylprednisolone (*n* = 12)	−2.04 (1.48)	−1.67 (−2.82 to −0.51)
Milligan, placebo (*n* = 8)	−0.25 (1.22)	
i.v. methylprednisolone (*n* = 13)	−2.04 (1.51)	−1.79 (−3.11 to −0.46)
Sellebjerg, placebo (*n* = 25)	−0.38 (0.81)	
Oral methylprednisolone (*n* = 26)	−0.94 (0.90)	−0.56 (−1.04 to −0.08)
Pooled difference:		−0.85 (standard error 0.21)

up to 24 weeks of follow-up. The relapse rate the following 2 years was also similar in the oral and i.v. treatment group [24]. A Class III study comparing the effect of i.v. and oral methylprednisolone (1000 mg daily for 5 days) in 40 patients found comparable effect of the two treatment regimens on magnetic resonance imaging (MRI) outcomes [25]. A recent Cochrane review concluded that oral and i.v. treatment are both efficacious with respect to clinical outcomes (relapse recovery and subsequent relapse activity), radiological outcomes, and bioavailability measures, but that there is still insufficient evidence to prove equivalence of oral and i.v. treatment [26].

Oral tapering doses of glucocorticoids are commonly used, but no randomized controlled studies have yet compared the outcome of a relapse in patients treated with tapering doses of glucocorticoids or placebo following short-term, high-dose methylprednisolone treatment. However, a recent Class III study found no difference in recovery rate in 152 patients treated with high-dose methylprednisolone followed by an oral prednisone taper and 112 patients treated with high-dose methylprednisolone only [27].

Three studies have compared i.v. methylprednisolone treatment given in different doses. One Class III study

found that recovery was faster after treatment with i.v. methylprednisolone (1 g once daily for 5 days) than after a single 1 g dose of i.v. methylprednisolone [28]. Two other studies (both Class III) have compared the effect of different doses of i.v. methylprednisolone in relapses of MS on a panel of different outcome measures. In the first study, treatment with i.v. methylprednisolone at a dose of 500 mg once daily for 5 days was compared to treatment with 2000 mg once daily for 5 days in 31 patients with a relapse of MS [29]. There was no difference in the efficacy of the low dose and the high dose of methylprednisolone in terms of clinical recovery or short-term suppression of MRI disease activity, but it was suggested that the high dose resulted in more pronounced suppression of MRI disease activity after 1 and 2 months. In the second study, i.v. methylprednisolone at a dose of 1 g or 2 g once daily for 5 days was compared in 24 patients who were followed up with clinical and neurophysiologic studies for 21 days after randomization to one of the two treatment arms [30]. This study showed no significant differences between the two methylprednisolone doses on the majority of diverse outcome measures, but a few favoured the higher dose over the lower dose. Two studies have compared the effect of treatment with different doses of methylprednisolone and dexamethasone in relapses of MS [31, 32]. Due to the small sample sizes and differences in the baseline characteristics of the patients randomized to the different treatment arms, the results of these two studies are difficult to interpret.

Glucocorticoid treatment of acute optic neuritis

In the North American Optic Neuritis Treatment Trial (ONTT), 457 patients were randomized to receive treatment with i.v. methylprednisolone (250 mg four times daily for 3 days followed by oral prednisone, 1 mg/kg for 11 days, 20 mg on day 15, and 10 mg on days 16 and 18), oral prednisone (1 mg/kg for 14 days, 20 mg on day 15, and 10 mg on days 16 and 18), or oral placebo [33]. Treatment allocation was not blinded in patients randomized to treatment with i.v. methylprednisolone, while prednisone treatment and placebo was given in a double-blind design. Thus, the study was a Class II study investigating the efficacy of methylprednisolone treatment, but a Class I study in the comparison of oral prednisone and placebo. The study found no significant effect of i.v. methylprednisolone or oral prednisone treatment on the recovery of visual acuity, but the recovery of contrast sensitivity and visual fields was significantly faster in patients treated with i.v. methylprednisolone. After 6 months, patients treated with i.v. methylprednisolone had still recovered slightly better than patients treated with placebo, but no significant treatment effect was seen at follow-up after 1 year [34]. Oral prednisone treatment had no effect on the recovery from acute optic neuritis in either the ONTT or a Danish Class I study of oral prednisolone versus placebo in 128 patients with acute optic neuritis ([33], J.L. Frederiksen, personal communication). Treatment with oral methylprednisolone (100 mg, 80 mg, 60 mg, 40 mg, 30 mg, 20 mg, 10 mg, and 5 mg daily for 3 days each) was not better than treatment with oral thiamine (100 mg daily for 24 days) on any of several outcome measures in a Class II study including 38 patients with acute optic neuritis [35].

Two additional studies (Class I) have compared the effect of treatment with high-dose methylprednisolone in acute optic neuritis. One study included 60 patients with acute optic neuritis who were treated with oral high-dose methylprednisolone (500 mg once daily for 5 days followed by 400, 300, 200, 100, 64, 48, 32, 16, 8, and 8 mg once daily the subsequent 10 days) or oral placebo [36].

Oral methylprednisolone treatment resulted in significantly better recovery of spatial visual function (visual acuity and contrast sensitivity), colour vision function, and visual symptoms after 1 week, but only borderline significant effects were observed after 3 weeks, and after 8 weeks there was no evidence of an effect of oral methylprednisolone treatment [36]. In a study of 66 patients with acute optic neuritis treatment with i.v. methylprednisolone (1 g once daily for 3 days) did not improve the outcome from acute optic neuritis after 26 weeks on either a panel of visual function and neurophysiologic variables or on MRI outcome measures [37].

A controversial finding in the ONTT was that patients treated with i.v. methylprednisolone appeared to have a lower risk of developing MS during 2 years of follow-up than patients treated with placebo. This was not statistically significant in the original trial report [33], but reached a significance level of $p = 0.03$ (not corrected for multiple comparisons) in a post hoc analysis where the baseline status of many patients had been reclassified [38, 39]. It was also suggested that oral prednisone treatment was associated with an increased risk of recurrent optic neuritis, but not an increased risk of subsequently developing MS [33, 38]. As there was no blinding to methylprednisolone treatment, and as the effect of treatment on MS risk was only observed after reanalysis and reclassification of the initial data, this part of the ONTT must be regarded as a Class III study. Another Class III study (a retrospective natural history study) has suggested that i.v. methylprednisolone treatment (1 g once daily for 3 days) could actually increase the risk of subsequently developing MS [40]. In the latter study, a surprisingly low risk of conversion to MS was, however, observed in the control group of untreated patients and patients treated with oral prednisone.

Glucocorticoid treatment in MS subgroups

Whether subgroups of patients with MS relapses may benefit more from glucocorticoid treatment has been addressed in only a few studies. It has been suggested that patients with more severe relapses are more likely to respond to treatment with i.v. methylprednisolone (Class IV evidence) [41]. Another uncontrolled (Class IV) study suggested that patients with high cerebrospinal fluid (CSF) concentrations of myelin basic protein (MBP) are more likely to improve after i.v. methylprednisolone treatment [42]. This finding was confirmed using 1-week follow-up data in a post hoc analysis of patients included in two randomized, placebo-controlled trials of oral high-dose methylprednisolone treatment [43]. However, the additional benefit of methylprednisolone treatment in patients with high CSF concentrations of MBP was not sustained at follow-up after 8 weeks, while patients who had an active gadolinium-enhanced MRI at baseline appeared to benefit from treatment even at follow-up after 8 weeks (Class III evidence) [43].

Side effects of glucocorticoid treatment

In the placebo-controlled trials serious adverse events were not observed after high-dose methylprednisolone treatment [10, 13, 15]. Milligan et al. did not report the precise frequency of adverse events, but noted that treatment was surprisingly free from serious adverse events [13]. Those most frequently reported were a slight reddening of the face, transient ankle swelling, and a metallic taste in the mouth during infusion. In the Cochrane review it was concluded that the oral administration of methylprednisolone is associated with a higher frequency of side effects (mainly gastrointestinal and psychic disorders), and that oral administration should be avoided for this reason [16]. In the study of Durelli et al. the incidence of elevated mood and insomnia increased during the study from two out of 11 patients (18%) treated with intravenous high-dose methylprednisolone at day 5 to five out of 11 patients (45%) at day 15 [10]. In the study of oral high-dose treatment with an oral tapering dose and a total treatment duration of 15 days, disturbed sleep was observed in 65% and slight mood changes in 23% [15], which is not significantly different from the frequency observed by Durelli and coworkers. Durelli and coworkers (1986) did not report gastrointestinal side effects, but all patients received prophylactic antacid treatment. In the study of oral high-dose methylprednisolone treatment, gastrointestinal side effects (mainly heartburn not requiring symptomatic treatment) were observed in 38% of patients treated with oral methylprednisolone and 8% in the placebo group [15]. The randomized comparisons of i.v. and oral treatment with methylprednisolone at equivalent doses found that the side effects of oral and i.v. methylprednisolone treatment were similar [22, 25]. This is supported by the results of a smaller, non-randomized

Class III study comparing treatment with i.v. methylprednisolone and oral prednisone at equivalent doses, which also failed to detect any difference in the side effects of oral and i.v. treatment [44].

In a review of 240 patients, who had been treated with one or more courses of i.v. methylprednisolone (1 g daily for 5 days followed by 10 days of oral prednisone treatment), minor infections were observed in four patients; one patient had a single seizure within 12 h of treatment, 11 patients were noted to have glucosuria during treatment, five had gastrointestinal symptoms that required antacid or H2 antagonist treatment, three patients had an exacerbation of acne, ankle oedema was recorded in two patients, and one patient was hypertensive during treatment. A feeling of wellbeing was common (frequency not given), and four patients had episodes of euphoria, whereas two patients were depressive. Transient facial flushing, a transient disturbance of taste, distal paraesthesia, insomnia, and mild weight gain occurred in a significant proportion of patients, but the exact frequency was not stated [45].

Severe side effects of methylprednisolone treatment are rare, but psychosis, acute pancreatitis, and anaphylactoid reactions to i.v. treatment have been reported [46–49]. Short-term methylprednisolone treatment in patients with MS appears to be safe in terms of long-term effects on bone mineralization, but pulsed methylprednisolone treatment has short-term effects on bone metabolism [50], and a recent study indicates that the risk of avascular bone necrosis after methylprednisolone treatment may not be negligible [51].

Other treatments

A single Class I crossover study of 22 patients with severe relapses of inflammatory demyelination (including 12 with MS) who were refractory to treatment with high-dose methylprednisolone suggested a beneficial effect of treatment with plasma exchange [52]. In this study there was 'moderate' or 'marked' improvement during plasma exchange treatment in eight out of 19 patients (42%), whereas such improvement was observed only after one out of 17 courses (6%) of sham treatment ($p = 0.01$). Open (Class IV) studies have also reported an effect of plasma exchange in patients with acute optic neuritis who had not improved after high-dose i.v. methylprednisolone treatment [53, 54]. One study found that an effect of plasma exchange that was sustained after 6 months was more likely when treatment was initiated early and in patients who had shown improvement already at hospital discharge [55].

Intravenous immunoglobulin (IVIg) treatment is widely used in a variety of neurological diseases. A single Class IV study of intravenous IVIg treatment in relapses of MS suggested that as many as 68% of patients improved within 24 h of treatment [56]. Two studies have investigated if IVIg treatment as add-on to therapy with high-dose i.v. methylprednisolone is superior to add-on placebo treatment [57, 58]. Both studies were negative on primary and secondary end-points.

A phase III study of IVIg treatment reported marked improvement in 23 patients with severe visual impairment after methylprednisolone treatment of optic neuritis, whereas there was no improvement in a control group comprising 24 patients treated with methylprednisolone only [59]. However, in this study spontaneous recovery in the control group was surprisingly poor, and a randomized Class I trial of treatment with IVIg or placebo in 68 patients with acute optic neuritis failed to detect any treatment effect [60].

Whereas treatment with natalizumab lowers the frequency of relapses in MS, natalizumab was not efficacious in the treatment of relapses in a randomized, placebo-controlled Class I study of 180 patients with an MS relapse [61].

A single Class II study compared the effect of multidisciplinary rehabilitation with the effect of 'standard therapy' in a randomized clinical trial design, where both treatment arms received i.v. methylprednisolone treatment. The study suggested that a multidisciplinary team rehabilitation programme results in better functional recovery after 3 months than does treatment with i.v. methylprednisolone in a 'standard' setting [62].

Treatment of relapses during pregnancy

There are no specific studies on relapse treatment in pregnant patients with MS, but short-term treatment with glucocorticoids is generally considered safe in pregnant women, and treatment may be considered in patients with a relapse of sufficient severity to warrant treatment, although treatment during the first trimester should probably be avoided (Class IV evidence [63]).

Recommendations

There is consistent evidence from several Class I studies and meta-analyses for a beneficial effect of glucocorticoid treatment in relapses of MS. Hence, treatment with intravenous or oral methylprednisolone in a dose of at least 500 mg daily for 5 days should be considered for treatment of relapses (Level A). Treatment with i.v. methylprednisolone (1 g once daily for 3 days with an oral tapering dose) may be considered for treatment of acute optic neuritis (Level B). Treatment with i.v. methylprednisolone (1 g once daily for 3 days) should be considered as an alternative treatment (GPP; [8]).

There is no evidence of major differences in the efficacy of methylprednisolone treatment given i.v. or orally in terms of clinical efficacy or side effects, but prolonged oral treatment may possibly be associated with a higher prevalence of side effects. Furthermore, due to the low number of patients included in the available clinical trials, some efficacy differences between the i.v. and oral route of administration cannot be excluded. The optimal dosage, the specific glucocorticoid to use, and whether to use a taper after initial pulse therapy, has not been adequately addressed in randomized controlled trials. This implies a need for new randomized studies assessing risk/benefit ratios and adverse effects of specific glucocorticoids, dose, and route of administration for treatment of MS relapses.

There is insufficient data to clearly define patient subgroups who are more likely to respond to methylprednisolone treatment, but treatment may be more efficacious in patients with clinical, MRI, or CSF evidence indicating higher disease activity (Level C recommendation). Home versus outpatient administration of i.v. steroids was evaluated in one clinical trial [64], and in one large French survey of home-based treatment of MS relapses with i.v. methylprednisolone [65]. The results of both studies indicate that treatment with i.v. steroids can be effectively and safely administered at home. Consideration may, however, sometimes be given to administering the first course of methylprednisolone as an inpatient (GPP).

In patients who fail to respond to therapy with methylprednisolone in the dose range used in the randomized, placebo-controlled trials [10, 11, 13, 15], treatment with higher doses (up to 2 g daily for 5 days) should be considered (Level C recommendation [8]).

There is insufficient data to support the use of IVIg therapy as monotherapy for relapses of MS. Treatment with IVIg as an add-on to treatment of MS relapses with methylprednisolone or as monotherapy for acute optic neuritis is not efficacious (Level A recommendation). Neither is natalizumab as monotherapy efficacious in MS relapses.

Patients with inflammatory demyelination, including patients with MS, who have not responded to treatment with methylprednisolone may benefit from plasma exchange treatment, but only about one-third of treated patients are likely to respond. This treatment regimen should probably be restricted to a subgroup of patients with severe relapses (Level B recommendation). A randomized controlled study specifically addressing the effect of plasma exchange and IVIg treatment in patients with severe relapses of MS not responding to methylprednisolone treatment would be desirable.

A more intense, interdisciplinary rehabilitation programme should be considered after treatment with i.v. methylprednisolone as evidence from a single trial suggests that this probably further improves recovery (Level B recommendation).

Conflicts of interest

Authors of this chapter have received the following: honoraria for lecturing, serving on advisory councils or trial steering committees; covering of travel expenses for attending meetings; or research grants from Almirall, Bayer Schering Pharma, Biogen Idec, EMD, Genentech, GenMab, Genzyme, Lundbeck, Merck Serono, Novartis, Novo Nordisk, Sanofi-aventis or Teva.

References

1. Confavreux C, Vukusic S, Moreau T, Adeleine P. Relapses and progression of disability in multiple sclerosis. *N Engl J Med* 2000;**343**(20):1430–8.
2. Lublin FD, Reingold SC. Defining the clinical course of multiple sclerosis: results of an international survey. National Multiple Sclerosis Society (USA) Advisory Committee on Clinical Trials of New Agents in Multiple Sclerosis. *Neurology* 1996;**46**(4):907–11.
3. McDonald WI, Compston A, Edan G, *et al*. Recommended diagnostic criteria for multiple sclerosis: guidelines from the International Panel on the diagnosis of multiple sclerosis. *Ann Neurol* 2001;**50**(1):121–7.
4. Polman CH, Reingold SC, Edan G, *et al*. Diagnostic criteria for multiple sclerosis: 2005 revisions to the 'McDonald Criteria'. *Ann Neurol* 2005;**58**(6):840–6.
5. Confavreux C, Vukusic S, Adeleine P. Early clinical predictors and progression of irreversible disability in multiple sclerosis: an amnesic process. *Brain* 2003;**126**(Pt 4):770–82.
6. Lublin FD, Baier M, Cutter G. Effect of relapses on development of residual deficit in multiple sclerosis. *Neurology* 2003;**61**(11):1528–32.
7. Goodin DS, Frohman EM, Garmany GP Jr, *et al*. Disease modifying therapies in multiple sclerosis: report of the Therapeutics and Technology Assessment Subcommittee of the American Academy of Neurology and the MS Council for Clinical Practice Guidelines. *Neurology* 2002;**58**(2): 169–78.
8. Rieckmann P, Toyka KV, Bassetti C, *et al*. Escalating immunotherapy of multiple sclerosis – new aspects and practical application. *J Neurol* 2004;**251**(11):1329–39.
9. Brainin M, Barnes M, Baron JC, *et al*. Guidance for the preparation of neurological management guidelines by EFNS scientific task forces – revised recommendations 2004. *Eur J Neurol* 2004;**11**(9):577–81.
10. Durelli L, Cocito D, Riccio A, *et al*. High-dose intravenous methylprednisolone in the treatment of multiple sclerosis: clinical-immunologic correlations. *Neurology* 1986;**36**(2): 238–43.
11. Filipovic SR, Drulovic J, Stojsavljevic N, Levic Z. The effects of high-dose intravenous methylprednisolone on event-related potentials in patients with multiple sclerosis. *J Neurol Sci* 1997;**152**(2):147–53.
12. Miller H, Newell DJ, Ridley A. Multiple sclerosis. Treatment of acute exacerbations with corticotrophin (A.C.T.H.). *Lancet* 1961;**2**(7212):1120–2.
13. Milligan NM, Newcombe R, Compston DA. A double-blind controlled trial of high dose methylprednisolone in patients with multiple sclerosis: 1. Clinical effects. *J Neurol Neurosurg Psychiatry* 1987;**50**(5):511–6.
14. Rose AS, Kuzma JW, Kurtzke JF, Namerow NS, Sibley WA, Tourtellotte WW. Cooperative study in the evaluation of therapy in multiple sclerosis. ACTH vs. placebo – final report. *Neurology* 1970;**20**(5):1–59.
15. Sellebjerg F, Frederiksen JL, Nielsen PM, Olesen J. Double-blind, randomized, placebo-controlled study of oral, high-dose methylprednisolone in attacks of MS. *Neurology* 1998;**51**(2):529–34.
16. Filippini G, Brusaferri F, Sibley WA *et al*. Corticosteroids or ACTH for acute exacerbations in multiple sclerosis. *Cochrane Database Syst Rev* 2000;(4):CD001331.
17. Brusaferri F, Candelise L. Steroids for multiple sclerosis and optic neuritis: a meta-analysis of randomized controlled clinical trials. *J Neurol* 2000;**247**(6):435–42.

18. Abbruzzese G, Gandolfo C, Loeb C. 'Bolus' methylprednisolone versus ACTH in the treatment of multiple sclerosis. *Ital J Neurol Sci* 1983;**4**(2):169–72.

19. Barnes MP, Bateman DE, Cleland PG, *et al.* Intravenous methylprednisolone for multiple sclerosis in relapse. *J Neurol Neurosurg Psychiatry* 1985;**48**(2):157–9.

20. Thompson AJ, Kennard C, Swash M, *et al.* Relative efficacy of intravenous methylprednisolone and ACTH in the treatment of acute relapse in MS. *Neurology* 1989;**39**(7):969–71.

21. Miller DM, Weinstock-Guttman B, Bethoux F, *et al.* A meta-analysis of methylprednisolone in recovery from multiple sclerosis exacerbations. *Mult Scler* 2000;**6**(4):267–73.

22. Alam SM, Kyriakides T, Lawden M, Newman PK. Methyl-prednisolone in multiple sclerosis: a comparison of oral with intravenous therapy at equivalent high dose. *J Neurol Neurosurg Psychiatry* 1993;**56**(11):1219–20.

23. Barnes D, Hughes RA, Morris RW, *et al.* Randomised trial of oral and intravenous methylprednisolone in acute relapses of multiple sclerosis. *Lancet* 1997;**349**(9056): 902–6.

24. Sharrack B, Hughes RA, Morris RW, *et al.* The effect of oral and intravenous methylprednisolone treatment on subsequent relapse rate in multiple sclerosis. *J Neurol Sci* 2000;**173**(1):73–7.

25. Martinelli V, Rocca MA, Annovazzi P, *et al.* A short-term randomized MRI study of high-dose oral vs intravenous methylprednisolone in MS. *Neurology* 2009;**73**(22):1842–8.

26. Burton JM, O'Connor PW, Hohol M, Beyene J. Oral versus intravenous steroids for treatment of relapses in multiple sclerosis. *Cochrane Database Syst Rev* 2009;(3):CD006921.

27. Perumal JS, Caon C, Hreha S, *et al.* Oral prednisone taper following intravenous steroids fails to improve disability or recovery from relapses in multiple sclerosis. *Eur J Neurol* 2008;**15**(7):677–80.

28. Bindoff L, Lyons PR, Newman PK, Saunders M. Methylpred-nisolone in multiple sclerosis: a comparative dose study. *J Neurol Neurosurg Psychiatry* 1988;**51**(8):1108–9.

29. Oliveri RL, Valentino P, Russo C, *et al.* Randomized trial comparing two different high doses of methylprednisolone in MS: a clinical and MRI study. *Neurology* 1998;**50**(6): 1833–6.

30. Fierro B, Salemi G, Brighina F, *et al.* A transcranial magnetic stimulation study evaluating methylprednisolone treatment in multiple sclerosis. *Acta Neurol Scand* 2002;**105**(3): 152–7.

31. La Mantia L, Eoli M, Milanese C, Salmaggi A, Dufour A, Torri V. Double-blind trial of dexamethasone versus methylprednisolone in multiple sclerosis acute relapses. *Eur Neurol* 1994;**34**(4):199–203.

32. Milanese C, La ML, Salmaggi A, *et al.* Double-blind randomized trial of ACTH versus dexamethasone versus methyl-prednisolone in multiple sclerosis bouts. Clinical, cerebrospinal fluid and neurophysiological results. *Eur Neurol* 1989;**29**(1):10–4.

33. Beck RW, Cleary PA, Anderson MM Jr, *et al.* A randomized, controlled trial of corticosteroids in the treatment of acute optic neuritis. The Optic Neuritis Study Group. *N Engl J Med* 1992;**326**(9):581–8.

34. Beck RW, Cleary PA. Optic neuritis treatment trial. One-year follow-up results. *Arch Ophthalmol* 1993;**111**(6):773–5.

35. Trauzettel-Klosinski S, Axman D, Diener HC. The Tübingen study on optic neuritis – a prospective, randomized and controlled trial. *Clin. Vis. Sci.* 1993. **8**:385–94.

36. Sellebjerg F, Nielsen HS, Frederiksen JL, Olesen J. A randomized, controlled trial of oral high-dose methylprednisolone in acute optic neuritis. *Neurology* 1999;**52**(7):1479–84.

37. Kapoor R, Miller DH, Jones SJ, *et al.* Effects of intravenous methylprednisolone on outcome in MRI-based prognostic subgroups in acute optic neuritis. *Neurology* 1998;**50**(1): 230–7.

38. Beck RW, Cleary PA, Trobe JD, *et al.* The effect of corticosteroids for acute optic neuritis on the subsequent development of multiple sclerosis. The Optic Neuritis Study Group. *N Engl J Med* 1993;**329**(24):1764–9.

39. Goodin DS. Perils and pitfalls in the interpretation of clinical trials: a reflection on the recent experience in multiple sclerosis. *Neuroepidemiology* 1999;**18**(2):53–63.

40. Herishanu YO, Badarna S, Sarov B, Abarbanel JM, Segal S, Bearman JE. A possible harmful late effect of methylpred-nisolone therapy on a time cluster of optic neuritis. *Acta Neurol Scand* 1989;**80**(6):569–74.

41. Nos C, Sastre-Garriga J, Borras C, Rio J, Tintore M, Montalban X. Clinical impact of intravenous methylpred-nisolone in attacks of multiple sclerosis. *Mult Scler* 2004; **10**(4):413–6.

42. Whitaker JN, Layton BA, Herman PK, Kachelhofer RD, Burgard S, Bartolucci AA. Correlation of myelin basic protein-like material in cerebrospinal fluid of multiple sclerosis patients with their response to glucocorticoid treatment. *Ann Neurol* 1993;**33**(1):10–7.

43. Sellebjerg F, Jensen CV, Larsson HB, Frederiksen JL. Gadolinium-enhanced magnetic resonance imaging predicts response to methylprednisolone in multiple sclerosis. *Mult Scler* 2003;**9**(1):102–7.

44. Metz LM, Sabuda D, Hilsden RJ, Enns R, Meddings JB. Gastric tolerance of high-dose pulse oral prednisone in multiple sclerosis. *Neurology* 1999;**53**(9):2093–6.

45. Lyons PR, Newman PK, Saunders M. Methylprednisolone therapy in multiple sclerosis: a profile of adverse effects. *J Neurol Neurosurg Psychiatry* 1988;**51**(2):285–7.

46. Chrousos GA, Kattah JC, Beck RW, Cleary PA. Side effects of glucocorticoid treatment. Experience of the

Optic Neuritis Treatment Trial. *JAMA* 1993;**269**(16): 2110–2.

47. Deruaz CA, Spertini F, Souza LF, Du Pasquier RA, Schluep M. Anaphylactic reaction to methylprednisolone in multiple sclerosis: a practical approach to alternative corticosteroids. *Mult Scler* 2007;**13**(4):559–60.

48. Pryse-Phillips WE, Chandra RK, Rose B. Anaphylactoid reaction to methylprednisolone pulsed therapy for multiple sclerosis. *Neurology* 1984;**34**(8):1119–21.

49. van den Berg JS, van Eikema Hommes OR, Wuis EW, Stapel S, van der Valk PG. Anaphylactoid reaction to intravenous methylprednisolone in a patient with multiple sclerosis. *J Neurol Neurosurg Psychiatry* 1997; **63**(6):813–4.

50. Dovio A, Perazzolo L, Osella G, *et al*. Immediate fall of bone formation and transient increase of bone resorption in the course of high-dose, short-term glucocorticoid therapy in young patients with multiple sclerosis. *J Clin Endocrinol Metab* 2004;**89**(10):4923–8.

51. Ce P, Gedizlioglu M, Gelal F, Coban P, Ozbek G. Avascular necrosis of the bones: an overlooked complication of pulse steroid treatment of multiple sclerosis. *Eur J Neurol* 2006;**13**(8):857–61.

52. Weinshenker BG, O'Brien PC, Petterson TM, *et al*. A randomized trial of plasma exchange in acute central nervous system inflammatory demyelinating disease. *Ann Neurol* 1999;**46**(6):878–86.

53. Ruprecht K, Klinker E, Dintelmann T, Rieckmann P, Gold R. Plasma exchange for severe optic neuritis: treatment of 10 patients. *Neurology* 2004;**63**(6):1081–3.

54. Trebst C, Reising A, Kielstein JT, Hafer C, Stangel M. Plasma exchange therapy in steroid-unresponsive relapses in patients with multiple sclerosis. *Blood Purif* 2009;**28**(2): 108–15.

55. Llufriu S, Castillo J, Blanco Y, *et al*. Plasma exchange for acute attacks of CNS demyelination: predictors of improvement at 6 months. *Neurology* 2009;**73**(12):949–53.

56. Soukop W, Tschabitscher H. Gamma globulin therapy in multiple sclerosis. Theoretical considerations and initial clinical experiences with 7S immunoglobulins in MS therapy. *Wien Med Wochenschr* 1986;**136**(18):477–80.

57. Sørensen PS, Haas J, Sellebjerg F, Olsson T, Ravnborg M. IV immunoglobulins as add-on treatment to methylprednisolone for acute relapses in MS. *Neurology* 2004;**63**(11): 2028–33.

58. Visser LH, Beekman R, Tijssen CC, *et al*. A randomized, double-blind, placebo-controlled pilot study of i.v. immune globulins in combination with i. v. methylprednisolone in the treatment of relapses in patients with MS. *Mult Scler* 2004;**10**(1):89–91.

59. Tselis A, Perumal J, Caon C, *et al*. Treatment of corticosteroid refractory optic neuritis in multiple sclerosis patients with intravenous immunoglobulin. *Eur J Neurol* 2008; **15**(11):1163–7.

60. Roed HG, Langkilde A, Sellebjerg F, *et al*. A double-blind, randomized trial of IV immunoglobulin treatment in acute optic neuritis. *Neurology* 2005;**64**(5):804–10.

61. O'Connor PW, Goodman A, Willmer-Hulme AJ, *et al*. Randomized multicenter trial of natalizumab in acute MS relapses: clinical and MRI effects. *Neurology* 2004;**62**(11): 2038–43.

62. Craig J, Young CA, Ennis M, Baker G, Boggild M. A randomised controlled trial comparing rehabilitation against standard therapy in multiple sclerosis patients receiving intravenous steroid treatment. *J Neurol Neurosurg Psychiatry* 2003;**74**(9):1225–30.

63. Ferrero S, Pretta S, Ragni N. Multiple sclerosis: management issues during pregnancy. *Eur J Obstet Gynecol Reprod Biol* 2004;**115**(1):3–9.

64. Chataway J, Porter B, Riazi A, *et al*. Home versus outpatient administration of intravenous steroids for multiple-sclerosis relapses: a randomised controlled trial. *Lancet Neurol* 2006;**5**(7):565–71.

65. Creange A, Debouverie M, Jaillon-Riviere V, *et al*. Home administration of intravenous methylprednisolone for multiple sclerosis relapses: the experience of French multiple sclerosis networks. *Mult Scler* 2009;**15**(9): 1085–91.

CHAPTER 28

Status epilepticus

H. Meierkord,[1] P. Boon,[2] B. Engelsen,[3] K. Göcke,[4] S. Shorvon,[5] P. Tinuper,[6] M. Holtkamp[1]

[1]Charité – Universitätsmedizin Berlin, Germany; [2]Ghent University Hospital, Belgium; [3]Haukeland University Hospital, and University of Bergen, Bergen, Norway; [4]Deutsche Epilepsievereinigung e.V., Berlin, Germany; [5]Institute of Neurology, University College London, UK; [6]University of Bologna, Italy

Background

Incidence, mortality, and morbidity

Generalised convulsive and non-convulsive status epilepticus (GCSE, NCSE) are important neurological conditions potentially associated with significant mortality and morbidity rates. Annual incidence rates of GCSE range from 3.6 to 6.6 per 100 000 and of NCSE from 2.6 to 7.8 per 100 000 [1–3]. Mortality and morbidity rates of SE are heavily influenced by the underlying aetiology and it is therefore difficult to give reliable figures for the condition itself [1, 4, 5]. In a recent large US sample including more than 11 000 patients, in-hospital mortality of GCSE was 3.5% [6]. Predictors of death were old age, mechanical ventilation, cerebrovascular disease, female sex, and a higher comorbidity index. In particular, mortality rates of NCSE after profound brain damage are high and usually due to the injury itself [5].

There is general agreement that immediate and effective treatment is required. First-line anticonvulsants like benzodiazepines and phenytoin fail to terminate SE in 30–50% of cases [7–9]. SE continuing after such failure is termed refractory status epilepticus (RSE) and represents an even more difficult clinical problem. Drug treatment approaches in this situation are based on prospective observational studies, retrospective series, case reports, and expert opinions. The goal of this paper is to summarise published treatment options for generalised convulsive and non-convulsive SE. Post-anoxic myoclonus is not considered in this guideline since there is no agreement regarding its epileptic nature. The focus of this article is on critical care situations in adults, and SE in children is not considered.

Mechanisms

The basic processes generating SE may be seen as a failure of the normal mechanisms that terminate seizures. Reduced inhibition and persistent excessive excitation create interactions that produce and sustain ongoing seizure activity. During prolonged seizure activity dynamic changes in gamma-aminobutyric acid (GABA)$_A$ and N-methyl-D-aspartate (NMDA) receptor function are seen that have been termed 'receptor trafficking' [10]. Ongoing seizure activity results in gradual reduction of GABA$_A$ receptors at the synaptic membrane following receptor internalisation into endocytotic vesicles and subsequent degradation [11]. This process results in erosion of endogenous GABAergic inhibition giving rise to sustained epileptic activity. Loss of postsynaptic GABA$_A$ receptors is a relevant pathophysiological factor on the way to progressive pharmacoresistance of drugs such as benzodiazepines, barbiturates, and propofol. In contrast, during ongoing epileptic activity NMDA receptors are progressively transported to the synaptic membrane, resulting in increasing numbers of excitatory NMDA receptors per synapse [12]. This process facilitates neuronal excitability and consecutively sustained SE. On the other hand, the enhanced expression of glutamate receptors may present a useful target in the pharmacological management of advanced stages of SE. Absence SE with 3-Hz spike-wave discharges are induced by excessive inhibition [13]. This form of SE does not lead to the neuronal injury seen with excessive excitation [14].

European Handbook of Neurological Management: Volume 1, 2nd edition. Edited by N. E. Gilhus, M. P. Barnes and M. Brainin.

Search strategy

One member of the task force panel (HM) searched available published reports from 1966 to 2005 and for the purpose of the current updated version from 2005 to 2009 using the database MEDLINE and EMBASE (last search in January 2009). The search was limited to papers published in English. The subject term 'status epilepticus' was combined with the terms 'controlled clinical trial', 'randomised controlled trial', 'multicentre study', 'meta-analysis', and 'crossover study'. Furthermore, the Cochrane Central Register of Controlled Trials (CENTRAL) was sought. Finally, the websites of the World Health Organization (WHO), the International League against Epilepsy (ILAE), and the American Neurological Association (ANA) were explored to look for additional information.

Evaluation of published literature

The evidence for therapeutic interventions (Class I–IV) and the rating of recommendations (level A–C) were classified by using the definitions previously reported [15].

Methods for reaching consensus

The other members of the task force read the first draft of the recommendations and discussed changes (informative consensus approach). Where there was a lack of evidence but consensus was clear we have stated our opinion as Good Practice Points (GPP).

Definitions

The time that has to evolve to define ongoing epileptic activity as 'status epilepticus' is as yet not generally agreed on. The Commission on Classification and Terminology of the International League Against Epilepsy defines SE as 'a seizure [that] persists for a sufficient length of time or is repeated frequently enough that recovery between attacks does not occur' [16]. Experimental studies have shown irreversible neuronal damage after about 30 min of continuing epileptic activity [17]. Therefore, this time window has been adopted by the majority of authors [1, 2, 18]. On the other hand, some clinical data indicate that spontaneous cessation of generalised convulsive seizures is unlikely after 5 min [19, 20] and therefore acute treat-

ment with anticonvulsants is required. Consequently, Lowenstein *et al.* have proposed an operational definition of SE that is based on a duration of 5 min [21]. Currently, clinical studies are based on 5 min [22], 10 min [8, 23], or 30 min [2, 24] of ongoing epileptic activity to define SE. The diagnosis of NCSE is based on changes in behaviour and/or mental processes from baseline associated with continuous epileptiform discharges in the EEG [25]. There is currently no generally accepted duration of electro-clinical alterations incorporated in the diagnostic criteria of NCSE.

NCSE includes the subtypes of absence status, complex partial, and subtle status epilepticus. Absence SE with 3-Hz spike-wave discharges is a benign type of NCSE, in most cases of which a small i.v. dose of lorazepam or diazepam will terminate the event. Therefore, absence SE is not further considered in this paper. CPSE represents the most frequent type and accounts for almost every second case of all forms of SE [2]. Subtle SE evolves from previously overt GCSE and is characterised by coma and ongoing electrographic seizure activity without any or with only subtle convulsive movements [23]. Subtle SE therefore is a form of NCSE that develops from GCSE if the latter has been treated insufficiently or has not been treated at all.

An appropriate definition of refractory SE also is still missing. The failure of two [8, 26] or three [27, 28] anticonvulsants has been suggested in combination with a minimal duration of the condition of 1 h [8, 29, 30] or 2 h [26, 31] or regardless of the time that has elapsed since onset [24, 27].

Results

Literature and data on treatment

Initial treatment of generalised convulsive status epilepticus

High-level evidence for the initial pharmacological treatment of GCSE has been given in some randomised controlled trials (RCTs) that are indicated below. In 384 patients with GCSE, intravenous (i.v.) administration of 0.1 mg/kg lorazepam was successful in 64.9% of cases, 15 mg/kg phenobarbital in 58.2% of cases, and 0.15 mg/kg diazepam directly followed by 18 mg/kg phenytoin in 55.8% of cases; the efficacy of these anticonvulsants was not significantly different [23] (Class I). The same trial has shown that in pairwise comparison initial monotherapy with 18 mg/kg phenytoin is significantly less effective than administration of lorazepam. Another RCT has focused on the pre-hospital treatment of GCSE performed by paramedics [22] (Class I). A total of 205 patients were administered 2 mg of i.v. lorazepam, 5 mg of i.v. diazepam, or placebo; the injection of identical doses of benzodiazepines was repeated when seizures continued for more than 4 min. Lorazepam terminated SE in 59.1% of cases and was as effective as diazepam (42.6%). Both drugs were significantly superior to the administration of placebo (21.1%). An earlier RCT on 81 episodes of all clinical forms of SE compared i.v. administration of 4 mg lorazeapm versus 10 mg diazepam, which were repeated when seizures continued or recurred after 10 min [32] (Class II). In episodes of GCSE with or without focal onset ($n = 39$), 13 episodes responded to lorazepam after the first administration and three after the second, while three episodes did not respond. With diazepam, 14 episodes responded to the first administration and two to the second, while four episodes did not respond. In a recent randomised open study, first-line anticonvulsant treatment of GCSE with 30 mg/kg valproic acid in 35 patients has been compared with 18 mg/kg phenytoin in another 33 cases [33] (Class III). Valproic acid terminated SE in 66% of cases, while phenytoin was successful in 42% ($p = 0.046$). Unfortunately, this study was underpowered, giving rise to cautious interpretation of the results. Also, the study was not limited to adults, but also included a significant number of children and adolescents in whom SE usually is less difficult to terminate. Another randomised open study on first-line treatment of SE compared valproic acid in 18 patients to phenytoin in nine cases using the same doses as in the latter above study [34] (Class III). Valproic acid (72%) was found to be as successful as phenytoin (78%). Unfortunately, this study too, did not yield data of major relevance for the treatment with first-line substances, since it also was underpowered and included patients with CGSE and CPSE, each of which is known to be associated with a different prognosis.

Initial treatment of complex partial status epilepticus

Currently, there are no studies available focusing exclusively on the initial anticonvulsant treatment of CPSE. Some trials included patients with CPSE but did not specify the success rate of anticonvulsant drugs in this form of SE [34, 35].

Initial treatment of subtle status epilepticus

The pharmacological treatment of subtle SE has been addressed in a RCT with 134 patients [23] (Class I). The i.v. administration of lorazepam (0.1 mg/kg), diazepam (0.15 mg/kg) followed by phenytoin (18 mg/kg), phenobarbital (18 mg/kg), and phenytoin (18 mg/kg) terminated SE in 8–24% of cases, only. Success rates were not significantly different between the drugs or drug combinations tested. However, the key criterion for study entry was the evidence of subtle SE at the time of evaluation, regardless of prior treatment. Though not further specified, it can be assumed that in some of the patients anticonvulsants have been administered before.

Side effects of initial treatment of status epilepticus

Safety issues of the common initial anticonvulsants have been compared in patients with overt GCSE as well as in patients with subtle SE [23] (Class I). In overt GCSE, hypoventilation was observed in 10–17% of cases, hypotension in 26–34%, and cardiac arrhythmias in 2–7%. These side effects were more frequent in subtle SE and ranged between 3 and 59% of cases. Distribution of side effects was not significantly different in patients treated with lorazepam, diazepam followed by phenytoin, phenobarbital, and phenytoin in overt and subtle SE. Out-of-hospital administration of benzodiazepines compared with placebo did not result in more complications such as arterial hypotension, cardiac arrhythmias, or respiratory depression requiring intervention [22] (Class I). These side effects occurred in 10.6% of patients treated with lorazepam, 10.3% treated with diazepam, and 22.5% given placebo.

Refractory generalised convulsive and non-convulsive SE

The rationale for treating refractory SE with anaesthetising anticonvulsants is to prevent both severe acute systemic and long-term neuronal consequences. Acute systemic complications such as pulmonary oedema and – potentially fatal – cardiac arrhythmias may occur early in the course of GCSE [36] but are rarely seen in CPSE. In experimental animal models, prolonged electrographic seizure activity results in brain damage [37, 38]. To what extent these findings can be translated to the human situation is not known. But it is for this reason that most authorities recommend general anaesthesia to obtain a burst suppression pattern on the EEG if initial therapy has not controlled SE within 1–2 h. However, there are no studies comparing anaesthetic therapy with continuing non-anaesthetising anticonvulsants. The therapeutic decision is based on the type of status epilepticus, age, comorbidity, and prognostic issues. This is of special relevance in patients with CPSE since the risks of anaesthesia (e.g. arterial hypotension, gastroparesis, immunosuppression, etc.) may be greater than the risks of ongoing non-convulsive epileptic activity [39]. In view of the lack of controlled studies, the decision on further treatment is based on a few retrospective studies and expert opinions. Retrospective studies have analysed the further treatment options after failure of initial anticonvulsants [8]. It should be noted that treatment pathways were naturally influenced by multiple variables such as aetiology, age, and comorbidity. In 26 episodes of RSE, after failure of first- and second-line drugs, 23 episodes were treated with a third-line drug that was non-anaesthetising in all but one case. In 12 of these episodes seizures were controlled, but 11 patients needed further more aggressive treatment [8] (Class IV). In another study, RSE was terminated by further non-anaesthetising anticonvulsants in 18 out of 35 episodes [40] (Class IV). However, data in both studies did not differentiate between GCSE and CPSE.

In view of the very few clinical studies, further available evidence has to be based on experts' opinions. Two surveys have been performed, one on the treatment of GCSE among American neurologists [41] and another on the management of refractory GCSE and CPSE among epileptologists and critical care neurologists in Austria, Germany, and Switzerland [42]. American neurologists did not agree on how to proceed in pharmacological treatment of SE after failure of benzodiazepines and phenytoin or fosphenytoin: more than 80% would not directly proceed to an anaesthetic (43% administer phenobarbital and 16% valproic acid), while 19% would directly administer anaesthetic [41] (Class IV). However, this survey did not include the management of refractory CPSE. The European survey revealed that after failure of benzodiazepines and phenytoin, two-thirds of the participants would administer in both GCSE and CPSE another non-anaesthetising anticonvulsant, the majority preferred phenobarbital. Immediate administration of an anaesthetic was preferred by 35% in GCSE and by 16%

in CPSE [42] (Class IV). Three-quarters of the experts did not administer anaesthetics in refractory CPSE at all, while all did at some time point in GCSE. Administration of anaesthetics was withheld in CPSE: more than 60% of the participants administer anaesthetics not earlier than 60 min after onset of status compared to only 21% of participants waiting that long in GCSE.

Further non-anaesthetising anticonvulsants
Though phenobarbital has been assessed in the initial anticonvulsant treatment [23] of SE, sufficient data on the efficacy of the substance after failure of benzodiazepines and phenytoin/fosphenytoin are missing. Doses of 20 mg/kg infused at a rate of 30–50 mg/min are used.

The role of i.v. valproic acid in the treatment of RSE is yet to be defined. Valproic acid is a non-sedating substance that has not caused hypotension or respiratory suppression and has been reported to be effective in generalised convulsive and complex partial RSE [43] (Class IV). In a randomised open study, SE refractory to diazepam administered in adequate doses was treated with valproic acid (20 mg/kg) or phenytoin (20 mg/kg) in 50 patients each [44] (Class III). Treatment success was 88 and 84% respectively. The clinical forms of SE that were included into the study are not reported, and approximately 30% of patients were younger than 18 years. In a retrospective study that included 63 patients with previously untreated or refractory GCSE, overall efficacy rates of 63% were reported, and valproic acid was even more successful in RSE [45] (Class IV). Loading doses of 25–45 mg/kg at infusion rates of up to 6 mg/kg/min have been suggested [46] (Class IV), and favourable tolerance of rapid administration ranging from 200 to 500 mg/min was reported [45] (Class IV).

Levetiracetam is a second-generation antiepileptic drug with proven oral efficacy in epilepsies with generalised and/or partial seizures. The substance is non-sedating and has almost no interactions with other drugs. In 2006, its i.v. formulation has been introduced into the market. Retrospective data describe treatment success in at least benzodiazepine-refractory SE in 16 out of 18 episodes with loading doses of i.v. levetiracetam between 250 and 1500 mg [47] (Class IV). A recent prospective observational study reported termination of 10 out of 11 episodes of various clinical forms of SE with i.v. levetiractam administered in a dose of 2500 mg in 5 min [48] (Class IV). In both studies, adverse effects of i.v. levetiracetam were negligible.

Lacosamide has been licensed in Europe and the US in autumn 2008 as oral and i.v. formulation for the adjunctive treatment of partial epilepsies. The pharmacokinetic profile is interesting for the treatment of SE as well; however, so far there has been only one report on its efficacy in a patient with non-convulsive predominantly aphasic SE [49].

Neither levetiracetam nor lacosamide is licensed for the treatment of SE.

Anaesthetising anticonvulsants

Most authorities recommend administration of anaesthetic agents to a depth of anaesthesia which produces a burst suppression pattern in the EEG [42] (Class IV) or an isoelectric EEG [50]. Studies are needed in this area, as these issues give rise to ethically highly problematic decisions.

Barbiturates, midazolam, and propofol are commonly used in refractory SE [42] (Class IV). There have been no RCTs comparing these treatment options. These substances have been assessed in prospective oberservational studies. Thiopental anaesthesia was induced in 10 patients with an initial bolus of 5 mg/kg and additional boluses of 1–2 mg/kg to achieve burst suppressions [51]. Thereafter, the infusion rate was started at 5 mg/kg/h and had to be increased to a median of 7 mg/kg/h to maintain burst suppression. In one patient, epileptic seizure activity reoccurred following tapering of thiopental after 12 h burst suppression. Mean arterial pressure decreased in all patients and required catecholamines in four. Nine patients were treated with antibiotics due to infection, indicating that high-dose thiopental anaesthesia may be immunosuppressive. Midazolam anaesthesia was induced in 19 patients with a bolus of 0.2 mg/kg followed by continuous infusion at a starting rate of 1 μg/kg/min [52] (Class IV). Infusion rate was increased to a median of 8 μg/kg/min to control clinical seizures. Seizure activity was terminated in all but one patient, and no patient developed haemodynamically relevant arterial hypotension or other important medical side effects. Propofol anaesthesia was induced in 10 consecutive patients with a bolus of 2–3 mg/kg, and further boluses of 1–2 mg/kg were given until a burst-suppression EEG pattern was achieved [53] (Class IV). Thereafter, an infusion of 4 mg/kg/h was initiated; however, the maintenance of a continuing burst suppression pattern was difficult to achieve and required incremental doses of propofol with a median maximum infusion rate of 9.5 mg/kg/h. The anaesthetic was tapered after 12 h of satisfactory burst suppression, and epileptic seizures reoccurred in three patients. Arterial hypotension was treated with fluid resuscitation in all patients, and seven patients received norepinephrine.

A systematic review of drug therapy for RSE including barbiturates, midazolam, and propofol assessed and compared data on 193 patients from 28 retrospective trials [54] (Class IV). Pentobarbital was more effective than either propofol or midazolam in preventing breakthrough seizures (12 versus 42%). However, in most studies barbiturates were titrated against an EEG burst suppression pattern while midazolam and propofol was administered to obtain EEG seizure cessation. Accordingly, side effects such as arterial hypotension were significantly more frequently seen with pentobarbital compared with midazolam and propofol (77 versus 34%). Overall mortality was 48% but there was no association between drug selection and the risk of death. A retrospective study assessed treatment aggressiveness on prognosis, revealing that outcome was independent of the specific coma-inducing agent used [9] (Class IV).

The above mentioned progressive loss of $GABA_A$ receptors with ongoing seizure activity limits the efficacy of anticonvulsants with predominantly GABAergic mechanisms of action. In advanced stages of SE when NMDA receptors are increasingly expressed, specific antagonists may be good candidates to be administered. Ketamine has been described in some case reports and patient series to terminate SE after failure of GABAergic anticonvulsants [55–57] (Class IV).

Recommendations

The use of an in-house protocol for the general management and specific pharmacological treatment of SE is highly recommended (GPP).

General initial management

General management approaches in generalised convulsive, complex partial, and subtle status epilepticus should include: assessment and control of the airways and of ventilation, arterial blood gas monitoring to see if there is metabolic acidosis and hypoxia requiring immediate treatment through airway management and supplemental oxygen, ECG and blood pressure monitoring. Other measures include: i.v. glucose and thiamine as required, emergency measurement of antiepileptic drug levels, electrolytes and magnesium, a full haematological screen, and measures of hepatic and renal function. The cause of the status should be identified urgently and may require treatment in its own right (GPP).

Initial pharmacological treatment for GCSE and NCSE

In GCSE, the preferred treatment pathway is i.v. administration of 4 mg lorazepam, this dose is repeated if seizures continue more than 10 min after first injection (Level A). If necessary, additional i.v. phenytoin (18 mg/kg) or equivalent fosphenytoin is recommended (Level A). Phenytoin should be loaded rapidly with an infusion rate at 50 mg/min; this regimen is as safe as anticonvulsant treatment using other drugs (Level A). Alternatively, 10 mg diazepam directly followed by 18 mg/kg phenytoin or equivalent fosphenytoin can be given, if seizures continue more than 10 min after first diazepam injection another 10 mg is recommended (Level A). If possible, pre-hospital treatment is recommended, and in GCSE i.v. administration of 2 mg lorazepam is as effective as 5 mg diazepam (Level A). Out-of-hospital i.v. administration of benzodiazepines in GCSE is as safe as placebo treatment (Level A). So far, available studies have not convincingly demonstrated a good enough efficacy of valproic acid to be included in the group of first-line substances for the treatment of generalised convulsive or other clinical forms of SE. Complex partial status epilepticus should be treated initially such as GCSE (GPP). Subtle status epilepticus evolving from previously overt GCSE in most cases will already have been treated with anticonvulsants. In the rare patients with previously untreated subtle SE, the initial anticonvulsant treatment should be identical to that of overt GCSE (GPP).

General management of refractory status epilepticus

GCSE that does not respond to initial anticonvulsant substances needs to be treated on an intensive care unit (GPP).

Pharmacological treatment for refractory GCSE and subtle status epilepticus

In GCSE and subtle status epilepticus, we suggest to proceed immediately to the infusion of anaesthetic doses of midazolam, propofol, or barbiturates because of the progressive risk of brain and systemic damage. Due to poor evidence we cannot recommend which of the anaesthetic substances should be the drug of choice. We recommend the titration of the anaesthetic against an EEG burst suppression pattern. This goal should be maintained for at least 24 h. Simultaneously, initiation of the chronic medication the patient will be treated with in future should begin (GPP).

Barbiturates Thiopental is started with a bolus of 3–5 mg/kg, then further boluses of 1–2 mg/kg every 2–3 min until seizures are controlled, thereafter continuous infusion at a rate of 3–7 mg/kg/h (GPP). Pentobarbital (the first metabolite of thiopental) is marketed in the US as the alternative to thiopental and is given as a bolus dose of 5–15 mg/kg over 1 h followed by an infusion of 0.5–1 mg/kg/h, increasing if necessary to 1–3 mg/kg/h (GPP).

Midazolam Effective initial i.v. doses of midazolam are a 0.2 mg/kg bolus, followed by continuous infusion at rates of 0.05–0.4 mg/kg/h (GPP).

Propofol Initial i.v. bolus of 2–3 mg/kg should be administered followed by further boluses at 1–2 mg/kg until seizure contol, then continuous infusion at 4–10 mg/kg/h (GPP).

In cases of elderly patients in whom intubation and artificial ventilation would not be justified, further non-anaesthetising anticonvulsants may be tried (see below) (GPP).

Pharmacological treatment for refractory complex partial status epilepticus

In complex partial status epilepticus, the time that has elapsed until termination of status is less critical compared to GCSE. Thus, general anaesthesia due to its possible severe complications should be postponed and further non-anaesthetising anticonvulsants may be tried before. Due to poor evidence and lack of any head-to-head comparison studies we cannot recommend which of the non-anaesthetising anticonvulsants should be the drug of choice (GPP).

Phenobarbital Initial i.v. bolus of 20 mg/kg i.v. at an infusion rate of 50 mg/min, administration of additional boluses requires intensive care conditions (GPP).

Valproic acid Intravenous bolus of 25–45 mg/kg infused at rates of up to 6 mg/kg/min (GPP).

Levetiracetam Intravenous bolus of 1000–3000 mg administered over a period of 15 min (GPP).

If the treatment regimen includes the administration of anaesthetics, the same protocol applies as described for refractory GCSE.

Conflicts of interest

The authors have reported conflicts of interest as follows.

H. Meierkord has declared no conflict of interest.

P. Boon has received Editorial/Advisory board fees from Cyberonics, Else-vier, Medtronic, Pfizer, Sanofi and UCB and speakersfees from Cyberonics, Medtronic and UCB.

B. Engelsen has declared no conflict of interest.

K. Göcke has declared no conflict of interest.

S. Shorvon has received Editorial/Advisoryboard fees from UCB and Speakers fees from UCB.

P. Tinuper has declared no conflict of interest.

M. Holtkamp has received speakers fees from UCB.

References

1. Coeytaux A, Jallon P, Galobardes B, Morabia A. Incidence of status epilepticus in French-speaking Switzerland: (EPISTAR). *Neurology* 2000;**55**:693–7.

2. Knake S, Rosenow F, Vescovi M, *et al.* Incidence of status epilepticus in adults in Germany: a prospective, population-based study. *Epilepsia* 2001;**42**:714–8.

3. Vignatelli L, Tonon C, D'Alessandro R. Incidence and short-term prognosis of status epilepticus in adults in Bologna, Italy. *Epilepsia* 2003;**44**:964–8.

4. Wu YW, Shek DW, Garcia PA, Zhao S, Johnston SC. Incidence and mortality of generalized convulsive status epilepticus in California. *Neurology* 2002;**58**:1070–6.

5. Shneker BF, Fountain NB. Assessment of acute morbidity and mortality in nonconvulsive status epilepticus. *Neurology* 2003;**61**:1066–73.

6. Koubeissi M, Alshekhlee A. In-hospital mortality of generalized convulsive status epilepticus: a large US sample. *Neurology* 2007;**69**:886–93.

7. Holtkamp M, Othman J, Buchheim K, Meierkord H. Predictors and prognosis of refractory status epilepticus treated in a neurological intensive care unit. *J Neurol Neurosurg Psychiatry* 2005;**76**:534–9.

8. Mayer SA, Claassen J, Lokin J, Mendelsohn F, Dennis LJ, Fitzsimmons BF. Refractory status epilepticus: frequency, risk factors, and impact on outcome. *Arch Neurol* 2002; **59**:205–10.

9. Rossetti AO, Logroscino G, Bromfield EB. Refractory status epilepticus: effect of treatment aggressiveness on prognosis. *Arch Neurol* 2005;**62**:1698–702.

10. Chen JW, Wasterlain CG. Status epilepticus: pathophysiology and management in adults. *Lancet Neurol* 2006; **5**:246–56.

11. Naylor DE, Liu H, Wasterlain CG. Trafficking of GABA(A) receptors, loss of inhibition, and a mechanism for pharmacoresistance in status epilepticus. *J Neurosci* 2005;**25**: 7724–33.

12. Wasterlain C, Liu H, Mazarati A, Baldwin R. NMDA receptor trafficking during the transition from single seizures to status epilepticus. *Ann Neurol* 2002;**52**(Suppl. 1):16.

13. Snead OC, III. Basic mechanisms of generalized absence seizures. *Ann Neurol* 1995;**37**:146–57.

14. Fountain NB. Status epilepticus: risk factors and complications. *Epilepsia* 2000;**41**(Suppl. 2):S23–30.

15. Brainin M, Barnes M, Baron JC, *et al.* Guidance for the preparation of neurological management guidelines by EFNS scientific task forces – revised recommendations 2004. *Eur J Neurol* 2004;**11**:577–81.

16. Proposal for revised clinical and electroencephalographic classification of epileptic seizures. From the Commission on Classification and Terminology of the International League Against Epilepsy. *Epilepsia* 1981;**22**:489–501.

17. Meldrum BS, Brierley JB. Prolonged epileptic seizures in primates. Ischemic cell change and its relation to ictal physiological events. *Arch Neurol* 1973;**28**:10–7.

18. Shorvon S. *Status Epilepticus: Its Clinical Features and Treatment in Children and Adults.* Cambridge: Cambridge University Press, 1994.

19. Theodore WH, Porter RJ, Albert P, *et al.* The secondarily generalized tonic-clonic seizure: a videotape analysis. *Neurology* 1994;**44**:1403–7.

20. Jenssen S, Gracely EJ, Sperling MR. How long do most seizures last? A systematic comparison of seizures recorded in the epilepsy monitoring unit. *Epilepsia* 2006;**47**:1499–503.

21. Lowenstein DH, Bleck T, Macdonald RL. It's time to revise the definition of status epilepticus. *Epilepsia* 1999; **40**:120–2.

22. Alldredge BK, Gelb AM, Isaacs SM, *et al.* A comparison of lorazepam, diazepam, and placebo for the treatment of out-of-hospital status epilepticus. *N Eng J Med* 2001; **345**:631–7.

23. Treiman DM, Meyers PD, Walton NY, *et al.* A comparison of four treatments for generalized convulsive status epilepticus. Veterans Affairs Status Epilepticus Cooperative Study Group. *N Eng J Med* 1998;**339**:792–8.

24. America's Working Group on Status Epilepticus. Treatment of convulsive status epilepticus. Recommendations of the Epilepsy Foundation of America's Working Group on Status Epilepticus. *JAMA* 1993;**270**:854–9. [Previous guidelines or recommendations].

25. Meierkord H, Holtkamp M. Non-convulsive status epilepticus in adults: clinical forms and treatment. *Lancet Neurol* 2007;**6**:329–39.

26. Prasad A, Worrall BB, Bertram EH, Bleck TP. Propofol and midazolam in the treatment of refractory status epilepticus. *Epilepsia* 2001;**42**:380–6.

27. Lowenstein DH, Alldredge BK. Status epilepticus. *N Eng J Med* 1998;**338**:970–6.

28. Cascino GD. Generalized convulsive status epilepticus. *Mayo Clin Proc* 1996;**71**:787–92.

29. Hanley DF, Kross JF. Use of midazolam in the treatment of refractory status epilepticus. *Clin Ther* 1998;**20**:1093–105.

30. Shorvon S, Baulac M, Cross H, Trinka E, Walker M. The drug treatment of status epilepticus in Europe: consensus document from a workshop at the first London Colloquium on Status Epilepticus. *Epilepsia* 2008;**49**:1277–85. [Previous guidelines or recommendations].

31. Stecker MM, Kramer TH, Raps EC, O'Meeghan R, Dulaney E, Skaar DJ. Treatment of refractory status epilepticus with propofol: clinical and pharmacokinetic findings. *Epilepsia* 1998;**39**:18–26.

32. Leppik IE, Derivan AT, Homan RW, Walker J, Ramsay RE, Patrick B. Double-blind study of lorazepam and diazepam in status epilepticus. *JAMA* 1983;**249**:1452–4.

33. Misra UK, Kalita J, Patel R. Sodium valproate vs phenytoin in status epilepticus: a pilot study. *Neurology* 2006;**67**:340–2.

34. Gilad R, Izkovitz N, Dabby R, *et al.* Treatment of status epilepticus and acute repetitive seizures with i.v. valproic acid vs phenytoin. *Acta Neurol Scand* 2008;**118**:296–300.

35. Peters CN, Pohlmann-Eden B. Intravenous valproate as an innovative therapy in seizure emergency situations including status epilepticus – experience in 102 adult patients. *Seizure* 2005;**14**:164–9.

36. Walton NY. Systemic effects of generalized convulsive status epilepticus. *Epilepsia* 1993;**34**(Suppl. 1):S54–8.

37. Holtkamp M, Matzen J, van Landeghem F, Buchheim K, Meierkord H. Transient loss of inhibition precedes spontaneous seizures after experimental status epilepticus. *Neurobiol Dis* 2005;**19**:162–70.

38. Walker MC, Perry H, Scaravilli F, Patsalos PN, Shorvon SD, Jefferys JG. Halothane as a neuroprotectant during constant stimulation of the perforant path. *Epilepsia* 1999;**40**:359–64.

39. Kaplan PW. No, some types of nonconvulsive status epilepticus cause little permanent neurologic sequelae (or: 'the cure may be worse than the disease'). *Neurophysiol Clin* 2000;**30**:377–82.

40. Holtkamp M, Othman J, Buchheim K, Masuhr F, Schielke E, Meierkord H. A 'malignant' variant of status epilepticus. *Arch Neurol* 2005;**62**:1428–31.

41. Claassen J, Hirsch LJ, Mayer SA. Treatment of status epilepticus: a survey of neurologists. *J Neurol Sci* 2003;**211**:37–41.

42. Holtkamp M, Masuhr F, Harms L, Einhaupl KM, Meierkord H, Buchheim K. The management of refractory generalised convulsive and complex partial status epilepticus in three

European countries: a survey among epileptologists and critical care neurologists. *J Neurol Neurosurg Psychiatry* 2003;**74**:1095–9.

43. Sinha S, Naritoku DK. Intravenous valproate is well tolerated in unstable patients with status epilepticus. *Neurology* 2000;**55**:722–4.

44. Agarwal P, Kumar N, Chandra R, Gupta G, Antony AR, Garg N. Randomized study of intravenous valproate and phenytoin in status epilepticus. *Seizure* 2007;**16**:527–32.

45. Limdi NA, Shimpi AV, Faught E, Gomez CR, Burneo JG. Efficacy of rapid IV administration of valproic acid for status epilepticus. *Neurology* 2005;**64**:353–5.

46. Venkataraman V, Wheless JW. Safety of rapid intravenous infusion of valproate loading doses in epilepsy patients. *Epilepsy Res* 1999;**35**:147–53.

47. Knake S, Gruener J, Hattemer K, *et al.* Intravenous levetiracetam in the treatment of benzodiazepine refractory status epilepticus. *J Neurol Neurosurg Psychiatry* 2008;**79**:588–9.

48. Uges JW, van Huizen MD, Engelsman J, *et al.* Safety and pharmacokinetics of intravenous levetiracetam infusion as add-on in status epilepticus. *Epilepsia* 2008;**50**:415–21.

49. Kellinghaus C, Berning S, Besselmann M. Intravenous lacosamide as successful treatment for nonconvulsive status epilepticus after failure of first-line therapy. *Epilepsy Behav* 2009;**14**:429–31.

50. Kaplan PW. Nonconvulsive status epilepticus. *Neurology* 2003;**61**:1035–6.

51. Parviainen I, Uusaro A, Kalviainen R, Kaukanen E, Mervaala E, Ruokonen E. High-dose thiopental in the treatment of refractory status epilepticus in intensive care unit. *Neurology* 2002;**59**:1249–51.

52. Ulvi H, Yoldas T, Mungen B, Yigiter R. Continuous infusion of midazolam in the treatment of refractory generalized convulsive status epilepticus. *Neurol Sci* 2002;**23**:177–82.

53. Parviainen I, Uusaro A, Kalviainen R, Mervaala E, Ruokonen E. Propofol in the treatment of refractory status epilepticus. *Intens Care Med* 2006;**32**:1075–9.

54. Claassen J, Hirsch LJ, Emerson RG, Mayer SA. Treatment of refractory status epilepticus with pentobarbital, propofol, or midazolam: a systematic review. *Epilepsia* 2002;**43**:146–53.

55. Bleck TP, Quigg M, Nathan BR, Smith TL, Kapur J. Electroencephalographic effects of ketamine treatment for refractory status epilepticus. *Epilepsia* 2002;**43**(Suppl. 1):282.

56. Sheth RD, Gidal BE. Refractory status epilepticus: response to ketamine. *Neurology* 1998;**51**:1765–6.

57. Pruss H, Holtkamp M. Ketamine successfully terminates malignant status epilepticus. *Epilepsy Res* 2008;**82**:219–22.

CHAPTER 29

Alcohol-related seizures

G. Bråthen,[1] E. Ben-Menachem,[2] E. Brodtkorb,[1] R. Galvin,[3] J. C. Garcia-Monco,[4] P. Halasz,[5] M. Hillbom,[6] M. A. Leone,[7] A. B. Young[8]

[1]Trondheim University Hospital, and Norwegian University of Science and Technology, Trondheim, Norway; [2]Institute of Clinical Neuroscience, SU/Sahlgrenska Hospital, Gothenburg, Sweden; [3]Cork University Hospital, Wilton, Cork, Ireland; [4]Hospital de Galdacano, Galdacano (Vizcaya), Spain; [5]National Institute of Psychiatry and Neurology, Epilepsy Center, Budapest, Hungary; [6]Oulu University Hospital, Oulu, Finland; [7]Ospedale Maggiore della Carità, Novara, Italy; [8]Dunsyre House, Dunsyre Carnwath, Lanark, UK

Background

It has been known since Hippocratic times that alcohol overuse causes epileptic seizures [1]. The nature of this relationship is complex and poorly understood. Despite being a considerable problem in neurological practice and responsible for one-third of seizure-related admissions [2–5], there is little consensus as to the optimal investigation and management of alcohol-related seizures. Furthermore, different treatment traditions and policies exist, and vary from country to country [6]. These guidelines summarize the current evidence for the diagnosis and management of alcohol-related seizures.

Methods

The task force systematically searched MEDLINE, EMBASE, the Cochrane databases, and several other sources for relevant trials related to a set of pre-defined key questions. Recent papers of high relevance were reviewed. Consensus was reached by discussions during meetings of the task force at EFNS congresses and at a workshop. The guideline was originally published in 2005 [7]. The literature search for the present update was performed in October 2009. The evidence (Class I–IV)

and recommendation levels (A–C) were applied in accordance with Brainin et al. [8]. Some important aspects of patient management that lack the evidence required for recommendations have been included; these are marked GPP, for 'Good Practice Points'.

Results

Diagnosis of alcohol-related seizures

History taking

Unless alcohol withdrawal symptoms are unequivocally present, the clinical diagnosis of an alcohol-related seizure can only be made by obtaining a drinking history that indicates alcohol overuse prior to the seizure. As patients frequently underreport true levels of alcohol consumption, there is a need to control for this bias. Therefore, whenever possible, a relative or friend should be asked about the recent alcohol intake.

Several other legal or illegal pharmacological agents may influence the tendency to have seizures, due either to withdrawal (e.g. benzodiazepines) or to a direct neurotoxic effect (e.g. antipsychotics, antidepressants, or stimulant drugs). These factors may complicate the clinical picture and should be considered in the diagnosis of alcohol-related seizures.

A good drinking history includes both the quantity and frequency of alcohol intake and changes in drinking pattern, at least during the previous 5 days, as well as the time of the last alcohol intake (GPP).

European Handbook of Neurological Management: Volume 1, 2nd edition. Edited by N. E. Gilhus, M. P. Barnes and M. Brainin.

Questionnaires

Structured questionnaires have been developed to reveal and grade excessive alcohol consumption as well as alcohol overuse and dependence. To be clinically useful a questionnaire needs to be both brief and reliable. The probably most commonly applied instrument is CAGE, which is the acronym for a simple four-question item. It is brief, easily memorized, and has reasonably fair accuracy [9]. However, it fails to detect binge drinking, which is probably best assessed by directly asking for the largest number of drinks in a single drinking occasion [10]. The Alcohol Use Disorders Identification Test (AUDIT) includes this item. It is a 10-item questionnaire which requires a 2–3 min interview and provides a fine-pitched grading (0–40) of alcohol use and overuse. For patient populations with lower drinking levels, it has higher accuracy than other questionnaires [11, 12] but is not easily memorized and may be perceived as too long for routine use in busy medical settings. A handful of brief versions, e.g. AUDIT-C, FAST, and AUDIT-PC, consisting of 3–5 AUDIT items, or Five-SHOT, a combination of AUDIT and CAGE items, have all shown good accuracy compared to AUDIT [13–16]. Other questionnaires, such as the Brief Michigan Alcoholism Screening Test (Brief MAST) [12] and the Munich Alcoholism Test (MALT) [17] have widespread use, but do not offer better accuracy than AUDIT or its brief versions, and their use in a routine clinical setting is more demanding.

Recommendation

Questionnaires offer high diagnostic accuracy for alcohol overuse (Level A recommendation). To identify patients with alcohol-related seizures and binge drinking, brief versions of AUDIT are recommended as they are accurate and easy to use in busy clinical settings (Level A recommendation).

Biomarkers

For detection of alcohol overuse, questionnaire-based interviews are reported to be more sensitive than any biomarker [18, 19]. However, in cases where information on recent alcohol consumption is unavailable or considered unreliable, markers of alcohol consumption can increase the accuracy of the clinical diagnosis [20, 21].

Carbohydrate-deficient transferrin (CDT) and gammaglutamyl transferase (GGT) are sensitive markers for alcohol overuse, although GGT is less specific than CDT. Systematic literature reviews have been inconclusive as to which marker is better [22, 23]. Both CDT and GGT show poor accuracy as screening instruments for alcohol-related seizures in unselected seizure populations [20]. Attempts to combine the tests have led to increased sensitivity [24–26]. As the current intoxication level is important information with potential treatment consequences [27], blood alcohol should be measured in patients with suspected alcohol-related seizures (GPP).

Recommendation

CDT and GT have a potential to support a clinical suspicion of alcohol overuse when the drinking history is inconclusive (Level A recommendation). Due to poor accuracy in unselected populations, biomarkers should not be applied as general screening instruments (Level C recommendation).

Patient examination and observation

The clinical examination should be focused on features distinctive of either epilepsy or withdrawal seizures (table 29.1). To predict the severity of alcohol withdrawal, the revised Clinical Institute Withdrawal Assessment Scale (CIWA-Ar) can be applied [30]. The CIWA-Ar takes 2–5 min to administer and grades withdrawal severity on a scale from 0 to 67 (available as appendix to this guideline on www.efns.org). More than 90% of alcohol withdrawal seizures occur within 48 h of cessation of a prolonged drinking bout [4, 31]. Patients should be observed in hospital for at least 24 h, after which a clinical risk assessment should be made with respect to development of symptoms of alcohol withdrawal (GPP).

For the general treatment of the alcohol withdrawal syndrome readers should refer to guidelines [32, 33, 34, 35].

Recommendation

The CIWA questionnaire can be applied to grade the severity of withdrawal symptoms and give support to the decision on whether to keep or discharge the patient (Level A recommendation).

Table 29.1 Early (<72 h) post-ictal signs and symptoms after seizures due to epilepsy and alcohol withdrawal seizures.

	Epilepsy	Early alcohol withdrawal
Consciousness level	Post-ictal sleep/ drowsiness	Sleeplessness
Mood	Calm	Anxiety, unrest, nightmares
Tremor	No	Yes
Sweating	No	Yes
Blood pressure	Normal	Elevated
Pulse rate	Normal	Elevated (>90)
Temperature	Normal/light fever	Fever
Arterial blood	Normal	Respiratory alkalosis[a]
EEG	Pathology[b]	Normal, low amplitude
Questionnaires	Normal scores	Normal or elevated scores

[a]Respiratory alkalosis may be masked by seizure-induced metabolic acidosis, but it will reappear within 2 h after cessation of convulsions ([29]).
[b]Initial post-ictal slowing in most patients. Interictal epileptiform discharges in approximately 50% ([28]).

Neuroimaging

The diagnostic yield of cerebral computed tomography (CT) after a first alcohol-related seizure is high, mainly because patients overusing alcohol have a high incidence of structural intracranial lesions [36, 37]. Seizures that occur later than 48 h after intake of the last drink may indicate other potential aetiologies than simple alcohol withdrawal, such as subdural haematoma, brain contusion, or mixed drug and alcohol overuse [38]. When patients present repeatedly with clinically typical alcohol-related seizures, re-imaging is not necessary, but changes in seizure type and frequency, seizure occurrence more than 48 h after cessation of drinking, or other unusual features should prompt repeat neuroimaging (GPP).

Recommendation

Although it may seem obvious that a given seizure is alcohol-related, if it is a first known seizure, the patient should have brain imaging (CT or MRI) without and with contrast (Level C recommendation).

Electroencephalography (EEG)

The incidence of EEG abnormalities (slow or epileptiform activity) is lower among patients with alcohol withdrawal seizures (AWS) than in those with seizures of other aetiology. Therefore, EEG pathology suggests that the seizure may not have been caused exclusively by alcohol withdrawal [31, 39].

Recommendation

EEG should be recorded after a first seizure. Subsequent to repeated AWS, EEG is considered necessary only if an alternative aetiology is suspected (Level C recommendation).

Patient management

Subsequent to the acute treatment of alcohol-related seizures, attention should be given to other potential complications of alcohol overuse such as thiamine deficiency, electrolyte disturbances, acute intracranial lesions, infections, and development of the alcohol withdrawal syndrome, potentially leading to delirium tremens. Apart from acute intracranial lesions, which fall outside the scope of these guidelines, these factors are addressed below.

Thiamine therapy

Prolonged heavy drinking causes reduced absorption and increased excretion of thiamine. Only 5–14% of patients with Wernicke's encephalopathy are diagnosed in life [40, 41]. The majority (~80%) of those who show CNS lesions caused by thiamine deficiency are chronic alcohol overusers [40, 42].

Thiamine is a comparatively harmless vitamin, the diagnosis of thiamine deficiency is difficult, and the consequences of not treating may be severe. Therefore, the threshold for starting therapy should be low. Oral administration is insufficient as the intestinal thiamine absorption may be severely impaired [43]. In a recent Cochrane review, only one sufficiently large randomized double-blind trial on the preventive effects of different doses of thiamine could be identified [44], from which it could only be concluded that a daily dose of 200 mg thiamine was better than 5 mg [45]. For the treatment of imminent or manifest Wernicke's encephalopathy, uncontrolled trials and empirical clinical practice suggest a daily dose of at least 200 mg thiamine parenterally for minimum 3–5 days. In our experience, patients with Wernicke's encephalopathy may benefit from continued treatment for more than 2 weeks (GPP).

> **Recommendation**
>
> Before starting any carbohydrate-containing fluids or food, patients presenting with known or suspected alcohol overuse should be given prophylactic thiamine in the emergency room (Level B recommendation).

Treatment of electrolyte disturbances

Due to large fluid intake (beer), hyponatraemia may develop in alcohol overusers. The serious disorder of central pontine myelinolysis is thought to be triggered by osmotic gradients in the brain, a situation that may well result from attempts to correct this electrolyte disturbance rapidly [46]. Hyponatraemia in alcohol overusers generally shows a benign clinical course [47], and usually repairs with cessation of alcohol intake and re-institution of a normal diet [48]. If infusion is considered necessary, according to a retrospective study the rate of serum sodium correction should not exceed 10 mmol/day [49]. The evidence is insufficient for treatment recommendations.

Hypomagnesaemia and respiratory alkalosis seem to be associated with alcohol withdrawal, and correction of hypomagnesaemia may raise the seizure threshold in the initial phase of alcohol withdrawal [50]. Unresponsiveness to parenteral thiamine therapy is a possible consequence of hypomagnesaemia [51]. However, there is not sufficient evidence to recommend routine correction of hypomagnesemia.

Should all patients with symptoms of alcohol withdrawal be offered seizure prophylactic treatment?

Patients with mild-to-moderate alcohol withdrawal symptoms (CIWA <10) can successfully be detoxified with supportive care only [52]. Supportive treatment includes a calm, reassuring atmosphere, dim light, coffee restriction, and hydration.

The mean incidence of seizures in patients receiving placebo during trials on drugs for prevention of AWS is approximately 8% [53]. These data originate from selected patients in need of treatment for alcoholism; the general seizure risk during uncomplicated alcohol withdrawal is probably lower. As seizures during previous detoxifications increase the risk for seizures during subsequent withdrawals [54, 55], patients with these characteristics will probably benefit from prophylactic treatment regardless of the current withdrawal symptom severity.

> **Recommendation**
>
> For patients with no history of withdrawal seizures and mild to moderate withdrawal symptoms, routine seizure preventive treatment is not recommended (Level B recommendation). Patients with severe alcohol withdrawal symptoms, regardless of seizure occurrence, should be treated pharmacologically (Level C recommendation).

Drug options for primary prevention of alcohol withdrawal seizures

An ideal drug for symptom relief during detoxification from alcohol should display fast loading, long duration, minor side effects, low toxicity, few interactions, minimal overuse potential, and high efficacy in preventing both withdrawal symptoms in general as well as seizures. Drugs should be available in more than one form, liquid being particularly useful for some patients. Apart from overuse potential, benzodiazepines (BZD) fulfil all the above listed criteria for an ideal drug. BZD are cheap, widely available, and have a well-documented safety profile.

In meta-analyses of controlled trials for primary prevention of AWS, a highly significant risk reduction for seizures with BZD compared with placebo have been demonstrated [53, 56]. Drugs with rapid onset of action (diazepam, lorazepam, alprazolam) seem to have higher overuse potential than those with slower onset of action (chlordiazepoxide, oxazepam, halazepam). For the purpose of reducing the risk of seizures due to BZD withdrawal and reducing rebound withdrawal symptoms after discontinuation, long-acting drugs should be preferred to short-acting ones [33, 53]. However, short-acting BZDs may have advantages for patients with respiratory insufficiency. Symptom-triggered treatment has been reported to be as effective as fixed-dose or loading therapy, resulting in lower doses and shorter treatment time [57, 58]. Lorazepam has some advantages over diazepam. Despite a shorter half-life it has longer duration of action because it is less accumulated in lipid stores. However, its onset of action is slightly slower than that of diazepam.

In a Cochrane review, the efficacy of anticonvulsants to prevent seizures did not reach statistical significance compared either to placebo, benzodiazepines or other drugs [59].

Many other drugs and drug combinations are being used, including chlormethiazole, gamma-hydroxybutyrate, and clonidine, all for which the documentation is insufficient [53, 57, 60, 61].

> **Recommendation**
>
> When pharmacological treatment is necessary, benzodiazepines should be chosen for the primary prevention of seizures in a person with alcohol withdrawal, as well as for treatment of the alcohol withdrawal syndrome. The drugs of choice are lorazepam and diazepam. Although lorazepam has some pharmacological advantages to diazepam, the differences are minor and, as i.v. lorazepam is largely unavailable in Europe, diazepam is recommended. Other drugs for detoxification should only be considered as add-ons (Level A recommendation).

Secondary prevention of withdrawal seizures

Following a withdrawal seizure, the recurrence risk within the same withdrawal episode is 13–24% [53]. Consequently, there is a good rationale for treating these patients as soon as possible in order to prevent subsequent seizures. Lorazepam reduces recurrence risk significantly [62]. Phenytoin did not prevent relapses in patients who had one or more seizures during the same withdrawal episode [53].

> **Recommendation**
>
> Benzodiazepines should be used for the secondary prevention of AWS (Level A recommendation). Phenytoin is not recommended for prevention of AWS recurrence (Level A recommendation). The efficacy of other antiepileptics for secondary prevention of AWS is undocumented.

Alcohol-related status epilepticus

Alcohol withdrawal is one of the commonest causes of status epilepticus (SE), and SE may be the first manifestation of alcohol-related seizures. Although SE has probably a better prognosis when alcohol related [63], it increases the risk for subsequent epilepsy [64]. One recent study indicates that lorazepam may be superior to diazepam for the treatment of out-of-hospital SE [65]. In another study comparing four treatments, lorazepam was considered easier to use but not more efficacious than diazepam, phenobarbital, or phenytoin [66].

> **Recommendation**
>
> For the initial treatment of alcohol-related status epilepticus, i.v. lorazepam is safe and efficacious. When unavailable, i.v. diazepam is a good alternative (Level A recommendation).

Management of epilepsy in patients with current alcohol overuse

The comprehensive management of these patients includes careful counselling and information about the seizure-precipitating effect of alcohol, particularly the concurrent withdrawal of alcohol and antiepileptic drugs (AEDs). Prescription of AEDs to alcohol overusers is often a fruitless undertaking, which may increase their seizure problems due to poor compliance, drug overuse, and drug-alcohol interactions [38]. The ideal drug for such patients should be well tolerated in combination with alcohol and have a benign side effect profile, including safety in overdose [67], and have a suppressive effect on drinking behaviour. In a few small studies, carbamazepine, valproic acid, gabapentin, and pregabalin have each been reported to reduce alcohol consumption [68–71], and topiramate has recently been shown to reduce craving for alcohol [72]. Prophylactic AED treatment should only be considered after recurrent epileptic seizures clearly unrelated to alcohol intake, following the usual guidelines for AED treatment. The available data do not allow for recommendations on this topic.

How much alcohol can a patient with epilepsy safely consume?

In various European countries, different advice has been given as to whether patients with epilepsy should abstain totally from alcohol [73]. Only one randomized controlled clinical study [74] has addressed this particular issue; an intake of one to three drinks each containing 9.8 g ethanol (standard alcohol units; see [75]) up to three times a week did not increase seizure susceptibility in treated patients with partial epilepsy. Another study suggested a seizure risk proportional to the alcohol intake level [76].

Alcohol sensitivity may vary between epilepsy syndromes. Generalized epilepsies, in particular juvenile myoclonic epilepsy, seem to be more sensitive to alcohol, sleep deprivation, and in particular the combination of these factors [77].

Recommendation

For the majority of patients with partial epilepsy and controlled seizures, and in the absence of any history of alcohol overuse, an intake of one to three standard alcohol units, one to three times a week, is safe (Level B recommendation).

Conflicts of interest

The present guidelines were developed without external financial support. None of the authors report conflicting interests.

References

1. Lloyd G. *Hippocratic Writings*. Middlesex, UK: Penguin Books, 1978; p. 222.
2. Earnest MP, Yarnell P. Seizure admissions to a city hospital: the role of alcohol. *Epilepsia* 1976;**17**:387–93.
3. Hillbom ME. Occurrence of cerebral seizures provoked by alcohol abuse. *Epilepsia* 1980;**21**:459–66.
4. Bråthen G, Brodtkorb E, Helde G, Sand T, Bovim G. The diversity of seizures related to alcohol use. A study of consecutive patients. *Eur J Neurol* 1999;**6**:697–703.
5. Jallon P, Smadja D, Cabre P, Le Mab G, Bazin M. EPIMART: prospective incidence study of epileptic seizures in newly referred patients in a french caribbean island (Martinique). *Epilepsia* 1999;**40**:1103–9.
6. Leone MA, Bråthen G. Treatment policies for alcohol-related seizures: a survey of European neurologists. *Eur J Neurol* 2007;**14**(3):e2–3.
7. Bråthen G, Ben-Menachem E, Brodtkorb E, *et al*. EFNS Guideline on the diagnosis and management of alcohol-related seizures: report of an EFNS task force. *Eur J Neurol* 2005;**12**:575–81.
8. Brainin M, Barnes M, Baron J-C, *et al*. Guidance for the preparation of neurological management guidelines by EFNS scientific task forces – revised recommendations. *Eur J Neurol* 2004;**11**:577–81.
9. Mayfield D, Mcleod G, Hall P. The CAGE questionnaire: validation of a new alcoholism screening instrument. *Am J Psychiatry* 1974;**131**(10):1121–3.
10. Matano RA, Koopman C, Wanat SF, Whitsell SD, Borgrefe A, Westrup D. Assessment of binge drinking of alcohol in highly educated employees. *Addict Behav* 2003;**28**: 1299–310.
11. Fiellin DA, Reid MC, O'Connor PG. Screening for alcohol problems in primary care: a systematic review. *Arch Intern Med* 2000;**160**(13):1977–89.
12. MacKenzie D, Langa A, Brown T. Identifying hazardous or harmful alcohol use in medical admissions: a comparison of Audit, CAGE and Brief MAST. *Alcohol Alcohol* 1996; **31**:591–9.
13. Bush K, Kivlahan DR, McDonnel MB, Fihn SD, Bradley KA. The AUDIT alcohol consumption questions (AUDIT-C): an effective brief screening test for problem drinking. *Arch Intern Med* 1998;**16**:1789–95.
14. Hodgson RJ, John B, Abbasi T, *et al*. Fast screening for alcohol misuse. *Addict Behav* 2003;**28**:1453–63.
15. Piccinelli M, Tessari E, Bortolomasi M, *et al*. Efficacy of the alcohol use disorders identification test as a screening tool for hazardous alcohol intake and related disorders in primary care: a validity study. *BMJ* 1997;**314**:420–7.
16. Seppa K, Lepisto J, Sillanaukee P. Five-shot questionnaire on heavy drinking. *Alcohol Clin Exp Res* 1998;**22**(8):1788–91.
17. Feuerlein W, Ringer C, Kufner H, Antons K. Diagnose des Alkoholismus. Der Münchner Alkoholismustest (MALT). *Munch Med Wschr* 1977;**119**:1275–86.
18. Aertgeerts B, Buntinx F, Ansoms S, Fevery J. Questionnaires are better than laboratory tests to screen for current alcohol abuse or dependence in a male inpatient population. *Acta Clin Belg* 2002;**57**:241–9.
19. Bernadt MW, Mumford J, Taylor C, Smith B, Murray RM. Comparison of questionnaire and laboratory tests in the detection of excessive drinking and alcoholism. *Lancet* 1982;**i**:325–8.
20. Bråthen G, Bjerve K, Brodtkorb B, Bovim G. Validity of carbohydrate-deficient transferrin and other markers as diagnostic aids in the detection of alcohol-related seizures. *J Neurol Neurosurg Psychiatry* 2000;**68**:342–8.
21. Martin MJ, Heyermann C, Neumann T, *et al*. Preoperative evaluation of chronic alcoholics assessed for surgery of

the upper digestive tract. *Alcohol Clin Exp Res* 2002; **26**:836–40.

22. Salaspuro M. Carbohydrate-deficient transferrin as compared to other markers of alcoholism: a systematic review. *Alcohol* 1999;**19**(3):261–71.

23. Scouller K, Conigrave KM, Macaskill P, Irwig L, Whitfield JB. Should we use carbohydrate-deficient transferrin instead of G-glutamyltransferase for detecting problem drinkers? A systematic review and metaanalysis. *Clin Chem* 2000;**46**: 1894–902.

24. Hietala J, Koivisto H, Anttila P, Niemelä O. Comparison of the combined marker GGT-CDT and the conventional laboratory markers of alcohol abuse in heavy drinkers, moderate drinkers and abstainers. *Alcohol Alcohol* 2006; **41**:528–33.

25. Bentele M, Kriston L, Clement HW, Härter M, Mundle G, Berner MM. The validity of the laboratory marker combinations DOVER and QUVER to detect physician's diagnosis of at-risk drinking. *Addict Biol* 2007;**12**:85–92.

26. Sillanaukee P, Olsson U. Improved diagnostic classification of alcohol abusers by combining carbohydrate-deficient transferrin and G-glutamyltransferase. *Clin Chem* 2001; **47**:681–5.

27. Savola O, Niemelä O, Hillbom M. Blood alcohol is the best indicator of hazardous alcohol drinking in young adults and working aged patients with trauma. *Alcohol Alcohol* 2004; **39**:340–5.

28. FIRST Group. Randomized clinical trial on the efficacy of antiepileptic drugs in reducing the risk of relapse after a first unprovoked tonic-clonic seizure. *Neurology* 1993;**43**: 478–83.

29. Orringer CE, Eustace JC, Wunsch CD, Gardner LB. Natural history of lactic acidosis after grand-mal seizures. A model for the study of an anion-gap acidosis not associated with hyperkalemia. *N Engl J Med* 1977;**297**:796–9.

30. Sullivan JT, Sykora K, Schneiderman J, Naranjo CA, Sellers EM. Assessment of alcohol withdrawal: the revised Clinical Institute Withdrawal Assessment for Alcohol scale (CIWA-AR). *Br J Addict* 1989;**84**:1353–7.

31. Victor M, Brausch C. The Role of Abstinence in the Genesis of Alcoholic Epilepsy. *Epilepsia* 1967;**8**:1–20.

32. Claassen CA, Adinoff B. Alcohol withdrawal syndrome. Guidelines for management. *CNS Drugs* 1999;**12**:279–91.

33. Mayo-Smith MF for the American Society of Addiction Medicine Working Group on Pharmacological Management of Alcohol Withdrawal. Pharmacological management of alcohol withdrawal. A meta-analysis and evidence-based practice guideline. *JAMA* 1997;**278**:144–51.

34. Mayo-Smith MF, Beecher LH, Fischer TL, *et al.* for the Working Group on the Management of Alcohol Withdrawal Delirium, Practice Guidelines Committee, American Society

of Addiction Medicine. Management of alcohol withdrawal delirium. An evidence-based practice guideline. *Arch Intern Med* 2004;**164**:1405–12.

35. Scottish Intercollegiate Guidelines Network (SIGN). *The Management of Harmful Drinking and Alcohol Dependence in Primary Care.* Edinburgh: SIGN, 2002; (SIGN publication No. 74).

36. Earnest MP, Feldman H, Marx JA, Harris BS, Biletch M, Sullivan LP. Intracranial lesions shown by CT in 259 cases of first alcohol related seizure. *Neurology* 1988;**38**:1561.

37. Schoenenberger RA, Heim SM. Indication for computed tomography of the brain in patients with first uncomplicated generalised seizure. *BMJ* 1994;**309**:986–9.

38. Hillbom ME, Hjelm-Jaeger M. Should alcohol withdrawal seizures be treated with anti-epileptic drugs? *Acta Neurol Scand* 1984;**69**:39–2.

39. Sand T, Bråthen G, Michler R, Brodtkorb E, Helde G, Bovim G. Clinical utility of EEG in alcohol-related seizures. *Acta Neurol Scand* 2002;**105**:18–24.

40. Torvik A, Lindboe CF, Rogde S. Brain lesions in alcoholics: a neuropathological study with clinical correlations. *J Neurol Sci* 1982;**56**:233–48.

41. Blansjaar BA, Van Dijk JG. Korsakoff-Wernicke syndrome. *Alcohol Alcohol* 1992;**27**:435–7.

42. Harper CG, Giles M, Finlay-Jones R. Clinical signs in the Wernicke-Korsakoff complex: a retrospective analysis of 131 cases diagnosed at necropsy. *J Neurol Neurosurg Psychiatry* 1986;**49**:341–5.

43. Holzbach E. Thiamine absorption in alcoholic delirium patients. *J Studies Alcohol* 1996;**57**:581–4.

44. Ambrose ML, Bowden SC, Whelan G. Thiamin treatment and working memory function of alcohol-dependent people: preliminary findings. *Alcohol Clin Exp Res* 2001; **25**:112–6.

45. Day E, Bentham P, Callaghan R, Kuruvilla T, George S. Thiamine for Wernicke-Korsakoff Syndrome in people at risk from alcohol abuse. *Cochrane Database of Systematic Reviews* 2004;(1):Art. No.: CD004033. DOI: 10.1002/14651858.CD004033.pub2.

46. Lampl C, Yazdi K. Central pontine myelinolysis. *Eur Neurol* 2002;**47**(1):3–10.

47. Mochizuki H, Masaki T, Miyakawa T, *et al.* Benign type of central pontine myelinolysis in alcoholism: clinical, neuroradiological and electrophysiological findings. *J Neurol* 2003;**250**:1077–83.

48. Kelly J, Wassif W, Mitchard J, Gardner WN. Severe hyponatremia secondary to beer potomania complicated by central pontine myelinolysis. *Int J Clin Pract* 1998;**52**:585–7.

49. Saeed BO, Beaumont D, Handley GH, Weaver JU. Severe hyponatremia: investigation and management in a district general hospital. *J Clin Pathol* 2002;**55**:893–6.

50. Victor M. The role of hypomagnesemia and respiratory alkalosis in the genesis of alcohol withdrawal symptoms. *Ann NY Acad Sci* 1973;**215**:235–48.

51. Traviesa DC. Magnesium deficiency: a possible cause of thiamine refractoriness in Wernicke-Korsakoff encephalopathy. *J Neurol Neurosurg Psychiatry* 1974;**37**:959–62.

52. Whitfield CL, Thompson G, Lamb A, Spencer V, Pfeifer M, Browning-Ferrando M. Detoxification of 1,024 alcoholic patients without psychoactive drugs. *JAMA* 1978;**239**(14): 1409–10.

53. Hillbom M, Pieninkeroinen I, Leone M. Seizures in alcohol-dependent patients. Epidemiology, pathophysiology and management. *CNS Drugs* 2003;**17**:1013–30.

54. Lechtenberg R, Worner T. Seizure risk with recurrent alcohol detoxification. *Arch Neurol* 1990;**47**:535–8.

55. Mayo-Smith MF, Bernard D. Late onset seizures in alcohol withdrawal. *Alcohol Clin Exp Res* 1995;**19**:656–9.

56. Ntais C, Pakos E, Kyzas P, Ioannidis JP. Benzodiazepines for alcohol withdrawal. *Cochrane Database Syst Rev* 2005;(3):Art. No.: CD005063. DOI: 10.1002/14651858. CD005063.pub2.

57. Saitz R, Mayo-Smith MF, Roberts MS, Redmond HA, Bernard DR, Calkins DR. Individualized treatment for alcohol withdrawal. A randomized double-blind controlled trial. *JAMA* 1994;**272**:519–23.

58. Jaeger TM, Lohr RH, Pankratz VS. Symptom-triggered therapy for alcohol withdrawal syndrome in medical inpatients. *Mayo Clin Proc* 2001;**76**:695–701.

59. Polycarpou A, Papanikolau P, Ionannidis JPA, Contopoulos Ioannidis D. Anticonvulsants for alcohol withdrawal. *Cochrane Database Syst Rev* 2005;(3):Art. No.: CD005064. DOI: 10.1002/14651858.CD005064.pub2.

60. Holbrook AM, Crowther R, Lotter A, Cheng C, King D. Meta-analysis of benzodiazepine use in the treatment of acute alcohol withdrawal. *CMAJ* 1999;**160**:649–55.

61. Robinson BJ, Robinson GM, Maling TJ, Johnson RH. Is clonidine useful in the treatment of alcohol withdrawal? *Alcohol Clin Exp Res* 1989;**13**:95–8.

62. D'Onofrio G, Rathlev NK, Ulrich AS, Fish SS, Freedland ES. Lorazepam for the prevention of recurrent seizures related to alcohol. *N Engl J Med* 1999;**340**:915–9.

63. Alldredge BK, Lowenstein DH. Status epilepticus related to alcohol abuse. *Epilepsia* 1993;**34**:1033–7.

64. Hesdorffer DC, Logroscino G, Cascino G, *et al.* Risk of unprovoked seizure after acute symptomatic seizure: effect of status epilepticus. *Ann Neurol* 1998;**44**:908–12.

65. Alldredge BK, Gelb AM, Isaacs SM, *et al.* A comparison of lorazepam, diazepam, and placebo for the treatment of out-of-hospital status epilepticus. *N Engl J Med* 2001;**345**: 631–7.

66. Treiman DM, Meyers PD, Walton NY, *et al.* A comparison of four treatments for generalized convulsive status epilepticus. Veterans Affairs Status Epilepticus Cooperative Study Group. *N Engl J Med* 1998;**339**:792–8.

67. Malcolm R, Myrick H, Brady KT, Ballenger JC. Update on anticonvulsants for the treatment of alcohol withdrawal. *Am J Addict* 2001;**10**(Suppl.):16–23.

68. Mueller TI, Stout RL, Rudden S, *et al.* A double-blind, placebo-controlled pilot study of carbamazepine for the treatment of alcohol dependence. *Alcohol Clin Exp Res* 1997;**21**(1):86–92.

69. Brower KJ, Myra Kim H, Strobbe S, Karam-Hage MA, Consens F, Zucker RA. A randomized double-blind pilot trial of gabapentin versus placebo to treat alcohol dependence and comorbid insomnia. *Alcohol Clin Exp Res* 2008;**32**(8):1429–38.

70. Salloum IM, Cornelius JR, Daley DC, Kirisci L, Himmelhoch JM, Thase ME. Efficacy of valproate maintenance in patients with bipolar disorder and alcoholism: a double-blind placebo-controlled study. *Arch Gen Psychiatry* 2005; **62**(1):37–45.

71. Martinotti G, Di Nicola M, Tedeschi D, Mazza M, Janiri L, Bria P. Efficacy and safety of pregabalin in alcohol dependence. *Adv Ther* 2008;**25**(6):608–18.

72. Johnson BA, Rosenthal N, Capece JA, *et al.* Topiramate for Alcoholism Advisory Board; Topiramate for Alcoholism Study Group. Topiramate for treating alcohol dependence: a randomized controlled trial. *JAMA* 2007;**298**(14): 1641–51.

73. Höppener RJ. The effect of social alcohol use on seizures in patients with epilepsy. In: Porter RJ, Mattson RH, Cramer JA, Diamond I (eds) *Alcohol and Seizures. Basic Mechanisms and Clinical Concepts.* Philadelphia: F.A. Davis Company, 1990; pp. 222–32.

74. Höppener RJ, Kuyer A, van der Lugt PJM. Epilepsy and alcohol: the influence of social alcohol intake on seizures and treatment in epilepsy. *Epilepsia* 1983;**24**: 459–71.

75. Turner C. How much alcohol is in a 'standard drink'? An analysis of 125 studies. *Br J Addict* 1990;**85**:1171–5.

76. Mattson RH, Fay ML, Sturman JK, Cramer JA, Wallace JD, Mattson EM. The effect of various patterns of alcohol use on seizures in patients with epilepsy. In: Porter RJ, Mattson RH, Cramer JA, Diamond I (eds) *Alcohol and Seizures. Basic Mechanisms and Clinical Concepts.* Philadelphia: F.A. Davis Company, 1990; pp. 233–40.

77. Pedersen SB, Petersen KA. Juvenile myoclonic epilepsy: clinical and EEG features. *Acta Neurol Scand* 1998;**97**: 160–3.

CHAPTER 30

Brain metastases

R. Soffietti,[1] P. Cornu,[2] J. Y. Delattre,[3] R. Grant,[4] F. Graus,[5] W. Grisold,[6] J. Heimans,[7] J. Hildebrand,[8] P. Hoskin,[9] M. Kalljo,[10] P. Krauseneck,[11] C. Marosi,[12] T. Siegal,[13] C. Vecht[14]

[1]San Giovanni Battista Hospital and University, Torino, Italy; [2]Pitié-Salpétrière and University, Paris, France; [3]Pitié-Salpétrière, Paris, France; [4]Western General Hospital and University, Edinburgh, UK; [5]Hospital Clinic, Villaroel, Barcelona Spain; [6]Kaiser-Franz-Josef Spital, Vienna Austria; [7]Academisch Ziekenhuis V.U., Amsterdam, The Netherlands; [8]Brussels, Belgium; [9]Mount Vernon Hospital and University, Northwood, Middlesex, UK; [10]University Hospital, Helsinki, Finland; [11]Neurologische Clinic, Bamberg, Germany; [12]Vienna General Hospital and University, Vienna, Austria; [13]Hadassah Hebrew University, Jerusalem, Israel; [14]Med Center Haaglanden, The Hague, The Netherlands

Objectives

The primary objective has been to establish evidence-based guidelines in regard to the management of patients with brain metastases. The secondary objective has been to identify areas where there are still controversies and clinical trials are needed.

Background

Brain metastases represent an important cause of morbidity and mortality for cancer patients and are more common than primary brain tumours. The incidence of brain metastases has increased over time as a consequence of the increase in overall survival for many types of cancer and the improved detection by magnetic resonance imaging (MRI). Brain metastases may occur in 20–40% of patients with cancer, being symptomatic during life in 60–75%. In adults, the primary tumours most likely to metastatize to the brain are located in the lung (minimum 50%), breast (15–25%), skin (melanoma) (5–20%), colon-rectum, and kidney, but any malignant tumour is able to metastatize to the brain. The primary site is unknown in up to 15% of patients. Brain metastases are more often diagnosed in patients with known malignancy (metachronous presentation). Less frequently (up to 30%) brain metastases are diagnosed either at the time of primary tumour diagnosis (synchronous presentation) or before the discovery of the primary tumour (precocious presentation). High performance status, absence of systemic metastases, controlled primary tumour, and younger age (<60–65 years) are the most important favourable prognostic factors. Based on these factors the Radiation Therapy Oncology Group (US) has identified subgroups of patients with different prognosis (recursive partitioning analysis (RPA) Class I, II, III) [1]. Recently, a new prognostic index, the grade prognostic assessment (GPA), that takes into account the number of brain metastases, in addition to age, KPS, and extracranial metastases, has been proposed [2]. Neurocognitive function is prognostically important as well [3]. The prognosis is similar for patients with both known and unknown primary tumour [4].

Search strategy

We searched: the Cochrane Library to date; MEDLINE–Ovid (January 1966 to date); MEDLINE–ProQuest; MEDLINE-EIFL; EMBASE–Ovid (January 1990 to date); CancerNet; Science Citation Index (ISI). We used specific and sensitive keywords, as well as combinations of keywords, and publications in any language of countries represented in the task force. We also collected guidelines from national and European multidisciplinary neuro-oncological societies and groups (from Italy, France,

European Handbook of Neurological Management: Volume 1, 2nd edition. Edited by N. E. Gilhus, M. P. Barnes and M. Brainin.

Table 30.1 Karnofsky Performance Status (KPS).

KPS 100	Normal; no complaints; no evidence of disease
KPS 90	Able to carry on normal activity; minor signs or symptoms of disease
KPS 80	Normal activity with effort; some signs or symptoms of disease
KPS 70	Cares for self; unable to carry on normal activity or to do active work
KPS 60	Requires occasional assistance, but is able to care for most personal needs
KPS 50	Requires considerable assistance and frequent medical care
KPS 40	Disabled; requires special care and assistance
KPS 30	Severely disabled; hospitalization is indicated, although death not imminent
KPS 20	Very sick; hospitalization necessary; active support treatment is necessary
KPS 10	Moribund; fatal processes progressing rapidly
KPS 0	Death

Netherlands, Germany, and the UK). Moreover, we performed an investigation (by email questionnaire) regarding the views of members of the task force on several critical issues, reflecting the different national situations (10 countries) and specializations (11 neurologists, one neurosurgeon, one radiation oncologist, one medical oncologist).

Method for reaching consensus

The scientific evidence of papers collected from the literature was evaluated and graded according to Brainin *et al.* (2004) [5], and recommendations were given according to the same paper. When sufficient evidence for recommendation A–C was not available, we considered a recommendation to be a 'Good Practice Point' (GPP) if agreed by all members of the task force. When analysing results and drawing recommendations at any stage, the differences were resolved by discussions.

Review of the evidence

Diagnosis

Headache (40–50%), focal neurological deficits (30–40%), and seizures (15–20%) are the most common presenting symptoms. A minority of patients have an acute

'stroke-like' onset, related to an intratumoural haemorrhage (in particular melanoma, choriocarcinoma, and renal carcinoma). Altered mental status or impaired cognition are seen in patients with multiple metastases and/or increased intracranial pressure, sometimes resembling a metabolic encephalopathy. Contrast-enhanced MRI is more sensitive than enhanced computed tomography (CT) (including double-dose delayed contrast) or unenhanced MRI in detecting brain metastases, particularly when located in the posterior fossa or very small [6] (Class II). Double or triple doses of gadolinium-based contrast agents are better than single doses, but increasing the dose may lead to an increased number of false-positive findings [7] (Class III).

There are no pathognomonic features on CT or MRI that distinguish brain metastases from primary brain tumours such as malignant gliomas and lymphomas or non-neoplastic conditions (abscesses, infections, demyelinating diseases, vascular lesions). A peripheral location, spherical shape, ring enhancement with prominent peritumoural oedema, and multiple lesions all suggest metastatic disease: these characteristics are helpful but not diagnostic, even in patients with a positive history of cancer. Diffusion-weighted (DW) MR imaging may be useful for the differential diagnosis of ring-enhancing cerebral lesions (restricted diffusion in abscesses compared to unrestricted diffusion in cystic or necrotic glioblastomas or metastases), but the findings are not specific [8, 9] (Class III). In patients with either histologically confirmed or radiologically suspected brain metastases and a negative history of cancer, chest CT is more sensitive than chest radiograph in detecting a synchronous lung tumour (more commonly a non-small-cell cancer) (Class III evidence). CT of the abdomen occasionally shows an unsuspected cancer. Further investigations are almost never fruitful without positive features in the patient's history or localizing signs on the physical examination to suggest a primary site [10] (Class III). Whole-body fluorodeoxyglucose positron emission tomography (FDG PET) is a sensitive tool for detecting a 'probable' primary tumour by visualizing foci of abnormal uptake, more often in the lung [11] (Class III), but the specificity in differentiating malignant tumours from benign or inflammatory lesions is relatively low.

Supportive care

Dexamethasone is commonly used to control cerebral oedema, because of the minimal mineralocorticoid effect and long half-life. Patients are generally managed with starting doses of 4–8 mg per day [12] (Class II). Up to 75% of patients show marked neurological improvement within 24–72 h after beginning dexamethasone. Any other corticosteroid is effective if given in equipotent doses. Side effects from chronic dexamethasone administration, including myopathy, are frequent and contribute to disability. When used as the sole form of treatment, dexamethasone produces about one month's remission of symptoms and slightly increases the 4–6-week median survival of patients who receive no treatment at all [13].

The need for anticonvulsant medication is clear in patients who have experienced a seizure by the time their brain tumour is diagnosed. The evidence does not support prophylaxis with antiepileptic drugs (AEDs) in patients with brain tumours, including metastases (Class I). Twelve studies, either randomized trials or cohort studies, investigating the ability of prophylactic AEDs (phenytoin, phenobarbital, valproic acid) to prevent first seizures have been examined and none has demonstrated efficacy [14]. Subtherapeutic levels of anticonvulsants were extremely common and the severity of side effects appeared to be higher (20–40%) in brain tumour patients than in the general population receiving anticonvulsants, probably because of drug interactions (Class II). Phenytoin, carbamazepine, and phenobarbital stimulate the cytochrome P450 system and accelerate the metabolism of corticosteroids and chemotherapeutic agents such as nitrosoureas, paclitaxel, cyclophosphamide, topotecan, irinotecan, thiotepa, adriamycin, and methotrexate, and thus reduce their efficacy. The role of prophylactic anticonvulsants remains to be addressed in some subgroups of patients who have a higher risk of developing seizures, such as those with metastatic melanoma, haemorrhagic lesions, and multiple metastases. For patients who underwent a neurosurgical procedure the efficacy of prophylaxis has not been proven [15] (Class II). The efficacy of novel AEDs (levetiracetam, topiramate, gabapentin, oxcarbazepine, lamotrigine) has not been extensively investigated.

Anticoagulant therapy is the standard treatment for acute venous thromboembolism (VTE) in cancer patients. For initial therapy subcutaneous low molecular weight heparin (LMWH) is as effective and safe as intravenous unfractionated heparin (UFH) [16] (Class I). LMWH is more effective than oral anticoagulant therapy (warfarin) in preventing recurrent VTE in cancer patients [17] (Class I). The duration of anticoagulant therapy has not been specifically addressed in cancer patients. A prophylaxis with either UFH or LMWH reduces the risk of VTE in patients undergoing major surgery for cancer (Class II).

Treatment of single brain metastasis

Surgery

Three randomized trials have compared surgical resection followed by WBRT with WBRT alone [18–20]. The first two studies have shown a survival benefit for patients receiving the combined treatment (median survival 9–10 months versus 3–6 months). In the Patchell study, patients who received surgery displayed a lower rate of local relapses (20% versus 52%) and a longer time of functional independence. The third study, which included more patients with an active systemic disease and a low Karnofsky performance status, did not show any benefit with the addition of surgery. Therefore, there is Class I evidence that the survival benefit of surgical resection is limited to the subgroup of patients with controlled systemic disease and good performance status. Surgical resection allows in the majority of patients an immediate relief of symptoms of intracranial hypertension, a reduction of focal neurological deficits and seizures, and a rapid steroid taper. Gross total resection of a brain metastasis can be achieved with lower morbidity using contemporary image-guided systems, such as preoperative functional MRI, intraoperative neuronavigation, and cortical mapping [21]. The combined resection of a solitary brain metastasis and a synchronous non-small-cell lung carcinoma (NSCLC) (stage I and II) yields a median survival of at least 12 months, with 10–30% of patients surviving at 5 years [22] (Class III). In patients with local brain relapse and good performance status, re-operation affords a neurological improvement and prolongation of survival [21] (Class III).

Leptomeningeal dissemination (LMD) can be a complication, especially for patients with posterior fossa metastases [23].

Stereotactic radiosurgery

Stereotactic radiosurgery (SRS) permits the delivery of a single high dose of radiation to a target of 3–3.5 cm of maximum diameter by using gamma-knife (multiple cobalt sources) or linear accelerator (Linac) through a stereotactic device. The rapid dose fall-off of SRS minimizes the risk of damage to the surrounding normal nervous tissue. Most brain metastases represent an ideal target for SRS, owing to the small size, spherical shape, and distinct radiographic and pathologic margins [24]. The dose is inversely related to tumour diameter and volume [25]. In patients with newly diagnosed brain metastases, a decrease of symptoms, a local tumour control (defined as shrinkage or arrest of growth) at 1 year of 80–90%, and a median survival of 6–12 months have been reported [26] (Class II). Metastases from radioresistant tumours, such as melanoma, renal cell carcinoma, and colon cancer, respond to SRS as well, as do metastases from radiosensitive tumours [27] (Class II). Radiosurgery allows the treatment of brain metastases in almost any location, including brainstem [28]. The type of radiosurgical procedure, gamma-knife or Linac-based, does not have an impact on the results. SRS combined with WBRT (radiosurgical boost) is superior to WBRT alone in terms of survival [29] (Class II). Survival following radiosurgery is comparable to that achieved with surgery [30, 31] (Class II). SRS is less invasive and can be accomplished in an outpatient setting, and thus offers cost-effectiveness advantages over surgery; on the other hand, patients with larger lesions may require chronic steroid administration. Radiosurgery is effective for patients with brain metastases that have recurred following WBRT [25] (Class II).

Acute (early) and chronic (late) complications following radiosurgery are reported in 10–40% of patients, serious complications being rare [32]. Acute reactions (due to oedema) occur more often within 2 weeks of treatment, and include headache, nausea and vomiting, worsening of pre-existent neurological deficits, and seizures. These reactions are generally reversible with steroids. Chronic complications consist of haemorrhage and radionecrosis (1–17%), requiring re-operation in up to 4% of patients. Radiographically, a transient increase in the size of the irradiated lesion, with increasing oedema and mass effect, with or without radionecrosis, cannot be distinguished from a tumour progression: FdG-PET [33] and MR spectroscopy [34] can give additional information .

Whole-brain radiotherapy alone

Median survival after WBRT alone is 3–6 months. Different fractionation schedules, ranging from 20 Gy in 1 week to 50 Gy in 4 weeks, yield comparable results [35, 36] (Class II). Nausea, vomiting, headache, fever, and transient worsening of neurological symptoms in the initial phase of therapy may be observed.

Whole-brain radiotherapy after surgery or radiosurgery (adjuvant WBRT)

It is still controversial whether adjuvant WBRT, which has a rationale of destroying microscopic metastatic deposits at the original tumour site or at distant locations, is necessary after complete surgical resection or radiosurgery. Time-consuming fractionated treatment, possible long-term neurotoxicity, and availability of effective salvage treatments at recurrence are the main arguments against WBRT [37], whereas the negative impact of central nervous system (CNS) progression on the neurologic and neurocognitive function when omitting initial WBRT, and the uncertainty regarding the value of salvage treatments in reversing the neurologic symptoms and signs are arguments in favour [38]. There are three randomized trials [39–41] showing that the omission of WBRT in patients with newly diagnosed brain metastases after either surgery or SRS results in significantly worse local and distant control in the brain on MRI, though it does not affect overall and functionally independent survival (Class I). WBRT may cause early adverse effects (fatigue, alopecia, eustachian tube dysfunction) and late neurotoxicity. Long-term survivors after WBRT frequently develop radiographic changes on CT or MRI, including cortical atrophy, hydrocephalus, and hyperintensity of the periventricular white matter in T2 and FLAIR images. Up to 11% of patients receiving hypofractionated schedules of radiotherapy (size fraction of 4–6 Gy) [42] have clinical symptoms such as memory loss progressing to dementia, frontal gait disorders, and urinary incontinence. Overall, aside from the risk of dementia after large fractions of WBRT, the true incidence of cognitive dysfunctions after conventional treatments (i.e. 30 Gy in 10 fractions) is not well understood, even if the deterioration of neurocognitive functions in long-term survivors (up to 36 months) could not be negligible [43].

The identification of patients with different risk of developing brain tumour relapse could be extremely important to define the most appropriate initial management [44].

Local forms of radiotherapy could be an alternative to WBRT after resection of a brain metastasis, because they target the most frequent site of tumour recurrence, that is the resection cavity. SRS to the resection cavity [45] and the Gliasite Radiation Therapy System (an intracavitary high-activity ^{125}I brachytherapy) [46] yield local control and local failure rates and survival in the range which is expected for patients in RPA Class 1 and 2, treated with either surgery + WBRT or SRS, alone or in association with WBRT. Radiation-induced neurocognitive deficits may result from radiation injury to proliferating neuronal progenitor cells in the subgranular zone of the hippocampus [47]. Conformal avoidance of the hippocampus during WBRT is a novel technique that allows treatment of the majority of the brain to full dose while keeping the radiation dose to the hippocampus relatively lower [48].

The treatment of multiple brain metastases

Median survival after WBRT alone is 2–6 months, with good palliation of neurological symptoms. Hypofractionated treatments are generally employed, most commonly 30 Gy in 10 fractions or 20 Gy in five fractions. In patients with poor prognostic factors, supportive care only is frequently prescribed. Radiosurgery is an alternative to WBRT in patients with up to three brain metastases. WBRT with radiosurgery boost improves functional independence but not survival in patients with two or three lesions [29] (Class I). Among new radiosensitizers, associated with WBRT, motexafin-gadolinium has shown a benefit in prolonging time to neurologic/neurocognitive progression in patients with brain metastases from NSCLC [49] (Class II) and efaproxiral has shown a benefit in prolonging survival and quality of life in patients with brain metastases from breast cancer [50] (Class II). When the number of brain metastases is limited (up to three), the lesions are accessible, and the patients are relatively young, in good neurological condition and with a controlled systemic disease, complete surgical resection yields results that are comparable to those obtained in single lesions [51] (Class III).

Chemotherapy

Chemotherapeutic agents are effectve in the treatment of brain metastases [30] (Class III): brain metastases are often as responsive as the primary tumour and extracranial metastases, but not always the intracranial response parallels the extracranial response; higher response rates are observed when newly diagnosed, chemotherapy-naïve patients are treated; response to chemotherapy of brain metastases from mostly chemosensitive tumours (small-cell lung carcinoma, germ cell tumours, lymphomas) is of the same order as that observed after radiotherapy. Novel cytotoxic drugs, such as temozolomide, capecitabine, and fotemustine, can be useful in brain metastases from lung cancers, breast cancers and melanoma respectively. The combination of radiotherapy and chemotherapy may improve the response rate and/or the progression-free survival, but not the overall survival [52, 53] (Class I).

Local chemotherapy after surgical resection (Gliadel wafers) could reduce the risk of local relapse [54] (Class III).

Targeted therapies

Molecularly targeted therapies have been increasingly investigated in recent years in patients with brain metastases [55]. Brain metastases from NSCLC can respond to the epidermal growth factor receptor (EGFR) inhibitors gefitinib and erlotinib [56, 57] (Class III). As with extracranial disease, the response of brain metastases to EGFR inhibitors appears to depend upon the presence of specific EGFR mutations [58]. The dual EGFR and HER-2 tyrosine kinase inhibitor lapatinib has shown modest activity in a recent phase II study on HER-2 + breast cancer patients with brain metastases following trastuzumab-based systemic chemotherapy and WBRT [59] (Class III).

Recommendations

Diagnosis

- When neurological symptoms and/or signs develop in a patient with known systemic cancer, brain metastases must always be suspected. Careful medical history and physical examination with emphasis on the presence/activity of the systemic disease and the general physical condition (estimation of the performance status) are recommended (GPP).

- CT is inferior to MRI (Level B), but it is sufficient when it shows multiple brain metastases.

- Contrast-enhanced MRI is indicated when: (a) surgery or radiosurgery are considered for one or two metastases on contrast-enhanced CT and a KPS ≥ 70; (b) contrast-enhanced CT is negative but the history is strongly suggestive for the presence of brain metastases in a patient with established malignant disease; (c) CT is not conclusive to eliminate non-neoplastic lesions (abscesses, infections, demyelinating diseases, vascular lesions) (GPP).

- Diffusion MRI is useful for the differential diagnosis of ring-enhancing lesions (Level C).

- EEG is indicated where there is suspicion of epilepsy, but there remains clinical uncertainty (GPP).

- Tissue diagnosis (by stereotactic or open surgery) should be obtained when: (a) the primary tumour is unknown; (b) the systemic cancer is well controlled and the patient is a long-term survivor; (c) lesions on MRI do not show the typical aspect of brain metastases; (d) there is clinical suspicion of an abscess (fever, meningism) (Level B). In patients with unknown primary tumour, CT of the chest/abdomen and mammography are recommended, but a further extensive evaluation is not appropriate in the absence of specific symptoms or indications from the brain biopsy (GPP). FDG PET can be useful for detecting the primary tumour (GPP). The histopathologic studies on the brain metastasis may provide valuable information in indicating a likely organ of origin and guiding further specialized diagnostic work-up: in this regard immunohistochemical staining to detect tissue-, organ-, or tumour-specific antigens is useful (GPP).

- CSF cytology and contrast enhanced MRI of the spine are needed when the coexistence of a carcinomatous meningitis is suspected (GPP).

Supportive care

- Dexamethasone is the corticosteroid of choice and twice-daily dosing is sufficient (GPP). Starting doses should not exceed 4–8 mg per day, but patients with severe symptoms, including impaired consciousness or other signs of increased intracranial pressure, may benefit from higher doses (≥16 mg/day) (Level B). An attempt to reduce the dose should be undertaken within 1 week of initiation of treatment; if possible, patients should be weaned off steroids within 2 weeks. If complete weaning off is not possible, the lowest possible dose should be looked for. Asymptomatic patients do not require steroids. Steroids may reduce the acute side effects of radiation therapy. All recommendations are Good Practice Points.

- AEDs should not be prescribed prophylactically (Level A). In patients who suffer from epileptic seizures and need a concomitant treatment with chemotherapeutics, enzyme-inducing antiepileptic drugs (EIAEDs) should be avoided (Level B).

- In patients with venous thromboembolism low molecular weight heparin is effective and well tolerated for both initial therapy and secondary prophylaxis (Level A). A duration of the anticoagulant treatment ranging from 3 to 6 months is recommended (GPP). Prophylaxis in patients undergoing surgery is recommended (Level B).

Treatment of single brain metastasis

- Surgical resection should be considered in patients with single brain metastasis in an accessible location, especially when the size is large, the mass effect is considerable, and an obstructive hydrocephalus is present (GPP). Surgery is recommended when the systemic disease is absent/controlled and the Karnofsky Performance score is 70 or more (Level A). When the combined resection of a solitary brain metastasis and a non-small-cell lung carcinoma (stage I and II) is feasible, surgery for the brain lesion should come first, with a maximum delay between the two surgeries not exceeding 3 weeks (GPP). Patients with disseminated but controllable systemic disease (i.e. bone metastases from breast cancer) or with a radioresistant primary tumour (melanoma, renal cell carcinoma) may benefit from surgery (GPP). Surgery at recurrence is useful in selected patients (Level C).

- Stereotactic radiosurgery should be considered in patients with metastases of a diameter of ≤3–3.5 cm and/or located in eloquent cortical areas, basal ganglia, brainstem, or with comorbidities precluding surgery (Level B). Stereotactic radiosurgery may be effective at recurrence after prior radiation (Level B).

- WBRT alone is the therapy of choice for patients with active systemic disease and/or poor performance status and should employ hypofractionated regimens such as 30 Gy in 10 fractions or 20 Gy in five fractions (Level B). For patients with poor performance status supportive care only can be employed (GPP).

- Following surgery or radiosurgery, in case of absent/controlled systemic disease and Karnofsky Performance score of 70 or more, one can either withhold adjuvant WBRT if close follow-up with MRI (every 3–4 months) is performed or deliver early WBRT with fractions of 1.8–2 Gy to a total dose of 40–55 Gy to avoid late neurotoxicity (GPP).

Treatment of multiple brain metastases

- In patients with up to three brain metastases, good performance status (KPS of 70 or more) and controlled systemic disease, stereotactic radiosurgery is an alternative to WBRT (Level B), while surgical resection is an option in selected patients (Level C).

- In patients with more than three brain metastases WBRT with hypofractionated regimens is the treatment of choice (Level B), whereas for patients with poor performance status supportive care only can be employed (GPP).

Chemotherapy

- Chemotherapy may be the initial treatment for patients with brain metastases from chemosensitive tumours, like small-cell lung cancers, lymphomas, germ cell tumours, and breast cancers, especially if asymptomatic, chemo-naïve, or an effective chemotherapy schedule for the primary is still available (GPP).

Targeted therapies

- Targeted therapies can be employed in patients with brain metastases recurrent after radiation therapy (GPP).

Conflicts of interest

None of the members of the task force, including the chairperson, had any form of conflict of interest.

References

1. Gaspar L, Scott C, Rotman M, *et al.* Recursive partitioning analysis (RPA) of prognostic factors in three Radiation Therapy Oncology Group (RTOG) brain metastases trials. *Int J Radiat Oncol Biol Phys* 1997;**37**:745–51.

2. Sperduto PW, Berkey B, Gaspar LE, *et al.* A new prognostic index and comparison to three other indices for patients with brain metastases: an analysis of 1960 patients in the RTOG database. *Int J Radiat Oncol Biol Phys* 2008;**70**: 510–4.

3. Meyers CA, Smith JA, Bezjak A. Neurocognitive function and progression in patients with brain metastases treated with whole brain radiation and motexafin gadolinium: results of a randomized phase III trial. *J Clin Oncol* 2004; **22**:157–65.

4. Rudà R, Borgognone M, Benech F, Vasario E, Soffietti R. Brain metastases from unknown primary tumor. *J Neurol* 2001;**248**:394–8.

5. Brainin M, Barnes M, Baron JC, *et al.* Guidance for the preparation of neurological management guidelines by EFNS scientific task forces – revised recommendations 2004. *Eur J Neurol* 2004;**11**:577–81.

6. Schellinger PD, Meinck HM, Thron A. Diagnostic accuracy of MRI compared to CT in patients with brain metastases. *J Neurooncol* 1999;**44**:275–81.

7. Sze G, Johnson C, Kawamura Y, *et al.* Comparison of single- and triple-dose contrast material in the MR screening of brain metastases. *AJNR* 1998;**19**:821–8.

8. Desprechins B, Stadnik T, Koerts G, *et al.* Use of diffusion-weighted MR imaging in the differential diagnosis between intracerebral necrotic tumors and cerebral abscesses. *AJNR Am J Neuroradiol* 1999;**20**:1252–7.

9. Hartmann M, Jansen O, Heiland S, *et al.* Restricted diffusion within ring enhancement is not pathognomonic for brain abscess. *AJNR Am J Neuroradiol* 2001;**22**:1738–42.

10. Van de Pol M, van Aalst VC, Wilmink JT, Twijnstra A. Brain metastases from an unknown primary tumor: which diagnostic procedures are indicated? *J Neurol Neurosurg Psychiatr* 1996;**61**:321–3.

11. Klee B, Law I, Hoigaard L, Kosteljanetz M. Detection of unknown primary tumours in patients with cerebral metastases using whole-body 18F-fluorodeoxyglucose positron emission tomography. *Eur J Neurol* 2002;**9**:657–62.

12. Vecht CJ, Hovestadt A, Verbiest HB, van Vliet JJ, van Putten WL. Dose-effect relationship of dexamethasone on Karnof-sky performance in metastatic brain tumors: a randomized study of doses of 4, 8, and 16 mg per day. *Neurology* 1996;**44**:675–80.

13. Cairncross JG, Posner JB. The management of brain metastases. In: Walker MD (ed.) *Oncology of the Nervous System* Boston: Martinus Nijhoff, 1983; pp. 342–77.

14. Glantz MJ, Cole BF, Forsyth PA, *et al.* Practice parameter: anticonvulsant prophylaxis in patients with newly diagnosed brain tumors. Report of the Quality Standards Subcommittee of the American Academy of Neurology. *Neurology* 2000;**54**:1886–93.

15. Kuijlen JM, Teernstra OP, Kessels AG, Herpers MJ, Beuls EA. Effectiveness of antiepileptic prophylaxis used with supratentorial craniotomies: a meta-analysis. *Seizure* 1996; **5**:291–8.

16. Gould MK, Dembitzer AD, Doyle RL, Hastie TJ, Garber AM. Low-molecular-weight heparins compared with unfractionated heparin for treatment of acute deep venous thrombosis. A meta-analysis of randomized, controlled trials. *Ann Intern Med* 1999;**130**:800–9.

17. Lee AY, Levine MN, Baker RI, *et al.* Low-molecular-weight heparin versus coumarin for the prevention of recurrent venous thromboembolism in cancer. *N Engl J Med* 2003;**349**:146–53.

18. Patchell RA, Tibbs PA, Walsh JW, *et al.* A randomized trial of surgery in the treatment of single metastases to the brain. *N Engl J Med* 1990;**322**:494–500.

19. Vecht CJ, Haaxma-Reiche H, Noordijk EM, *et al.* Treatment of single brain metastasis: radiotherapy alone or combined with neurosurgery? *Ann Neurol* 1993;**33**:583–90.

20. Mintz AH, Kestle J, Rathbone MP, *et al.* A randomized trial to assess the efficacy of surgery in addition to radiotherapy in patients with a single cerebral metastasis. *Cancer* 1996;**78**:1470–6.

21. Vogelbaum MA, Suh JH. Resectable brain metastases. *J Clin Oncol* 2006;**24**:1289–94.

22. Kelly K, Bunn PA. It is time to reevaluate our approach to the treatment of brain metastases in patients with non-small cell lung cancer? *Lung Cancer* 1998;**20**:85–91.

23. Suki D, Abouassi H, Patel AJ, *et al.* Comparative risk of leptomeningeal disease after resection or stereotactic radiosurgery for solid tumor metastasis to the posterior fossa. *J Neurosurg* 2008;**108**:248–57.

24. Baumert BG, Rutten I, Dehing-Oberije C, *et al.* A pathology-based substrate for target definition in radiosurgery of brain metastases. *Int J Radiat Oncol Biol Phys* 2006;**66**:187–94.

25. Shaw E, Scott C, Souhami L, *et al.* Single dose radiosurgical treatment of recurrent previously irradiated primary brain tumors and brain metastases: final report of RTOG protocol 90-05. *Int J Radiat Oncol Biol Phys* 2000;**47**:291–8.

26. Mehta MP, Tsao MN, Whelan TJ, *et al.* The American Society for Therapeutic Radiology and Oncology (ASTRO)

evidence-based review of the role of radiosurgery for brain metastases. *Int J Radiat Oncol Biol Phys* 2005;**63**: 37–46.

27. Manon R, O'Neill A, Knisely J, *et al*. Phase II trial of radiosurgery for one to three newly diagnosed brain metastases from renal cell carcinoma, melanoma, and sarcoma: an Eastern Cooperative Oncology Group study (E 6397). *J Clin Oncol* 2005;**23**:8870–6.

28. Fuentes S, Delsanti C, Metellus P, *et al*. Brainstem metastases: management using gamma knife radiosurgery. *Neurosurgery* 2006;**58**:37–42.

29. Andrews DW, Scott CB, Sperduto PW, *et al*. Whole brain radiation therapy with or without stereotactic radiosurgery boost for patients with one to three brain metastases: phase III results of the RTOG randomised trial. *Lancet* 2004; **363**:1665–72.

30. Soffietti R, Costanza A, Laguzzi E, Nobile M, Rudà R. Radiotherapy and chemotherapy of brain metastases. *J Neuro-Oncol* 2005;**75**:1–12.

31. Rades D, Kueter JD, Veninga T, Gliemroth J, Schild SE. Whole brain radiotherapy plus stereotactic radiosurgery (WBRT+SRS) versus surgery plus whole brain radiotherapy (OP+WBRT) for 1–3 brain metastases: results of a matched pair analysis. *Eur J Cancer* 2009;**45**:400–4.

32. Williams BJ, Suki D, Fox BD, *et al*. Stereotactic radiosurgery for metastatic brain tumors: a comprehensive review of complications. *J Neurosurg* 2009;**111**:439–48.

33. Chao ST, Suh JH, Raja S, Lee SY, Barnett G. The sensitivity and specificity of FDG PET in distinguishing recurrent brain tumor from radionecrosis in patients treated with stereotactic radiosurgery. *Int J Cancer* 2001;**96**:191–7.

34. Rock JP, Scarpace L, Hearshen D, *et al*. Associations among magnetic resonance spectroscopy, apparent diffusion coefficients, and image-guided histopathology with special attention to radiation necrosis. *Neurosurgery* 2004;**54**: 1111–7.

35. Borgelt BB, Gelber RD, Kramer S, *et al*. The palliation of brain metastases: final results of the first two studies by the Radiation Therapy Oncology Group. *Int J Radiat Oncol Biol Phys* 1980;**6**:1–9.

36. Hoskin PJ, Brada M. Radiotherapy for brain metastases. *Clin Oncol* 2001;**13**:91–4.

37. Sneed PK, Suh JH, Goetsch SJ, *et al*. A multi-institutional review of radiosurgery alone vs. radiosurgery with whole brain radiotherapy as the initial management of brain metastases. *Int J Radiat Oncol Biol Phys* 2002;**53**:519–26.

38. Regine WF, Huhn JL, Patchell RA, *et al*. Risk of symptomatic brain tumor recurrence and neurologic deficit after radiosurgery alone in patients with newly diagnosed brain metastases: results and implications. *Int J Radiat Oncol Biol Phys* 2002;**52**:333–8.

39. Patchell RA, Tibbs PA, Regine WF, *et al*. Postoperative radiotherapy in the treatment of single brain metastases to the brain. *JAMA* 1998;**280**:1485–9.

40. Aoyama H, Shirato H, Tago M, *et al*. Stereotactic radiosurgery plus wholebrain radiation therapy vs stereotactic radiosurgery alone for treatment of brain metastases: a randomized controlled trial. *JAMA* 2006;**295**:2483–91.

41. Muller RP, Soffietti R, Abacioglu MU, *et al*. Adjuvant whole-brain radiotherapy versus observation after radiosurgery or surgical resection of 1–3 cerebral metastases: results of the EORTC 22952-26001 study. *J Clin Oncol* 2009; **27**:89s.

42. De Angelis LM, Delattre JY, Posner JB. Radiation-induced dementia in patients cured of brain metastases. *Neurology* 1989;**39**:789–96.

43. Aoyama H, Tago M, Kato N, *et al*. Neurocognitive function of patients with brain metastasis who receieved either whole brain radiotheraphy plus stereotactic radiosurgery or radiosurgery alone. *Int J Radiat Oncol Biol Phys* 2007;**68**: 1388–95.

44. Sawrie SM, Guthrie BL, Spencer SA, *et al*. Predictors of distant brain recurrence for patients with newly diagnosed brain metastases treated with stereotactic radiosurgery alone. *Int J Radiat Oncol Biol Phys* 2007;**70**:181–6.

45. Soltys SG, Adlwer JR, Lipani JD, *et al*. Stereotactic radiosurgery of the postoperative resection cavity for brain metastases. *Int J Radiat Oncol Biol Phys* 2007;**70**:187–93.

46. Rogers LR, Rock JP, Sills AK, *et al*. Results of a phase II trial of the GliaSite Radiation Therapy System for treatment of newly diagnosed, resected single brain metastases. *J Neurosurg* 2006;**105**:375–84.

47. Monje ML, Palmer T. Radiation injury and neurogenesis. *Curr Opin Neurol* 2003;**16**:129–34.

48. Gutiérrez AN, Westerly DC, Tomé WA, *et al*. Whole brain radiotherapy with hippocampal avoidance and simultaneously integrated brain metastases boost: a planning study. *Int J Radiat Oncol Biol Phys* 2007;**69**:589–97.

49. Mehta MP, Shapiro WR, Phan SC, *et al*. Motexafin gadolinium combined with prompt whole brain radiotherapy prolongs time to neurologic progression in non-small-cell lung cancer patients with brain metastases: results of a phase III trial. *Int J Radiat Oncol Biol Phys* 2009;**73**:1069–76.

50. Scott C, Suh J, Stea B, *et al*. Improved survival, quality of life, and quality-adjusted survival in breast cancer patients treated with efaproxiral (Efaproxyn) plus whole-brain radiation therapy for brain metastases. *Am J Clin Oncol* 2007;**30**:580–7.

51. Pollock BE, Brown PD, Foote RL, *et al*. Properly selected patients with multiple brain metastases may benefit from aggressive treatment of their intracranial disease. *J Neuro Oncol* 2003;**61**:73–80.

52. Antonadou D, Paraskevaidis M, Sarris G, *et al.* Phase 2 randomized trial of temozolomide and concurrent radiotherapy in patients with brain metastases. *J Clin Oncol* 2002;**20**:3644–50.

53. Verger E, Gil M, Yaya R, *et al.* Temozolomide and concomitant whole brain radiotherapy in patients with brain metastases: a phase 2 trial. *Int J Radiation Oncology Biol Phys* 2005;**61**:185–91.

54. Ewend MG, Brem S, Gilbert M, *et al.* Treatment of single brain metastasis with resection, intracavity carmustine polymer wafers, and radiation therapy is safe and provides excellent local control. *Clin Cancer Res* 2007;**13**:3637–41.

55. Soffietti R, Rudà R, Trevisan E. Brain metastases: current management and new developments. *Curr Opin Oncol* 2008;**20**:676–84.

56. Ceresoli G, Cappuzzo F, Gregorc V, Bartolini S, Crinò L, Villa E. Gefitinib in patients with brain metastases from non-small cell lung cancer: a prospective trial. *Ann Oncol* 2004;**15**:1042–7.

57. Fekrazad MH, Ravindranathan M, Jones DV Jr. Response of intracranial metastases to erlotinib therapy. *J Clin Oncol* 2007;**25**:5024–6.

58. Shimato S, Mitsudomi T, Kosaka T, *et al.* EGFR mutations in patients with brain metastases from lung cancer: association with the efficacy of gefitinib. *Neurooncology* 2006;**8**:137–44.

59. Lin NU, Diéras V, Paul D, *et al.* Multicenter phase II study of lapatinib in patients with brain metastases from HER2-positive breast cancer. *Clin Cancer Res* 2009;**15**:1452–9.

CHAPTER 31

Paraneoplastic neurological syndromes

C. A. Vedeler,[1] J. C. Antoine,[2] B. Giometto,[3] F. Graus,[4] W. Grisold,[5] J. Honnorat,[6] P. A. E. Sillevis Smitt,[7] J. J. G. M. Verschuuren,[8] R. Voltz[9] for the Paraneoplastic Neurological Syndrome Euronetwork

[1]Haukeland University Hospital and University of Bergen, Norway; [2]Hopital Bellevue, Saint Etienne, France; [3]University of Padua, Italy; [4]Institut d'Investigacio Biomedica August Pi I Sunyer (IDIBAPS), Hospital Clinic, University of Barcelona, Spain; [5]Kaiser Franz Josef hospital and Ludwig Boltzmann Institute for Neurooncology, Vienna, Austria; [6]Hospital Neurologique, Lyon, France; [7]Erasmus University Medical Center, Rotterdam, The Netherlands; [8]Leiden University Medical Center, The Netherlands; [9]University of Cologne, Germany

Background

Paraneoplastic neurological syndromes (PNS) were initially defined as neurological syndromes of unknown cause that often antedate the diagnosis of an underlying, usually not clinically evident, cancer. In the past two decades, the discovery that many PNS are associated with antibodies against neural antigens expressed by the tumour (onconeural antibodies) has suggested that some PNS are immune mediated. PNS are rare and occur in less than 1% of patients with cancer, although convincing epidemiologic data are missing. However, the diagnosis and treatment is important because the disability caused by the PNS is often severe and the correct diagnosis usually leads to the discovery of a small tumour with a chance of being cured (table 31.1). Recommended diagnostic criteria for PNS have been published by the PNS Euronetwork [1]. In this paper, the European Federation of Neurological Societies (EFNS) task force, as part of the PNS Euronetwork, has outlined guidelines for the management of classical PNS.

Methods

The task force considered the different syndromes known as paraneoplastic and chose to focus on classical PNS [1]:

European Handbook of Neurological Management: Volume 1, 2nd edition. Edited by N. E. Gilhus, M. P. Barnes and M. Brainin. © 2011 Blackwell Publishing Ltd.

paraneoplastic limbic encephalitis (PLE), subacute sensory neuronopathy (SSN), paraneoplastic cerebellar degeneration (PCD), and paraneoplastic opsoclonus-myoclonus (POM), as well as Lambert-Eaton myasthenic syndrome (LEMS) and paraneoplastic peripheral nerve hyperexcitability (PPNH). Myasthenia gravis has not been included as it has been reported together with a broader overview of LEMS and PNH in a separate task force report on treatment of neuromuscular disorders [2]. Paraproteinemic neuropathies have previously been evaluated by another EFNS task force [3]. Paraneoplastic retinopathy and dermatomyositis have not been included in this report.

Search strategies have included English literature from the following databases: Cochrane Library, Medline, PubMed (last search August 2009). The keywords used for the search included 'limbic encephalitis', 'sensory neuronopathy', 'cerebellar ataxia', 'opsoclonus-myoclonus', 'Lambert-Eaton myasthenic syndrome', 'neuromyotonia' in combination with 'investigation' and 'therapy'. All evidence available was evaluated as Class IV – case reports, case series, and expert opinion [4]. Thus, no recommendations reach Level A, B, or C [4]. However, Good Practice Points (GPP) were agreed by consensus.

Paraneoplastic limbic encephalitis

Clinical features

Paraneoplastic limbic encephalitis (PLE) is characterized by the acute, or subacute, onset of symptoms that suggest

Table 31.1 Treatment of paraneoplastic neurological syndromes.

Paraneoplastic syndrome	Common associated tumours	Onconeural antibodies	Response to symptomatic treatment	Response to immunotherapy	Response to tumour therapy

Limbic encephalitis	SCLC
	Testicular
	Breast
	Hodgkin's
	Ovarian
	  teratoma
	Thymoma
		Hu, CV2/CRMP5,
		  amphiphysin,
		  AMPAR, VGKC
		Ma2
		AMPAR
		None
		NMDAR, not specific
		  for paraneoplasia
		CV2/CRMP5, GAD,
		  AMPAR, VGKC,
		  but not specific
		  for paraneoplasia
			Yes	Good in patients
				  with NMDAR
				  or VGKC
				  antibodies. Bad
				  in patients with
				  onconeural
				  antibodies
				  other than
				  Ma2
					Yes, patients
					  often stabilize
					  if treated early

Subacute sensory
  neuronopathy
	SCLC
	Breast
	Ovarian sarcoma
	Hodgkin's
		Hu
		CV2/CRMP5
			Yes	Rare	Yes, especially
					  when treated
					  early

Cerebellar
  degeneration
	Ovary
	Breast
	SCLC
	Hodgkin's
		Yo
		Hu
		Tr
		CV2/CRMP5 VGCC,
		  but not specific
		  for paraneoplasia
			Yes	Rare	Yes, especially in
					  Hodgkin's

Opsoclonus-
  myoclonus
	Lung
	Breast
	Gynaecological
	  tumours
	Melanoma
	Histocytoma
	Neuroblastoma
	  in children
		Ri
		Hu
		Ma2
		Amphiphysin
		Often none,
		  especially in
		  children
			Yes	Occasionally in
				  adults. Often in
				  children
					Yes

Lambert-Eaton
  myasthenic
  syndrome
	SCLC	VGCC, but not
		  specific for
		  paraneoplasia
			Yes	Yes	Yes

Peripheral nerve
  hyperexcitability
  syndromes
	Thymoma
	SCLC
	Non-SCLC
	Hodgkin's
	Plasmacytoma
		VGKC, but not
		  specific for
		  paraneoplasia
			Yes	Yes	Yes

involvement of the limbic system. Patients may develop short-term memory loss or amnesia, become disoriented, or may show psychosis including visual or auditory hallucinations, or paranoid obsession. Confusion, depression, and anxiety are also common. Generalized or partial complex seizures are seen in about 50% of patients. In the majority of patients, the symptoms antedate the diagnosis of a tumour by a mean of 3–5 months. PLE is preferentially associated with small-cell lung cancer (SCLC) (40%), germ cell tumours of the testis (20%), breast cancer (8%), Hodgkin's lymphoma, thymoma, and immature teratoma [5].

Investigation

Magnetic resonance imaging (MRI) alterations in PLE are seen in about 60% of patients, but the figure is probably much higher if fluid attenuation inversion recovery (FLAIR) sequences are included in the study. The MRI features are most evident on coronal sections and typically consist of abnormal high-signal intensity on T2 sequences in one or both medial temporal lobe(s). On T1 sequences the temporal-limbic area may be hypointense and atrophic and rarely enhance with contrast injection [6]. In the absence of MRI abnormalities, fluorodeoxyglucose-positron emission tomography (FDG-PET) studies should show an increased tracer activity in the medial temporal lobe, which may reflect an acute stage of the inflammatory process [7]. In 45% of patients, electroencephalogram (EEG) reveals epileptic abnormalities from the temporal lobe, but in the majority of patients it shows unilateral or bilateral temporal slow waves. Cerebrospinal fluid (CSF) examinations show inflammatory signs (e.g. pleocytosis, oligoclonal bands) in about 60% of patients.

Antineuronal antibodies may be found in the serum and CSF of about 60% of patients with PLE. Two types of antibodies have been characterized: (1) onconeural antibodies that target intracellular antigens and are tightly associated with the presence of an underlying tumour, and (2) antibodies against surface receptors that are present in patients with limbic encephalitis that may or may not be paraneoplastic.

The most frequent onconeuronal antibodies are: anti-Hu, anti-Ma2 (with or without anti-Ma1), anti-CV2/CRMP5, and anti-amphiphysin. Seventy-eight per cent of patients with PLE and anti-Hu have symptoms that suggest a dysfunction in areas of the nervous system other than the limbic system. In fact, PLE may be the presenting or the predominant disorder of patients with paraneoplastic encephalomyelitis (PEM) or the 'anti-Hu syndrome'. These patients usually are older than 40 years, and the related tumour is a SCLC. Patients with only Ma2 antibodies are usually male, younger than 40 years, and clinically present with symptoms of diencephalic and upper brainstem dysfunction. The MRI evaluation is more likely to present abnormalities in medial temporal lobes, hypothalamus, basal ganglia, thalamus, or upper brainstem collicular region [8]. CV2/CRMP5 antibodies are instead detected in patients with thymoma or SCLC [9].

Three types of antibodies against different surface neuronal receptors have been identified in patients with PLE.

(1) Voltage-gated potassium channel (VGKC) antibodies can be associated with PLE and thymoma and SCLC, although the great majority of patients with these antibodies present with non-paraneoplastic LE [10–12]. (2) Anti-N-methyl-D-aspartate (NMDA) receptor-associated encephalitis is a recently described disorder that usually affects young women. A few days after prodromic fever or headache, most patients develop a syndrome that predictably evolves in stages, including prominent psychiatric symptoms (agitation, delusional thoughts, hallucinations) or less frequently short-term memory loss, seizures, progressive unresponsiveness (catatonia-like stage), central hypoventilation, autonomic instability (fluctuations of blood pressure, temperature, and cardiac rhythm), orofacial dyskinesias, and limb choreoathetosis and dystonia. Intensive care support and ventilation may be required for several weeks or many months. The majority of patients do not fulfil the criteria of classical LE and only 50% have an underlying ovarian teratoma or more rarely other tumours such as SCLC [13]. (3) A recent study reported the presence of antibodies against the GLUR1 or 2 subunits of the α-amino-3-hydroxy-5-methyl-4-isoxazoleproprionic acid receptor (AMPAR) of glutamate. The 10 patients described had classical LE. The median age was 60 years (38–87 years) and nine were women. Seven had tumours of the lung, breast, or thymus [14]. An important practical point is that patients with PLE may harbour both onconeural and anti-receptor antibodies [15].

Patients older than 40 years, smokers, and with Hu antibody have to be investigated for the presence of a SCLC. Anti-Hu-positive patients could also have extrathoracic tumours, but these can be considered responsible for PLE only when they express Hu antigens [16]. The absence of Hu antibody does not rule out the presence of SCLC; however, in patients older than 40 years, and without onconeural antibodies, the more frequently associated tumours are: breast cancer, non-SCLC tumours, and thymoma. Imaging studies to detect SCLC include high-resolution computed tomography (CT) of the chest and PDG-PET if the CT scan is negative [17, 18]. Special attention must be addressed to abnormal lymph nodes in the mediastinum. Bronchoscopy is usually negative. In male patients younger than 40 years, the detection of Ma2 antibodies suggests the presence of testicular cancer, which should be evaluated with ultrasound.

Therapy

Early detection and treatment of the underlying tumour is the approach that offers the greatest chance for neurological improvement or symptom stabilization. In men with only Ma2 antibodies, elective orchidectomy and serial examination of the testicle to rule out in situ carcinomas is indicated in patients at high risk of testicular cancer, suggested by the presence of calcifications or undescended testicle. The increasing evidence that PLE is immune-mediated has prompted the use of immune-modulating therapies. There are no reports that indicate which kind of immune therapy should be used. Patients are usually treated with one or more of the following: intravenous immunoglobulin, plasma exchange, or steroids [5]. Patients with antibodies against surface antigens usually respond to immunotherapy. PLE without onconeural antibodies and those with Ma2 antibodies (with or without anti-Ma1) may also respond to immune therapy [5]. Symptomatic therapy of PLE is directed against epilepsy and psychiatric symptoms.

Subacute sensory neuronopathy

Clinical features

Several neuropathies have been reported as paraneoplastic, but only subacute sensory neuronopathy (SSN) is regarded as a classical PNS [1]. SSN is associated with SCLC in 70–80% of cases, but may also occur with breast cancer, ovarian cancer, sarcoma, or Hodgkin's disease [19]. SSN precedes the overt clinical manifestations of the cancer with a median delay of 4.5 months [16]. The onset of SSN is usually subacute and rapidly progressive over weeks before a plateau phase is reached. The distribution is frequently multifocal or asymmetrical. Symptoms consist of pain and paraesthesiae [16]. Upper limbs are usually affected first or almost invariably involved with the evolution. Sensory loss, especially affecting deep sensation, often leads to severe sensory ataxia and tendon reflexes are absent. Sensory loss may also affect the face, chest, or abdomen. Many patients become bedridden, but also an indolent course has been reported [20]. SSN occurs in 74% of patients with PEM and is predominant in 50–60% and clinically pure in 24% [16]. Autonomic neuropathy including digestive pseudo-obstruction is frequent. These features were used to propose diagnosis criteria of paraneoplastic SSN [1] that have proved to be efficient [21].

Investigation

CSF analysis may show elevated protein concentration, pleocytosis, and sometimes oligoclonal bands. Electrophysiologically, the hallmark is a severe and diffuse alteration of sensory nerve action potentials that are either absent or markedly reduced [22]. Motor conduction velocities can be mildly altered. Nerve biopsy is usually not necessary, but may sometimes be helpful to distinguish SSN from multiple mononeuropathy due to vasculitis [23].

Hu antibodies are most often associated with SSN. Their estimated specificity in the diagnosis of cancer in patients suspected to have SSN is 99%, but the sensitivity is 82% [24]. The absence of Hu antibodies does not exclude the presence of an underlying cancer. CV2/CRMP5 antibodies also occur with peripheral neuropathies [25, 26]. In this setting, the neuropathy is usually sensory or sensori-motor, in which upper limbs are less frequently involved, but often associated with cerebellar ataxia [9, 27]. The electrophysiological pattern is axonal or mixed axonal and demyelinating. SCLC, neuroendocrine tumours, and thymoma are usually associated with CV2/CRMP5 antibodies. When high-resolution CT of the chest is negative, FDG-PET is recommended [17, 18].

Therapy

In a retrospective study of 200 patients with PEM/SSN, treatment of the tumour was an independent predictor of improvement and stabilization of the neurological disorder [16], arguing that an early diagnosis of the cancer may give the patients the best chance of stabilizing the neurological disorder. Several uncontrolled trials using intravenous immunoglobulin, steroids, plasma exchange, rituximab, or cyclophosphamide have been performed in small series of patients with PNS including SSN [28–31]. The effect of these treatments is difficult to assess, but patients with neuropathy or a recent onset of the PNS may sometimes show benefits. However, a larger series failed to demonstrate a clear benefit of intravenous immunoglobulin, steroids, plasma exchange, or cyclophosphamide, alone or in combination [29]. Symptomatic treatment is directed against neuropathic pain, sensory ataxia, and dysautonomic manifestation, such as orthostatic hypotension.

Paraneoplastic cerebellar degeneration

Clinical features

Paraneoplastic cerebellar degeneration (PCD) is characterized by subacute development of a severe pancerebellar dysfunction. Cerebellar signs usually begin with gait ataxia and, over a few weeks or months, progress to severe, usually symmetrical truncal and limb ataxia, with dysarthria and often nystagmus [32]. Occasionally, the onset is rapid, within a few hours or days. Vertigo is common, and many patients complain of diplopia. The cerebellar deficit usually stabilizes, but, the patient is then often severely incapacitated and most become bed-bound in the first 3 months after diagnosis. PCD is preferentially associated with ovarian cancer, breast cancer, SCLC, or Hodgkin's disease.

Investigation

Brain MRI studies are initially normal, but can demonstrate cerebellar atrophy in the latter stages of the disease. CSF examination shows inflammatory signs without cancer cells (e.g. pleocytosis, oligoclonal bands) in about 60% of PCD patients.

Yo antibodies are most frequently associated with PCD. These patients are mainly female with an average age of 61 years. The associated cancer is ovary, breast, or other gynaecological malignancies. Patients with Hu antibodies differ from those with anti-Yo in terms of a frequent association with SCLC, the same frequency in male and female, and often other neurological manifestations as part of PEM [16]. Between 13 and 20% of patients with Hu antibodies present with a subacute cerebellar syndrome that, in the initial stage, cannot be differentiated from PCD [16]. Neuropathy is observed in 60% of patients with PCD and CV2/CRMP5 antibodies [9, 27] and such antibodies are observed in about 7% of patients with PCD [33]. Patients with CV2/CRMP5 antibodies are mainly male (70%) with an average age of 62 years. The most frequently associated tumour is SCLC (60%). Tr antibodies are markers of patients with PCD and Hodgkin's disease, which is the third most common associated cancer with PCD, after SCLC and ovarian cancer. Unlike other antibodies, anti-Tr usually disappears after treatment of the tumour or, in a few patients, is only found in the CSF [34]. Ri antibodies are mainly observed in patients with cerebellar ataxia and paraneo-

plastic opsoclonus-myoclonus (POM). The associated cancers are breast or lung cancer. Some cases of PCD have been reported in association with antibodies against amphiphysin, Ma2, Zic4, mGluR1, or VGCC [1, 35]. When VGCC antibodies are present, LEMS can be associated with PCD [33, 36]. The absence of onconeural antibodies cannot rule out the diagnosis of PCD, as only 50% of patients with PCD harbour such antibodies [33].

If a SCLC is suspected, the tumour is generally demonstrated by high-resolution CT of the chest. Special attention must be addressed to abnormal lymph nodes in the mediastinum. Bronchoscopy is usually negative. The use of FDG-PET should be reserved for patients with onconeural antibodies when conventional imaging fails to identify a tumour [17, 18]. In patients without onconeural antibodies, the sensitivity and specificity of FDG-PET is poorer. If a gynaecological tumour is suspected, careful breast and pelvic examination, mammography, and pelvic CT are recommended. If no malignancy is revealed with this initial work-up, surgical exploration and removal of the ovaries may be warranted, particularly in postmenopausal women with Yo antibodies [32].

Therapy

The best chance to at least stabilize the syndrome is to treat the underlying tumour [35]. Immune therapy is rarely effective, and only few patients have been reported with improvement after intravenous immunoglobulin, steroids, or plasmapheresis [29, 30, 37]. Patients with anti-Tr and Hodgkin's disease are more likely to improve than those with other antibodies [34]. In patients with Yo antibodies, the prognosis is worse in patients with ovarian cancer and better in patients with breast cancer [38]. The prognosis is also better in PCD patients without onconeural antibodies than in patients with Hu antibodies [33]. Symptomatic treatment of cerebellar ataxia includes neurorehabilitation with speech and swallowing therapy, and modest additional gains can be seen with propranolol or antiepileptic drugs.

Paraneoplastic opsoclonus-myoclonus

Clinical features

Opsoclonus means involuntary eye movements in any direction. It does not remit in darkness and with eyes closed, and may occur intermittently or, if more severe, constantly. In paraneoplastic opsoclonus-myoclonus (POM), opsoclonus is often accompanied by cerebellar signs such as gait ataxia and limb myoclonus, the so-called dancing eyes, dancing feet syndrome, and encephalopathy [39–41]. In contrast to most paraneoplastic syndromes, the course of POM may be remitting and relapsing [39, 42].

In infants, the most common associated tumour is neuroblastoma [43, 44]. In adults, it is lung cancer, breast cancer, or a gynaecological cancer such as ovary or uterus [45–47]. The association with other tumours on a single-case basis has been reported, such as melanoma [48, 49], malignant fibrous histiocytoma [50], ovarian teratoma [51], esthesioneuroblastoma [52], renal adenocarcinoma [53], and non-Hodgkin's lymphoma [54, 55].

Investigation

Brain MRI studies are generally normal, while examination of the CSF may show mild pleocytosis and protein elevation. Most infant [56, 57] and adult patients do not harbour a clearly defined onconeural antibody [45, 58]. In those who do, anti-Hu, anti-amphiphysin, anti-Ri, or anti-Ma2 may be found [45, 59–61].

In children, the search for an occult neuroblastoma should include imaging of the chest and abdomen (CT scan or MRI), urine catecholamine measurements (VMA and HVA), and metaiodobenzylguanidine (MIBG) scan [62]. When negative, the evaluation should be repeated after several months [63].

Initial investigation in adult patients suspected of POM should be directed at tumours associated with this condition, that is, high-resolution CT of the chest and abdomen, and gynaecological examination and mammography in women [45]. When this evaluation is negative, FDG-PET should be considered [17, 18].

Therapy

Tumour therapy is the mainstay of management [45]. In the paediatric population, POM may improve following treatment with adrenocorticotropic hormone (ACTH), steroids, or intravenous immunoglobulin, but residual CNS signs are frequent [43, 63–66]. In contrast to idiopathic OM, no clear advantage of immune therapy has been demonstrated in adult POM [45]. Improvement following steroids, cyclophosphamide, azathioprine,

intravenous immunoglobulin, plasma exchange, or plasma filtration with a protein A column has been described in single cases [42, 61, 67, 68]. Symptomatic therapy of nystagmus and oscillopsia includes the use of various anti-epileptic drugs, baclofen, or propranolol [41]. Myoclonus can be treated with anti-epileptic drugs. In children, trazodone may improve sleep disturbances and rage attacks [69].

Lambert-Eaton myasthenic syndrome

Clinical features

In more than 90% of the patients, muscle weakness starts proximal in the legs. Weakness can spread to other skeletal muscles in a caudo-cranial order, but only rarely leads to need for artificial respiration. Ptosis, ophthalmoplegia, and diplopia tend to be less frequent and milder than in myasthenia gravis [61]. Autonomic dysfunction is characterized by the presence of a dry mouth, dryness of the eyes, blurred vision, impotence, constipation, impaired sweating, or orthostatic hypotension [70]. The autonomic dysfunction is mostly mild to moderate, in contrast to the severe disabling autonomic dysfunction sometimes found in SSN/PEM. In less than 10% of cases, patients with Lambert-Eaton myasthenic syndrome (LEMS) and SCLC develop PCD [33, 36, 71].

Investigation

Electrophysiological studies show a reduced amplitude of the compound muscle action potential (CMAP) after nerve stimulation with decrement at low-frequency stimulation (3 Hz) of more than 10%, and an increment of more than 100% after maximum voluntary contraction of the muscle for 15 s. Increment is in fact normalization of the initial low CMAP. Thus, increment will not be found if the initial CMAP is normal. High-frequency stimulation at >20 Hz also produces an increased increment, but is painful and not usually necessary. Anti-P/Q-type VGCC antibodies are present in the serum of at least 85% of the patients [72]. These antibodies are found in both forms of LEMS, with or without SCLC. Antibodies to N-type VGCC have also been found in the serum, but their contribution to the muscle weakness or autonomic dysfunction is probably small. They are not used for diagnostic purposes.

In half of the LEMS patients, a SCLC will be found. The SCLC is detected within 1 year in 96% of the patients [71]. A retrospective study of 77 patients with LEMS showed that patients who had been smoking and were HLA-B8-negative had a 69% chance of developing SCLC. On the other hand, none of 24 patients who never smoked and were HLA-B8-positive developed SCLC [73]. Recently, a new serum antibody was described that appears to be very specific for the presence of a SCLC in patients with LEMS. This SOX antibody is present in 64% of the patients with LEMS and SCLC, and in 22% of the patients with SCLC and no clinical paraneoplastic syndrome [74]. Thus, although the specificity is high (95%), the sensitivity is moderate (65%), as the antibody is absent in about one-third of LEMS patients with a SCLC [75].

It is recommended that all patients are examined by high-resolution chest CT, and PDG-PET if the CT scan is negative. A bronchoscopy has no additional diagnostic value if both these investigations are negative [71]. If chest CT and PDG-PET scan are available, repeated screening every 6 months for 2 years is probably sufficient. If no further risk factors for a tumour (smoking, older age, HLA-B8, other paraneoplastic syndromes) are present, screening can most likely stop after two rounds of screening at a 6-month interval [71].

Therapy

For patients with a SCLC it is important to treat the tumour. Specific tumour therapy in a small retrospective series resulted in recovery from the neurological syndrome within 6–12 months [76]. One patient remained tumour-free after radiotherapy and local resection at 12 years. Chemotherapy, which is the first choice of tumour treatment, will also have an immunosuppressive effect on LEMS. It has been shown that the presence of LEMS in patients with SCLC improves survival [77]. Symptomatic treatment consists of 3,4-diaminopyridine [78]. A recent double-blind crossover trial with intravenous administration of 3,4-DAP, pyridostigmin, or both confirmed the therapeutic value of 3,4-DAP, but could not demonstrate an additional role for pyridostigmin [79]. If this treatment is not sufficient, steroids, azathioprine, plasma exchange, and intravenous immunoglobulin should be considered.

Paraneoplastic peripheral nerve hyperexcitability syndromes

Clinical features

The commonest form of peripheral nerve hyperexcitability (PNH) (neuromyotonia, Isaacs' syndrome) is autoimmune and often caused by antibodies to VGKC [80]. Paraneoplastic PNH (PPNH) is present in up to 25% of the patients and can predate the detection of a tumour by up to 4 years [81]. In a study of 60 patients, seven (12%) had a thymoma with myasthenia gravis (MG), two (3%) had a thymoma without clinical MG, four (7%) had a SCLC, and one (2%) had a lung adenocarcinoma [81]. PPNH can also occur with Hodgkin's disease [82, 83] and plasmacytoma [84].

The clinical hallmark of PNH is spontaneous and continuous skeletal muscle overactivity, usually presenting as twitching and painful cramps and often accompanied by various combinations of stiffness, pseudomyotonia, pseudotetany, and weakness [85]. About 33% of patients also have sensory features and up to 50% have hyperhidrosis, suggesting autonomic involvement. CNS features can occur, ranging from personality change and insomnia to a psychosis with delusions, hallucinations, and autonomic disturbance (Morvan's syndrome).

Investigation

EMG helps to confirm PNH and excludes other causes of continuous muscle overactivity such as stiff limb syndromes [85]. Nerve conduction studies may characterize an underlying peripheral neuropathy [81, 85].

There is no antibody that indicates whether PNH is paraneoplastic. VGKC antibodies are found in about 35% of all acquired PNH patients, although this rises to 80% in those with thymoma [80]. VGKC antibodies can also be associated with PLE and thymoma without PNH, or with non-paraneoplastic LE [10–12]. Hu antibodies can be helpful as one PPNH patient had SCLC [86]. Serum and urine screening for a paraprotein can help identify a plasmacytoma [84].

Most adults warrant a post-contrast CT mediastinum scan as up to 15% of patients have a thymoma, sometimes in the absence of MG or AChR antibodies [81]. This is combined with a high-resolution CT of the chest, as about 10% of PNH patients will have a SCLC or adenocarcinoma [81]. Chest CT may also help detect

Hodgkin's disease [82, 83]. When the initial tumour screen is negative and malignancy is still suspected, PDG-PET is the investigation of choice. Monitoring for up to 4 years is indicated in those at risk of lung cancer [81].

Treatment

PPNH often improves and can remit after treatment of cancer [82, 84–86]. The demonstration that most cases of PNH are autoimmune has led to trials of immuno-modulatory therapies in patients, including a few with thymoma [85, 87] whose symptoms are debilitating or refractory to symptomatic therapy. Plasma exchange often produces useful clinical improvement lasting about 6 weeks, accompanied by a reduction in EMG activity [85] and a fall in VGKC antibody titres [88]. Experience suggests that intravenous immunoglobulin can also help [89] despite reports that it worsened PNH in one patient [90] and was less effective than plasma exchange in another [91]. By analogy with LEMS, selected patients with severe PPNS refractory to other treatments may benefit from immunomodulatory therapy.

Prednisolone, with or without azathioprine or metho-trexate, has been useful in selected autoimmune PNH patients [85, 92] including a few patients with thymoma-associated PPNH who did not improve after thymectomy [85]. All forms of PNH, including paraneoplastic, usually improve with symptomatic treatment using various anti-epileptic drugs [85].

Recommendations

- Patients with PNS most often present with neurological symptoms before an underlying tumour is detected. Onconeural antibodies should be sought in sera from patients with suspected PNS. The antibodies are important for the diagnosis and tumour search.

- Radiological investigations for tumours, such as high-resolution CT for the detection of SCLC, are important, but should be followed by PDG-PET if no tumour is found.

- Patients should be followed at regular intervals, for example every 6 months for up to 4 years, to search for tumour in cases where the initial tumour screen was negative.

- Early detection and treatment of the tumour is the approach that offers the greatest chance for PNS stabilization. This should be done in cooperation with an oncologist,

pulmologist, gynaecologist, or paediatrician, depending on the associated tumour.

- Immune therapy (steroids, plasma exchange, or intravenous immunoglobulin) usually has no or only modest effect on PLE, SSN, or PCD.

- Children with POM may respond to immune therapy, whereas no evidence for the effect of such therapy has been shown in adults with POM.

- Patients with LEMS or PPNH should be treated with immune therapy if symptomatic therapy does not give sufficient improvement.

- Symptomatic therapy should be offered to all patients with PNS.

Acknowledgements

This study was supported by grant QLG1-CT-2002-01756 of the European Commission. Ian Hart has previously contributed to this chapter. We thank Maarten Titulaer for help in preparing part of the text.

Conflicts of interest

The authors have reported no conflicts of interest relevant to this manuscript.

References

1. Graus F, Delattre JY, Antoine JC, et al. Recommended diagnostic criteria for paraneoplastic neurological syndromes. *J Neurol Neurosurg Psychiatry* 2004;**75**:1135–40.

2. Skeie GO, Apostolski S, Evoli A, et al. Guidelines for the treatment of autoimmune neuromuscular transmission disorders. *Eur J Neurol* 2006;**13**:691–9.

3. Willison HJ, Ang W, Gilhus NE, et al. EFNS Task force report: a questionairre-based survey on the service provision and quality assurance for determiniation of diagnostic autoantibody tests in European neuroimmunology centres. European Federation of Neurological Societies. *Eur J Neurol* 2000;**7**:625–8.

4. Brainin M, Barnes M, Baron J-C, et al. Guidance for the preparation of neurological management guidelines by EFNS scientific task forces – revised recommendations 2004. *Eur J Neurol* 2004;**11**:577–81.

5. Gultekin SH, Rosenfeld MR, Voltz R, et al. Paraneoplastic limbic encephalitis: neurological symptoms, immunological findings and tumor association in 50 patients. *Brain* 2000;**123**:1481–94.

6. Dirr LY, Elster AD, Donofrio PD, Smith M. Evolution of brain abnormalities in limbic encephalitis. *Neurology* 1990;**40**:1304–6.

7. Provenzale JM, Barboriak DP, Coleman RE. Limbic encephalitis: comparison of FDG PET and MRI findings. *Am J Roentgenol* 1998;**18**:1659–60.

8. Dalmau J, Graus F, Villarejo A, *et al*. Clinical analysis of anti-Ma2-associated encephalitis. *Brain* 2004;**127**:1831–44.

9. Yu Z, Kryzer TJ, Grisemann GE, *et al*. CRMP-5 neuronal autoantibody: marker of lung cancer and thymoma-related autoimmunity. *Ann Neurol* 2001;**49**:146–54.

10. Buckley C, Oger J, Clover L, *et al*. Potassium channel antibodies in two patients with reversible limbic encephalitis. *Ann Neurol* 2001;**50**:74–9.

11. Pozo-Rosich P, Clover L, Saiz A, *et al*. Voltage-gated potassium channel antibodies in limbic encephalitis. *Ann Neurol* 2003;**54**:530–3.

12. Vincent A, Buckley C, Schott JM, *et al*. Potassium Channel antibody-associated encephalopathy: a potentially immunotherapy-responsive form of encephalitis. *Brain* 2004;**127**:701–12.

13. Dalmau J, Gleichman AJ, Hughes EG, *et al*. Anti-NMDA-receptor encephalitis:case series and analysis of the effects of antibodies. *Lancet Neurol* 2008;**7**:1091–8.

14. Lai M, Hughes EG, Peng X, *et al*. AMPA receptor antibodies in limbic encephalitis alter synaptic receptor location. *Ann Neurol* 2009;**65**:424–34.

15. Graus F, Saiz A, Lai M, *et al*. Neuronal surface antigen antibodies in limbic encephalitis: clinical-immunologic associations. *Neurology* 2008;**71**:930–6.

16. Graus F, Keime-Guibert F, Reòe R, *et al*. Anti-Hu-associated paraneoplastic encephalomyelitis: analysis of 200 patients. *Brain* 2001;**124**:1138–48.

17. Linke R, Schroeder M, Helmberger T, Voltz R. Antibody-positive paraneoplastic neurologic syndromes: value of CT and PET for tumor diagnosis. *Neurology* 2004;**63**:282–6.

18. Younes-Mhenni S, Janier MF, Cinotti L, *et al*. FDG-PET improves tumour detection in patients with paraneoplastic neurological syndromes. *Brain* 2004;**127**:2331–8.

19. Horwich MS, Cho L, Porro RS, Posner JB. Subacute sensory neuropathy: a remote effect of carcinoma. *Ann Neurol* 1977;**2**:7–19.

20. Graus F, Bonaventura I, Uchya M, *et al*. Indolent anti-Hu-associated paraneoplastic sensory neuropathy. *Neurology* 1994;**44**:2258–61.

21. Camdessanché JP, Jousserand G, Ferraud K, *et al*. The pattern and diagnostic criteria of sensory neuronopathy. The pattern and diagnostic criteria of sensory neuronopathy. A case control study. *Brain* 2009;**132**:1723–33.

22. Camdesssance JP, Antoine JC, Honnorat J, *et al*. Paraneoplastic peripheral neuropathy associated with anti-Hu antibodies. A clinical and electrophysiological study of 20 patients. *Brain* 2002;**125**:166–75.

23. Younger DS, Dalmau J, Inghirami G, *et al*. Anti-Hu-associated peripheral nerve and muscle microvasculitis. *Neurology* 1994;**44**:181–3.

24. Molinuevo JL, Graus F, Serrano C, *et al*. Utility of anti-Hu antibodies in the diagnosis of paraneoplastic sensory neuropathy. *Ann Neurol* 1998;**4**:976–80.

25. Antoine JC, Honnorat J, Camdesssance JP, *et al*. Paraneoplastic anti-CV2 antibodies react with peripheral nerve and are associated with a mixed axonal and demyelinating peripheral neuropathy. *Ann Neurol* 2001;**49**:214–21.

26. Honnorat J, Cartalat-Carel S, Ricard D, *et al*. Onco-neural antibodies and tumour type determine survival and neurological symptoms in paraneoplastic neurological syndromes with Hu or CV2/CRMP5 antibodies. *J Neurol Neurosurg Psychiatry* 2009;**80**:412–6.

27. Honnorat J, Antoine JC, Derrington E, *et al*. Antibodies to a subpopulation of glial cells and a 66 kDa developmental protein in patients with paraneoplastic neurological syndromes. *J Neurol Neurosurg Psychiatry* 1996;**61**:270–8.

28. Uchuya M, Graus F, Vega F, *et al*. Intravenous immunoglobulin treatment in paraneoplastic neurological syndromes with antineuronal autoantibodies. *J Neurol Neurosurg Psychiatry* 1996;**60**:388–39.

29. Keime-Guibert F, Graus F, Fleury A, *et al*. Treatment of paraneoplastic neurological syndromes with antineuronal antibodies (anti-Hu, anti-Yo) with a combination of immunoglobulins, cyclophosphamide, and methylprednisolone. *J Neurol Neurosurg Psychiatry* 2000;**68**:479–82.

30. Vernino S, O'Neill BP, Marks RS, *et al*. Immunomodulatory treatment trial for paraneoplastic neurological disorders. *Neuro-Oncol* 2004;**6**:55–62.

31. Shams'ili S, de Beukelaar J, Gratama JW, *et al*. An uncontrolled trial of rituximab for antibody associated paraneoplastic neurological syndromes. *J Neurol* 2006;**253**:16–20.

32. Peterson K, Rosenblum MK, Kotanides H, Posner JB. Paraneoplastic cerebellar degeneration. I. A clinical analysis of 55 anti-Yo antibody-positive patients. *Neurology* 1992;**42**:1931–7.

33. Mason WP, Graus F, Lang B, *et al*. Small-cell lung cancer, paraneoplastic cerebellar degeneration and the Lambert-Eaton myasthenic syndrome. *Brain* 1997;**120**:1279–300.

34. Bernal F, Shams'ili S, Rojas I, *et al*. Anti-Tr antibodies as markers of paraneoplastic cerebellar degeneration and Hodgkin's disease. *Neurology* 2003;**60**:230–4.

35. Shams'ili S, Grefkens J, de Leeuw B, *et al*. Paraneoplastic cerebellar degeneration associated with antineuronal antibodies: analysis of 50. *Patients Brain* 2003;**126**:1409–18.

36. Fukuda T, Motomura M, Nakao Y, *et al*. Reduction of P/Q-type calcium channels in the postmortem cerebellum of

paraneoplastic cerebellar degeneration with Lambert-Eaton myasthenic syndrome. *Ann Neurol* 2003;**53**:21–8.

37. Widdess-Walsh P, Tavee JO, Schuele S, Stevens GH. Response to intravenous immunoglobulin in anti-Yo associated paraneoplastic cerebellar degeneration: case report and review of the literature. *J Neurooncol* 2003;**63**:187–90.

38. Rojas I, Graus F, Keime-Guibert F, *et al.* Long-term clinical outcome of paraneoplastic cerebellar degeneration and anti-Yo antibodies. *Neurology* 2000;**55**:713–5.

39. Anderson NE, Budde-Steffen C, Rosenblum MK, *et al.* Opsoclonus, myoclonus, ataxia, and encephalopathy in adults with cancer: a distinct paraneoplastic syndrome. *Medicine* 1988;**67**:100–9.

40. Buttner U, Straube A, Handke V. Opsoclonus and ocular flutter. *Nervenarzt* 1997;**68**:633–7.

41. Straube A, Leigh RJ, Bronstein A, *et al.* EFNS task force-therapy of nystagmus and oscillopsia. *Eur J Neurol* 2004;**11**:83–9.

42. Dropcho EJ, Kline LB, Riser J. Antineuronal (anti-Ri) antibodies in a patient with steroid-responsive opsoclonus-myoclonus. *Neurology* 1993;**43**:207–11.

43. Mitchell WG, Davalos-Gonzalez Y, Brumm VL, *et al.* Opsoclonus-ataxia caused by childhood neuroblastoma: developmental and neurologic sequelae. *Pediatrics* 2002;**109**:86–98.

44. Gambini C, Conte M, Bernini G, *et al.* Neuroblastic tumors associated with opsoclonus-myoclonus syndrome: histological, immunohistochemical and molecular features of 15 Italian cases. *Virchows Arch* 2003;**442**:555–62.

45. Bataller L, Graus F, Saiz A, Vilchez JJ. Clinical outcome in adult onset idiopathic or paraneoplastic opsoclonus-myoclonus. *Brain* 2001;**124**:437–43.

46. Voltz R. Paraneoplastic neurological syndromes: an update on diagnosis, pathogenesis, and therapy. *Lancet Neurol* 2002;**1**:294–305.

47. Darnell JC, Posner JB. Paraneoplastic syndromes involving the nervous system. *N Engl J Med* 2003;**349**:1543–54.

48. Berger JR, Mehari E. Paraneoplastic opsoclonus-myoclonus secondary to malignant melanoma. *J Neurooncol* 1999;**41**:43–5.

49. Jung KY, Youn J, Chung CS. Opsoclonus-myoclonus syndrome in an adult with malignant melanoma. *J Neurol* 2006;**253**:942–3.

50. Zamecnik J, Cerny R, Bartos A, *et al.* Paraneoplastic opsoclonus-myoclonus syndrome associated with malignant fibrous histiocytoma: neuropathological findings. *Cesk Patol* 2004;**40**:63–7.

51. Fitzpatrick AS, Gray OM, McConville J, McDonnell GV. Opsoclonus-myoclonus syndrome associated with benign ovarian teratoma. *Neurology* 2008;**70**:1292–3.

52. Van Diest D, De Raeve H, Claes J, *et al.* Paraneoplastic opsoclonus-myoclonus-ataxia (OMA) syndrome in an

adult patient with esthesioneuroblastoma. *J Neurol* 2008;**255**:594–6.

53. Vigliani MC, Palmucci L, Polo P, *et al.* Paraneoplastic opsoclonus-myoclonus associated with renal cell carcinoma and responsive to tumour ablation. *J Neurol Neurosurg Psychiatry* 2001;**70**:814–5.

54. Kumar A, Lajara-Nanson WA, Neilson RW Jr. Paraneoplastic opsoclonus-myoclonus syndrome: initial presentation of non-Hodgkins lymphoma. *J Neurooncol* 2005;**73**:43–5.

55. Ducrocq X, Petit J, Taillandier L, *et al.* Paraneoplastic opsoclonus-myoclonus syndrome revealing T-cell lymphoma. *Presse Med* 1999;**28**:330–3.

56. Antunes NL, Khakoo Y, Matthay KK, *et al.* Antineuronal antibodies in patients with neuroblastoma and paraneoplastic opsoclonus-myoclonus. *J Pediatr Hematol Oncol* 2000;**22**:315–20.

57. Pranzatelli MR, Tate ED, Wheeler A, *et al.* Screening for autoantibodies in children with opsoclonus-myoclonus-ataxia. *Pediatr Neurol* 2002;**27**:384–7.

58. Bataller L, Rosenfeld MR, Graus F, Vilchez JJ, *et al.* Autoantigen diversity in the opsoclonus-myoclonus syndrome. *Ann Neurol* 2003;**53**:347–53.

59. Prestigiacomo CJ, Balmaceda C, Dalmau J. Anti-Ri-associated paraneoplastic opsoclonus-ataxia syndrome in a man with transitional cell carcinoma. *Cancer* 2001;**91**:1423–8.

60. Wong AM, Musallam S, Tomlinson RD, *et al.* Opsoclonus in three dimensions: oculographic, neuropathologic and modelling correlates. *J Neurol Sci* 2001;**189**:71–81.

61. Wirtz PW, Sotodeh M, Nijnuis M, *et al.* Difference in distribution of muscle weakness between myasthenia gravis and the Lambert-Eaton myasthenic syndrome. *J Neurol Neurosurg Psychiatry* 2002;**73**:766–8.

62. Swart JF, de Kraker J, van der Lely N. Metaiodobenzylguanidine total-body scintigraphy required for revealing occult neuroblastoma in opsoclonus-myoclonus syndrome. *Eur J Pediatr* 2002;**161**:255–8.

63. Hayward K, Jeremy RJ, Jenkins S, *et al.* Long-term neurobehavioral outcomes in children with neuroblastoma and opsoclonus-myoclonus-ataxia syndrome: relationship to MRI findings and anti-neuronal antibodies. *J Pediatr* 2001;**139**:552–9.

64. Rudnick E, Khakoo Y, Antunes NL, *et al.* Opsoclonus-myoclonus-ataxia syndrome in neuroblastoma: clinical outcome and antineuronal antibodies – a report from the Children's Cancer Group Study. *Med Pediatr Oncol* 2001;**36**:612–22.

65. Ertle F, Behnisch W, Al Mulla NA, *et al.* Treatment of neuroblastoma-related opsoclonus-myoclonus-ataxia syndrome with high-dose dexamethasone pulses. *Pediatr Blood Cancer* 2008;**50**:683–7.

66. Catsman-Berrevoets CE, Aarsen FK, van Hemsbergen ML. Improvement of neurological status and quality of

life in children with opsoclonus myoclonus syndrome at long-term follow-up. *Pediatr Blood Cancer* 2009;**53**:1048–53.

67. Nitschke M, Hochberg F, Dropcho E. Improvement of paraneoplastic opsoclonus-myoclonus after protein A column therapy. *N Engl J Med* 1995;**332**:192.

68. Jongen JL, Moll WJ, Sillevis Smitt PA, *et al.* Anti-Ri positive opsoclonus-myoclonus-ataxia in ovarian duct cancer. *J Neurol* 1988;**245**:691–2.

69. Pranzatelli MR, Tate ED, Dukart WS, *et al.* Sleep disturbance and rage attacks in opsoclonus-myoclonus syndrome: response to trazodone. *J Pediatr* 2005;**147**:372–8.

70. O'Neill JH, Murray NM, Newsom-Davis J. The Lambert-Eaton myasthenic syndrome. A review of 50 cases. *Brain* 1988;**111**:577–96.

71. Titulaer MJ, Wirtz PW, Willems LNA, *et al.* Screening for small cell lung cancer: a follow-up study of patients with Lambert-Eaton myasthenic syndrome. *J Clin Oncol* 2008;**26**:4276–81.

72. Motomura M, Johnston I, Lang B, *et al.* An improved diagnostic assay for Lambert-Eaton myasthenic syndrome. *J Neurol Neurosurg Psychiatry* 1995;**58**:85–7.

73. Wirtz PW, Willcox N, van der Slik AR, *et al.* HLA and smoking in prediction and prognosis of small cell lung cancer in autoimmune Lambert-Eaton myasthenic syndrome. *J Neuroimmunol* 2005;**159**:230–7.

74. Sabater L, Titulaer M, Saiz A, *et al.* SOX1 antibodies are markers of paraneoplastic Lambert Eatonmyasthenic syndrome. *Neurology* 2008;**70**:924–8.

75. Titulaer MJ, Klooster R, Potman M, *et al.* SOX antibodies in small-cell lung cancer and Lambert-Eaton myasthenic syndrome: frequency and relation with survival. *J Clin Oncol* 2009;**27**:4260–7.

76. Chalk CH, Murray NM, Newsom-Davis J, O'Neill JH, Spiro SG. Response of the Lambert-Eaton myasthenic syndrome to treatment of associated small-cell lung carcinoma. *Neurology* 1990;**40**:1552–6.

77. Maddison P, Newsom-Davis J, Mills KR, Souhami RL. Favourable prognosis in Lambert-Eaton myasthenic syndrome and small-cell lung carcinoma. *Lancet* 1999;**353**:117–8.

78. McEvoy KM, Windebank AJ, Daube JR, Low PA. 3,4-Diaminopyridine in the treatment of Lambert-Eaton myasthenic syndrome. *N Engl J Med* 1989;**321**:1567–71.

79. Wirtz PW, Verschuuren JJ, van Dijk JG, *et al.* Efficacy of 3,4-diaminopyridine and pyridostigmine in the treatment of Lambert–Eaton myasthenic syndrome: a randomized,

double-blind, placebo-controlled, crossover study. *Clin Pharmacol Ther* 2009;**86**:44–8.

80. Hart IK, Waters C, Vincent A, *et al.* Autoantibodies detected to expressed potassium channels are implicated in neuromyotonia. *Ann Neurol* 1997;**41**:238–46.

81. Hart IK, Maddison P, Newsom-Davis J, *et al.* Phenotypic variants of peripheral nerve hyperexcitability. *Brain* 2002;**125**:1887–95.

82. Caress JB, Abend WK, Preston DC, Logigian EL. A case of Hodgkin's lymphoma producing neuromyotonia. *Neurology* 1997;**49**:258–9.

83. Lahrmann H, Albrecht G, Drlicek M, *et al.* Acquired neuromyotonia and peripheral neuropathy in a patient with Hodgkin's disease. *Muscle Nerve* 2001;**24**:834–8.

84. Zifko U, Drlicek M, Machacek E, *et al.* Syndrome of continuous muscle fiber activity and plasmacytoma with IgM paraproteinemia. *Neurology* 1994;**44**:560–1.

85. Newsom-Davis J, Mills KR. Immunological associations of acquired neuromyotonia (Isaacs' syndrome). Report of five cases and literature review. *Brain* 1993;**116**:453–69.

86. Toepfer M, Schroeder M, Unger JM, *et al.* Neuromyotonia, myoclonus, sensory neuropathy and cerebellar symptoms in a patient with antibodies to neuronal nucleoproteins (anti-Hu-antibodies). *Clin Neurol Neurosurg* 1999;**101**:207–9.

87. Hayat GR, Kulkantrakorn K, Campbell WW, Giuliani MJ. Neuromyotonia: autoimmune pathogenesis and response to immune modulating therapy. *J Neurol Sci* 2000;**181**:38–43.

88. Shillito P, Molenaar PC, Vincent A, *et al.* Acquired neuromyotonia: evidence for autoantibodies directed against K^+ channels of peripheral nerves. *Ann Neurol* 1995;**38**:714–22.

89. Alessi G, De Reuck J, De Bleecker J, Vancayzeele S. Successful immunoglobulin treatment in a patient with neuromyotonia. *Clin Neurol Neurosurgery* 2000;**102**:173–5.

90. Ishii A, Hayashi A, Ohkoshi N, *et al.* Clinical evaluation of plasma exchange and high dose intravenous immunoglobulin in a patient with Isaacs' syndrome. *J Neurol Neurosurg Psychiatry* 1994;**57**:840–2.

91. van den Berg JS, van Engelen BG, Boerman RH, de Baets MH. Acquired neuromyotonia: superiority of plasma exchange over high-dose intravenous human immunoglobulin. *J Neurol* 1999;**246**:623–5.

92. Nakatsuji Y, Kaido M, Sugai F, *et al.* Isaacs' syndrome successfully treated by immunoadsorption plasmapheresis. *Acta Neurol Scand* 2000;**102**:271–3.

CHAPTER 32

Nystagmus and oscillopsia

A. Straube,[1] A. Bronstein,[2] D. Straumann[3]

[1]University of Munich, Germany; [2]Imperial College of Science, Technology and Medicine, London, UK; [3]University of Zurich, Switzerland

Introduction

One function of the ocular motor system is to stabilize images during eye and head movements on the retina (especially the central fovea). Involuntary or abnormal eye movements cause excessive motion of images on the retina without a corresponding efference copy (or corollary discharge) [1], leading to blurred vision and to the illusion that the seen world is moving (oscillopsia). This leads to spatial disorientation, impaired postural balance and vertigo. In clinical practice, the identification of specific eye movement abnormalities is often useful in the topological diagnosis of a broad range of disorders that affect the brain. Although we now know quite a lot about the anatomy, physiology, and pharmacology of the ocular motor system, our treatment options for abnormal eye movements remain fairly limited. Most drug treatments are based on case reports. Only recently several small controlled trials have been published, and they were all based on a small number of subjects, and not all patients always respond positively to the treatment. Thus, all treatment recommendations have to be classified as Class C [2]. The goal of the paper is to summarize all published treatment options for nystagmus and oscillopsia as well as to provide a short overview on definitions and pathomechanisms of certain distinct ocular motor syndromes.

A large part of this review concerns nystagmus, which is defined as repetitive, to-and-fro involuntary eye movements that are initiated by slow drifts of the eye. Physiological nystagmus occurs during rotation of the body in space or during ocular following of moving scenes and acts to *preserve* clear vision (vestibular and optokinetic nystagmus respectively). In contrast, pathological nystagmus causes the eyes to drift away from the visual target, thus degrading vision. Most commonly, nystagmus consists of an alternation of unidirectional drifts away from the target, e.g. due to a vestibular imbalance, and their correction by fast movements (saccades), which temporarily bring the visual target back to the fovea; this is jerk nystagmus. Another rarer form, pendular nystagmus, consists of to-and-fro quasi-sinusoidal eye oscillations. Nystagmus should be distinguished from inappropriate saccades that prevent steady fixation (e.g. ocular flutter). Saccades are fast movements, and the smeared retinal signal due to these movements remains largely unperceived. However, patients in whom abnormal saccades repeatedly misdirect the fovea often complain of difficulty in reading. In general most of the later in life acquired nytagmus syndromes as well as saccadic oscillations cause oscillopsia and vertigo; in contrast, most of the congenital or in early youth acquired nystagmus syndromes are not accompanied by oscillopsia. The recommendations are a revised and extended version of the 2004 guidelines [3].

Methods

One member of the task force panel (AS) searched through all available published information using the database MEDLINE (last search September 2009). The search was restricted to papers published in English, French, or German. The key words used for the search included the following sequences: 'nystagmus and therapy', 'treatment of ocular motor disorders', and

European Handbook of Neurological Management: Volume 1, 2nd edition. Edited by N. E. Gilhus, M. P. Barnes and M. Brainin.

'treatment of double vision'. All published papers were included, as only a limited number of controlled studies are available. The other members of the task force read the first draft of the recommendation and discussed changes (informative consensus approach).

Supranuclear ocular motor disorders

Central vestibular disorders

The vestibulo-ocular reflex (VOR) normally generates compensatory eye rotations of short latency and in the same plane but opposite direction to the head rotation that elicits them. Disorders of the vestibular *periphery* cause nystagmus in a direction that is determined by the pattern of the involved labyrinthine semicircular canals. The complete, unilateral loss of one labyrinth causes a mixed horizontal-torsional nystagmus that is suppressed by visual fixation. *Central* vestibular disorders may also cause an imbalance of these reflexes, leading to upbeat, downbeat, or torsional nystagmus (see below); typically a straight horizontal beating nystagmus (e.g. no rotational component) or nystagmus beats not in the direction of the stimulated semicircular canal (e.g. crosscoupling) is due to a central vestibular lesion. Another consequence of vestibular disease is a change in the size (gain = eye velocity divided by head velocity) of the overall dynamic VOR response. As a result of this change, patients complain of oscillopsia during rapid head movements. A VOR gain larger than 1 (i.e. eye velocity exceeds head velocity) results from a disinhibition of the brainstem circuits responsible for the VOR and is caused by central, vestibulo-cerebellar dysfunction. Loss of peripheral vestibular function causes impaired vision and oscillopsia during locomotion, due to the inability to compensate for the high-frequency head perturbations that occur with each footstep, i.e. the gain of the VOR remains too low for gaze stabilization after peripheral vestibular lesions. The treatment of oscillopsia due to bilateral vetibular failure (e.g. idiopathic, gentamycin intoxication, postmeningitic, due to autoimmune diseases, and idiopathic [4]) is vestibular rehabilitation including head-eye coordination exercises.

Downbeat nystagmus

Downbeat nystagmus (DBN) is a central vestibular nystagmus, present when the eyes are close or in the primary gaze position; it usually increases on down gaze and especially on lateral gaze. It also often becomes evident or is increased by placing the patient in a head-hanging position, or by tipping the head forward. In many patients with vestibulo-cerebellar atrophy, the drift velocity increases in prone position and is minimal in supine position [5]. As a result, many cerebellar patients report better reading capability when lying on their back. In other patients, the gravity-dependence of DBN is opposite or missing [6]. Visual fixation has little effect on its slow-phase speed; convergence may suppress or enhance it in some patients. In general, the nystagmus is accompanied by a vestibulocerebellar (vermal) ataxia with a tendency to fall backwards [7]. The pathomechanism of downbeat nystagmus remains unclear. Hypotheses conjectured various deficits such as an imbalance of central vertical vestibular [8], asymmetric impairment of vertical SP pathways [9] or dissociation between internal coordinate systems for vertical saccade generation and gaze holding [10]. DBN and associated ocular motor signs (impaired vertical smooth pursuit, gaze-evoked nystagmus, and gravity dependence of the upward drift) can be explained by damage of the inhibitory vertical gaze-velocity-sensitive Purkinje cells in the cerebellar flocculus [11]. These cells show spontaneous activity and a physiological asymmetry in that most of them exhibit downward on-directions. A loss of floccular Purkinje cells therefore leads to disinhibition of their brainstem target neurons and, consequently, to spontaneous upward drift.

Aetiology

The most common cause of downbeat nystagmus is cerebellar degeneration (hereditary, sporadic, or paraneoplastic). Other important causes are Chiari malformation and drug intoxication (especially the anticonvulsants and lithium). Multiple sclerosis (MS) is an uncommon cause, and a congenital form is rare [12]. In practice, cerebellar atrophy, Arnold-Chiari malformation, various cerebellar lesions (MS, vascular, tumours), and idiopathic causes account for approximately 25% of the cases each [6]. In a recent study about one-third were classified as idiopathic and about a half of these patients showed a combination of bilateral vestibulopathy, peripheral polyneuropathy, and/or cerebellar signs [13]. There seems to be no change over long time of the DBN [14]. Downbeat nystagmus occurs in the channelopathy episodic ataxia type 2, for which a new treatment option has recently been developed [15].

Upbeat nystagmus

Upbeat nystagmus (UBN) is present with the eyes close to the central position and usually increases on up gaze. Vertical smooth pursuit is usually disrupted by the nystagmus. In some patients the upbeat nystagmus changes to downbeat nystagmus during convergence. UBN can appear as a result of a pontine lesion along the ventral tegmental tract, which originates in the superior vestibular nucleus. The associated relative hypoactivity of the drive to the motoneurons of the elevator muscles results in a downward drift.

Aetiology

The main causes are MS, tumours of the brainstem, Wernicke's encephalopathy, cerebellar degeneration, and intoxication (e.g. nicotine), which may be the causes for lesions in the ascending pathways from the anterior canals (and/or the otoliths) at the pontomesencephalic or pontomedullary junction, near the perihypoglossal nuclei [16]. Upbeat nystagmus is most often seen after medullary lesions [17], but can also be seen after pontine lesion along the ventral tegmental tract, which originates in the superior vestibular nucleus [18].

Recommmendations

Downbeat nystagmus. No studies on the natural course of downbeat nystagmus are available. In non-placebo-controlled studies with a limited number of patients, administration of the GABA-A agonist clonazepam (0.5 mg per os (p.o.) three times daily [19], the GABA-B agonist baclofen (10 mg p.o. three times daily) [20], and gabapentin (probably calcium channel blocker) [21] had positive effects and reduced downbeat nystagmus. Intravenous injection of the cholinergic drug physostigmine (Ach-esterase inhibitor) worsened downbeat nystagmus in five patients. This effect was partially reversed in one patient by the anticholinergic drug biperiden, suggesting that anticholinergic drugs might be beneficial, as was shown in a double-blind study on intravenous scopolamine [22]. In isolated patients with a craniocervical anomaly, a surgical decompression by removal of part of the occipital bone in the region of the foramen magnum was beneficial [23–25]; personal observation). Recent placebo-controlled studies have suggested that the potassium channel blockers 3,4-diaminopyridine (3x20mg/day) and 4-aminopyridine (3 × 10 mg/day) may be effective in reducing downbeat nystagmus [26] and in improving the VOR and smooth pursuit [27]. A further study in 11 patients with DBN due to cerebellar degeneration confirmed this effect and showed that 3,4-diaminopyridine especially reduce the gravity-independent velocity bias [28]. As downbeat nystagmus is generally less pronounced in upward gaze, base-down prisms sometimes help to reduce oscillopsia during reading in some patients.

Upbeat nystagmus. Treatment with baclofen (5–10 mg p.o. three times daily) resulted in an improvement in several patients [20]. There are some observations that 10 mg 4-aminopyridine three times a day reduces upbeat nystagmus [29].

Seesaw nystagmus

Seesaw nystagmus is a rare pendular or jerk oscillation. One half-cycle consists of elevation and intorsion of one eye with synchronous depression and extorsion of the other eye. During the next half-cycle there is a reversal of the vertical and torsional movements. The frequency is lower in the pendular (2–4 Hz) than in the jerk variety.

Aetiology

Jerk hemi-seesaw nystagmus has been attributed to unilateral meso-diencephalic lesions [30], affecting the interstitial nucleus of Cajal and its vestibular afferents from the vertical semicircular canals [31, 32]. The pendular form is associated with lesions affecting the optic chiasm. Loss of crossed visual input seems to be the crucial element in the pathophysiology of pendular seesaw nystagmus [17].

Recommendations

Alcohol had a beneficial effect (1.2 g/kg body weight) in two patients [33, 34], but this cannot be recommended as treatment, as did clonazepam [35]. Recently, Averbruch-Heller *et al.* [21]reported on three patients with a seesaw component to their pendular nystagmus, who improved on gabapentin.

Periodic alternating nystagmus

Periodic alternating nystagmus is a spontaneous horizontal beating nystagmus, the direction of which changes periodically. Periods of oscillation range from 1 s to 4 min, typically 1–2 min. When the nystagmus amplitude gradually decreases, the nystagmus reverses its direction, and then the amplitude increases again. During the nystagmus patients often complain of increasing/decreasing oscillopsia.

Aetiology

Patients with periodic alternating nystagmus commonly have vestibulocerebellar lesions. Their nystagmus also disrupts visual fixation, being present also during normal viewing. These observations and animal experiments support the idea that this type of nystagmus is caused by lesions of the inferior cerebellar vermis (nodulus and uvula), leading to a disinhibition of the GABA-ergic velocity-storage mechanism, which is mediated in the vestibular nuclei [36, 37]. The underlying aetiologies are craniocervical anomalies, MS, cerebellar degenerations or tumours, brainstem infarction, anticonvulsant therapy, and bilateral visual loss.

disease), as a component of the syndrome of oculopalatal tremor (myoclonus), and in Whipple's disease [53]; the two more common aetiologies in the adult are MS and brainstem stroke [51]. On the basis of observations that the nystagmus is often dissociated and that eye movements other than optokinetic nystagmus and voluntary saccades are also disturbed, a lesion in the brainstem near the oculomotor nuclei has been suggested [48]. Alternatively, an inhibition of the inferior olive due to lesions of the 'Mollaret triangle' [51] or an instability of the gaze-holding network (neural integrator) has been proposed; this suggestion has received experimental modelling support [54] and has led to the proposal of potential therapies [17].

Recommmendations

In general, periodic alternating nystagmus (PAN) does not improve spontaneously. Several case reports of acquired as well as congenital PAN describe a positive effect of baclofen, a GABA-B agonist, in a dose of 5–10 mg p.o. three times daily [35, 38–42]. Furthermore, phenothiazine and barbiturates have been found to be effective in single cases [40, 43]. Recently, also memantine was described as effective [44]. Periodic alternating nystagmus due to bilateral visual loss resolves if vision is restored [45, 46]. In a case of PAN associated to a Chiari-malformation a surgical decompression resolved the PAN [47].

Non-vestibular supranuclear ocular motor disorders

Acquired pendular nystagmus

Acquired pendular nystagmus (APN) is a quasi-sinusoidal oscillation that may have a predominantly horizontal, vertical, or mixed trajectory (i.e. circular, elliptical, or diagonal); it can be predominantly monocular or binocular [48–51]. The frequency of this type of nystagmus is 2–7 Hz [52], and often the nystagmus is associated with head titubation (not synchronized with the nystagmus), trunk and limb ataxia, palatal myoclonus, or visual impairment.

Aetiology

Acquired pendular nystagmus occurs with several disorders of myelin (MS, toluene abuse, Pelizaeus Merzbacher

---

Recommmendations

Most reports (case reports or case series) state that anticholinergic treatment with trihexyphenidyl (20–40 mg p.o. daily) is effective [55, 56], but in a double-blind study by Leigh et al. [57] only one of six patients showed improvement from this oral treatment, whereas three patients showed a decrease in nystagmus and improvement of visual acuity during treatment with tridihexethyl chloride (a quaternary anticholinergic that does not cross the blood–brain barrier). In contrast, Barton et al. [22] found in a double-blind trial that scopolamine (0.4 mg intravenous (i.v.)) decreased the nystagmus in all five tested patients with acquired pendular nystagmus. However, there are even observations that scopolamine may make the pendular nystagmus worse in some patients [58]. In three other patients the combination with lidocaine (100 mg i.v.) decreased nystagmus [48, 59]. Recently, Starck et al. [60] reported an improvement in three of 10 patients who received a scopolamine patch (containing 1.5 mg scopolamine, released at a rate of 0.5 mg per day). The same authors failed to observe further improvement when scopolamine and mexiletine (400–600 mg p.o. daily) were given in combination. The most effective substance in their study was memantine, a glutamate antagonist, which significantly improved the nystagmus in all nine tested patients (15–60 mg p.o. daily). Two patients responded to clonazepam (3 × 0.5–1.0 mg p.o. daily), a GABA-A agonist [60]. In a further crossover study Starck and co-workers [61] showed that memantine as well as gabapentin was able not only to reduce the nystagmus but also to improve visual acuity. Two other groups have reported benefit with GABA-ergic drugs. Traccis et al. [49] showed improvement in one of three patients with APN and cerebellar ataxia due to MS when treated with isoniazid (800–1000 mg p.o. daily) and glasses with prisms that induced convergence. This observation was not confirmed by other investigators [62]. Gabapentin substantially improved the nystagmus (and visual acuity) in 10 of 15 patients [21]. Gabapentin was superior to vigabatrin in a small series of patients [63]. Interestingly, Mossman et al. [64] described two patients who benefited from intake of alcohol but not from other substances. Recently, a beneficial effect of cannabis was also reported [65, 66].

Practically, treatment should start with memantine in a dosage of 15–60 mg p.o. or alternatively 300–400 mg gabapentin three times daily. If there is no or only a small effect, benzodiazepines like clonazepam (0.5–1.0 mg p.o. three times daily) can be tried. Further possibilities are scopolamine patches or trihexyphenidyl.

Opsoclonus and ocular flutter

Opsoclonus consists of repetitive bursts of conjugate saccadic oscillations, which have horizontal, vertical, and torsional components. During each burst of these high-frequency oscillations, the movement is continuous, without any intersaccadic interval. These oscillations are often triggered by eye closure, convergence, pursuit, and saccades; amplitudes range up to 2–15° (overview in [53]). In ocular flutter, the same pattern is restricted to the horizontal plane. The ocular symptoms are often accompanied by cerebellar signs, such as gait and limb myoclonus (the 'dancing feet, dancing eyes syndrome').

Aetiology

A functional disturbance of active saccadic suppression by the pontine omnipause neurons is the most probable pathophysiological mechanism. As histological abnormalities of these neurons have not been shown [67], a functional lesion of the glutaminergic cerebellar projections from the fastigial nuclei to the omnipause cells is a likely cause for their disinhibition. In a functional magnetic resonance imaging (fMRI) study, an increased activation of the fastigial region during opsoclonus was shown [68]. Ramat and colleagues suggested that the lesion of the fastigial nucleus interrupts the local feedback loop through the cerebellum but not the brainstem interconnections [69]. Opsoclonus can be observed in benign cerebellar encephalitis (post-viral, e.g. coxsackie B37; post-vaccinal), or as a paraneoplastic symptom (infants, neuroblastoma; adults, carcinoma of the lung, breast, ovary, or uterus).

Recommmendations

In addition to therapy for any underlying process such as tumour or encephalitis, treatment with immunoglobulins or prednisolone may be occasionally effective [70]. Four of five patients with square-wave oscillations, probably a related fixation disturbance, showed an improvement on therapy with valproic acid [71] or in patients with hereditary spinocerebellar atxia on therapy with memantine 20 mg/daily [72]. In single cases an improvement has been observed during treatment with propranolol (40–80 mg p.o. three times daily), nitrazepam (15–30 mg p.o. daily), and clonazepam (0.5–2.0 mg p.o. three times daily) (overview in [35, 73]. Nausieda et al. [74] reported a dramatic improvement in one patient after the administration of 200 mg thiamine i.v.

Congenital nystagmus

Congenital nystagmus is a fixational nystagmus and is characterized by gaze-dependent involuntary to and fro eye movements, which can be pendular, jerky, or elliptic. Typically the patients report little or no oscillopsia or visual blurring, compared to the fast nystagmus velocities seen. The prevalence of congenital nystagmus is estimated to be 1/1000.

Aetiology

The aetiology is in most cases not known. Most probably it is a congenital disturbance of the fixational system [75]; this idea is in agreement with the observation that the congenital nystagmus can be regularly seen in patients with albinism and retinal diseases [75].

Recommmendations

In most cases therapy not necessary. Besides surgical inventions [77] only a few reports on medical treatment trials are reported. Baclofen [78], cannabis [79], and especially memantine and gabapentin are described. In a study with 47 patients, memantine (up to 40 mg) as well as gabapentine (up to 2400 mg) were shown to be superior to placebo and both also improved visual acuity [76]. A similar result was in a retrospective study of 23 patients with acquired as well as congenital nystagmus reported [80, 81].

Nuclear and infranuclear ocular disorders

Superior oblique myokymia

Superior oblique myokymia consists of paroxysmal monocular high-frequency oscillations. In the primary gaze position and in abduction, these oscillations are mainly torsional, but when the eyes are in adduction the oscillations have a vertical component. Voluntary eye movements, as when looking down, can provoke the oscillations. The patients usually complain of oscillopsia during these paroxysmal attacks.

Aetiology

The pathophysiology of this condition is not entirely clear. In analogy to hemifacial spasm and trigeminal neuralgia, vascular compression of the IV nerve [82–84], or alternatively spontaneous discharges in the IV nerve nucleus [85] or of the superior oblique muscle may be responsible [86].

Recommmendations

Spontaneous remissions, which can last for days up to years, are typical of superior oblique myokymia but there are several reports that anticonvulsants, especially carbamazepine, have a therapeutic effect. Carbamazepine (200–400 mg p.o. three or four times daily) or, less often, phenytoin (250–400 mg p.o. daily) are recommended [87, 88]). Gabapentin has also been reported to be effective [89]. Rosenberg and Glaser [88] described a decrease in the efficacy of the treatment after a month in some patients. Beta-blockers, even topically, have been reported to be effective [90, 91]. In chronic cases that did not improve with anticonvulsants, tenotomy of the superior oblique muscle was performed, but usually it necessitates inferior oblique surgery as well [92, 93]. Surgical decompression of the IV nerve has also been reported to be beneficial but may result in superior oblique palsy [94, 95]. Practically, treatment should be started with carbamazepine (200–400 mg p.o. three to four times daily) or phenytoin (250–400 mg p.o. daily).

Paroxysmal vestibular episodes

Clinically, the patients describe short, repeated, paroxysmal attacks of to-and-fro vertigo and unsteadiness of stance or gait lasting usually seconds (to maximally minutes), which can sometimes be provoked by particular head positions. Other symptoms can be tinnitus, hyperacusis, or facial contractions during the attacks. In some patients, such attacks can be triggered by head turning [96]. Clinical examination between the attacks may reveal signs of permanent vestibular deficit, hypoacusis, or facial paresis on the affected side [97, 98]. Mild vestibular deficits can be found with caloric testing in about 70% of the patients [96].

Aetiology

High-resolution magnetic resonance imaging may show the compression of the VIII nerve by an artery (most often AICA) or seldom a vein in the region of the root entry zone of the vestibular nerve in some patients, but this can also be seen in subjects without symptoms. The neuropathological mechanism may be peripheral ephaptic transmission that takes place in the part of the cranial nerve still containing central myelin (derived from oligodendroglia), if the nerve has direct contact with a blood vessel. This hypothesis is supported by the analysis of epidemiological data that show a correlation of the incidence of the syndrome with the anatomical length of the central myelin [99]. Another theory is that the pulsation of the blood vessel causes an afferent sensory inflow that then causes a false central response.

Recommendations

As initial therapy, an anticonvulsant should be given [100]. Mean dosages of carbamazepine of about 600 mg/daily and of oxacarbazepine of about 900 mg/daily led to a reduction of the attack frequency of about 90% [95]. In general, a positive response to antiepileptic drugs can be achieved with low dosages. If the symptoms do not cease, a surgical approach may be considered [101]. There are no satisfactory follow-up studies, and the diagnostic criteria have not yet been fully established.

Conflicts of interest

The present guidelines were developed without external financial support. None of the authors reports conflicting interests.

References

1. Grüsser OJ. Some recent studies on the quantitative analysis of efference copy mechanisms in visual perception. *Acta Psychol (Amst)* 1986;**63**(1–3):49–62.

2. Hilgers R-D. Qualitätsbeurteilung von Studien zur klinischen Effektivität. In: Lauterbach KW, Schrappe M (eds) *Gesundheitsökonomie, Qualitätsmanagement Und Evidence-Based Medicine*. Stuttgart: Schattauer, 2001; pp. 89–95.

3. Straube A, Leigh RJ, Bronstein A, *et al*. EFNS task force – therapy of nystagmus and oscillopsia. *Eur J Neurol* 2004;**11**(2):83–9.

4. Rinne T, Bronstein AM, Rudge P, Gresty MA, Luxon LM. Bilateral loss of vestibular function: clinical findings in 53 patients. *J Neurol* 1998;**245**(6–7):314–21.

5. Marti S, Palla A, Straumann D. Gravity dependence of ocular drift in patients with cerebellar downbeat nystagmus. *Ann Neurol* 2002;**52**:712–21.

6. Bronstein AM, Miller DH, Rudge P, Kendall BE. Down beating nystagmus: magnetic resonance imaging and neuro-otological findings. *J Neurol Sci* 1987;**81**:173–84.

7. Büchele W, Brandt T, Degner D. Ataxia and oscillopsia in downbeat-nystagmus vertigo syndrome. *Adv Otorhinolaryngol* 1983;**30**:291–7.

8. Baloh RW, Spooner JW. Downbeat nystagmus. A type of central vestibular nystagmus. *Neurology* 1981;**31**:304–10.

9. Zee DS, Friendlich AR, Robinson DA. The mechanism of downbeat nystagmus. *Arch Neurol* 1974;**30**(3):227–37.

10. Glasauer S, Hoshi M, Kempermann U, Eggert T, Büttner U. Three-dimensional eye position and slow phase velocity in humans with downbeat nystagmus. *J Neurophysiol* 2003;**89**:338–54.

11. Marti S, Straumann D, Büttner U, Glasauer S. A model-based theory on the origin of downbeat nystagmus. *Exp Brain Res* 2008;**188**(4):613–31.

12. Halmagyi MG, Rudge P, Gresty MA, Sanders MD. Down-beating nystagmus. A review of 62 cases. *Arch Neurol* 1983;**40**:777–84.

13. Wagner JN, Glaser M, Brandt T, Strupp M. Downbeat nystagmus: aetiology and comorbidity in 117 patients. *J Neurol Neurosurg Psychiatry* 2008;**79**(6):672–7.

14. Wagner J, Lehnen N, Glasauer S, Strupp M, Brandt T. Prognosis of idiopathic downbeat nystagmus. *Ann N Y Acad Sci* 2009;**1164**:479–81.

15. Strupp M, Schüler O. Improvement of downbeat nystagmus and postural imbalance by 3,4-diaminopyridine, a prospective, placebo-controlled study. *J Vestib Res* 2002;**11**:226.

16. Fisher A, Gresty M, Chambers B, Rudge P. Primary position upbeating nystagmus: a variety of central positional nystagmus. *Brain* 1983;**106**:949–64.

17. Stahl JS, Averbuch-Heller L, Leigh RJ. Acquired nystagmus. *Arch Ophthalmol* 2000;**118**:544–9.

18. Pierrot-Deseilligny C, Milea D. Vertical nystagmus: clinical facts and hypotheses. *Brain* 2005;**128**:(Pt 6):1237–46.

19. Currie J, Matsuo V. The use of clonazepam in the treatment of nystagmus induced oscillopsia. *Ophthalmology* 1986;**93**: 924–32.

20. Dieterich M, Straube A, Brandt T, Paulus W, Büttner U. The effects of baclofen and cholinergic drugs on upbeat and downbeat nsytagmus. *J Neurol Neurosurg Psychiatry* 1991; **54**:627–32.

21. Averbuch-Heller L, Tusa RJ, Fuhry L, *et al*. A double-blind controlled study of gabapentin and baclofen as treatment for acquired nystagmus. *Ann Neurol* 1997;**41**:818–25.

22. Barton JJS, Huaman AG, Sharpe JA. Muscarinic antagonists in the treatment of acquired pendular and downbeat nystagmus: a double-blind, randomized trial of three intravenous drugs. *Ann Neurol* 1994;**35**:319–25.

23. Pedersen RA, Troost BT, Abel LA, Zorub D. Intermittent down beat nystagmus and oscillopsia reversed by suboccipital craniectomy. *Neurology* 1980;**30**:1232–42.

24. Spooner JW, Baloh RW. ArnoldChiari malformation. Improvement in eye movements after surgical treatment. *Brain* 1981;**104**:51–60.

25. Liebenberg WA, Georges H, Demetriades AK, Hardwidge C. Does posterior fossa decompression improve oculomotor and vestibulo-ocular manifestations in Chiari 1 malformation? *Acta Neurochir (Wien)* 2005;**147**(12):1239–40.

26. Strupp M, Schüler O, Krafczyk S, *et al*. Treatment of downbeat nystagmus with 3,4-diaminopyridine a prospective, placebo-controlled, double-blind study. *Neurology* 2003; **61**:165–70.

27. Kalla R, Glasauer S, Schautzer F, *et al*. 4-aminopyridine improves downbeat nystagmus, smooth pursuit, and VOR gain. *Neurology* 2004;**62**(7):1228–9.

28. Sprenger A, Rambold H, Sander T, *et al*. Treatment of the gravity dependence of downbeat nystagmus with 3,4-diaminopyridine. *Neurology* 2006;**67**(5):905–7.

29. Glasauer S, Kalla R, Büttner U, Strupp M, Brandt T. 4-aminopyridine restores visual ocular motor function in upbeat nystagmus. *J Neurol Neurosurg Psychiatry* 2005; **76**(3):451–3.

30. Halmagyi GM, Aw ST, Dehaene I, Curthoys IS, Todd MJ. Jerk-waveform see-saw nystagmus due to unilateral mesodiencephalic lesion. *Brain* 1994;**117**:775–88.

31. Endres M, Heide W, Kompf D. See-saw nystagmus. Clinical aspects, diagnosis, pathophysiology: observations in 2 patients. *Nervenarzt* 1996;**67**:484–9.

32. Rambold H, Helmchen C, Büttner U. Unilateral muscimol inactivations of the interstitial nucleus of Cajal in the alert rhesus monkey do not elicit seesaw nystagmus. *Neurosci Lett* 1999;**272**:75–8.

33. Frisèn L, Wikkelso C. Posttraumatic seesaw nystagmus abolished by ethanol ingestion. *Neurology* 1986;**36**: 841–4.

34. Lepore FE. Ethanol-induced resolution of pathologic nystagmus. *Neurology* 1987;**37**:877.

35. Carlow TJ. Medical treatment of nystagmus and ocular motor disorders. *Int Ophthalmol Clin* 1986;**26**:251–64.

36. Waespe W, Cohen B, Raphan T. Dynamic modification of the vestibuloocular reflex by the nodulus and uvula. *Science* 1985;**228**:199–202.

37. Furman JMR, Wall C, Pang D. Vestibular function in periodic alternating nystagmus. *Brain* 1990;**113**:1425–39.

38. Halmagyi MG, Rudge P, Gresty MA. Treatment of periodic alternating nystagmus. *Ann Neurol* 1980;**8**:609–11.

39. Larmande P, Larmande A. Action du baclofene sur le nystagmus alternant periodique. *Bull Mem Soc Fr Ophtalmol* 1983;**94**:390–3.

40. Isago H, Tsuboya R, Kataura A. A case of periodic alternating nystagmus: with special reference to the efficacy of baclofen treatment. *Auris Nasus Larynx* 1985;**12**:15–21.

41. Nuti D, Ciacci G, Giannini F, Rossi A, Frederico A. Aperiodic alternating nystagmus: report of two cases and treatment by baclofen. *Ital J Neurol Sci* 1986;**7**:453–9.

42. Comer RM, Dawson EL, Lee JP. Baclofen for patients with congenital periodic alternating nystagmus. *Strabismus* 2006;**14**(4):205–9.

43. Nathanson M, Bergman PS, Bender MB. Visual disturbances as the result of nystagmus on direct forward gaze. Effect of amobarbital sodium. *Arch Neurol Psychiatry* 1953;**69**:427–35.

44. Kumar A, Thomas S, McLean R, et al. Treatment of acquired periodic alternating nystagmus with memantine: a case report. *Clin Neuropharmacol* 2009;**32**(2):109–10.

45. Cross SA, Smith JL, Norton EW. Periodic alternating nystagmus clearing after vitrectomy. *J Clin Neuroophthalmol* 1982;**2**:511.

46. Jay WM, Williams BB, De Chicchis A. Periodic alternating nystagmus clearing after cataract surgery. *J Clin Neuroophthalmol* 1985;**5**:149–52.

47. Al-Awami A, Flanders ME, Andermann F, Polomeno RC. Resolution of periodic alternating nystagmus after decompression for Chiari malformation. *Can J Ophthalmol* 2005;**40**(6):778–80.

48. Gresty M, Ell JJ, Findley LJ. Acquired pendular nystagmus: its characteristics, localising value and pathophysiology. *J Neurol Neurosurg Psychiatry* 1982;**45**:431–9.

49. Traccis S, Rosati G, Monaco MF, Aiello IN, Agnetti V. Successful treatment of acquired pendular elliptical nystagmus in multiple sclerosis with isoniazid and base-out prisms. *Neurology* 1990;**40**:492–4.

50. Leigh RJ, Tomsak RL, Grant MP, et al. Effectiveness of botulinum toxin administered to abolish acquired nystagmus. *Ann Neurol* 1992;**32**:633–42.

51. Lopez LI, Bronstein AM, Gresty MA, Du Boulay EP, Rudge P. Clinical and MRI correlates in 27 patients with acquired pendular nystagmus. *Brain* 1996;**119**: 465–72.

52. Zee DS. Mechanisms of nystagmus. *Am J Otolaryngol* 1985;(Suppl.):30–4.

53. Leigh RJ, Zee DS. *The Neurology of Eye Movements*, 3rd edn. New York: Oxford University Press, 1999.

54. Das VE, Oruganti P, Kramer PD, Leigh RJ. Experimental tests of a neural-network model for ocular oscillations caused by disease of central myelin. *Exp Brain Res* 2000; **133**:189–97.

55. Herishanu Y, Louzoun Z. Trihexyphenidyl treatment of vertical pendular nystagmus. *Neurology* 1986;**36**: 82–4.

56. Jabbari B, Rosenberg M, Scherokman B, Gunderson CH, McBurney JW, McClintock W. Effectiveness of trihexyphenidyl against pendular nystagmus and palatal myoclonus: evidence of cholinergic dysfunction. *Mov Disord* 1987; **2**:93–8.

57. Leigh RJ, Burnstine TH, Ruff RL, Kasmer RJ. The effect of anticholinergic agents upon acquired nystagmus: a double-blind study of trihexyphenidyl and tridihexethyl chloride. *Neurology* 1991;**41**:1737–41.

58. Kim JI, Averbuch-Heller L, Leigh RJ. Evaluation of transdermal scopolamine as treatment for acquired nystagmus. *J Neuro-Ophthalmol* 2001;**21**:188–92.

59. Ell J, Gresty M, Chambers BR, Frindley L. Acquired pendular nystagmus: characteristics, pathophysiology and pharmacological modification. In: Roucoux A, Crommeilinck M (eds) *Physiological and Pathological Aspects of Eye Movements*. The Hague, Boston, and London: Dr W. Junk Publ., 1982; pp. 89–98.

60. Starck M, Albrecht H, Pöllmann W, Straube A, Dieterich M. Drug therapy of acquired nystagmus in multiple sclerosis. *J Neurol* 1997;**244**:916.

61. Starck M, Albrecht H, Pöllmann W, Dieterich M, Straube A. Acquired pendular nystagmus in multiple sclerosis: an examiner-blind cross-over treatment study of memantine and gabapentin. *J Neurol* 2010;**257**(3): 322–7.

62. Leigh RJ, Averbuch-Heller L, Tomsak RL, Remler BF, Yaniglos SS, Dell'Osso LF. Treatment of abnormal eye movements that impair vision: strategies based on current concepts of physiology and pharmacology. *Ann Neurol* 1994;**36**:129–41.

63. Bandini F, Castello E, Mazzella L, Mancardi GL, Solaro C. Gabapentin but not vigabatrin is effective in the treatment of acquired nystagmus in multiple sclerosis: how valid is the GABAergic hypothesis? *J Neurol Neurosurg Psychiatry* 2001;**71**:107–10.

64. Mossman SS, Bronstein AM, Rudge P, Gresty MA. Acquired pendular nystagmus suppressed by alcohol. *Neuro-Ophthalmol* 1993;**13**:99–106.

65. Schon F, Hart PE, Hodgson TL, *et al.* Suppression of pendular nystagmus by smoking cannabis in a patient with multiple sclerosis. *Neurology* 1999;**53**:2209–10.

66. Dell'Osso LF. Suppression of pendular nystagmus by smoking cannabis in a patient with multiple sclerosis. *Neurology* 2000;**13**:2190–1.

67. Ridley A, Kennard C, Scholtz CL, Büttner-Ennever JA, Summers B, Turnbull A. Omnipause neurons in two cases of opsoclonus associated with oat cell carcinoma of the lung. *Brain* 1987;**110**:1699–709.

68. Helmchen C, Rambold H, Sprenger A, Erdmann C, Binkofski F; fMRI study. Cerebellar activation in opsoclonus: an fMRI study. *Neurology* 2003;**61**(3):412–5.

69. Ramat S, Leigh RJ, Zee DS, Optican LM. What clinical disorders tell us about the neural control of saccadic eye movements. *Brain* 2007;**130**:10–35.

70. Pless M, Ronthal M. Treatment of opsoclonus-myoclonus with high-dose intravenous immunoglobulin. *Neurology* 1996;**46**:583–4.

71. Traccis S, Marras MA, Puliga MV, *et al.* Square-wave jerks and square-wave oscillations: treatment with valproic acid. *Neuro-Ophthalmol* 1997;**18**:51–8.

72. Serra A, Liao K, Martinez-Conde S, Optican LM, Leigh RJ. Suppression of saccadic intrusions in hereditary ataxia by memantine. *Neurology* 2008; **70**(10):810–12.

73. Leopold HC. Opsoklonus- und Myoklonie-Syndrom. Klinische und elektronystagmographische Befunde mit Verlaufsstudien. *Fortschr Neurol Psychiatr* 1985;**53**:42–54.

74. Nausieda PA, Tanner CM, Weiner WJ. Opsoclonic cerebellopathy. A paraneoplastic syndrome responsive to thiamine. *Arch Neurol* 1981;**38**:780–2.

75. Tusa RJ. Nystagmus: diagnostic and therapeutic strategies. *Semin Ophthalmol* 1999;**14**:65–73.

76. McLean R, Proudlock F, Thomas S, Degg C, Gottlob I. Congenital nystagmus: randomized, controlled, double-masked trial of memantine/gabapentin. *Ann Neurol* 2007;**61**(2):130–8.

77. Hertle RW, Yang D. Clinical and electrophysiological effects of extraocular muscle surgery on patients with Infantile Nystagmus Syndrome (INS). *Semin Ophthalmol* 2006;**21**(2):103–10.

78. Yee RD, Baloh RW, Honrubia V. Effect of baclofen on congenital nystagmus. In: Lennerstrand G, Zee DS, Keller E (eds) *Functional Basis of Ocular Motility*. Oxford: Pergamon, 1982; pp. 151–8.

79. Pradeep A, Thomas S, Roberts EO, Proudlock FA, Gottlob I. Reduction of congenital nystagmus in a patient after smoking cannabis. *Strabismus* 2008;**16**(1):29–32.

80. Shery T, Proudlock FA, Sarvananthan N, McLean RJ, Gottlob I. The effects of gabapentin and memantine in acquired and congenital nystagmus: a retrospective study. *Br J Ophthalmol* 2006;**90**(7):839–43.

81. Sarvananthan N, Proudlock FA, Choudhuri I, Dua H, Gottlob I. Pharmacologic treatment of congenital nystagmus. *Arch Ophthalmol* 2006;**124**(6):916–8.

82. Lee JP. Superior oblique myokymia: a possible etiologic factor. *Arch Ophthalmol* 1984;**102**:1178–9.

83. Hashimoto M, Ohtsuka K, Hoyt WF. Vascular compression as a cause of superior oblique myokymia disclosed by thin-slice magnetic resonance imaging. *Am J Ophthalmol* 2001; **31**:676–7.

84. Yousry I, Dieterich M, Naidich TP, Schmid UD, Yousry TA. Superior oblique myokymia: magnetic resonance imaging support for the neurovascular compression hypothesis. *Ann Neurol* 2002;**51**:361–8.

85. Hoyt WF, Keane JR. Superior oblique myokymia: report and discussion of five cases of benign intermittent uniocular microtremor. *Arch Ophthalmol* 1962;**84**:461–7.

86. Leigh RJ, Tomsak RL, Seidman SH, Dell'Osso LF. Superior oblique myokymia. Quantitative characteristics of the eye movements in three patients. *Arch Ophthalmol* 1991;**109**:1710–3.

87. Susac JO, Smith JL, Schatz NJ. Superior oblique myokymia. *Arch Neurol* 1973;**29**:432–4.

88. Rosenberg MI, Glaser JS. Superior oblique myokymia. *Ann Neurol* 1983;**13**:667–9.

89. Tomsak RL, Kosmorsky GA, Leigh RJ. Gabapentin attenuates superior oblique myokymia. *Am J Ophthalmol* 2002; **133**:721–3.

90. Tyler RD, Ruiz RS. Propranolol in the treatment of superior oblique myokymia. *Arch Ophthalmol* 1990;**108**:175–6.

91. Bibby K, Deane JS, Farnworth D, Cappin J. Superior oblique myokymia: a topical solution? *Br J Ophthalmol* 1994;**78**:882.

92. Palmer EA, Shults WT. Superior oblique myokymia: preliminary results of surgical treatment. *J Pediatr Ophthalmol Strabismus* 1984;**21**:91–101.

93. Brazis PW, Miller NR, Henderer JD, Lee AG. The natural history and results of treatment of superior oblique myokymia. *Arch Ophthalmol* 1994;**112**:1063–7.

94. Samii M, Rosahl SK, Carvalho GA, Krzizok T. Microvascular decompression for superior oblique myokymia: first experience. *J Neurosurg* 1998;**89**:1020–4.

95. Scharwey K, Krzizok T, Samii M, Rosahl SK, Kaufmann H. Remission of superior oblique myokymia after microvascular decompression. *Ophthalmologica* 2000;**214**:426–8.

96. Hüfner K, Barresi D, Glaser M, *et al.* Vestibular paroxysmia: diagnostic features and medical treatment. *Neurology* 2008;**71**(13):1006–14.

97. Brandt T, Dieterich M. Vestibular paroxysmia: vascular compression of the eighth nerve? *Lancet* 1994;**26**:798–9.

98. Straube A, Büttner U, Brandt T. Recurrent attacks with skew deviation, torsional nystagmus and contraction of the left frontalis muscle. *Neurology* 1994;**44**:177–8.

99. De Ridder D, Moller A, Verlooy J, Cornelissen M, De Ridder L. Is the root entry/exit zone important in micro-vascular compression syndromes? *Neurosurgery* 2002;**51**: 427–33.

100. Brandt T. *Vertigo. Its Multisensory Syndromes*, 2nd edn. London: Springer-Verlag, 1999.

101. Jannetta PJ, Møller MD, Møller AR. Disabling positional vertigo. *N Engl J Med* 1984;**310**:1700–5.

CHAPTER 33

Orthostatic hypotension

H. Lahrmann,[1] P. Cortelli,[2] M. Hilz,[3] C. J. Mathias,[4] W. Struhal,[5] M. Tassinari[2]

[1]Kaiser Franz Josef Hospital and L. Boltzmann Institute for Neurooncology, Vienna, Austria; [2]University of Bologna, Italy; [3]University Erlangen-Nuremberg, Erlangen, Germany, and New York University, School of Medicine, NY, USA; [4]Imperial College London at St Mary's Hospital, and National Hospital for Neurology and Neurosurgery, Queen Square, and Institute of Neurology, University College London, UK; [5]General Hospital (AKH), Linz, Austria

Background

Orthostatic (postural) hypotension (OH) is a frequent cause of syncope and may contribute to morbidity, disability and even death, because of the potential risk of substantial injury [1]. It may be the initial sign of autonomic failure and cause major symptoms in many primary and secondary diseases of the autonomic nervous system (ANS) (e.g. pure autonomic failure (PAF), multiple system atrophy (MSA), Parkinson's disease, dementia with Lewy bodies, pure autonomic failure, autoimmune autonomic ganglionopathy, amyloidosis, and diabetic autonomic neuropathy). It occurs frequently in elderly patients because of therapy (vasoactive drugs, dopamine and agonists, antidepressants), reduced fluid intake, and decreased ANS function. The prevalence of OH in patients 65 years and older has been reported to range from 5 to 30% [2]. In Parkinson's disease the prevalence of OH may be as high as 60% [3]. Characteristic symptoms of OH include light-headedness, visual blurring, dizziness, generalized weakness, fatigue, cognitive slowing, leg buckling, coat-hanger ache, and gradual or sudden loss of consciousness. Falls with injuries may result. However, a recent study demonstrated that one-third of patients with severe OH (blood pressure falls > 60 mmHg systolic) are asymptomatic during head-up tilt test [4].

Orthostatic hypotension is defined by consensus as a fall in blood pressure (BP) of at least 20 mmHg systolic and/or 10 mm Hg diastolic within 3 min in the upright position [5]. This reduces perfusion pressure of organs, especially above heart level, such as the brain. Neurogenic OH results from impaired cardiovascular adrenergic function. The lesion can be postganglionic as in PAF, or preganglionic as in MSA. Other causes of OH are low intravascular volume (blood or plasma loss, fluid or electrolyte loss), impaired cardiac function due to structural heart disease, and vasodilatation, due to drugs, alcohol, heat [1].

Objectives

Orthostatic hypotension is an under-diagnosed disorder. Many new treatment options, pharmacological and non-pharmacological, have been published in recent years. Evidence-based guidelines for clinical and laboratory diagnostic work-up, and therapeutic management of OH are provided for physicians involved in the care of such patients.

Methods

Electronic search strategies used the following databases: Cochrane library, MEDLINE, Pub Med, and various internet search routines, for English publications. Key search terms included 'orthostatic hypotension', 'syncope', 'hypotension' and 'therapy', 'treatment', and 'diagnosis', and first-year availability of each referenced literature database until October 2009. References classified by evidence levels were selected by one individual and checked by another investigator. Where there was a lack of evidence but consensus was clear, we have stated our opinion as Good Practice Points (GPP) [6].

European Handbook of Neurological Management: Volume 1, 2nd edition. Edited by N. E. Gilhus, M. P. Barnes and M. Brainin. © 2011 Blackwell Publishing Ltd.

Diagnostic strategies

Tests to investigate OH are considered here and not general investigations of the ANS. A limitation is a paucity of randomized and blind studies. The wide variation of test methods, protocols, and equipment in autonomic laboratories make comparison of results difficult [7].

The history is of particular importance and has a high diagnostic value (pre-existing disease, detailed description of sequence of symptoms). The initial clinical evaluation should include a detailed physical and neurological examination, 12-lead ECG recording, routine laboratory testing, and BP measurements while supine and upright. Non-neurogenic causes of OH must be considered, as they can exacerbate neurogenic OH.

The cardiovascular responses to standing may be investigated by recording BP and heart rate while supine and for up to 3 min while upright. Passive head-up tilt testing (HUT) is recommended if the active standing test is negative, especially if the history is suggestive of OH, and in patients with motor impairment, as in Parkinson's disease, MSA, and spinal cord lesions. Tilt tables with foot board support, and if available, devices providing non-invasive, automatic, and ideally continuous heart rate and BP measurements are recommended [8].

Protocol:
• Orthostatic testing should take place in a quiet room, at a temperature between 20 and 24°C. The patient should rest while supine for ideally 5 min before HUT is started. Emptying the bladder before testing is recommended.
• Passive HUT to an angle between 60 and 80° for 3 min is recommended for the diagnosis of OH [9, 10].
• HUT is considered positive if systolic BP falls below 20 mmHg and diastolic BP below 10 mmHg of baseline. If symptoms occur, the patient should be tilted back to the supine position immediately.
• Measurement of plasma noradrenaline levels while supine and upright may be of value.
• In contrast with cardiologic guidelines pharmacological provocation with sublingual nitro-glycerine or intravenous isoproterenol is not recommended to diagnose OH as it reduces sensitivity and will result in false-positive outcomes [9].
• Combination of HUT and physiological measures, such as lower body negative pressure application, as used in neurally-mediated syncope, is not recommended for diagnosis of OH.

HUT is a safe procedure for the diagnosis of OH [11]. However, as syncope and arrhythmias have been described, the investigating staff should be adequately trained to recognize such problems. Resuscitation equipment and a team experienced in cardiac life support should be available at short notice (GPP).

Recommendations

All Level C
• Structured history taking.
• Detailed physical examination.
• 12-lead ECG recording.
• Routine laboratory testing.
• BP measurements while supine and upright.
• Cardiologic referral, if heart disease or abnormal ECG is present or suspected.
• Active standing or HUT, ideally with continuous assessment of BP and HR for 3 min.
• Further ANS screening tests, with other appropriate investigations, depending on the possible aetiology of the underlying disorder [1].

Management

Many new treatment options for OH have been studied in the past decade. Controlled trials have been performed for drugs and physical therapy. However, many of these studies included only small groups of patients with a variety of disorders that cause OH, and different diagnostic criteria have been used. If not noted otherwise, studies are classified as Class IV [6].

General principles
In addition to head up postural change, BP is influenced by many stimuli in everyday life. These include a hot environment, carbohydrate-rich meals, and exercise. The physiological mechanisms and individual strategies to avoid OH and syncope should be explained to the patients and caregivers. The following recommendations are mainly a result of panel consensus and qualified as GPP.

Elevated environmental temperatures, a hot bath or shower, and sauna should be avoided as they cause venous pooling. Prolonged recumbence during daytime and sudden head-up postural change, particularly in the morning, when BP may be lowered by nocturnal polyuria, should be avoided [12]. Postprandial hypotension may increase OH (vasodilatation in splanchnic vessels). Large meals, especially carbohydrate-rich, and alcohol should be avoided. A carefully controlled and individualized exercise training (swimming, aerobics, and, if possible, cycling and walking) often improves OH.

Supine hypertension

Supine hypertension may be a problem, resulting from medication and/or being part of the disease. Therefore, 24 h measurement of BP is best before and if needed after starting a new therapy. Patients may self-monitor BP, daily at about the same time, and when they experience symptoms. Pressor medications should be avoided after 6pm and the bed head elevated (20–30 cm). On occasion, short-acting antihypertensive drugs may be considered (e.g. nitro-glycerine sublingual).

Non-pharmacological treatment

Avoidance of factors that may induce OH is recommended first line, particularly in mild forms. Educating the patients and carers on the mechanisms of OH is important. The next step includes a range of non-pharmacological strategies.

Patients should be advised to move to head-up position slowly, sit on the edge of the bed for some minutes after recumbence, and activate calf muscles while supine. Physical counter manoeuvres can be applied immediately at the onset of presyncopal symptoms. They need to be explained and trained individually. In case of motor disabilities and compromised balance, as in the cerebellar forms of MSA, programmes with appropriate aids have to be developed. Leg crossing with tension of the thigh, buttock, and calf muscles (party position), bending over forward to reduce the orthostatic difference between the heart and brain and compress the splanchnic vessels by increasing abdominal pressure, squatting to reduce blood pooling are effective in temporarily reducing OH [13–17]. Not all patients can perform these manoeuvres, and sitting or lying down, and using a cane that can be folded into a tripod chair [16], are useful. Elastic stockings and abdominal compression bands reduce venous pooling and have been shown to be effective in small studies [18, 19]. Sleeping with elevation of the head-end of the bed

(20–30 cm), particularly in combination with low dose fludrocortisone, improves OH [20].

To compensate for renal salt loss a liberal intake of salt, at least 8 g (150 mmol) of sodium chloride daily, if needed as salt tablets (starting dose 500 mg t.i.d.), are recommended. Water repletion (2–2.5 l/day) is important, while 500 ml of water is effective in raising BP immediately [21].

Cardiac pacing is not recommended in neurogenic OH [22].

Pharmacological treatment

Plasma expansion

Fludrocortisone

Fludrocortisone acetate is a synthetic mineralocorticoid with minimal glucocorticoid effects. It increases renal sodium reabsorbtion and expands plasma volume. Sensitization of alpha-adrenoceptors may augment the action of noradrenaline. After oral administration, fludrocortisone is readily absorbed and peak plasma levels are reached within 45 min. Elimination half-life is around 7 h.

Review of clinical studies No Class I and II studies were identified. One Class III [23] and one Class IV [24] study have shown an increase in BP and improvement of symptoms.

Recommendations
All Level C

• Fludrocortisone as first-line drug monotherapy of OH (0.1–0.2 mg per day).

• Full benefit requires a high dietary salt and adequate fluid intake.

• Combination of a high salt diet, head-up tilt sleeping (20–30 cm) and a low dose of fludrocortisone (0.1–0.2 mg) is an effective means of improving OH [20].

Mild dependent oedema can be expected and fludrocortisone should be used with caution in patients with a low serum albumin. Higher doses of fludrocortisone can result in fluid overload and congestive heart failure, severe supine hypertension and hypokalaemia [25]. To prevent hypokalaemia food rich in potassium such as fruits, vegetables, poultry, fish and meat is advisable. Headache may occur, especially while supine.

Alpha receptor agonists

There are many sympathomimetic drugs that act on alpha-adrenoceptors. Midodrine has been investigated extensively. Adrenaline (epinephrine) and noradrenaline (norepinephrine) are inactive when administered orally, and rapidly inactivated in the body after infusion. Common adverse effects of sympathomimetics with a central action such as ephedrine, are tachycardia, anxiety, restlessness, insomnia, and tremor. Dry mouth, impaired circulation to the extremities, supine hypertension, and cardiac arrhythmias may occur.

Midodrine

Midodrine is a prodrug with an active metabolite, desglymidodrine, that is a peripherally acting alpha-1-adrenoceptor agonist. It increases BP via vasoconstric-

tion. Midodrine does not cross the blood–brain barrier after oral administration and does not increase heart rate. The absolute bioavailability is 93% and the elimination half-life of desglymidodrine is 2–3 h. The duration of action of midodrine is approximately 4 h. It is excreted mainly in urine.

Review of clinical studies Class I: One dose-response study [26] and two studies with a total number of 259 patients investigating the efficacy, safety, and tolerability of long-term midodrine application [27, 28] were identified. An increase in orthostatic BP and decrease in OH-related symptoms were reported.

Class III: Efficacy and safety were higher with midodrine than with ephedrine [29].

Class IV: Midodrine reduced exercise induced OH in PAF [30].

Recommendations

All Level A

- Midodrine is recommended for mono- or combined therapy (e.g. with fludrocortisone).

- Initial dosage is 2.5 mg orally two to three times daily increasing gradually up to 10 mg t.i.d.

- Supine hypertension is a common (25%) adverse effect and may be severe. The last dose should be administered at least 4 h before going to sleep and BP should be monitored.

- Adverse effects are piloerection (goose bumps, 13%), scalp

or general pruritus (10 and 2%), scalp or general paraesthesia (9% each), urinary retention (6%), and chills (5%).

Some patients worsen on midodrine, maybe due to adrenoceptor desensitization [31]. It should be administered with caution in patients with hepatic dysfunction and is contraindicated in severe heart disease, acute renal failure, urinary retention, phaeochromocytoma, and thyrotoxicosis [32].

DOPS

Dihydroxyphenylserine (DOPS) is a prodrug which is converted by dopadecarboxylase to noradrenaline.

Review of clinical studies Class I: Administration of 200 mg and 400 mg L-DOPS daily improved OH symptoms in 146 chronic haemodialysis patients [33]. In short-term (4 weeks, $n = 86$) and long-term studies (24–52 weeks, $n = 74$) the efficacy of L-DOPS (400 mg/day) for OH after dialysis was demonstrated [34].

Class III: In 20 patients with familial amyloid neuropathy, L-threo-DOPS effectively improves orthostatic tolerance [35]. DL-DOPS improved OH in 10 patients with central and peripheral ANS disorders [36]. In 19 patients with severe OH, L-DOPS improved BP and orthostatic tolerance [37]. In 26 MSA and six PAF patients, the dosage of 300 mg twice daily L-threo-DOPS was effective in controlling symptomatic OH [38].

Recommendations

Level A

In a dosage between 200 mg and 400 mg per day, L-DOPS reduces OH. It is the only effective treatment of dopamine beta-hydroxylase deficiency. In all studies reviewed, no major side effects were reported. Future studies will have to investigate which patient groups benefit most from this drug.

Octreotide

The somatostatin analogue octreotide inhibits release of gastrointestinal peptides, some of which have vasodilatatory properties. It is administered subcutaneously starting with 25–50 μg.

Review of clinical studies Four Class III studies were identified: In 18 PAF patients octreotide reduced postural, postprandial, and exertion-induced hypotension without causing or increasing nocturnal hypertension [39]. Octreotide improved OH in MSA patients after acute and chronic administration [40, 41]. The combination of midodrine and octreotide was more effective in reducing OH than either drug alone [42].

Recommendations

Level C

Subcutaneous doses of 25–150 μg 30 min before a meal may be used to reduce postprandial OH. It does not increase supine hypertension. Nausea and abdominal cramps may occur.

Other treatment options

For the drugs listed below there is no clear evidence for use in OH. Many are recommended as GPP and warrant future studies.

Ephedrine, which acts on alpha- and beta-adrenergic receptors, is recommended by the authors, as it reduces OH in many patients, particularly with central lesions like MSA (15 mg t.i.d.). *Yohimbine*, an alpha-2-adrenoceptor antagonist with central and peripheral effects, has been used in refractory OH (6 mg daily) [43], Class III). Dihydroergotamine (DHE), a direct alpha-adrenoceptor agonist stimulating constriction of venous capacity vessels, has shown some benefit and may be used in severe OH (3–5 mg t.i.d. oral) (Level C: [44], Class III; [45], Class III; [46], Class IV). *Desmopressin*, a vasopressin analogue, acts on renal tubular vasopressin-2 receptors, diminishing nocturnal polyuria, and may be applied as nasal spray (10–40 μg) or orally (100–400 μg) at night [12], Class IV). *Erythropoietin* is recommended in anaemic patients [47–49], particularly in familial amyloidosis [50]. *Indomethacin*, a prostaglandin synthetase inhibitor, has been used in severe OH (75–150 mg/day) [51], Class IV, [43], Class III). *Pyridostigmine* may be effective in the treatment of OH through potentiation of sympathetic cholinergic ganglionic transmission, leading to increased vascular tone in the upright position [52]. In a double-blind, randomized, four-way crossover study the acute effects of 60 mg pyridostigmine bromide on supine and upright BP were tested against midodrine and placebo. Pyridostigmine significantly improved standing BP without worsening supine hypertension [53]. However, further studies on the long-term efficacy and on possible adverse effects have to be performed before this treatment can be evaluated.

Summary

- OH is defined as fall in BP within 3 min of active standing or HUT.
- The key to managing OH is individually tailored therapy. The goal of treatment is to improve the patient's functional capacity and quality of life, preventing injury, rather than to achieve a target BP.
- Management of patients with OH consists of education, advice, and training on various factors that influence blood pressure, and special aspects that have to be avoided (foods, habits, positions, and drugs).
- Physical measures include leg crossing, squatting, elastic abdominal binders and stockings, and careful exercise (GPP).
- Increased water (2–2.5 l/day) and salt ingestion (>8 g or 150 mmol per day) effectively improve OH.
- Fludrocortisone is a valuable starter drug (0.1–0.2 mg per day, Level C). Second-line drugs include sympathomimetics, such as midodrine (start with 2.5 mg b.i.d and increase to 10 mg t.i.d, Level A) or ephedrine (15 mg t.i.d., GPP). DOPS (200–400 mg daily, Level A) reduces OH with only minor side effects. It is an effective treatment in dopamine beta-hydroxylase deficiency.
- Supine hypertension has to be considered.
- Individual testing with a series of drugs, based on the risk of side effects, pharmacological interactions and probability of response in the individual patient, may be considered when the measures shown here should not be satisfactory.

Need of update

These guidelines will be updated when substantial new data pertaining to the management of OH become available.

Conflicts of interest

The present guidelines were developed without external financial support. None of the authors reports conflicting interests.

References

1. Mathias CJ. Autonomic diseases: clinical features and laboratory evaluation. *J Neurol Neurosurg Psychiatry* 2003; **74**(Suppl. 3):iii31–41.

2. Low PA. Prevalence of orthostatic hypotension. *Clin Auton Res* 2008;**18**(Suppl. 1):8–13.

3. Senard JM, Brefel-Courbon C, Rascol O, Montastruc JL. Orthostatic hypotension in patients with Parkinson's disease: pathophysiology and management. *Drugs Aging* 2001;**18**:495–505.

4. Arbogast SD, Alshekhlee A, Hussain Z, McNeeley K, Chelimsky TC. Hypotension unawareness in profound orthostatic hypotension. *Am J Med* 2009;**122**(6):574–80.

5. Schatz IJ, Bannister R, Freeman RL, *et al.* Consensus statement on the definition of orthostatic hypotension, pure autonomic failure, and multiple system atrophy. *Neurology* 1996;**46**:1470.

6. Brainin M, Barnes M, Baron JC, *et al.* Guidance for the preparation of neurological management guidelines by EFNS scientific task forces – revised recommendations 2004. *Eur J Neurol* 2004;**11**:577–81.

7. Lahrmann H, Magnifico F, Haensch CA, Cortelli P. Autonomic nervous system laboratories: a European survey. *Eur J Neurol* 2005;**12**:375–9.

8. Mathias CJ, Bannister R. Investigation of autonomic disorders. In: Mathias CJ, Bannister R (eds) *Autonomic Failure. A Textbook of Clinical Disorders of the Autonomic Nervous System*, 4th edn. Oxford: Oxford Univ. Press, 2002; pp. 169–95.

9. Ravits JM. AAEM minimonograph #48: autonomic nervous system testing. *Muscle Nerve* 1997;**20**:919–37.

10. Chandler MP, Mathias CJ. Haemodynamic responses during head-up tilt and tilt reversal in two groups with chronic autonomic failure: pure autonomic failure and multiple system atrophy. *J Neurol* 2002;**249**:542–8.

11. Brignole M, Alboni P, Benditt D, *et al.* Guidelines on management (diagnosis and treatment) of syncope. *Eur Heart J* 2001;**22**:1256–306.

12. Mathias CJ, Fosbraey P, da Costa DF, Thornley A, Bannister R. The effect of desmopressin on nocturnal polyuria, overnight weight loss, and morning postural hypotension in patients with autonomic failure. *Br Med J (Clin Res Ed)* 1986;**293**:353–4.

13. Bouvette CM, McPhee BR, Opfer-Gehrking TL, Low PA. Role of physical countermaneuvers in the management of orthostatic hypotension: efficacy and biofeedback augmentation. *Mayo Clin Proc* 1996;**71**:847–53.

14. ten Harkel AD, van Lieshout JJ, Wieling W. Effects of leg muscle pumping and tensing on orthostatic arterial pressure: a study in normal subjects and patients with autonomic failure. *Clin Sci (Lond)* 1994;**87**:553–8.

15. Wieling W, van Lieshout JJ, van Leeuwen AM. Physical manoeuvres that reduce postural hypotension in autonomic failure. *Clin Auton Res* 1993;**3**:57–65.

16. Smit AA, Wieling W, Opfer-Gehrking TL, Emmerik-Levelt HM, Low PA. Patients' choice of portable folding chairs to reduce symptoms of orthostatic hypotension. *Clin Auton Res* 1999;**9**:341–4.

17. van Dijk N, de Bruin IG, Gisolf J, *et al.* Hemodynamic effects of leg crossing and skeletal muscle tensing during free standing in patients with vasovagal syncope. *J Appl Physiol* 2005;**98**(2):584–90.

18. Denq JC, Opfer-Gehrking TL, Giuliani M, Felten J, Convertino VA, Low PA. Efficacy of compression of different capacitance beds in the amelioration of orthostatic hypotension. *Clin Auton Res* 1997;**7**:321–6.

19. Tanaka H, Yamaguchi H, Tamai H. Treatment of orthostatic intolerance with inflatable abdominal band. *Lancet* 1997;**349**:175.

20. van Lieshout JJ, ten Harkel AD, Wieling W. Fludrocortisone and sleeping in the head-up position limit the postural decrease in cardiac output in autonomic failure. *Clin Auton Res* 2000;**10**:35–42.

21. Mathias CJ, Young TM. Water drinking in the management of orthostatic intolerance due to orthostatic hypotension, vasovagal syncope and postural tachycardia syndrom. *Eur J Neurol* 2004;**11**:613–9.

22. Sahul ZH, Trusty JM, Erickson M, Low PA, Shen WK. Pacing does not improve hypotension in patients with severe orthostatic hypotension – a prospective randomized crossover pilot study. *Clin Auton Res* 2004;**14**:255–8.

23. Campbell IW, Ewing DJ, Clarke BF. 9-Alpha-fluorohydrocortisone in the treatment of postural hypotension in diabetic autonomic neuropathy. *Diabetes* 1975;**24**:381–4.

24. Hoehn MM. Levodopa-induced postural hypotension. Treatment with fludrocortisone. *Arch Neurol* 1975;**32**:50–1.

25. Schatz IJ, Miller MJ, Frame B. Corticosteroids in the management of orthostatic hypotension. *Cardiology* 1976; **61**(Suppl. 1):280–9.

26. Wright RA, Kaufmann HC, Perera R, *et al.* A double-blind, dose response study of midodrine in neurogenic orthostatic hypotension. *Neurology* 1998;**51**:120–4.

27. Jankovic J, Gilden JL, Hiner BC, *et al.* Neurogenic orthostatic hypotension: a double-blind, placebo-controlled study with midodrine. *Am J Med* 1993;**95**:38–48.

28. Low PA, Gilden JL, Freeman R, Sheng KN, McElligott MA. Efficacy of midodrine vs placebo in neurogenic orthostatic hypotension: a randomized, double-blind multicenter study. *JAMA* 1997;**277**:1046–51. Correction. ibid.; 278: 388.

29. Fouad-Tarazi FM, Okabe M, Goren H. Alpha sympathomimetic treatment of autonomic insufficiency with orthostatic hypotension. *Am J Med* 1995;**99**:604–10.

30. Schrage WG, Eisenach JH, Dinenno FA, *et al.* Effects of midodrine on exercise-induced hypotension and blood pressure recovery in autonomic failure. *J Appl Physiol* 2004;**97**:1978–84.

31. Kaufmann H, Brannan T, Krakoff L, Yahr MD, Mandeli J. Treatment of orthostatic hypotension due to autonomic failure with a peripheral alpha-adrenergic agonist (midodrine). *Neurology* 1988;**38**:951–6.

32. McClellan KJ, Wiseman LR, Wilde MI. Midodrine: a review of its therapeutic use in the management of orthostatic hypotension. *Drugs Aging* 1998;**12**:76–86.

33. Akizawa T, Koshikawa S, Iida N, *et al.* Clinical effects of L-threo-3,4-dihydroxyphenylserine on orthostatic hypotension in hemodialysis patients. *Nephron* 2002;**90**: 384–90.

34. Iida N, Koshikawa S, Akizawa T, *et al.* Effects of L-threo-3,4-dihydroxyphenylserine on orthostatic hypotension in hemodialysis patients. *Am J Nephrol* 2002;**22**:338–46.

35. Carvalho MJ, van den Meiracker AH, Boomsma F, *et al.* Improved orthostatic tolerance in familial amyloidotic polyneuropathy with unnatural noradrenaline precursor L-threo-3,4-dihydroxyphenylserine. *J Auton Nerv Syst* 1997; **62**:63–71.

36. Freeman R, Landsberg L, Young J. The treatment of neurogenic orthostatic hypotension with 3,4-DL-threo-dihydroxyphenylserine: a randomized, placebo-controlled, crossover trial. *Neurology* 1999;**53**:2151–7.

37. Kaufmann H, Saadia D, Voustianiouk A, *et al.* Norepinephrine precursor therapy in neurogenic orthostatic hypotension. *Circulation* 2003;**108**:724–8.

38. Mathias CJ, Senard JM, Braune S, *et al.* L-theo-dihydroxphenylserine (L-threo-DOPS, droxidopa) in the management of neurogenic orthostatic hypotension: a multi-national, multi-centre, dose-ranging study in multiple system atrophy and pure autonomic failure. *Clin Auton Res* 2001;**11**: 235–42.

39. Alam M, Smith G, Bleasdale-Barr K, Pavitt DV, Mathias CJ. Effects of the peptide release inhibitor, octreotide, on daytime hypotension and on nocturnal hypertension in primary autonomic failure. *J Hypertens* 1995;**13**: 1664–9.

40. Bordet R, Benhadjali J, Libersa C, Destee A. Octreotide in the management of orthostatic hypotension in multiple system atrophy: pilot trial of chronic administration. *Clin Neuropharmacol* 1994;**17**:380–3.

41. Bordet R, Benhadjali J, Destee A, Belabbas A, Libersa C. Octreotide effects on orthostatic hypotension in patients with multiple system atrophy: a controlled study of acute administration. *Clin Neuropharmacol* 1995;**18**:83–9.

42. Hoeldtke RD, Horvath GG, Bryner KD, Hobbs GR. Treatment of orthostatic hypotension with midodrine and octreotide. *J Clin Endocrinol Metab* 1998;**83**:339–43.

43. Jordan J, Shannon JR, Biaggioni I, Norman R, Black BK, Robertson D. Contrasting actions of pressor agents in severe autonomic failure. *Am J Med* 1998;**105**:116–24.

44. Conte JJ, Fournie GJ, Maurette MH. Dihydroergotamine: an effective treatment for postural hypotension due to antihypertensive drugs (ganglion-blocking agents excepted). *Cardiology* 1976;**61**(Suppl. 1):342–9.

45. Lubke KO. A controlled study with Dihydergot on patients with orthostatic dysregulation. *Cardiology* 1976;**61**(Suppl. 1):333–41.

46. Victor RG, Talman WT. Comparative effects of clonidine and dihydroergotamine on venomotor tone and orthostatic tolerance in patients with severe hypoadrenergic orthostatic hypotension. *Am J Med* 2002;**112**:361–8.

47. Hoeldtke RD, Streeten DH. Treatment of orthostatic hypotension with erythropoietin. *N Engl J Med* 1993;**329**: 611–5.

48. Biaggioni I, Robertson D, Krantz S, Jones M, Haile V. The anemia of primary autonomic failure and its reversal with recombinant erythropoietin. *Ann Intern Med* 1994; **121**:181–6.

49. Perera R, Isola L, Kaufmann H. Effect of recombinant erythropoietin on anemia and orthostatic hypotension in primary autonomic failure. *Clin Auton Res* 1995;**5**:211–3.

50. Beirão I, Lobato L, Moreira L, *et al.* Long-term treatment of anemia with recombinant human erythropoietin in familial amyloidosis TTR V30M. *Amyloid* 2008;**15**(3):205–9.

51. Kochar MS, Itskovitz HD. Treatment of idiopathic orthostatic hypotension (Shy-Drager syndrome) with indomethacin. *Lancet* 1978;**1**:1011–4.

52. Singer W, Opfer-Gehrking TL, McPhee BR, Hilz MJ, Bharucha AE, Low PA. Acetylcholinesterase inhibition: a novel approach in the treatment of neurogenic orthostatic hypotension. *J Neurol Neurosurg Psychiatry* 2003;**74**:1294–8.

53. Singer W, Sandroni P, Opfer-Gehrking TL, *et al.* Pyridostigmine treatment trial in neurogenic orthostatic hypotension. *Arch Neurol* 2006;**63**(4):513–8.

CHAPTER 34

Cerebral venous and sinus thrombosis

K. Einhäupl,[1] J. Stam,[2] M.-G. Bousser,[3] S. F. T. M. de Bruijn,[4] J. M. Ferro,[5] I. Martinelli,[6] F. Masuhr[1]

[1]Charité-Universitätsmedizin Berlin, Germany; [2]Academic Medical Centre Amsterdam, The Netherlands; [3]Hôpital Lariboisière, Paris, France; [4]Haga Hospital The Hague and LUMC, Leiden, The Netherlands; [5]Hospital Santa Maria, Lisboa, Portugal; [6]A. Bianchi Bonomi Hemophilia and Thrombosis Center, IRCCS Maggiore Hospital, University of Milan, Italy

Background and objectives

Cerebral venous and sinus thrombosis (CVST) is a rare condition that accounts for less than 1% of all strokes. The exact incidence in adults is unknown since population-based studies are not available, but one can expect five to eight cases per year in a tertiary care centre [1, 2]. A Canadian study reported an incidence of 0.67 cases per 100 000 children below 18 years and 43% of the reported cases were seen in neonates [3]. The peak incidence in adults is in their third decade with a male/female ratio of 1.5–5 per year [2, 4]. Diagnosis is still frequently overlooked or delayed due to the wide spectrum of clinical symptoms and the often subacute or lingering onset. Headache is the most frequent symptom of CVST and occurs in almost 90% of all cases [5]. The headache may be of acute onset (thunderclap headache) and may be clinically indistinguishable from headache in patients with subarachnoid haemorrhage [6]. Focal or generalized seizures are far more frequently seen in CVST than in arterial stroke and occur in 40% of all patients, with an even higher incidence (76%) in peripartum CVST [5, 7]. Focal neurological signs (including focal seizures) are the most common finding in CVST. They include central motor and sensory deficits, aphasia, or hemianopsia and occur in 40–60% of all cases. In patients with focal deficits together with headache, seizures, or an altered consciousness, CVST should always be considered. The syndrome of isolated intracranial hypertension (IIH) with head-

ache, vomiting, and blurred vision due to papilloedema is the most homogeneous pattern of clinical presentation accounting for 20–40% of CVST cases. Stupor or coma are found in 15–19% of patients at hospital admission [5, 8] and are usually seen in cases with extensive thrombosis or affection of the deep venous system with bilateral thalamic involvement. Of all clinical signs reported in CVST, coma at admission is the most consistent and strongest predictor of a poor outcome [4, 5].

Intra-arterial four-vessel angiography has long been the gold standard for establishing the diagnosis of CVST, but today magnetic resonance imaging (MRI) and magnetic resonance angiography (MRA) are regarded the best tools both for the diagnosis and follow-up of CVST (for review see [9]). Cranial computed tomography (CCT) alone is not sufficient but diagnosis can be established in combination with CT angiography, although the use of iodinated contrast fluid and ionizing radiation remains a disadvantage which makes it inappropriate for follow-up examinations.

Current therapeutic measures used in clinical practice include the use of anticoagulants such as dose-adjusted intravenous heparin or body weight-adjusted subcutaneous low-molecular-weight heparin, the use of thrombolysis, and symptomatic therapy including control of seizures and elevated intracranial pressure. The use of heparin has long been a matter of debate. Whereas anticoagulation is effective in the treatment and prevention of extracerebral venous thrombosis, the high rate of spontaneous intracranial haemorrhages seen in patients with CVST make many physicians hesitate to administer heparin because of safety concerns. The introduction of local thrombolysis has stirred the discussion about the optimal therapy of patients with CVST [10].

European Handbook of Neurological Management: Volume 1, 2nd edition. Edited by N. E. Gilhus, M. P. Barnes and M. Brainin.
© 2011 Blackwell Publishing Ltd.

The aim of the present task force was to review the strength of evidence to support these interventions and the preparation of recommendations on the therapy of CVST based on the best available evidence for the efficacy and safety of anticoagulant therapy, thrombolysis, and symptomatic therapy.

Materials and methods

Search strategy

MEDLINE 1966–2009 and EMBASE 1966–2009 were examined with appropriate MESH and free subject terms: cerebral venous and sinus thrombosis, cerebral venous thrombosis, cortical vein thrombosis, intracranial thrombosis.

These were combined with the terms: treatment, medication, therapy, controlled clinical trial, randomized controlled trial, multicentre study, meta analysis, anticoagulation, thrombolysis, local thrombolysis, antiepileptic therapy, intracranial pressure, steroids, hyperventilation, osmotic diuretics, craniectomy, decompressive surgery.

The Cochrane Central Register of Controlled Trials (CENTRAL) and the Cochrane Library and references of selected articles were also searched. Review articles and book chapters were also included if they were considered to provide comprehensive reviews of the topic. The search included reports of research in human beings only and in English language. The task force included six neurologists and one specialist in internal medicine with an expertise in the field of haemostasis and thrombosis (I.M.). The literature search was performed by K.E. and F.M., who also prepared a first draft of the manuscript. The manuscript was sent via email and was reviewed by all members of the task force and suggestions and corrections were incorporated. Recommendations were reached by consensus of all task force members and were also based on our own awareness and clinical experience. Where there was a lack of evidence but consensus was clear we stated our opinion as Good Practice Points (GPP). The final draft of the manuscript was approved by all members of the task force. All necessary steps for the preparation of the presented recommendation were performed via email correspondence.

The classification for evidence levels for therapeutic interventions were made according to the guidance for the preparation of neurological management guidelines by EFNS scientific task forces [11].

Treatment

Heparin therapy

The rationale of anticoagulant therapy in CVST is to avoid thrombus extension, to favour spontaneous thrombus resolution, and to prevent pulmonary embolism, particularly in patients with concomitant extracranial deep vein thrombosis. At the same time anticoagulation (AC) may promote or worsen intracranial haemorrhage (ICH), which occurs in 40–50% of patients with CVST [5, 12] and which may be the main reason to withhold AC. In addition, anticoagulation is always associated with an increased risk for extracranial bleeding complications.

There are only two small controlled trials that compared the efficacy and safety of AC with placebo for the treatment of CVST. Both trials chose an unfavourable outcome as the main criterion to evaluate the efficacy of AC instead of a good outcome (e.g. Rankin Scale 0–1), which might have been a better choice in a condition with a much better prognosis than arterial stroke. In addition, the 3 months' follow-up for the evaluation of the functional outcome may have been too short since major improvement of the patients with CVST can be observed far beyond.

The first study [13] compared dose-adjusted intravenous heparin with placebo in 20 patients (10 patients in each treatment group) (Class II evidence). Eight patients in the heparin group recovered completely and none died, whereas only one patient in the placebo group recovered fully and three patients died. Treatment assessment was performed by using a specially developed CVST severity scale that contained the items headache, focal signs, seizures, and level of consciousness. Using this scale, there was a significant difference between the two groups after 3 days in favour of the active treatment and the difference remained significant after 3 months. Three patients with previous ICH recovered completely and no new haemorrhages occurred in the heparin group whereas in the placebo group two patients with pretreatment ICH died and two new haemorrhages were observed. There were no major extracranial haemorrhages in the heparin group and one probable case of fatal pulmonary embolism in the control group.

The outcome assessment was criticized [14] because the CVST severity scale was not validated as a final outcome measure in neurological patients. Using death and dependency as clearly defined outcome parameters, the difference between the two groups would not be significant. Nevertheless, the study did show some benefit and even more important suggested the safety of AC in patients with CVST.

The second randomized trial compared body weight-adjusted subcutaneous low-molecular-weight heparin (LMWH) with placebo in 60 patients with CVST [12] (Class I evidence). A poor outcome – defined as death or Barthel index < 15 – was observed after 3 weeks in six of the 30 patients treated with LMWH (20%) compared to seven of the 29 controls (24%). After three months, three patients (10%) in the LMWH group and six patients (21%) in the placebo group had a poor outcome which corresponded to a non-significant absolute risk reduction of 11% in favour of the active treatment. No new ICH or secondary worsening of the 15 patients with pretreatment haemorrhage was observed in the LMWH group. There was one major extracerebral haemorrhage in the heparin group and one probable case of fatal pulmonary embolism in the control group.

A meta-analysis of these two trials showed that the use of AC led to an absolute risk reduction in death or dependency of 13% (confidence interval −30 to +3%) with a relative risk reduction of 54% [15]. Although this difference did not reach statistical significance, both trials showed a consistent and clinically meaningful trend in favour of AC and demonstrated the safety of anticoagulant therapy. Thus, data from controlled trials favour the use of anticoagulation in patients with CVST because it may reduce the risk of a fatal outcome and severe disability and does not promote ICH, at least in the small number of patients in the trials. In patients with isolated intracranial hypertension (and proven CVST) and threatened vision with the need for repeated lumbar punctures to remove cerebrospinal fluid (CSF) in order to obtain a normal closing pressure, AC should be withheld until 24 h after the last lumbar puncture.

It is unclear, whether treatment with full-dose intravenous heparin or subcutaneously applied LMWH is equally effective for CVST. A meta-analysis that compared the efficacy of fixed-dose subcutaneous LMWH versus adjusted-dose unfractionated heparin for extracerebral venous thromboembolism found a superiority for

LMWH and significantly fewer major bleeding complications [16]. Further advantages include the route of administration, which increases the mobility of patients, and the lack of laboratory monitoring and subsequent dose adjustments. A possible advantage of dose-adjusted intravenous heparin therapy particularly in critical ill patients may be the fact that the activated partial thromboplastin time normalizes within 1–2 h after discontinuation of the infusion if complications occur or surgical intervention is necessary.

Recommendation

Current evidence shows that patients with CVST without contraindications for anticoagulation should be treated either with body weight-adjusted subcutaneous low-molecular-weight heparin or dose-adjusted intravenous heparin with an at least doubled activated partial thromboplastin time (Level B recommendation). Concomitant intracranial haemorrhage related to CVST is not a contraindication for heparin therapy. For the reasons mentioned above, LMWH should be preferred in uncomplicated CVST cases.

Thrombolysis

There is currently no evidence from randomized controlled trials about the efficacy and safety of either systemic or local thrombolytic therapy in patients with CVST. Thrombolytic therapy has the potential to provide faster restitution of venous outflow, and positive effects of local thrombolytic treatment of CVST have increasingly been reported from uncontrolled series [17–20] (Class IV evidence). Patients were treated with either heparin and urokinase or heparin and recombinant tissue plasminogen activator (rtPA) which may result in fewer bleeding complications due to its clot selectiveness and shorter half-life. Two uncontrolled studies that used rtPA in combination with dose-adjusted intravenous heparin included a total of 21 patients [18, 19]. In the Korean study [18], which included nine patients, a mean total dose of 135 mg (range 50–300 mg) rtPA was used compared to 46 mg (range 23–128 mg) in the American study [19], which included 12 patients. Both studies placed a microcatheter directly into the thrombus via the transfemoral vein and performed a bolus injection of rtPA followed by continuous infusion. In the two studies combined, rapid (mean time of 20 h in the Korean and 29 h in the American study) and complete recanalization was achieved in 15 of 21 patients, and 14 of 21 patients showed a complete clinical recovery. However, there were two extracerebral bleeding complications in the Korean study and two patients with pre-treatment ICH in the American study worsened because of increased intracerebral bleeding, which required surgery in one case. Thus, although recanalization was rapidly achieved, local thrombolysis may carry a higher risk of bleeding complications compared to anticoagulant therapy, particularly if pre-treatment ICH is present [10]. Trials that compare heparin therapy and local thrombolysis are lacking and there is no evidence that clinical outcome is better than with heparin alone. Currently, local thrombolysis may be a therapeutic option for patients at high risk for a poor outcome despite heparin therapy. The International Study on Cerebral Vein and Dural Sinus Thrombosis (ISCVT) identified coma on admission and thrombosis of the deep venous system apart from underlying causes as the most important predictors for a poor clinical outcome [5]. More than 80% of the included 624 adult patients were treated with AC. Comatose patients may define a subgroup of patients with CVST who are at high risk of death despite AC [8]. Under this particular condition, the effect of AC may come too late to prevent irreversible brain damage and these patients may possibly benefit from thrombolytic therapy. A systematic review on the use of thrombolytics in CVST suggested a possible benefit in such severe cases [21]. Thirty-eight of the reported patients were comatose at the start of thrombolytic therapy, of whom six (16%) died. Intracranial haemorrhage occurred in 17% and was associated with clinical deterioration in 5% of cases. In comparison, a retrospective analysis found that eight (53%) of the 15 patients with stupor or coma at the start of dose-adjusted intravenous heparin therapy died [8]. In the ISCVT, 12 (38%) of the 31 comatose patients died [5]. However, the results of the review were based on case reports and uncontrolled case series and there are as yet no established clinical criteria for the use of thrombolytics in CVST (Class IV evidence). In a recent prospective study [22] of 20 patients treated with endovascular thrombolysis alone or in combination with endovascular thrombectomy (15 patients), 12 patients recovered, two survived with handicaps, and six (30%) died. Twelve were comatose and 14 had haemorrhagic infarcts before thrombolysis. Large haemorrhagic infarcts before treatment were associated with a

fatal outcome and five patients had increased ICH after thrombolysis. Patients with large infarcts and impending herniation did not benefit (Class IV evidence).

A controlled randomized trial is warranted to further study the efficacy and safety of thrombolysis in CVST. However, such a trial will be difficult to perform in single centres because of the small number of severe patients, particularly in countries and centres with early diagnosis of CVST. Only an international multicentre trial may be able to clarify the role of thrombolysis in the treatment of CVST.

Recommendation

There is insufficient evidence to support the use of either systemic or local thrombolysis in patients with CVST. If patients deteriorate despite adequate anticoagulation and other causes of deterioration have been ruled out, thrombolysis may be a therapeutic option in selected cases, possibly in those without intracranial haemorrhage or impending herniation from large haemorrhagic infarcts (GPP). The optimal substance, dosage, route (systemic or local), or method of administration (repeated bolus or bolus plus infusion) are not known.

Oral anticoagulation

Controlled data about the benefit and optimal duration of oral anticoagulant therapy (OAT) in patients with CVST are not available, but most authors recommend continued anticoagulation after the acute phase. In the ISCVT, median time on OAT after discharge was 7.7 months [5]. A MRI follow-up study of 33 patients suggested that recanalization occurs within the first 4 months after CVST irrespective of further OAT [23]. These data may provide some guidance on the duration of OAT, but whether incomplete or absent recanalization increases the risk of recurrence is not known (Class IV evidence). No recurrences occurred in two follow-up studies which showed incomplete or no recanalization in more than 40% of the patients [23, 24].

Analogous to patients with extracerebral venous thrombosis, OAT with a target INR of 2.0–3.0 may be given for 3 months if CVST was secondary to a transient (reversible) risk factor and for 6–12 months if it was idiopathic [25]. However, the risk of recurrence of CVST may be lower than that of extracerebral venous thrombosis. In the ISCVT, 2.2% of all patients had a recurrent sinus thrombosis with a median follow-up of 16 months

[5], and prolonged OAT may expose some patients to an unnecessary bleeding risk, although there was also a risk of 4.3% for other thrombotic events during follow-up including 2.5% of pelvic or limb venous thrombosis and 0.5% of pulmonary embolism.

OAT is also recommended for 6–12 months in patients with extracerebral venous thrombosis and 'mild' thrombophilia (heterozygous factor V Leiden or prothrombin G20210A mutation, and high plasma levels of factor VIII) [26]. Long-term treatment should be considered for patients with 'severe' thrombophilia associated with a high risk of recurrence (antithrombin, protein C or protein S deficiency, homozygous factor V Leiden or protormbin G20210A mutation, antiphospholipid antibodies, and combined abnormalities) [26]. Indefinite OAT is also recommended in patients with two or more episodes of idiopathic objectively documented extracerebral venous thrombosis [25]. Thus, in the absence of controlled data the decision on the duration of anticoagulant therapy must be based on individual hereditary and precipitating factors as well as on the potential bleeding risks of long-term OAT. Regular follow-up visits should be performed after discontinuation of OAT and patients should be informed about early signs (headache) indicating a possible relapse.

Recommendation

There are insufficient data about the optimal duration of OAT in patients with CVST. Analogous to patients with a first episode of extracerebral venous thrombosis, OAT may be given for 3 months if CVST was secondary to a transient risk factor, for 6–12 months in patients with idiopathic CVST and in those with 'mild' thrombophilia. Indefinite OAT should be considered in patients with two or more episodes of CVST and in those with one episode of CVST and 'severe' thrombophilia (GPP).

Symptomatic treatment

Symptomatic therapy includes the use of antiepileptic drugs, management of increased intracranial pressure, the control of psychomotor agitation, and analgesic treatment.

Control of seizures

There are no data regarding the effectiveness of a prophylactic use of antiepileptic drugs (AED) in patients with CVST. Whereas some authors recommend prophylactic treatment [27] because of the high incidence of seizures (and series of seizures or even status epilepticus) and their possible detrimental effects on the metabolic situation during the acute phase of the disease, others restrict the use of anticonvulsants to patients with seizures [28]. One study identified focal sensory deficits and the presence of focal oedema or ischaemic/haemorrhagic infarcts on admission CCT/MRI as significant predictors of early symptomatic seizures [29]. Another study [30] identified cortical vein thrombosis, ICH, and focal motor deficits as independent predictors for early epileptic seizures (Class IV evidence). Patients with supratentorial lesions and presenting seizures had the highest risk for recurrent seizures in the ISCVT that was significantly decreased by AED use [31] (Class III evidence).

Although data are insufficient to give recommendations, these findings suggest that prophylactic treatment with AED may be a therapeutic option for those patients, whereas it is not warranted when there are no focal neurological deficits and no supratentorial lesions on brain scan (e.g. patients with isolated intracranial hypertension). If no antiepileptic treatment has been performed before the first seizure occurs, effective concentrations of AEDs should be achieved rapidly because series of seizures frequently occur in patients with CVST.

The risk of residual epilepsy after CVST is low compared to the high rate of patients with early seizures. Reported incidences range from 5 to 10.6% [5, 29, 32]. In the Portuguese series [29], all late seizures occurred within the first year. A haemorrhagic lesion in the acute brain scan was the strongest predictor of postacute seizures. In all series together, late seizures were more common in patients with early symptomatic seizures than in those patients with none. Thus, prolonged treatment with AED for 1 year may be reasonable for patients with early seizures and haemorrhagic lesions on admission brain scan, whereas in patients without these risk factors AED therapy may be tapered off gradually after the acute stage.

Recommendation

Prophylactic antiepileptic therapy may be a therapeutic option in patients with focal neurological deficits and supratentorial lesions on admission CT/MRI (GPP). The optimal duration of treatment for patients with seizures is unclear.

Treatment of elevated intracranial pressure

Although brain swelling is observed in about 50% of all patients with CVST on CCT, minor brain oedema needs no other treatment than AC, which improves the venous outflow sufficiently to reduce intracranial pressure in most patients [27, 28]. In patients with isolated intracranial hypertension and threatened vision, a lumbar puncture with sufficient cerebrospinal fluid (CSF) removal to obtain a normal closing pressure should be performed before starting AC 24 h after the puncture. There are no controlled data, but acetazolamide may be considered in patients with persistent papilloedema. In few patients vision continues to deteriorate despite repeated lumbar punctures and/or acetazolamide. In these cases shunting procedures (lumboperitoneal, ventriculoperitoneal shunts, or optic nerve fenestration) should be considered.

Anti-oedema treatment is necessary in only 20% of patients and should be carried out according to general principles of therapy of raised intracranial pressure (head elevation at about 30 degrees, hyperventilation with a target $PaCO_2$ pressure of 30–35 mmHg, intravenous application of osmotic diuretics). However, one should keep in mind, that osmotic substances might be harmful in venous outflow obstruction, since they are not as quickly eliminated from the intracerebral circulation as in other conditions. The use of tris–hydroxy-methly-aminomethane (THMA), which decreases ICP after intravenous administration via an alkalotic vasoconstriction, may be a therapy option in ventilated patients. Restricted volume intake for treatment of brain oedema must be avoided, since these measures can cause an additional deterioration of blood viscosity. Steroids cannot be recommended for treatment of elevated intracranial pressure. No benefit was found in a case-control study of the ISCVT [33] and the use of steroids was associated with a detrimental effect in patients without parenchymal lesions (Class III evidence).

The most frequent cause of death in patients with CVST is transtentorial brain herniation [34]. In severe cases with impending herniation due to a unilateral large haemorrhagic infarct, decompressive surgery may be the only way to save the patient's life. Local thrombolysis seems no treatment option in such cases because of the incalculable risk of further ICH extension with an additional detrimental effect on ICP. Stefini and co-workers

[35] reported three patients with fixed dilated pupils due to transtentorial herniation who underwent decompressive surgery, two of whom recovered with only minor neurological sequelae (Class IV evidence). Coutinho and co-workers [36] reported three consecutive cases treated with decompressive hemicraniectomy, of whom two patients had an excellent outcome and one died. Reviewing the literature, the authors found another seven cases of severe CVST treated with decompressive surgery, of whom all survived with a favourable outcome (mRS ≤ 3) (Class IV evidence). The haemorrhagic infarct should not be removed because neuronal damage is often less pronounced in CVST-related haemorrhage, explaining the possible reversibility of even severe clinical symptoms [37].

Recommendations

In patients with isolated intracranial hypertension and threatened vision, possible therapeutic measures may include one or more lumbar punctures, acetazolamide, and incidentally CSF-shunting procedures. There are no controlled data about the risks and benefits of certain therapeutic measures to reduce an elevated intracranial pressure in patients with CVST. However, based on the available evidence, steroids seem not to be useful and should be avoided (GPP). Anti-oedema treatment should be carried out according to general principles of therapy of raised intracranial pressure. In a small subgroup of patients with severe CVST and impending herniation attributable to large haemorrhagic infarcts, decompressive craniectomy can be life-saving (GPP).

Conflicts of interest

The authors have reported no conflicts of interest relevant to this manuscript.

K. Einhäupl was the principal investigator of the treatment trial with unfractionated heparin [13]. J. Stam and S.T.F.M. de Bruijn were principal investigators of the CVST Study Group Trial [12].

References

1. Bousser MG, Chiras J, Bories J, Castaigne P. Cerebral venous thrombosis – a review of 38 cases. *Stroke* 1985;**16**:199–213.

2. Einhäupl KM, Villringer A, Haberl RL, *et al.* Clinical spectrum of sinus venous thrombosis. In: Einhäupl K, Kempski O, Baethmann A (eds) *Cerebral Sinus Thrombosis. Experimental and Clinical Aspects.* New York: Plenum Press, 1990; pp. 149–55.

3. deVeber G, Andrew M, Adams C, for the Canadian Pediatric Ischemic Stroke Study Group. Cerebral sinovenous thrombosis in children. *N Engl J Med* 2001;**345**:417–23.

4. De Bruijn SFTM, de Haan RJ, Stam J, for the Cerebral Venous Sinus Thrombosis Study Group. Clinical features and prognostic factors of cerebral venous and sinus thrombosis in a prospective series of 59 patients. *J Neurol Neurosurg Psychiatry* 2001;**70**:105–8.

5. Ferro JM, Canhão P, Stam J, Bousser MG, Barinagarrementeria F, for the ISCVT Investigators. Prognosis of cerebral vein and dural sinus thrombosis. Results of the International Study on Cerebral Vein and Dural Sinus Thrombosis (ISCVT). *Stroke* 2004;**35**:664–70.

6. De Bruijn SFTM, Stam J, Kapelle LJ, for the Cerebral Venous Sinus Thrombosis Study Group. Thunderclap headache as first symptom of cerebral venous sinus thrombosis. *Lancet* 1996;**348**:1623–5.

7. Cantu C, Barinagarrementeria F. Cerebral venous thrombosis associated with pregnancy and puerperium. Review of 67 cases. *Stroke* 1993;**24**:1880–4.

8. Mehraein S, Schmidtke K, Villringer A, Valdueza JM, Masuhr F. Heparin treatment in cerebral sinus and venous thrombosis: patients at risk of fatal outcome. *Cerebrovasc Dis* 2003;**15**:17–21.

9. Masuhr F, Mehraein S, Einhäupl K. Cerebral venous and sinus thrombosis. *J Neurol* 2004;**251**:11–23.

10. Bousser MG. Cerebral venous thrombosis. Nothing, heparin, or local thrombolysis? *Stroke* 1999;**30**:481–3.

11. Brainin M, Barnes M, Baron J-C, *et al.* Guidance for the preparation of neurological management guidelines by EFNS scientific task forces – revised recommendations 2004. *Eur J Neurol* 2004;**11**:577–81.

12. De Bruijn SFTM, Stam J, for the Cerebral Venous Sinus Thrombosis Study Group. Randomized, placebo-controlled trial of anticoagulant treatment with low-molecular-weight heparin for cerebral sinus thrombosis. *Stroke* 1999;**30**: 484–8.

13. Einhäupl KM, Villringer A, Meister W, *et al.* Heparin treatment in sinus venous thrombosis. *Lancet* 1991;**338**: 597–600.

14. Stam J, Lensing AWA, Vermeulen M, Tijssen JGP. Heparin treatment for cerebral venous and sinus thrombosis. *Lancet* 1991;**338**:1154.

15. Stam J, de Bruijn SFTM, deVeber G. Anticoagulation for cerebral sinus thrombosis. *Cochrane Database Syst Rev* 2001;Art. No.(4):CD002005.

16. Van Dongen CJJ, van den Belt AGM, Prins MH, Lensing AWA. Fixed dose subcutaneous low molecular weight heparins versus adjusted dose unfractionated heparin for venous thromboembolism. *Cochrane Database Syst Rev* 2004;Art. No.(4):CD001100.

17. Horowitz M, Purdy P, Unwin H, *et al.* Treatment of dural sinus thrombosis using selective catheterisation and urokinase. *Ann Neurol* 1995;**38**:58–67.

18. Kim SY, Suh JH. Direct endovascular thrombolytic therapy for dural sinus thrombosis: infusion of alteplase. *Am J Neuroradiol* 1997;**18**:639–45.

19. Frey IL, Muro GJ, McDougall CG, Dean BL, Jahnke HK. Cerebral venous thrombosis. Combined intrathrombus rtPA and intravenous heparin. *Stroke* 1999;**30**:489–94.

20. Wasay M, Bakshi R, Kojan S, Bobustuc G, Dubey N, Unwin DH. Nonrandomized comparison of local urokinase thrombolysis versus systemic heparin anticoagulation for superior sagittal sinus thrombosis. *Stroke* 2001;**32**:2310–7.

21. Canhão P, Falcão F, Ferro JM. Thrombolytics for cerebral sinus thrombosis. A systematic review. *Cerebrovasc Dis* 2003;**15**:159–66.

22. Stam J, Majoie CBLM, van Delden OM, van Lienden KP, Reekers JA. Endovascular thrombectomy and thrombolysis for severe cerebral sinus thrombosis: a prospective study. *Stroke* 2008;**39**:1487–90.

23. Baumgartner RW, Studer A, Arnold M, Georgiadis D. Recanalisation of cerebral venous thrombosis. *J Neurol Neurosurg Psychiatry* 2003;**74**:459–61.

24. Strupp M, Covi M, Seelos K, Dichgans M, Brandt T. Cerebral venous thrombosis: correlation between recanalization and clinical outcome – a long-term follow-up of 40 patients. *J Neurol* 2002;**249**:1123–4.

25. Kearon C, Kahn SR, Agnelli G, Goldhaber S, Raskob GE, Comerota AJ. Antithrombotic therapy for venous thromboembolic disease. The 8th ACCP conference on antithrombotic and thrombolytic therapy. *Chest* 2008;**133**: 454S–545S.

26. Lijfering WM, Brouwer L-LP, Veeger NJGM, *et al.* Selective testing for thrombophilia in patients with first venous thrombosis: results from a retrospective family cohort study on absolute thrombotic risk for currently known thrombophilic defects in 2479 relatives. *Blood* 2009;**113**: 5314–22.

27. Einhäupl KM, Masuhr F. Cerebral venous and sinus thrombosis – an update. *Eur J Neurol* 1994;**1**:109–26.

28. Ameri A, Bousser MG. Cerebral venous thrombosis. *Neurol Clin* 1992;**10**:87–111.

29. Ferro JM, Correia M, Rosas MJ, Pinto AN, Neves G, for the Cerebral Venous Thrombosis Portuguese Collaborative Study Group. Seizures in cerebral vein and dural sinus thrombosis. *Cerebrovasc Dis* 2003;**15**:78–83.

30. Masuhr F, Busch M, Amberger N, *et al*. Risk and predictors of early epileptic seizures in acute cerebral venous and sinus thrombosis. *Eur J Neurol* 2006;**13**:852–6.

31. Ferro JM, Canhão P, Bousser MG, Stam J, Barinagarrementeria F, for the ISCVT Investigators. Early seizures in cerebral vein and dural sinus thrombosis: risk factors and role of antiepileptics. *Stroke* 2008;**39**:1152–8.

32. Preter M, Tzourio C, Ameri A, Bousser MG. Long-term prognosis in cerebral venous thrombosis – follow-up of 77 patients. *Stroke* 1996;**27**:243–6.

33. Canhão P, Cortesão A, Cabral M, *et al.*, for the ISCVT Investigators. Are steroids useful to treat cerebral venous thrombosis? *Stroke* 2008;**39**:105–10.

34. Canhão P, Ferro JM, Lindgren AG, Bousser MG, Stam J, Barinagarrementeria F, for the ISCVT Investigators. Causes and predictors of death in cerebral venous thrombosis. *Stroke* 2005;**36**:1720–5.

35. Stefini R, Latronico N, Cornali C, Rasulo F, Bollati A. Emergent decompressive craniectomy in patients with fixed dilated pupils due to cerebral venous and dural sinus thrombosis: report of three cases. *Neurosurgery* 1999;**45**:626–9.

36. Coutinho JM, Majoie CBLM, Coert BA, Stam J. Decompressive hemicraniectomy in cerebral sinus thrombosis. Consecutive case series and review of the literature. *Stroke* 2009;**40**:2233–5.

37. Villringer A, Mehraein S, Einhäupl KM. Pathophysiological aspects of cerebral sinus venous thrombosis. *J Neuroradiol* 1994;**21**:72–80.

CHAPTER 35

Cerebral vasculitis

N. J. Scolding,[1] H. Wilson,[2] R. Hohlfeld,[3] C. Polman,[4] M. I. Leite,[5] N. E. Gilhus[6]

[1]Institute of Clinical Neurosciences, University of Bristol, Frenchay Hospital, Bristol, UK; [2]Royal Free Hospital, London, UK; [3]Klinikum Grosshadern, Munich, Germany; [4]VU Medical Center, MB Amsterdam, The Netherlands; [5]John Radcliffe Hospital, University of Oxford, UK; [6]University of Bergen and Department of Neurology, Haukeland University Hospital, Bergen, Norway

Introduction

Cerebral vasculitis is an uncommon disorder that offers unusual problems for the neurologist. It is notoriously difficult to recognize, producing a wide range of possible neurological symptoms and signs with no typical or characteristic features [1–3]. Potential clinical patterns that might facilitate recognition have been proposed [4] but have not been tested prospectively on large numbers of patients, and their value in consequence remains to be substantiated.

Suspicion of the disorder having been entertained, confirmation or exclusion of cerebral vasculitis presents a second serious set of problems. There are no serological or other blood or spinal fluid laboratory tests of any sensitivity or specificity; imaging by computed tomography (CT) or magnetic resonance imaging (MRI) is likewise lacking in sensitivity; angiography is of questionable use [4–10]. Finally, while intuitively this is a disorder most neurologists would regard as eminently treatable, there remains a complete absence of any therapeutic trials to provide an evidence base for this assumption.

This combination of difficulties in recognition and in diagnosis, in a disorder that is serious and indeed not uncommonly fatal, and yet (probably) highly treatable, emphasizes the importance of attempting to address the clinical problem of cerebral vasculitis [11]. It is, however, an uncommon disorder – there are no epidemiological data, but an estimate has been hazarded of an incidence of 1–2 million per year – creating additional difficulties;

even two or three neurological centres collaborating are unlikely to accumulate sufficient numbers of patients within a workable time frame for useful studies.

Methods

The European Federation of Neurological Societies (EFNS) Scientist Panel on Neuroimmunology considered that a European collaborative cohort might offer a powerful means of beginning to address the problems outlined above. A task force on cerebral vasculitis was established to improve the recognition, diagnosis, and management of cerebral vasculitis throughout Europe. This will be achieved by providing guidelines whose confirmation will ultimately depend on the establishment of a sound evidence base. A European-wide survey of current clinical practice was included.

A simple 10-point questionnaire covering various aspects of the diagnosis and management of cerebral vasculitis was sent to 51 expert neurologists in 26 European countries. Replies were received from 29 (57%) experts from 15 countries.

Statements about diagnosis and treatment were discussed among the task force members. Evidence was classified according to the EFNS guidelines [12]. As very few relevant controlled studies exist on the topic, the recommendations given should be regarded as Good Practice Points (GPP) [12], where advice is given on the basis of consensus in our group and available evidence.

Results of survey

The cumulative number of patients given the diagnosis of cerebral vasculitis by the 29 responding expert

European Handbook of Neurological Management: Volume 1, 2nd edition. Edited by N. E. Gilhus, M. P. Barnes and M. Brainin.
© 2011 Blackwell Publishing Ltd.

neurologists is approximately 140 per year, a mean of 4.8 cases per neurologist per year.

Dependence on cerebral angiography varied widely, but 11 of 29 neurologists (38%) based this diagnosis on angiography in more than 75% of cases; a mean of 50% of patients throughout Europe had been diagnosed as having cerebral vasculitis based on angiography. Only three neurologists depended on cerebral biopsy in 80% or more of cases; conversely 12 of 25 neurologists (48%) based diagnosis on biopsy in more than 20% of cases. Most neurologists committed between 0 and five patients to biopsy per year, a mean of 2.3 biopsies per year. Thirteen of 29 neurologists (45%) only recommended biopsy if there was an identifiable lesion. Of the remainder, most used non-dominant frontal or temporal open biopsy, usually ensuring that parenchymal and meningeal tissue were included.

Eighty per cent of the patients with the diagnosis of cerebral vasculitis received steroids (orally or intravenously) alone as 'first-line treatment', and cyclophosphamide only if steroids failed. Most of the remaining neurologists used cyclophosphamide as first-line therapy. Fourteen used cyclophosphamide as second line treatment, others using azathioprine (three), intravenous immunoglobulin (two), methotrexate (one), and other 'potent immunosuppressive' agents (two). Only four respondents treated patients with potent immunosuppressive agents 'only if biopsy-proven', 84% administering such treatment without tissue confirmation of the diagnosis. All acknowledged the difficulties of assessing the therapeutic response – variably relying on clinical imaging, spinal fluid tests, and blood tests, particularly erythrocyte sedimentation rate (ESR) and C-reactive protein levels.

All 29 neurologists were interested in participating in further collaborative European research.

Conclusions and Discussion

Even European neurologists with particular interest in cerebral vasculitis see only a handful of cases per year. Nevertheless, the cumulative experience of some 140 cases per year emphasizes the potential power of the pooled response. A large prospective study would offer a number of valuable opportunities.

First, an analysis of the clinical features may provide means of improving the recognition of cerebral

Table 35.1 Cerebral vasculitis: suggested clinical patterns of presentation that might facilitate recognition [4].

- Acute or sub-acute encephalopathy, with headache with an acute confusional state, progressing to drowsiness and coma.
- Intracranial mass lesion -with headache, drowsiness, focal signs and (often) raised intracranial pressure.
- Superficially resembling atypical multiple sclerosis (MS-plus) in phenotype -with a relapsing-remitting course, and features such as optic neuropathy and brain stem episodes, but also accompanied by other features less common in multiple sclerosis: seizures, severe and persisting headaches, encephalopathic episodes, or stroke-like episodes.

vasculitis. Three clinical patterns have been previously suggested [4]]. First, patients may present with acute, subacute, or recurrent encephalopathy; the second is presentation with features of a focal, space-occupying lesion (a presentation recently re-emphasized and separately analysed [13]). Third, patients may exhibit a clinical picture that in many ways resembles multiple sclerosis – a relapsing, remitting course, often including brainstem episodes and optic neuropathy, and often with multifocal white matter lesions on MRI scanning and oligoclonal bands on cerebrospinal fluid (CSF) analysis (table 35.1), but which usually includes atypical features. However, these patterns were suggested from an analysis of only 10–12 cases, and though reference to retrospective case series suggests the patterns might accommodate virtually all cases of cerebral vasculitis, their true value remains to be proven by large prospective studies. In the past, stroke-like presentation of CNS vasculitis has often been suggested, but a critical analysis suggests this may in fact be extremely uncommon [14]]. Whether these or indeed better patterns might usefully aid recognition of cerebral vasculitis cannot be determined on the basis of small studies on pooled retrospective series with the case-selection biases they carry.

The value of a number of laboratory or imaging investigative procedures similarly requires a prospective study. Specifically, the negative predictive power of tests such as a normal ESR, or normal C-reactive protein [4], or normal spinal fluid analysis [4–6], together with the positive predictive power of these tests – or combinations of various test results with particular clinical and/or imaging features – all these also require prospective studies including relatively large numbers of patients.

There was particular variation in relation to the diagnostic weight given to cerebral angiography. In many instances, there was radiological uncertainty concerning the distinction between 'vasculopathy' and 'vasculitis'. Angiography is a test limited in both sensitivity and specificity in the diagnosis of cerebral vasculitis: retrospective series suggest a sensitivity of only 24–33% [5, 6, 8, 15, 16], with a specificity of a similar order – a number of inflammatory, metabolic, malignant, or other vasculopathies can accurately mimic angiitis. Reversible cerebral vasoconstriction syndrome has in particular received recent attention [17].

There was a corresponding limited reliance on brain biopsy for diagnosis. Sometimes this was explained by local factors, such as difficulties in access to neurosurgical intervention. This test too is, of course, limited in sensitivity, and necessarily entails some iatrogenic risk [18, 19]. However, a retrospective study of some 61 patients biopsied for suspected cerebral vasculitis has usefully illuminated this topic [16]. No patient suffered any significant morbidity as a result of the procedure. Thirty-six per cent of the patients were confirmed as having cerebral vasculitis, but no less usefully and importantly, 39% biopsies showed an alternative, unsuspected diagnosis – lymphoma (six cases), multiple sclerosis (two cases), or infection (seven cases, including toxoplasmosis, herpes, and also two cases of cerebral abscess). Biopsy failed to yield a clear diagnosis in 25% of patients in this study, though even here, biopsy might arguably not be described as 'non-contributory', at least helping exclude some of the alternative diagnoses mentioned above.

This valuable retrospective study also provided some evidence first that biopsy of normal-appearing tissue was no less likely to yield diagnostic information than biopsy targeted upon discrete lesions [16]. The numbers (20 biopsies of normal appearing tissue, 40 of radiologically apparent lesions) were not very large and again a more substantial prospective study would be useful.

What lessons may be learnt, and does this preliminary and rather informal survey yield any provisional recommendations? First, the results confirm the relative uncommonness of the disorder, while emphasizing the potential strength of a collaborative effort, in which, additionally, there emerged considerable enthusiasm. According to current practice, 140 patients are given this diagnosis annually by the 29 responding neurologists, with perhaps 20–40 of these having biopsy confirmation. Expanding the collaborating neurologist pool – and

several regional specialists have, since this survey, expressed interest in joining – would yet further increase the power of any prospective study of both diagnostic approaches and of therapy.

Second, the wide variation in current clinical practice is of interest. The very limited sensitivity and specificity of cerebral angiography has arguably been under-emphasized in the past; some series of cerebral vasculitis patients have indeed rested wholly on this investigation for diagnosis. There has also perhaps been historically an over-emphasis on the value of steroids. While there have been no prospective placebo-controlled trials of immunosuppressive treatment in cerebral vasculitis, large retrospective series of patients with systemic Wegener's granulomatosis, or with microscopic polyangiitis, provide clear support for their use [20–23]. There is some merit in the argument that the absence of tissue confirmation properly directs neurologists away from prescribing cyclophosphamide and towards steroids, but responding neurologists in this survey indicated that it was not this factor that inhibited their use of potent immunosuppressives; only three of 29 neurologists used cyclophosphamide as part of their first-line therapeutic regimen.

Whether cyclophosphamide is best given by intravenous pulses or continuous oral therapy is not established [21, 24], and this question could of course usefully be incorporated into a large prospective study. Most regimes recommend an induction course of between 10 and 16 g cumulative dose; (retrospective) studies of patients with systemic vasculitis and other inflammatory disorders suggest that bladder carcinoma, perhaps the most notorious and serious toxic effect of cyclophosphamide, may be restricted very largely to patients who have received cumulative dose in excess of 100 g [25].

From a practical perspective, we now feel able to propose the diagnostic approach outlined in figure 35.1, and a pragmatic approach to therapy [26, 27]] when a tissue diagnosis of cerebral vasculitis has been confirmed (table 35.2). These represent, in our view, reasonable syntheses emerging from the currently available evidence, but this evidence is not adequate for formal recommendations [11, 12]]. We suggest therefore that a further prospective pan-European study of cerebral vasculitis is needed and could carry sufficient power to confirm or improve this management approach; it is also likely to yield valuable insights into the recognition, diagnosis, and treatment of this difficult, unusual, and often very serious neurological disorder.

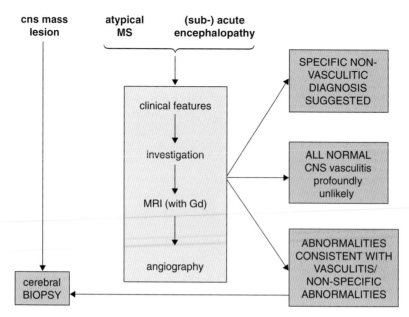

Figure 35.1 A diagnostic approach to suspected cerebral vasculitis

Table 35.2 Cerebral vasculitis: a common treatment regime.

Induction regime (3 months)	Maintenance regime (continued for a further 10 months)
High-dose steroids	Alternate-day steroids 10–20 mg prednisolone
Intravenous methyl prednisolone, 1 g/day for 3 days	
Plus	Plus
Oral* cyclophosphamide 2.0 mg/kg§ (max 200 mg/day)	Azathioprine[a] (2 mg/kg/day) instead of cyclophosphamide
Then	
Oral prednisolone 60 mg/day (after intravenous methyl prednisolone), decreasing at weekly intervals by 10 mg increments to 10 mg/day if possible	

[a]Methotrexate (10–25 mg once weekly) is an alternative to azathioprine.

Conflicts of interest

The authors have reported no conflicts of interest relevant to this manuscript.

References

1. Moore PM, Fauci AS. Neurologic manifestations of systemic vasculitis. A retrospective and prospective study of the clinicopathologic features and responses to therapy in 25 patients. *Am J Med* 1981;**71**:517–24.
2. Moore PM. Central nervous system vasculitis. *Curr Opin Neurol* 1998;**11**:241–6.
3. Scolding NJ. Central nervous system vasculitis. *Semin Immunopathol* 2009 Nov 12. [Epub ahead of print].
4. Scolding NJ, Jayne DR, Zajicek JP, Meyer PAR, Wraight EP, Lockwood CM. The syndrome of cerebral vasculitis: recognition, diagnosis and management. *Q J Med* 1997;**90**:61–73.
5. Calabrese LH, Mallek JA. Primary angiitis of the central nervous system. Report of 8 new cases, review of the literature, and proposal for diagnostic criteria. *Medicine* 1988;**67**:20–39.
6. Hankey G. Isolated angiitis/angiopathy of the CNS. Prospective diagnostic and therapeutic experience. *Cerebrovasc Dis* 1991;**1**:2–15.
7. Greenan TJ, Grossman RI, Goldberg HI. Cerebral vasculitis: MR imaging and angiographic correlation. *Radiology* 1992;**182**:65–72.
8. Vollmer TL, Guarnaccia J, Harrington W, Pacia SV, Petroff OAC. Idiopathic granulomatous angiitis of the central nervous system: diagnostic challenges. *Arch Neurol* 1993;**50**:925–30.

9. Alhalabi M, Moore PM. Serial angiography in isolated angiitis of the central nervous system. *Neurology* 1994;**44**:1221–6.

10. Stone JH, Pomper MG, Roubenoff R, Miller TJ, Hellmann DB. Sensitivities of noninvasive tests for central nervous system vasculitis: a comparison of lumbar puncture, computed tomography, and magnetic resonance imaging. *J Rheumatol* 1994;**21**:1277–82.

11. Joseph FG, Scolding NJ. Cerebral vasculitis – a practical approach. *Pract Neurol* 2002;**2**:80–93.

12. Brainin M, Barnes M, Baron JC, et al. Guidance for the preparation of neurological management guidelines by EFNS scientific task forces – revised recommendations 2004. *Eur J Neurol* 2004;**11**:577–81.

13. Molloy ES, Singhal AB, Calabrese LH. Tumour-like mass lesion: an under-recognised presentation of primary angiitis of the central nervous system. *Ann Rheum Dis* 2008;**67**:1732–5.

14. Scolding N. Vasculitis and stroke. Chapter 44, *Handb Clin Neurol* 2008;**93**:873–86.

15. Koo EH, Massey EW. Granulomatous angiitis of the central nervous system: protean manifestations and response to treatment. *J Neurol Neurosurg Psychiatry* 1988;**51**:1126–33.

16. Alrawi A, Trobe J, Blaivas M, Musch DC. Brain biopsy in primary angiitis of the central nervous system. *Neurology* 1999;**53**:858–60.

17. Santos E, Zhang Y, Wilkins A, Renowden S, Scolding N. Reversible cerebral vasoconstriction syndrome presenting with haemorrhage. *J Neurol Sci* 2009;**276**(1–2):189–92.

18. Barza M, Pauker SG. The decision to biopsy, treat, or wait in suspected herpes encephalitis. *Ann Intern Med* 1980;**92**:641–9.

19. Chu CT, Gray L, Goldstein LB, Hulette CM. Diagnosis of intracranial vasculitis: a multi-disciplinary approach. *J Neuropathol Exp Neurol* 1998;**57**:30–8.

20. Hoffman GS, Kerr GS, Leavitt RY, et al. Wegener granulomatosis: an analysis of 158 patients. *Ann Intern Med* 1992;**116**:488–98.

21. Adu D, Pall A, Luqmani RA, et al. Controlled trial of pulse versus continuous prednisolone and cyclophosphamide in the treatment of systemic vasculitis. *QJM* 1997;**90**:401–9.

22. Scolding NJ. Systemic inflammatory diseases and the nervous system. In: Scolding NJ (ed.) *New Treatments in Neurology*. Oxford: Butterworth Heinemann, 2000; pp. 187–215.

23. Hoffman GS, Leavitt RY, Fleisher TA, Minor JR, Fauci AS. Treatment of Wegener's granulomatosis with intermittent high-dose intravenous cyclophosphamide. *Am J Med* 1990;**89**:403–10.

24. Cupps TR. Cyclophosphamide: to pulse or not to pulse? [editorial; comment]. *Am J Med* 1990;**89**:399–402.

25. Talar WC, Hijazi YM, Walther MM, et al. Cyclophosphamide-induced cystitis and bladder cancer in patients with Wegener granulomatosis. *Ann Intern Med* 1996;**124**:477–84.

26. Savage CO, Harper L, Adu D. Primary systemic vasculitis. *Lancet* 1997;**349**:553–8.

27. Jayne D, Rasmussen N, Andrassy K, et al. A randomized trial of maintenance therapy for vasculitis associated with anti-neutrophil cytoplasmic autoantibodies. *N Engl J Med* 2003;**349**:36–44.

CHAPTER 36

Neurological problems in liver transplantation

M. Guarino,[1] J. Benito-León,[2] J. Decruyenaere,[3] E. Schmutzhard,[4] K. Weissenborn,[5] A. Stracciari[1]

[1]S. Orsola-Malpighi University Hospital, Bologna, Italy; [2]University Hospital 12 de Octubre, Madrid, Spain and Centro de Investigación Biomédica en Red sobre Enfermedades Neurodegenerativas (CIBERNED), Madrid, Spain; [3]Ghent University Hospital, Belgium; [4]Innsbruck Medical University, Austria; [5]Hannover Medical School, Germany

Introduction

Neurological problems are reported in 13–47% of patients after orthotopic liver transplantation (LT) [1, 2], with a significantly lower incidence in living donor liver transplantation versus patients who receive a cadaveric graft [3]. Most neurological complications occur early after surgery and increase morbidity, mortality, and hospital stays [4–6].

In 1999, a Task Force was set up under the auspices of the European Federation of Neurological Societies (EFNS) to devise guidelines to prevent and manage neurological problems in LT [4]. We considered six key topics in clinical practice: immunosuppression neurotoxicity, seizures, central pontine myelinolysis (CPM), neuromuscular disorders, cerebrovascular disorders, and central nervous system (CNS) infections. Attention focused on problems emerging in the first 6 months after surgery.

The present article is an update and revision of the previous guidelines.

Search strategy

Each member of the Task Force was assigned one of the six selected topics and systematically reviewed the relevant literature through the MEDLINE database of the National Library of Medicine from January 2005 to June 2009, the Cochrane Library, existing guidelines (National Clinical Clearinghouse, Scottish Intercollegiate Guidelines Network, National Institute of Clinical Excellence) and textbooks.

Data collection and analysis of evidence was performed independently by each participant according to the above assignment.

On the basis of the single reports, A.S. produced a first draft of the updated guidelines, which was then submitted several times for the approval of all the members until any discrepancies on each topic were solved and a consensus was reached.

Grading of recommendations

The literature is analysed giving the class of evidence (I–IV) according to EFNS guidelines [7].

The recommendation section includes statements classified in levels A–C derived from Classes I–III of evidence according to EFNS guidelines when feasible. For those clinical areas exhibiting Class IV scientific evidence, recommendations were based on the agreement obtained and indicated in the text as Good Practice Points (GPP).

Results

Immunosuppression neurotoxicity

The most widely used immunosuppressants in LT are the calcineurin inhibitors ciclosporin (CS) and

European Handbook of Neurological Management: Volume 1, 2nd edition. Edited by N. E. Gilhus, M. P. Barnes and M. Brainin.
© 2011 Blackwell Publishing Ltd.

tacrolimus (FK506). Mycophenolate mofetil, sirolimus (or rapamycin), and its derivate everolimus have recently been introduced. Corticosteroids, OKT3, and antithymocyte globulin complete the immunosuppressive regimen. Neurotoxicity is mainly associated with CS and FK506, amounting to 10–30% for CS and up to 32% for FK506 [4, 6]. Sirolimus, everolimus, and mycophenolate mofetil lack the neurotoxicity of calcineurin inhibitors [4, 8, 9]. Neurotoxicity often occurs early after surgery, not always related to high drug plasma levels. Manifestations vary and mainly affect the CNS. They are usually distinguished in minor (tremor, headache, insomnia, paraesthesiae) and major (encephalopathy, akinetic mutism, seizures, speech disorders, polyneuropathy, myopathy).

Several predisposing factors have been advocated for the neurotoxicity of calcineurin inhibitors: hypocholesterolaemia, hypomagnesaemia, hypertension, and hepatic encephalopathy [4, 10] (Class III). New oral formulations of CS (Neoral) [11] and delayed starting and low-dosage regimens [12] seem to attenuate the severity of neurotoxicity, whereas it may be exacerbated by concomitant treatments (e.g. metoclopramide) [13, 14] (Classes III and IV). Magnetic resonance imaging (MRI) may disclose non-enhancing high-resolution T2 images mainly involving the posterior white matter. However, CS- and FK506-related pontine abnormalities, similar to CPM, have also been reported, sometimes associated with an insidious speech disorder that may rapidly evolve into mutism and locked-in syndrome [4]. Given its sensitivity in revealing cerebral white matter abnormalities, MRI supports the diagnosis of neurotoxicity [15–17] (Classes II and IV).

To treat neurotoxicity, a reduction of dose and switching from CS to FK506 and vice versa have been suggested [18, 19] (Class IV).

The recent use of novel drug combinations (calcineurin inhibitors plus mycophenolate mofetil or sirolimus) allows lower dosages of CS and FK506 [20] without weakening the immunosuppression efficacy (Class IV). The same occurs with the implementation of so-called CS- and FK506-sparing regimens by switching to mycophenolate mofetil or sirolimus [4, 21] (Class IV).

In most cases, these approaches lead to a resolution of symptoms [22, 23] (Class IV) and a reversal of neuroimaging abnormalities [15, 16, 24, 25] (Class IV). However, some patients with irreversible deficits are occasionally seen [26, 27] (Class IV), especially if the immunosuppressive regimen is not changed promptly.

Minor side effects are usually transient and self-limiting. Headache, tremor, paraesthesiae, and insomnia are successfully managed with symptomatic conventional treatment [1] (Class IV). However, a change in the immunosuppressive regimen has occasionally been necessary in refractory headache [28–30] (Class IV). Recently, a favourable prophylactic effect of riboflavin on post-transplant headache has been reported [31] (Class IV).

OKT3 neurotoxicity usually presents with headache, rarely with transient aseptic meningitis, and exceptionally with a diffuse encephalopathy. The use of lower doses or pre-treatment with steroids, antihistaminic drugs, or indomethacin may decrease the severity of symptoms [32] (Class IV). Acute side effects of corticosteroids include behavioural and mood disorders, while chronic use may lead to myopathy, both reversible with adjustment of therapy [33] (Class IV).

Recommendations

CS and tacrolimus neurotoxicity: prevention requires minimum efficacious doses, oral administration as soon as possible, strict monitoring of plasma levels (including metabolites), electrolyte imbalance (e.g. hypomagnesaemia), hypertension check and correction, and attention to pharmacological interactions (Level C). Brain MRI is the choice diagnostic tool (Level B) and should be performed as soon as severe neurotoxicity is suspected (GPP). In case of major side effects, prompt switching to a non-calcineurin inhibitor (e.g. sirolimus) is indicated (GPP). Secondary options include conversion from CS to tacrolimus and vice versa (GPP). Minor complications require switching only in case of intractable and invalidating symptoms. Generally, their treatment should follow the guidelines for

these disorders, administering drugs lacking both hepatotoxicity and interference with immunosuppressants (e.g. gabapentin for paraesthesiae, riboflavin for migraine prophylaxis) (GPP).

OKT3 neurotoxicity: prevention consists of administering minimal dosages and premedication with corticosteroids (GPP). Aseptic meningitis does not need treatment because it is usually self-limiting. Encephalopathy requires antioedema agents and very rarely OKT3 withdrawal (GPP).

Corticosteroid neurotoxicity: severe acute behavioural disorders may be treated by a temporary reduction and/or withdrawal of intravenous steroid administration. Brief regimens of low-dose neuroleptics may be considered (GPP).

Seizures

Seizures occur in 0–40% of LT recipients [4, 6, 34], with a tendency to lower numbers in the more recent reports. Most are generalized tonic-clonic seizures. Convulsive or non-convulsive status epilepticus is rare. Seizures occur most often early after surgery, due to drugs, acute metabolic derangement, hypoxic–ischaemic injury, cerebral lesions, sudden withdrawal of narcotic agents, or inadvertent discontinuation or changes in anticonvulsant drugs in patients with epilepsy. Immunosuppressant toxicity is the main aetiology [4].

Preventive measures mainly focus on the control of metabolic parameters and correct drug management. The diagnostic approach includes a wide spectrum of tests to cover all possible causes [35, 36] (Class IV). Cerebral MRI is the investigation of choice to search for seizure aetiology in the general population [37] (Class II) and also seems applicable in LT patients, as MRI can detect immunosuppressant-related brain damage, CNS infection, metabolic lesions, stroke, or CNS tumours.

No randomized controlled trials are available on the use of antiepileptic drugs in liver-transplanted patients. Treatment can be problematic because of both the interference between most antiepileptics and immunosuppressants, and the frequent need for intravenous therapy. Switching between tacrolimus and CS has been described to be effective for seizure control in immunosuppressant-induced cases [38] (Class IV). Among intravenous anticonvulsants, phenytoin was preferred in the past [35] (Class IV).

Considering the pharmacokinetic properties of levetiracetam (no protein-binding, no dependence upon liver cytochrome P450, renal excretion, no known active metabolites, no drug–drug interactions) and initial clinical experiences [39], this new antiepileptic drug can be recommended as a first-line therapy for seizure control in LT patients, although data from controlled studies are lacking (Class IV). Among oral antiepileptics, gabapentin, pregabalin and levetiracetam [36, 40, 41] are of interest for both their efficacy and lack of hepatic induction (Class IV). However, doses should be reduced in patients with concomitant renal dysfunction, while in patients on dialysis supplemental doses must be given after dialysis.

Some antiepileptic drugs can produce clinically relevant interactions with the immunosuppressants used after LT. Carbamazepine, oxcarbazepine, phenobarbital and phenytoin may reduce CS, tacrolimus and corticosteroid blood levels, with a delayed effect of up to 10 days. Prognostic studies report a favourable outcome for both survival and absence of seizure recurrence after a short period of therapy (1–3 months) if seizures are induced by metabolic derangements or calcineurin inhibitors [34, 35, 41] (Classes III and IV). Seizures due to cerebrovascular events, sepsis or organ rejection have a poor prognosis [34].

Recommendations

Seizure prevention requires close monitoring of metabolic parameters and immunosuppressant levels, and caution in managing discontinuation or adjustment of epileptogenic drugs (GPP). The diagnostic approach should routinely include laboratory tests, EEG, and neuroimaging. Cerebrospinal fluid (CSF) examination is indicated when CNS infection is suspected (GPP). Brain MRI is the current standard of reference (Level B). When MRI is not available or is contraindicated, computed tomography (CT) can be applied (Level C).

The first-line intravenous antiepileptic drug is levetiracetam at a dose of 500 mg twice daily (up to 1000 mg twice daily) (Class IV). Alternatively, phenytoin could be used dosed to target a level between 10 and 20 μg/ml (GPP). When oral administration is possible, gabapentin, pregabalin, or levetiracetam should be considered (GPP). Status epilepticus management must be managed according to guidelines for the general population (GPP). In most cases, antiepileptic therapy can be suspended after 3 months (Level C).

Central pontine myelinolysis (CPM)

CPM is usually seen in alcoholic and malnourished patients, attributed to a rapid correction of hyponatraemia. CPM has been reported in 1–8% of LT recipients [4]. The high incidence in LT is likely to be favoured by the usual hyponatraemic state of patients with cirrhosis and by the large replacement of fluids during the operation, leading to a sharp increase in plasma levels of sodium. CPM occurs early after surgery. The clinical picture can vary considerably from paucisymptomatic pictures to misleading presentations or severe signs characterized by dysarthria, paraparesis, or quadriparesis [4]. A high mortality rate has been reported [42, 43].

Hyponatraemia and an abrupt rise in serum sodium (>18 mM/l per 24–48 h) are significantly related to CPM in LT recipients [42, 43] (Class IV). Other risk factors may be the plasma osmolality increase after surgery, the duration of the operation, and high CS levels [43] (Class IV).

There is no definite therapy for CPM. Sporadic suggestions include the use of steroids or plasmapheresis [44] alone or in combination with intravenous immunoglobulins [45] (Class IV). Re-inducing hyponatraemia in the very early phase of CPM has also been proposed [46] (Class IV). Prevention is based on a slow correction of perioperative hyponatraemia [42, 43], not exceeding 8 mM/l per day [47]. Transplantation at an early stage of the liver disease has also been suggested [43] (Class IV). MRI is currently the best investigation [48] (Class IV).

The large-scale introduction of MRI has increasingly facilitated the ante mortem diagnosis of CPM, although the radiological findings lag behind and do not necessarily correlate with the clinical picture. Serial MRI could be needed because the appearance of the lesion may be delayed [49] (Class IV). Magnetic resonance spectroscopy and perfusion of CPM have rarely been described. In an earlier phase, pontine lesions may show high-signal intensity on diffusion-weighted imaging (DWI) with decreased apparent diffusion coefficient value, decreased N-acetylaspartate (NAA)/creatine (Cr) ratio, increased choline (Cho)/Cr ratio, and increased perfusion on the cerebral blood volume map. In a chronic phase, the lesion may show isosignal intensity on DWI, a further decreased NAA/Cr ratio, an increased Cho/Cr ratio, and decreased perfusion [50] (Class IV).

Recommendations

Given enough time before LT, hyponatraemia should be corrected slowly. The variations in serum sodium concentration must be carefully monitored and controlled before and during surgery to avoid major fluctuations (GPP). If the patient is hyponatraemic when undergoing LT, a perioperative hourly correction rate at or below 0.5 mM/l per hour should be maintained. The correction rate should not exceed 8 mM/l per day (GPP). MRI should be performed early and repeated if negative (GPP).

Neuromuscular disorders

Neuromuscular disorders present with focal or generalized weakness [4]. *Focal weakness* includes mononeuropathies, with an incidence of 2–13%, and brachial plexopathy (1–5.8%). Axonal involvement is common. Invasive procedures, perioperative positioning and rarely

compressive masses (e.g. haematoma) are the main causes. *Generalized weakness* occurs in 1.5–10% of patients and consists of axonal or demyelinating polyneuropathy and necrotizing myopathy, mainly related to immunosuppression neurotoxicity and critical illness. Guillain–Barré syndrome and chronic inflammatory demyelinating polyneuropathy are also reported [4].

No systematic studies have analysed the risk factors for neuromuscular complications in LT. Diabetes and alcoholism do not seem to increase the risk of perioperative mononeuritis [51] (Class III). High doses of corticosteroids and the use of non-depolarizing neuromuscular blocking agents are reported to favour quadriplegia after LT [51, 52] (Class III). Diagnosis is mainly based on conventional electrophysiological study, muscular enzyme assessment and CSF examination. Nerve or muscle biopsy should also be considered. The prognosis is usually good [52–54] (Class IV), but some patients need mechanical supports to walk.

The prevention of perioperative neuropathy is focused on careful perioperative nursing [55] (Class IV). Minimizing the use of corticosteroids and neuromuscular blocking agents in a critical illness setting has proved to be of help in preventing neuromuscular disorders [56] (Class IV). Treatment includes a change of immunosuppression when neurotoxicity is the cause [57, 58] (Class IV), and conventional therapy in case of Guillain–Barré syndrome [59] or chronic inflammatory demyelinating polyneuropathy [60] (Class II). No specific treatment exists for critical illness neuromuscular disorders. In monocentre studies, intensive insulin therapy with the aim of strict glycaemic control showed a significant reduction in morbidity, mortality, and critical illness neuropathy [61]. However, further trials, including a recent large multicentre randomized study in 6104 patients, could not confirm these results, and therefore strict glycaemia control with target levels between 81 and 108 mg/dl are no longer recommended [62].

Recommendations

Perioperative mononeuropathies: prevention implies caution during catheterization, and avoiding blinded cannulations and external compressions by blood pressure cuffs or tourniquets (GPP).

To reduce perioperative malpositioning, it is indicated to maintain the arms at less than 90° of abduction, to maintain the arms at less than 30° of extension when combined with abduction, padding the exposed nerves (i.e. at the level of fibular head, popliteal space, calcaneus, under the forearms, under the hands) with frequent repositioning during prolonged surgery. Patients should be instructed to avoid postures potentially compressing or stretching the nerves (GPP).

Generalized weakness: prevention requires avoiding when possible the prolonged use of non-depolarizing neuromuscular blocking agents, and minimizing the use of high-dose intravenous corticosteroids (Level C). In case of calcineurin inhibitor toxicity, prompt switching to a different agent (e.g. sirolimus) is recommended (GPP). Customary general treatment for critical illness and conventional management of Guillain–Barré syndrome and chronic inflammatory demyelinating polyneuropathy are indicated (Level B).

Recommendations

Prevention includes correction of coagulopathies before surgery (e.g. administration of platelets and blood products, but with caution due to the risk of consumptive coagulopathy), avoiding perioperative cerebral hypoperfusion, and control of cerebrovascular risk factors after LT (especially hypertension) (GPP). According to general guidelines, CT scanning is the preferred diagnostic test in the early phases of acute cerebrovascular disorders, especially to detect haemorrhage (Level C). Despite its greater sensitivity, MRI is often not tolerated or is not applicable immediately after LT, but should be considered to characterize vascular lesions or to rule out other aetiologies (GPP).

A search for bacteriaemia or fungaemia to detect infection should be routinely applied (GPP). The general treatment of cerebrovascular disorders in LT should not differ from that applied in the general population (GPP). Concomitant antifungal treatment should be given in the presence of angiopathy related to CNS infections (Level C).

Cerebrovascular disorders

Acute cerebrovascular disorders occur in 2–6.5% of LT recipients, mostly with cerebral haemorrhage, usually within 2 months after surgery [4, 63, 64]. Focal deficits may be obscured by diffuse encephalopathy. Several risk factors are recognized, those directly associated with hepatic failure such as coagulation disturbances, and those secondary to immunosuppressive therapy such as hypercholesterolaemia, diabetes, and hypertension [65–68]. Perioperative events, such as cerebral hypoperfusion and massive transfusion, may also favour cerebrovascular injury. Causes of cerebral bleeding include *Aspergillus* angiopathy and mycotic aneurysms. Older age and systemic infection may be possible risk factors of in-hospital intracranial haemorrhage [64].

Adjustment of cerebrovascular risk factors before, during, and after LT is the main preventive measure [65, 67] (Class IV).

Diagnosis and treatment are similar to those adopted in the general population. Attention is paid to the search for infection as a cause of acute cerebrovascular disorders, in order to institute prompt systemic antibiotic/antifungal therapy once infection occurs, especially in elderly patients [64, 65] (Class III–IV). Effective measures should be taken to prevent post-transplant infection, such as improvement of patient's systemic condition, bacteriological surveillance, and infection control measures.

CNS infections

CNS infections in LT recipients are favoured by immunosuppression, the incidence being estimated to reach 5% [69, 70], with a high mortality [49, 71]. It seems reasonable to differentiate CNS infections after LT into those clinically relevant within 1 month after organ transplantation and those infections with the highest risk of occurring 1–6 months after LT.

Infections leading to CNS disease within 1 month are usually caused by the fact that the pathogenic agent was already present before transplantation, was acquired through the transplanted organ, occurred as a complication of surgery, or represents an intensive care complication (e.g. invasive catheter-associated infection, etc.) [71, 72]. Beside staphylococci, LT recipients have an immediate post-surgery risk of infection with enteric organisms, i.e. Gram-negative bacteria, enterococci or *Candida*.

The highest risk of developing a post-transplant CNS infection is seen 1–6 months after LT. In this period of time, parasites, fungi, and viruses of the family of herpesviridae (herpes simplex virus type 1 and type 2, human herpes virus 6, cytomegalovirus, varicella zoster virus) act as opportunistic pathogenic agents [72, 73]. Opportunistic infections presenting beyond 6 months after LT are frequently seen in patients with a chronic rejection reaction, namely in those patients needing high-dose immunosuppression, particularly if they need additional immunosuppressive therapeutics.

Beside infections with members of the herpesviridae family (cytomegalovirus, Epstein–Barr virus), hepatitis B or C virus infections may already be seen affecting the central and peripheral nervous systems. In addition, such patients may develop the Epstein–Barr virus-associated B-cell lymphoproliferative disease [72]. Clinical patterns include meningitis, encephalitis, abscesses, a combination of all three, or even septic embolism.

Neuroimaging, spinal tap after excluding increased intracranial pressure, and a search for signs of systemic infection are the core of diagnosis. Brain biopsy can be performed in individual cases [69, 74] (Class IV). CSF polymerase chain reaction is crucial in detecting

viral infections [75] (Class I). Prevention focuses on eradicating infection in donor, recipient, or both, and optimizing intensive care management, mainly avoiding nosocomial contamination, during both surgery and post-surgery intensive care management [69, 72, 76, 77] (Class III). No prospective data are available suggesting the need for specific prophylactic antimicrobial strategies for CNS infection in transplanted patients. Treatment is based on guidelines for immunocompromised patients [71, 72, 75, 78–82] and LT centres' experience [69, 72, 83] (Class III). Antimicrobial agents can interfere with drugs used in liver-transplanted patients (e.g. voriconazole with tacrolimus and sirolimus, phenytoin and carbamazepine; amphotericin B with CS) [84].

Recommendations

An early in-depth diagnostic approach is advocated, including brain CT/MRI, lumbar puncture and possibly brain biopsy, and the search for extracerebral sources of infection (GPP). CSF polymerase chain reaction is essential for viral infections (Level A). Prompt administration of therapy on suspicion of the diagnosis without definitive proof is needed to control infection (GPP). An exhaustive search for latent infection in donor and recipient is required, including close monitoring for intestinal strongyloidiasis in patients who have lived for long periods in tropical or subtropical countries (Level C). Exposure to hospital contamination must be avoided (Level C). Specific drug protocols to prevent brain infections are not required (GPP).

Treatment of neurolisteriosis consists of prolonged administration of ampicillin intravenously; the second choice includes trimethoprim-sulfamethoxazole (Level C). For brain nocardiosis, prolonged administration of trimethoprim-sulfamethoxazole is suggested (Level C).

For brain aspergillosis, the first choice drug is voriconazole: initially, 6 mg/kg intravenously every 12 h in two doses, then 4 mg/kg intravenously every 12 h, switching to oral dosing (the same dosage) as tolerated and clinically justified; the

maintenance regimen consists of 200–300 mg orally every 12 h. The duration of intravenous therapy should be between 6 and 27 days, followed by oral administration for 4–24 weeks (Level A). In cases of intolerance, contraindications, or therapy failure, use liposomal amphotericin B (1–5 mg/kg per day) or caspofungin 50 mg/day (with a loading dose of 70 mg on day 1) or itraconazole (except after voriconazole) (Level B). Surgical resection may be considered. Rhinocerebral mucormycosis needs maximally dosed liposomal amphotericin B (5–10 mg/kg per day).

First-line treatment for cryptococcal meningitis is a combination of (liposomal) amphotericin B plus 5-flucytosine. Schedule treatment includes: induction with amphotericin B (0.7 mg/kg per day) and flucytosine (150 mg/kg per day) for 2 weeks, followed by consolidation with fluconazole for 8–10 weeks (400–800 mg/day), followed by 6–12 months at lower doses of fluconazole (200 mg/day) (Level A). Treatment for herpesvirus-6 and cytomegalovirus encephalitis is ganciclovir and foscarnet, either alone or in combination (Level C). For progressive multifocal leukoencephalopathy, cidofovir is an option (GPP).

Conflicts of interest

We declare that we have no conflict of interest in connection with this paper.

References

1. Stracciari A, Guarino M. Neuropsychiatric complications of liver transplantation. *Metab Brain Dis* 2001;**16**:3–11.
2. Saner FH, Nadalin S, Radtke A, *et al.* Liver transplantation and neurological side effects. *Metab Brain Dis* 2009;**24**:183–7.
3. Saner FH, Gu Y, Minouchehr S, *et al.* Neurological complications after cadaveric and living donor liver transplantation. *J Neurol* 2006;**253**:612–17.
4. Guarino M, Benito-Leon J, Decruyenaere J, Schmutzhard E, Weissenborn K, Stracciari A. EFNS guidelines on management of neurological problems in liver transplantation. *Eur J Neurol* 2006;**13**:2–9.
5. Kim BS, Kim BS, Lee SG, *et al.* Neurologic complications in adult living donor liver transplant recipients. *Clin Transplant* 2007;**21**:544–7.

6. Saner FH, Sotiropoulos GC, Gu Y, *et al.* Severe neurological events following liver transplantation. *Arch Med Res* 2007;**38**:75–9.

7. Brainin M, Barnes M, Baron J-C, *et al.* Guidance for the preparation of neurological management guidelines by EFNS scientific task forces – revised recommendations. *Eur J Neurol* 2004;**11**:577–81.

8. Jiménez-Pérez M, Lozano Rey JM, Marin Garcia D, *et al.* Efficacy and safety of monotherapy with mycophenolate mofetil in liver transplantation. *Transplant Proc* 2006;**38**:2480–1.

9. Di Benedetto F, Di Sandro S, De Ruvo N, *et al.* Sirolimus monotherapy in liver transplantation. *Transplant Proc* 2007;**39**:1930.

10. Dhar R, Young GB, Marotta P. Perioperative neurological complications after liver transplantation are best predicted by pre-transplant hepatic encephalopathy. *Neurocrit Care* 2008;**8**:253–8.

11. Wijdicks EFM, Dahlke LJ, Wiesner RH. Oral cyclosporine decreases severity of neurotoxicity in liver transplant recipients. *Neurology* 1999;**52**:1708–10.

12. Gomez R, Moreno E, Loinaz C, *et al.* Liver transplantation with a twenty-four delay and an initial low dose of cyclosporine. *Hepato-Gastroenterology* 1996;**43**:435–9.

13. Trzepacz PT, Gupta B, Di Martini A. Pharmacologic issues in organ transplantation: psychopharmacology and neuropsychiatric medication side effects. In: Trzepacz PT, Di Martini A (eds) *The Transplant Patient.* Cambridge, UK: Cambridge University Press, 2000; pp. 187–213.

14. Prescott WA Jr, Callahan BL, Park JM. Tacrolimus toxicity associated with concomitant metoclopramide therapy. *Pharmacotherapy* 2004;**24**:532–7.

15. Appignani BA, Bhadella RA, Blacklow SC, Wang AK, Roland SF, Freeman RB. Neuroimaging findings in patients on immunosuppressive therapy: experience with tacrolimus toxicity. *Am J Roentgenol* 1996;**166**:683–8.

16. Bianco F, Fattaposta F, Locuratolo N, *et al.* Reversible diffusion MRI abnormalities and transient mutism after liver transplantation. *Neurology* 2004;**62**:981–3.

17. Zivkovic S. Neuroimaging and neurologic complications after organ transplantation. *J Neuroimaging* 2007;**17**:210–23.

18. Pratschke J, Neuhaus R, Tullius SG, *et al.* Treatment of cyclosporine-related adverse effects by conversion to tacrolimus after liver transplantation. *Transplantation* 1997;**64**:938–40.

19. Abouljoud MS, Kumar MS, Brayman KL, Emre S, Bynon JS; OLN Study Group. Neoral rescue therapy in transplant patients with intolerance to tacrolimus. *Clin Transplant* 2002;**16**:168–72.

20. McAlister VC, Peltekian KM, Malatjalian DA, *et al.* Orthotopic liver transplantation using low-dose tacrolimus and sirolimus. *Liver Transpl* 2001;**7**:701–8.

21. Yu S, He X, Yang L, *et al.* A retrospective study of conversion from tacrolimus-based to sirolimus-based immunosuppression in orthotopic liver transplant recipients. *Exp Clin Transplant* 2008;**6**:113–17.

22. Forgacs B, Merhav HJ, Lappin J, Mieles L. Successful conversion to rapamycin for calcineurin inhibitor-related neurotoxicity following liver transplantation. *Transplant Proc* 2005;**37**:1912–14.

23. Al Masri O, Fathallah W, Quader S. Recovery of tacrolimus-associated brachial neuritis after conversion to everolimus in a pediatric renal transplant recipient – case report and review of the literature. *Pediatr Transplant* 2008;**12**:914–17.

24. Ravaioli M, Guarino M, Stracciari A, *et al.* Speech disorder related to tacrolimus-induced pontine myelinolysis after orthotopic liver transplantation. *Transpl Int* 2003;**16**:605–7.

25. Bartynski WS, Tan HP, Boardman JF, Shapiro R, Marsh JW. Posterior reversible encephalopathy syndrome after solid organ transplantation. *Am J Neuroradiol* 2008;**29**:924–30.

26. Casanova B, Prieto M, Deya E, *et al.* Persistent cortical blindness after cyclosporine leukoencephalopathy. *Liver Transpl Surg* 1997;**3**:638–40.

27. De Weerdt A, Claeys KG, De Jonghe P, *et al.* Tacrolimus-related polyneuropathy: case report and review of the literature. *Clin Neurol Neurosurg* 2008;**110**:291–4.

28. Rozen TD, Wijdicks EFM, Hay JH. Treatment-refractory cyclosporine-associated headache. Relief with conversion to FK-506. *Neurology* 1996;**47**:1347.

29. Kiemeneij IM, de Leeuw FE, Ramos LM, van Gijn J. Acute headache as a presenting symptom of tacrolimus encephalopathy. *J Neurol Neurosurg Psychiatry* 2003;**74**:1126–7.

30. Toth CC, Burak K, Becker W. Recurrence of migraine with aura due to tacrolimus therapy in a liver transplant recipient successfully treated with sirolimus substitution. *Headache* 2005;**45**:245–54.

31. Stracciari A, D'Alessandro R, Baldin E, Guarino M. Post-transplant headache: benefit from riboflavin. *Eur Neurol* 2006;**56**:201–3.

32. Rossi SJ, Schroeder TJ, Hariharan S, First MR. Prevention and management of the adverse effects associated with immunosuppressive therapy. *Drug Saf* 1993;**9**:104–31.

33. Rosener M, Martin E, Zipp F, Dichgans J, Martin R. Neurological side-effects of pharmacologic corticoid therapy. *Nervenarzt* 1996;**67**:983–6.

34. Choi EJ, Kang JK, Lee SA, Kim KH, Lee SG, Andermann F. New-onset seizures after liver transplantation: clinical

implications and prognosis in survivors. *Eur Neurol* 2004;**52**:230–6.

35. Wijdicks EFM, Plevak DJ, Wiesner RH, Steers JL. Causes and outcome of seizures in liver transplant recipients. *Neurology* 1996;**47**:1523–5.

36. Wszolek ZK, Steg RE. Seizures after orthotopic liver transplantation. *Seizure* 1997;**6**:31–9.

37. Scottish Intercollegiate Guidelines Network – SIGN. *Diagnosis and management of epilepsy in adults*, 2004.

38. Sevmis S, Karakayali H, Emiroglu R, Akkoc H, Haberal M. Tacrolimus-related seizure in the early postoperative period after liver transplantation. *Transplant Proc* 2007;**39**:1211–13.

39. Glass GA, Stankiewicz J, Mithoefer A, Freeman R, Bergethon PR. Levetiracetam for seizures after liver transplantation. *Neurology* 2005;**64**:1084–5.

40. Chabolla DR, Harnois DM, Meschia JF. Levetiracetam monotherapy for liver transplant patients with seizures. *Transplant Proc* 2003;**35**:1480–1.

41. Chabolla DR, Wszolek ZK. Pharmacologic management of seizures in organ transplant. *Neurology* 2006;**67**:S34–8.

42. Abbasoglu O, Goldstein RM, Vodapally MS, *et al.* Liver transplantation in hyponatremic patients with emphasis on central pontine myelinolysis. *Clin Transplant* 1998;**12**:263–9.

43. Yu J, Zheng SS, Liang TB, Shen Y, Wang WL, Ke QH. Possible causes of central pontine myelinolysis after liver transplantation. *World J Gastroenterol* 2004;**10**:2540–3.

44. Bibl D, Lampl C, Gabriel C, *et al.* Treatment of central pontine myelinolysis with therapeutic plasmapheresis. *Lancet* 1999;**353**:1155.

45. Saner FH, Koeppen S, Meyer M, *et al.* Treatment of central pontine myelinolysis with plasmapheresis and immunoglobulins in liver transplant patient. *Transpl Int* 2008;**21**:390–1.

46. Oya S, Tsutsumi K, Ueki K, Kirino T. Reinduction of hyponatremia to treat central pontine myelinolysis. *Neurology* 2001;**57**:1931–2.

47. Martin RJ. Central pontine and extrapontine myelinolysis: the osmotic demyelination syndromes. *J Neurol Neurosurg Psychiatry* 2004;**75**(Suppl. 3):22–8.

48. Ruzek KA, Campeau NG, Miller GA. Early diagnosis of central pontine myelinolysis with diffusion-weighted imaging. *Am J Neuroradiol* 2004;**25**:210–13.

49. Bronster DJ, Emre S, Boccagni P, Sheiner PA, Schwartz ME, Miller CM. Central nervous system complications in liver transplant recipients – incidence, timing, and long-term follow-up. *Clin Transplant* 2000;**14**:1–7.

50. Guo Y, Hu JH, Lin W, Zheng KH. Central pontine myelinolysis after liver transplantation: MR diffusion, spectroscopy and perfusion findings. *Magn Reson Imaging* 2006;**24**:1395–8.

51. Campellone JV, Lacomis D. Neuromuscular disorders. In: Wijdicks EFM (ed.) *Neurologic Complications in Organ Transplant Recipients*. Oxford, UK: Butterworth-Heinemann, 1999; pp. 169–92.

52. Mirò O, Salmeron JM, Masanes F, *et al.* Acute quadriplegic myopathy with myosin-deficient muscle fibres after liver transplantation. *Transplantation* 1999;**67**:1144–51.

53. Wijdicks EFM, Litchy WJ, Wiesner RH, Krom RA. Neuromuscular complications associated with liver transplantation. *Muscle Nerve* 1996;**19**:696–700.

54. Rezaiguia-Delclaux S, Lefaucher JP, Zakkouri M, Duvoux C, Duvaldestin P, Stephan F. Severe acute polyneuropathy complicating orthotopic liver allograft failure. *Transplantation* 2002;**74**:880–2.

55. Warner MA. Perioperative neuropathies. *Mayo Clin Proc* 1998;**73**:567–74.

56. Motomura M. Critical illness polyneuropathy and myopathy. *Rinsho Shinkeigaku* 2003;**43**:802–4.

57. Ayres RCS, Dousset B, Wixon S, Buckels JAC, McMaster P, Mayer AD. Peripheral neuropathy with tacrolimus. *Lancet* 1994;**343**:862–3.

58. Bronster DJ, Yonover P, Stein J, Scelsa SN, Miller CM, Sheiner PA. Demyelinating sensorimotor polyneuropathy after administration of FK506. *Transplantation* 1995;**59**:1066–8.

59. El-Sabrout RA, Radovancevic B, Ankoma-Sey V, Van Buren C. Guillain-Barré syndrome after solid organ transplantation. *Transplantation* 2001;**71**:1311–16.

60. Taylor BV, Wijdicks EFM, Poterucha JJ, Weisner RH. Chronic inflammatory demyelinating polyneuropathy complicating liver transplantation. *Ann Neurol* 1995;**38**:828–31.

61. Van den Berghe G, Wouters P, Weekers F, *et al.* Intensive insulin treatment reduced mortality and morbidity in critically ill patients. *N Engl J Med* 2001;**345**:1359–67.

62. The NICE-SUGAR investigators. Intensive versus Conventional Glucose Control in Critically Ill Patients. *N Engl J Med* 2009;**360**:1283–97.

63. Borg MAJP, van der Wouden E-J, Sluiter WJ, *et al.* Vascular events after liver transplantation: a long-term follow-up study. *Transpl Int* 2007;**21**:74–80.

64. Ling L, He X, Zeng J, Liang Z. In-hospital cerebrovascular complications following orthotopic liver transplantation: a retrospective study. *BMC Neurol* 2008;**8**:52.

65. Adair JC. Cerebrovascular disorders. In: Wijdicks EFM (ed.) *Neurologic Complications in Organ Transplant Recipients*. Oxford, UK: Butterworth-Heinemann, 1999; pp. 193–216.

66. Singh N, Yu VL, Gayowski T. Central nervous system lesions in adult liver transplant recipients: clinical review with implications for management. *Medicine* 1994;**73**:110–18.

67. Wang WL, Yang ZF, Lo CM, Liu CL, Fan ST. Intracerebral hemorrhage after liver transplantation. *Liver Transpl* 2000;**6**:345–8.

68. Laryea M, Watt KD, Molinari M. Metabolic syndrome in liver transplant recipients: prevalence and association with major vascular events. *Liver Transpl* 2007;**13**:1109–14.

69. Tolkoff-Rubin NE, Hovingh KG, Rubin RH. Central nervous system infections. In: Wijdicks EFM (ed.) *Neurologic Complications in Organ Transplant Recipients.* Boston: Butterworth Heinemann, 1999; pp. 141–68.

70. Singh N, Husain S. Infections of the central nervous system in transplant recipients. *Transpl Infect Dis* 2000;**2**:101–11.

71. Roos KL. Infection in solid organ and bone marrow transplant recipients. In: Noseworth JH (ed.) *Neurological Therapeutics – Principles and Practice*, 2nd edn. Abingdon, Oxon: Informa Health Care, 2006; pp. 1185–95.

72. Schmutzhard E, Pfausler B. Infektionen des ZNS beim immunkompetenten Patienten. *Nervenarzt* 2008;**79**:93–112.

73. Noguchi T, Mihara F, Yoshiura T, *et al.* MR imaging of human herpesvirus-6 encephalopathy after hematopoietic stem cell transplantation in adults. *Am J Neuroradiol* 2006;**27**:2191–5.

74. Bonham CA, Dominguez EA, Fukui MB, *et al.* Central nervous system lesions in liver transplant recipients: prospective assessment of indications for biopsy and implications for management. *Transplantation* 1998;**66**:1596–604.

75. Portegies P, Solod L, Cinque P, *et al.* Guidelines for the diagnosis and management of neurological complications of HIV infection. *Eur J Neurol* 2004;**11**:297–304.

76. Stone WJ, Schaffner W. Strongyloides infections in transplant recipients. *Semin Respir Infect* 1990;**5**:58–64.

77. Soave R. Prophylaxis strategies for solid organ transplantation. *Clin Infect Dis* 2001;**33**(Suppl. 1):26–31.

78. Saag MS, Graybill RJ, Larsen RA, *et al.* Practice guidelines for the management of cryptococcal disease. *Clin Infect Dis* 2000;**30**:710–8.

79. Ascioglu S, Rex JH, de Pauw B, *et al.* Defining opportunistic invasive fungal infections in immunocompromised patients with cancer and hematopoietic stem cell transplants: an international consensus. *Clin Infect Dis* 2002;**34**:7–14.

80. Bohme A, Ruhnke M, Buchheidt DT, *et al.* Treatment of fungal infections in hematology and oncology – guidelines of the Infectious Diseases Working Party (AGIHO) of the German Society of Hematology and Oncology (DGHO). *Ann Hematol* 2003;**82**(Suppl. 2):S133–40.

81. Dewhurst S. Human herpesvirus type 6 and human herpesvirus type 7 infections of the central nervous system. *Herpes* 2004;**11**(Suppl. 2):105A–11A.

82. Ruhnke M, Kofla G, Otto K, *et al.* CNS aspergillosis, recognition, diagnosis and management. *CNS Drugs* 2007;**21**:659–67.

83. Wu G, Vilchez RA, Eidelman B, *et al.* Cryptococcal meningitis: an analysis among 5521 consecutive organ transplant recipients. *Transpl Infect Dis* 2002;**4**:183–8.

84. Venkataramanan R, Zang S, Gayowski T, Singh N. Voriconazole inhibition of the metabolism of tacrolimus in a liver transplant recipient and in human liver microsomes. *Antimicrob Agents Chemother* 2002;**46**:3091–3.

CHAPTER 37

Fatty acid mitochondrial disorders

*C. Angelini,[1] A. Federico,[2] H. Reichmann,[3] A. Lombes,[4] C. Verney Saban,[5]
P. Chinnery,[6] J. Vissing[7]*

[1]University of Padova, Padova, Italy; [2]University of Siena, Siena, Italy; [3]University Clinic Carl Gustav Carus, Dresden, Germany;
[4]Institute of Myology, Paris, France; [5]Hôpital de Lyon, France; [6]Newcastle University Medical School, Newcastle-upon-Tyne, UK;
[7]University of Copenhagen, Copenhagen, Denmark

Introduction

Lipid storage myopathies (LSMs) represent various disease entities whose biochemical defects are heterogeneous [1]; these disorders might be due either to defects of the carnitine membrane carrier or to enzymatic defects in beta-oxidation of long-chain fatty acid (LCFA). L-carnitine, carnitine palmitoyltransferase I (CPT I), carnitine acyltransferase, and CPT II provide a mechanism whereby long-chain fatty acyl-CoA molecules are transferred from the cytosol across the outer and inner mitochondrial membrane to the mitochondrial matrix, where they undergo beta-oxidation [2]. A series of enzymes bound to the mitochondrial inner membrane or dissolved in the matrix transform fatty acyl-CoA into acetyl-CoA (figure 37.1). A mitochondrial trifunctional protein associated to the inner mitochondrial membrane has been identified that performs three different enzymatic activities during LCFA oxidation. The description of the disorders has been organized according to the pathway of LCFA transfer and oxidation.

Search strategy

The task force for metabolic disorders systematically searched the MEDLINE database using key words, and examined textbooks and existing guidelines. According to the guidance for the preparation of neurological management by European Federation of Neurological Societies task force [3], articles were included if they contained data that could be rated according to grades of recommendation for treatment classified in terms of evidence-based medicine. Most guideline recommendations in this document are derived from case reports (Class IV evidence), as no large trials have been conducted in fatty acid disorders. These guidelines reflect consensus in the opinions of experts in the field (Good Practice Points). The consensus was reached by analysing series of treated patients and discussing pre-existing guidelines.

Results

CPT II deficiency

In the most typical presentations, CPT II deficiency is seen in young adults (table 37.1) experiencing episodes of muscle pain and rhabdomyolysis triggered by prolonged exercise, fasting, cold, or a combination of these. The disease is autosomal recessive and is mostly seen in males, but intolerance to exercise might be observed also in carriers of CPT II mutations, suggesting a dominant negative effect of this tetrameric protein [4]. The rhabdomyolytic attacks are associated with pain, stiffness without cramps, and highly elevated creatine kinase levels (about 50 000 U or maybe even up to 200,000 U), reflecting muscle necrosis. This may lead to acute renal failure.

*European Handbook of Neurological Management: Volume 1,
2nd edition. Edited by N. E. Gilhus, M. P. Barnes and M. Brainin.
© 2011 Blackwell Publishing Ltd.*

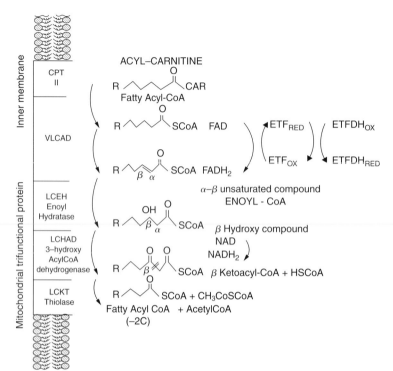

Figure 37.1. Pathway of long-chain fatty acid oxidation by enzymes in the inner mitochondrial membrane. CPT II, carnitine palmitoyltransferase II; VLCAD, very-long-chain acyl-CoA dehydrogenase; FAD, flavine adenine dinucleotide; FADH$_2$, reduced form of FAD; ETF, electron-transferring flavoprotein (RED, reduced; OX, oxidized); ETFDH, electron transfer flavoprotein dehydrogenase (RED, reduced; OX, oxidized); LCEH, long-chain enoyl hydratase; LCHAD, long-chain beta-hydroxy acyl-CoA-dehydrogenase; NAD, nicotinamide adenine dinucleotide (NADH$_2$, reduced form of NAD); LCKT, long-chain beta-keto thiolase; CAR, carnitine; CoA, coenzyme A. The other co-factors and enzymes are in either the cytosol or the mitochondrial matrix.

Table 37.1 Carnitine palmitoyltransferase (CPT) II deficiency.

Young adults
Paroxysmal myoglobinuria
Residual: malonyl-CoA insensitive CPT activity
CPT gene is located in chromosome 1
Serine 113 to leucine is the most common missense
  mutation 6% cases (429C > T)

Diagnosis

CPT II deficiency was routinely diagnosed by the determination of enzyme activity in muscle biopsies involving the time-dependent conversion of radiolabelled CPT II substrates by the isotope-exchange assay. Now, when available, the diagnosis can be made on the basis of genetic analysis (figure 37.2) and acylcarnitine profile.

Analysis of acylcarnitines in the blood, using tandem mass spectrometry, was developed in the late 1980s, allowing the diagnosis of most inborn errors of fatty acid metabolism, including CPT II defects. A characteristic profile of blood acylcarnitines has been reported [5]:

CPT II deficiency leads to an increase of serum palmitoylcarnitine (C16:0) and oleoylcarnitine (C18:1), whereas short- and medium-chain acylcarnitines are normal (figure 37.3), and in attacks free carnitine is low. Only a small amount of plasma (100 µl) or blood spotted onto filter paper (Guthrie card) is required. It is important to collect samples from patients when they are acutely ill, since a non-significant profile can be observed when patients are metabolically well equilibrated.

It is noteworthy that CPT II patients show the same elevated long-chain acyl-carnitine profile in plasma as carnitine/acylcarnitine translocase (CACT) deficiency. These disorders can easily be distinguished by their clinical presentation. However, the clinical presentation of the severe hepato-cardio-muscular form of CPT II deficiency can significantly overlap with that of CACT deficiency. In most cases, a direct measurement of enzymatic activity is required to differentiate between these two metabolic defects. Tandem mass spectrometry of serum acylcarnitines is a rapid screening test that should be included early in the diagnostic work-up of patients with recurrent myoglobinuria, recurrent muscular weakness, and myalgia. In

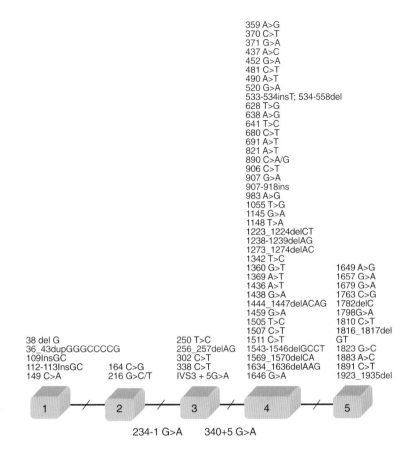

					359 A>G
					370 C>T
					371 G>A
					437 A>C
					452 G>A
					481 C>T
					490 A>T
					520 G>A
					533-534insT; 534-558del
					628 T>G
					638 A>G
					641 T>C
					680 C>T
					691 A>T
					821 A>T
					890 C>A/G
					906 C>T
					907 G>A
					907-918ins
					983 A>G
					1055 T>G
					1145 G>A
					1148 T>A
					1223_1224delCT
					1238-1239delAG
					1273_1274delAC
					1342 T>C

1360 G>T 1649 A>G
1369 A>T 1657 G>A
1436 A>T 1679 G>A
1438 G>A 1763 C>G
1444_1447delACAG 1782delC
1459 G>A 1798G>A
1505 T>C 1810 C>T
1507 C>T 1816_1817del

38 del G   250 T>C   1511 C>T   GT
36_43dupGGGCCCCG 256_257delAG 1543-1546delGCCT 1823 G>C
109InsGC   302 C>T   1569_1570delCA   1883 A>C
112-113InsGC 164 C>G 338 C>T 1634_1636delAAG   1891 C>T
149 C>A   216 G>C/T IVS3 + 5G>A 1646 G>A   1923_1935del

Figure 37.2. Structural organization and mutational spectrum of the carnitine palmitoyltransferase II gene.

234-1 G>A   340+5 G>A

particular, in young children suspected of CPT II deficiency, it is desirable to avoid a diagnostic muscle biopsy. Further evaluation will clarify whether the typical clinical phenotype together with a characteristic mass spectrum is sufficient to establish the diagnosis of a CPT II defect without performing tissue enzymatic assay.

The acylcarnitine profile has also demonstrated its high value as a fast and non-invasive method for the presymptomatic detection of inborn errors of fatty acid oxidation in newborn screening. Overnight fasting is useful but may lead also to unexpected hypoglycaemic episodes.

Recommendations

Preventing episodes of myoglobinuria is important, and this can be achieved by avoiding strenuous exercise during fasting or cold. During an attack, infusion of a 5% glucose solution is useful as an alternative metabolic fuel. According to published guidelines, a standard treatment protocol for myoglobinuria [6] is intravenous infusion of hypotonic sodium chloride and sodium bicarbonate (sodium chloride 110 mmol/l, sodium bicarbonate 40 mmol/l) in 5% glucose solution to which 10 g of mannitol per litre is added in a 20% solution. In a person weighing 75 kg, the solution should be infused at a rate of 12 l/day in order to obtain a dieresis of 8 l/day and keep the pH above 6.5. This therapeutic regimen will control both

hyperkalaemia and acidosis, and therefore might prevent acute renal failure.

In general, patients with CPT II deficiency must avoid triggering factors of metabolic crisis such as fasting, cold, or prolonged exercise under fasting or stress-fuel conditions. However, a high-carbohydrate diet (20% fat, 15% protein, 65% carbohydrate) improves exercise tolerance, as indicated by a lowering of perceived exertion and an increased duration of exercise [7]. An anaplerotic diet using medium odd-chain triglycerides (triheptanoin) might improve cardiomyopathy, muscle weakness, and rhabdomyolysis. This kind of therapy is based on the concept that triheptanoin as an anaplerotic compound provides an alternative substrate for both the tricarboxylic cycle and the electron transport chain, and may thus restore energy production [8–10].

A potential new therapy is being investigated using peroxisome proliferator-activated receptor (PPAR)-delta agonists, such as bezafibrate, which has the ability to partially or totally restore fatty acid oxidation in patients with the adult form of CPT II deficiency. A basic study [11] showed that bezafibrate treatment of mild-type CPT II-deficient fibroblasts resulted in a time- and dose-dependent increase in CPT II mRNA and residual enzyme activity, and led to a normalization of 3H-palmitate and 3H-myristate cellular oxidation rates, suggesting that PPARs could be therapeutic targets for the correction of hereditary beta-oxidation defects. Bezafibrate did not correct fatty acid oxidation in fibroblasts from patients with a severe CPT II-deficient phenotype.

A French group [12] evaluated the efficacy of bezafibrate as a treatment in six adults with the mild adult form of CPT II

deficiency. After bezafibrate treatment, the palmitoyl L-carnitine oxidation levels and the CPT II mRNA in skeletal muscle increased significantly, the episodes of rhabdomyolysis decreased, and the quality of life (evaluated with the use of the 36-Item Short-Form General Health Survey) improved considerably. The results of this pilot trial showed a therapeutic efficacy of bezafibrate, suggesting that further study of this agent for the pharmacological treatment of the mild form of CPT II deficiency might be of interest.

Bezafibrate has been prescribed for more than 25 years as a hypolipidaemic agent, in large cohorts of adults, and is generally considered to have a good safety profile. Occasionally, a drug-induced increase in plasma levels of creatine phosphokinase can be observed. However, bezafibrate-induced rhabdomyolysis is extremely rare and has only been reported in patients with renal insufficiency who tend to accumulate the drug.

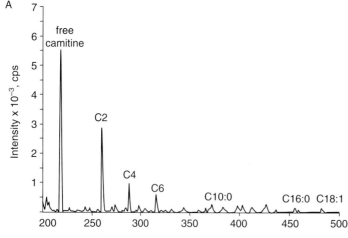

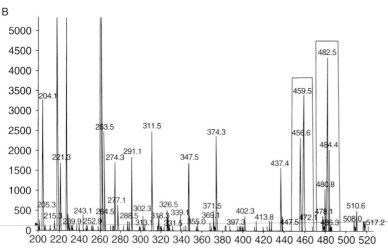

Figure 37.3. Tandem mass acyl-carnitine spectra of serum of a normal subject (A) and a CPTII-deficient patient (B). In CPTII deficiency a characteristic elevation of palmitoyl-carnitine (C_{16}) and oleoyl-carnitine ($C_{18:1}$) can be observed. 227 Da: free carnitine, 263 Da: acetyl-carnitine, 291 Da: butyryl-carnitine, 311 Da: isovaleryl-carnitine, 347 Da: octanoyl-carnitine, 437 Da: myristoyl-carnitine, 459 Da: palmitoyl-carnitine. The peaks related to palmitoyl-carnitine and oleoyl-carnitine are enclosed in boxes.

Carnitine transport defects

Primary L-carnitine deficiency syndromes are rare biochemical disorders and can be classified on the basis of clinical and biochemical criteria into muscle carnitine deficiency and systemic carnitine deficiency. A carnitine deficiency syndrome should be suspected in a patient with LSM when the following symptoms are present: hypoglycaemia, with or without ketoacidosis with a Reye-like syndrome, myalgias, weakness, abnormal fatigability, and cardiomyopathy with left axis deviation [13, 14]. Primary systemic carnitine deficiency is a well-recognized treatable entity of childhood (table 37.2) characterized by progressive cardiomyopathy, LSM, attacks of hypoglycaemia, and hepatomegaly with a Reye-like syndrome that may lead to permanent brain damage [15].

Diagnosis

In several cases, a defect of the carnitine 'high-affinity' transport organic cation transporter 2 (*OCTN2*) gene has been demonstrated in cultured fibroblasts, and genomic DNA can be screened for mutations [16, 17].

Guidelines for therapy

Carnitine supplementation corrects cardiomyopathy and other clinical signs [13]. In some cases, this treatment may prevent the need for cardiac transplantation. The L-carnitine dose may vary from 100 to 600 mg/kg per day on the basis of the calculated carnitine depletion from muscle, liver, heart, and kidney. Individually adjusted dosing may require plasma level measurements. No side effects are noted for L-carnitine supplementation except

occasional diarrhoea or a fishy body odour. In some cases, a medium-chain triglyceride diet may be added (Class IV evidence).

Muscle carnitine deficiency

In primary muscle carnitine deficiency, the clinical syndrome is confined to skeletal muscle [18, 19]; the clinical features are episodes of fluctuating muscle weakness, affecting mostly the limb and neck muscles, and severe myalgia.

Diagnostic guidelines and therapy

The patients show appropriate ketogenesis on fasting and on a fat-rich diet. Biochemical features are low muscle carnitine (below 15%) and absence of organic aciduria. Carnitine concentrations in the plasma and liver are normal. There is *in vitro* stimulation by L-carnitine of labelled palmitate and oleate oxidation. Although much is known about the mechanisms of carnitine transport, data on muscle-specific transport (low affinity) in human muscle carnitine deficiency cases are still scanty. In a childhood case, an abnormal low-affinity carnitine transport [19] was found in cultured muscle. This could be due to either a delayed maturation or an abnormal carnitine carrier protein. The available evidence indicates that the low muscle content is the result of a genetic defect in the sarcolemmal carnitine transporter. Therefore, muscle carnitine deficiency could be caused by an abnormal low-affinity carrier or by a low amount of sarcolemmal carnitine carriers. It is distinguished from carnitine insufficiency by the absence of acylcarnitine elevation in plasma or urine.

Treatment with an L-carnitine replacement and medium chain triglyceride diet has been successful in a number of cases (Class IV evidence).

Defects of beta-oxidation

Defects of fatty acid oxidation may affect muscle alone or in conjunction with other tissue manifestations, i.e. liver and heart (table 37.3). For most of the different enzyme deficiencies, the clinical features are similar. In some patients, this is reflected by exercise-induced muscle pain and rhabdomyolysis. The diagnosis is often suggested by characteristic patterns of organic acids excreted in the urine, which are specific for various enzymatic blocks.

Enzymatic and immunochemical analysis performed in fibroblasts and/or in muscle and liver mitochondria

---

Table 37.2 Primary systemic carnitine deficiency.

Inheritance: autosomal recessive
Gene: OCTN2 organic cation transporter
Clinical presentation
    Progressive cardiomyopathy
    Muscle weakness
    Fasting hypoglycaemia
    Urine: normal organic acid pattern
    Low total carnitine in plasma, urine and muscle
    Normal ratio carnitine/acyl-carnitines
    Molecular biology: several point mutations reported

OCTN2, organic cation transporter 2.

Table 37.3 Clinical features in metabolic defects of fatty acids disorders.

	Cramps	Myoglobinuria	Myalgia	Weakness	Heart	Metabolic crisis
Systemic carnitine transporter	−	−	−	−	+	+
Muscle carnitine	−	−	+	+	−	−
CPT II	+	+	+	−	−	−
VLCAD	−	+	−	−	+	+
Trifunctional protein	−	+	−	−	+	+
MCAD	−	−		−	−	+
SCAD	−	−	+	+	−	+
RR-MAD	−	−	−	+	−	+

CPT II; carnitine palmitoyltransferase deficiency, VLCAD; very long-chain acyl-CoA deficiency, MCAD; medium-chain acyl-CoA deficiency, SCAD; short-chain acyl-CoA deficiency, RR-MAD; riboflavin-responsive multiple acyl-CoA-dehydrogenase.

were used to confirm the diagnosis The use of acylcarnitine and genetics has completely changed the way in which we diagnose the inborn errors of beta-oxidation, which are:

• very long-chain acyl-CoA dehydrogenase (LCHAD or VLCAD) deficiency;
• trifunctional enzyme deficiency;
• medium-chain acyl-CoA dehydrogenase (MCAD) deficiency;
• short-chain acyl-CoA dehydrogenase (SCAD) deficiency;
• riboflavin-responsive disorders of β-oxidation (RR-MADD).

Guidelines for the laboratory diagnosis of fatty acid oxidation defects

Dicarboxylic aciduria is a distinct finding associated with a metabolic block of beta-oxidation. The substrates are converted to dicarboxylic acids by the combined action of omega-oxidation in the endoplasmic reticulum and by peroxisomal beta-oxidation.

The metabolic intermediates accumulating behind the enzymatic block can be detected in urine and blood. Often, they are formed only during a metabolic crisis. The qualitative and quantitative study of the organic acids produced in the patients is indicated by gas chromatography–mass spectrometry (GC–MS) analysis. Acylcarnitines can be revealed in patients with organic aciduria due to the activity of acylcarnitine transferase,

and their pattern of appearance in plasma and urine is a useful diagnostic test [2]. They are especially important in the diagnosis of beta-oxidation blocks such as VLCAD or MCAD deficiencies.

Other secondary metabolites, produced by enzymatic reactions that free CoA from acyl residues, can be detected in patients' urine. Glycine derivatives like hexanoyl-glycine or phenylpropionyl-glycine are pathognomonic of MCAD deficiency. The presence of glycine or acylcarnitine derivatives in the urine indicates an increased accumulation of acyl-CoA in the mitochondria. Glutaric aciduria type 2 is pathognomonic of riboflavin-responsive LSM. Fat accumulation in a muscle biopsy depends upon diet and activity level. Analysis of metabolites is a crucial investigation, and can be combined with a study of labelled fatty acid oxidation and appropriate enzyme studies in fibroblasts.

VLCAD deficiency

VLCAD deficiency has mostly been described in children [20]. The patients reported so far can be grouped according to their clinical course: a first group has an onset in the first few months of life and shows a high mortality; a second group is characterized by recurrent episodes of coma after fasting, but presents no cardiomyopathy; a third group presents with late-onset rhabdomyolysis and myalgia after muscle exercise.

Deficient patients cannot oxidize C18 to C16 fatty acids, whereas the oxidation of shorter fatty acids (shorter than C14) is normal. The disease is inherited as an auto-somal recessive trait. The common mutation for long-chain beta-hydroxy acyl-CoA-dehydrogenase (LCHAD) deficiency is 1538 G>C. The onset of symptoms is in the first year of life, characterized by intermittent hypogly-caemia, lethargy, and coma. The typical presentation is a progressive lethargy, evolving into coma during fasting or during a febrile episode associated with vomiting and diarrhea that induces a catabolic state. Hepatomegaly, cardiomyopathy, and muscle weakness are usually observed. Exercise-induced myoglobinuria is a possible presentation [21, 22]. Cardiological involvement is fre-quent. Other distinctive laboratory findings include hypoglycaemia, hypoketonuria, high serum ammonia, and a slight elevation of serum aminotransferases. Low ketones during severe hypoglycaemia strongly suggests a specific defect of fatty acid oxidation. Liver biopsy, when performed, reveals an increase in both macro- and microvesicular fat and mitochondrial abnormalities.

Trifunctional enzyme deficiency

Three adult patients from a family with recurrent rhab-domyolysis and peripheral neuropathy were reported [23]. A low-fat/high-carbohydrate diet was beneficial in one patient, reducing the frequency of rhabdomyolysis.

MCAD deficiency

MCAD deficiency (OMIM number 201450) is the most common error of fatty oxidation found in the USA, UK, and Northern Europe. Patients present with recurrent somnolence, vomiting, coma, hypoglycaemia, fatty infil-tration of the liver, and dicarboxylic aciduria. The crises are often precipitated by infections. Patients cannot oxidize the medium-chain fatty acids (C12 to C6). The disorder becomes life-threatening during episodes of stress or fasting (table 37.4), which result in decreased caloric intake or increased catabolism.

MCAD deficiency has been found in cases of Reye-like syndrome, and in some cases of sudden infant death syn-drome. The first episodes of the disorder occur in the first 12–18 months of life. Incidence in the two sexes is similar. The mortality rate is 25%, but can reach 60% in cases with a later onset (second year of life). In half the families, there was a high incidence of death in infancy.

Hepatomegaly due to fatty liver has been described in some cases. Seizures have been reported, but patients may have normal development and growth, and no clinical

Table 37.4 Medium-chain acyl-CoA-dehydrogenase deficiency.

Children
Reye-like syndrome
Fasting hypoglycaemia, non-ketotic
Episodes of coma
Low total plasma carnitine
Decreased tissue carnitine
Decreased octanoic oxidation in fibroblasts
Medium-chain dicarboxylic aciduria
Chromosome lp31
Common mutation 329 lysine to glutamic acid 90% of
cases (986 A > G, K304E)

sign of cardiomyopathy or myopathy. During the crisis, all patients develop hypoketotic hypoglycaemia, with an increased ratio of free fatty acids to ketone bodies, ele-vated serum aminotransferases, and mild hyperam-monaemia, probably due to increased proteolysis. Plasma and tissue carnitine is low (25% of controls in liver and muscle), with an increased acyl/free carnitine ratio. The secondary carnitine insufficiency observed in MCAD-deficient patients is due not only to an increased excre-tion of acylcarnitines, with depletion of tissue carnitine, but also to defective reabsorption in the kidney.

Molecular biology

Several laboratories have identified the molecular aetiol-ogy of MCAD deficiency as a common point mutation in the locus 1p31 (chromosome 1). The mutation, an A to G transition at nucleotide 985, leads to a substitution of lysine by glutamic acid in the mature protein dehydro-genase. It has been observed that patients with MCAD synthesize a normally size MCAD precursor, which is usually targetted to the mitochondria. A small group (10%) of mutation carriers is completely asymptomatic.

Treatment Recommendations

The treatment is similar in LCHAD and MCAD deficiency: fasting and long intervals between meals should be avoided, a high-carbohydrate, low-fat diet should be administered, and L-carnitine supplementation can be useful in preventing secondary carnitine insufficiency (Class IV evidence). Prevention is important, considering the high incidence of the disease (1 in 8930 in a newborn screening programme in Pennsylvania, USA) and the good prognosis in patients under adequate dietary control. The best prevention is the identification of patients during the asymptomatic period, possibly at birth. Screening of all newborns can be achieved by searching for the typical metabolites in the urine. In Pennsylvania [24], a dry blood spot test on Guthrie cards of newborn babies has been proposed to analyse blood acylcarnitines using GC–MS. On peripheral blood DNA, the identification of the A to G mutation, present in 90% of patients, is obtained by restriction analysis (NcoI) of the relevant sequence amplified by the polymerase chain reaction. Data obtained after the initial screening indicate that there is a high prevalence of the mutated allele in babies of German and British heritage, whereas this mutation is rarely found in newborns from the Mediterranean area. The data suggest that the mutation occurred in a single progenitor in Germany. Prenatal diagnosis is possible using the same molecular analysis.

Table 37.5 Riboflavin-responsive multiple acyl-CoA-dehydrogenase deficiency.

Myopathic form
Adult onset
Lipid storage myopathy
Low SCAD, MCAD
Low free carnitine, increased acyl-carnitines, glutaric
 aciduria type 2
Riboflavin responsive

SCAD, short-chain acyl-CoA deficiency; MCAD, medium-chain acyl-CoA deficiency.

SCAD deficiency

Few patients with SCAD deficiency have been described. In SCAD deficiency, the dicarboxylic aciduria is not striking. Many shorter-chain fatty acid residues are seen, such as ethylmalonic, butyric, and methylsuccinic acids. In these patients, the oxidation of C4 to C6 fatty acids is compromised. As MCAD catalyses 50% of C4 dehydrogenation, the diagnosis may be difficult and may require inhibition of MCAD with specific antisera. SCAD deficiency is associated with different clinical phenotypes: a severe infantile form [25] and a late-onset myopathic picture.

Riboflavin-responsive multiple acyl-CoA dehydrogenase defects (RR-MADD)

This is a relatively common LSM presenting in adult life with fluctuating episodes of profound weakness, associated with carnitine insufficiency and glutaric aciduria, and usually underdiagnosed, that responds dramatically to riboflavin [26–28]. Both SCAD and MCAD activity are low in the skeletal muscle and mitochondria of these patients who present with an LSM [26, 27]. Therefore this entity is called riboflavin-responsive multiple acyl-CoA dehydrogenase deficiency (RR-MADD) (table 37.5).

It is difficult to explain the improvement of patients and the enzyme changes observed during riboflavin treatment. Riboflavin deficiency may be due to different mechanisms. Riboflavin enters as a coenzyme not only in acyl-CoA dehydrogenase, but also in complex I and complex II of the respiratory chain. Possible mechanisms of riboflavin deficiency include: (1) decreased cellular riboflavin uptake and decreased flavin adenine dinucleotide (FAD) synthesis; (2) decreased FAD transport into mitochondria; (3) abnormal binding of FAD to apoenzymes; and (4) increased catabolism of FAD for increased FADPase. A biochemical study of mitochondrial and muscle FAD and flavin mononucleotide (FMN) levels reveals different mechanisms in patients with riboflavin deficiency [28]. Most of these patients have shown to have electron-transferring flavoprotein dehydrogenase (ETFDH) deficiency [29, 30].

Diagnosis

The presence of the characteristic organic acid pattern in urine and blood from a newborn with non-ketotic hypoglycaemia and metabolic acidosis establishes the diagnosis as glutaric aciduria type II. Urinary organic acid analysis by GC–MS shows an increase in lactic acid, malonic acid, ethylmalonic acid, glutaric acid, adipic acid, 2-hydroxyglutaric acid, suberic acid, sebacic acid, and dodecanedioic acid. The finding of 2-hydroxyglutaric aciduria in such patients is a useful diagnostic point and distinguishes the condition from glutaric aciduria type I (glutaryl-coA dehydrogenase deficiency), in which 3-hydroxyglutaric is excreted.

Diagnosis in the late-onset cases may be considerably more difficult because metabolic acidosis, the usual indication for examining urine organic acids, may not be

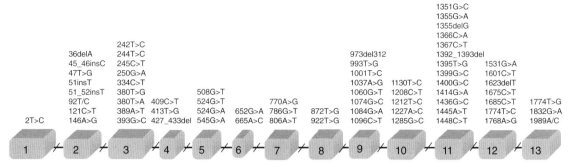

Figure 37.4. Structural organization and mutational spectrum of the ETFDH gene.

present. Furthermore, the organic aciduria in such patients is considerably less pronounced and is often intermittent, being present only during acute episodes. A wider use of blood acylcarnitine analysis should reduce the number of missed diagnoses. Acylcarnitine analysis can reveal a combined elevation of short-chain (<C6), medium-chain (C6–C14), and long-chain (>C14) acyl-carnitines. In RR-MADD, free carnitine in serum is decreased because of the increased acylcarnitine levels.

Other RR-MADD cases can be diagnosed by enzymatic assay and mutation analysis (figure 37.4) of ETFDH, the most frequently involved enzyme [29].

Recommendations

It is important to recognize these patients as they improve after riboflavin treatment (100–200 mg/day). Several cases of LSM-associated beta-oxidation defects have been reported, because of multiple acyl-CoA-dehydrogenase deficiency, that were riboflavin responsive (Class IV evidence). Evidence that a biochemical defect involving the oxidation of short-chain fatty acids causes a deficiency of SCAD, MCAD, and FAD, as well as depletion of FMN co-factors in muscle mitochondria should be sought in most cases, especially in those who are riboflavin responsive [28].

Therapy with riboflavin and a low-fat, low-protein diet is beneficial, although the long-term treatment of patients with late-onset glutaric aciduria type II is still challenging. The emerging consensus is that riboflavin prescription is the first-line treatment for RR-MADD patients. Most reports have advocated combination therapy with riboflavin and carnitine as more effective, although a few reports have noted the ineffectiveness of carnitine. Interestingly, the clinical manifestations of primary carnitine deficiency are sometimes similar to those of RR-MADD, especially during metabolic crisis. Accordingly, supplementation of riboflavin together with carnitine is reasonable for the patients suspected of having RR-MADD, but not yet diagnosed. A more recent study [30] suggested that combination therapy with riboflavin and CoQ$_{10}$ resulted in some cases in a better long-term outcome compared with riboflavin plus carnitine in patients with the myopathic form of CoQ$_{10}$ deficiency due to ETFDH mutations. Other drugs, such as glycine, prednisolone, and insulin, have also been studied, but their effectiveness remains uncertain.

Good Practice Points for the treatment of fatty acids disorders

The main caution in defects of mitochondrial beta-oxidation is the avoidance of fasting (Class IV evidence). By not allowing patients with such disorders to become dependent on beta-oxidation, the accumulation of toxic intermediate metabolites is avoided and the development of the most critical symptoms is minimized. Fat consumption should be restricted to 25% of total calories, and the amount of LCFA should be reduced (Class IV evidence). Increased caloric intake from carbohydrates may be necessary during intermittent illness because of increased metabolic demands on the body. A low-fat, high-carbohydrate diet is beneficial in reducing the frequency of rhabdomyolysis in several disorders of fatty acid metabolism, including CPT II deficiency [31] and trifunctional enzyme deficiency [23]. The current dietary treatment of LCFA defects (high carbohydrates with medium even-chain triglycerides, and reduced long-chain fats) is based on evidence provided by experts' opinion alone or from descriptive case series without controls. It is difficult to perform double-blind studies to prevent cardiomyopathy, rhabdomyolysis, and muscle weakness.

Conflicts of interest

The authors have no conflict of interest.

Acknowledgements

This paper was prepared as a part of a European Biobank Network.

References

1. Bruno C, Dimauro S. Lipid storage myopathies. *Curr Opin Neurol* 2008;**21**:601–6.

2. Angelini C, Vergani L, Martinuzzi A. Clinical and biochemical aspects of carnitine deficiency and insufficiency: transport defects and inborn errors of beta-oxidation. *Crit Rev Clin Lab Sci* 1992;**29**:217–42.

3. Brainin M, Barnes M, Baron JC, *et al.* Guidance for the preparation of neurological management guidelines by EFNS scientific task forces – revised recommendations 2004. *Eur J Neurol* 2004;**11**:577–81.

4. Orngreen MC, Duno M, Ejstrup R, *et al.* Fuel utilization in subjects with carnitine palmitoyltransferase 2 gene mutations. *Ann Neurol* 2005;**57**:60–6.

5. Gempel K, Kiechl S, Hofmann S, *et al.* Screening for carnitine palmitoyltransferase II deficiency by tandem mass spectrometry. *J Inherit Metab Dis* 2002;**25**:17–27.

6. Better OS, Stein GH. Early management of shock and prophylaxis of acute renal failure in traumatic rhabdomyolysis. *N Engl J Med* 1990;**322**:825–9.

7. Vorgerd M. Therapeutic options in other metabolic myopathies. *Neurotherapeutics* 2008;**5**:579–82.

8. Roe CR, Mochel F. Anaplerotic diet therapy in inherited metabolic disease: therapeutic potential. *J Inherit Metab Dis* 2006;**29**:332–40.

9. Roe CR, Roe DS, Wallace M, *et al.* Choice of oils for essential fat supplements can enhance production of abnormal metabolites in fat oxidation disorders. *Mol Genet Metab* 2007;**92**:346–50.

10. Roe CR, Yang BZ, Brunengraber H, *et al.* Carnitine palmitoyltransferase deficiency: successful anaplerotic diet therapy. *Neurology* 2008;**71**:260–4.

11. Djouadi F, Aubey F, Schlemmer D, *et al.* Bezafibrate increases very-long-chain acyl-CoA dehydrogenase protein and mRNA expression in deficient fibroblasts and is a potential therapy for fatty acid oxidation disorders. *Hum Mol Genet* 2005;**14**:2695–703.

12. Bonnefont JP, Bastin J, Behin A, *et al.* Bezafibrate for an inborn mitochondrial beta-oxidation defect. *N Engl J Med* 2009;**360**:838–40.

13. Tein I, De Vivo C, Brieman F, *et al.* Impaired skin fibroblast carnitine uptake in primary systemic carnitine deficiency manifested by childhood carnitine-responsive cardiomyopathy. *Pediatr Res* 1990;**28**:247–55.

14. Nezu J, Tamai I, Oku A, *et al.* Primary systemic carnitine deficiency is caused by mutations in a gene encoding sodium ion-dependent carnitine transporter. *Nat Genet* 1999;**21**:91–4.

15. Chapoy PR, Angelini C, Brown WJ, *et al.* Systemic carnitine deficiency: a treatable inherited lipid storage disease presenting as recurrent Reye's syndrome. *N Engl J Med* 1980;**303**:1389–94.

16. Tang NL, Ganapathy V, Wu X, *et al.* Mutations of OCTN2, an organic cation/carnitine transporter, lead to deficient cellular carnitine uptake in primary carnitine deficiency. *Hum Mol Genet* 1999;**8**:655–60.

17. Longo N, Arnat di San Filippo C, Pasquali M. Disorders of carnitine transport and the carnitine cycle. *Am J Med Genet C Semin Med Genet* 2006;**142**:77–85.

18. Engel AG, Angelini C. Carnitine deficiency of human skeletal muscle with associated lipid storage myopathy: reports of a new syndrome. *Science* 1973;**179**:899–902.

19. Vergani L, Angelini C. Infantile lipid storage myopathy with nocturnal hypoventilation shows abnormal low-affinity muscle carnitine uptake *in vitro. Neuromuscl Disord* 1999;**5**:320–2.

20. Hale DE, Batshaw MC, Coates P, *et al.* Long-chain acyl-coenzyme A dehydrogenase deficiency: an inherited cause of no ketotic hypoglycemia. *Pediatr Res* 1985;**19**:666–71.

21. Olgivie I, Pourfarzam M, Jackson S, *et al.* Very long-chain acyl-coenzyme A dehydrogenase deficiency presenting with exercise induced myoglobinuria. *Neurology* 1994;**44**:463–73.

22. Orngreen MC, Norgaard MG, Sacchetti M, *et al.* Fuel utilization in patients with very-long-chain acyl-CoA dehydrogenase deficiency. *Ann Neurol* 2004;**56**:279–83.

23. Schaefer J, Jackson S, Dick DJ, *et al.* Trifunctional enzyme deficiency: adult presentation of a usually fatal beta-oxidation defect. *Ann Neurol* 1996;**40**:597–602.

24. Ziadeh R, Hoffman EP, Finegold DN, *et al.* Medium-chain acyl-CoA dehydrogenase deficiency in Pennsylvania: neonatal screening shows high incidence and unexpected mutation frequencies. *Pediatr Res* 1995;**37**:675–8.

25. Coates PM, Acili DE, Finocchiaro G, *et al.* Genetic deficiency of short chain acyl-coenzyme A dehydrogenase in cultured fibroblasts from a patient with muscle carnitine deficiency and severe skeletal muscle weakness. *J Clin Invest* 1988;**81**: 171–5.

26. Antozzi C, Garavaglia B, Mora M, *et al.* Late-onset riboflavin responsive myopathy with combined multiple acyl-CoA dehydrogenase and respiratory chain deficiency. *Neurology* 1994;**44**:2153–8.

27. Vergani L, Angelini C, Pegoraro E, *et al.* Hereditary protein C deficiency associated with riboflavin responsive lipid storage myopathy. *Eur J Neurol* 1996;**3**:61–5.

28. Vergani L, Barile M, Angelini C, *et al.* Riboflavin therapy: biochemical heterogeneity in two adult lipid storage myopathies. *Brain* 1999;**122**:2401–11.

29. Olsen RK, Olpin SE, Andresen BS, *et al.* ETFDH mutations as a major cause of riboflavin-responsive multiple acyl-CoA dehydrogenation deficiency. *Brain* 2007;**130**: 2045–54.

30. Gempel K, Topaloglu H, Talim B, *et al.* The myopathic form of coenzyme Q10 deficiency is caused by mutations in the electron-transferring-flavoprotein dehydrogenase (ETFDH) gene. *Brain* 2007;**130**:2037–44.

31. Orngreen MC, Ejstrup R, Vissing J. Effect of diet on exercise tolerance on carnitine palmitoyltransferase II deficiency. *Neurology* 2003;**61**:559–61.

CHAPTER 38

Management of narcolepsy in adults

M. Billiard,[1] Y. Dauvilliers,[2] L. Dolenc-Grošelj,[3] G.J. Lammers,[4] G. Mayer,[5] K. Sonka[6]

[1]University of Montpellier, France; [2]Gui de Chauliac Hospital, Montpellier, France; [3]University Medical Center, Ljubljana, Slovenia; [4]Leiden University Medical Center, The Netherlands; [5]Department of Neurology, Schwalmstadt-Treysa, Germany; [6]Charles University, Prague, Czech Republic

Introduction

The treatments used for narcolepsy, either pharmacological or behavioural, are diverse. However, the quality of the published pieces of clinical evidence supporting them varies widely, and studies comparing the efficacy of different substances are lacking. Several treatments are used on an empirical basis, especially antidepressants for cataplexy, as these medications are already used widely in depressed patients, leaving little motivation from the manufacturers to investigate their efficacy in relatively rare indications. On the other hand, modafinil and sodium oxybate have been evaluated in large randomized placebo-controlled trials. Our objective was to reach a consensus on the use of these two drugs and of other available medications.

Narcolepsy is a disabling syndrome, first described by Westphal [1] and Gelineau [2]. Excessive daytime sleepiness is the main symptom of narcolepsy. It includes a feeling of sleepiness waxing and waning throughout the day, and episodes of irresistible sleep recurring daily or almost daily. Cataplexy is the second most common symptom of narcolepsy and the most specific one. It is defined as a sudden loss of voluntary muscle tone with preserved consciousness triggered by emotion. Its frequency is extremely variable, from one or fewer per year to several per day. Other symptoms, referred to as auxiliary symptoms, are less specific and not essential for the diagnosis. These include hypnagogic and hypnopompic hallucinations – visual perceptual experiences occurring at sleep onset or on awakening; sleep paralysis – a transient generalized inability to move or to speak during the transition from wakefulness to sleep or vice versa; and disturbed nocturnal sleep with frequent awakenings and parasomnias. Obesity, headache, memory/concentration difficulties, and depressed mood are additional common features of narcolepsy.

The prevalence of narcolepsy is estimated at around 25–40 per 100 000 in Caucasian populations. It is often extremely incapacitating, interfering with every aspect of life, in work and social settings.

Excessive daytime sleepiness is lifelong, although it diminishes with age as assessed by the multiple sleep latency test (MSLT), an objective test of sleepiness based on 20-min polygraphic recording sessions repeated every 2 h, four or five times a day. Cataplexy may vanish after a certain time, spontaneously or with treatment. Hypnagogic hallucinations and sleep paralysis are often temporary. Disturbed nocturnal sleep has no spontaneous tendency to improve with time.

In the revised International Classification of Sleep Disorders [3], three forms of narcolepsy are distinguished: narcolepsy with cataplexy, narcolepsy without cataplexy, and narcolepsy due to a medical condition. The essential diagnostic criteria of narcolepsy with cataplexy are:

A. The patient has a complaint of excessive daytime sleepiness occurring almost daily for at least 3 months.

B. A definite history of cataplexy, defined as sudden and transient episodes of loss of muscle tone triggered by emotions, is present.

C. The diagnosis of narcolepsy with cataplexy should, whenever possible, be confirmed by nocturnal polysomnography followed by an MSLT. The mean sleep latency on the MSLT is less than or equal to 8 min, and two or more sleep-onset rapid eye movement periods

European Handbook of Neurological Management: Volume 1, 2nd edition. Edited by N. E. Gilhus, M. P. Barnes and M. Brainin.

(SOREMPs) are observed following sufficient nocturnal sleep (minimum 6h) during the night prior to the test. Alternatively, hypocretin-1 levels in the cerebrospinal fluid (CSF) are less than or equal to 110 pg/ml, or one-third of mean normal control values.

D. The hypersomnia is not better explained by another sleep disorder, medical or neurological disorder, mental disorder, medication use, or substance use disorder.

The diagnostic criteria of narcolepsy without cataplexy include the same criteria A and D, while criteria B and C are as follows:

B. Typical cataplexy is not present, although doubtful or atypical cataplexy-like episodes may be reported.

C. The diagnosis of narcolepsy without cataplexy must be confirmed by nocturnal polysomnography followed by an MSLT. In narcolepsy without cataplexy, the mean sleep latency on the MSLT is less than or equal to 8 min, and two or more SOREMPs are observed following sufficient nocturnal sleep (minimum 6h) during the night prior to the test.

The diagnostic criteria of narcolepsy due to a medical condition include the same criteria A and D, while criteria B and C are as follows:

B. One of the following is observed:

i. A definite history of cataplexy, defined as sudden and transient episodes of loss of muscle tone (muscle weakness) triggered by emotions is present.

ii. If cataplexy is not present or is very atypical, polysomnographic monitoring performed over the patient's habitual sleep period followed by an MSLT must demonstrate a mean sleep latency on the MSLT of less than 8 min, with two or more SOREMPs despite sufficient nocturnal sleep prior to the test (minimum 6h).

iii. Hypocretin-1 levels in the CSF are less than 110 pg/ml (or 30% of normal control values), provided the patient is not comatose.

C. A significant underlying medical or neurological disorder accounts for the daytime sleepiness.

Recent years have been characterized by several breakthroughs in the understanding of the pathophysiology of the condition. First, there have been the discoveries of a mutation of the hypocretin type 2 receptor in the autosomal recessive canine model of narcolepsy [4], and of a narcoleptic phenotype in orexin (hypocretin) knockout mice [5]. Then came the observation of lowered or undetectable levels of hypocretin-1 in the CSF of most human narcoleptics [6, 7] and the finding that sporadic narcolepsy, in dogs and humans, may also be related to a deficiency in the production of hypocretin-1 ligands [8]. The undetectable hypocretin-1 levels seem to be the consequence of a selective degeneration of hypocretin cells in the lateral hypothalamus. An autoimmune aetiology is hypothesized. However, direct evidence for such a mechanism is still lacking.

Compared with these advances, no revolutionary new treatments have been developed for excessive daytime sleepiness or cataplexy in the last few years, except for the recent trials with intravenous immunoglobulin (IVIg). However, there are several reasons for updating the European Federation of Neurological Societies (EFNS) guidelines on the management of narcolepsy [9]. First, modafinil has been used successfully in Europe for the last 10–15 years, decreasing the need to use amphetamine and amphetamine-like stimulants. Second, sodium oxybate has been approved by the European Medicines Agency (EMEA) for the treatment of narcolepsy with cataplexy and by the Food and Drug Administration (FDA) for the treatment of cataplexy and excessive daytime sleepiness in patients with narcolepsy. Third, the newer antidepressants are now widely used in the treatment of cataplexy.

The first effort in standardizing the treatment of narcolepsy was the 'Practice parameters for the use of stimulants in the treatment of narcolepsy' [10]. Seven years later, an update of these practice parameters for the treatment of narcolepsy, grading the evidence available and modifying the 1994 practice parameters, was published – 'Practice parameters for the treatment of narcolepsy: an update for 2000' [11]. Then came the guidelines on the diagnosis and management of narcolepsy in adults and children prepared for the UK [12], the EFNS guidelines on management of narcolepsy [9], and finally 'Practice parameters for the treatment of narcolepsy and other hypersomnias of central origin' [13], 'Treatment of narcolepsy and other hypersomnias of central origin' [14], and 'Therapies for narcolepsy with or without cataplexy: evidence based review' [15].

Methods and search strategy

The best available evidence to address each question was sought, with the classification scheme by type of study design according to the EFNS guidance document [16]. If the highest level of evidence was not sufficient or required updating, the literature search was extended to the lower adjacent level of evidence. Several databases were used, including the Cochrane Library, MEDLINE, EMBASE, and Clinical Trials until September 2005. Previous guidelines for treatment were sought. Each member of the task force was assigned a special task, primarily based on symptoms of narcolepsy (excessive daytime sleepiness and irresistible episodes of sleep, cataplexy, hallucinations and sleep paralysis, disturbed nocturnal sleep, parasomnias) and also on associated features (obstructive sleep apnoea hypopnoea syndrome, periodic limb movements during sleep, neuropsychiatric symptoms) and special treatments (behavioural and experimental).

Methods for reaching consensus

Each member of the task force was first invited to send his own contribution to the chairman. A meeting gathering seven of the nine members of the task force was then scheduled during the Vth International Symposium on Narcolepsy in Ascona, Switzerland, 10–15 October 2004. A draft of the guidelines was then prepared by the chairman and circulated among all members of the task force for comments. On receipt of these comments, the chairman prepared the final version that was circulated again among members for endorsement.

The current revision of the EFNS guidelines was prepared by the chairman based on the same databases until November 2009 and circulated among members for endorsement.

Results

Excessive daytime sleepiness and irresistible episodes of sleep

Modafinil is approved for the treatment of excessive daytime sleepiness in narcolepsy by both the EMEA and the FDA; sodium oxybate is approved for the treatment of narcolepsy with cataplexy in adults by the EMEA, and for the treatment of excessive daytime sleepiness and cataplexy in patients with narcolepsy by the FDA. Methylphenidate is approved for the treatment of excessive

daytime sleepiness at the national agency level in Belgium, Denmark, Germany, France, and Switzerland, and by the FDA. All other drugs are 'off-label'.

Modafinil (N06BA07) and armodafinil (FDA approved, EMEA not submitted)

Modafinil is a (2-[(diphenylmethyl) sulfinyl] acetamide) chemically unrelated to central nervous system (CNS) stimulants such as amphetamine and methylphenidate.

Modafinil may enhance the activity of wake-promoting neurons by increasing the extracellular concentration of dopamine [17, 18]. This rise in extracellular dopamine may be caused by blockade of the dopamine transporter (DAT) [19]. Modafinil may also reduce the activity of sleep-promoting (VLPO) neurons by inhibiting the norepinephrine transporter (NET) presynaptically [20]. In addition, modafinil could increase the extracellular concentration of 5-hydroxytryptamine in different brain areas [18, 21, 22] as well as the extracellular concentration of histamine [23]. On the other hand, modafinil does not seem to act as an alpha-agonist [24], to have a direct effect on the reuptake of glutamate or the synthesis of gamma-aminobutyric acid (GABA) or glutamate [25], or to require orexin/hypocretin to act on alertness [26].

Modafinil reaches peak bioavailability in about 2 h. The main metabolic pathway is its transformation at the hepatic level into inactive metabolites that are eliminated at the renal level. The elimination half-life is 9–14 h. The steady state is reached after 2–4 days.

Co-administration of modafinil with drugs such as diazepam, phenytoin, propranolol, warfarin, some tricyclic antidepressants, and selective serotonin reuptake inhibitors (SSRIs) may increase the circulatory levels of those compounds due to the inhibition of certain cytochrome P 450 (CYP) hepatic enzymes. On the other hand, modafinil may reduce plasma levels of oral contraceptives due to the induction of some CYP hepatic enzymes [27]. Hence, women should be advised to use a product containing 50 µg or more of ethinylestradiol or an alternative method of contraception while using modafinil.

Armodafinil is the *R*-enantiomer of modafinil. It primarily affects areas of the brain involved in controlling wakefulness. Despite similar half-lives, plasma concentration following armodafinil administration is higher late in the day than that following modafinil administration, resulting in a more prolonged effect during the day and a potential improvement in sleepiness in the late afternoon in patients with narcolepsy [28].

Two Class II evidence studies ([29], 50 patients; [30], 70 patients) and two Class I evidence studies ([31] and [32], 285 and 273 patients, respectively) have shown the efficacy of modafinil on excessive daytime sleepiness at doses of 300, 200, and 400 mg/day. The key points of these studies were: a reduction in daytime sleepiness, an overall benefit noted by physicians as well as by patients, and a significant improvement in maintaining wakefulness measured by the Maintenance of Wakefulness Test (MWT) with the 300 mg/day dose [29]; a significant decrease in the likelihood of falling asleep measured by the Epworth Sleepiness Scale (ESS), a reduction of severe excessive daytime sleepiness and irresistible episodes of sleep as assessed by the sleep log, and a significant improvement in maintaining wakefulness measured with the MWT, with both 200 and 400 mg/day doses [30]; consistent improvements in subjective measures of sleepiness (ESS) and in clinician-assessed change in the patient's condition (Clinical Global Impression), and significant improvement in maintaining wakefulness (MWT) and in decreasing sleepiness judged on the MSLT with both the 200 and the 400 mg/day doses [31, 32].

Three further studies have dealt with open-label extension data. Beusterien et al. [33] reported significantly high scores on 10 of 17 health-related quality of life scales in 558 narcoleptic patients on a modafinil 400 mg/day dose, with positive treatment effects sustained over the 40-week extension period. Moldofsky et al. [34] reported on 69 patients who entered a 16-week open-label extension trial, followed by a 2-week randomized placebo-controlled period of assessment. Mean sleep latencies on the MWT were 70% longer in the modafinil group compared with placebo. The latency to sleep decreased from 15.3 to 9.7 min in the group switched from modafinil to placebo, and the ESS score increased from 12.9 to 14.4. Mitler et al. [35] reported on 478 patients who were enrolled in two 40-week open-label extension studies. The majority of patients (75%) received modafinil 400 mg daily. Disease severity improved in over 80% of patients throughout the 40-week study.

According to a Class I evidence study [36] in which the efficacy of modafinil 400 mg once daily, 400 mg given in a split dose, or 200 mg once daily was compared, the 400 mg split-dose regimen improved wakefulness significantly in the evening compared with the 200 mg and 400 mg once-daily regimen (both $p < 0.05$). In addition, a Class IV evidence study [37] has indicated that, in patients switched from amphetamine or methylphenidate to modafinil, the frequency of cataplexy may increase due to the mild anticataplectic effect of the latter.

The most frequently reported adverse effects are headache (13%), nervousness (8%), and nausea (5%). Most adverse effects are mild to moderate in nature [35].

There is no reported evidence that tolerance develops to the effects of modafinil on excessive daytime sleepiness, although some clinicians have observed it. Similarly, it is generally accepted that modafinil has a low abuse potential [38]. On rare occasions, worsening of cataplexy with modafinil has been observed.

The FDA classifies drugs as A (controlled studies in humans have shown no risk), B (controlled studies in animals have shown no risk), C (controlled studies in animals have shown risk), and D (controlled studies in humans have shown risk) according to their embryotoxic and teratogenic effects. In the case of modafinil, teratology studies performed in animals did not provide any evidence of harm to the fetus (FDA category B). However, modafinil is not recommended in narcoleptic pregnant women as clinical studies are still insufficient.

A single Class I evidence study was performed in 196 patients randomized to receive armodafinil 150 mg, armodafinil 250 mg, or placebo once daily for 12 weeks [39]. Efficacy was assessed using the Maintenance of Wakefulness test and subjective tests. Compared with baseline measurements, the mean change from baseline at the final visit for armodafinil was an increase of 1.3, 2.6, and 1.9 min in the 150 mg, 250 mg, and combined groups respectively, compared with a decrease of 1.9 min for placebo ($p < 0.01$ for all three comparisons). However, this study did not provide a comparison of modafinil and armodafinil.

Sodium oxybate (N07XX04)

Sodium oxybate is the sodium salt of gammahydroxybutyrate (GHB), a natural neurotransmitter/neuromodulator that may act through its own receptors and via stimulation of GABA-B receptors. However, the mechanism of action of GHB that accounts for its utility in treating the symptoms of narcolepsy is still poorly understood. In particular, it is rather puzzling that although most of the behavioural effects of GHB appear to be mediated by GABA-B receptors, the prototypical

GABA-B receptor agonist baclofen is not active against excessive daytime sleepiness and cataplexy [40], suggesting that GHB and baclofen act at different subtypes of GABA-B receptor [41].

Regarding its pharmacokinetics, sodium oxybate is rapidly absorbed following oral administration, and a plasma peak is reached within 25–75 min of ingestion. Its half-life is 90–120 min, but the effects of sodium oxybate last much longer compared with its half-life. Significant pharmacological interactions have not been described, nor has induction or inhibition of hepatic enzymes.

Two Class I evidence studies [42, 43] and two Class IV evidence studies [44, 45] have shown reduced excessive daytime sleepiness and increased level of alertness, and a more recent Class I evidence study [46] has shown sodium oxybate and modafinil to be equally active for the treatment of excessive daytime sleepiness, producing additive effects when used together.

At doses ranging from 3 to 9 g nightly, adverse effects were dose-related and included dizziness in 23.5–34.3%, nausea in 5.9–34.3%, headache in 8.8–31.4%, confusion in 3.0–14.3%, enuresis in 0–14.3%, and vomiting in 0–11.4% of the cases [42].

Of concern is the abuse potential of GHB. GHB is misused in athletes for its metabolic effects (growth hormone-releasing effect), and it has been used as a 'date rape' drug because of its rapid sedating effect. However, a risk management programme in the US permits the safe handling and distribution of the compound and minimizes the risk for diversion [47]. A post-marketing surveillance study involving 26 000 patients from 16 different countries revealed only 10 cases (0.039%) meeting DSM-IV abuse criteria, 4 cases (0.016%) meeting DSM-IV dependence criteria, and 2 cases (0.008%) of sodium oxybate-facilitated sexual assault, indicating that abuse potential in patients with narcolepsy receiving sodium oxybate is very low [48]. Also of concern are the reports implicating sodium oxybate with several cases of worsening sleep-related breathing disturbances [49] or even death [50], although in the latter case patient number 2 died while not using his continuous positive airway pressure device [51]. According to a recent study [52], the administration of 9 g sodium oxybate to patients with mild to moderate obstructive sleep apnoea syndrome does not negatively impact on sleep-disordered breathing, but it might increase central apnoeas in some individuals and should be used with caution.

Animal studies have shown no evidence of teratogenicity (FDA category B). However, the potential risk for humans is unknown, and sodium oxybate is not recommended during pregnancy.

Amphetamines and amphetamine-like CNS stimulants

Amphetamine (N06BA01)

Amphetamines, including d,l-amphetamine, d-amphetamine (sulphate), and metamphetamine (chlorhydrate), have been used for narcolepsy since the 1930s [53].

At low doses, the main effect of amphetamine is to release dopamine and to a lesser extent norepinephrine through reverse efflux, via monoaminergic transporters, the DAT and NET transporters. At higher doses, monoaminergic depletion and inhibition of reuptake occurs. The d-isomer of amphetamine is more specific for dopaminergic transmission and is a better stimulant compound. Methamphetamine is more lipophilic than d-amphetamine and therefore has more central and fewer peripheral effects than d-amphetamine. The elimination half-life of these drugs is between 10 and 30 h.

Five reports concerned the use of amphetamines. Three Class II evidence studies [54, 55] showed that d-amphetamine and methamphetamine are effective treatments of excessive daytime sleepiness in short-term use (up to 4 weeks) at starting doses of 15–20 mg increasing up to 60 mg/day. One Class IV evidence study [56] showed that long-term drug treatment would result in only a minor reduction in irresistible sleep episode propensity.

The main adverse effects are minor irritability, hyperactivity, mood changes, headache, palpitations, sweating, tremors, anorexia, and insomnia [57], but doses of over 120% of the maximum recommended by the American Academy of Sleep Medicine are responsible for a significantly higher occurrence of psychosis, substance misuse, and psychiatric hospitalizations [58].

Tolerance to amphetamine effect may develop in up to one-third of patients [59]. There is little or no evidence of abuse and addiction in narcoleptic patients [60].

Dextroamphetamine, with a FDA category D classification, and methamphetamine, with a FDA category C classification, are contraindicated during conception and pregnancy.

Amphetamines are controlled drugs.

Methylphenidate (N06BA04)

Similar to the action of amphetamine, methylphenidate induces dopamine release, but, in contrast, it does not have any major effect on monoamine storage. The clinical effect of methylphenidate is supposed to be similar to that of amphetamines. However, clinical experience would argue for a slight superiority of amphetamines. In comparison with amphetamine, methylphenidate has a much shorter elimination half-life (2–7 h), and the daily dose may be divided into two or three parts. A sustained-release form is available and can be useful for some patients.

There were five reports on the use of methylphenidate. There was only one Class II evidence study showing a significant improvement for all dosages (10, 30, 60 mg/day) compared with baseline [61]. According to a Class IV evidence study [62], methylphenidate conveyed a good to excellent response in 68% of cases and according to another one [63] methylphenidate produced marked to moderate improvement in 90% of cases. On the MWT, the sleep latencies were increased up to 80% of controls with a 60 mg daily dose [64].

Adverse effects are the same as with amphetamines. However, methylphenidate probably has a better therapeutic index than d-amphetamine, with less reduction of appetite or increase in blood pressure [65]. Moreover, in a study assessing the neuronal toxicity of methamphetamine and methylphenidate, methylphenidate failed to induce sensitization to hyperlocomotion, while methamphetamine clearly induced behavioural sensitization [66].

Tolerance may develop. Abuse potential is low in narcoleptic patients.

Methylphenidate has no FDA classification because no adequate animal or human studies have been performed. It is contraindicated in pregnant women.

Other compounds

Mazindol (A08AA06)

Mazindol is an imidazolidine derivative with pharmacological effects similar to the amphetamines. It is a weak releasing agent for dopamine, but it also blocks dopamine and norepinephrine reuptake with high affinity. Its elimination half-life is around 10 h.

There were five reports on the use of mazindol in treating excessive daytime sleepiness in narcoleptic patients.

According to a Class II evidence study [54] mazindol was effective in reducing sleepiness at a dose of 2 + 2 mg/day (during 4 weeks) in 53–60% of subjects. In addition, several Class IV evidence studies [67–70] have shown a significant improvement of sleepiness in 50–75% of patients. Clinical experience suggests to start treatment at a low dosage of 1 mg/day, which may be effective in individual patients.

Adverse effects include dry mouth, nervousness, constipation, and less frequently nausea, vomiting, headache, dizziness, tachycardia and excessive sweating. Rare cases of pulmonary hypertension and cardiac valvular regurgitation have been reported. For this reason, it has been withdrawn from the market in several countries. Its use in narcolepsy is still warranted according to most experts, but as a third-line treatment and with close monitoring. Tolerance is uncommon, and abuse potential may be low [67]. Mazindol is classified as FDA category B without controlled studies in humans. It is contraindicated in pregnant women.

Selegiline (N04B0D1)

Selegiline is a potent irreversible monoamine oxidase B selective inhibitor. It is metabolically converted to desmethyl selegiline, amphetamine, and methamphetamine. The elimination half-life of the main metabolites is variable – 2.5 h for desmethyl selegiline, 18 h for amphetamine, and 21 h for methamphetamine. According to one Class II evidence study [71], selegiline, 10–40 mg daily, reduced irresistible episodes of sleep and sleepiness by up to 45%, and according to another [72], selegiline at a dose of at least 20 mg/day caused a significant improvement of daytime sleepiness and a reduction in irresistible episodes of sleep, as well as a dose-dependent rapid eye movement (REM) suppression during night-time sleep and naps. The results were similar in a Class IV evidence study [73] showing an improvement in 73% of patients. The use of selegiline is limited by potentially sympathomimetic adverse effects and interaction with other drugs. Co-administration of triptans and serotonin specific reuptake inhibitors is contraindicated. Abuse potential is low [71, 72].

Selegiline is another FDA category B drug without controlled studies in humans. It is contraindicated in pregnant women.

Pemoline (N06BA05)

Pemoline, an oxazolidine derivative with long half-life (12 h) and mild action, selectively blocks dopamine reuptake and only weakly stimulates dopamine release.

There were two reports on the use of pemoline in narcoleptic patients: a Class II evidence study [60] using three dosages (18.75, 56.25, and 112.50 mg/day), which did not show an improvement of wakefulness, and a Class IV evidence study [74], which showed a moderate to marked improvement in sleepiness in 65% of narcoleptic patients. However, due to potential lethal hepatotoxicity, the medication has been withdrawn from the market in most countries.

Behavioural treatments

Although non-pharmacological treatments of narcolepsy have more or less always been part of an integrative treatment concept, only a few systematic studies have been performed investigating the impact of such approaches on the symptoms of narcoleptic patients.

Class II and III evidence studies investigated the effects of various sleep–wake schedules on excessive daytime sleepiness and sleep in narcoleptic patients. However, most of these studies were extremely heterogeneous, and only two studies [75, 76] looked at the effects of a behavioural regime in a clinically meaningful time range (2–4 weeks). In the latter study, involving 29 treated narcoleptic patients randomly assigned to one of three treatment groups – (1) two 15-min naps per day, (2) a regular schedule for nocturnal sleep, and (3) a combination of scheduled naps and regular bedtimes – the best response was found in the third treatment group. All other studies considered only acute (1–2 days) manipulations. Among those, a study by Mullington and Broughton [77] tested two napping strategies: a single long nap placed 180 degrees out of phase with the nocturnal mid-sleep time (i.e. with the mid-nap point positioned 12 h after the nocturnal mid-sleep time), and five naps positioned equidistantly throughout the day, with the mid-nap time of the third nap set at 180 degrees out of phase with the nocturnal mid-sleep and the others equidistant between the hours of morning awakening and evening sleep onset. The two protocols tested resulted in a reaction time improvement, but no difference between long and multiple naps was disclosed. Most experts agree that patients should live a regular life: go to bed at the same hour each night and rise at the same time each day and, essentially, take one or more naps during the day.

Recommendations

The first-line pharmacological treatment of excessive daytime sleepiness and irresistible episodes of sleep is not unequivocal. In cases when the most disturbing symptom is excessive daytime sleepiness, modafinil should be prescribed based on its efficacy, limited adverse effects, and easiness of manipulation. Modafinil can be taken in variable doses from 100 to 400 mg/day, given in one dose in the morning or two doses, one in the morning and one early in the afternoon. However, it is possible to tailor the schedule and dose of administration according to the individual needs of the patient. On the other hand, when excessive daytime somnolence coexists with cataplexy and poor sleep, sodium oxybate may be prescribed, based on its well-evidenced efficacy on the three symptoms. However, this benefit should be balanced with its more delicate manipulation: the dose should be carefully titrated up to an adequate level over several weeks; the drug should not be used in association with other sedatives, respiratory depressants and muscle relaxants; vigilance should be held for the possible development of sleep-disordered breathing; and depressed patients should not be treated with this drug. Sodium oxybate should be given at a starting dose of 4.5 g/night, increasing by increments of 1.5 g at 4-week intervals. Adverse effects may require to reduce the dose and titrate more slowly. The optimal response on excessive daytime sleepiness may take as long as 8–12 weeks. Supplementation with modafinil is generally more successful than sodium oxybate alone. Methylphenidate may be an option in case modafinil is insufficiently active and sodium oxybate is not recommended. Moreover, the short-acting effect of methylphenidate is of interest when modafinil needs to be supplemented at a specific time of the day, or in situations where maximum alertness is required. Methylphenidate LP and mazindol may be of interest in a limited number of cases.

Behavioural treatment measures are always advisable. Essentially, the studies available support on a B Level the recommendation to have regular nocturnal sleep times and to take planned naps during the day, as naps temporarily decrease sleep tendency and shorten reaction time. Because of varying performance demands and limitations on work or home times for taking them, naps are best scheduled on a patient-by-patient basis.

Cataplexy

Sodium oxybate is the single drug approved for cataplexy by the EMEA and the FDA. In addition, tricyclic antidepressants have the indication 'cataplexy' at the national agency level in Italy, Spain, Sweden, Switzerland, and the United Kingdom, as do SSRIs in Belgium, Denmark, France, Germany, and Switzerland. All other medications are 'off-label'.

Sodium oxybate (N07XX04)

A Class I evidence study [42] and a Class IV evidence study [45] have shown a significant dose-dependent reduction of the number of cataplectic attacks in large samples of patients (136 in the first study and 118 in the second) using doses of sodium oxybate 3–9 g nightly in two doses, which were significant at 4 weeks and maximal after 8 weeks. In addition, the Class I evidence study [78] was conducted to demonstrate the long-term efficacy of sodium oxybate for the treatment of cataplexy. Fifty-five narcoleptic patients with cataplexy who had received continuous treatment with sodium oxybate for 7–44 months (mean 21 months) were enrolled in a double-blind treatment withdrawal paradigm. During the 2-week double-blind phase, the abrupt cessation of sodium oxybate therapy in the placebo group resulted in a significant increase in the number of cataplectic attacks compared with the patients who remained on sodium oxybate. Ultimately, the Xyrem International Study Group [79] conducted a Class I evidence study with 228 adult narcolepsy with cataplexy patients randomized to receive 4.5, 6, or 9 g sodium oxybate nightly or placebo for 8 weeks. Compared with placebo, doses of 4.5, 6, and 9 g sodium oxybate for 8 weeks resulted in statistically significant median decreases in weekly cataplexy attacks of 57.0, 65.0, and 84.7%, respectively.

Adverse effects and abuse potential have been dealt with above.

Non-specific monoamine uptake inhibitors (N06AA)

The first use of tricyclics for treating cataplexy dates back to 1960, with imipramine [80]. This was followed by desmethylimipramine [81], clomipramine [82], and protriptyline [83].

Clomipramine, a drug that is principally a serotoninergic reuptake inhibitor but metabolizes rapidly into desmethyl clomipramine, an active metabolite with principally adrenergic reuptake inhibitory properties, has been the most widely evaluated for cataplexy, with one Class III evidence study [84] and four Class IV evidence studies [56, 82, 85, 86]. All these studies have shown a complete abolition or decrease in severity and frequency of cataplexy at doses of 25–75 mg daily. However, low doses of 10–20 mg daily are often very effective, and it is always advisable to start with these.

Adverse effects consist of anticholinergic effects including dry mouth, sweating, constipation, tachycardia, weight increase, hypotension, difficulty in urinating, and impotence. One trial [86] mentioned the development of tolerance after 4.5 months. Patients may experience with tricyclics a worsening or *de novo* onset of REM sleep behaviour disorder. Moreover, there is a risk, if the tricyclics are suddenly withdrawn, of a marked increase in the number and severity of cataplectic attacks, a situation referred to as 'rebound cataplexy', or even 'status cataplecticus'. Tolerance to the effects of tricyclics may develop.

Animal studies have not shown teratogenic properties, and epidemiological studies performed in a limited number of women have not shown any risk of malformation in the fetus (FDA category B). However, the newborns of mothers submitted to longstanding treatment with high doses of antidepressants may show symptoms of atropine intoxication. Thus, if cataplexy is mild, it is advisable to cease the anticataplectic drug before conception. When cataplexy is severe, the risk of injury during pregnancy may be greater than the risks caused to the infant by the drug.

Newer antidepressants

Selective serotonin reuptake inhibitors (SSRIs) (N06AB)

These compounds are much more selective than tricyclic antidepressants towards the serotoninergic transporter. However it has been shown that their activity against cataplexy is correlated with the levels of their active noradrenergic metabolites [87]. In comparison with tricyclics, higher doses are required, and the effects are less pronounced [88].

According to a Class II evidence study [89], femoxetine, 600 mg/day, reduced cataplexy. In addition, two Class III evidence studies [90, 91] have shown fluoxetine (20–60 mg/day), and one Class III evidence study [84] has shown fluvoxamine (25–200 mg/day), to be mildly active on cataplexy. In Class IV evidence studies, citalopram, a very selective serotonin uptake inhibitor, proved active in three cases of intractable cataplexy [92], and escitalopram, the most selective serotonin uptake inhibitor, led to a significant decline in the number of cataplectic attacks per week while excessive daytime sleepiness remained unchanged [93].

Adverse effects are less pronounced than with tricyclics. They include CNS excitation, gastrointestinal upset, movement disorders, and sexual difficulties. The risk of a marked increase in number and severity of cataplectic attacks has been documented after discontinuation of SSRIs [94]. Tolerance to SSRIs does not develop.

Studies performed in animals did not provide any evidence of malformation (FDA category B). However, clinical studies are not sufficient to assess a possible risk for the human fetus. Thus, the use of SSRIs is not recommended in narcoleptic pregnant women.

Norepinephrine reuptake inhibitors
In a Class III evidence study [95], viloxazine (N06AX09) at a 100 mg dose daily significantly reduced cataplexy. The main advantage of this compound rests in its limited adverse effects (nausea and headache in one subject only out of 22).

In a Class IV evidence study [96], reboxetine (N06AX18) at a daily dose of 2–10 mg significantly reduced cataplexy. Treatment was generally well tolerated, with only minor adverse effects being reported (dry mouth, hyperhydrosis, constipation, restlessness). Atomoxetine (N06BA09) (36–100 mg/day) has been used anecdotally with success in cataplexy [97]. Of note, however, atomoxetine has been shown to slightly but significantly increase heart rate and blood pressure in large samples. Thus caution is needed.

Norepinephrine/serotonin reuptake inhibitors
Venlafaxine (N06AX16) (150–375 mg/day), was given to four subjects for a period of 2–7 months [98]. An initial improvement in both excessive daytime sleepiness and cataplexy was reported by all subjects. No subjective adverse effects were observed apart from slight insomnia in two subjects. Venlafaxine's main adverse effects are gastrointestinal. Increased heart rate and blood pressure may be observed at doses of 300 mg or more. Tolerance was reported in one subject. Venlafaxine is not recommended in pregnant narcoleptic women.

Recently, a pilot study on duloxetine, a new norepinephrine and serotonin reuptake inhibitor, was conducted in three patients who had narcolepsy with cataplexy. A rapid anticataplectic activity associated with excessive daytime sleepiness improvement was observed [99].

Other compounds

Mazindol (A08AA06)
Mazindol has an anticataplectic property in addition to its alerting effect. According to a Class II evidence study [54], mazindol at a dose of 2 + 2 mg/day (over 4 weeks) did not alter the frequency of cataplexy. On the other hand, in one Class IV evidence study [70], the 'percentage of efficacy' was 50%, and in another Class IV evidence study [68], 85% of subjects reported a significant improvement in terms of cataplexy.

Potential adverse effects have been reviewed above.

Selegiline (N04B0D1)
Selegiline has a potent anticataplectic effect in addition to its relatively good alerting effect. According to one Class I evidence study, selegiline reduced cataplexy up to 89% at a dose of 10–40 mg [71], and, according to a second, reduced cataplexy significantly at a dose of 10 mg × 2 [72]. Adverse effects and interaction with other drugs have been referred to above.

Amphetamine (N06BA01)
As previously indicated, the main effect of amphetamines is to release dopamine and, to a lesser extent, norepinephrine and serotonin. The effect of amphetamine on norepinephrine neurons, in particular, may help to control cataplexy. This may be an important factor in patients who switch from amphetamine to modafinil and find that their mild cataplexy is no longer controlled.

Behavioural therapy
The single non-pharmacological approach known to specifically reduce the frequency and severity of cataplexy, which however has not been empirically studied, is to avoid precipitating factors. Because cataplexy is tightly linked to strong, particularly positive, emotions, the most important precipitating factor is social contact. Indeed, social withdrawal is frequently seen in narcolepsy and is helpful in reducing cataplexy, but it can hardly be considered as a recommendation or 'treatment'.

Recommendations

Based on several Class I evidence (Level A rating) studies, the first-line pharmacological treatment of cataplexy is sodium oxybate at a starting dose of 4.5 g/night divided into two equal doses of 2.25 g/night. The dose may be increased to a maximum of 9 g/night, divided into two equal doses of 4.5 g/night, by increments of 1.5 g at 2-week intervals. Adverse effects may need the dose to be reduced and titrated more slowly. Most patients will start to feel better within the first few days, but the optimal response at any given dose may take as long as 8–12 weeks. As indicated above, the drug should not be used in association with other sedatives, respiratory depressants, and muscle relaxants, vigilance should be held for the possible development of sleep-disordered breathing, and depressed patients should not be treated with the drug. Second-line pharmacological treatments are antidepressants. Tricyclic antidepressants, particularly clomipramine (10–75 mg), are potent anticataplectic drugs. However, they have the drawback of anticholinergic adverse effects. The starting dosage should always be as low as possible. SSRIs are slightly less active but have fewer adverse effects. The norepinephrine/serotonin reuptake inhibitor venlafaxine is widely used today but lacks any published clinical evidence of efficacy. The norepinephrine reuptake inhibitors, such as reboxetine and atomoxetine, also lack published clinical evidence. Given the well-evidenced efficacy of sodium oxybate and antidepressants, the place for other compounds is fairly limited. There is no accepted behavioural treatment of cataplexy.

Hallucinations and sleep paralysis

The treatment of hallucinations and sleep paralysis is considered as a treatment of REM-associated phenomena. Most studies have focused much more on the treatment of cataplexy. An improvement in cataplexy is most often associated with a reduction in hallucinations and sleep paralysis. A Class I evidence study [42] did not reveal any significant differences in hypnagogic hallucinations and sleep paralysis when compared with placebo. However, this study was not powered to detect a difference in hypnagogic hallucinations. On the other hand, a Class IV evidence study [44] with 21 narcoleptic patients administered increasing nightly doses of sodium oxybate up to 9 g showed an increasing number of patients reporting fewer hypnagogic hallucinations and less sleep paralysis. There is no report on any attempt to modify the occurrence of hypnagogic hallucinations or sleep paralysis by behavioural techniques.

Recommendations

Recommendations are as for cataplexy.

Poor sleep

Benzodiazepines (N05CD) and non-benzodiazepines (N05CF)

A single Class III evidence study [100] has shown an improvement in sleep efficiency and overall sleep quality with triazolam 0.25 mg given for two nights only. Adverse effects were not recorded. No effect of improved sleep in excessive daytime sleepiness was recorded. No study has been performed with either zopiclone or zolpidem or zaleplon.

Sodium oxybate (N07XX04)

The US Xyrem studies have shown a significant decrease in the number of night-time awakenings, with sodium oxybate 9 g [42] and a significant improvement of nocturnal sleep quality ($p = 0.001$) characterized by increased slow wave sleep [45]. Most importantly, a recent Class I evidence study in patients receiving sodium oxybate and sodium oxybate/modafinil evidenced a median increase in stages 3 and 4 and delta power, and a median decrease in nocturnal awakenings [101]. Interestingly, clinical experience suggests that poor sleep is the first symptom to improve with sodium oxybate, and that efficacy on poor sleep foresees efficacy on the other symptoms.

The adverse effects are the same as already listed.

Modafinil (N06BA07)

In the US Modafinil in Narcolepsy Multicenter Study Group [32] a small improvement in sleep consolidation was evidenced through increased sleep efficiency. Thus, it is always advisable to wait for the effects of modafinil before prescribing a special treatment for disturbed nocturnal sleep in narcoleptic patients.

Behavioural therapy

No study has ever been conducted to investigate the effects of behavioural treatments on night-time sleep in narcoleptic patients, in clinically relevant settings.

Recommendations

According to recent studies with sodium oxybate, this agent appears as the most appropriate to treat poor sleep (Level A). Benzodiazepine or non-benzodiazepine hypnotics may be effective in consolidating nocturnal sleep (Level C). Unfortunately, objective evidence is lacking over intermediate or long-term follow-up. The improvement in poor sleep reported by some patients once established on modafinil is noteworthy.

Parasomnias

Narcoleptic patients often display vivid and frightening dreams and REM sleep behaviour disorder (RBD). Given the beneficial effects of sodium oxybate on disturbed nocturnal sleep, this medication might be of interest in the case of disturbed dreams. However, no systematic study of sodium oxybate on dreams of individuals with narcolepsy has ever been conducted.

In the case of RBD, its occurrence in narcoleptic patients is remarkable for three reasons. First, the age of onset of RBD in narcoleptic patients is younger than in the other forms of chronic RBD. Second, the frequency of the episodes is less marked and RBD events are usually less violent than in the other forms of RBD. Third, RBD may precede narcolepsy by several years.

There is no available report of any prospective, double-blind, placebo-controlled trial of any drug specific for RBD in narcoleptic subjects, and only a few case reports of narcoleptic subjects with RBD. The use of clonazepam was reported as successful in two cases [102, 103]. In one case [100], clonazepam led to the development of obstructive sleep apnoea syndrome. An alternative treatment is needed when patients affected with RBD do not respond or are intolerant to clonazepam. In a recent study involving 14 patients, two of whom had narcolepsy, melatonin was used successfully in 57% of cases at a dose of 3–12 mg per night [104]. Adverse effects such as sleepiness, hallucination, and headache were recorded in one third of patients.

Recommendations

Based on the available information, it is difficult to provide guidance for prescribing in parasomnias associated with narcolepsy other than to recommend conventional medications.

Associated features

Obstructive sleep apnoea/hypopnoea syndrome

According to several publications [105, 106], the prevalence of obstructive sleep apnoea/hypopnoea syndrome (OSAHS) is greater in narcoleptic patients than in the general population. One potential explanation is the frequency of obesity in narcolepsy, which could predispose to OSAHS. Only one Class IV study has described the effect of continuous positive airway pressure (CPAP) in narcolepsy patients with OSAHS: excessive daytime sleepiness did not improve in 11 of the 14 patients treated with CPAP [107].

Periodic limb movements in sleep

Periodic limb movements in sleep (PLMS) are more prevalent in narcolepsy than in the general population [106, 108]. This applies particularly to young narcoleptic patients. L-Dopa [109], GHB [110], and bromocriptine [111] are effective treatments of PLMS in narcolepsy patients. However, there is no documented effect on excessive daytime sleepiness.

Neuropsychiatric symptoms

No higher rate of psychotic manifestations has been evidenced in narcoleptic patients. On the other hand, depression is more frequent in narcoleptic patients than in the general population [112–115].

Antidepressant drugs and psychotherapy are indicated. However, there is no systematic study of these therapeutic procedures in depressed narcoleptic patients.

Recommendations

OSAHS should be treated no differently in narcoleptic patients than the general population, although it has been shown that CPAP does not improve excessive daytime sleepiness in most narcolepsy subjects. There is usually no need to treat PLMS in narcoleptic patients. Antidepressants and psychotherapy should be used in depressed narcoleptic patients (Level C) as in non-narcoleptic depressed patients.

Psychosocial support and counselling

Patients' groups

Interaction with those who have narcolepsy is often of great benefit to the patient and his or her spouse regarding the recognition of symptoms and possible countermeasures. Here are the website addresses of four important patient support groups:

- France : http://perso.wanadoo.fr/anc.paradoxal/
- Germany : http://dng-ev.org
- NL : http://www.narcolepsie.nl
- UK : http://www.narcolepsy.org.uk

Social workers

Social workers can provide support and counselling in various important areas such as career selection, adjustments at school or at work, and when financial or marital problems exist.

Recommendations

Interaction with narcoleptic patients and counselling from trained social workers are recommended (Level C).

Good Practice Points

A prerequisite before implementing a potentially life-long treatment is to establish an accurate diagnosis of narcolepsy with or without cataplexy, and to check for possible comorbidity. Following a complete interview, the patient should undergo an all-night polysomnography followed immediately by a MSLT. HLA typing is rarely helpful. CSF hypocretin-1 measurement may be of help and is added as diagnostic test in the revised International Classification of Sleep Disorders [3], particularly if the MSLT cannot be used or provides conflicting information. Levels of CSF hypocretin are significantly reduced or absent in cases of narcolepsy with cataplexy. In the absence of cataplexy, the value of measuring hypocretin is debatable.

Once diagnosed, patients must be given as much information as possible about their condition (the nature of the disorder, genetic implications, medications available, their potential adverse effects) to help them cope with a potentially debilitating condition.

Regular follow-up is essential to monitor response to treatment, adapt the treatment in case of insufficient response or adverse effects, and above all encourage the patient to persist with a management plan. Another polysomnographic evaluation of patients should be considered in case of worsening of symptoms or development of other symptoms, but not for evaluating treatment in general.

Future treatments

Current treatments for human narcolepsy are symptomatically based. However, given the major developments in understanding the neurobiological basis of the condition, new therapies are likely to emerge. It is imperative that neurologists remain aware of future developments, because of the implications for treating a relatively common and debilitating disease.

There are three focuses for future therapy:

- Symptomatic endocrine/transmitter-modulating therapies, including thyrotrophin-releasing hormone and thyrotrophin-releasing hormone agonists; slow-wave sleep enhancers (selective GABA-B agonists), and histaminergic H3 receptor antagonists/inverse agonists. Several histaminergic compounds are currently being studied for the treatment of excessive daytime sleepiness. A published pilot study has shown encouraging results [116].
- Hypocretin-based therapies: hypocretin agonists, hypocretin cell transplantation, and gene therapy.
- Immune-based therapies, particularly IVIg. These therapies are given close to disease onset and are supposed to modulate the presumed but not proven autoimmune process that causes the hypocretin deficiency. A beneficial effect in particular on cataplexy has been claimed [117]. Note, however, that all the studies were small and not blinded, that possible spontaneous fluctuations may have influenced outcome, and that the placebo effect may be large [118].

Conclusion

The recommendations expressed in these guidelines are based on the best currently available knowledge. However, developments in the field of narcolepsy are rapidly advancing, and the use of new symptomatic treatments and of treatments directed at replacing hypocretin or even preventing the loss of neurons containing the neuropeptide may become a reality in the near future.

Conflicts of interest

Dr Billiard was a member of the Xyrem (UCB Pharma) advisory board and received honoraria from UCB for invited talks.

Dr Dauvilliers was involved in a clinical trial with Cephalon and another one with Orphan. He is a member of the Xyrem (UCB Pharma) advisory board and has recently received honoraria from Cephalon.

Dr Dolenc-Groselj received honoraria from Medis (the Slovenian representative for Xyrem) for invited talks.

Dr Lammers is a member of the Xyrem (UCB Pharma) advisory board and has received honoraria from UCB for invited talks.

Dr Mayer received honoraria from Cephalon and UCB Pharma for invited talks. He was involved in one trial with Cephalon and two trials with Orphan drugs. He is a member of the Xyrem advisory board.

Dr Sonka was involved in two trials with Orphan and is currently involved in a trial with Cephalon. Dr Sonka is also a member of the Xyrem advisory board.

References

1. Westphal C. Eigentümliche mit Einschlafen verbundene Anfälle. *Arch Psychiatr Nervenkr* 1877;**7**:631–5.

2. Gelineau J. De la narcolepsie. *Gaz des Hôp (Paris)* 1880;**55**:626–8, 635–7.

3. American Academy of Sleep Medicine. *ICSD-2 – International Classification of Sleep Disorders: Diagnostic and Coding Manual*, 2nd edn. Westchester, IL: American Academy of Sleep Medicine, 2005.

4. Lin L, Faraco J, Li R, *et al*. The sleep disorder canine narcolepsy is caused by a mutation in the hypocretin (orexin) receptor 2 gene. *Cell* 1999;**98**:365–76.

5. Chemelli RM, Willie JT, Sinton CM, *et al*. Narcolepsy in orexin knockout mice: molecular genetics of sleep regulation. *Cell* 1999;**98**:437–51.

6. Nishino S, Ripley B, Overeem S, *et al*. Low CSF hypocretin (orexin) and altered energy homeostasis in human narcolepsy. *Ann Neurol* 2001;**50**:380–8.

7. Nishino S, Ripley B, Overeem S, Lammers GL, Mignot E. Hypocretin (orexin) deficiency in human narcolepsy. *Lancet* 2000;**355**(9197):39–40.

8. Ripley B, Fujiki N, Okura M, Mignot E, Nishino S. Hypocretin levels in sporadic and familial cases of canine narcolepsy. *Neurobiol Dis* 2001;**8**:525–34.

9. Billiard M, Bassetti C, Dauvilliers Y, *et al*. EFNS guidelines on management of narcolepsy. *Eur J Neurol* 2006;**13**:1035–48.

10. Standards of Practice Committee of the American Sleep Disorders Association. Practice parameters for the use of stimulants in the treatment of narcolepsy. *Sleep* 1994;**17**:348–51.

11. Littner M, Johnson SF, McCall WV, *et al*. Practice parameters for the treatment of narcolepsy: an update for 2000. *Sleep* 2001;**24**:451–66.

12. Britton T, Hansen A, Hicks J, *et al*. *Guidelines on the diagnosis and management of narcolepsy in adults and children. Evidence-based guidelines for the UK with graded recommendations*. Ashtead: Taylor Patten Communications, 2002.

13. Morgenthaler TI, Kapur VK, Brown T, *et al*, Standards of Practice Committee of the AASM. Practice parameters for the treatment of narcolepsy and other hypersomnias of central origin. *Sleep* 2007;**30**:1705–11.

14. Wise MS, Arand DL, Auger RR, Brooks SN, Watson NF. Treatment of narcolepsy and other hypersomnias of central origin. *Sleep* 2007;**30**:1712–27.

15. Keam S, Walker MC. Therapies for narcolepsy with or without cataplexy: evidence based review. *Curr Opin Neurol* 2007;**20**:699–703.

16. Brainin M, Barnes M, Baron JC, *et al*. Guidance for the preparation of neurological management guidelines by EFNS scientific task forces–revised recommendations 2004. *Eur J Neurol* 2004;**11**:577–81.

17. Ferraro L, Tanganelli S, O'Connor WT, Antonelli T, Rambert FA, Fuxe K. The vigilance promoting drug modafinil increases dopamine release in the rat nucleus accumbens via the involvement of a local GABAergic mechanism. *Eur J Pharmacol* 1996;**306**:33–9.

18. De Saint-Hilaire Z, Orosco M, Rouch C, Blanc G, Nicolaidis S. Variations in extracellular monoamines in the prefrontal cortex and medial hypothalamus after modafinil administration: a microdialysis study in rats. *Neuroreport* 2001;**12**:3533–7.

19. Wisor JP, Nishino S, Sora I, Uhl GH, Mignot E, Edgar DM. Dopaminergic role in stimulant-induced wakefulness. *J Neurosci* 2001;**21**:1787–94.

20. Gallopin T, Luppi PH, Rambert FA, Frydman A, Fort P. Effect of the wake-promoting agent modafinil on sleep-promoting neurons from the ventrolateral preoptic nucleus: an in vitro pharmacologic study. *Sleep* 2004;**27**:19–25.

21. Tanganelli S, Fuxe K, Ferraro L, Janson AM, Bianchi C. Inhibitory effects of the psychoactive drug modafinil on gamma-aminobutyric acid outflow from the cerebral cortex of the awake freely moving guinea-pig. Possible involvement of 5-Hydroxytryptamine mechanisms. *Naunyn Schmiedebergs Arch Pharmacol* 1992;**345**:461–5.

22. Ferraro L, Fuxe K, Tanganelli S, Tomasini MC, Rambert FA, Antonelli T. Differential enhancement of dialysate serotonin levels in distinct brain regions of the awake rat by modafinil: possible relevance for wakefulness and depression. *J Neurosci Res* 2002;**68**:107–12.

23. Ishizuka T, Sakamoto Y, Sakurai T, Yamatodani A. Modafinil increases histamine release in the anterior hypothalamus of rats. *Neurosci Lett* 2003;**339**:143–6.

24. Mignot E, Nishino S, Guilleminault C, Dement WC. Modafinil binds to the dopamine uptake carrier site with low affinity. *Sleep* 1994;**17**:436–7.

25. Ferraro L, Antonelli T, Tanganelli S, *et al.* The vigilance promoting drug modafinil increases extracellular glutamate levels in the medial preoptic area and the posterior hypothalamus of the conscious rat: prevention by local GABAA receptor blockade. *Neuropsychopharmacology* 1999;**20**:346–56.

26. Willie J, Renthal W, Chemelli RM, *et al.* Modafinil more effectively induces wakefulness in orexin-null mice than in wild-type littermates. *Neuroscience* 2005;**130**:983–95.

27. Palovaara S, Kivisto KT, Tapanainen P, Manninen P, Neuvonen PJ, Laine K. Effect of an oral contraceptive preparation containing ethinylestradiol and gestodene on CYP3A4 activity as measured by midazolam 1-hydroxylation. *Br J Clin Pharmacol* 2000;**50**:333–7.

28. Darwish M, Kirby M, Hellriegel ET, Robertson P Jr. Armodafinil and modafinil have substantially different pharmacokinetic profiles despite having the same terminal half-lives: analyses from three randomized, single dose, pharmacokinetic studies. *Clin Drug Investig* 2009;**29**: 613–23.

29. Billiard M, Besset A, Montplaisir J, *et al.* Modafinil: a double-blind multicenter study. *Sleep* 1994;**17**:(Suppl.): 107–12.

30. Broughton RJ, Fleming JAE, George CFP, *et al.* Randomized, double-blind, placebo-controlled crossover trial of modafinil in the treatment of excessive daytime sleepiness in narcolepsy. *Neurology* 1997;**49**:444–51.

31. U.S. Modafinil in Narcolepsy Multicenter Study Group. Randomized trial of modafinil for the treatment of pathological somnolence in narcolepsy. *Ann Neurol* 1998;**43**:88–97.

32. U.S. Modafinil in Narcolepsy Multicenter Study Group. Randomized trial of modafinil as a treatment for the excessive daytime somnolence of narcolepsy. *Neurology* 2000;**54**:1166–75.

33. Beusterien KM, Rogers AE, Walsleben JA, *et al.* Health-related quality of life effects of modafinil for treatment of narcolepsy. *Sleep* 1999;**22**:757–65.

34. Moldofsky H, Broughton RJ, Hill JD. A randomized trial of the long-term, continued efficacy and safety of modafinil in narcolepsy. *Sleep Med* 2000;**1**:109–16.

35. Mitler MM, Hirsh J, Hirshkowitz M, Guilleminault C. Long-term efficacy and safety of modafinil (PROVIGIL®) for the treatment of excessive daytime sleepiness associated with narcolepsy. *Sleep Med* 2000;**1**:231–43.

36. Schwartz JR, Feldman NT, Bogan RK, Nelson MT, Hughes RJ. Dosing regimen of modafinil for improving daytime wakefulness in patients with narcolepsy. *Clin Neuropharmacol* 2003;**26**:252–7.

37. Guilleminault C, Aftab FA, Karadeniz D, Philip P, Leger D. Problems associated with switch to modafinil – a novel alerting agent in narcolepsy. *Eur J Neurol* 2000;**7**:381–4.

38. Jasinski DR, Kovacevi-Ristanovi R. Evaluation of the abuse liability of modafinil and other drugs for excessive daytime sleepiness associated with narcolepsy. *Clin Neuropharmacol* 2000;**23**:149–56.

39. Harsh JR, Hayduk R, Rosenberg R, *et al.* The efficacy and safety of armodafinil as treatment for adults with excessive sleepiness associated with narcolepsy. *Curr Med Res Opin* 2006;**22**:761–74.

40. Carter LP, Koek W, France CP. Behavioral analyses of GHB: receptor mechanisms. *Pharmacol Ther* 2009;**121**:100–14.

41. Koek W, Carter LP, Lamb RJ, *et al.* Discriminative stimulus effects of gamma-hydroxybutyrate (GHB) in rats discriminating GHB from baclofen and diazepam. *J Pharmacol Exp Ther* 2005;**314**:170–9.

42. U.S. Xyrem® Multicenter Study Group. A randomized, double-blind, placebo-controlled multicenter trial comparing the effects of three doses of orally administered sodium oxybate with placebo for the treatment of narcolepsy. *Sleep* 2002;**25**:42–9.

43. Xyrem International Study Group. Further evidence supporting the use of sodium oxybate for the treatment of cataplexy: a double -blind, placebo-controlled study in 228 patients. *Sleep Med* 2005;**6**:415–21.

44. Mamelak M, Black J, Montplaisir J. A pilot study on the effects of sodium oxybate on sleep architecture and daytime alertness in narcolepsy. *Sleep* 2004;**27**:1327–34.

45. U.S. Xyrem® Multicenter Study Group. A 12-month, open-label multi-center extension trial of orally administered sodium oxybate for the treatment of narcolepsy. *Sleep* 2003;**26**:31–5.

46. Black J, Houghton WC. Sodium oxybate improves excessive daytime sleepiness in narcolepsy. *Sleep* 2006;**29**:939–46.

47. Fuller DE, Hornfeldt CS, Kelloway JS, Stahl PJ, Anderson TF. The Xyrem risk-management program. *Drug Saf* 2004;**27**:293–306.

48. Wang YG, Swick TJ, Carter LP, Thorpy MS, Benowitz NL. Safety overview of postmarketing and clinical experience of sodium oxybate (Xyrem): abuse, misuse, dependence and diversion. *J Clin Sleep Med* 2009;**5**:365–71.

49. Seeck-Hirschner M, Baier PC, Von Freier A, Aldenhoff J, Göder R. Increase in sleep-related breathing disturbances after treatment with sodium oxybate in patients with narcolepsy and mild obstructive sleep apnea syndrome: two case reports. *Sleep Med* 2009;**10**:154–5.

50. Zvosec DL, Smith SW, Hall BJ. Three deaths associated with use of Xyrem. *Sleep Med* 2009;**10**:490–3.

51. Lammers GJ, Bassetti C, Billiard M, , et al. Sodium oxybate is an effective and safe treatment for narcolepsy. *Sleep Med* 2010;**11**:105–6.

52. George CFP, Feldman N, Inhaber N, et al. A safety trial of sodium oxybate in patients with obstructive sleep apnea: acute effects on sleep-disordered breathing. *Sleep Med* 2009;**11**:38–42.

53. Prinzmetal M, Bloomberg W. The use of benzedrine for the treatment of narcolepsy. *JAMA* 1935;**105**:2051–4.

54. Shindler J, Schachter M, Brincat S, Parkes JD. Amphetamine, mazindol, and fencamfamin in narcolepsy. *BMJ* 1985;**290**:1167–70.

55. Mitler MM, Hajdukovic R, Erman M. Treatment of narcolepsy with methamphetamine. *Sleep* 1993;**16**:306–17.

56. Chen SY, Cloift SJ, Dahlitz MJ, Dunn G, Parkes JD. Treatment in the narcoleptic syndrome: self assessment of the action of dexamphetamine and clomipramine. *J Sleep Res* 1995;**4**:113–18.

57. Mitler MM, Aldrich MS, Koob GF, Zarcone V. Narcolepsy and its treatment with stimulants (ASDA standards of practice). *Sleep* 1994;**17**:352–71.

58. Auger RR, Goodman SH, Silber MH, Krahn LE, Pankratz VS, Slocumb NL. Risks of high-dose stimulants in the treatment of disorders of excessive somnolence: a case-control study. *Sleep* 2005;**28**:667–72.

59. Guilleminault C. Amphetamines and narcolepsy: use of the Stanford database. *Sleep* 1993;**16**:199–201.

60. Parkes JD, Dahlitz M. Amphetamine prescription. *Sleep* 1993;**16**:201–3.

61. Mitler MM, Shafor R, Hajdukovik R, Timms RM, Browman CP. Treatment of narcolepsy: objective studies on methylphenidate, pemoline, and protriptyline. *Sleep* 1986;**9**:260–4.

62. Yoss RE, Daly D. Treatment of narcolepsy with Ritalin. *Neurology* 1959;**9**:171–3.

63. Honda Y, Hishikawa Y, Takahashi Y. Long-term treatment of narcolepsy with methylphenidate (Ritalin®). *Curr Ther Res* 1979;**25**:288–98.

64. Mitler MM, Hajdukovic R, Erman M, Koziol JA. Narcolepsy. *J Clin Neurophysiol* 1990;**7**:93–118.

65. Guilleminault C, Carskadon MA, Dement WC. On the treatment of rapid eye movement narcolepsy. *Arch Neurol* 1974;**30**:90–3.

66. Narita M, Asato M, Shindo K, Kuzumaki N, Suzuki T. Differences in neuronal toxicity and molecular mechanisms in methamphetamine and methylphenidate. *Nihon Shinkei Seishin Yakurigaku Zasshi* 2009;**29**:115–20.

67. Parkes JD, Schachter M. Mazindol in the treatment of narcolepsy. *Acta Neurol Scand* 1979;**60**:250–4.

68. Vespignani H, Barroche G, Escaillas JP, Weber M. Importance of mazindol in the treatment of narcolepsy. *Sleep* 1984;**7**:274–5.

69. Alvarez B, Dahlitz M, Grimshaw J, Parkes JD. Mazindol in long-term treatment of narcolepsy. *Lancet* 1991;**337**:1293–4.

70. Iijima S, Sugita Y, Teshima Y, Hishikawa Y. Therapeutic effects of mazindol on narcolepsy. *Sleep* 1986;**9**:265–8.

71. Hublin C, Partinen M, Heinonen E, Puuka P, Salmi T. Selegiline in the treatment of narcolepsy. *Neurology* 1994;**44**:2095–101.

72. Mayer G, Meier-Ewert K. Selegiline hydrochloride treatment in narcolepsy. A double-blind, placebo-controlled study. *Clin Neuropharmacol* 1995;**18**:306–19.

73. Reinish LW, MacFarlane JG, Sandor P, Shapiro CM. REM changes in narcolepsy with selegiline. *Sleep* 1995;**18**:362–7.

74. Honda Y, Hishikawa Y. A long-term treatment of narcolepsy and excessive daytime sleepiness with pemoline (Bentanamin®). *Curr Ther Res* 1980;**27**:429–41.

75. Rogers AE, Aldrich MS. The effect of regularly scheduled naps on sleep attacks and excessive daytime sleepiness associated with narcolepsy. *Nurs Res* 1993;**42**:111–7.

76. Rogers AE, Aldrich MS, Lin X. Comparison of three different sleep schedules for reducing daytime sleepiness in narcolepsy. *Sleep* 2001;**24**:385–91.

77. Mullington J, Broughton R. Scheduled naps in the management of daytime sleepiness in narcolepsy-cataplexy. *Sleep* 1993;**16**:444–56.

78. U.S. Xyrem® Multicenter Study Group. Sodium oxybate demonstrates long-term efficacy for the treatment of cataplexy in patients with narcolepsy. *Sleep Med* 2004;**5**:119–23.

79. The Xyrem International Study Group. A double-blind, placebo-controlled study demonstrates sodium oxybate is effective for the treatment of excessive daytime sleepiness in narcolepsy. *J Clin Sleep Med* 2005;**1**:391–7.

80. Akimoto H, Honda Y, Takahashi Y. Pharmacotherapy in narcolepsy. *Dis Nerv Syst* 1960;**21**:1–3.

81. Hishikawa Y, Ida H, Nakai K, Kaneko Z. Treatment of narcolepsy with imipramine (tofranil) and desmethylimipramine (pertofran). *J Neurol Sci* 1965;**3**:453–61.

82. Passouant P, Baldy-Moulinier M. Données actuelles sur le traitement de la narcolepsie. Action des imipraminiques. *Concours Med* 1970;**92**:1967–70.

83. Schmidt HS, Clark RW, Hyman PR. Protriptyline: an effective agent in the treatment of the narcolepsy-cataplexy syndrome and hypersomnia. *Am J Psychiatry* 1977;**134**:183–5.

84. Schachter M, Parkes JD. Fluvoxamine and clomipramine in the treatment of cataplexy. *J Neurol Neurosurg Psychiatry* 1980;**43**:171–4.

85. Shapiro CM. Treatment of cataplexy with clomipramine. *Arch Neurol* 1975;**32**:653–6.

86. Guilleminault C, Raynal D, Takahashi S, Carkadon M, Dement W. Evaluation of short-term and long-term

treatment of the narcolepsy syndrome with clomipramine hydrochloride. *Acta Neurol Scand* 1976;**54**:71–87.

87. Nishino S, Arrigoni J, Shelton J, Dement WC, Mignot E. Desmethyl metabolites of serotonergic uptake inhibitors are more potent for suppressing canine cataplexy than their parent compounds. *Sleep* 1993;**16**:706–12.

88. Nishino S, Mignot E. Pharmacological aspects of human and canine narcolepsy. *Prog Neurobiol* 1997;**52**:27–78.

89. Schrader H, Kayed K, Bendixen Markset AC, Treidene HE. The treatment of accessory symptoms in narcolepsy: a double-blind cross-over study of a selective serotonin reuptake inhibitor (femoxetine) versus placebo. *Acta Neurol Scand* 1986;**74**:297–303.

90. Langdon N, Bandak S, Shindler J, Parkes JD. Fluoxetine in the treatment of cataplexy. *Sleep* 1986;**9**:371–2.

91. Frey J, Darbonne C. Fluoxetine suppresses human cataplexy: a pilot study. *Neurology* 1994;**44**:707–9.

92. Thirumalai SS, Shubin RA. The use of citalopram in resistant cataplexy. *Sleep Med* 2000;**1**:313–16.

93. Sonka K, Kemlink D, Pretl M. Cataplexy treated with escitalopram – clinical experience. *Neuroendocrinol Lett* 2006;**27**:174–6.

94. Poryazova R, Siccoli M, Werth E, Bassetti C. Unusually prolonged rebound cataplexy after withdrawal of fluoxetine. *Neurology* 2005;**65**:967–8.

95. Guilleminault C, Mancuso J, Salva MA, *et al.* Viloxazine hydrochloride in narcolepsy: a preliminary report. *Sleep* 1986;**9**: 275–9.

96. Larrosa O, de la Liave Y, Barrio S, Granizo JJ, Garcia-Borreguero D. Stimulant and anticataplectic effects of reboxetine in patients with narcolepsy. *Sleep* 2001;**24**:282–5.

97. Niederhofer H. Atomoxetine also effective in patients suffering from narcolepsy. *Sleep* 2005;**28**:1189.

98. Smith M, Parkes JD, Dahlitz M. Venlafaxine in the treatment of the narcoleptic syndrome. *J Sleep Res* 1996;**5**(Suppl. 1):217.

99. Izzi F, Placidi F, Marciani MG. Effective treatment of narcolepsy-cataplexy with duloxetine. A report of 3 cases. *Sleep Med* 2009;**10**:153–4.

100. Thorpy MJ, Snyder M, Aloe FS, Ledereich PS, Starz KE. Short-term triazolam use improves nocturnal sleep of narcoleptics. *Sleep* 1992;**15**:212–16.

101. Black J, Pardi D, Hornfeldt CS, Inhaber N. The nightly administration of sodium oxybate results in significant reduction in the nocturnal sleep disruption of patients with narcolepsy. *Sleep Med* 2009;**10**:829–35.

102. Schuld A, Kraus T, Haack M, Hinze-Selch D, Pollmächer T. Obstructive sleep apnea syndrome induced by clonazepam in a narcoleptic patient with REM-sleep-behavior disorder. *J Sleep Res* 1999;**8**:321–2.

103. Yeh SB, Schenck CH. A case of marital discord and secondary depression with attempted suicide resulting from REM sleep behavior disorder in a 35-year-old woman. *Sleep Med* 2004;**5**:151–4.

104. Boeve BF, Silber MH, Ferman TJ. Melatonin for treatment of REM sleep behaviour disorder in neurologic disorders: results in 14 patients. *Sleep Med* 2003;**4**:281–4.

105. Baker TL, Guilleminault C, Nino-Murcia G, Dement WC. Comparative polysomnographic study of narcolepsy and idiopathic central nervous system hypersomnia. *Sleep* 1986;**9**:232–42.

106. Mayer G, Kesper K, Peter H, Ploch T, Leinweber T, Peter JH. Comorbidity in narcoleptic patients. *Dtsch Med Wochenschr* 2002;**127**:1942–6.

107. Sansa G, Iranzo A, Santamaria J. Obstructive sleep apnea in narcolepsy. *Sleep Med* 2010;**11**:93–5.

108. Montplaisir J, Michaud M, Denesle R, Gosselin A. Periodic leg movements are not more prevalent in insomnia or hypersomnia but are specifically associated with sleep disorders involving a dopaminergic impairment. *Sleep Med* 2000;**1**:163–7.

109. Boivin DB, Montplaisir J, Poirier G. The effects of L-dopa on periodic leg movements and sleep organization in narcolepsy. *Clin Neuropharmacol* 1989;**16**:339–45.

110. Bedard MA, Montplaisir J, Godbout R, Lapierre O. Nocturnal gamma-hydroxybutyrate. Effect on periodic leg movements and sleep organization of narcoleptic patients. *Clin Neuropharmacol* 1989;**12**:29–36.

111. Boivin DB, Lorrain D, Montplaisir J. Effects of bromocriptine on periodic limb movements in human narcolepsy. *Neurology* 1993;**43**:2134–6.

112. Roth B, Nevsimalova S. Depression in narcolepsy and hypersomnia. *Schweiz Arch Neurol Psychiatr* 1975;**116**:291–300.

113. Broughton RJ, Ghanem Q, Hishikawa Y, Sugita Y, Nevsimalova S, Roth B. Life effects of narcolepsy in 180 patients from North America, Asia and Europe compared to matched controls. *Can J Neurol Sci* 1981;**8**:299–304.

114. Kales A, Soldatos CR, Bixler EO, *et al.* Narcolepsy-cataplexy. II. Psychosocial consequences and associated psychopathology. *Arch Neurol* 1982;**39**:169–71.

115. Vourdas A, Shneerson JM, Gregory CA, *et al.* Narcolepsy and psychopathology; is there an association? *Sleep Med* 2002;**3**:353–60.

116. Lin JS, Dauvilliers Y, Arnulf I, *et al.* An inverse agonist of the histamine H(3) receptor improves wakefulness in narcolepsy. Studies in orexin –/– mice and patients. *Neurobiol Dis* 2008;**30**:74–83.

117. Dauvilliers Y. Follow-up of four narcolepsy patients treated with intravenous immunoglobulins. *Ann Neurol* 2006;**60**:153.

118. Fronczek R, Verschuuren J, Lammers GJ. Response to intravenous immunoglobulins and placebo in a patient with narcolepsy with cataplexy. *J Neurol* 2007;**254**: 1607–8.

CHAPTER 39
Sleep disorders in neurodegenerative disorders and stroke

P. Jennum,[1] J. Santamaria Cano,[2] C. Bassetti,[3] P. Clarenbach,[4] B. Högl,[5] J. Mathis,[6] R. Poirrier,[7] K. Sonka,[8] E. Svanborg,[9] L. Dolenc Groselj,[10] D. Kaynak,[11] M. Kruger,[12] A. Papavasiliou,[13] Z. Zahariev[14]

[1]Glostrup Hospital, University of Copenhagen, Denmark; [2]Hospital Clinic of Barcelona, Spain; [3]University Hospital Zurich, Switzerland; [4]Evangelisches Johannes-Krankenhaus, Germany; [5]Medical University of Innsbruck, Austria; [6]University Hospital, Inselspital, Bern, Switzerland; [7]CHU Sart Tilman, Liège, Belgium; [8]Charles University of Prague, Czech Republic; [9]Division of Clinical Neurophysiology, Linköping, Sweden; [10]University Medical Centre, Ljubljana, Slovenia; [11]Dokuz Eylu l University, Izmir, Turkey; [12]Hôpital de la Ville, Luxembourg; [13]Palia Pendeli Children's Hospital, Athens, Greece; [14]High Medical School, Plovdiv, Bulgaria

Introduction

Sleep is an active process generated and modulated by a complex set of neural systems located mainly in the hypothalamus, brainstem, and thalamus. Sleep is altered in many neurological diseases due to several mechanisms: lesions of the brain areas that control sleep and wakefulness, lesions or diseases that produce pain, reduced mobility, and treatments. Excessive daytime sleepiness (EDS), sleep fragmentation, insomnia, sleep-disordered breathing (SDB), nocturnal behavioural phenomena such as rapid eye movement (REM) sleep behaviour disorder or nocturnal seizures, restless legs syndrome, and periodic leg movement syndrome (PLMS) are common symptoms and findings in neurological disorders. Sleep disorders may precede and influence the disease course in neurological diseases, involving daytime functioning, quality of life, morbidity, and mortality.

Diagnostic and treatment procedures and the treatment of sleep disorders have developed considerably in recent years. There are thus increased opportunities for the management of sleep disorders associated with neurological diseases.

European Handbook of Neurological Management: Volume 1, 2nd edition. Edited by N. E. Gilhus, M. P. Barnes and M. Brainin.
© 2011 Blackwell Publishing Ltd.

The current guideline will focus on *neurodegenerative disorders* and *stroke*, with an emphasis on *sleep breathing disorders* in neurological disease, and is an update from a former review [1] in accordance to European Federation of Neurological Societies (EFNS) guidelines [2].

The review will cover three main areas:
1. tauopathies (Alzheimer's disease, progressive supranuclear palsy, and corticobasal degeneration);
2. synucleinopathies (Parkinson's disease, multiple system atrophy [MSA], and dementia with Lewy bodies [DLB]);
3. stroke, amyotrophic lateral sclerosis (ALS), myotonic dystrophy, myasthenia gravis, and spinocerebellar ataxias.

Search strategy

The literature search included PUBMED and the Cochrane Database. These were searched until 2009 or over as much of this range as possible, looking for the different sleep disorders and symptoms in each of the most frequent or relevant degenerative neurological disorders and stroke. Language of writing was restricted to European languages. Studies considered for inclusion were, when possible, randomized controlled trials of adult patients, in any setting, suffering a neurodegenerative disorder (motor neuron disease, Parkinson's disease, Alzheimer's disease) or stroke. There had to be an explicit complaint of insomnia, parasomnia, or hypersomnia in the study participants. We also included observational studies. Abstracts were selected by the chairmen and independently inspected by individual members of the task force; full papers were obtained where necessary. A classification of the different studies according to evidence levels for therapeutic interventions and diagnostic measures will be done in accordance with the guidance [2]. The panel will discuss what possible diagnostic tests and health care interventions could be recommended in each particular disease.

Method for reaching consensus

Where there was uncertainty, further discussion was sought by the panel. Data extraction and quality assessments were undertaken independently by the panel reviewers.

Sleep disorders

Classification of sleep disorders

The International Classification of Sleep Disorders version 2 (ICSD-2) lists 95 sleep disorders [3]. The ISCD-2 has eight major categories:

1. Insomnias
2. Sleep-related breathing disorders
3. Hypersomnias not due to a sleep-related breathing disorder
4. Circadian rhythm sleep disorders
5. Parasomnias
6. Sleep-related movement disorders
7. Isolated symptoms
8. Other sleep disorders.

Only a selected number of the sleep disorders related to neurological diseases will be mentioned in this paper.

Insomnia

Insomnias are defined by a complaint of repeated difficulties with sleep initiation, sleep maintenance, duration, consolidation, or quality that occurs despite adequate time and opportunity for sleep, and that result in some form of daytime impairment.

Insomnias can be divided into acute and chronic forms. The acute form, also termed adjustment insomnia,

can usually be attributed to a well-defined circumstance, while chronic insomnia is often a consequence of conditional (psychophysiological) factors, is idiopathic, or is found in patients with psychiatric, medical, or neurological disorders. The latter may be due to degeneration or dysfunction of the central nervous system areas involved in sleep regulation, or due to motor or sensory symptoms produced by the disease (pain, reduced nocturnal mobility, nocturnal motor activity, etc.) that lower the threshold for arousal from sleep. Finally, insomnia may be caused by the alerting effects of the drugs employed in the treatment of neurological diseases.

Sleep-disordered breathing (SDB)

These disorders are characterized by disordered breathing during sleep. A uniform syndrome recommendation was suggested in 1999 by the American Academy of Sleep Medicine [4], which is included in ICSD-2:

1. Obstructive sleep apnoea syndrome (OSAS)
2. Central sleep apnoea–hypopnoea syndrome (CSAHS)
3. Cheyne–Stokes breathing syndrome (CSBS)
4. Sleep-related hypoventilation/hypoxaemic syndromes (SHVS).

For a more thorough review of SDB, see the EFNS guideline [1].

EDS not due to a sleep-related breathing disorder

Hypersomnias (EDS) is defined by the inability to stay fully alert and awake during the day, resulting in unintended lapses into sleep. EDS should be separated from fatigue, which refer to physical or mental weariness. The most common disorders in this group are narcolepsy, idiopathic hypersomnia, insufficient sleep, and the use of sedating medication. EDS is also commonly reported in patients with neurological disease including neurodegeneration, post-stroke, inflammation, tumour, injury, or brain trauma, and may be caused by degeneration of the sleep–wake centres, sleep fragmentation, or medication. Hypersomnia in a narrow sense is describing a prolonged major sleep episode, usually beyond 10 hours. This phenomenon is typical in "'idiopathic hypersomnia with prolonged sleep time', but is also reported in 'non-organic hypersomnia' (ICSD-2). The diagnostic work-up should always consider the possibility of sleep insufficiency syndrome or poor sleep hygiene.

Circadian rhythm disorders

Circadian rhythm disorders are defined as a misalignment between the patient's sleep pattern and the pattern that is desired or regarded as the societal norm. Most of the conditions observed in this group are associated with external factors like shift work, jet lag or social habits, but in relation to neurological diseases, conditions that destruct the neural input to the suprachiasmatic nucleus (e.g. complete bilateral retinal, optic nerve, chiasm, or hypothalamic lesions) may induce a condition that resembles circadian disorders.

Parasomnias

Parasomnias are undesirable sensorimotor events that appear exclusively during sleep. Parasomnias are disorders of arousal, partial arousal, and sleep stage transition. These disorders do not primarily cause a complaint of insomnia or excessive sleepiness, but frequently involve abnormal behaviours during sleep. Many of the disorders are common in children, but some are also present in adults. Parasomnias are subdivided into the following groups:

1. disorders of arousal from non-REM sleep: confusional arousal, sleep walking, and sleep terror;

2. parasomnias usually associated with REM sleep: REM sleep behaviour disorder (RBD), recurrent isolated sleep paralysis, and nightmare disorder;

3. Other parasomnias, such as enuresis, sleep-related groaning (catathrenia), exploding head syndrome, sleep-related hallucinations, and eating disorders.

Of these parasomnias, RBD has a particular relationship to neurodegenerative diseases.

REM sleep behaviour disorder (RBD)

This disorder is characterized by vigorous movements occurring during REM sleep associated with an abnormal absence of the physiological muscle atonia and with increased phasic electromyographic (EMG) activity during REM sleep [5–7]. Diagnostic criteria are:

• the presence of REM sleep without atonia: the EMG finding of excessive amounts of sustained or intermittent elevation of fragmented EMG tone, or excessive phasic submental or (upper or lower extremity) EMG twitching;

• one or both of the following:

   a. sleep-related injuries, potentially injurious, or disruptive behaviours in the history;

b. abnormal REM sleep behaviours documented during polysomnography (PSG) monitoring;

• an absence of electroencephalographic (EEG) epileptiform activity during REM sleep unless RBD can be clearly distinguished from any concurrent REM sleep-related seizure disorder;

• the sleep disturbance not being better explained by another sleep disorder, medical or neurological disorder, mental disorder, or medication use or substance use disorder.

The patient and those sharing the bed can be injured. RBD is observed in the majority of patients with MSA, in DLB, and in a significant proportion of patients with Parkinson's disease. RBD is also commonly observed in diffuse Lewy body (DLB) and Machado–Joseph disease [8–19]. Patients with isolated RBD have a significant risk of developing Parkinson's disease, DLB, or MSA, especially if other brainstem manifestations such as changes reduced smell, depression, mild cognitive impairment, or incontinence are present [6, 10, 20]. The occurrence of hallucinations in Parkinson's disease is related to the presence of RBD [8]. Reduced striatal dopamine transporters have been observed in these patients [21]. RBDs are strongly linked to narcolepsy with cataplexy, especially in patients with hypocretin deficiency [22], and are further observed in a number of other diseases, for example stroke and multiple sclerosis. A confident diagnosis relies on a full PSG recording, preferably with a synchronized audiovisual recording.

There is a need for further clarification of the EMG abnormalities in RBD, with special emphasis on muscle tone, motor activity (number of movements, duration, and intensity), and their relation to sleep stages. These are is currently undergoing clarification and evaluation.

Sleep-related movement disorders

Sleep-related movement disorders are characterized by relatively simple, usually stereotypic movements that disturb sleep to complex movements of different intensity, duration and periodicities or lack of it. Periodic limb movements (PLM), restless legs syndrome (RLS), bruxism, leg cramps, rhythmic movement disorders and other sleep-related movement disorders are classified under this group. Of these RLS and PLM are of particular interest in patients with neurodegenerative disorders. Of special focus is subdivision into different types of stage dependent movements during sleep, as observed in the majority of neurodegenerative disorders, RBD and in patients with narcolepsy with cataplexy. This area is currently undergoing clarification and evaluation.

Sleep disorders associated with neurological disease

Tauopathies

Patients with progressive supranuclear palsy, Alzheimer's disease, and corticobasal degeneration may complain of significant sleep-related circadian disturbances, as well as sleep–wake and daytime problems [5, 23–29].

• Sleep/wake disturbances and disruption are commonly observed in Alzheimer's disease, with daytime sleep, sleep attack and episodes of microsleep.

• Insomnia (sleep fragmentation and difficulties maintaining sleep) is common, as are nocturnal wandering, nocturnal confusion, 'sundowning' psychosis, and nocturia.

• EDS, sleep attacks, and episodes of microsleep during the daytime may be associated with cognitive problems.

• Sleep-related disorders such as RBD, RLS, PLMS, nocturnal complex and dystonic movements, and cramps may occur in progressive supranuclear palsy and corticobasal degeneration, but are rare in Alzheimer's disease.

• Sleep breathing disorders are common in Alzheimer's disease and are associated with disease progression and a poorer prognosis; however, the clinical significance of diagnosing and treating them in this group of patients is questionable.

Recommendations

Sleep disorders are commonly observed in patients with tauopathies, and there should be an increased awareness of these disorders. It is recommended to perform a detailed medical history of sleep disorders in tauopathies, i.e. insomnia, EDS, motor and dreaming activity, and SDB. PSG recording, preferably with audiovisual recording, is suggested for the diagnosis, especially when RBD and/or SDB are suspected disorders (Level C).

Synucleinopathies

Parkinson's disease, MSA, and DLB are often associated with major sleep–wake disorders [13, 17, 28, 30–38]:

• Parkinson's disease-related motor symptoms including nocturnal akinesia, early-morning dystonia, painful cramps, tremor, and difficulties turning in bed;

• treatment-related nocturnal disturbances (e.g. insomnia, confusion, hallucinations, and motor disturbances);

• sleep-related symptoms such as hallucinations and vivid dreams (nightmares), insomnia (sleep fragmentation and difficulties maintaining sleep), nocturia, psychosis, and panic attacks;

• EDS, sleep attacks, and episodes of microsleep during waking hours;

• sleep-related disorders including RBD, RLS, PLMS, nocturnal dystonic movements, cramps, and SDB. The presence of RBD in Parkinson's disease is associated with cognitive and autonomic changes;

• laryngeal stridor and obstructive sleep apnoea, which are commonly observed in patients with MSA and are associated with a poorer prognosis. Continuous positive airway pressure (CPAP) ventilation may improve respiration and prognosis (Class III).

Recommendations

The majority of patients with synucleinopathies experience one or more sleep disorders. It is recommended to perform a detailed medical history of sleep disorders in tauopathies, i.e. insomnia, EDS, motor, and dreaming activity, and SDB PSG recording, preferably with audiovisual recording, is suggested for the diagnosis, especially when RBD and/or SDB is suspected (Level B).

Stroke

Patients with strokes, primarily infarctions, may suffer from several sleep disorders and disturbances. Their occurrence and manifestations may vary depending on the specific neurological deficits [39–50]:

• SDB, especially OSAS and nocturnal oxygen desaturations, have commonly (>50%) been found in patients with acute stroke as well as after neurological recovery. OSAS is a risk factor for stroke, and co-existing OSAS in stroke patients may increase the risk of a further stroke. The presence of SDB, especially OSAS, may worsen the prognosis and increase the stroke re-occurrence risk. SDB may be provoked by stroke, especially, after damage to the respiratory centres in the brainstem or bulbar/pseudobulbar paralysis due to brainstem. Pre-existing sleep apnoea prior to stroke may present a risk factor for stroke, with comorbid obesity, diabetes, coronary artery disease and hypertension, and other cerebrovascular risk factors. There are several haemodynamic changes in sleep apnoea that may play a role in the pathogenesis of stroke development. Stroke and SDB are both common and are associated with significant morbidity and mortality.

• CPAP treatment for OSAS in may reduce the risk of cardio- and cerebrovascular complications (Class I) and potential re-occurrence of stroke, but the compliance is poor to moderate compared with the compliance in OSAS patients who have not had a stroke (B).

• Sleepiness and fatigue are commonly reported in patients after stroke and are often disabling symptoms.

• Other sleep disorders, such as insomnia, RBD, and PLMS, may be observed as part of or after stroke.

Recommendations

Sleep disorders, especially SDB, occur often in stroke patients. Screening for SDB and other sleep disorders is recommended as part of the stroke evaluation programme, especially in ischaemic stroke patients (Level A).

Motor neuron, motor end plate, and muscle diseases

SDB is observed in several neuromuscular diseases, including muscular dystrophy, myotonic dystrophy, myasthenia gravis, ALS, and post-polio syndrome. Although there may be differences, some general observations can be made. Hypoxaemia, especially during REM sleep, is commonly found. Severity is correlated to respiratory strength, and sleep-related hypoventilation is usually non-obstructive [51, 52].

Patients with ALS and other severe motor neuron diseases have progressive motor deterioration with progressive respiratory insufficiency. This may manifest primarily during sleep, where the motor drive is reduced. This is especially true for patients with the bulbar form of ALS or involvement of C3–C5 in the anterior horn [53, 54]. The prognosis is closely related to respiratory muscle strength [55]. Of note, sudden nocturnal death often occurs during sleep. Respiratory indices such as low nocturnal oxygen saturation are associated with a poorer prognosis [56, 57]. Patients with diaphragmatic involvement may have significantly reduced REM sleep [58]. The

primary SDB in patients with ALS – as in other neuromuscular diseases – is therefore a sleep hypoventilation syndrome (SHVS), whereas OSAS is rare [53].

Management of these patients should therefore include relevant questions regarding symptoms suspicious for SDB. Common symptoms of nocturnal hypoventilations include insomnia, headache, and daytime somnolence [59].

Oximetry has been suggested for the identification of and screening for sleep-related hypoventilation in patients with ALS, but its value is limited to identifying nocturnal desaturations that may occur during non-REM and REM sleep [57, 60, 61]. Care should be taken because pCO may increase before desaturations are observed, especially in patients with additional chronic obstructive lung disease. Nocturnal oximetry has been suggested as valuable for screening and for evaluating the treatment effect [53, 57]. There has been no validation of the diagnostic yield between a full PSG, respiratory polygraphy, and nocturnal oximetry in these patients. It is, however, important to identify early symptoms of respiratory failure in sleep, as these patients are able to compensate their hypercapnia during wakefulness for a long time. This is the at which one should bring in a regular measurement of respiratory parameters [62–66].

Recommendations

SDB often occurs in patients with motor neuron, motor end plate, and muscle diseases, and should be considered in all patients. Minimum evaluation should include PSG eventually combined with additional carbon dioxide analysis, and eventually supplied with serial polygraphy or oximetry measures for the identification of sleep-related hypoventilation during the disease course (Level B).

Genetic neurodegenerative disorders

Other neurodegenerative disorders of genetic cause may present several sleep disturbances. Subjects with SCA-3 (Machado–Joseph disease) may also complain of RLS, periodic leg movements, vocal cord paralysis, and RBD [9, 11, 18, 67, 68]. In patients with Huntington's disease, the involuntary movements tend to diminish during sleep [69]. Sleep disturbances, including disturbed sleep pattern with an increased sleep onset latency, reduced sleep efficiency, frequent nocturnal awakenings, and more time spent awake with less slow wave sleep, have been reported. These abnormalities correlate in part with the duration of illness, severity of clinical symptoms, and degree of atrophy of the caudate nucleus [70]. The sleep phenotype of Huntington's disease may also include insomnia, advanced sleep phase, periodic leg movements, RBDs, and reduced REM sleep, but not narcolepsy. Reduced REM sleep may precede chorea. Mutant huntingtin may exert an effect on REM sleep and motor control during sleep [71]. However, other studies have not reported specific sleep disorders in Huntington patients [72].

Recommendations

Sleep disorders occur in several genetic neurological diseases. The patients should be questioned, and further evaluation of these disorders should rely on a clinical judgement (Level C).

Management of sleep disorders in neurological diseases

Diagnostic techniques in sleep disorders

Diagnostic procedures for sleep diagnosis include PSG, partial time PSG, partial polygraphy (or respiratory polygraphy), and limited channel polygraphy: oximetry determining arterial oxygen saturation/pulse and actimetry. Daytime sleepiness may be evaluated with the Multiple Sleep Latency Test (MSLT) or Maintenance of Wakefulness Test (MWT). Many of the tests are increasingly easy to perform in or outside hospital due to technological advantages. Consequently, diagnostic procedures may be more easily performed as part of the diagnostic program for neurological patients. An overview of these tests is presented in table 39.1.

Treatment of SDB in neurological diseases

Treatment of OSAS

CPAP is a well-documented treatment for moderate and severe OSAS (apnoea–hyperpnoea index ≥15/h) and improves nocturnal respiratory abnormalities, daytime function, and cognitive problems [73–78] (Class I). There is no significant difference regarding treatment effect or changes in subjective variables between fixed-pressure CPAP and auto-adjusted CPAP [79, 80] (Class I).

CPAP and bi-level positive airway pressure ventilation is potentially useful in patients with SDB in stroke [40], despite negative reports [81]. The evidence on whether this influences quality of life, daytime symptoms, rehabilitation, morbidity, and mortality is, however, limited, which needs further clarification [49] (Class II).

Severe SDBs, including laryngeal stridor in patients with MSA, may be treated with CPAP/bi-level CPAP. Recent studies suggest that treatment with CPAP for MSA patients with laryngeal stridor showed high CPAP tolerance, no recurrence of stridor, no major side effects, and a subjective improvement in sleep quality, and that there is an increased survival time for MSA patients without stridor [31, 82]. CPAP is therefore an effective, non-invasive, long-term therapy for nocturnal stridor (Level C) and may prevent worsening of stridor under increasing dopaminergic dosages.

In some patients, for example those with neuromuscular disorders, CPAP may be difficult to accept, and bi-level positive airway pressure ventilation may be used [83] (Class IV).

There is evidence suggesting that oral appliance use improves subjective sleepiness and SDB compared with controls in patients with OSAS without neurological disease (Level B). Nasal CPAP is apparently more effective in improving SDB than oral appliance use (Level B). There are no data regarding the use of oral appliances in patients with neurological diseases, so caution should be applied concerning the use of oral appliances in patients with OSAS [84, 85] (Level C).

Surgical treatment has a limited effect on OSA [86, 87] (Class III). There are no studies suggesting that surgery in the upper airway has any effect on OSAS in patients with neurological diseases.

Drug treatments have no positive effect on OSAS [88] (Class II). There is no study available indicating that medication has any treatment effect for OSAS in patients with neurological diseases

Although some patients with OSAS present an increased weight and a negative lifestyle profile (in terms of tobacco, alcohol, and physical activity), no controlled

Table 39.1 Methods for the diagnosis of sleep disorders in neurological disease.

Type of PSG	Definition	Indication	Advantage/disadvantage
Routine PSG	Multi-channel EEG, EOG, submental EMG, ECG, respiration, +/– tibial EMG	Routine screening for sleep disorders: SDB, PLMS, chronic insomnia	Gold standard. May be performed in or outside hospital. Standard method
Extended PSG	Routine PSG + extra physiological channels, e.g. EMG, intraoesophageal pressure, carbon dioxide	Special indications: oesophageal reflux, myoclonias, etc. Depends on selected channels	Moderately expensive, time-consuming, staff-demanding
Video-PSG	PSG + video recording	Motor and behavioural phenomena during sleep	A video signal is present. Full physiological recording. Includes audiovisual channels
Full EEG–PSG	Full 10–20 EEG + PSG	Motor and behavioural disturbances for the differential diagnosis of epilepsies	Full diagnostic procedures are obtained. The difference between the methods is primarily the number of EEG channels. Expensive, time-consuming, staff-demanding
MSLT	Multiple (≥4) trials per day of PSG determination of sleep latencies of intended sleep	Central hypersomnias including narcolepsy, distinction between tiredness and EDS. Supportive for EDS in neurological diseases	Supportive for the diagnosis of hypersomnia and narcolepsy/sensitive to foregoing sleep loss and discontinuation of REM sleep-inhibiting drugs
MWT	Multiple (≥4) trials per day of PSG determination of sleep latencies of intended sleep inhibition	Determination of ability to stay awake	Supportive for wakefulness capabilities, useful for driving ability and treatment effects
Partial channel polygraphy			
Respiratory polygraphy	Monitoring of respiration + arterial oxygen saturation +/– cardiac measures, e.g. pulse	OSAS	Easy, inexpensive. Moderate to good sensitivity and specificity for OSAS; the validity for other SDBs is not known
Oximetry	Monitoring of arterial oxygen saturation	Monitoring or screening for severe SDB	Easy, inexpensive. Low sensitivity and specificity for SDB. Exclusion of SDB not possible
Actigraphy	Determination of motor activity (days–months)	Sleep–wake disturbances	Inexpensive. Limited clinical usefulness

ECG, electrocardiography; EOG, Electrooculography. See text for other abbreviations.

studies have evaluated the effect of intervention against these factors [89] (Class IV). No studies have addressed the effect of lifestyle interventions on OSAS in patients with neurological diseases.

Treatment of CSAHS

Case series have shown that CPAP treatment does not influence the carbon dioxide response in CSAHS, despite a reduction in apnoeas, an increase in paO_3, and a reduction in subjective sleepiness [90–92] (Class IV). Probably

due to the rareness of the disease, there are no randomized studies regarding CSAHS and treatment. Drug treatment with acetazolamide and theophylline has furthermore been suggested [93], but the evidence for their use is poor (Class IV).

Treatment of CSBS

Initially, CPAP was used in patients with central apnoea/CSBS and cardiac insufficiency [94–97], but in recent years adaptive ventilation has been found to be effective, probably via an increased preload in patients with significant cardiac failure, and to reduce the respiratory abnormalities, although the long-term prognosis is not known [98, 99] (Class IV). A recent randomized controlled study suggests that the use of non-invasive adaptive ventilation may improve daytime function and respiratory and cardiac measures [100] (Class II). The experience with the use of adaptive ventilation, CPAP or bi-level CPAP in patients with Cheyne–Stokes respiration due to central respiratory failure, for example brainstem lesions, is sparse, and the evidence level is poor (Class C).

Treatment of sleep hypoventilation syndrome

Treatment includes nasal intermittent positive-pressure ventilation (NIPPV) with bi-level positive airways pressure (variable positive airways pressure), non-invasive volumetric ventilation, and eventually invasive ventilation, under the control of nocturnal respiratory parameters [101] (Class IV). CPAP is not the primary treatment, as the motor effort is mostly reduced in these patients, which may lead to worsening of the SDB. NIPPV may reduce sleep disturbances, increase cognitive function, and prolong the period to tracheostomy [102, 103] (Class IV). Current evidence about the therapeutic benefit of mechanical ventilation is weak but consistent, suggesting alleviation of the symptoms of chronic hypoventilation in the short term. Evidence from a single randomized trial of non-invasive ventilation with a limited number of participant suggests a prolonged survival and improved quality of life in people with ALS, especially among those with minor bulbar involvement, but not in patients with severe bulbar impairment [104, 105] (Class III).

Follow-up

Although there is no evidence on when and how the follow-up of treatment with CPAP and NIPPV should be executed, we recommend regular follow-up of the treatment with control of compliance and treatment effect (Class IV).

Ethical aspects

Treatment of patients with severe neurological diseases such as ALS and MSA with NIPPV includes medical and ethical problems that should be addressed. Adequate involvement of the patients and family, and the treatment, its use, and its limitations, should be carefully discussed early in the course of the disease. It is important to clarify the limitations of the treatment, and the discussion should include careful debate regarding whether such treatment should be offered, its initiation, the need for tracheotomy, whether invasive ventilation should be offered, and discontinuation [106, 107].

Drug treatment

Treatment of EDS in neurological diseases

Several groups of patients with neurological diseases commonly complain of EDS. The aetiology may be secondary to the neurological disease or its medication (dopaminergic or benzodiazepine drugs), or the consequence of concomitant sleep disorders such as sleep apnoea, nocturnal motor phenomena, etc. In patients in whom these factors cannot be modified, stimulants such as methylphenidate or modafinil may be used as symptomatic therapy. Modafinil was primarily introduced to treat EDS in narcolepsy [108–113]. Case studies [114, 115] and double-blind controlled studies [116, 117] suggest that modafinil reduces EDS in Parkinson's patients (Class B-II) despite the fact that Ondo *et al.*'s study did not prove the long-term effect of modafinil in Parkinson's disease [118]. Modafinil has also been suggested in ALS [119] and post-stroke depression [120, 121], but no controlled studies are available (Class IV). Furthermore, modafinil has been used for the treatment of residual EDS in OSAS undergoing CPAP treatment without neurological comorbidity [122]. There is some evidence that other centrally acting drugs such ass methylphenidate may have similar effects [123], but there have been no comparisons between modafinil and methylphenidate. EDS in Parkinson's disease was successfully reduced by sodium oxybate [124] (Class II).

Other drug and non-pharmacological treatment of sleep disorders in neurological diseases

Treatment of sleep disorders in neurodegenerative diseases is often complex and may involve different strategies. Parkinson's disease-related motor symptoms can be treated with long-acting DA agonists to obtain continuous DA receptor stimulation during the night. On the other hand, nocturnal disturbances may be related to treatment, and therefore continued monitoring of treatment effect should offered.

Some sleep disorders, such as RLS and PLMS, may be controlled by DA agents, and others, such as insomnia and EDS, may be improved by reducing dopaminergic stimulation (Class IV).

Clonazepam or donepezil, possibly prescribed with melatonin, has been suggested based on case series for the treatment of RBD. No controlled studies are available [33, 125].

Patients with dementias often present circadian disturbances that may be relieved by melatonin and light therapy [126–142] (Class IV).

In selected cases, treatment with hypnotics are mentioned to be useful, but the evidence is limited and care should be undertaken in terms of chronic use, the risk of falls, daytime sedation, confusion, and the risk of worsening of SDB in the elderly.

Recommendations

1. Patients with neurological diseases often have significant sleep disorders that affect sleep and daytime function, with increased morbidity and even mortality. Many of these disorders are treatable. Therefore, increased awareness should be directed toward sleep disorders in patients with neurodegenerative, cerebrovascular, and neuromuscular diseases. Despite this, there are limited number of studies with a high evidence level.

2. PSG is a diagnostic minimum for the diagnoses of sleep disorders in patients with neurological diseases.

3. In patients with nocturnal motor and/behaviour manifestations, a full video-PSG/video-EEG–PSG is recommended.

4. Respiratory polygraphy has a moderate sensitivity and specificity in the diagnosis of OSAS without neurological diseases, but its value for the diagnosis of other SDBs or in neurological patients with suspected OSAS has not been evaluated compared with the gold standard of PSG. Consequently, respiratory polygraphy may be used as a method for detecting OSAS, but the value of its use for SDB in patients with neurological diseases needs further validation.

5. Oximetry has a poor sensitivity/specificity for the identification of OSAS in patients without neurological diseases. Oximetry cannot differentiate between obstructive and central sleep apnoea and is insufficient to identify stridor. Oximetry alone is not recommended for the diagnosis of SDB in neurological disorders.

6. Patients with SDB, muscle weakness, and cardiac or pulmonary comorbidity may present a sleep hypoventilation syndrome that manifests early as increased carbon dioxide. $paCO$ should be measured in such cases during sleep recordings.

7. Fixed-pressure CPAP/auto-adjusted CPAP is the most effective treatment for OSAS. This probably also includes patients with OSAS and neurological diseases. However, there is a need for further evaluation of the effect of CPAP in patients with OSAS and neurological diseases.

8. Bi-level/variable positive-airway pressure ventilation, NIPPV, and volumetric ventilation are useful for SDBs such as central apnoeas, Cheyne-Stokes breathing, and alveolar hypoventilation.

9. There is a clear need for further studies focusing on the diagnostic procedures and treatment modalities in neurological patients with sleep disorders.

Conflicts of interest

None reported.

References

1. Jennum P, Santamaria J, Clarenbach P, *et al*. Report of an EFNS task force on management of sleep disorders in neurological disease (degenerative neurological disorders and stroke). *Eur J Neurol* 2007;**14**(11):1189–2005.

2. Brainin M, Barnes M, Baron JC, *et al*. Guidance for the preparation of neurological management guidelines by EFNS scientific task forces–revised recommendations 2004. *Eur J Neurol* 2004;**11**(9):577–81.

3. American Academy of Sleep Medicine. *International Classification of Sleep Disorders. Diagnostic and Coding Manual*, 2nd edn. Westchester, IL: American Academy of Sleep Medicine, 2005.

4. American Academy of Sleep Medicine Task Force. Sleep-related breathing disorders in adults: recommendations for syndrome definition and measurement techniques in clinical research. The Report of an American Academy of Sleep Medicine Task Force. *Sleep* 1999;**22**(5):667–89.

5. Schenck CH, Mahowald MW, Anderson ML, Silber MH, Boeve BF, Parisi JE. Lewy body variant of Alzheimer's

disease (AD) identified by postmortem ubiquitin staining in a previously reported case of AD associated with REM sleep behavior disorder. *Biol Psychiatry* 1997;**42**(6): 527–8.

6. Schenck CH, Bundlie SR, Mahowald MW. Delayed emergence of a parkinsonian disorder in 38% of 29 older men initially diagnosed with idiopathic rapid eye movement sleep behaviour disorder. *Neurology* 1996;**46**(2):388–93.

7. Schenck CH, Mahowald MW. REM sleep behavior disorder: clinical, developmental, and neuroscience perspectives 16 years after its formal identification in SLEEP. *Sleep* 2002;**25**(2):120–38.

8. Onofrj M, Thomas A, D'Andreamatteo G, et al. Incidence of RBD and hallucination in patients affected by Parkinson's disease: 8-year follow-up. *Neurol Sci* 2002;**23**(Suppl. 2):S91–4.

9. Friedman JH, Fernandez HH, Sudarsky LR. REM behavior disorder and excessive daytime somnolence in Machado-Joseph disease (SCA-3). *Mov Disord* 2003;**18**(12):1520–2.

10. Iranzo A, Molinuevo JL, Santamaria J, et al. Rapid-eye-movement sleep behaviour disorder as an early marker for a neurodegenerative disorder: a descriptive study. *Lancet Neurol* 2006;**5**(7):572–7.

11. Syed BH, Rye DB, Singh G. REM sleep behavior disorder and SCA-3 (Machado-Joseph disease). *Neurology* 2003;**60**(1):148.

12. Uchiyama M, Isse K, Tanaka K, et al. Incidental Lewy body disease in a patient with REM sleep behavior disorder. *Neurology* 1995;**45**(4):709–12.

13. Boeve BF, Silber MH, Ferman TJ. REM sleep behavior disorder in Parkinson's disease and dementia with Lewy bodies. *J Geriatr Psychiatry Neurol* 2004;**17**(3):146–57.

14. Turner RS. Idiopathic rapid eye movement sleep behavior disorder is a harbinger of dementia with Lewy bodies. *J Geriatr Psychiatry Neurol* 2002;**15**(4):195–9.

15. De Cock VC, Vidilhet M, Leu S, et al. Restoration of normal motor control in Parkinson's disease during REM sleep. *Brain* 2007;**130**:450–6.

16. Iranzo A, Santamaria J, Tolosa E. The clinical and pathophysiological relevance of REM sleep behavior disorder in neurodegenerative diseases. *Sleep Med Rev* 2009;**13**(6):385–401.

17. Boeve BF, Silber MH, Ferman TJ, Lucas JA, Parisi JE. Association of REM sleep behavior disorder and neurodegenerative disease may reflect an underlying synucleinopathy. *Mov Disord* 2001;**16**(4):622–30.

18. Iranzo A, Munoz E, Santamaria J, Vilaseca I, Mila M, Tolosa E. REM sleep behavior disorder and vocal cord paralysis in Machado-Joseph disease. *Mov Disord* 2003;**18**(10):1179–83.

19. De Cock VC, Lannuzel A, Verhaeghe S, et al. REM sleep behavior disorder in patients with guadeloupean parkinsonism, a tauopathy. *Sleep* 2007;**30**(8):1026–32.

20. Postuma RB, Gagnon JF, Vendette M, Fantini ML, Massicotte-Marquez J, Montplaisir J. Quantifying the risk of neurodegenerative disease in idiopathic REM sleep behavior disorder. *Neurology* 2009;**72**:1296–300.

21. Eisensehr I, Linke R, Tatsch K, et al. Increased muscle activity during rapid eye movement sleep correlates with decrease of striatal presynaptic dopamine transporters. IPT and IBZM SPECT imaging in subclinical and clinically manifest idiopathic REM sleep behavior disorder, Parkinson's disease, and controls. *Sleep* 2003;**26**(5):507–12.

22. Knudsen S, Gammeltoft S, Jennum P. The association between hypocretin-1 deficiency, cataplexy, and REM sleep behaviour disorder (RBD) in narcolepsy. *Brain* 2010 in press

23. De Bruin VS, Machado C, Howard RS, Hirsch NP, Lees AJ. Nocturnal and respiratory disturbances in Steele-Richardson-Olszewski syndrome (progressive supranuclear palsy). *Postgrad Med J* 1996;**72**(847):293–6.

24. Pareja JA, Caminero AB, Masa JF, Dobato JL. A first case of progressive supranuclear palsy and pre-clinical REM sleep behavior disorder presenting as inhibition of speech during wakefulness and somniloquy with phasic muscle twitching during REM sleep. *Neurologia* 1996;**11**(8):304–6.

25. Kimura K, Tachibana N, Aso T, Kimura J, Shibasaki H. Subclinical REM sleep behavior disorder in a patient with corticobasal degeneration. *Sleep* 1997;**20**(10):891–4.

26. Janssens JP, Pautex S, Hilleret H, Michel JP. Sleep disordered breathing in the elderly. *Aging (Milano)* 2000;**12**(6):417–29.

27. Volicer L, Harper DG, Manning BC, Goldstein R, Satlin A. Sundowning and circadian rhythms in Alzheimer's disease. *Am J Psychiatry* 2001;**158**(5):704–11.

28. Ferman TJ, Smith GE, Boeve BF, et al. DLB fluctuations: specific features that reliably differentiate DLB from AD and normal aging. *Neurology* 2004;**62**(2):181–7.

29. Reynolds CF III, Kupfer DJ, Taska LS, et al. Sleep apnea in Alzheimer's dementia: correlation with mental deterioration. *J Clin Psychiatry* 1985;**46**(7):257–61.

30. Silber MH, Levine S. Stridor and death in multiple system atrophy 10. *Mov Disord* 2000;**15**(4):699–704.

31. Iranzo A, Santamaria J, Tolosa E. Continuous positive air pressure eliminates nocturnal stridor in multiple system atrophy. Barcelona Multiple System Atrophy Study Group. *Lancet* 2000;**356**(9238):1329–30.

32. Gilman S, Chervin RD, Koeppe RA, et al. Obstructive sleep apnea is related to a thalamic cholinergic deficit in MSA. *Neurology* 2003;**61**(1):35–9.

33. Massironi G, Galluzzi S, Frisoni GB. Drug treatment of REM sleep behavior disorders in dementia with Lewy bodies. *Int Psychogeriatr* 2003;**15**(4):377–83.

34. Yamaguchi M, Arai K, Asahina M, Hattori T. Laryngeal stridor in multiple system atrophy. *Eur Neurol* 2003; **49**(3):154–9.

35. Barone P, Amboni M, Vitale C, Bonavita V. Treatment of nocturnal disturbances and excessive daytime sleepiness in Parkinson's disease. *Neurology* 2004;**63**(8 Suppl. 3): S35–8.

36. Vendette M, Gagnon JF, Décary A, *et al.* REM sleep behavior disorder predicts cognitive impairment in Parkinson disease without dementia. *Neurology* 2007;**69**: 1843–9.

37. Ferman TJ, Boeve BF, Smith GE, *et al.* Dementia with Lewy bodies may present as dementia and REM sleep behavior disorder without parkinsonism or hallucinations. *J Int Neuropsychol Soc* 2002;**8**(7):907–14.

38. Gilman S, Koeppe RA, Chervin RD, *et al.* REM sleep behavior disorder is related to striatal monoaminergic deficit in MSA. *Neurology* 2003;**61**(1):29–34.

39. Bassetti C, Mathis J, Gugger M, Lovblad KO, Hess CW. Hypersomnia following paramedian thalamic stroke: a report of 12 patients. *Ann Neurol* 1996;**39**(4):471–80.

40. Harbison J, Ford GA, Gibson GJ. Nasal continuous positive airway pressure for sleep apnoea following stroke. *Eur Respir J* 2002;**19**(6):1216–17.

41. Cherkassky T, Oksenberg A, Froom P, Ring H. Sleep-related breathing disorders and rehabilitation outcome of stroke patients: a prospective study. *Am J Phys Med Rehabil* 2003;**82**(6):452–5.

42. McArdle N, Riha RL, Vennelle M, *et al.* Sleep-disordered breathing as a risk factor for cerebrovascular disease: a case-control study in patients with transient ischemic attacks. *Stroke* 2003;**34**(12):2916–21.

43. Nachtmann A, Stang A, Wang YM, Wondzinski E, Thilmann AF. Association of obstructive sleep apnea and stenotic artery disease in ischemic stroke patients. *Atherosclerosis* 2003;**169**(2):301–7.

44. Palomaki H, Berg A, Meririnne E, *et al.* Complaints of poststroke insomnia and its treatment with mianserin. *Cerebrovasc Dis* 2003;**15**(1-2):56–62.

45. Kang SY, Sohn YH, Lee IK, Kim JS. Unilateral periodic limb movement in sleep after supratentorial cerebral infarction. *Parkinsonism Relat Disord* 2004;**10**(7):429–31.

46. Mohsenin V. Is sleep apnea a risk factor for stroke? A critical analysis. *Minerva Med* 2004;**95**(4):291–305.

47. Parra O, Arboix A, Montserrat JM, Quinto L, Bechich S, Garcia-Eroles L. Sleep-related breathing disorders: impact on mortality of cerebrovascular disease. *Eur Respir J* 2004; **24**(2):267–72.

48. Brown DL, Chervin RD, Hickenbottom SL, Langa KM, Morgenstern LB. Screening for obstructive sleep apnea in stroke patients: a cost-effectiveness analysis. *Stroke* 2005; **36**(6):1291–3.

49. Hermann DL, Basetti C. Sleep-related breathing and sleep-wake disturbances in ischemic stroke. *Neurology* 2009; **73**(16):1313–22.

50. Harbison J, Ford GA, James OF, Gibson GJ. Sleep-disordered breathing following acute stroke. *QJM* 2002; **95**(11):741–7.

51. Hukins CA, Hillman DR. Daytime predictors of sleep hypoventilation in Duchenne muscular dystrophy. *Am J Respir Crit Care Med* 2000;**161**(1):166–70.

52. Dedrick DL, Brown LK. Obstructive sleep apnea syndrome complicating oculopharyngeal muscular dystrophy. *Chest* 2004;**125**(1):334–6.

53. Ferguson KA, Strong MJ, Ahmad D, George CF. Sleep-disordered breathing in amyotrophic lateral sclerosis. *Chest* 1996;**110**(3):664–9.

54. Kimura K, Tachibana N, Kimura J, Shibasaki H. Sleep-disordered breathing at an early stage of amyotrophic lateral sclerosis. *J Neurol Sci* 1999;**164**(1): 37–43.

55. Lyall RA, Donaldson N, Polkey MI, Leigh PN, Moxham J. Respiratory muscle strength and ventilatory failure in amyotrophic lateral sclerosis. *Brain* 2001;**124**(Pt 10): 2000–13.

56. Velasco R, Salachas F, Munerati E, *et al.* Nocturnal oxymetry in patients with amyotrophic lateral sclerosis: role in predicting survival. *Rev Neurol (Paris)* 2002;**158**(5 Pt 1):575–8.

57. Pinto A, de Carvalho M, Evangelista T, Lopes A, Sales-Luis L. Nocturnal pulse oximetry: a new approach to establish the appropriate time for non-invasive ventilation in ALS patients. *Amyotroph Lateral Scler Other Motor Neuron Disord* 2003;**4**(1):31–5.

58. Arnulf I, Similowski T, Salachas F, *et al.* Sleep disorders and diaphragmatic function in patients with amyotrophic lateral sclerosis. *Am J Respir Crit Care Med* 2000;**161**(3 Pt 1):849–56.

59. Takekawa H, Kubo J, Miyamoto T, Miyamoto M, Hirata K. Amyotrophic lateral sclerosis associated with insomnia and the aggravation of sleep-disordered breathing. *Psychiatry Clin Neurosci* 2001;**55**(3):263–4.

60. Elman LB, Siderowf AD, McCluskey LF. Nocturnal oximetry: utility in the respiratory management of amyotrophic lateral sclerosis. *Am J Phys Med Rehabil* 2003;**82**(11): 866–70.

61. Bach JR, Bianchi C, Aufiero E. Oximetry and indications for tracheotomy for amyotrophic lateral sclerosis. *Chest* 2004;**126**(5):1502–7.

62. Budweiser S, Murbeth RE, Jorres RA, Heinemann F, Pfeifer M. Predictors of long-term survival in patients with restrictive thoracic disorders and chronic respiratory failure undergoing non-invasive home ventilation. *Respirology* 2007;**12**(4):S551–9.

63. Ragette R, Mellies U, Schwake C, Voit T, Teschler H. Patterns and predictors of sleep disordered breathing in primary myopathies. *Thorax* 2002;**57**:724–8.

64. Storre JH, Steurer B, Kabitz H, Dreher M, Windisch W. Transcutaneous PCO2 monitoring during initiation of noninvasive ventilation. *Chest* 2007;**132**(6):S1810–6.

65. Ward S, Chatwin M, Heather S, Simonds AK. Randomised controlled trial of non-invasive ventilation (NIV) for nocturnal hypoventilation in neuromuscular and chest wall disease patients with daytime normocapnia. *Thorax* 2005;**60**(12):S1019–24.

66. Fauroux B, Lofaso F. Non-invasive mechanical ventilation: when to start for what benefit? *Thorax* 2005;**60**(12):979–80.

67. Schols L, Haan J, Riess O, Amoiridis G, Przuntek H. Sleep disturbance in spinocerebellar ataxias: is the SCA3 mutation a cause of restless legs syndrome? *Neurology* 1998;**51**(6):1603–7.

68. Fukutake T, Shinotoh H, Nishino H, *et al*. Homozygous Machado-Joseph disease presenting as REM sleep behaviour disorder and prominent psychiatric symptoms. *Eur J Neurol* 2002;**9**(1):97–100.

69. Fish DR, Sawyers D, Allen PJ, Blackie JD, Lees AJ, Marsden CD. The effect of sleep on the dyskinetic movements of Parkinson's disease, Gilles de la Tourette syndrome, Huntington's disease, and torsion dystonia. *Arch Neurol* 1991;**48**(2):210–14.

70. Wiegand M, Moller AA, Lauer CJ, *et al*. Nocturnal sleep in Huntington's disease. *J Neurol* 1991;**238**(4):203–8.

71. Arnulf I, Nielsen J, Lohmann E, *et al*. Rapid eye movement sleep disturbances in Huntington disease. *Arch Neurol* 2008;**65**(4):482–8.

72. Emser W, Brenner M, Stober T, Schimrigk K. Changes in nocturnal sleep in Huntington's and Parkinson's disease. *J Neurol* 1988;**235**(3):177–9.

73. Wright J, Johns R, Watt I, Melville A, Sheldon T. Health effects of obstructive sleep apnoea and the effectiveness of continuous positive airways pressure: a systematic review of the research evidence. *BMJ* 1997;**314**(7084):851–60.

74. Douglas NJ. Systematic review of the efficacy of nasal CPAP. *Thorax* 1998;**53**(5):414–15.

75. McMahon JP, Foresman BH, Chisholm RC. The influence of CPAP on the neurobehavioral performance of patients with obstructive sleep apnea hypopnea syndrome: a systematic review. *WMJ* 2003;**102**(1):36–43.

76. Sanchez AI, Martinez P, Miro E, Bardwell WA, Buela-Casal G. CPAP and behavioral therapies in patients with obstructive sleep apnea: effects on daytime sleepiness, mood, and cognitive function. *Sleep Med Rev* 2009;**13**:223–33.

77. McDaid C, Griffin S, Weatherly H, *et al*. Continuous positive airway pressure devices for the treatment of obstructive sleep apnoea-hypopnoea syndrome: a systematic review and economic analysis. *Health Technol Assess* 2009;**13**:iii–xiv, 1.

78. Giles TL, Lasserson TJ, Smith BH, White J, Wright J, Cates CJ. Continuous positive airways pressure for obstructive sleep apnoea in adults. *Cochrane Database Syst Rev* 2006;(3):CD001106.

79. Berry RB, Parish JM, Hartse KM. The use of auto-titrating continuous positive airway pressure for treatment of adult obstructive sleep apnea. An American Academy of Sleep Medicine review. *Sleep* 2002;**25**(2):148–73.

80. Noseda A, Andre S, Potmans V, Kentos M, de Maertelaer V, Hoffmann G. CPAP with algorithm-based versus titrated pressure: a randomized study. *Sleep Med* 2009;**10**(9):988–92.

81. Hsu CY, Vennelle M, Li HY, Engleman HM, *et al*. Sleep-disordered breathing after stroke: a randomised controlled trial of continuous positive airway pressure. *J Neurol Neurosurg Psychiatry* 2006;**77**:1143–9.

82. Iranzo A, Santamaria J, Tolosa E, *et al*. Long-term effect of CPAP in the treatment of nocturnal stridor in multiple system atrophy. *Neurology* 2004;**63**(5):930–2.

83. Randerath WJ, Galetke W, Ruhle KH. Auto-adjusting CPAP based on impedance versus bilevel pressure in difficult-to-treat sleep apnea syndrome: a prospective randomized crossover study. *Med Sci Monit* 2003;**9**(8):CR353–8.

84. Lim J, Lasserson TJ, Fleetham J, Wright J. Oral appliances for obstructive sleep apnoea. *Cochrane Database Syst Rev* 2003;(4):CD004435.

85. Cohen R. Limited evidence supports use of oral appliances in obstructive sleep apnoea. *Evid Based Dent* 2004;**5**(3):76.

86. Bridgman SA, Dunn KM. Surgery for obstructive sleep apnoea. *Cochrane Database Syst Rev* 2000;(2):CD001004.

87. Sundaram S, Bridgman SA, Lim J, Lasserson TJ. Surgery for obstructive sleep apnoea. *Cochrane Database Syst Rev* 2005;(4):CD001004.

88. Smith I, Lasserson T, Wright J. Drug treatments for obstructive sleep apnoea. *Cochrane Database Syst Rev* 2002;(2):CD003002.

89. Shneerson J, Wright J. Lifestyle modification for obstructive sleep apnoea. *Cochrane Database Syst Rev* 2001;(1):CD002875.

90. Yu L, Huang XZ, Wu QY. Management of nocturnal nasal mask continuous positive airway pressure in central hypoventilation in patients with respiratory diseases. *Zhonghua Jie He He Hu Xi Za Zhi* 1994;**17**(1):38–40.

91. Hommura F, Nishimura M, Oguri M, *et al*. Continuous versus bilevel positive airway pressure in a patient with idiopathic central sleep apnea. *Am J Respir Crit Care Med* 1997;**155**(4):1482–5.

92. Verbraecken J, Willemen M, Wittesaele W, van de Heyning HP, De Backer W. Short-term CPAP does not influence the increased CO_2 drive in idiopathic central sleep apnea. *Monaldi Arch Chest Dis* 2002;**57**(1):10–18.

93. American Thoracic Society. Idiopathic congenital central hypoventilation syndrome: diagnosis and management. American Thoracic Society. *Am J Respir Crit Care Med* 1999;**160**(1):368–73.

94. Bradley TD. Hemodynamic and sympathoinhibitory effects of nasal CPAP in congestive heart failure. *Sleep* 1996;**19**(10):S232–5.

95. Granton JT, Naughton MT, Benard DC, Liu PP, Goldstein RS, Bradley TD. CPAP improves inspiratory muscle strength in patients with heart failure and central sleep apnea. *Am J Respir Crit Care Med* 1996;**153**(1): 277–82.

96. Sin DD, Logan AG, Fitzgerald FS, Liu PP, Bradley TD. Effects of continuous positive airway pressure on cardiovascular outcomes in heart failure patients with and without Cheyne-Stokes respiration. *Circulation* 2000; **102**(1):61–6.

97. Krachman SL, Crocetti J, Berger TJ, Chatila W, Eisen HJ, D'Alonzo GE. Effects of nasal continuous positive airway pressure on oxygen body stores in patients with Cheyne-Stokes respiration and congestive heart failure. *Chest* 2003;**123**(1):59–66.

98. Teschler H, Dohring J, Wang YM, Berthon-Jones M. Adaptive pressure support servo-ventilation: a novel treatment for Cheyne-Stokes respiration in heart failure. *Am J Respir Crit Care Med* 2001;**164**(4):614–19.

99. Arzt M, Floras JS, Logan AG, *et al*; CANPAP Investigators. Suppression of central sleep apnea by continuous positive airway pressure and transplant-free survival in heart failure: a post hoc analysis of the Canadian Continuous Positive Airway Pressure for Patients with Central Sleep Apnea and Heart Failure Trial (CANPAP). *Circulation* 2007;**115**(25):3173–80.

100. Pepperell JC, Maskell NA, Jones DR, *et al*. A randomized controlled trial of adaptive ventilation for Cheyne-Stokes breathing in heart failure. *Am J Respir Crit Care Med* 2003;**168**(9):1109–14.

101. Gonzalez MM, Parreira VF, Rodenstein DO. Non-invasive ventilation and sleep. *Sleep Med Rev* 2002;**6**(1):29–44.

102. Newsom-Davis IC, Lyall RA, Leigh PN, Moxham J, Goldstein LH. The effect of non-invasive positive pressure ventilation (NIPPV) on cognitive function in amyotrophic lateral sclerosis (ALS): a prospective study. *J Neurol Neurosurg Psychiatry* 2001;**71**(4):482–7.

103. Butz M, Wollinsky KH, Wiedemuth-Catrinescu U, *et al*. Longitudinal effects of noninvasive positive-pressure ventilation in patients with amyotrophic lateral sclerosis. *Am J Phys Med Rehabil* 2003;**82**(8):597–604.

104. Annane D, Orlikowski D, Chevret S, Chevrolet JC, Raphael JC. Nocturnal mechanical ventilation for chronic hypoventilation in patients with neuromuscular and chest wall disorders. *Cochrane Database Syst Rev* 2007;(4): CD001941

105. Radunovic A, Annane D, Jewitt K, Mustfa N. Mechanical ventilation for amyotrophic lateral sclerosis/motor neuron disease. *Cochrane Database Syst Rev* 2009;**7**(4): CD004427.

106. Bourke SC, Gibson GJ. Non-invasive ventilation in ALS: current practice and future role. *Amyotroph Lateral Scler Other Motor Neuron Disord* 2004;**5**(2):67–71.

107. Mast KR, Salama M, Silverman GK, Arnold RM. End-of-life content in treatment guidelines for life-limiting diseases. *J Palliat Med* 2004;**7**(6):754–73.

108. Besset A, Chetrit M, Carlander B, Billiard M. Use of modafinil in the treatment of narcolepsy: a long term follow-up study. *Neurophysiol Clin* 1996;**26**(1):60–6.

109. Narcolepsy Multicenter Study Group. Randomized trial of modafinil as a treatment for the excessive daytime somnolence of narcolepsy: US Modafinil in Narcolepsy Multicenter Study Group. *Neurology* 2000;**54**(5):1166–75.

110. Mitler MM, Harsh J, Hirshkowitz M, Guilleminault C. Long-term efficacy and safety of modafinil (PROVIGIL((R)) for the treatment of excessive daytime sleepiness associated with narcolepsy. *Sleep Med* 2000;**1**(3):231–43.

111. Moldofsky H, Broughton RJ, Hill JD. A randomized trial of the long-term, continued efficacy and safety of modafinil in narcolepsy. *Sleep Med* 2000;**1**(2):109–16.

112. Schwartz JR, Nelson MT, Schwartz ER, Hughes RJ. Effects of modafinil on wakefulness and executive function in patients with narcolepsy experiencing late-day sleepiness. *Clin Neuropharmacol* 2004;**27**(2):74–9.

113. Narcolepsy Multicenter Study Group. Randomized trial of modafinil for the treatment of pathological somnolence in narcolepsy. US Modafinil in Narcolepsy Multicenter Study Group. *Ann Neurol* 1998;**43**(1):88–97.

114. Rabinstein A, Shulman LM, Weiner WJ. Modafinil for the treatment of excessive daytime sleepiness in Parkinson's disease: a case report. *Parkinsonism Relat Disord* 2001; **7**(4):287–8.

115. Nieves AV, Lang AE. Treatment of excessive daytime sleepiness in patients with Parkinson's disease with modafinil. *Clin Neuropharmacol* 2002;**25**(2):111–14.

116. Hogl B, Saletu M, Brandauer E, *et al*. Modafinil for the treatment of daytime sleepiness in Parkinson's disease: a double-blind, randomized, crossover, placebo-controlled polygraphic trial. *Sleep* 2002;**25**(8):905–9.

117. Adler CH, Caviness JN, Hentz JG, Lind M, Tiede J. Randomized trial of modafinil for treating subjective daytime sleepiness in patients with Parkinson's disease. *Mov Disord* 2003;**18**(3):287–93.

118. Ondo WG, Fayle R, Atassi F, Jankovic J. Modafinil for daytime somnolence in Parkinson's disease: double blind, placebo controlled parallel trial. *J Neurol Neurosurg Psychiatry* 2005;**76**(12):1636–9.

119. Sternbach H. Adjunctive modafinil in ALS. *J Neuropsychiatry Clin Neurosci* 2002;**14**(2):239.

120. Smith BW. Modafinil for treatment of cognitive side effects of antiepileptic drugs in a patient with seizures and stroke. *Epilepsy Behav* 2003;**4**(3):352–3.

121. Sugden SG, Bourgeois JA. Modafinil monotherapy in post-stroke depression. *Psychosomatics* 2004;**45**(1):80–1.

122. Kingshott RN, Vennelle M, Coleman EL, Engleman HM, Mackay TW, Douglas NJ. Randomized, double-blind, placebo-controlled crossover trial of modafinil in the treatment of residual excessive daytime sleepiness in the sleep apnea/hypopnea syndrome. *Am J Respir Crit Care Med* 2001;**163**(4):918–23.

123. Morgenthaler TI, Kapur VK, Brown T, *et al.* Practice parameters for the treatment of narcolepsy and other hypersomnias of central origin. Standards of Practice Committee of the American Academy of Sleep Medicine. *Sleep* 2007;**30**(12):1705–11.

124. Ondo WG, Perkins T, Swick T, *et al.* Sodium oxybate for excessive daytime sleepiness in Parkinson disease: an open-label polysomnographic study. *Arch Neurol* 2008;**65**(10): 1337–40.

125. Boeve BF, Silber MH, Ferman TJ. Melatonin for treatment of REM sleep behavior disorder in neurologic disorders: results in 14 patients. *Sleep Med* 2003;**4**(4):281–4.

126. Mishima K, Okawa M, Hozumi S, Hishikawa Y. Supplementary administration of artificial bright light and melatonin as potent treatment for disorganized circadian rest-activity and dysfunctional autonomic and neuroendocrine systems in institutionalized demented elderly persons. *Chronobiol Int* 2000;**17**(3):419–32.

127. Lovell BB, Ancoli-Israel S, Gevirtz R. Effect of bright light treatment on agitated behavior in institutionalized elderly subjects. *Psychiatry Res* 1995;**57**(1):7–12.

128. McGaffigan S, Bliwise DL. The treatment of sundowning. A selective review of pharmacological and nonpharmacological studies. *Drugs Aging* 1997;**10**(1):10–17.

129. Van Someren EJ, Kessler A, Mirmiran M, Swaab DF. Indirect bright light improves circadian rest-activity rhythm disturbances in demented patients. *Biol Psychiatry* 1997; **41**(9):955–63.

130. Okumoto Y, Koyama E, Matsubara H, Nakano T, Nakamura R. Sleep improvement by light in a demented aged individual. *Psychiatry Clin Neurosci* 1998;**52**(2): 194–6.

131. Koyama E, Matsubara H, Nakano T. Bright light treatment for sleep-wake disturbances in aged individuals with dementia. *Psychiatry Clin Neurosci* 1999;**53**(2): 227–9.

132. Lyketsos CG, Lindell VL, Baker A, Steele C. A randomized, controlled trial of bright light therapy for agitated behaviors in dementia patients residing in long-term care. *Int J Geriatr Psychiatry* 1999;**14**(7):520–5.

133. Yamadera H, Ito T, Suzuki H, Asayama K, Ito R, Endo S. Effects of bright light on cognitive and sleep-wake (circadian) rhythm disturbances in Alzheimer-type dementia. *Psychiatry Clin Neurosci* 2000;**54**(3):352–3.

134. Haffmans PM, Sival RC, Lucius SA, Cats Q, van Gelder L. Bright light therapy and melatonin in motor restless behaviour in dementia: a placebo-controlled study. *Int J Geriatr Psychiatry* 2001;**16**(1):106–10.

135. Sheehan B, Keene J. Sunlight levels and behavioural disturbance in dementia. *Int J Geriatr Psychiatry* 2002;**17**(8): 784–5.

136. Fetveit A, Skjerve A, Bjorvatn B. Bright light treatment improves sleep in institutionalised elderly–an open trial. *Int J Geriatr Psychiatr* 2003;**18**(6):520–6.

137. Fontana GP, Krauchi K, Cajochen C, *et al.* Dawn-dusk simulation light therapy of disturbed circadian rest-activity cycles in demented elderly. *Exp Gerontol* 2003; **38**(1–2):207–16.

138. Luijpen MW, Scherder EJ, Van Someren EJ, Swaab DF, Sergeant JA. Non-pharmacological interventions in cognitively impaired and demented patients–a comparison with cholinesterase inhibitors. *Rev Neurosci* 2003;**14**(4): 343–68.

139. Skjerve A, Bjorvatn B, Holsten F. Light therapy for behavioural and psychological symptoms of dementia. *Int J Geriatr Psychiatry* 2004;**19**(6):516–22.

140. Sutherland D, Woodward Y, Byrne J, Allen H, Burns A. The use of light therapy to lower agitation in people with dementia. *Nurs Times* 2004;**100**(45):32–4.

141. Mishima K, Okawa M, Hishikawa Y, Hozumi S, Hori H, Takahashi K. Morning bright light therapy for sleep and behavior disorders in elderly patients with dementia. *Acta Psychiatr Scand* 1994;**89**(1):1–7.

142. Mishima K, Hishikawa Y, Okawa M. Randomized, dim light controlled, crossover test of morning bright light therapy for rest-activity rhythm disorders in patients with vascular dementia and dementia of Alzheimer's type. *Chronobiol Int* 1998;**15**(6):647–54.

143. American Thoracic Society. Clinical indications for noninvasive positive pressure ventilation in chronic respiratory failure due to restrictive lung disease, COPD, and noctur-

nal hypoventilation – a consensus conference report. *Chest* 1999;**116**(2):521–34.

144. Carvalho BS, Waterhouse J, Edwards B, Simons R, Reilly T. The use of actimetry to assess changes to the rest-activity cycle. *Chronobiol Int* 2003;**20**(6):1039–59.

145. Chesson AL Jr, Ferber RA, Fry JM, *et al.* The indications for polysomnography and related procedures. *Sleep* 1997; **20**(6):423–87.

146. Chesson AL Jr, Wise M, Davila D, *et al.* Practice parameters for the treatment of restless legs syndrome and periodic limb movement disorder. An American Academy of Sleep Medicine Report. Standards of Practice Committee of the American Academy of Sleep Medicine. *Sleep* 1999; **22**(7):961–8.

147. Chesson AL Jr, Berry RB, Pack A. Practice parameters for the use of portable monitoring devices in the investigation of suspected obstructive sleep apnea in adults. *Sleep* 2003;**26**(7):907–13.

148. Hayward P. News from the European Neurological Society meeting. *Lancet Neurol* 2004;**3**(8):449.

149. Jennum P, Sjøl A. Snoring, sleep apnea and cardiovascular risk factors in a 30-60 year-old population. The MONICA II study. *Int J Epidemiol* 1993;**22**(3):439–44.

150. Johns MW. Sensitivity and specificity of the multiple sleep latency test (MSLT), the maintenance of wakefulness test and the Epworth sleepiness scale: failure of the MSLT as a gold standard. *J Sleep Res* 2000;**9**(1):5–11.

151. Le Bon O, Hoffmann G, Tecco J, *et al.* Mild to moderate sleep respiratory events: one negative night may not be enough. *Chest* 2000;**118**(2):353–9.

152. Middelkoop HA, van Dam EM, Smilde-van den Doel DA, Van Dijk G. 45-hour continuous quintuple-site actimetry: relations between trunk and limb movements and effects of circadian sleep-wake rhythmicity. *Psychophysiology* 1997;**34**(2):199–203.

153. Olson EJ, Boeve BF, Silber MH. Rapid eye movement sleep behaviour disorder: demographic, clinical and laboratory findings in 93 cases. *Brain* 2000;**123**(Pt 2):331–9.

154. Reyner LA, Horne JA, Reyner A. Gender- and age-related differences in sleep determined by home-recorded sleep logs and actimetry from 400 adults. *Sleep* 1995;**18**(2): 127–34.

155. Ross SD, Allen IE, Harrison KJ, Kvasz M, Connelly J, Sheinhait IA. *Systematic Review of the Literature Regarding the Diagnosis of Sleep Apnea*, 1999.

156. Ruehland WR, Rochford PD, O'Donoghue FJ, Pierce RJ, Singh P, Thornton AT. The new AASM criteria for scoring hypopneas: impact on the apnea hypopnea index. *Sleep* 2009;**32**(2):150–7.

157. Sforza E, Johannes M, Claudio B. The PAM-RL ambulatory device for detection of periodic leg movements: a validation study. *Sleep Med* 2005;**6**(5):407–13.

158. Skjerve A, Holsten F, Aarsland D, Bjorvatn B, Nygaard HA, Johansen IM. Improvement in behavioral symptoms and advance of activity acrophase after short-term bright light treatment in severe dementia. *Psychiatry Clin Neurosci* 2004;**58**(4):343–7.

159. Young T, Palta M, Dempsey J, Skatrud J, Weber S, Badr S. The occurrence of sleep-disordered breathing among middle-aged adults. *N Engl J Med* 1993;**328**(17):1230–5.

CHAPTER 40

Cognitive rehabilitation

S.F. Cappa,[1] T. Benke,[2] S. Clarke,[3] B. Rossi,[4] B. Stemmer,[5] C.M. van Heugten[6]

[1]Vita-Salute University and San Raffaele Scientific Institute, Milan, Italy; [2]Clinic for Neurology, Innsbruck, Austria; [3]Division of Neuropsychology, Lausanne, Switzerland; [4]University of Pisa, Italy; [5]University of Montreal, Canada; [6]Maastricht University, The Netherlands

Introduction

The rehabilitation of disorders of cognitive functions (language, spatial perception, attention, memory, calculation, praxis), following acquired neurological damage of different aetiology (in particular, stroke and traumatic brain injury [TBI]), is an expanding area of neurological rehabilitation, and has been the focus of considerable research interest in recent years. In 1999, a Task Force on Cognitive Rehabilitation was set up under the auspices of the European Federation of Neurological Societies (EFNS). The aim was to evaluate the existing evidence for the clinical effectiveness of cognitive rehabilitation in stroke and TBI, and provide recommendations for neurological practice. The results were published in 2003 in the *European Journal of Neurology* [1] and updated in 2005 [2]. The present chapter is an update and a revision of these guidelines.

For these guidelines, we have limited ourselves to a review of studies dealing with the rehabilitation of non-progressive neuropsychological disorders due to stroke and TBI. As a consequence, several important areas of 'cognitive rehabilitation' have been excluded, such as the rehabilitation of dementia, psychiatric, and developmental disorders. In addition, we have not considered studies of pharmacological treatments.

The prevalence and relevance of cognitive rehabilitation for stroke and TBI patients require the establishment of recommendations for the practice of cognitive rehabilitation, and these have been formally recognized by a

subcommittee of the Brain Injury Interdisciplinary Special Interest Group of the American Congress of Rehabilitation Medicine. The initial recommendations of the Committee were published in 1992 as the 'Guidelines for cognitive rehabilitation' [3] and were based on so-called expert opinion that did not take into account empirical evidence on the effectiveness of cognitive rehabilitation. More recently, a review of the scientific literature for cognitive rehabilitation in patients with TBI published from January 1988 through August 1998 (including 11 randomized clinical trials [RCTs]) noted that data on the effectiveness of cognitive rehabilitation programmes were limited by the heterogeneity of subjects, interventions, and outcomes studied [4].

As a preliminary consideration, we wish to underline that the present status of studies on the effectiveness of cognitive rehabilitation is still not satisfactory. We are fully convinced that the standards required for the evaluation of pharmacological and surgical interventions also apply to rehabilitation. In particular, it is necessary to show that rehabilitation is effective not only in modifying the impairment, but also in having sustained effects at the disability level. Unfortunately, the majority of RCTs in this area are of poor methodological quality, have insufficient sample size, and fail to assess the outcome at the disability level. Many other studies fail to compare intervention with placebo or sham treatment.

Before recommendations are advanced, a word of caution is necessary to alert the reader to the fact that there are differences in the classification schemes and rating systems used by different professional societies. Consequently, reviews and recommendations based on such systems may not always be directly comparable. Furthermore, inherent to each classification schema are grey zones, leeway of interpretation, and difficulties

European Handbook of Neurological Management: Volume 1, 2nd edition. Edited by N. E. Gilhus, M. P. Barnes and M. Brainin.
© 2011 Blackwell Publishing Ltd.

comparing studies due to their heterogeneous approaches. (For a helpful discussion on issues pertaining to classification schemes and recommended guidelines, see [5].) As communicated by Cicerone [6], increasing national and international collaboration among the various societies and organizations should lead to more consensus on the best practice of cognitive rehabilitation.

Search strategy

Each member of the task force was assigned an area of cognitive rehabilitation (S.F.C., aphasia; S.C./S.F.C., unilateral neglect; B.R., attention; B.S., memory; C.M.v.H., apraxia; T.B., acalculia) and systematically searched the Evidence-Based Medicine Reviews/Cochrane Central Register of Controlled Trials, MEDLINE and PsycINFO databases using the appropriate key words, and searched textbooks and existing guidelines. The general consensus was to include articles only if they contained data that could be rated according to the grades of recommendation for management, classified in terms of level of evidence following the revised guidance statement for neurological management guidelines of the EFNS [7].

Method for reaching consensus

Data collection and analysis of evidence were performed independently by each participant according to the assignment mentioned above. On the basis of the single reports, S.F.C. produced a first draft of the guidelines that was circulated several times among the task force members until the discrepancies in each topic were solved and a consensus was reached.

Results

Rehabilitation of aphasia

The rehabilitation of speech and language disorders following brain damage is the area of intervention for acquired cognitive deficits with the longest tradition, dating back to the nineteenth century [8]. A variety of approaches have been applied to the rehabilitation of aphasia, from stimulation approaches to the recent attempts to establish theory-driven treatment pro-

grammes based on the principles of cognitive neuropsychology [9]. The need to establish the effectiveness of aphasia rehabilitation has stimulated a number of investigations, dating back to the period after the Second World War, and has been based on a variety of methodologies. A meta-analysis of studies dealing with the effectiveness of language rehabilitation, limited to aphasia as a result of stroke, has been made available by the Cochrane collaboration. The review covers articles about speech and language rehabilitation after stroke up to January 1999 [10]. The conclusion of the review is that 'speech and language therapy treatment for people with aphasia after a stroke has not been shown either to be clearly effective or clearly ineffective within an RCT. Decisions about the management of patients must therefore be based on other forms of evidence. Further research is required to find out if speech and language therapy for aphasic patients is effective. If researchers choose to do a trial, this must be large enough to have adequate statistical power, and be clearly reported'. This conclusion is based on a limited number of RCTs (12), all of which were considered of poor quality.

The reviews by Cicerone *et al.* [11] (updated in 2005) reached a different conclusion, i.e. that 'cognitive-linguistic therapies' can be considered as Practice Standard for aphasia after stroke; similar, positive conclusions for TBI are based on limited and less consistent evidence. The reasons for this discrepancy can be found in the different criteria used in the two reviews. Several studies classified as Class I by Cicerone *et al.* [11, 12] were excluded by the Cochrane reviewers. For example, one study by Hagen [13] was excluded because of the lack of true randomization (the patients being sequentially assigned to treatment or no treatment). Another study [14] was probably excluded because it dealt only with computer-assisted reading rehabilitation. Two small RCTs [15, 16], which reported positive treatment effects, were excluded from the Cochrane Review because they were devoted to communication disorders after TBI.

By definition, all Class II and III evidence is not included in the Cochrane review. This resulted in the exclusion of the three large studies by Basso *et al.* [17], Shewan and Kertesz [18] and Poeck *et al.* [19], all indicating significant benefits of treatment. An additional small Class II study by Carlomagno *et al.* [20] supported the usefulness of writing rehabilitation in patients in the post-acute stage. Additional evidence for treatment effects comes from investigations on small patient samples (Class II). A study comparing group communication treatment with 'deferred treatment' indicated positive effects on both linguistic and communication measures [21]. A randomized study compared semantic with phonological treatment of anomia. Both treatments resulted in a significant improvement in functional communication [22].

Single-case studies are also not considered in the Cochrane Reviews. This is particularly relevant because most of the treatment studies based on the cognitive neuropsychological approach make use of the single-case methodology. A review paper by Robey *et al.* [23] critically discussed this approach and concluded that generally large treatment effects have been found in aphasic patients. Moss and Nicholas [24] analysed the single-case studies in chronic aphasic patients, and did not find a relationship between treatment response and time post-onset.

Some of the available RCTs comparing therapy with unstructured stimulation were based on a very limited number of treatment sessions. Recent studies have addressed the crucial issue of the role of intensity and length of treatment. A meta-analysis by Bhogal *et al.* [25] showed that studies reporting a significant treatment effect provided 8.8 h of therapy per week for 11.2 weeks, while the negative studies only provided approximately 2 h per week for 22.9 weeks. The total length of therapy was significantly inversely correlated with a mean change in the Porch Index of Communicative Abilities scores. The number of hours of therapy provided in a week was significantly correlated to greater improvement on the Porch Index of Communicative Abilities and the Token Test. These results suggest that an intense therapy programme provided over a short amount of time can improve outcomes of speech and language therapy for stroke patients with aphasia (see, however, [26]). A small RCT comparing intensive (5 h/week) with conventional (2 h/week) intervention found similar effects of the two treatment schedules at 6 months [27]. On a similar line, several studies have assessed the effectiveness of 'constraint-induced' aphasia therapy (CIT), i.e. an approach based on the intensive stimulation of language modality, constraining the use of non-verbal communication strategies. A small RCT comparing 'massed' with conventional treatment showed a significant superiority of the 'massed' intervention [28]. A further study by Meinzer

et al. [29] indicates that a similar programme is associated with a persistent improvement at a 6 months follow-up. The results of a small-scale, Class III study comparing CIT with a comparable schedule of multiple-modality treatment suggest that the effectiveness of the approach is more related to 'massed practice' than to the forced use of language modality [30]. A recent Class I study [31] compared the effectiveness of CIT alone, memantine alone, or combined CIT and pharmacological treatment. The best outcome, assessed with a functional communication scale, was found in the combined treatment group, and was persistent at long-term follow-up.

The use of computerized training as an adjunct to aphasia treatment is supported by the results of several Class III studies [12]. In particular, a study by Laganaro *et al.* [32] suggested that the number of treatment items rather than the number of repetitions plays an important role in recovery of naming. Additional data have been reported by Fridriksson *et al.* [33] (positive effects of visual speech training on naming abilities) and Manheim *et al.* [34] (positive effects of intensive computerized home training on communication abilities).

Recommendations

The conclusions of the Cochrane Review of aphasia rehabilitation after stroke are not compatible with Level A for aphasia therapy. Considerable evidence from Class II and III studies, as well as from rigorous single-case studies supports its probable effectiveness (Level B). There is a need for further investigations in the field, based on the definition of specific language targets (i.e. word comprehension, sentence production) in homogeneous samples of patients submitted to well-defined treatment approaches.

Rehabilitation of unilateral spatial neglect

The presence of hemineglect beyond the acute stage is associated with poor outcome in terms of independence [35, 36], and considerable effort is therefore devoted to its rehabilitation. Several reviews on the effectiveness of unilateral spatial neglect (ULN) rehabilitation are available [37–44].

A Cochrane Review [45] reported data from 12 studies and found evidence that cognitive rehabilitation resulted in significant and persisting improvements in performance in cancellation and line bisection tests. There was, however, insufficient evidence to confirm or exclude an effect of cognitive rehabilitation at the level of disability, or on destination following discharge from hospital.

There is evidence for the effectiveness of multiple approaches in reducing ULN manifestations. *Combined training of visual scanning, reading, copying, and figure description* yielded a statistically significant improvement in neglect symptoms in one Class II [46] and two Class III studies [47, 48]. Visual scanning training alone was shown to improve neglect significantly in one Class I study [49]. *Spatiomotor or visuo-spatiomotor cueing* improved neglect significantly in one Class I [50] and two Class III studies [51, 52]. *Visual cueing with kinetic stimuli* was found to bring a significant, albeit transient, improvement in three Class III studies [53–55]. However, the use of optokinetic stimulation did not improve neglect in a recent Class I study [56]. *Video feedback* [57] and *visuo-motor feedback* [58] were shown to improve significantly performance on trained tasks in Class III and II studies, respectively. *Training of sustained attention, increasing of alertness or cueing of spatial attention* was shown to significantly improve neglect in Class III studies [59–62].

Several studies investigated the effects of *influencing multisensory representations*. These studies in general demonstrated transient effects, lasting little longer than the end of the appropriate stimulation. Vestibular stimulation by cold water infusion into the left outer ear canal showed significant effects on different aspects of the unilateral neglect in five Class III studies [63–66]. Galvanic vestibular stimulation significantly improved neglect symptoms in one Class III study [67]. Transcutaneous electrical stimulation of the left neck muscles showed significant effects in four Class III studies [68–71], and neck muscle vibration demonstrated an effect in one Class II study [72]. The latter is the only study of this group that showed a persistent effect after 2 months. Changes in trunk orientation had significantly positive effects in one Class II study [73].

The use of *prism goggles* deviating by 10 degrees to the right, introduced relatively recently, was shown to improve significantly, in a transient fashion, neglect symptoms in two Class II [74, 75] and one Class III study [76]. A Class III study applied the prism goggle treatment for a 2-week period and obtained statistically significant improvement in the long term [77]. Two further Class III studies [78, 79] have shown a persistence of the effects at, respectively, 3 and 6 months.

The *forced use of the left visual hemifield or left eye* showed a relative benefit in neglect in one Class II [80] and three Class III studies [81–83]. A negative result was reported by Fong *et al.* [84].

Computer training yielded mixed results. One Class I [85] and one Class III [86] study reported an absence of significantly positive effects, while a more recent Class II study showed a statistically significant improvement in wheelchair mobility [87].

Recommendations

Several methods of neglect rehabilitation were investigated in Level I or II studies. The Cochrane Review concludes that, while there is evidence of persisting improvements in ULN symptoms, insufficient evidence is available to confirm or exclude an effect of cognitive rehabilitation at the functional level. With this caveat in mind, present evidence confers Level A recommendation to visual scanning training and to visuo-spatiomotor training, and Level B recommendation to the combined training of visual scanning, reading, copying, and figure description; to trunk orientation; to neck vibration; to forced use of the left eye; to the use of prism goggles; and to video feedback. Level B–C recommendation was made for training of sustained attention and alertness. Level C of recommendation is valid for transient effects due to caloric or galvanic vestibular stimulations, as well as transcutaneous electrical stimulation of the neck muscles.

Rehabilitation of attention disorders

Attention deficits follow many types of brain damage, including stroke and TBI [88, 89]. A pioneering study by Ben-Yishay *et al.* [90] explored the treatment of deficits in focusing and sustaining attention in 40 brain-injured adults. There was not only an improvement in the attention-training tasks, but also a generalization to other psychometric measures of attention, both maintained at 6-month follow-up. Using a multiple-baseline design, with patients at 4–6 years after head injury, Wood [91] found that contingent token reinforcement was effective in increasing patients' ability to sustain attention on a task. Several studies [92–94] have explicitly incorporated and evaluated therapeutic interventions such as feedback, reinforcement, and strategy teaching into the attention rehabilitation programmes.

The Cochrane Review by Lincoln *et al.* [95], having searched for controlled trials of attention training in stroke, identified only the study of Schoettke [96] showing the efficacy of attention training in improving sustained attention.

Thirteen studies were reviewed by Cicerone *et al.* [11], including three prospective RCTs [93, 94, 97], four Class II controlled studies [90, 96–98], and six Class III studies [91, 101–105]. Most controlled studies compared attention training with an alternative treatment without including a no-treatment condition; a very important distinction is between studies conducted in the acute and post-acute stage. Cicerone *et al.* [11] concluded that evidence from two RCTs [93, 97] with a total of 57 subjects, and two controlled studies [98, 100] with a total of 49 subjects, supports the effectiveness of attention training beyond the effects of non-specific cognitive stimulation for subjects with TBI or stroke during the post-acute phase of recovery and rehabilitation. Cicerone *et al.* [11] recommended such a form of intervention as a practice guideline for these individuals. Interventions should include not only training with different stimulus modalities and complexity, but also therapist activities such as monitoring subjects' performance, providing feedback, and teaching strategies. Attention training appears to be more effective when directed at improving the subject's performance on more complex, functional tasks. However, the effects of treatment may be relatively small or task-specific, and an additional need exists to examine the impact of attention treatment on activities of daily living (ADLs) or functional outcomes.

Cicerone *et al.* [12] updated their previous evidence-based recommendations of the Brain Injury Interdisciplinary Special Interest Group of the American Congress of Rehabilitation Medicine for cognitive rehabilitation of people with TBI and stroke, based on a systematic review of the literature from 1998 through 2002 . They identified five further studies on rehabilitation of attention deficits after TBI. Two were Class I prospective randomized studies [106, 107] comparing attention treatment with alternative treatments; one was a Class II study [108] that compared attention treatment with no treatment; and two were Class III studies [109, 110]. Sohlberg *et al.* [106] used a crossover design to compare the effectiveness of 'attention process training' (APT) brain injury education and support for 14 patients with acquired brain injury. Self-reported changes in attention and memory functioning, as well as an improvement on neuropsychological measures of attention-executive functioning, were greater after APT than after therapeutic support. The

second Class I study [107] taught 22 patients with severe TBI to compensate for slowed information-processing and the experience of 'information overload' in daily tasks. Participants were randomly assigned to receive either time pressure management or an alternative treatment of generic 'concentration' training. Participants receiving time pressure management showed a significantly greater use of self-management strategies and a greater improvement in attention and memory functioning than did participants who received the alternative treatment. Although the precise nature of the interventions in these 2 Class I studies differs, they share a common emphasis on the development of strategies to compensate for residual cognitive deficits ('strategy training') rather than attempting to directly restore the underlying impaired function ('restitution training'). The results of these two studies and of an additional small Class II study [108] are therefore consistent with a strategy training model for attention deficits after TBI.

Stablum *et al.* [111] in a Class III study reported that the shift cost was greater for patients with severe TBI than for controls: treatment consisted of five sessions, in which an endogenous task shift paradigm was used. When a subject is engaged in two speeded tasks, not simultaneously but with some form of alternation, the response is slower to an item of task A if it is preceded by an item of task B than if it was preceded by an item of task A. This shift cost is small when subjects can prepare in advance for the new task (endogenous task shift), whereas the cost is much greater when preparation is not possible (exogenous task shift). A significant reduction of the endogenous shift cost from assessment to retest was found. The reduction remained stable at the 4-month follow-up session. It seems that these results were not simply due to retesting, as the control patients did not show any improvement at retest. Interestingly, no reduction of exogenous task shift cost was found. The results showed also that the beneficial effect of the treatment generalizes to other executive functions.

TBI patients who successfully completed attentional training showed changes in attentional network activation on functional magnetic resonance imaging, namely decreased frontal lobe activity together with increased function of the anterior cingulated cortices and precuneus in comparison with the pre-training neuroimaging data showing, in the same patients, more activation in the frontal and temporoparietal lobes, and less activation in the anterior cingulate gyrus and temporo-occipital regions compared with the healthy subjects [112]. Spontaneous blinking is considered to be influenced by basic cognitive processes, among them vigilance and attention. Therefore, from a methodological point of view, the monitoring of spontaneous blinking in chronic patients affected by various degrees of consciousness deficit after TBI and stroke has been shown to be useful to define the outcome of the syndrome [113].

Acute studies

One Class I and two Class II studies evaluated the effectiveness of attention treatment during the acute period of rehabilitation. The Class I study of Novack [94] compared the effectiveness of focused treatment consisting of sequential, hierarchical interventions directed at specific attention mechanisms versus unstructured intervention consisting of non-sequential, non-hierarchical activities requiring memory or reasoning skills. Both groups improved, but there were no intergroup differences: the observed improvements are probably due to spontaneous recovery. One Class II study [92] used a multiple baseline design across subjects and evaluated a programme for the remediation of processing speed deficits in 10 patients with severe TBI (6–34 weeks post-injury). The authors reported no benefit or generalization of effects of attention training; however, improvement did occur in some patients when practice on attention training tasks was combined with therapist feedback and praise. In the other Class II study [99], 35 subjects with lateralized stroke showed beneficial effects of attention training on five of 14 outcome measures, especially on measures of perceptual speed and selective attention in left hemisphere lesions.

Cicerone et al. [12], updating their previous review [11], stated that there was insufficient evidence to support the use of specific interventions for attention deficits during acute rehabilitation.

Post-acute studies

Two Class I and two Class II studies assessed the attention treatment effectiveness during the post-acute period of rehabilitation. Gray et al. [97] treated 31 patients with attention dysfunction, randomly assigned to receive either computerized attention retraining or an equivalent amount of recreational computer use. Immediately after training, the experimental group showed marked improvement on two measures of attention (although when premorbid intelligence score and time since injury were added as covariates, the treatment effect was no longer significant); at 6-month follow-up, the treatment group showed continued improvement and superior performance compared with the control group on tests involving auditory–verbal working memory. The authors suggested that the improvement, continuing over the follow-up period, was consistent with a strategy training model as it becomes increasingly automated and integrated into a wider range of behaviours [99]. In the second post-acute Class I study [93], community-dwelling patients with moderate to severe brain injury were screened for orientation, vision, aphasia, and psychiatric illness. The experimental attention training group improved significantly more than the alternative (memory) treatment group on four attention measures administered throughout the treatment period, although the effects did not generalize to the second set of neuropsychological measures.

Sohlberg and Mateer [100] employed a Class II multiple-baseline design with four patients to evaluate the effectiveness of a specific, hierarchical attention training programme. All subjects showed gain on a single attention outcome measure administered after the start of attention training but not after training on visuospatial processing; this improvement also generalized to cognitive and everyday problems. Strache [98] conducted a prospective Class II study on patients with mixed trauma and vascular aetiologies, and compared two closely related interventions for concentration with subjects in an untreated control group receiving general rehabilitation. After 20 treatment sessions, both attention treatments resulted in significant improvement on attention measures in respect of control subjects, with some generalization to memory and intelligence measures. Rath et al. [114], in three interrelated Class II controlled studies, examined the construct of problem-solving as it relates to the assessment of deficits in higher level outpatients with traumatic brain damage. The difference between the groups were significant first for timed attention tasks, then for psychosocial and problem-solving self-report inventories, then for patients' self-report problem-solving, and also in self-report inventory. It means that it is necessary to have many different approaches to the construct of problem-solving (multidimensional approach) to obtain good rehabilitation.

Several attempts were made to establish the differential role for effectiveness of training of specific components of attention. Rios *et al.* [115] in a Class II controlled study on TBI consider attention as a basic cognitive function, a prerequisite for other cognitive processes. It is divided into four different subprocesses – cognitive flexibility, speed of processing, interference, and working memory – which must be taken into consideration. The results of the work support the view that these different subprocesses of attentional control can be differentiated between high and low level processes and may have implications for neuropsychological assessment and rehabilitation.

Cicerone *et al.* [12] reported evidence from two Class I studies [106, 107] with 36 subjects that supports the effectiveness of attention training for subjects with TBI during the post-acute period of rehabilitation. Considering such evidence, along with Cicerone *et al.*'s previous recommendation based on two Class I studies with 57 subjects [11], strategy training for attention deficits exhibited by subjects with TBI has been recommended as a practice standard during the post-acute period of rehabilitation [12]. Results of studies in this area suggest greater benefits on complex tasks requiring the regulation of attention, rather than on basic aspects of attention (e.g. reaction time, vigilance). These findings are consistent with the emphasis on strategy training to compensate for attention deficits in functional situations.

Pero *et al.* [116] evaluated the effectiveness of the Sohlberg and Mateer's APT using a comprehensive assessment of different attentional processes. Two TBI patients were given the APT in a chronic phase: both showed some degree of recovery, particularly in attentional tasks with a selective component; lesser improvement was observed in tasks related to the intensity dimension of attention, namely those concerning alertness or vigilance. This Class IV study further supports selective training effects of APT on attentional deficits of patients with TBI.

Improvements in speed of processing appear to be less robust than improvements in non-speeded tasks [92, 101, 105]. Moreover, several studies also suggest greater benefits of attention training on more complex tasks requiring selective or divided attention than on basic tasks of reaction time or vigilance [97, 99, 105]. Wilson and Robertson [104], implementing a series of individualized interventions intended to facilitate voluntary control over attention during functional activities,

effectively decreased the attention lapses that the subject experienced when reading novels and texts.

Rohling *et al.* [117] recently provided a meta-analysis of cognitive rehabilitation literature that was originally reviewed by Cicerone *et al.* [11, 12] for the purpose of providing evidence-based practice guidelines for TBI patients. The meta-analysis revealed sufficient evidence for the effectiveness of attention training after TBI.

Recommendations

During the acute period of recovery and inpatient rehabilitation, evidence is insufficient to distinguish the effects of specific attention training from spontaneous recovery or more general cognitive interventions for patients with moderate to severe TBI and stroke. Therefore, specific interventions for attention during the period of acute recovery are not recommended. On the other hand, the availability of Class I evidence for attention training in the post-acute phase after TBI is compatible with a Level A recommendation. Moreover, the available evidence suggests that cognitive rehabilitation has differential effects on various components of attention; therefore, more research is needed to clarify the differential effects of interventions, and new methodologies are required for the assessment of related neural processes.

Rehabilitation of memory

Memory impairment is a well-documented sequel following TBI. Nearly a fourth (25%) of those who have sustained TBI suffer from memory problems, and more than a third of patients who have suffered a stroke show cognitive impairments in one or more cognitive domains such as attention, memory, orientation, language, and executive functions. Generally, approaches to memory rehabilitation are either oriented towards restoring or optimizing damaged or residual functions, or focus on compensating for lost or deficient functions. Within these approaches, training techniques are oriented towards alleviating memory problems such as difficulties of learning and retrieval, or everyday functioning. Others focus on training specific contents such as orientation, dates, names, faces, routines, or appointments. Still others target specific memory systems such as working, episodic, declarative, or prospective memory, or modality-specific impairments such as visual or verbal problems. As cognitive domains frequently overlap, general cognitive training has also been attempted in order to enhance various cognitive functions, including memory. The training techniques that have been investigated systematically include practice and rehearsal, domain-specific learning, mnemonics, and other strategies as well as the use of external memory aids and environmental supports. Whatever the technique used, the main question is how effective and long-lasting it is.

The current report on memory rehabilitation updates our previous reviews [118], literature from 2005 to January 2009, and considers various review or summary papers [12, 119–122]. Although we will not review pharmacological treatment, we would like to point the reader to some valuable reviews of the effects of pharmacological treatment in TBI [121, 123–126].

Studies targetting intervention strategies without the use of external memory aids

Early studies on the general use of compensatory memory strategies previously reported on showed partially contradictory findings, and it was difficult to draw a clear conclusion (for details, see [118]. For example, Doornhein and de Haan [127] did not find positive effects on memory impairment in stroke patients using compensatory strategies, whereas Berg *et al.* [128] reported positive effects, and Ryan and Ruff [129] found a training effect only for mild memory impairment. Later studies include a case report on three patients with TBI that found improved prospective memory and diary use using self-awareness and compensatory strategy training ([130]; Class IV study). A Class II study compared a control group receiving low-dose memory training with two high-frequency training groups that included process-oriented memory training and compensatory strategy training [131]. The study investigated 62 patients of mixed aetiologies with mild to moderate memory disorders; no conclusions can thus be drawn for specific pathologies or disease severity. The frequency or intensity with which a group was trained affected the degree to which verbal memory performance improved. Compared with strategy training, process-oriented memory training improved verbal memory performance and decreased the forgetting rate in the intensive memory trainings groups.

A series of Class III studies and a Class IV study targetting more specific memory strategies reported an advantage of errorless learning techniques (in which people are prevented from making errors) over errorful tech-

niques (such as trial and error) in people with memory impairments. TBI and stroke patients benefited most when learning without errors was encouraged [132–134]. Findings indicated that any benefit of errorless learning may depend on the type of task used, the way in which memory is tested, and the severity of the memory impairment. Furthermore, pre-exposure to the target stimuli seemed to enhance the benefit of errorless learning [135–137]. Findings of a more recent Class II study also emphasized the dependency of the learning technique on the nature of the task. Mount and colleagues [138] investigated the effectiveness of errorless learning and trial and error learning for teaching ADLs during acute stroke rehabilitation in 33 patients with different levels of memory impairment. They did not find a difference between the two learning techniques when used to acquire two specific ADL skills (use of wheelchair and use of donning-sock). Only one of the techniques – the trial and error approach but not the errorless learning method – led to a carry-over effect of learning in one type of ADL task (the sock-donning task). It was also found that explicit memory impairment did not affect the effectiveness of either learning method. It is noteworthy that this study showed the effectiveness of the learning techniques in a natural instead of a 'laboratory' setting.

Another technique of learning and retaining information is based on a spacing effect that has been shown to improve learning and memory performance when information is distributed over time. Two Class III studies reported improved recall and recognition performance and learning of new information in TBI patients with different severity statuses when the material was presented in repeated trials distributed over time [139, 140]. Comparing spaced retrieval training with didactic strategy instructions (both over the telephone) in 38 severely impaired TBI patients, Bourgeois *et al.* [141] found that both techniques reduced memory problems but that the spaced retrieval technique was more effective (Class II study). However, these effects did not have an impact on quality of life measures.

The use of visual imagery to enhance memory performance has been reported by Kaschel *et al.* [142]. This Class III study compared nine target group patients with 12 control group patients of mixed aetiologies and in rehabilitation centres across different countries. The target group received imagery-based training, while the control group was trained with the standard programme in their respective rehabilitation centre. Positive effects of visual imagery training on memory functioning were reported at post-training and were maintained at the 3-month follow-up assessment.

In healthy people, memory performance is improved if items to be learned are self-generated. Two studies investigated the efficacy of self-generation in patients with TBI. Comparing 18 moderate to severe TBI patients with 18 healthy controls, Lengenfelder *et al.* [143] showed that self-generation of verbal material improved both subsequent recall and recognition compared with words that were provided to the subjects (Class III study). Another Class II study compared self-generation of verbal material with didactic presentation of material in two groups of 20 patients with TBI. The authors reported improvements in recognition memory but not in free recall [144]. Furthermore, self-generation procedures only improved recall performance when the newly learned material was supplemented with specific reminder cues.

A Class IV study has focused on a specific sequel frequently observed in patients with TBI – associating faces with names in a real-world context [145]. Five single cases with severe TBI were first trained with a traditional training programme (using name restating, phonemic cuing and visual imagery) followed by real-world training (actual, to-be-named people). Four of the five patients showed an improved recall of names, especially in real-world contexts, regardless of the type of cuing strategy. Unfortunately, the findings of this study are difficult to interpret as the effects of the traditional training and real-world training cannot be teased apart. It is also not clear whether any of the patients had visual or gnostic difficulties, which are frequently observed after TBI.

A Class III study investigated the effects of intense, adaptive working memory training in stroke patients. Fifteen patients who had had a mild to severe stroke (age 34–65 years, seen 12–36 months after the event) were divided into a treatment and a passive control group [146]. The treatment group was trained with a battery of visuospatial and auditory working memory tasks at home on a computer for 40 min daily for 5 days over 5 weeks. Eight neuropsychological tests served as baseline and outcome measures. Working memory and attention improved in the training but not the passive stroke group.

While the studies previously discussed generally focused on using some type of memory training to improve learning and specific aspects of memory, there are also studies that address a broader range of cognitive functions, motivated by the fact that patients with TBI often show impairments of several functional systems (such as attention, memory, executive functions, etc.) and the mounting problems to provide resources to treat all patients individually, Thickpenny-Davis and Barker-Collo [147] investigated the impact of eight learning modules (60-min sessions twice a week over 4 weeks) in a structured group format memory rehabilitation programme (Class III). The learning module consisted of didactic teaching about memory and memory strategies, small group activities, discussions, problem-solving, and practice implementing memory strategies. Ten patients with moderate to severe TBI and two stroke patients were divided into a waiting group and a memory group. Patients in the memory group showed an increased use of memory aids and strategies, an improved knowledge about memory and memory strategies, reduced self-rated behaviors indicative of memory impairment, and an improvement on neuropsychological assessment of memory. The improvements were maintained at 1-month follow-up assessment.

Another study aimed at improving planning skills in patients with TBI through a self-instructional technique involving self-cueing to recall specific autobiographical experiences [148]; Class II study). Thirty patients with severe TBI were randomly allocated to an (active) control group and a training group. While the control group was engaged in conversation, the experimental group underwent training in a procedure aimed at prompting autobiographical memory to support planning skills. Compared with the control group, the training group improved their planning skills, although the effect size indicated only a modest intervention effect. In addition, the authors found an effective increase in the number of specific memories recalled.

A Class I study evaluated the effect of everyday music listening on the recovery of cognitive functions and mood in 54 stroke patients at baseline and 3 and 6 months after the stroke [149]. Compared with a group listening to a non-music audio book or a group without listening material, patients who listened to their favourite music showed a greater improvement in focused attention and verbal memory, and were in a less depressed and confused mood.

In summary, there is some evidence that the frequency with which memory training is applied plays a role in having an effect on mild to moderate memory impairment. A process-oriented training approach is effective and improves verbal and prospective memory. It is, however, not clear whether patients who have had a TBI or stroke profit to the same degree from such training. Within the framework of specific training techniques, errorless learning is probably an effective intervention (Level B) in TBI and stroke patients. The effectiveness, however, depends on the nature of the task to be learned and the type of memory impairment. Exploiting the spacing effect to improve learning and memory performance is another probably effective intervention (Level B) in TBI patients, although other techniques, such as training visual-imagery strategies in patients of mixed aetiology, training working memory in stroke patients, using a wide variety of intervention material in structured group intervention, and training autobiographical memory, have shown beneficial effects. For these individual approaches, more evidence is, however, needed for a clear recommendation. Other approaches going beyond the mere training of memory functions have also shown beneficial effects on memory as well as on other cognitive functions. Regularly listening to music during the early recovery phase of stroke patients is an effective intervention technique (Level A) that improves attention and verbal memory. There is also evidence that training memory through self-instructional recall techniques affects not only memory, but also planning skills, and is evaluated as probably effective (Level B).

Studies targeting intervention techniques using non-electronic external memory aids

Keeping external aids such as a notebook or a diary is a common way to improve memory performance. Two Class III studies and a series of single-case Class IV studies support the use of external non-electronic memory aids such as a notebook or diary as a possibly effective (Level C) intervention [101, 150–155]. There is some indication that a combined treatment using an external memory aid (diary) with internal strategy training increases efficacy.

The use of assistive electronic technologies

The increasing availability of computers, the Internet, wireless connections, and other electronic devices opens a wide range of possibilities to incorporate these technologies into memory rehabilitation (for a review on assistive technology for cognition devices, see [156].

Two Class III studies [157, 158] and some Class IV studies [159, 160] showed improved memory performance in patients with TBI after using computer-based memory training software. A comparison of computer-assisted memory training with a therapist memory training group and a control group without memory training in 37 patients with TBI showed that memory training was superior to no training but there was no difference in memory improvement between the computer and therapist training group [161]. Interpretation of this study is, however, difficult as the level of TBI severity is not clear, the group being very heterogeneous in terms of age and time post-surgery, and there also seem to be discrepancies in the reported results in the text and tables. Although there is (Level C) evidence that computer-based memory training is possibly effective, there is currently not sufficient evidence showing its superiority over non-computer-assisted training.

Besides computers, portable paging systems have been used to enhance memory performance. A randomized crossover-designed study [162] (Class III) showed the effectiveness of a portable externally programmed paging system (NeuroPage) in a large number of patients who were memory- and executive function-impaired as a result of TBI, stroke, and other aetiologies. Two studies followed using the same patient pool but separated out different aetiologies and controlled for demographic variables, thus upgrading the quality of the studies to Class II [163, 164]. Reporting on 36 patients with stroke [163] and 63 with TBI [164], it was shown that the paging system was effective in compensating for everyday memory and planning problems in the two patient groups. Comparing the stroke group with the TBI group at follow-up (cessation of pager use), it was found that the stroke group's benefit had returned to baseline while the TBI group continued to profit from the system [163]. The authors suggested that this decline may have been due to poorer executive functions in the stroke group.

Another electronic memory aid device is the portable voice organizer. This device can be trained to recognize a patient's individual speech patterns, store messages dictated by the user, and replay messages at prespecified time periods. It was shown that such a system facilitated the free and cued recall of therapy goals and plans in a controlled within-subject design study with TBI patients [165] (Class III study). The efficacy of the voice organizer has also been demonstrated in a Class IV study with patients of different aetiologies, including TBI [166].

Several single-case studies with TBI patients (Class IV) using personal digital assistants (PDAs) with data transmission via the mobile phone network [167], an alphanumeric paging system [168], and mobile phones that can be programmed to remind individuals to perform tasks at specific times [169] have shown mixed results concerning the successful use of these system.

In summary, portable paging systems are probably effective (Level B) systems to enhance memory performance, while the effectiveness of other electronic memory devices (PDAs, mobile phones) still needs more empirical support.

The usefulness of a virtual environment for specific memory or learning skills has been investigated in two Class III studies [170, 171]; for a review of the use and possibilities of virtual reality in memory rehabilitation, see [172]. As reported previously, the studies indicated that patients with stroke or TBI could improve on spatial memory performance or verbal and visual learning in virtual environments, and memory training in virtual environments was rated as possibly effective (Level C evidence) (for details, see [118]). There are currently no newer controlled studies available that would update the previous findings.

Recommendations

Memory strategy training is one of the most common intervention techniques, and has been evaluated as effective for subjects with mild memory impairments after TBI or stroke by Cicerone and colleagues [12]. Comper and colleagues [119] arrive at a different conclusion. Reviewing the efficacy of cognitive training for patients with mild TBI, they concluded that there is very little evidence suggesting that cognitive rehabilitation therapy is effective in treating individuals with mild TBI. The differences in evaluation may be due to the heterogeneity of the patients and the types of cognitive function investigated. Besides severity of the TBI, other factors to consider are the frequency of training and the specific strategic approach applied. Errorless learning, spaced recall techniques, self-instructional recall techniques, and process-oriented training are supported by Level B evidence and are thus recommended as probably effective. Other techniques, such as training visual-imagery strategies in patients of mixed aetiology, training working memory in stroke patients, using structured group intervention with a wide variety of intervention material, and training autobiographical memory, have also shown positive effects. However, more supportive evidence for these individual techniques is needed before clear recommendations can be made. The use of non-electronic external memory aids such as a notebook or diary has shown a benefit and is evaluated as possibly effective (Level C).

A non-specific intervention approach to improve cognitive abilities after stroke has shown advantages in the cognitive as well as emotional domain. Regularly listening to music during the early recovery phase of stroke patients has shown effectiveness in improving attention and verbal memory (Level A evidence).

Computer-assisted memory training is also possibly effective, although there is currently insufficient evidence to judge whether it is superior to non-computer-assisted training. Generally, the use of electronic external memory devices such as paging systems and portable voice systems is recommended as possibly effective (Level B evidence) in patients after stroke and TBI. Still more empirical support is, however, needed on the specific use of PDAs or mobile phones with reminder functions to arrive at evidence-based recommendation.

Memory training in virtual environments has shown positive effects on verbal, visual, and spatial learning in patients with stroke and TBI, and is rated as possibly effective (Level C evidence). A direct comparison of performing learning and memory training in virtual environments versus non-virtual environments is still lacking, and no recommendation can be made on the specificity of the technique.

More stringently controlled studies have appeared in recent years and thus facilitated evidence-based recommendations. There is, however, still a need to tease apart the effects that cognitive training has on specific aetiologies, the role that the severity of the impairment plays within these aetiologies, the lasting effect of the training and its ecological validity, and the effect of other non-memory-oriented intervention on memory functions (for a discussion, see [121]). It is conceivable that the type and intensity of training has different effects depending on the neural circuits damaged, the functional impairment profile, the age and gender of the patient, the time that has passed since injury, the education level of the patient, and other external factors (such as social and vocational situation). It would also be important to know whether a combination of interventions (including pharmacological therapy) is beneficial, and if so what the best combination would be. The number of variables involved makes generalization across individuals difficult and favours training programmes tailored to the individual circumstances.

Rehabilitation of apraxia

Although the incidence of apraxia after acquired brain damage is considerable, the literature on recovery and treatment is minimal. Several reasons for this lack of evidence can be identified [173]. First, patients with apraxia often seem to be unaware of their deficit and rarely complain; second, many researchers believe that recovery from apraxia is spontaneous and treatment is not necessary; third, some authors believe that apraxia only occurs when performance is requested of patients in testing situations, and that correct behaviour is displayed in natural settings. By now, however, there is agreement that apraxia hinders independence in ADLs. Goldenberg et al. [174] assessed complex ADLs in patients with apraxia and controls. They found that apraxic patients had more difficulties than patients with left brain damage without apraxia and healthy controls. In two other studies, comparable results were found: Hanna-Paddy et al. [175] found a significant relationship between severity of apraxia and dependency in physical functioning; Walker et al. [176] studied the impact of cognitive impairments on upper body dressing difficulties after stroke using video analysis – those patients who failed shirt-dressing showed neglect and apraxia at follow-up. Recently, the impact of apraxia on the dependence of patients with stroke in their ADLs has again been confirmed [177]. These results suggest that treatment of apraxia should be part of the overall neurorehabilitation programme after brain damage.

Recently, a Cochrane Review has been published that has determined which therapeutic interventions are effective for targeting disabilities due to motor apraxia following stroke [178]. The literature search was carried out up to November 2006 and revealed only three trials including a total of 132 participants [179–181]. The authors of the review conclude, on the basis of these three trials, that there is insufficient evidence to support or refute the effectiveness of specific interventions for motor apraxia following stroke. However, since there are more therapy studies conducted than the strict methodology of the Cochrane Collaboration for RCTs allows, a broader set of studies examining the effectiveness of treating apraxia will be reviewed in this brief summary. The studies are labelled either observational or experimental, and the quality of the studies is described. The reader is also referred to Buxbaum et al. [182] for a review on the treatment of limb apraxia.

There are two recent RCTs on the rehabilitation of apraxia. As the study by Edmans et al. [179] was on the treatment of perceptual problems, it will not be discussed here. Smania et al. [180] assessed in an RCT the effectiveness of a rehabilitative training programme for patients with limb apraxia. Thirteen patients with acquired brain injury and limb apraxia (lasting more than 2 months) as a result of lesions in the left cerebral hemisphere participated in the study. The study group underwent an experimental training for limb apraxia consisting of a behavioural training programme with gesture-production exercises. The control group received conventional treatment for aphasia. Assessments involved neuropsychological tests of aphasia, verbal comprehension, general intelligence, oral apraxia, and constructional apraxia, and three tests concerning limb praxic function (ideational and ideomotor apraxia and gesture recognition). Everyday activities related to each test were used to measure the outcome. The patients in the study group achieved a significant improvement of performance in both the ideational and ideomotor apraxia tests. They also showed a significant reduction of errors in ideational and ideomotor apraxia tests. The change in performance was not significant for the control group. The results show the possible effectiveness of a specific training programme for the treatment of limb apraxia.

Donkervoort et al. [181] determined in a controlled study the efficacy of strategy training in left hemisphere stroke patients with apraxia. A total of 113 patients who had suffered a stroke in the left hemisphere stroke and had apraxia were randomly assigned to two treatment groups: (1) strategy training integrated into the usual occupational therapy; and (2) usual occupational therapy only. The primary outcome measure was a standardized ADL observation by a blinded research assistant. Additional ADL measures were used as secondary outcome measures (Barthel ADL index, ADL judgement by occupational therapists and by patients). After 8 weeks of treatment, patients who received strategy training ($n = 43$) improved significantly more than patients in the usual treatment group ($n = 39$) on the ADL observations. This reflects a small to medium effect (effect size 0.37) of strategy training on ADL functioning. With respect to the secondary outcome measures, a medium effect (effect size 0.47) was found on the Barthel ADL index. No beneficial effects of strategy training were found after 5 months (at follow-up).

In addition, we performed secondary analyses on the data of Donkervoort et al. [181] to examine the transfer of the effects of cognitive strategy training for stroke patients with apraxia from trained to non-trained tasks. The analyses showed that, in both treatment groups, the scores on the ADL observations for non-trained tasks improved significantly after 8 weeks of training compared with the baseline score. Change scores of non-trained activities were larger in the strategy training group compared with the usual treatment group. These results suggest that transfer of training is possible, although further research should confirm these exploratory findings [183]. Recently, we performed a study specifically aiming to measure the transfer effects of the cognitive strategy training for apraxia [184]. In this study, we showed that patients performed trained and non-trained tasks at the same level of independency at the rehabilitation centre as well as at home, indicating a transfer of training effects that remained stable over time.

A promising approach has been brought forward by Sunderland et al. [185]. In a single-blind, ramdomized, multiple-baseline experiment, they showed that an ecological and individualized approach for dressing behaviour had a significant treatment effect for right hemisphere patients but not for left hemisphere patients; the benefits of this approach to dressing therapy are currently being evaluated further.

Several Class II studies also support the efficacy of apraxia rehabilitation. Goldenberg and Hagman [186] studied a group of 15 patients with apraxia who made fatal errors in ADLs: an error was rated as fatal if the patient could not proceed without help or if the error prohibited the patient from accomplishing the task successfully. The study design was as follows: each week an ADL test was performed; between tests, the patient was trained in one of three activities, whereas support, but no therapeutic advice, was given for two other activities. Each week, the patient was trained in a further activity, while the other activities were performed in daily life. Thus, in the following week, training was done in the second activity, and in the third week the remaining activity was trained. In case fatal errors were still seen during performance, another cycle of therapy was run. At the end of the therapy, 10 patients could perform all three activities without fatal errors. Three patients made only one fatal error. No generalization of training effects was found from trained to non-trained activities. Seven

patients were re-examined after 6 months: only those patients who kept practising the activities in their daily life still showed the positive results of the training.

Van Heugten et al. [187] performed a study evaluating a therapy programme for teaching patients strategies to compensate for the presence of apraxia. The outcome was studied in a pre/post test design; measurements were conducted at baseline and after 12 weeks of therapy. Thirty-three stroke patients with apraxia were treated in occupational therapy departments in general hospitals, rehabilitation centres, and nursing homes. The patients showed considerable improvement in ADL functioning on all measures and slight improvements on the apraxia test and motor functioning test. The effect sizes for the disabilities, ranging from 0.92 to 1.06, were large compared with the effect sizes for apraxia (0.34) and motor functioning (0.19). The significant effect of treatment is also seen when individual improvement and subjective improvement are considered. These results suggest that the programme seems to be successful in teaching patients compensatory strategies that enable them to function more independently, despite the lasting presence of apraxia.

Poole [188] published a study examining the ability of participants with a left hemisphere stroke to learn one-handed shoe-tying. Participants with a left hemisphere stroke with and without apraxia and control participants were taught how to tie their shoelaces with one hand. Retention was assessed after a 5-min interval during which participants performed other tasks. All groups differed significantly with regard to the number of trials to learn the task. However, on the retention task, the control adults and the stroke patients without apraxia required a similar numbers of trial, whereas the participants with apraxia required significantly more trials than the other two groups. All groups required fewer trials on the retention task than on the learning task.

Further evidence is provided by single-case studies. Wilson [189] studied a female adolescent with extensive damage to her brain following an anaesthetic accident. One of the most disabling consequences of the damage was apraxia, which made her almost completely dependent in daily life. Wilson concluded that the step-by-step programme was successful in teaching the patient some tasks, but generalization to new tasks was not found at follow-up. Maher et al. [190] studied the effects of treatment on a 55-year-old man with ideomotor apraxia and preserved gesture recognition. One-hour therapy sessions were given daily during a 2-week period. During therapy sessions, many cues were offered that were withdrawn systematically, while feedback and correction of errors were given as well. The production of gestures improved qualitatively. Ochipa *et al.* [191] subsequently developed a treatment programme aimed at specific error types. Praxis performance was studied in two stroke patients. It appeared that both patients achieved a considerable improvement in performance, but the observed effects were treatment specific: treatment of a specific error type did not improve across untreated gestures. Jantra *et al.* [192] studied a 61-year-old man with a right-sided stroke followed by apraxic gait. After 3 weeks of gait training supplemented with visual cues, the patient became independent with safe ambulating. Pilgrim and Humphreys [193] presented the case of a left-handed head injured patient with ideomotor apraxia of his left upper limb. The patient's performance on the 10 objects was measured before and after training in three different modalities. A mixed-design analysis of variance was carried out showing a positive effect of therapy but little carry-over to everyday life. Bulter [194] presents a case study that explores the effectiveness of tactile and kinaesthetic stimulation as an intervention strategy, in addition to visual and verbal mediation, in the rehabilitation of a man with ideational and ideomotor apraxia following a head injury. The results indicated some improvement after a training period and limited evidence of the effectiveness of additional sensory input.

Goldenberg *et al.* [174] conducted a therapy study with six apraxic patients in which two methods of treatment were compared: direct training of the activity based on the guided performance of the whole activity, and exploration training aimed at teaching the patient the structure–function relationships underlying correct performance but not involving actual completion of the activity. Exploration training had no effect on performance, whereas direct training of the activity reduced errors and the need for assistance. Training effects were largely preserved at follow-up, but the rate of errors increased when the trained activities were tested with a partially different set of objects. Performance improved with repeated testing of untrained activities during initial baseline, but there was no reduction of errors or amount of assistance required for untrained activities during the training of other activities. As therapeutic results were

restricted to trained activities and to some degree to trained objects, the authors concluded that therapy should be tailored to the specific needs of patients and their family and should be linked closely to the normal routines of daily life.

Recently, a single-case study was executed in which repetition of a newly designed facilitation exercise was used in a patient with corticobasal degeneration, leading to a decrease of difficulties in ADL performance [195].

Recommendations

There is Level A evidence for the effectiveness of apraxia treatment with compensatory strategies. Treatment should focus on functional activities that are structured and practised using errorless learning approaches. As transfer of training is difficult to achieve, training should focus on specific activities in a specific context close to the patients' normal routines. Recovery of apraxia should not be the goal for rehabilitation.

Rehabilitation of acalculia

Acquired disorders of number processing and calculation (DNPC) are manifold and may occur after many types of brain damage. Depending on the underlying disease and lesion location, the frequency of calculation disorders in patients with neurological disorders has been estimated to range between 10% and 90% [196]. As with other cognitive deficits, subsets of number and calculation knowledge may be individually affected, requiring a profound assessment to define the profile of impairment. A review summarising the remediation of DNPC has to account for the variety of its clinical presentations and underlying causes [197], the frequent association with aphasia or other cognitive impairments, and the limited knowledge regarding its spontaneous recovery [198].

Most research designs and statistical evaluation procedures are taken from the field of single-subject research [199, 200]. Outcome measures typically consist of a comparison of an individual's pre- and post-treatment performance, the decrease of error rates and response latencies, the confirmation of generalization or transfer, and the use of prior learning in new context. The amount of functional disability in daily life is rarely assessed or estimated in this corpus of studies. As a literature search based on databanks was unsatisfactory, the authors reviewed the existing literature themselves and used a pre-existing overview related to the topic [201, 202].

Two main types of treatment rationale have been applied to DNPC. One, the 'reconstitution' or 're-teaching' approach, consists of improvements to lost or damaged abilities by way of extensive practice and drill in order to improve efficiency and speed. The other, indirect approach promotes the use of 'back-up' strategies based on the patient's residual resources [201]. In this case, the treatment would work not merely to restore the functionality of the impaired component, but rather to exploit preserved abilities to compensate for the deficit. Both types of remediation employ step-by-step training consisting of a presentation of problems of increasing difficulty, facilitation cues, and other types of assistance that eventually fade with progressive recovery; in all cases, direct feedback is provided to patients on their accuracy and errors.

Studies have been mostly 'quasi-experimental' using a single-case or small-group approach guided by the principles of cognitive neuropsychology [203–206] and single-subject research (Class II, III, and IV evidence). Group studies using control groups are considered inadequate by most authors due to known reasons (problems with patient selection, group homogeneity, heterogeneity of subjacent deficit and premorbid functional level). The group study of Gauggell and Billino [207] deals with the effects of motivation rather than of specific treatment.

Rehabilitation of DNPC may be grouped into several areas of intervention [208]. Rehabilitation of *transcoding ability* (the ability to translate numerical stimuli between different formats) has been successfully performed in several studies [209–213], mostly by re-teaching the patient the required set of rules. Impairments of *arithmetical facts* (simple multiplication, addition, subtraction, or division solved directly from memory) were the target of several rehabilitation studies [208, 214–220]. In all studies, extensive practice with the defective domain of knowledge, i.e. multiplication tables, determined significant improvement. A positive outcome was also reached by a rehabilitation programme based on the strategic use of the patient's residual knowledge of arithmetic [215]. This specific case suggests that the integration of declarative, procedural, and conceptual knowledge critically mediates the reacquisition process. Miceli and Capasso [214] have successfully rehabilitated a patient with deficient *arithmetical procedures* (the knowledge required to solve multidigit calculations). Deficient *arithmetical problem-solving* (the ability to provide a solution

for complex, multistep arithmetical text problems) has also been treated in one study [221]. The study was rated as partly successful by the authors, as patients benefited from the cueing procedure, engaged and generated a higher number of correct solution steps, but did not show a prominent effect on the actual execution process.

Recommendations

Overall, the available evidence suggests that rehabilitation procedures used to treat selected variants of DNPC have been successful (Level C). Notably, significant improvements were observed even in severely impaired and chronic patients. Several caveats, however, need to be mentioned in this context. At present, little is known about the prognosis and spontaneous recovery of DNPC; thus, the effects of different interventions in the early stages of numerical disorders may be difficult to evaluate. Moreover, different underlying neurological disorders (e.g. stroke, dementia, trauma) have only partly been compared in terms of their specific effects on DNPC. Furthermore, it has not been studied in detail how impairments of attention or executive functions influence the rehabilitation process of DNPC.

General recommendations

In our opinion, there is enough overall evidence to award a grade A, B, or C recommendation to some forms of cognitive rehabilitation in patients with neuropsychological deficits in the post-acute stage after a focal brain lesion (stroke, TBI). This general conclusion is based on a limited number of RCTs, and is supported by a considerable amount of evidence coming from Class II, III, and IV studies. In particular, the use of a rigorous single-case methodology has been considered by the present reviewers as a source of acceptable evidence in this specific field, in which the application of the RCT methodology is difficult for a number of reasons, related to the lack of consensus on the target of treatment, the methodology of the intervention, and the assessment of the outcomes. Similar conclusions were reached on the basis of a meta-analysis of effect sizes reported by Rohling *et al.* [117].

Future developments

There is clearly a need for large-scale RCTs evaluating well-defined methodologies of intervention in common clinical conditions (e.g. assessment of the efficacy of an intervention for ULN after right hemispheric stroke on long-term motor disability). The main difficulty of this approach lies in the highly heterogeneous nature of cognitive deficits. For example, it is hard to believe that the same standardized aphasia treatment may be effective for a patient with a fluent neologistic jargon and another with agrammatic nonfluent production. Research in neuropsychology has focused on the assessment of specific, theoretically driven treatments in well-defined areas of impairment, usually by means of single-case methodology (e.g. the effect of a linguistically driven intervention compared with simple stimulation on the ability to retrieve lexical items belonging to a defined class). To the present panel, both approaches represent potentially fruitful avenues for research in this field.

Future studies should also aim at a better clinical and pathological definition of the patients included in the trials. The gross distinction between stroke and traumatic brain damage used in the present review is clearly insufficient: a separation of the main categories of cerebrovascular pathology and a subdivision on pathological grounds of the survivors of traumatic brain damage can be expected to improve the quality of rehabilitation studies.

Conflicts of interest

The authors report no conflicts of interest in connection with this chapter.

Acknowledgements

The authors contributed to the reviews as follows: A. Bellmann, ULN; C. Bindschaedler, ULN; L. Bonfiglio, attention rehabilitation; P. Bongioanni, attention rehabilitation; S. Chiocca, attention rehabilitation; M. Delazer, acalculia; L. Girelli, acalculia.

References

1. Cappa SF, Benke T, Clarke S, Rossi B, Stemmer B, van Heugten C. EFNS guidelines on cognitive rehabilitation. *Eur J Neurol* 2003;**10**:11–23.

2. Cappa SF, Benke T, Clarke S, Rossi B, Stemmer B, van Heugten CM. Task Force on Cognitive Rehabilitation; European Federation of Neurological Societies. EFNS guidelines on cognitive rehabilitation: report of an EFNS task force. *Eur J Neurol* 2005;**12**:665–80.

3. Harley JP, Allen C, Braciszeski TL, Cicerone KD, Dahlberg C, Evans S. Guidelines for cognitive rehabilitation. *Neurol Rehabil* 1992;**2**:62–7.

4. NIH Consensus Development Panel on Rehabilitation of Persons with Traumatic Brain Injury. Rehabilitation of persons with traumatic brain injury. *J Am Med Assoc* 1999;**282**:974–83.

5. French J, Gronseth G. Lost in the jungle of evidence. *Neurology* 2008;**71**:1634–8.

6. Cicerone KD. *Evidence-based guidelines for cognitive rehabilitation: a European perspective [Electronic Version]*. Published online 16.02.2006 by the International Brain Injury Association, 2006. Available at: http://internationalbrain. org/news.php?dep=3&page=3&list=5.

7. Brainin MBM, Baron J-C, Gilhus NE, Hughes R, Selmaj K, Waldema G. Guidance for the preparation of neurological management guidelines by EFNS scientific task forces – revised recommendations 2004. *Eur J Neurol* 2004;**11**:1–6.

8. Howard D, Hatfield FM. *Aphasia Therapy: Historical and Contemporary Issues*. Hove: Lawrence Erlbaum, 1987.

9. Basso A. *Aphasia and its Therapy*. Oxford: Oxford University Press, 2003.

10. Greener J, Enderby P, Whurr R. Speech and language therapy for aphasia following stroke. *Cochrane Database Syst Rev* 2000;(4):CD000425.

11. Cicerone KD, Dahlberg C, Kalmar K, *et al*. Evidence-based cognitive rehabilitation: recommendations for clinical practice. *Arch Phys Med Rehabil* 2000;**81**:1596–615.

12. Cicerone KD, Dahlberg C, Malec JF, *et al*. Evidence-based cognitive rehabilitation: updated review of the literature from 1998 through 2002. *Arch Phys Med Rehabil* 2005;**86**:1681–92.

13. Hagen C. Communication abilities in hemiplegia: effect of speech therapy. *Arch Phys Med Rehabil* 1973;**54**:454–63.

14. Katz RC, Wertz RT. The efficacy of computer-provided reading treatment for chronic aphasic adults. *J Speech Lang Hear Res* 1997;**40**:493–507.

15. Helffenstein D, Wechsler R. The use of interpersonal process recall (IPR) in the remediation of interpersonal and communication skill deficits in the newly brain injured. *Clin Neuropsychol* 1982;**4**:139–43.

16. Thomas-Stonell NP, Johnson P, Schuller R. *et al.* Evaluation of a computer-based program for cognitive-communication skills. *J Head Trauma Rehabil* 1994;**9**:25–37.

17. Basso A, Capitani E, Vignolo LA. Influence of rehabilitation on language skills in aphasic patients. A controlled study. *Arch Neurol* 1979;**36**:190–6.

18. Shewan CM, Kertesz A. Effects of speech language treatment on recovery from aphasia. *Brain Lang* 1985;**23**:272–99.

19. Poeck K, Huber W, Willmes K. Outcome of intensive language treatment in aphasia. *J Speech Hear Disord* 1989;**54**:471–9.

20. Carlomagno S, Pandolfi M, Labruna L, Colombo A, Razzano C. Recovery from moderate aphasia in the first year post-stroke: effect of type of therapy. *Arch Phys Med Rehabil* 2001;**82**:1073–80.

21. Elman RJ, Bernstein-Ellis E. The efficacy of group communication treatment in adults with chronic aphasia. *J Speech Lang Hear Res* 1999;**42**:411–19.

22. Doesborgh SJ, van de Sandt-Koenderman MW, Dippel DW, van Harskamp F, Koudstaal PJ, Visch-Brink EG. Effects of semantic treatment on verbal communication and linguistic processing in aphasia after stroke: a randomized controlled trial. *Stroke* 2004;**35**:141–6.

23. Robey RR, Schultz MC, Crawford AB, Sinner CA. Single-subject clinical-outcome research: designs, data, effect sizes, and analyses. *Aphasiology* 1999;**13**:445–73.

24. Moss A, Nicholas M. Language rehabilitation in chronic aphasia and time postonset: a review of single-subject data. *Stroke* 2006;**37**(12):3043–51.

25. Bhogal SK, Teasell R, Speechley M. Intensity of aphasia therapy, impact on recovery. *Stroke* 2003;**34**:987–93.

26. Marshall RC. The impact of intensity of aphasia therapy on recovery. *Stroke* 2008;**39**(2):e48.

27. Bakheit AM, Shaw S, Barrett L, *et al.* A prospective, randomized, parallel group, controlled study of the effect of intensity of speech and language therapy on early recovery from poststroke aphasia. *Clin Rehabil* 2007;**21**(10):885–94.

28. Pulvermueller F, Neininger B, Elbert T, *et al.* Constraint-induced therapy of chronic aphasia after stroke. *Stroke* 2001;**32**:1621–6.

29. Meinzer M, Djundja D, Barthel G, Elbert T, Rockstroh B. Long-term stability of improved language functions in chronic aphasia after constraint-induced aphasia therapy. *Stroke* 2005;**36**(7):1462–6.

30. Maher LM, Kendall D, Swearengin JA, *et al.* A pilot study of use-dependent learning in the context of constraint induced language therapy. *J Int Neuropsychol Soc* 2006;**12**(6):843–52.

31. Berthier ML, Green C, Lara JP, *et al.* Memantine and constraint-induced aphasia therapy in chronic poststroke aphasia. *Ann Neurol* 2009;**65**(5):577–85.

32. Laganaro M, Di Pietro M, Schnider A. Computerised treatment of anomia in acute aphasia: treatment intensity and training size. *Neuropsychol Rehabil* 2006;**16**(6):630–40.

33. Fridriksson J, Baker JM, Whiteside J, *et al.* Treating visual speech perception to improve speech production in nonfluent aphasia. *Stroke* 2009;**40**(3):853–8.

34. Manheim LM, Halper AS, Cherney L. Patient-reported changes in communication after computer-based script training for aphasia. *Arch Phys Med Rehabil* 2009;**90**(4):623–7.

35. Denes G, Semenza C, Stoppa E, Lis A. Unilateral spatial neglect and recovery from hemiplegia: a follow-up study. *Brain* 1982;**105**:543–52.

36. Stone SP, Patel P, Greenwood RJ, Halligan PW. Measuring visual neglect in acute stroke and predicting its recovery: the visual neglect recovery index. *J Neurol Neurosurg Psychiatry* 1992;**55**:431–6.

37. Robertson IH, Hawkins K. Limb activation and unilateral neglect. *Neurocase* 1999;**5**:153–60.

38. Robertson IH. Cognitive rehabilitation: attention and neglect. *Trends Cogn Sci* 1999;**3**:385–93.

39. Diamond PT. Rehabilitative management of post-stroke visuospatial inattention. *Disabil Rehabil* 2001;**23**:407–12.

40. Pierce SR, Buxbaum LJ. Treatments of unilateral neglect: a review. *Arch Phys Med Rehabil* 2002;**83**:256–68.

41. Kerkhoff G. Modulation and rehabilitation of spatial neglect by sensory stimulation. *Prog Brain Res* 2003;**142**:257–71.

42. Paton A, Malhortra P, Husain M. Hemispatial neglect. *J Neurol Neurosurg Psychiatry* 2004;**75**:13–21.

43. Pizzamiglio L, Guariglia C, Antonucci G, Zoccolotti P. Development of a rehabilitative program for unilateral neglect. *Restor Neurol Neurosci* 2006;**24**(4–6):337–45.

44. Luaute J, Halligan P, Rode G, Rossetti Y, Boisson D. Visuo-spatial neglect: a systematic review of current interventions and their effectiveness. *Neurosci Biobehav Rev* 2006;**30**(7):961–82.

45. Bowen A, Lincoln NB. Cognitive rehabilitation for spatial neglect following stroke. *Cochrane Database Syst Rev* 2007;(2):CD003586.

46. Antonucci A, Guariglia C, Judica A, *et al.* Effectiveness of neglect rehabilitation in a randomized group study. *J Clin Exp Neuropsychol* 1995;**17**:383–9.

47. Pizzamiglio L, Antonucci G, Judica A, Montenero P, Razzano C, Zoccolotti P. Cognitive rehabilitation of the hemineglect disorder in chronic patients with unilateral right brain damage. *J Clin Exp Neuropsychol* 1992;**14**:901–23.

48. Vallar G, Guariglia C, Magnotti L, Pizzamiglio L. Dissociation between position sense and visual-spatial components of hemineglect through a specific rehabilitation treatment. *J Clin Exp Neuropsychol* 1997;**19**:763–71.

49. Weinberg J, Diller L, Gordon WA, *et al.* Visual scanning training effect on reading-related tasks in acquired right brain damage. *Arch Phys Med Rehabil* 1977;**58**:479–86.

50. Kalra L, Perez I, Gupta S, Wittink M. The influence of visual neglect on stroke rehabilitation. *Stroke* 1997;**28**:1386–91.

51. Lin K-C, Cermark SA, Kinsbourne M, Trombly CA. Effects of left-sided movements on line bisection in unilateral neglect. *J Int Neuropsychol Soc* 1996;**2**:404–11.

52. Frassinetti F, Rossi M, Ladavas E. Passive limb movements improve visual neglect. *Neuropsychologia* 2001;**39**:725–33.

53. Butter CM, Kirsch NL, Reeves G. The effect of lateralized dynamic stimuli on unilateral spatial neglect following right hemisphere lesions. *Restor Neurol Neurosci* 1990;**2**:39–46.

54. Pizzamiglio L, Frasca R, Guariglia C, Incoccia C, Antonucci G. Effect of optokinetic stimulation in patients with visual neglect. *Cortex* 1990;**26**:535–40.

55. Butter CM, Kirsch N. Effect of lateralized kinetic visual cues on visual search in patients with unilateral spatial neglect. *J Clin Exp Neuropsychol* 1995;**17**:856–67.

56. Pizzamiglio L, Fasotti L, Jehkonen M, *et al.* The use of optokinetic stimulation in rehabilitation of the hemineglect disorder. *Cortex* 2004;**40**:441–50.

57. Tham K, Tegnér R. Video feedback in the rehabilitation of patients with unilateral neglect. *Arch Phys Med Rehabil* 1997;**78**:410–13.

58. Harvey M, Hood B, North A, Robertson IH. The effects of visuomotor feedback training on the recovery of hemispatial neglects symptoms: assessment of a 2-week and follow-up intervention. *Neuropsychologia* 2003;**41**:886–93.

59. Ladavas E, Menghini G, Umilta C. A rehabilitation study of hemispatial neglect. *Cogn Neuropsychol* 1994;**11**:75–95.

60. Robertson IH, Tegnér R, Tham K, Lo A, Nimmo-Smith I. Sustained attention training for unilateral neglect: theoretical and rehabilitation implications. *J Clin Exp Neuropsychol* 1995;**17**:416–30.

61. Kerkhoff G. Rehabilitation of visuospatial cognition and visual exploration in neglect: a cross-over study. *Restor Neurol Neurosci* 1998;**12**:27–40.

62. Hommel M, Peres B, Pollack P, *et al.* Effects of passive tactile and auditory stimuli on left visual neglect. *Arch Neurol* 1990;**47**:573–6.

63. Rode G, Perenin MT. Temporary remission of representational hemineglect through vestibular stimulation. *Neurol Report* 1994;**5**:869–72.

64. Rode G, Tiliket C, Charopain P, Boisson D. Postural asymmetry reduction by vestibular caloric stimulation in left hemiparetic patients. *Scand J Rehabil Med* 1998;**30**:9–14.

65. Bottini G, Paulesu E, Gandola M, *et al.* Left caloric vestibular stimulation ameliorates right hemianesthesia. *Neurology* 2005;**65**(8):1278–83.

66. Adair JC, Na DL, Schwartz RL, Heilman KM. Caloric stimulation in neglect: evaluation of response as a function of neglect type. *J Int Neuropsychol Soc* 2003;**9**(7):983–8.

67. Rorsman I, Magnusson M, Johansson BB. Reduction of visuo-spatial neglect with vestibular galvanic stimulation. *Scand J Rehabil Med* 1999;**31**:117–24.

68. Vallar G, Rusconi ML, Barozzi S, *et al.* Improvement of left visuo-spatial hemineglect by left-sided transcutaneous electrical stimulation. *Neuropsychologia* 1995;**33**:73–82.

69. Guariglia C, Lippolis G, Pizzamiglio L. Somatosensory stimulation improves imagery disorders in neglect. *Cortex* 1998;**34**:233–41.

70. Perennou DA, Leblond C, Amblard B, Micallef JP, Herisson C, Pelissier JY. Transcutaneous electric nerve stimulation reduces neglect-related postural instability after stroke. *Arch Phys Med Rehabil* 2001;**82**:440–8.

71. Johannsen L, Ackermann H, Karnath HO. Lasting amelioration of spatial neglect by treatment with neck muscle vibration even without concurrent training. *J Rehabil Med* 2003;**35**(6):249–53.

72. Schindler I, Kerkhoff G, Karnath HO, Keller I, Goldenberg G. Neck muscle vibration induces lasting recovery in spatial neglect. *J Neurol Neurosurg Psychiatry* 2002;**73**:412–19.

73. Wiart L, Bon Saint Côme A, Debelleix X, *et al.* Unilateral neglect syndrome rehabilitation by trunk rotation and scanning training. *Arch Phys Med Rehabil* 1997;**78**:424–9.

74. Rossetti Y, Rode G, Pisella L, *et al.* Prism adaptation to rightward optical deviation rehabilitates left hemispatial neglect. *Nature* 1998;**395**:166–9.

75. Angeli V, Benassi MG, Ladavas E. Recovery of oculomotor bias in neglect patients after prism adaptation. *Neuropsychologia* 2004;**42**:1223–34.

76. Farne A, Rossetti Y, Toniolo S, Ladavas E. Ameliorating neglect with prism adaptation: visuo-manual and visuo-verbal measures. *Neuropsychologia* 2002;**40**:718–29.

77. Frassinetti F, Angeli V, Meneghello F, Avanzi S, Ladavas E. Long-lasting amelioration of visuospatial neglect by prism adaptation. *Brain* 2002;**125**:608–23.

78. Serino A, Bonifazi S, Pierfederici L, Ladavas E. Neglect treatment by prism adaptation: what recovers and for how long. *Neuropsychol Rehabil* 2007;**17**:657–87.

79. Serino A, Angeli V, Frassinetti F, Ladavas E. Mechanisms underlying neglect recovery after prism adaptation. *Neuropsychologia* 2006;**44**(7):1068–78.

80. Beis J-M, André J-M, Baumgarten A, Challier B. Eye patching in unilateral spatial neglect: efficacy of two methods. *Arch Physical Med Rehabil* 1999;**80**:71–6.

81. Butter CM, Kirsch N. Combined and separate effects of eye patching and visual stimulation on unilateral neglect following stroke. *Arch Phys Med Rehabil* 1992;**73**:1133–9.

82. Walker R, Young AW, Lincoln NB. Eye patching and the rehabilitation of visual neglect. *Neuropsychol Rehabil* 1996;**6**:219–31.

83. Zeloni G, Farnè A, Baccini M. Viewing less to see better. *J Neurol Neurosurg Psychiatry* 2002;**73**(2):195–8.

84. Fong KN, Chan MK, Ng PP, *et al.* The effect of voluntary trunk rotation and half-field eye-patching for patients with unilateral neglect in stroke: a randomized controlled trial. *Clin Rehabil* 2007;**21**(8):729–41.

85. Robertson IH, Gray J, Pentland B, Waite LJ. Microcomputer-based rehabilitation for unilateral left visual neglect: a randomized controlled trial. *Arch Phys Med Rehabil* 1990;**71**:663–8.

86. Bergego C, Azouvi P, Deloche G, *et al.* Rehabilitation of unilateral neglect: a controlled multiple-baseline-across-subjects trial using computerised training procedures. *Neuropsychol Rehabil* 1997;**7**(4):279–93.

87. Webster JS, McFarland PT, Rapport LJ, Morrill B, Roades LA, Abadee PS. Computer-assisted training for improving wheelchair mobility in unilateral neglect patients. *Arch Phys Med Rehabil* 2001;**82**:769–75.

88. Bruhn P, Parsons O. Continuous reaction time in brain damage. *Cortex* 1971;**7**:278–91.

89. Van Zomeren AH, Van DenBurg W. Residual complaints of patients two years after severe head injury. *J Neurol Neurosurg Psychiatry* 1985;**48**:21–8.

90. Ben-Yishay Y, Diller L, Rattok J. *A Modular Approach to Optimizing Orientation, Psychomotor Alertness and Purposive Behaviour in Severe Head Trauma Patients.* Rehabilitation Monograph No. 59. New York: New York University Medical Centre, 1978; pp. 63–7.

91. Wood RL. Rehabilitation of patients with disorders of attention. *J Head Trauma Rehabil* 1986;**1**:43–53.

92. Ponsford JL, Kinsella G. Evaluation of a remedial programme for attentional deficits following closed-head injury. *J Clin Exp Neuropsychol* 1988;**10**:693–708.

93. Niemann H, Ruff RM, Baser CA. Computer assisted attention retraining in head injured individuals: a controlled efficacy study of an out-patient program. *J Consult Clin Psychol* 1990;**58**:811–17.

94. Novack TA, Caldwell SG, Duke LW, Bergquist TF. Focused versus unstructured intervention for attention deficits after traumatic brain injury. *J Head Trauma Rehabil* 1996;**11**:52–60.

95. Lincoln NB, Majid MJ, Weyman N. Cognitive rehabilitation for attention deficits following stroke. *Cochrane Database Syst Rev* 2000;(4):CD002842.

96. Schoettke H. Rehabilitation von Aufmerksamkeitsstörungen nach einem Schlaganfall. Effektivität eines verhaltensmedizinisch-neuropsychologischen Aufmerksamkeitstrainings. *Verhaltenstherapie* 1997;**7**:21–3.

97. Gray JM, Robertson I, Pentland B, Anderson S. Microcomputer-based attentional retraining after brain damage: a randomised group controlled trial. *Neuropsychol Rehabil* 1992;**2**:97–115.

98. Strache W. Effectiveness of two modes of training to overcome deficits of concentration. *Int J Rehabil Res* 1987;**10**(S5):141S–5S.

99. Sturm W, Wilmes K. Efficacy of a reaction training on various attentional and cognitive functions in stroke patients. *Neuropsychol Rehabil* 1991;**1**:259–80.

100. Sohlberg MM, Mateer CA. Training use of compensatory memory books: a three stage behavioral approach. *J Clin Exp Neuropsychol* 1989;**11**:871–91.

101. Ethier M, Braun CMJ, Baribeau JMC. Computer-dispensed cognitive-perceptual training of closed head injury patients after spontaneous recovery. Study 1: speeded tasks. *Can J Rehabil* 1989;**2**:223–33.

102. Gray JM, Robertson I. Remediation of attentional difficulties following brain injury: 3 experimental single case studies. *Brain Inj* 1989;**3**:163–70.

103. Gansler DA, McCaffrey RJ. Remediation of chronic attention deficits in traumatic brain-injured patients. *Arch Clin Neuropsychol* 1991;**6**:335–53.

104. Wilson B, Robertson IH. A home based intervention for attentional slips during reading following head injury: a single case study. *Neuropsychol Rehabil* 1992;**2**:193–205.

105. Sturm W, Wilmes K, Orgass B. Do specific attention deficits need specific training? *Neuropsychol Rehabil* 1997;**7**:81–103.

106. Sohlberg MM, McLaughlin KA, Pavese A, Heidrich A, Posner MI. Evaluation of attention process training and brain injury education in persons with acquired brain injury. *J Clin Exp Neuropsychol* 2000;**22**:656–76.

107. Fasotti L, Kovacs F, Eling PA, Brouwer WH. Time pressure management as a compensatory strategy training after closed head injury. *Neuropsychol Rehabil* 2000;**10**:47–65.

108. Cicerone KD. Remediation of 'working attention' in mild traumatic brain injury. *Brain Inj* 2002;**16**:185–95.

109. Palmese CA, Raskin SA. The rehabilitation of attention in individuals with mild traumatic brain injury: using the APT-II programme. *Brain Inj* 2000;**14**:535–48.

110. Park NW, Proulx GB, Towers WM. Evaluation of the attention process training programme. *Neuropsychol Rehabil* 1999;**9**:135–54.

111. Stablum F, Umiltà C, Mazzoldi M, Pastore N, Magon S. Rehabilitation of endogenous task shift processes in closed head injury patients. *Neuropsychol Rehabil* 2007;**17**: 1–33.

112. Kim YH, Yoo WK, Ko MH, Park CH, Kim ST, Na DL. Plasticity of the attentional network after brain injury and cognitive rehabilitation. *Neurorehabil Neural Repair* 2009;**23**:468–77.

113. Bonfiglio L, Carboncini MC, Bongioanni P, *et al.* Spontaneous blinking behaviour in persistent vegetative and minimally conscious states: relationship with evolution and outcome. *Brain Res Bull* 2005;**68**:163–70.

114. Rath JF, Langenbahn DM, Simon D, Sherr RL, Fletcher J, Diller L. The construct of problem solving in higher level neuropsychological assessment and rehabilitation. *Arch Clin Neuropsychol* 2004;**19**:613–35.

115. Rios M, Perianez JA, Munoz-Cespedes JM. Attentional control and slowness of information processing after severe traumatic brain injury. *Brain Inj* 2004;**18**:257–72.

116. Pero S, Incoccia C, Caracciolo B, Zoccolotti P, Formisano R. Rehabilitation of attention in two patients with traumatic brain injury by means of 'attention process training'. *Brain Inj* 2006;**20**:1207–19.

117. Rohling ML, Faust ME, Beverly B, Demakis G. Effectiveness of cognitive rehabilitation following acquired brain injury: a meta-analytic re-examination of Cicerone *et al.*'s (2000, 2005) systematic reviews. *Neuropsychology* 2009;**23**:20–39.

118. Cappa SF, Benke T, Clarke S, Rossi B, Stemmer B, van Heugten CMV. Cognitive rehabilitation. In: Hughes R, Brainin M, Gilhus NE (eds) *European Handbook of Neurological Management*, 1st edn. Chichester: Wiley-Blackwell/EFNS, 2007; pp. 592–612.

119. Comper P, Bisschop SM, Carnide N, Tricco A. A systematic review of treatments for mild traumatic brain injury. *Brain Inj* 2005;**19**(11):863–80.

120. das Nair R, Lincoln N. Cognitive rehabilitation for memory deficits following stroke. *Cochrane Database Syst Rev* 2007;Art. No.(3):CD002293.

121. Gordon WA, Zafonte R, Cicerone K, *et al.* Traumatic brain injury rehabilitation. State of the science. *Am J Phys Med Rehabil* 2008;**85**:343–82.

122. Teasell R, Bayona N, Marshall S, *et al.* A systematic review of the rehabilitation of moderate to severe acquired brain injuries. *Brain Inj* 2007;**21**(2):107–12.

123. Arciniegas DB, Silver JM. Pharmacotherapy of posttraumatic cognitive impairments. *Behav Neurol* 2006;**17**:25–42.

124. DeMarchi R, Bansal V, Hung A, *et al.* Review of awakening agents. *Can J Neurol Sci* 2005;**32**:4–17.

125. Poole NA, Agrawal N. Cholinomimetic agents and neurocognitive impairment following head injury: a systematic review. *Brain Inj* 2008;**22**(7–8):519–34.

126. Tenovuo O. Pharmacological enhancement of cognitive and behavioral deficits after traumatic brain injury. *Curr Opin Neurol* 2006;**19**:528–33.

127. Doornhein K, de Haan EHF. Cognitive training for memory deficits in stroke patients. *Neuropsychol Rehabil* 1998;**8**:393–400.

128. Berg I, Koning-Haanstra M, Deelman B. Long term effects of memory rehabilitation. A controlled study. *Neuropsychol Rehabil* 1991;**1**:97–111.

129. Ryan TV, Ruff RM. The efficacy of structural memory retraining in a group comparison of head trauma patients. *Arch Clin Neuropsychol* 1988;**3**:165–79.

130. Fleming JM, Shum D, Strong J, Lightbody S. Prospective memory rehabilitation for adults with traumatic brain injury: a compensatory training programme. *Brain Inj* 2005;**19**(1):1–10.

131. Hildebrandt H, Bussmann-Mork B, Schwendemann G. Group therapy for memory impaired patients: a partial remediation is possible. *J Neurol* 2006;**253**:512–9.

132. Baddeley A, Wilson BA. When implicit learning fails: amnesia and the problem of error elimination. *Neuropsychologia* 1994;**32**:53–68.

133. Squires EJ, Hunkin NM, Parkin AJ. Errorless learning of novel associations in amnesia. *Neuropsychologia* 1997;**35**:1103–11.

134. Hunkin NM, Squires EJ, Parkin AJ, Tidy JA. Are the benefits of errorless learning dependent on implicit memory? *Neuropsychologia* 1998;**36**:25–36.

135. Kalla T, Downes JJ, van den Broek M. The pre-exposure technique: enhancing the effects of errorless learning in the acquisition of face-name associations. *Neuropsychol Rehabil* 2001;**11**(1):1–16.

136. Kessels RPC, de Haan EHF. Implicit learning in memory rehabilitation: a meta-analysis on errorless learning and vanishing cues methods. *J Clin Exp Neuropsychol* 2003;**25**:805–14.

137. Riley GA, Sotiriou D, Jaspal S. Which is more effective in promoting implicit and explicit memory: the method of vanishing cues or errorless learning without fading? *Neuropsychol Rehabil* 2004;**14**(3):257–83.

138. Mount J, Pierce SR, Parker J, DiEgidio R, Woessner R. Trial and error versus errorless learning of functional skills in patients with acute stroke. *NeuroRehabilitation* 2007;**22**:123–32.

139. Schacter DL, Rich SA, Stampp MS. Remediation of memory disorders: experimental evaluation of the spaced retrieval techniques. *J Clin Exp Neuropsychol* 1985;**7**:79–96.

140. Hillary FG, Schultheis MT, Challis BH, Millis SR, Carnevale GJ. Spacing of repetitions improves learning and memory after moderate and severe TBI. *J Clin Exp Neuropsychol* 2003;**25**(1):49–58.

141. Bourgeois MS, Lenius K, Turkstra L, Camp C. The effects of cognitive teletherapy on reported everyday memory behaviours of persons with chronic traumatic brain injury. *Brain Inj* 2007;**21**(12):1245–57.

142. Kaschel R, Della Sala S, Cantagallo A, Fahlbock A, Laaksonen R, Kazen M. Imagery mnemonics for the rehabilitation of memory: a randomised group controlled trial. *Neuropsychol Rehabil* 2002;**12**:127–53.

143. Lengenfelder J, Chiaravalloti ND, DeLuca J. The efficacy of the generation effect in improving new learning in persons with traumatic brain injury. *Rehabil Psychol* 2007;**52**(3):290–6.

144. Schefft BK, Dulay MF, Fargo JD. The use of a self-generation memory encoding strategy to improve verbal memory and learning in patients with traumatic brain injury. *Appl Neuropsychol* 2008;**15**(1):61–8.

145. Manasse NJ, Hux K, Snell J. Teaching face-name associations to survivors of traumatic brain injury: a sequential treatment approach. *Brain Inj* 2005;**19**(8):633–41.

146. Westerberg H, Jacobaeus H, Hirvikoski T, *et al.* Computerized working memory training after stroke: a pilot study. *Brain Inj* 2007;**21**(1):21–9.

147. Thickpenny-Davis KL, Barker-Collo SL. Evaluation of a structured group format memory rehabilitation program for adults following brain injury. *J Head Trauma Rehabil* 2007;**22**(5):303–13.

148. Hewitt J, Evans JJ, Dritschel B. Theory driven rehabilitation of executive functioning: improving planning skills in people with traumatic brain injury through the use of an autobiographical episodic memory cueing procedure. *Neuropsychologia* 2006;**44**(8):1468–74.

149. Särkämö T, Tervaniemi M, Laitinen S, *et al.* Music listening enhances cognitive recovery and mood after middle cerebral artery stroke. *Brain* 2008;**131**(3):866–76.

150. Burke J, Danick J, Bemis B, Durgin C. A process approach to memory book training for neurological patients. *Brain Inj* 1994;**8**:71–81.

151. Evans JJ, Wilson BA, Needham P, Brentnall S. Who makes good use of memory aids? Results of a survey of people with acquired brain injury. *J Int Neuropsychol Soc* 2003;**9**:925–35.

152. Ownsworth TL, McFarland K. Memory remediation in long-term acquired brain injury: two approaches in diary training. *Brain Inj* 1999;**13**:605–26.

153. Schmitter-Edgecombe M, Fahy J, Whelan J, Long C. Memory remediation after severe closed head injury. Notebook training versus supportive therapy. *J Consult Clin Psychol* 1995;**63**:484–9.

154. Squires EJ, Hunkin NM, Parkin AJ. Memory notebook training in a case of severe amnesia: generalizing from paired associate learning to real life. *Neuropsychol Rehabil* 1996;**6**:55–65.

155. Zencius A, Wesolowski MD, Burke WH. A comparison of four memory strategies with traumatically brain-injured clients. *Brain Inj* 1990;**4**:33–8.

156. LoPresti EF, Mihailidis A, Kirsch N. Assistive technology for cognitive rehabilitation: state of the art. *Neuropsychol Rehabil* 2004;**14**(1/2):5–39.

157. Kerner MJ, Acker M. Computer delivery of memory retraining with head injured patients. *Cogn Rehabil* 1985;26–31.

158. Tam S-F, Man W-K. Evaluating computer-assisted memory retraining programmes for people with post-head injury amnesia. *Brain Inj* 2004;**18**(5):461–70.

159. Glisky EL, Glisky ML. Learning and memory impairments. In: Eslinger PJ (ed.) *Neuropsychological Interventions: Clinical Research and Practice*. New York: Guilford Press, 2002; pp. 137–62.

160. Kapur N, Glisky EL, Wilson BA. Technological memory aids for people with memory deficits. *Neuropsychol Rehab* 2004;**14**(1/2): 41–60.

161. Dou ZL, Man DWK, Ou HN, Zheng JL, Tam SF. Computerized errorless learning-based memory rehabilitation for Chinese patients with brain injury: a preliminary quasi-experimental clinical design study. *Brain Injury* 2006; **20**: 219–25.

162. Wilson BA, Emslie HC, Quirk K, Evans JJ. Reducing everyday memory and planning problems by means of a paging system: a randomised control crossover study. *J Neurol Neurosurg Psychiatry* 2001;477–82.

163. Fish J, Manly T, Emslie H, Evans JJ, Wilson BA. Compensatory strategies for acquired disorders of memory and planning: differential effects of a paging system for patients with brain injury of traumatic versus cerebrovascular aetiology. *J Neurol Neurosurg Psychiatry* 2008;**79**(8):930–5.

164. Wilson BA, Emslie H, Quirk K, Evans J, Watson P. A randomized control trial to evaluate a paging system for people with traumatic brain injury. *Brain Inj* 2005;**19**(11):891–4.

165. Hart T, Hawkey K, Whyte J. Use of a portable voice organizer to remember therapy goals in traumatic brain injury rehabilitation: a within-subjects trial. *J Head Trauma Rehabil* 2002;**17**(6):556–70.

166. van den Broek MD, Downes J, Johnson Z, Dayus B, Hilton N. Evaluation of an electronic memory aid in the neuropsychological rehabilitation of prospective memory deficits. *Brain Inj* 2000;**14**:455–62.

167. Inglis E, Szymkowiak A, Gregor P, *et al.* Issues surrounding the user-centred development of a new interactive memory aid. In: Keates S, Langdon P, Clarkson PJ, Robinson P (eds) *Universal Access and Assistive Technology*. Proceedings of the Cambridge Workshop on UA and AT '02. New York: Springer, 2002; pp. 171–8.

168. Kirsch NL, Shenton M, Rowan J. A generic, 'in-house', alphanumeric paging system for prospective activity impairments after traumatic brain injury. *Brain Inj* 2004;**18**(7):725–34.

169. Stapleton S, Adams M, Atterton L. A mobile phone as a memory aid for individuals with traumatic brain injury: a preliminary investigation. *Brain Inj* 2007;**21**(4):401–11.

170. Grealy MA, Johnson DA, Rushton SK. Improving cognitive function after brain injury: the use of exercise and virtual reality. *Arch Phys Med Rehabil* 1999;**80**:661–7.

171. Rose FD, Brooks BM, Attree EA, *et al.* A preliminary investigation into the use of virtual environments in memory

retraining after vascular brain injury: indications for future strategy? *Disabil Rehabil* 1999;**21**:548–54.

172. Brooks B, Rose F. The use of virtual reality in memory rehabilitation: current findings and future directions. *Neurol Rehabil* 2003;**18**(2):147–57.

173. Maher ML, Ochipa C. Management and treatment of limb apraxia. In: Rothi LJG, Heilman KM (eds) *Apraxia: The Neuropsychology of Action*. Hove: Psychology Press, 1997; 75–91.

174. Goldenberg G, Daumuller M, Hagman S. Assessment and therapy of complex activities of daily living in apraxia. *Neuropsychol Rehabil* 2001;**11**(2):147–69.

175. Hanna-Paddy B, Heilman KM, Foundas AL. Ecological implications od ideomotor apraxia: evidence from physical activities of daily living. *Neurology* 2003;**60**(1):487–90.

176. Walker CM, Sunderland A, Sharma J, Walker MF. The impact of cognitive impairments on upper body dressing difficulties after stroke: a video analysis of patterns of recovery. *J Neurol Neurosurg Psychiatry* 2004;**75**:43–8.

177. Unsal-Delialioglu S, Kurt M, Kaya K, Culna C, Ozel S. Effects of ideomotor apraxia on functional outcome in patients with right hemiplegia. *Int J Rehabil Res* 2008;**31**(2):177–80.

178. West C, Bowen A, Hesketh A, Vail A. Interventions for motor apraxia following stroke. *Cochrane Database Syst Rev* 2008;(1):CD004132.

179. Edmans JA, Webster J, Lincoln NB. A comparison of two approaches in the treatment of perceptual problems after stroke. *Clin Rehabil* 2000;**14**:230–43.

180. Smania N, Girardi F, Domenciali C, Lora E, Aglioti S. The rehabilitation of limb apraxia: a study in left brain damaged patients. *Arch Phys Med Rehabil* 2000;**81**:379–88.

181. Donkervoort M, Dekker J, Stehmann-Saris J, Deelman BG. Efficacy of strategy training in left-hemisphere stroke patients with apraxia: a randomized clinical trial. *Neuropsychol Rehabil* 2001;**11**:549–66.

182. Buxbaum LJ, Haaland KY, Hallett M, *et al.* Treatment of limb apraxia; moving forward to improved action. *Am J Phys Med Rehabil* 2008;**87**:149–61.

183. Geusgens C, van Heugten CM, Donkervoort M, van den Ende E, Jolles J, van den Heuvel W. Transfer of training effects in stroke patients with apraxia: an exploratory study. *Neuropsychol Rehabil* 2005;**16**(2):213–29.

184. Geusgens CA, van Heugten CM, Cooijmans JP, Jolles JJ, van den Heuvel WJ. Transfer efects of a cognitive strategy training for stroke patients with apraxia. *J Clin Exp Neuropsychol* 2007;**29**(8):831–41.

185. Sunderland A, Walker CM, Walker MF. Action errors and dressing disability after stroke: an ecological approach to neuropsychological assessment and intervention. *Neuropsychol Rehabil* 2006;**16**(6):666–83.

186. Goldenberg G, Hagman S. Therapy of activities of daily living in patients with apraxia. *Neuropsychol Rehabil* 1998;**8**:123–41.

187. Van Heugten CM, Dekker J, Deelman BG, van Dijuk AJ, Stehmann-Saris JC, Kinebanian A. Outcome of strategy training in stroke patients: a phase-II study. *Clin Rehabil* 1998;**2**:294–303.

188. Poole J. Effect of apraxia on the ability to learn one-handed shoe tying. *Occup Ther J Res* 1998;**18**:275–91.

189. Wilson BA. Sarah: learning some self-care skills after an anaesthetic accident. In: Wilson B (ed) *Case Studies in Neuropsychological Rehabilitation*. Oxford: Oxford University Press, 1999; 37–52.

190. Maher LM, Rothi LJG, Greenwald ML. Treatment of gesture impairment: a single case. *Am Speech Hear Assoc* 1991;**33**:195.

191. Ochipa C, Maher LM, Rothi LJG. Treatment of ideomotor apraxia. *Int J Neuropsychol Soc* 1995;**2**:149.

192. Jantra P, Monga TN, Press JM, Gervais BJ. Management of apraxic gait in a stroke patient. *Arch Phys Med Rehabil* 1992;**73**:95–7.

193. Pilgrim E, Humphreys GW. Rehabilitation of a case of ideomotor apraxia. In: Riddoch MJ, Humphreys GW (eds) *Cognitive Neuropsychology and Cognitive Rehabilitation*. Hove: Lawrence Erlbaum, 1994; 275–91.

194. Bulter J. Intervention effectiveness: evidence from a case study of ideomotor and ideational apraxia. *Br J Occup Ther* 1997;**60**:491–7.

195. Kawahira K, Noma T, Liyama J, Etoh S, Ogata A, Shimodozono M. Improvements in limb kinetic apraxia by repetition of a newly designed facilitation exercise in a patient with cortico-basal degeneration. *Int J Rehabil Res* 2009;**32**(2):178–83.

196. Jackson M, Warrington EK. Arithmetic skills in patients with unilateral cerebral lesions. *Cortex* 1986;**22**:611–20.

197. Willmes K. Acalculia. In: Goldenberg G, Miller B (eds) *Handbook of Clinical Neurology*, Vol. **88**, Chapter 17. Amsterdam: Elsevier, 2008; pp. 339–58.

198. Basso A, Caporall A, Faglioni P. Spontaneous recovery from aphasia. *J Int Neuropsychol Soc* 2005;**11**:99–107.

199. Kratochwill TR, Levin LR (eds) *Single-case Research Design and Analysis*. Hove: Lawrence Erlbaum, 1992.

200. Randall RR, Schultz MC, Crawford AB, Sinner CA. Single-subject clinical outcome research: designs, data, effect sizes, and analyses. *Aphasiology* 1999;**13**:445–73.

201. Girelli L, Seron X. Rehabilitation of number processing and calculation skills. *Aphasiology* 2001;**15**:695–712.

202. Lochy A, Domahs F, Delazer M. Rehabilitation of acquired calculation and number processing disorders. In: Campbell JID (ed.) *Handbook of Mathematical Cognition*, Chapter 27. New York: Psychology Press, 2005; pp. 469–85.

203. Shallice T. Case-study approach in neuropsychological research. *J Clin Neuropsychol* 1979;**1**:183–211.

204. Caramazza A. Cognitive neuropsychology and rehabilitation: an unfulfilled promise? In: Seron X, Deloche G (eds) *Cognitive Approach in Neuropsychological Rehabilitation.* Hillsdale, NJ: Lawrence Erlbaum Associates Ltd, 1989; 383–98.

205. Seron X. Effectiveness and specificity in neuropsychological therapies: a cognitive point of view. *Aphasiology* 1997;**11**:105–23.

206. Riddoch MJ, Humphreys GW. *Cognitive Neuropsychology and Cognitive Rehabilitation.* Hove: Lawrence Erlbaum, 1994.

207. Gauggel S, Billino J. The effects of goal-setting on arithmetic performance of brain damaged patients. *Arch Clin Neuropsychol* 2002;**17**:283–94.

208. Girelli L, Delazer M. Subtraction bugs in an alcalculic patient. *Cortex* 1996;**32**:547–55.

209. Deloche G, Ferrand I, Naud E, Baeta E, Vendrell J, Claros-Salinas D. Differential effects of covert and overt training of the syntactic component of verbal processing and generalisations to other tasks: a single-case study. *Neuropsychol Rehabil* 1992;**2**:257–81.

210. Jacquemin A, Calicis F, van der Linden M, Wyns C, Noël MP. Evaluation et prise en charge des déficits cognitifs dans les états déments. In: de Partz MP, Leclercq M (eds) *La rééducation neuropsychologique de l'adulte.* Paris: Edition de la Société de Neuropsychologie de Langue Française, 1991; 131–51.

211. Sullivan KS, Macaruso P, Sokol SM. Remediation of Arabic numeral processing in a case of development dyscalculia. *Neuropsychol Rehabil* 1996;**6**:27–53.

212. Ablinger I, Weniger D, Willmes K. Treating number transcoding difficulties in a chronic aphasic patient. *Aphasiology* 2006;**20**:37–58.

213. Deloche G, Seron X, Ferrand I. Reeducation of number transcoding mechanisms: a procedural approach. In: Seron X, Deloche G (eds) *Cognitive Approach in Neuropsychological Rehabilitation.* Hillsdale, NJ: Lawrence Erlbaum, 1989; 249–87.

214. Miceli G, Capasso R. *I disturbi del calcolo. diagnosi e riabilitazione.* Milano: Masson, 1991.

215. Girelli L, Bartha L, Delazer M. Strategic learning in the rehabilitation of semantic knowledge. *Neuropsychol Rehabil* 2002;**12**:41–61.

216. Domahs F, Lochy A, Eibl G, Delazer M. Adding colour to multiplication: rehabilitation of arithmetical fact retrieval in a case of traumatic brain injury. *Neuropsychol Rehabil* 2004;**14**:303–28.

217. Zaunmüller L, Domahs F, Dressel K, *et al.* Rehabilitation of arithmetic fact retrieval. *Neuropsychol Rehabil* 2009;**19**:422–43.

218. Domahs F, Bartha L, Delazer M. Rehabilitation of arithmetical abilities: different intervention strategies for multiplication. *Brain Lang* 2003;**87**:165–6.

219. Hittmair-Delazer M, Semenza C, Denes G. Concepts and facts in calculation. *Brain* 1994;**117**:715–28.

220. Whetstone T. The representation of arithmetic facts in memory: results from retraining a brain-damaged patient. *Brain Cogn* 1998;**36**:290–309.

221. Delazer M, Bodner T, Benke T. Rehabilitation of arithmetical text problem solving. *Neuropsychol Rehabil* 1998;**8**:401–12.

Index